MISSION ONCOLOGY for MCh

Authentic Answers with Explanations

SECOND EDITION

KANTAMANI BALA TEJA MS, MCh

Peepee Publishers and Distributors (P) Ltd.®

Mission Oncology for MCh

Published by
Pawaninder P. Vij and Anupam Vij

Peepee Publishers and Distributors (P) Ltd.
Head Office: 160, Shakti Vihar, Pitam Pura, Delhi-110 034 (India)

Correspondence Address:

7/31, First Floor, Ansari Road, Daryaganj
New Delhi-110 002 (India)

Ph: 41512412, 23246245, 9811156083

e-mail: peepee160@yahoo.co.in

e-mail: peepee160@gmail.com

www.peepeepub.com

join us on facebook.com/pp.publishers

First Edition: 2017

Second Edition: 2020

ISBN: 978-81-8445-276-1

Dedicated to

My beloved parents and family

K. V. RAGHAVULU – Father

K. PANITHA LAKSHMI – Mother

K. BHANU TEJA (Brother) and K. RAMA LAKSHMI

PREFACE

On viewing the pattern of many MCh Oncology Exam patterns, I felt that there is no book available in the market for the best preparation to crack the exam. Many of the exams had repeats all the time. This book is started with sole purpose of clearing various aspects of Oncology and guide aspirants for their preparation. These questions had been solved by experts of India from reputed institutes. For controversial question, every attempt has been made to trace the source and solve the questions.

I have included Tablets, Magical Points, Illustrations and Flowcharts for the better understanding.

I have highlighted all repeat questions so that aspirants will concentrate on them.

I would like to concentrate all the contributors for their commitment and hard work.

The only short cut for success in our exam is hard work.

Have faith in you, your parents and Almighty God.

All the best!

To NEET aspirants, you can solve all multiple choice questions of gastroenterology of NEET exam, based on this book practice papers. Remember one point, every MCQ counts in nationwide pattern exams. So, read every book regarding concerned specialty and excel in exams.

Dr. Kantamani Bala Teja

ACKNOWLEDGEMENTS

There is long list of people whom I want to thank for their contributions. A simple thank you does not suffice to show my gratitude for their work.

I would like to thank the following persons for their contributions:

Dr. Mahendra, Dr. Kaustab Gaur, Dr. Kaushik Rao, Dr. Amita Sekhar Padhy, Dr. Rajyalakshmi, Dr. Pavitra, Dr. Chandana, Dr. Dipinjan Biswas, Dr. Madan Gupta, Dr. Ankit Mahuvakar, Dr. Kartik Krishnan, Dr. Rachit Mathur, Dr. Muddasir Bhati, Dr. Lohit Arora, Dr. Teertha Shetty, Dr. Tejas Vispute, Dr. Aravind Guru, Dr. Shravan Nadkarni, Dr. Nishit Shrivastav, Dr. Nityanand, Dr. Rigved, Dr. Prudhvi, Dr. Preethi, Dr. Sahil, Dr. Siddharth Nekkanti.

I would also like to thank my friends who molded me into who I'm today.

Dr. Ram Prakash, Dr. Rajesh, Dr. Rakesh, Dr. Kishore, Dr. Mahesh, Dr. Venkateswarulu, Dr. Pavan, Dr. Ashok, Dr. Satish.

I thank Mr. Pawaninder Paul Vij, Director of Peepee Publishers and Distributors (P) Ltd., who has always been with me and supported me. I would also like to thank entire publishing team for their efforts in bringing this excellent book to this stage.

Note: ***Book abides to the rules of NEET/DNB Non disclosure agreement (NDA). If MCQs simulate the NEET pattern, they are just mere resemblance and are handpicked questions from standard textbooks by the author.***

HOW TO USE THIS BOOK

Start from Part 1, End with Part 6 (At the end of preparation, just before NEET please only revise the latest pattern papers rather than the whole book).

Please keep standard textbook aside to review every now and then for extra points.

This book cannot replace them in preparation.

REFERENCES

1. ***Devita, 11th Edition***
2. ***Sabiston, 20th Edition***
3. ***Schwartz, 11th Edition***
4. ***Casciato Manual***
5. ***Bethedsa Handbook***
6. ***Washington Manual of Oncology***
7. ***Harrison Manual of Oncology***
8. ***Stell and Maren Textbook***
9. ***MD Anderson Handbook of Oncology***

NOTE: The references for every question has been given below along with page number so that the reader can search and read for extra information.

This Book is made by Group of Experts only not by Single person/Association/Coaching centre

"He who makes us understand is not the teacher, but who molds us to the best is the one."

These words played a crucial role in my life I expect the same in yours too.

CONTENTS

PART ONE	**CHAPTER-WISE THEORY: GI ONCOLOGY – I**	
	1. Carcinoma Esophagus	1-6
	2. Gastric Cancer	7-14
	3. Gastric Lymphoma	15-17
	4. GIST	18-20
	5. Small Bowel Malignancies	21-25
	6. Hereditary CRC	26-33
	7. Colorectal Cancer	34-46
	8. Appendiceal Tumors	47-48
	9. Tumors of Anal Canal and Margin	49-50
PART ONE	**GI ONCOLOGY – II**	
	10. Liver Tumors	51-65
	11. Gallbladder Cancer	66-71
	12. Cholangiocarcinoma	72-79
	13. Pancreatic Cancers	80-88
PART ONE	**GENITOURINARY ONCOLOGY**	
	14. Renal Cell Carcinoma *Internist's Tumor, Grawitz Tumor, Hypernephroma, Renal Adenocarcinoma*	89-97
	15. Bladder Carcinoma	98-103
	16. Penile Cancer	104-109
	17. Prostate Cancer	110-115
	18. Testicular Cancers	116-121
PART ONE	**HEAD AND NECK ONCOLOGY**	
	19. Basics and Molecular Biology of Head and Neck Cancer	122-124
	20. Staging	125-127
	21. Oral Cavity	128-140
	22. Sinonasal Malignancies	141-147
	23. Nasopharyngeal Carcinoma *Guangdong Tumor*	148-153
	24. Oropharyngeal Tumors	154-160
	25. Hypopharyngeal Tumors	161-169
	26. Laryngeal Tumors	170-178
	27. Rehabilitation of Voice	179-180
	28. Carcinoma of Unknown Primary (CUP)	181-183
	29. Benign Salivary Gland Tumors	184-186
	30. Malignant Salivary Gland Tumors	187-190
	31. Parapharyngeal Tumors	191-193
	32. Temporal Bone Tumors	194-199
PART ONE	**NEURO-ONCOLOGY**	
	33. Neuro-Oncology	200-214
PART ONE	**ENDOCRINE ONCOLOGY**	
	34. Thyroid Malignancies	215-223
	35. Parathyroid Carcinoma	224-226
	36. Adrenocortical Carcinoma	227-232
	37. Men Syndrome	233-235
	38. Pancreatic Neuroendocrine Tumors	236-241
	39. Carcinoid Tumors and NET	242-245
PART ONE	**THORACIC ONCOLOGY (LUNG AND CHEST WALL)**	
	40. Carcinoma Lung	246-260
	41. Miscellaneous	261-263

PART ONE	**MUSCULOSKELETAL ONCOLOGY**	
	42. Bone Tumors	264-277
	43. Soft Tissue Sarcoma	278-285
PART ONE	**DERMATO-ONCOLOGY**	
	44. Melanoma	286-296
	45. Non Melanomatous Skin Cancer – SCC AND BCC	297-301
	46. Other Malignant Skin Cancers *Most Frequently Asked Topics in Institute Based Exams*	302-303
	47. Malignant Mucosal Melanoma	304
PART ONE	**BREAST CANCER**	
	48. Breast Cancer	305-323
PART ONE	**PEDIATRIC ONCOLOGY**	
	49. Neuroblastoma	324
	50. Wilm's Tumor	325-326
	51. Hepatoblastoma	327
	52. Retinoblastoma	328-330
PART ONE	**MISCELLANEOUS**	
	53. Radiotherapy	331-337
	54. Anticancer Drugs	338-346
	55. Miscellaneous	347-360
	Must Read	361-377
PART TWO	**CHAPTER-WISE MCQs**	
	56. Basics of Oncology *Genetics, Radiation, Chemotherapy, Molecular Biology and Allied Aspects*	378-432
	57. Genitourinary Oncology *NEET SS Pattern MCQs*	433-438
	58. Thoracic Oncology *Multiple Choice Questions*	439-447
	59. Bone and STS *Multiple Choice Questions*	448-449
	60. Endocrine Oncology *Multiple Choice Questions*	450-455
	61. Breast Cancer *Multiple Choice Questions*	456-462
	62. Head and Neck *Multiple Choice Questions*	463-472
PART THREE	**PREVIOUS MCQs**	
	63. Multiple Choice Questions (Papers)	473-505
PART FOUR	**PRACTICE PAPERS**	
	64. Multiple Choice Questions (Papers)	506-609
PART FIVE	**RECENT MODEL PAPERS**	
	65. Multiple Choice Questions	610-753
PART SIX	**GENERAL SURGERY REVIEW**	
	66. General Surgery *NEET SS Pattern*	754-787
PART SEVEN	**CHARTS AND TABLES FOR FINAL REVISION**	
	67. Tables and Charts for Final Review	788-799
PART EIGHT	**STATISTICS**	
	68. Statistics	800-818
PART NINE	**LATEST PATTERN QUESTIONS**	
	69. Latest Pattern Questions and Miscellaneous	819-884

PART ONE: CHAPTER-WISE THEORY
GI ONCOLOGY - I

CHAPTER 1
CARCINOMA ESOPHAGUS

- Overall, Most common site – Middle 3rd
- Squamous cell carcinoma – Upper 2/3rd
- Adenocarcinoma – Lower 1/3rd

INTRODUCTION

- ***Squamous cell carcinoma usually affects upper two-thirds; adenocarcinoma usually lower-third***
- Incidence of adenocarcinoma is increasing
- Male > Female
- Most common–5th Decade
- ***Most common type–Exophytic***
- Lymph node involvement is a bad prognostic factor
- Dysphagia is the most common presenting symptom, but is a late feature
- Accurate pretreatment staging is essential in patients thought to be fit to undergo 'curative' treatment

Predisposing factors for Squamous Cell Carcinoma		
HPV Infections	**Mucosal damage**	**Premalignant lesions**
• Excess nitrates in drinking water • Opium smoking • Fungal toxins in pickled vegetables • Dietary deficiency: Vitamin A, Molybdenum, Zinc • Head and neck cancer • Celiac sprue	• **Hot beverages** • **Lye ingestion** • **Radiation** • Corrosives • Bulimia	• **Tylosis Palmaris et plantaris (40-60% develop cancers)** • **Achalasia cardia (30%)** • **Esophageal web** (20%) Strictures and diverticula • **Plummer Vinson syndrome (10%)**

Squamous Cell Carcinoma	Adenocarcinoma
• Most common type worldwide • More common in blacks • Most common in China, Southeast Asia • Male to female ratio–3:1	• More common in whites • Most common in Western countries • Male to female ratio – **15:1**

RISK FACTORS

Squamous Cell Carcinoma	Adenocarcinoma
• Smoking • Nitrites • Lye ingestion • Chronic achalasia • Alcohol	• Barrett's esophagus • Chronic GERD • Smoking

Contd.

Contd.

• HIV • Radiation strictures • PV syndrome • Tylosis • Deficiency of Mo, Zn, Vit A	

- ***Obesity is protective against SCC***
- ***CAG-A strain is protective against Adenocarcinoma***
- ***Most common site of distant metastasis is LIVER***

GENETICS

• CA 19 – 9 : Response to therapy and recurrence • EGF DNA for metastasis • Cyclin D1 – over amplified • P53 mutation • CD 44 gene – dysplasia of SCC

Comparison of two types of esophageal cancer

	Squamous cell carcinoma	**Adenocarcinoma**
Site	Upper two-thirds	Lower one-third
Predisposing factors	Smoking alcohol	Barrett's esophagus–GORD
Behaviour	Less aggressive	More aggressive
Incidence	Less common	More common
Achalasia cardia	Is the predisposing factor	Does not give rise to adenocarcinoma
Chemoradiation	It can be an alternate treatment	Not alternate to surgery
Surgery	Can be the first choice or chemoradiation	Surgery is the first choice–unfit patient, chemotherapy
Dietary carcinogens	A. Elevated nitrates in drinking water B. Food containing fungi–Geotrichum candidum–pickles, corn C. Baked bread	Consumption of meat Alcohol

- **Barrett esophagus** is the single most important risk factor for **Adenocarcinoma**
- **Bisphosphonates** increase the risk in patients with Barrett esophagus

CLINICAL FEATURES

- **Progressive Dysphagia** (initially for solids, later for semisolids and liquids) is the most common symptom
- **Short term weight loss** is also a common symptom
- Since difficulty in swallowing does not occur until **>60%** of the esophageal circumference is infiltrated with cancer
- **Advanced malignancy:** RLN paralysis, Horner's syndrome, chronic spinal pain and diaphragmatic paralysis

INVESTIGATIONS

- **Endoscopy and Biopsy–Investigation of choice**
- Barium swallow–**Shouldering sign and irregular filling defect**
- Fluoroscopy – **Rat tail appearance**
- **PET** – Distant, regional lymph nodes, organ mets
- **EUS** – T and N staging

Endoscopic Ultrasound

- High frequency (5-30 MHz) transducer
- To determine depth of spread of a malignant tumor through Esophageal wall
- Involvement of adjacent organs
- Metastasis to lymph nodes
- Also detects contiguous spread ***downward into cardia***
- Can detect metastasis in the liver
- Can also detect small lymph nodes which are <5 mm (which can't be detected by CT scan also)
- If 'Endoscopic sonography' detects ***more than 5 lymph nodes***, it is not a case for curative resection

CHROMOENDOSCOPY

- Chromoendoscopy involves the topical application of stains or pigments to improve tissue localisation, characterisation, or diagnosis during endoscopy
- **Absorptive stains** (e.g., Lugol's solution and methylene blue) diffuse or are preferentially absorbed across specific epithelial cell membranes
- **Contrast stains** (e.g., indigocarmine) highlight surface topography and mucosal irregularities by permeating mucosal crevices
- **Reactive stains** (e.g., Congo red and phenol red) undergo chemical reactions with specific cellular constituents, resulting in a colour change

STAGING

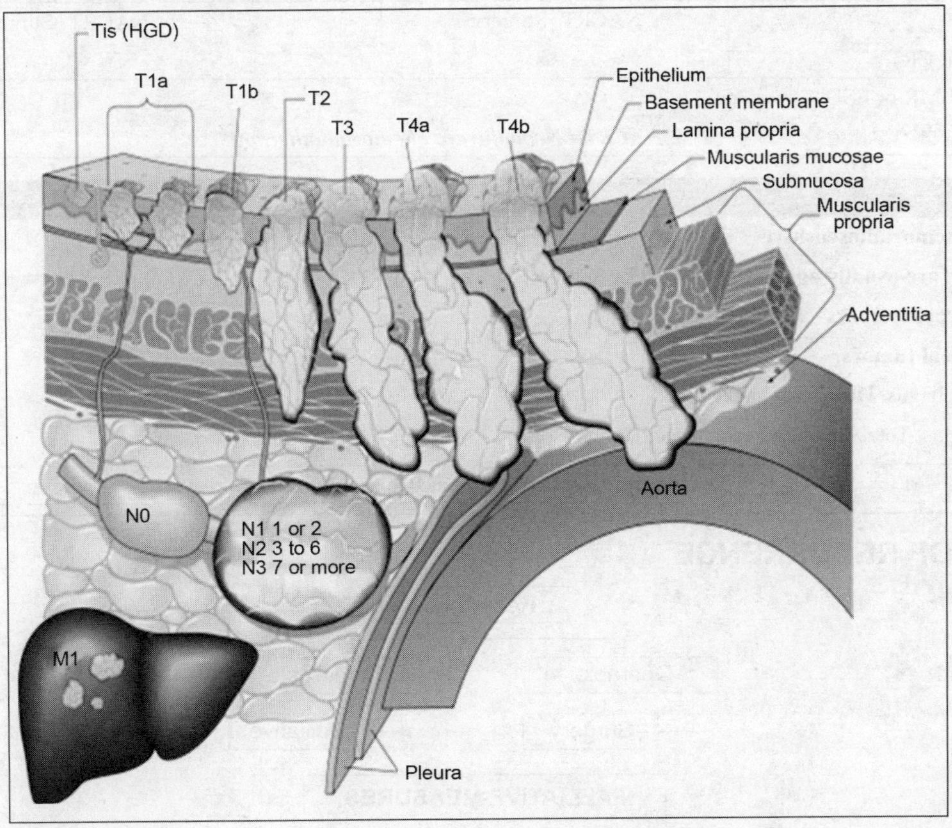

MANAGEMENT

- ***SCC–multifocal potential***
- **Radical esophagectomy** is the most important aspect of curative treatment **Trans Hiatal**
- **ORRINGERS (incision made are two one in the abdomen and the other in the neck)**
- **Surgery–Gold standard primary treatment for local and regional tumors of esophagus**

- Aim of the surgery is **Ro Resection** (complete macroscopic and microscopic removal)
- ***For SCC: Esophagectomy* (Proximal 10 cm and distal 5 cm resection** from macroscopic tumor)
- ***Partial esophagectomy***–Tumors of lower 2/3rd of esophagus (Excluding cancer cardia)
- Adeno carcinoma curative resection should include 10 cm proximal and distal margins as a part of en-bloc resection
- **Post cricoid carcinoma and upper 3rd growth – radiotherapy**

Herkovic Regimen
• 50 Gy of radiation delivered in (25 fractions) 6 weeks with Cisplatinum and 5 FU+ Paclitaxel
• High response rate in metastatic esophageal cancer which also acts as radiation sensitizer
• Useful adjuvant to RT

PALLIATIVE TREATMENT

- Endoscopic laser treatment ND YAG laser
- Brachytherapy Intracavitary irradiation with caesium or iridium pellets loaded into an applicator placed inside the lumen
- SEMS–Self expanding metallic stents
- Ethanol injection

SUMMARY

Stage 1	Stage 2	Stage 3
Surgery alone If N+ then Adjuvant CRT	NACRT+Surgery	NACRT+Surgery
T1–Surgery alone/EMR or ESD *NACRT= Neoadjuvant chemoradiotherapy*		

Must Remember
• **SCC is more Chemoradiosensitive**
• **Cervical tumors are usually aggressive**–NACRT+ Surgery
• **Upper/Mid thoracic tumors**–Near total Esophagectomy
• **Lower Esophageal tumors:** No Barrett's esophagus–Distal esophagectomy Barrett's esophagus–Total/Near total esophagectomy
Margin for resection is 10 cm Proximal and 5 cm distal

MANAGEMENT OF RECURRENCE

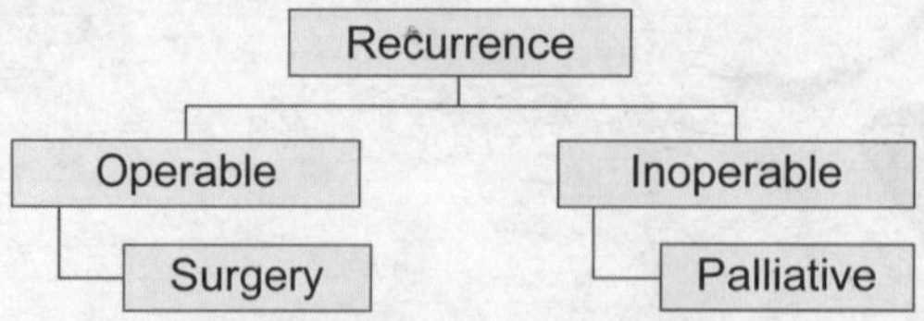

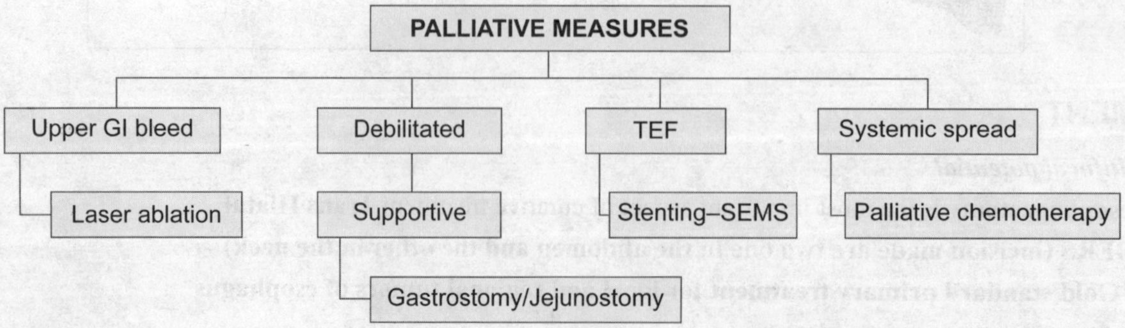

CHARTS

Primary tumor (T)*	
TX	Primary tumor cannot be assessed
T0	No evidence of primary tumor
Tis	High-grade dysplasia**
T1	Tumor invades lamina propria, muscularis mucosae, or submucosa
T1a	Tumor invades lamina propria or muscularis mucosa
T1b	Tumor invades submucosa
T2	Tumor invades muscularis propria
T3	Tumor invades adventitia
T4	Tumor invades adjacent structures
T4a	Resectable tumor invading pleura, pericardium, or diaphragm
T4b	Unresectable tumor invading other adjacent structures such as aorta, vertebral body, trachea, etc.
Regional lymph nodes (N)*	
NX	Regional lymph nodes cannot be assessed
N0	No regional lymph nodes metastasis
N1	Metastasis in 1-2 regional lymph nodes
N2	Metastasis in 3-6 regional lymph nodes
N3	Metastasis in $\geq$ 7 regional lymph nodes

SQUAMOUS CELL CARCINOMA ESOPHAGUS

Stage	T	N	M	Grade	Location
0	Tis	N0	M0	1, X	Any
IA	T1	N0	M0	1, X	Any
IB	T1	N0	M0	2-3	Any
	T2-3	N0	M0	1, X	Lower, X
IIA	T2-3	N0	M0	1, X	Upper, middle
	T2-3	N0	M0	2-3	Lower, X
IIB	T2-3	N0	M0	2-3	Upper, middle
	T1-2	N1	M0	Any	Any
IIIA	T1-2	N2	M0	Any	Any
	T3	N1	M0	Any	Any
	T4a	N0	M0	Any	Any
IIIB	T3	N2	M0	Any	Any
IIIC	T4a	N1-2	M0	Any	Any
	T4b	Any	M0	Any	Any
	Any	N3	M0	Any	Any
IV	Any	Any	M1	Any	Any

ADENOCARCINOMA ESOPHAGUS

Stage	T	N	M	Grade
0	Tis	N0	M0	1, X
IA	T1	N0	M0	1-2, X
IB	T1	N0	M0	3
	T2	N0	M0	1-2, X
IIA	T2	N0	M0	3
IIB	T3	N0	M0	Any
	T1-2	N1	M0	Any

Contd.

Contd.

IIIA	T1-2	N2	M0	Any
	T3	N1	M0	Any
	T4a	N0	M0	Any
IIIB	T3	N2	M0	Any
IIIC	T4a	N1-2	M0	Any
	T4b	Any	M0	Any
	Any	N3	M0	Any
IV	Any	Any	M1	Any

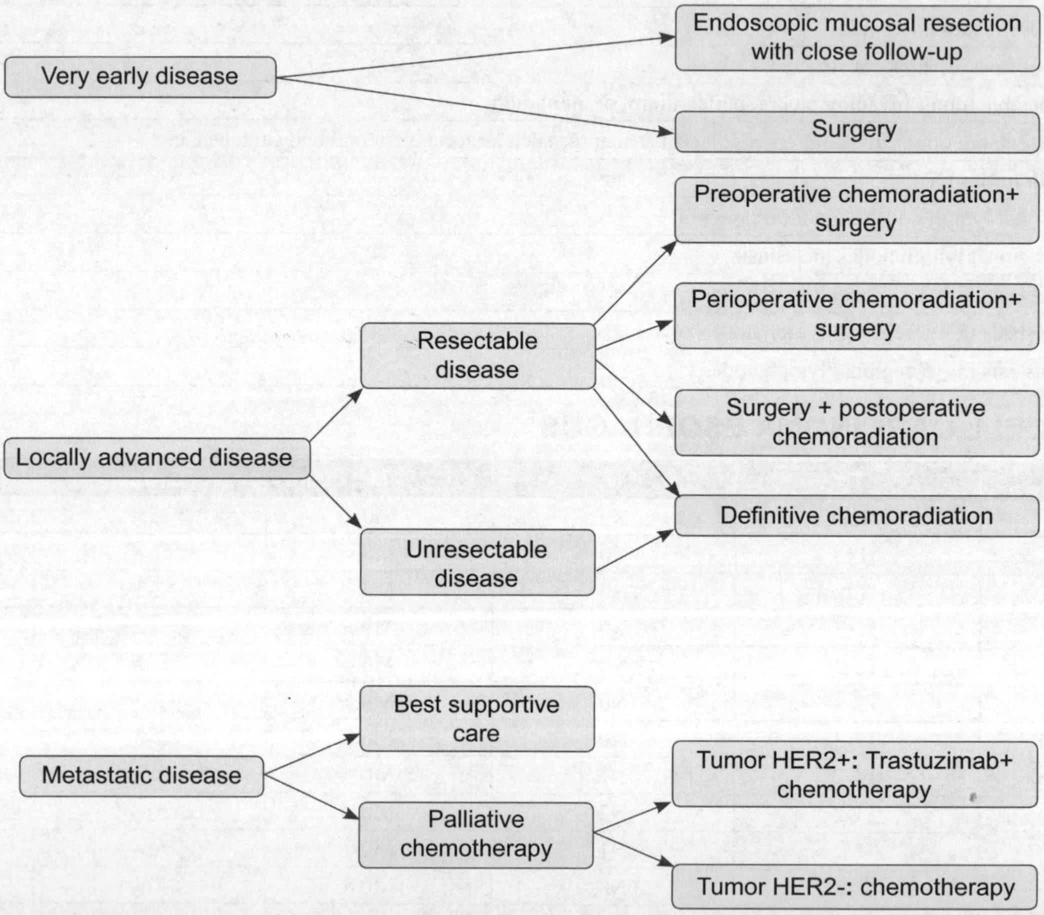

Stage	Treatment
Tis-T1a	Endoscopic mucosal resection, photodynamic therapy, radiofrequency ablation, or esophagectomy alone
T1b	Esophagectomy alone
T2-T4, node positive	Neoadjuvant chemoradiation followed by esophagectomy
Distant metastasis	Palliative chemotherapy, radiation, or chemoradiation, esophageal dilation and stenting

Prognostic factors	Tumor related	Host related	Treatment related
Essential	Depth of invasion Lymph node involvement Presence of lymphovascular invasion (LVI)	Performance status Age Nutritional status	Quality of surgery Multimodality approach
Additional	Tumor grading Tumor location	Economic status	Nutritional support
New and promising	CEA VEGF-C HER2		

CHAPTER 2

GASTRIC CANCER

ETIOLOGY

Risk Factors	Genetic and Familial	Premalignant Lesions
• **Smoking,** alcohol • Spicy foods, high salt diet • Smoked meat or fish • EBV, *H. pylori* • Low animal fat and proteins • High nitrate consumption • High complex carbohydrate • Lack of fresh fruits, vegetables • Deficiency of antioxidant vitamins • Rubber and coal workers • Low socioeconomic status	• **E cadherin gene** mutation – **CDH1** (90% risk) • TP53 mutation • BRCA1 mutation • APC gene mutation • β-catenin mutation • BAX mutation • *CDKN2A mutation* • Blood group A • HNPCC • Li Fraumeni syndrome	• **Chronic Atrophic gastritis** – Most common precursor lesion • Adenomatous polyps (FAP) • Hyperplastic polyps • **Chronic gastric ulcer** • Pernicious anemia • **Intestional metaplasia (H. pylori)** • **Menetrier's disease** • **Stomach remnant (stump carcinoma)** after Billroth II GI or Vagotomy GI

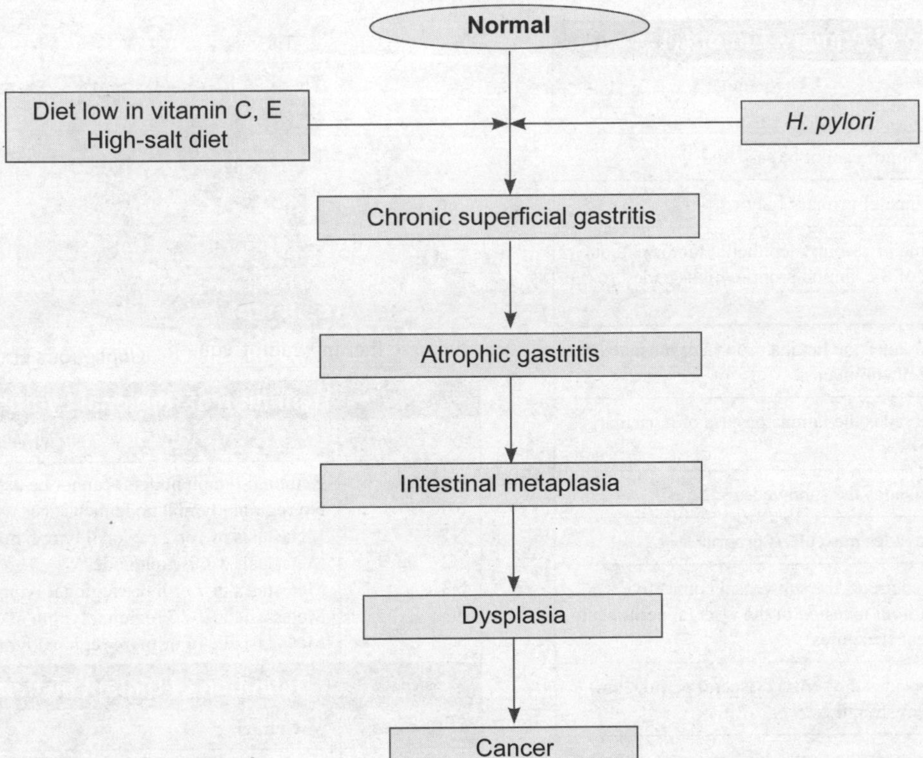

Gastric carcinogenesis

Factors that decrease the risk of gastric cancer
• *Fresh fruits and vegetables* • *Diet rich in vitamin C and E* • *Aspirin* • *History of duodenal ulcer*

- Most common type of gastric cancer–***Adenocarcinoma***

Lauren's (DIO) Classification	
Intestional type	**Diffuse type**
• Favorable prognosis • Frequently ulcerative • Common in **H pylori** induced • Well differentiated	• Poor prognosis • Blood group A, familial type, young people, females • Poorly differentiated • Early gastric wall penetration and lymphatic spread • **Linitis plastica**

Depending on the depth of invasion	
Early gastric cancer	**Advanced gastric cancer**
• Involvement of mucosa and/or sub-mucosa only, with or without lymph node involvement (T1 + any N) • Overall cure rate with gastric resection and lymphadenectomy–95% **Japanese classification** • Protruded • Superficial • Excavated	• Involvement of muscularis and serosa with or without lymph node involvement **Borrmann's classification** I–single polypoid carcinoma II–ulcerated carcinoma with clear cut margins III–ulcerated carcinoma without clear cut margins IV–diffuse carcinoma, Linitis plastic V–unclassified

TNM STAGING

Definition of Primary Tumor (T)

T Category	T Criteria
Tx	Primary tumor cannot be assessed
T0	No evidence of primary tumor
Tis	Carcinoma *in situ:* intraepithelial tumor without invasion of the lamina propria, high-grade dysplasia
T1	Tumor invades the lamina propria or muscularis mucosae or submucosa
T1a	Tumor invades the lamina propria or muscularis mucosae
T1b	Tumor invades the submucosa
T2	Tumor invades muscularis propria[a]
T3	Tumor penetrates the subserosal connective tissue without invasion of the visceral peritoneum or adjacent structures[b,c]
T4	Tumor invades the serosa (visceral peritoneum) or adjacent structures[b,c]
T4a	Tumor invades the serosa (visceral peritoneum)
T4b	Tumor invades adjacent structures/organs

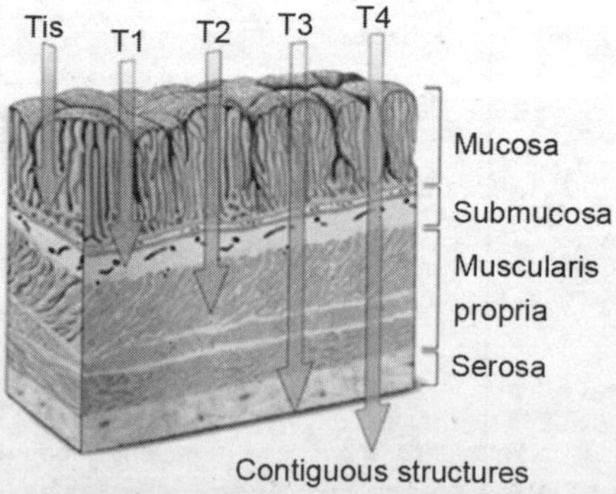

Definition of Regional Lymph Node (N)

N Category	N Criteria
Nx	Regional lymph node(s) cannot be assessed
N0	No regional lymph node metastasis
N1	Metastasis in 1or 2 regional lymph nodes
N2	Metastasis 3-6 lymph nodes
N3	Metastasis in 7 or more regional lymph nodes
N3a	Metastasis in 7-15 regional lymph nodes
N3b	Metastasis in 16 or more regional lymph nodes

Definition of Distant Metastasis (M)

M Category	M Criteria
M0	No distant metastasis
M1	Distant metastasis

	N0	N1	N2	N3	M+
T1	IA	IB	IIA	IIB	IV
T2	IA	IIA	IIB	IIIA	
T3	IIA	IIB	IIIA	IIIB	
T4a	IIB	IIIA	IIIB	IIIC	
T4b	IIIB	IIIB	IIIC	IIIC	

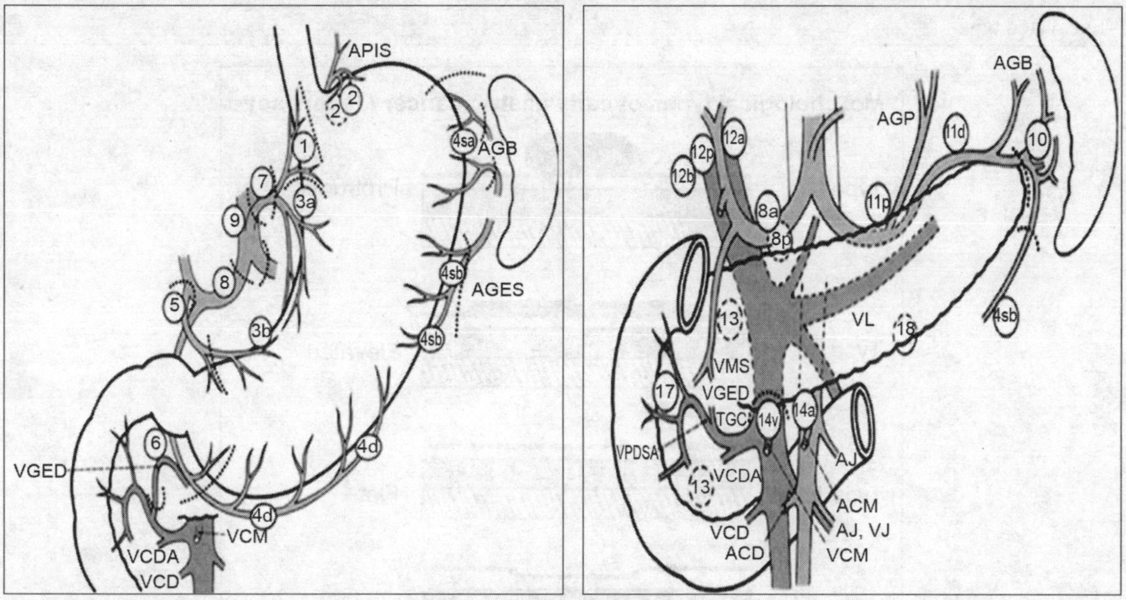

No. 1	Right paracardial LN
No. 2	Lest paracardial LN
No. 3a	LN along the left gastric vessels
No. 3b	LN along the right gastric vessels
No. 4sa	LN along the short gastric vessels
No. 4sb	LN along the left gastroepiploic vessels
No. 4d	LN along the right gastropiploic vessels
No. 5	Suprapyloric LN
No. 6	Infrapyloric LN
No. 7	LN along the left gastric artery
No. 8a	LN along the common hepatic artery (anterosuperior group)
No. 8b	LN along the common hepatic artery (posterior group)
No. 9	LN along the celiac artery
No. 10	LN at the splenic hilum
No. 11p	LN along the proximal splenic artery
No. 11d	LN along the distal splenic artery
No. 12a	LN in the hepatoduodenal ligament (along the hepatic artery)
No. 12b	LN in the hepatoduodenal ligament (along the bile duct)
No. 12p	LN in the hepatoduodenal ligament (behind the portal vein)
No. 13	LN on the posterior surface of the pancreatic head
No. 14v	LN along the superior mesenteric vein
No. 14a	LN along the superior mesenteric artery
No 15	LN along the middle colic vessels
No. 16a1	LN in the aortic hiatus
No. 16a2	LN around the abdominal aorta (from the upper margin of the celiac trunk to the lower margin of the left renal vein)
No. 16b1	LN around the abdominal aorta (from the lower margin of the left renal vein to the upper margin of the inferior mesenteric artery)
No. 16b2	LN around the abdominal aorta (from the upper margin of the inferior mesenteric artery to the aortic bifurcation)
No. 17	LN on the anterior surface of the pancreas head
No. 18	LN along the inferior margin on the pancreas
No. 19	Infradiaphragmatic LN
No. 20	LN in the esophageal hiatus of the diaphragm
No. 110	Paraesophageal LN in the lower thorax
No. 111	Supradiaphragmatic LN
No. 112	Posterior mediastinal LN

EARLY GASTRIC CANCER

- ***Cancer limited to mucosa and submucosa*** 30–40% in Japan

> - **Type I**–Protruding - > twice the thickness of normal mucosa
> - **Type IIa**–Superficial elevated upto twice thickness of that of normal mucosa
> - **Type IIb**–Flat type
> - **Type IIc**–Superficial depressed type
> - **Type III**–Excavated type

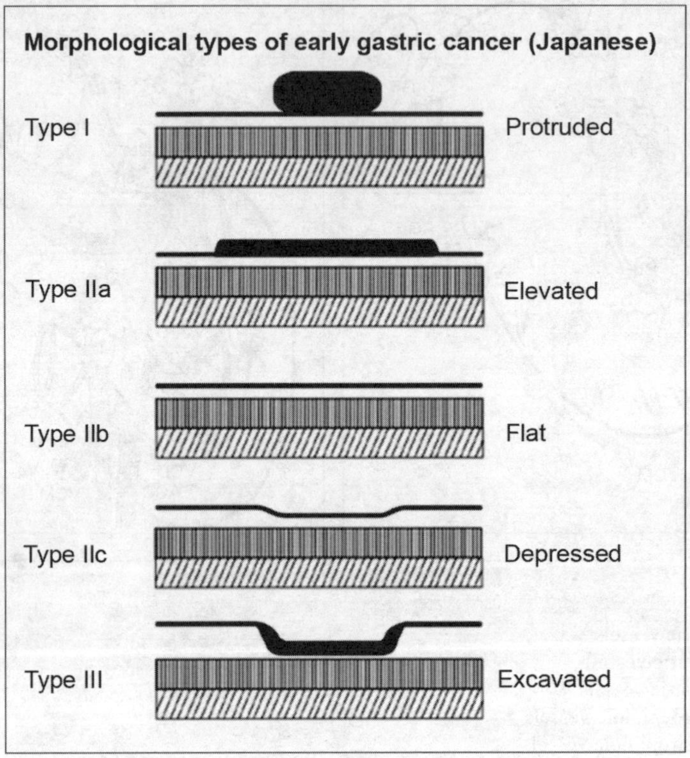

- Estimated median duration of early gastric cancer is 37 months
- 5 Years survival rates exceedingly 80% after adequate resection

ADVANCED GASTRIC CANCER

- **Polypoid fungating:**
  – Occurs in 10% of tumor with nodular polypoid surface with superficial ulceration
  – Relatively good prognosis after aggressive surgical management – well differentiated adenocarcinoma.
- **Ulcerating or penetrating:**
  – Cancer occurs in more than 50% – tumor in sessile and may look like benign gastric ulcer
- **Superficial spreading:**
  – More unusual (6%)
  – Diffusely infiltrates over wide area, predominantly confined to mucosa and submucosa. 50% metastasized to the perigastric lymph nodes at the time of presentation
- **Linitis plastica:**
  – Extensive infiltration of the submucosa/muscular layers with a marked fibroblastic/desmoplastic reaction around columns of malignant cells
  – Extensions into the esophagus and mesentery may occur

- Superficial erosions are common
- Poor prognosis
- Mucosa only biopsy may prove negative. 25% can cross pyloric ring and into first part of the duodenum with poor prognosis

Linitis Plastica (Scirrhous Carcinoma/Brinton's Disease

- Type IV gastric carcinoma (poorly differentiated mucin-producing carcinoma cells that infiltrates the muscle wall)
- **LEATHER BOTTLE STOMACH**
- Aggressive diffuse type with proliferation of fibrous tissue of submucosa which is thickened ***(Mother of Pearl appearance)***
- Mucosa appears normal
- Barium meal: Small sized stomach
- **Poor prognosis**
- Total gastrectomy with Esophagojejunal anastomosis is the treatment

Metastasis

- **Virchow's node – enlarged left supraclavicular nodes (Troisier's sign)**
- **Irish nodes –** Palpable ipsilateral axillary lymph nodes
- **Lymph node groups** (Nodal involvement does not imply systemic dissemination)

Group I: *Perigastric nodes*
Group II: *Along the root of major vessels*
Group III: *At root of SMA and hepatoduodenal ligament*
Group IV: *Distant lymph nodes*

- Blood borne metastasis mostly to **liver**
- **Transperitoneal spread** – best identified by **laparoscopy**
- **Sister Mary Joseph's node** (umbilical secondaries)
- **Blummer's shelf** (rectal secondaries)
- **Krukenberg's tumor** – Ovaries (commonly in colloid carcinoma of stomach)

CLINICAL FEATURES

- Vague epigastric discomfort after food (earliest symptom)
- Pain – non-radiating, unresolved by food particles
- Weight loss (most common symptom), anorexia, fatigue, vomiting
- Melena, Hematemesis
- Proximal Tumors – Dysphagia
- Distal tumors – Gastric outlet obstruction

INVESTIGATIONS

- Endoscopy and biopsy is the investigation of choice (6-8 biopsies taken)
- PET-CT is most useful for detecting distant metastasis and recurrent gastric cancer
- Laparoscopy US is very sensitive to see nodes and liver metastasis
- Endoscopic ultrasound–90% accuracy in detecting T staging and 80% in nodal staging

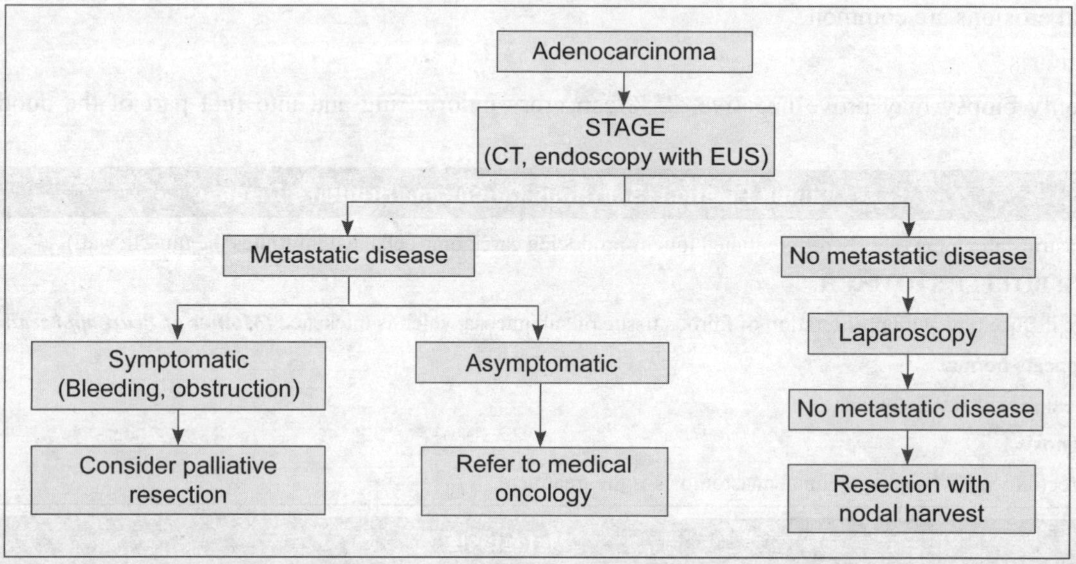

Barium Meal Findings in CA Stomach
• Irregular filling defect
• Loss of rugosity
• Delayed emptying
• Dilation of stomach in carcinoma pylorus
• Decreased stomach capacity in Linitis plastica
• Margin of lesion projects outward from the ulcer/lesion into the gastric lumen – ***Carmanns meniscus sign***

- **Tetracycline fluorescence test:** Gastric cancer cells take up tetracycline given orally which appears yellow under UV light
- **CA 72-4** is an important tumor marker to evaluate the relapse

Paraneoplastic Syndromes
• Trousseau syndrome (migratory thrombophlebitis)
• Acanthosis nigricans (hyper pigmentation of axilla and groin)
• Microangiopathic hemolytic anemia
• Diffuse Seborrheic keratoses (Leser-Trélat sign)

TREATMENT

- Surgical resection of the stomach is only curative treatment
- Tumors < 2 cm, elevated, well differentiated, without nodal disease: ***Endoscopic mucosal resection (EMR)***
- ***Growth in the body, proximal stomach, Linitis plastica*** – Total radical Gastrectomy with Oesophagogastric anastomosis
- ***Growth in pylorus*** – Lower radical gastrectomy with proximal 5 cm clearance, distal 2 cm clearance, nodal clearance, removal of greater and lesser omentum and later, Bilroth II anastomosis.
- ***Inoperable patients*** should undergo a course of Neo-adjuvant chemotherapy: epirubicin + cisplatinum + 5-FU infusion or oral capecitabine
- ***Radiotherapy*** – Gastric cancer are relatively radio resistant
- ***Proximal margin***–Needed for resection is 6 cm
- ***NCCN guidelines***–Atleast 4 cm margin required
- ***Distal margin***–1st part of duodenum

Dissection (D)	Regional Lymph Node Groups Removed
D0	None
D1	Perigastric
D2	D1 plus nodes along hepatic, left gastric, celiac and splenic arteries; splenic hilar nodes; +/- splenectomy
D3[a]	D2 plus periaortic and portahepatis

Operable–Subtotal/Total radical gastrectomy

Inoperable–Palliative resection

SURGICAL RESECTION

- R0 – Incomplete removal of perigastric nodes
- R1 – Complete removal of perigastric nodes
- R2 – R1 + removal of nodes along normal vessels
- R3 – R2 + removal of N3 nodes

	R1	R2
Upper 1/3 lesion	1-4	1-11 + paraesophageal
Middle 1/3 lesion	1, 3-6	1-11
Lower 1/3 lesion	3-6	1, 3-9

Signs of Inoperability

- Ascites, Liver secondaries, Para-aortic lymph nodes
- Adherent to pancreas, colon or mesocolon
- Blummer shelf, Left supraclavicular nodes, Sister Mary Joseph nodule, Irish node (Left axillary node secondaries)
- Palpable mass is incurable but resectable surgically

Prophylactic total gastrectomy is advised for those having

E cadherin gene mutation (90% risk)

Deletion/inactivation of p53

Over expression of COX-2

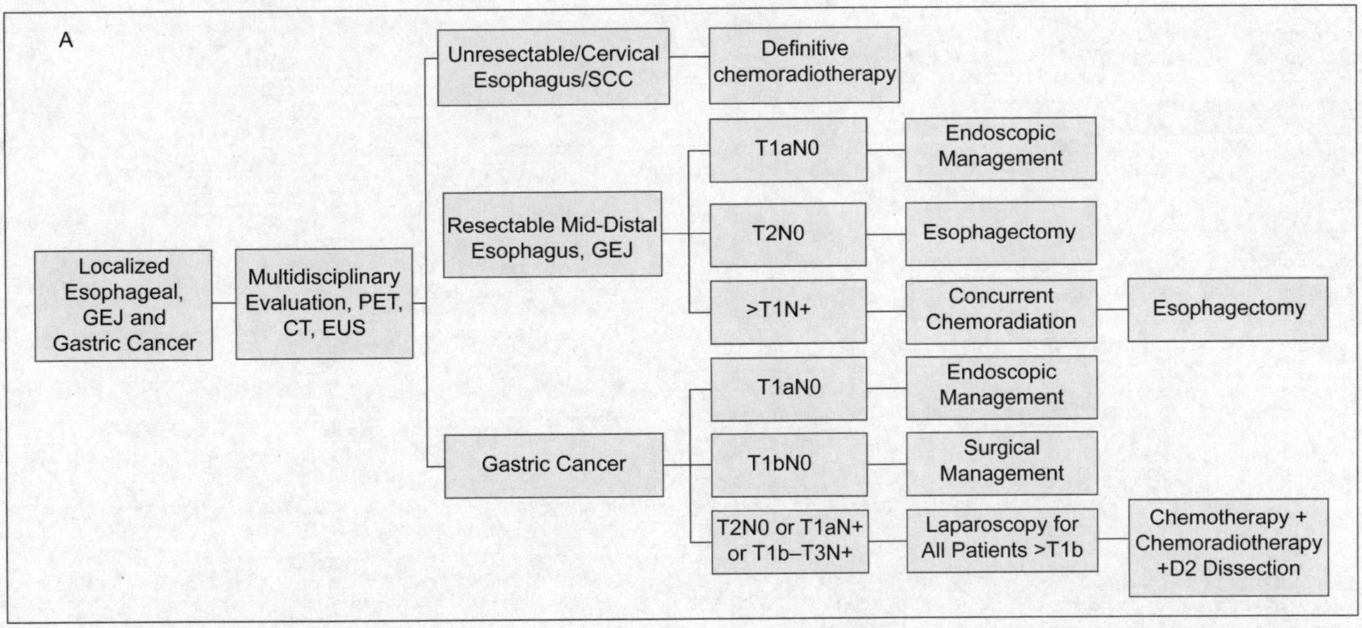

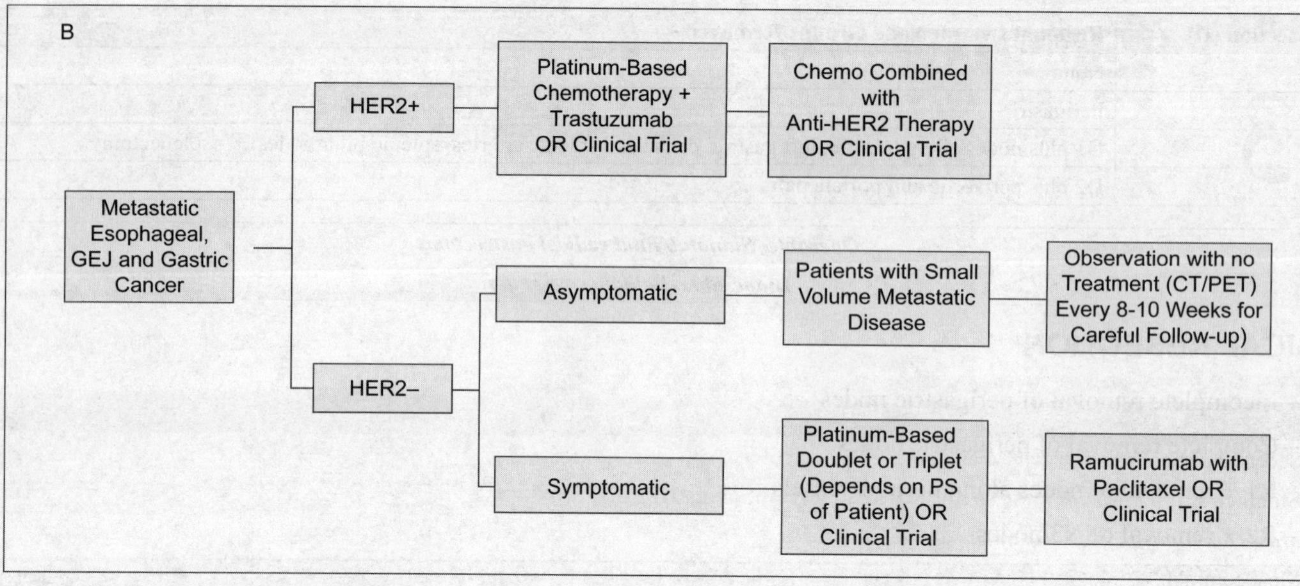
B
Metastatic Esophageal, GEJ and Gastric Cancer
HER2+
Platinum-Based Chemotherapy + Trastuzumab OR Clinical Trial
Chemo Combined with Anti-HER2 Therapy OR Clinical Trial
HER2–
Asymptomatic
Patients with Small Volume Metastatic Disease
Observation with no Treatment (CT/PET) Every 8-10 Weeks for Careful Follow-up)
Symptomatic
Platinum-Based Doublet or Triplet (Depends on PS of Patient) OR Clinical Trial
Ramucirumab with Paclitaxel OR Clinical Trial

CHAPTER 3

GASTRIC LYMPHOMA

One Liners

- Second most common primary malignancy of stomach
- **Stomach is the most common site of extranodal lymphoma (JIPMER SS)**
- ***Most common site is gastric antrum***
- Most common histological type of GI lymphoma is Diffuse large B cell lymphoma
- ***Diagnosis is made by endoscopic biopsy***
- EUS is most sensitive technique for per gastric lymphatic involvement
- ***Most common site of GI lymphoma is stomach***
- Origin of GI lymphoma is submucosal lymphoid tissue
- Associated with HIV, H. pylori and long term immunosuppression

Marker for GI lymphoma is CD20

- Treatment of choice in GI lymphoma is subtotal gastrectomy, chemotherapy with/without radiation based on extent of disease
- **Chemotherapy regimen for diffuse large B cell lymphoma is CHOP**
- MALToma is 2nd most common gastric lymphoma
- MALToma is associated with H. pylori infection
- **Remission of MALToma occurs with anti H. pylori therapy in many cases**

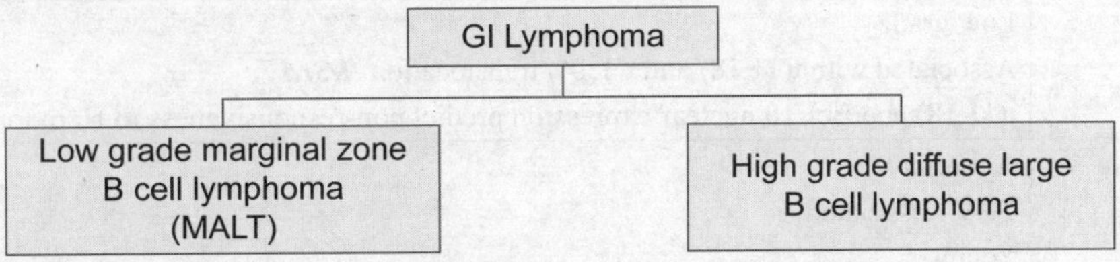

- Rarest lymphoma of all primary GI lymphoma–***Rectal***
- Constitute 20% of all lymphoma

Dawson's Criteria

- Absence of clinically enlarged lymph nodes on physical examination
- Absence of enlarged mediastinal lymph nodes on chest X-ray
- Normal hematologic values and bone marrow biopsy
- Normal spleen and liver

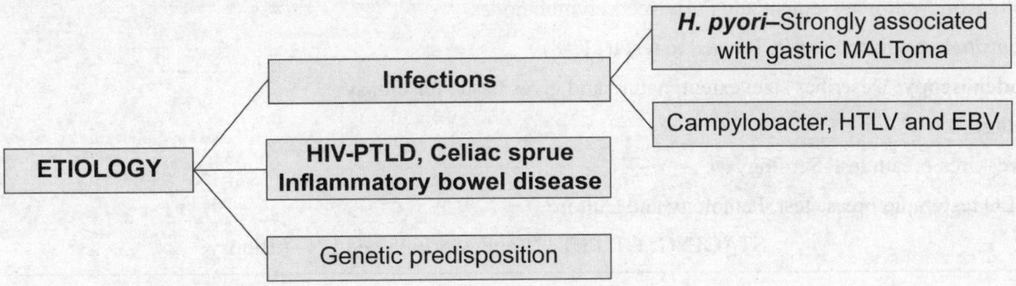

Pathology
• DLBCL • MALToma • Follicular cell lymphoma • Mantle cell lymphoma • Burkitt's lymphoma

ANN Arbor Staging
IE–Confined to GIT
IIE–Spread to regional lymph nodes
IIIE–Other abdominal organs
IVE–Beyond abdomen–chest, bone marrow
Lugano staging–GI lymphoma

Staging Systems for Primary Gastrointestinal Non-Hodgkin Lymphoma

Stage			
ANN ARBOR	**RAO ET AL**	**MUSSHOFF**	**Description**
IE	IE	IE	Tumor confined to GI tract
IIE	IIE	IIE	Tumor with spread to regional lymph nodes
IIE	IIIE	IIE	Tumor with nodal involvement beyond regional lymph nodes (para-aortic, iliac)
IIIE-IV	IVE	IIIE-IV	Tumor with spread to other intra-abdominal organs (liver, spleen) or beyond abdomen (chest, bone marrow)

Gastric Lymphoma

- Most common site for GI lymphoma
- Most common GI lymphoma–DLBCL
- Most common site–ANTRUM
- 6th decade
- Primary→ 5%
- Males
- ***H. pylori–Most important etiologic factor***

DLBCL	Most common type Aggressive Can arise Denovo and also from CLL-SLL, Follicular lymphoma and MALToma
MALToma	Low grade Associated with t(11,18) and t(1,14) translocation–***1/3rd*** t(11,18) and Bcl-10 nuclear expression predict non-responsiveness to H. pylori eradication
Burkitt's lymphoma	Aggressive EBV Associated Younger Cardia/Body **Endemic**–Children, Africa

- Epigastric Pain–Most common symptom
- Early satiety
- Anemia–Very common (>50%)

Investigations

Investigation of choice–Endoscopy and Biopsy

- **EUS**–Depth of gastric wall involvement and Perivisceral lymoh nodes
- Fluorescence *in situ* hybridization or PCR–used to test t(11,18)
- **Esophagoduodenoscopy:** Describes size, extent, nature and gives tissue for biopsy
- **H. pylori testing:**

  Non invasive–Urea breath test, Serology

  Invasive–CLO test–rapid urease test, Pathology and Culture

STAGING: CT, PET-CT and Any enlarged LN→ Biopsy

Treatment

- ***Chemotherapy***–Mainstay of treatment
- CHOP-R regimen
- **Indications of surgery:** Symptomatic recurrence, Associated with complications and Limited gastric disease
- **Complications:** Bleeding, Obstruction
- Patients with localized disease (Stage I and II) have lower relapse rates with addition of consolidation radiotherapy
- **Relapse**–High dose chemotherapy followed by autologous stem cell transplantation

Management of Gastric Maltoma	
Early stage with no t(11,18) or Bcl 10 expression	***H. pylori eradication with careful follow up*** Repeat endoscopy every 2 months to ensure infection clearance Biannual surveillance for 3 years to look for tumor regression
Transmural invasion *Nodal disease* *Large cell phenotypic transformation* *T (11,18)* *Bcl- 10 expression* *H. pylori –ve*	Predicts failure after H. pylori eradication Suggests poor prognosis ***Chemoradiation +/- Surgery***
If persistent MALT lymphoma after H. pylori therapy If without evidence of H. pylori infection	*External beam Radiotherapy–Best response* *If RT contraindicated Rituximab is advised*
Median time for remission–15 Months	

Small Intestinal Lymphoma

- Most common neoplasia in children <10 years
- ***Most common site–Ileum***

Treatment

- Asymptomatic–Chemotherapy
- Symptomatic–Surgical resection
- B cell lymphoma–More chemosensitive
- T cell lymphoma–Surgical resection

CHAPTER 4

GIST

- Gastrointestinal stromal tumors (GIST) are mesenchymal tumors of GI tract
- Cell of origin–Interstitial Cells of Cajal (pacemaker cells of GI tract)
- They have a incidence of 1.5 per 100000
- 1% of all GI tumors
- Most common mesenchymal tumor of GI tract
- Third common tumor in GI tract next to adenocarcinoma and lymphomas
- Slightly predominant in male
- Occurs in all age group
- Median age 60 – 65
- Those which occur in young have Wild Type (WT) mutations

SITE OF OCCURRENCE

- > 50% – STOMACH
- 25% – SMALL BOWEL
- 5% from the rectum
- Small minority from the esophagus

MUTATIONS IN GIST

- KIT–Stem cell factor or STEEL factor
- PDGFRA–Platelet derived growth factor alpha
- ***Downstream pathways:*** RAS/MAPK, P13/AKT/Mammalian taget of rapamycin Mtor

KIT Oncogene Mutations

- Exon 11–70% (Juxta membrane location)
- Exon 9–10% –Predominantly found in small intestine, Extra cellular Domain
- Exon 13 and 17–Intracellular Domain

PDGFRA Oncogene Mutations

- Predominantly found in stomach
- Exons 12,14 and 18
- 70% in exon 18D842V (Known for its insensitivity to Imatinib)

WT-KIT AND PDGFRA

- 10 to 15% of GIST have WT KIT or PDGFRA
- They have different pathogenesis and natural history

- **Classification:**
  - SDH deficient
  - Neurofibromatosis NF1 related
  - BRAF related

Succinate Dehydrogenase Deficient GIST

- Absence of KIT and PDGFRA mutations
- Arise exclusively in Stomach
- Associated with resistance to imatinib
- Great majority of tumors arise in childhood
- Immunohistochemically they are negative for SDH B

Carney's Triad	Carney Stratakis Syndrome
• GIST • Pulmonary Chondromas • Paragangliomas	• GIST • Paragangliomas
Young Children and Young adult females Spread to lymph nodes and Indolent course	Negative for SDH A Indolent course

Natural History

- Indolent tumors
- Frequently metastasize to liver
- Rarely spread to lymph nodes (SDH deficient)
- Never spreads to lungs

Clinical Presentation

- One-fourth of GISTs are diagnosed in a clinical emergency (Overt bleeding)
- One-fourth of GISTs are discovered incidentally during diagnostic assessments
- Rest presents with symptoms of compression from an abdominal mass, or chronic anemia, fatigue

Histopathology

- Spindle cells or Epitheloid cells or both
- No clinical implications
- Epithelioid variety is common in stomach
- No histological features to distinguish malignancy from benign
- All GIST are considered malignant

Immunophenotyping

- 95 % are positive for C-kit (CD117)
- 60-70% positive for CD34
- Negative for alpha-smooth muscle actin (SMA) (leiomyoma)
- Negative for S100 protein (Schwannoma)
- Negative for Desmin (desmoids)

STAGING

- Conventional staging system is seldom used

- Aim of evaluation is to distinguish between local and metastatic
- TNM classification is available

Risk stratification
• Mitotic index • Size of the tumor • Site of the tumor *Armed Forces Institute of Pathology AFIP* *MSKCC nomograms* *CONTOUR maps*

MANAGEMENT

- Localized Early stage tumors – Resect
- Locally Advanced – Preoperative Tyrosine kinase inhibitors

Surgical Principles

- Simple excision with negative surgical margin
- Tumor rupture to be avoided
- R0 better than R1 better than R2
- R1 in rectum should be resected
- Other sites consideration to be given to resect
- If surgical procedure is going to be morbid consider Preoperative TKI
- Unresectable consider preoperative TKI

IMATINIB MESYLATE

- Imatinib mesylate is a protein-tyrosine kinase inhibitor that inhibits the Bcr-Abl tyrosine kinase
- Imatinib is also an inhibitor PDGF and c-kit
- *In vitro,* imatinib inhibits proliferation and induces apoptosis in (GIST) cells, which express an activating c-kit mutation

> - **Imatinib:**
>   - 400 mg by mouth daily
>   - Possibly 800 mg by mouth daily, in case of: Exon 9 KIT-mutated GIST, Progression on imatinib 400 mg
> - **Sunitinib:**
>   - 50 mg by mouth daily for 4 weeks every 6 weeks
>   - 37.5 mg by mouth daily continuously
> - **Regorafenib:**
>   - 160 mg by mouth daily for 3 weeks every 4 weeks

Adjuvant Setting

- Imatinib to be given for Intermediate and High risk group
- To be given for 3 years

Metastatic

- Indefinite TKI

CHAPTER 5

SMALL BOWEL MALIGNANCIES

- Small intestine accounts for 75% of the length of GIT
- Small bowel malignancies encompass <5% of all GI cancers

Less incidence of malignancy
• Secretion of protective factors of small intestine • Stool quality • Low levels of carcinogenic factors • Secretion of Immunoglobulin A

- Adenocarcinoma accounts for 30% to 50% of small bowel malignancies
- Carcinoid 20% to 30%, and lymphomas and stromal tumors 15% each
- ***Carcinoids are more common in the ileum***
- ***Adenocarcinomas are more often found in the proximal small intestine***
- ***Sarcomas and lymphomas are most commonly seen in the distal small bowel but can be found throughout***

Associated familial inherited syndromes
• Familial adenomatous polyposis • Peutz–Jeghers • Lynch syndrome • Cowden syndrome • Von Recklinghausen neurofibromatosis • Crohn's disease *"High proportion of ileal tumors are seen in Cystic fibrosis"*

CLINICAL FEATURES

- Most common symptom–Abdominal pain
- Duodenal cancers can present with jaundice if ampulla is involved
- **Bowel perforation is presenting symptom in 10% of patients and is more often seen with lymphoma or sarcoma**

INVESTIGATIONS

CT imaging carries sensitivity of 80% for small bowel lesions and increases to 85% to 95% with CT or MR enterography

- For carcinoid tumors, radiolabeled somatostatin analog [^{111}In-DTPA] octreotide scintigraphy ***(OctreoScan)***→Used as an adjunct for identification of the primary and extraabdominal lesions, carrying a sensitivity of 88% and specificity of 97%
- **Enteroclysis:** Test of choice for detection of distal small bowel tumors (90% sensitivity)
- VCE–used to evaluate small intestine has poor diagnostic yield when used in patients with delayed gastric emptying, previous abdominal operations and poor bowel preparation

Adenocarcinoma

30% to 50% of all small bowel malignancies

>50% arise in the duodenum

Adenocarcinoma of Crohns disease is most common in Ileum

FAP

- APC gene is mutated in 10% to 18% of SBA compared to 80% of sporadic CRC
- Germline mutations in APC gene are found in FAP.
- ***FAP patients develop duodenal adenomas in 80% of cases with 4% developing adenocarcinoma.***

Lynch Syndrome

- ***MLH1, MSH2, MSH6 and PMS2 mismatch repair genes germ line inactivation is found in >90% of Lynch syndrome***
- Sporadic mutations, particularly in MLH1 can occur with overall inactivation of MMR system occurring in 15% of CRC
- 4% life time risk of adenocarcinoma
- SBA have deficiency in MMR in up to 35% of cases, much higher than that in CRC
- ***SBA patients with dMMR are more likely to have lesions localized to proximal (duodenum, jejunum)*** *rather than distal small intestines*
- Proteins frequently mutated in SBA are KRAS and p53 with mutation rates as high as 53% and 52%, respectively
- ***Ki ras mutations are seen in half of the tumors***

Duodenal tumors tend to be polypoidal

Jejunal and Ileal tumors are large and annular

Clinical Features

- >50% of patients present with stage III or IV disease
- Typically 50-70 years age
- Commoner in males
- Compared to carcinoid, lymphoma, and stromal tumors, SBA have a poorer prognosis
- LN metastasis–35% of patients at the time of diagnosis
- 20% have distant metastasis–***Liver is most common location***
- Patients with primary small bowel carcinoma should be monitored for development of 2nd malignant tumor (Most commonly colon)

CEA elevated in 30% of patients

CA 19-9 elevated in 40% of patients

Duodenal lesions

- **Proximal duodenal lesions- Pancreaticoduodenectomy with locoregional lymphadenectomy**
- **Distal duodenal lesions- Wide excision with lymphadenectomy**

Primary treatment for SBA–Complete resection with locoregional lymphadenectomy

Jejunal and ileal lesions–Wide excision and regional LN dissection

Ileal lesions close to cecum–Right colectomy or ileocecectomy to obtain -ve margins

T1a	Invades Lamina propria (LP)
T1b	Invades Submucosa (SM)
T2	Invades Muscularis propria (MP)
T3	Invades through Muscularis propria into Subserosa Or Extends into Non-peritonealized Perimuscular tissue (Mesentry/Retroperitoneum)
T4	Perforates visceral peritoneum or directly invades other loops of small intestine, mesentery of adjacent bowel loops and abdominal wall by way of serosa ***Duodenum–Invasion of pancreas/bile duct***
N1	Metastasis in 1 or 2 Lymph nodes
N2	Metastasis in 3 or more Lymph nodes

	N0	N1	N2	M1
T1	I	IIIA	IIIB	IV
T2	I	IIIA	IIIB	IV
T3	IIA	IIIA	IIIB	IV
T4	IIB	IIIA	IIIB	IV

Adjuvant Therapy

5-fluorouracil–based chemotherapy is standard for patients with high risk SBA (+LN)

HIPEC

- Hyperthermic intraperitoneal chemotherapy with cytoreductive surgery is standard of care for pseudomyxoma peritonei, peritoneal mesothelioma and colorectal cancer with peritoneal only metastases

Metastatic disease–Systemic chemotherapy is primary treatment

(CAPOX/FOLFOX)

- Duodenal tumors <1 cm should be treated by polypectomy
- Lesions >2 cm are treated by endoscopic removal
- Tumors located near ampulla of vater (at 2nd part of duodenum)–Pancreaticoduodenectomy

CARCINOIDS

- Peak incidence of carcinoid tumors is in the seventh to eighth decades
- Jejunal/ileal NETs occur at higher rates occur in males
- Small bowel carcinoids account for 42% of NETs of GIT
- Malignant nature of carcinoids is based on LN Status and Presence of metastasis
- Associated with 10% MEN1 and NF1

Most commonly arise from terminal ileum

RISK FACTORS

- Family history of Prostate or Colorectal cancer among any first-degree relatives, tongue or mouth cancer in siblings and endometrial, kidney, skin, or NHL in parents
- Smoking increases risk of small bowel carcinoids

Mid Gut Grading System				
Grade	Differentiation	Traditional	WHO	Criteria
Low	Well differentiated	Carcinoid tumor	Grade 1	<2 mitoses/10 HPF or <3% Ki 67 index
Intermediate	Well differentiated	Carcinoid tumor	Grade 2	2-20 mitoses/10 HPF or 3-20% Ki 67 index
High	Poorly differentiated	Small cell carcinoma Large cell neuroendocrine carcinoma	Grade 3	>20 mitoses/10 HPF or >20% Ki 67 index

T1	Invades lamina propria/submucosa and size less than or equal to 1cm
T2	Invades muscularis propria or size >1cm
T3	Invades through muscularis propria into subserosal tissue without penetration of overlying serosa
T4	Invades visceral peritoneum or other organs or adjacent structures
N1	Regional lymph node metastasis <12 nodes
N2	***Large mesenteric masses >2 cm and extensive nodal deposits (12/more) especially that encase superior mesenteric vessels***
M1a	Confined to liver
M1b	At least 1 extrahepatic disease–Lung, ovary, non-regional lymph node, peritoneum, bone
M1c	Both hepatic and extrahepatic metastases

- Regional LN→ ***70% of patients***
- Liver metastasis→ ***50% of patients***
- 20-30% of patients can present with carcinoid syndrome
- Carcinoid syndrome–Flushing (94%), DiAarrhea (80%)–Triggered by alcohol, blue cheese, chocolate or red wine
- Long-term carcinoid syndrome leads to Right sided heart failure
- ***Most extreme manifestation of carcinoid syndrome–Carcinoid crisis***
- Carcinoid crisis can be triggered by surgery and therefore all patients with NETs should be given Octreotide preoperatively
- **Chromogranin A**–Polypeptide present in secretory granules of neuroendocrine cells, Elevated in 60-100% of patients.

False elevations of CgA
Renal/Liver Failure, Chronic gastritis, Taking PPI's (Stop PPI's 2 weeks before CgA evaluation)
False elevations of 5HIAA
After recent alcohol consumption, Nuts, Tomatoes, Cold/Cough remedies

- CgA and 5HIAA are reflective of tumor burden and detects tumor recurrence after initial resection
- MRI–Carcinoids on T1 weighted images→ Hypointense/Isointense, Liver metastasis→Bright on T2 weighted images
- Can create desmoplastic reaction resulting in contraction and foreshortening of mesentery
- If localized disease–Complete resection of primary tumor with regional lymphadenopathy
- Metastatic disease–Complete resection of all lesions is possible
- Unresectable metastatic disease–Surveillance
- Somatostatin analogues–Symptom relief and Disease stabilization
- Somatostatin refractory cases–Interferon alpha is used to treat diarrhea in 50% of cases
- PROMID Study→Octreotide and
- RADIANT 2→Everolimus
- Overall 5 years survival→ Resectable metastatic disease 68% and Unresectable metastatic disease 38%
- ***Liver transplantation***→ Can be considered for patients with liver limited high burden disease
- ***Hepatic artery embolization***→ Palliate painful refractory liver metastasis

SARCOMAS

- Constitute 8% of small intestinal malignancies
- Most common type–Leiomyosarcoma and GIST
- Most common site–Jejunum
- Most common symptom–Abdominal pain
- ***Risk factors–EBV, Radiation, Li Fraumeni syndrome and Hereditary retinoblastoma***
- Heterogenous mass with presence of necrosis if tumor has out grown blood supply
- Treatment–Complete resection
- No lymphadenectomy required
- Metastatic disease and Bleeding/Obstruction–Palliative resection/Enteric bypass

LYMPHOMA

- 15% of all primary small intestinal malignancies
- Affects 60-70 years of age
- **Risk factors**–Celiac disease, HIV, PTLD, Wegener's granulomatosis, Wiskott Aldrich syndrome, SCID, X-linked agamma pylori and IPSID

Lymphoma of Celiac Disease is T cell Lymphoma (Jejunal)

- Most common site–Ileum (60-65%)
- Predominantly NHL (B cell)
- Multifocal with skip lesions upto 15% cases
- Most common mode of presentation–Partial small bowel obstruction
- Forms 25% of GI Lymphomas
- 25% present with perforation
- CHOP regimen
- **Surgery**–Bleeding, Obstruction and Perforation

METASTATIC MALIGNANCIES

- Most common malignancy of small bowel–Metastatic lesions
- Primary tumors that often spread to small bowel–Colon, Ovary, Lung and Melanoma
- Melanoma–Can spread to mesenteric LN and therefore during time of resection local lymphadenectomy is recommended.
- Tumor that extreme propensity to spread to small bowel–Melanoma

CHAPTER 6

HEREDITARY CRC

Gene mutations that promote colorectal cancer		
Mutation Type	**Genes Involved**	**Type of Disease Caused**
Germline	*APC*	Familial adenomatous polyposis
	MMR	HNPCC (Lynch syndrome)
Somatic	**Oncogenes:** *myc, ras, src, erbB*	Sporadic disease
	Tumor suppressor genes: *TP53, DCC, APC* **MMR genes:** *bMSH2, bMLH1, bPMS1, bPMS2, bMSH6, bMSH3*	
Genetic polymorphism	*APC*	Familial colon cancer in Ashkenazi Jews

Pathogenesis and Molecular Aspects
APC Gene • APC gene–Tumor suppressor gene • Chromosome 5q21– ***Germ line truncation mutation*** • Forms cytoplasmic complex with GSK 3 beta, beta catenin and axin • APC gene defects are known to be present in 80% of sporadic CRC • When APC is mutated, ***Beta catenin levels rise and Wnt is activated*** • Mutations in ***both alleles*** are necessary to initiate polyp formation • Majority of mutations are premature stop codons that result in Truncated APC protein
APC Inactivation alone doesn't result in Carcinoma
K Ras • Signaling molecule in EGFR pathway • Most commonly involved gene in CRC– K ras • Proto oncogene • ***Mutation of only 1 allele*** • K ras gene product is a G protein involved in Intracellular signal transduction – When active K ras binds GTP, hydrolysis of GTP to GDP then inactivates G protein – Mutation of K ras results in inability of hydrolyze GTP thus leaving G protein permanently active leading to uncontrolled cell division **MYH Gene** • Occurs on chromosome 1p • MYH is base excision repair gene • Biallelic deletion • Expressed in AR
P53–75% of Colorectal cancer

Contd.

Contd.

DCC

- Tumor suppressor gene and Loss of both alleles is required for Malignant degeneration
- ***Present in >70% of CRC***
- May negatively impact prognosis
- DPC4 gene–Located on chromosome 18q

SMAD4

- Signaling cascade of TGF beta and Beta catenin
- Downstream effector of APC gene
- Chromosome 18q
- SMAD 2 and 4–Associated with 5-10% of Sporadic CRC

Genetic Pathways

LOH Pathway

- Characterized by Chromosomal deletions and tumor aneuploidy
- 80% CRC arise
- *Tend to occur more in distal colon and associated with poor prognosis*

Microsatellite Instability

- Tumors associated with MSI appear to have different biologic characteristics than do tumors that result from LOH pathway
- **MSI**–*Right colon and possess diploid DNA and associated with better prognosis*

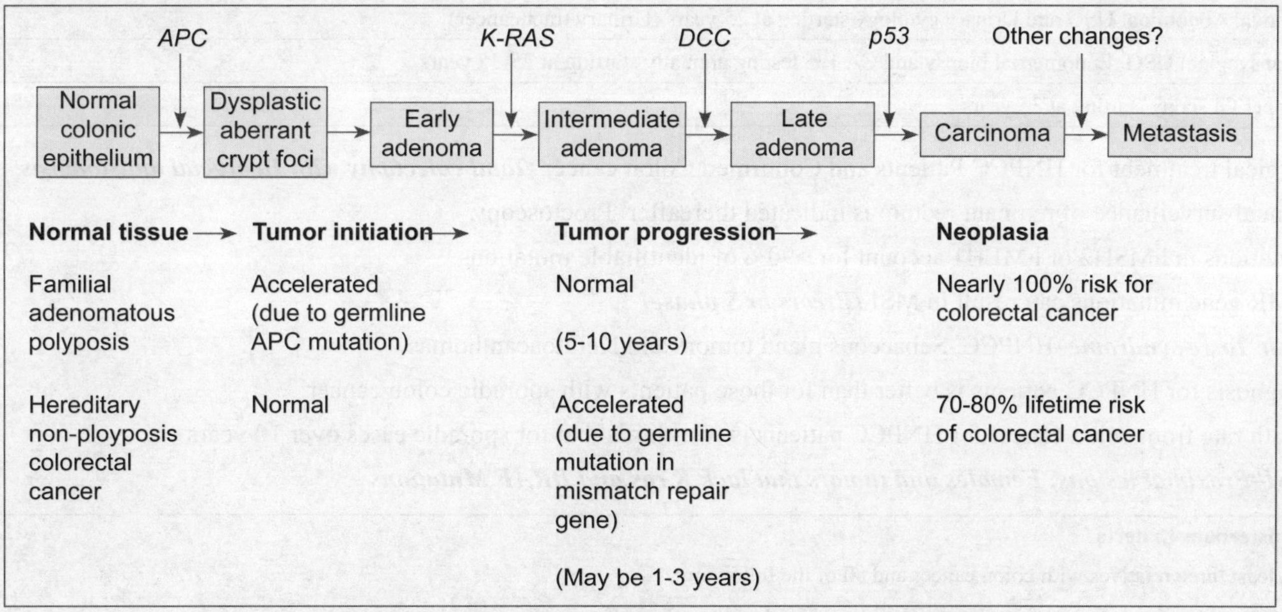

***Tubular adenoma:** <1cm→<5% and >2 cm→35%*

***Villous adenoma:** >2 cm→ 50%*

HNPCC (LYNCH SYNDROME)

- Most commonly inherited rectal cancer syndrome
- Approximately 3% of all CRC
- Accounts for approximately 15% of cancers in patients with family history of colorectal cancer
- *Autosomal dominant*
- *Germline mutations in DNA mismatch repair genes (Care taker genes)*
- Molecular signature of MMR mutations–MSI finding

- MLH1 and MSH2 account for 90% of all mutations
- Penetrance varies from 30-70%
- One allele from germline mutation of MMR gene

Relatively young (44 years), Proximal distribution (70% of cancers located in right colon), predominantly mucinous or poorly differentiated (Signet ring) adenocarcinoma with increased synchronous and metachronous cancers

- ***Life time Risk of developing CRC by 4th or 5th decade is approximately 80%***
- Increased risk of Endometrial, Gastric, Ovarian and Hepatobiliary cancers
- 20% of patients have synchronous tumors
- 20-60% of patients develop metachronous CRC if subtotal colectomy is not performed
- Possibility of Lynch syndrome–Adenomatous Polyps at Early age
- Most common extracolonic cancer–Endometrial cancer
- PMS2/MSH6–More attenuated forms of HNPCC
- ***MSH6 Inactivation***–Associates with higher risk of Endometrial cancer

Mostly right sided cancers (60-70% proximal to splenic flexure)

Screening Protocol
Screening colonoscopy in affected individuals should begin by 20-25 years or 10 years younger than youngest age at diagnosis in family whichever comes 1st and should be repeated every 2 years until 35 years
Annual Abdominal USG and Urinary cytology starting at 25 years (Urinary tract cancer)
Transvaginal USG, Endometrial biopsy and CA 125 testing annually starting at 25-35 years
Upper GI scopy starting at 35 years

- Surgical treatment for HNPCC Patients and Confirmed Colon cancer–***Total colectomy with Ileorectal anastomosis***
- Annual surveillance of remnant rectum is indicated thereafter–Proctoscopy
- Mutations in hMSH2 or hMLH1 account for >90% of identifiable mutations
- MMR gene mutations can result in MSI ***(Errors in S phase)***
- ***Muir Torre syndrome***–HNPCC, Sebaceous gland tumors and Keratoacanthomas
- Prognosis for HNPCC patients is better than for those patients with sporadic colon cancer
- Death rate from colon cancer for HNPCC patients is two-thirds that for sporadic cases over 10 years
- ***MSI–Proximal lesions, Females and tumors that lack K ras and BRAF Mutations***

Amsterdam Criteria

At least three relatives with colon cancer and all of the following:

- One affected person is a first-degree relative of the other two affected persons
- Two successive generations affected
- At least one case of colon cancer diagnosed before the age of 50 years
- FAP excluded

Modified Amsterdam Criteria

Same as the Amsterdam criteria, except that cancer must be associated with HNPCC (colon, endometrium, small bowel, ureter, renal pelvis) instead of specifically colon cancer

Bethesda Criteria

The Amsterdam criteria or one of the following:

- Two cases of HNPCC-associated cancer in one patient, including synchronous or metachronous cancer

Contd.

Contd.

- Colon cancer and a first-degree relative with HNPCC-associated cancer and/or colonic adenoma (one case of diagnosed before age 45 years and adenoma diagnosed before age 40 years)
- Colon or endometrial cancer diagnosed before age 45 years
- Right-sided colon cancer that has an undifferentiated pattern (solid, cribriform) or signet cell histopathologic characteristics diagnosed before age 45 years
- Adenomas diagnosed before age 40 years

FAP

- Accounts for 1% of all CRC
- Autosomal dominant disorder with APC germline mutations (5q21)–***Gatekeeper gene***
- Gene is expressed in 100% of patients with mutation
- ***Life time risk of CRC in FAP is 100%***
- CRC develops in nearly 100% by 40 years of age
- Present with strong history of early colon cancers in 1st/2nd degree relatives
- 90% of patients develop polyps in upper GIT particularly ***Duodenum***
- 5% of duodenal polyps progress to Invasive carcinoma
- ***Gastric and Duodenal polyps occur in approximately 50% of affected individuals***
- Most patients of FAP die of colon cancer by their 5th decade
- ***APC mutation testing +ve →75% cases***
- Occurs in codon 1250 to 1464 at 3' end of codon
- FAP patients will have known family history and up to 25% present without other affected family members
- Average age of new patient with FAP is 29 years
- Average age of newly discovered CRC related to FAP–39 years
- Flexible sigmoidoscopy of 1st degree relatives of FAP patients begins at age 10-15 years
- ***If APC testing is +ve in a relative of patient with known APC mutation***→Annual flexible sigmoidoscopy beginning at age 10-15 years is done until polyps are identified
- ***If APC testing is –ve***→ relative can be screened starting at 50 years per average risk guidelines
- ***If APC testing is refused/unavailable or if mutation can't be identified***–Annual flexible sigmoidoscopy beginning at age 10-15 years is performed until 24 years
- Screening flexible sigmoidoscopy is then done every 2 years until 34 years age, every 3 years until 44 years age and then every 3 to 5 years
- Most common site of adenomas other than colorectal region–Duodenum
- Upper GI endoscopy is recommended for surveillance every 1-3 years beginning at age 25-30 years
- COX 2 inhibitors may slow or prevent development of polyps
- Celecoxib and sulindac caused regression of adenomatous polyps in FAP
- Earliest pathological change–***Abberant crypt formation***

Risk of rectal cancer is almost 3 times higher in FAP with mutation after codon 1250 than before this codon.

Associated with

- **CHRPE**–75% of affected individuals
- **Desmoids**
  - Present in Retroperitoneum and Abdominal wall of affected patients usually after surgery
  - Often locally invasive

Contd.

Contd.

- – Direct invasion of mesenteric vessels, ureters or walls of small intestine
- – ***Small desmoids***– Confined to abdominal wall is appropriately treated by resection
- – *Initial treatment is usually with sulindac or tamoxifen* (Hormone responsive to treatment with Tamoxifen)
- **Gardner syndrome** (DOD)–Epidermoid cysts, Mandibular osteoma and Periampullary neoplasms
  - – ***Osteomas***–Usually palpable prominences in skull, mandible and tibia
  - – ***Almost always Benign***
  - – Bone cysts, Supernumerary and Impacted molars or congenital absent teeth
- **Turcot syndrome**–CNS Tumors, Colonic polyps

AFAP

- Autosomal dominant
- Attenuated adenomatous polyposis coli is less aggressive variant of FAP
- Develop fewer polyps
- Confined typically to proximal colon–***Right colon***
- ***Mutations close to 5' end if gene produce a short truncated protein***

"Rarely affects rectum"

- CRC manifests later in ***5th decade***–More than 50%
- APC mutation seen in only 30% of patients
- Genetic counseling and testing–Mutation unknown→ Screening colonoscopy at 13-15 years then every 4 years to 28 years and then every 3 years

MAP

- MYH associated polyposis is an ***Autosomal recessive disorder***
- Results from biallelic germline mutations in MYH (Base excision repair gene)
- No detectable APC mutation
- Most develop CRC before 60 years

FAMILIAL CRC

- Non-syndromic familial CRC–Accounts for 10-15% of CRC
- Life time risk of developimg CRC increases with family history of disease
- With no family history of– 6%, 1st degree relative affected–12%, Two 1st degree relatives affected–36%
- Screening colonoscopy every 5 years beginning at age 40 or beginning 10 years before age of earliest diagnosed patient in pedigree
- No associated genetic abnormalities–*LOH/MSI*

SPORADIC CRC

- Loss of APC and P53 with accumulation of chromosomal instability over time
- Loss of DNA Mismatch repair and acquired MLH1 methylation
- BRAF (Serrated/Methylator pathway)–Characterized by methylation of CpG islands that cause silencing of critical tumor suppressor genes resulting CIMP (CpG island methylator phenotype) tumors

	Hereditary Adenomatous Polyposis Syndromes		Hereditary Hamartomatous Polyposis Syndromes			
Hereditary Nonpolyposis Colon Cancer	**Familial Adenomatous Polyposis (FAP) ϕ Gardner Syndrome**	**Turcot Syndrome**	**Cowden Disease**	**Familial Juvenile Polyposis**	**Peutz-Jeghers Syndrome**	**Ruvalcaba-Myhre-Smith Syndrome (Bannayan-Zonana Syndrome)**
GI Features						
Small number of colorectal polyps	Hundreds to thousands of colorectal polyps; duodenal adenomas and gastric polyps, usually fundic gland	Colorectal polyps, which may be few or resemble classic FAP	Polyps most commonly of colon and stomach	Juvenile polyps mostly in colon but throughout GI tract; defined by $\geq$10 juvenile polyps	Small number of polyps throughout GI tract but most common in small intestine	Hamartomatous GI polyps, usually lipomas, hemangiomas, or lymphangiomas
Other Clinical Features						
Muir-Torre variant: Sebaceous adenomas, keratoacanthomas, sebaceous epitheliomas, and basal cell epitheliomas	Osteomas, desmoids tumors, epidermoid cysts, and congenital hypertrophy of retinal epithelium	Brain tumors, including cerebellar medulloblastoma and glioblastomas	Mucocutaneous lesions, thyroid adenomas and goiter, fibroadenomas and fibrocystic disease of the breast, uterine leiomyomas, macrocephaly	Cogenital abnormalities in at least 20%, including malrotation, hydrocephalus, cardiac lesions, Meckel's diverticulum, mesenteric lymphangioma	Pigmented lesions of skin; benign and malignant genital tumors	Dysmorphic facial features macrocephaly, seizures, intellectual impairment, pigmented macules of shaft and glans of penis
Malignancy Risk						
70%-80% lifetime risk for colorectal cancer; 30%-60% lifetime risk for endometrial cancer, ↑ risk for ovarian cancer, gastric carcinoma, transitional cell carcinoma of the ureters and renal pelvis, small bowel cancer, and sebaceous carcinomas	Colorectal cancer risk approaches 100%; ↑ risk for periampullary malignant disease, thyroid carcinoma, central nervous system tumors, heptoblastoma	Colorectal carcinoma and brain tumors	10% risk for thyroid cancer and up to 50% risk for adenocarcinoma of breast in affected women	9% to 25% risk for colorectal cancer; ↑ risk for gastric, duodenal, and pancreatic cancer	↑Risk for GI malignant disease and pancreatic cancer and adenoma malignum of cervix; unknown risk for breast cancer	Malignant GI tumors identified but lifetime risk for malignant disease unknown
Screening Recommendations						
Clonoscopy at age 20-25 years; repeat every 1-3 years; transvaginal ultrasound or endometrial aspiration at age 20-25 years; repeat annually (expert opinion only)	Flexible proctosigmoidoscopy at age 10-12 years; repeat every 1-2 years until age of 35 years; after the age of 35 years, repeat every 3 years; upper GI endoscopy every 1-3 years starting when polyps first identified	Same as for FAP, also consider imaging of the brain	Annual physical examination with special attention to thyroid; mammography at age 30 years or 5 years before earliest breast cancer case in the family, routine colon cancer surveillance (expert opinion only)	Screening by age 12 years if symptoms have not yet arisen; colonoscopy with multiple random biopsy specimens every several years (expert opinion only)	Upper GI endoscopy, small bowel radiography, colonoscopy every 2 years; pancreatic ultrasound and hemoglobin levels annually; gynecologic examination, cervical smear, pelvic ultrasound annually; clinical breast examination and mammography at age 25 years; clinical testicular	No known published re-commendations

Contd.

Contd.

					examination and testicular ultrasound in males with feminizing features (expert opinion only)	
Genetic Basis						
AD	AD	AD	AD	AD inheritance in some families	AD	AD
MLH1 (chromosome 3p) MSH2 (chromosome 2p) MSH6/GTMP (chromosome 2p) PMS1 (chromosome 2q) PMS2 (chromosome 7q)	*APC* (chromosome 5q)	*APC* mutations identified predominantly in families with cerebellar medulloblastoma *MLH1, PMS2* mutations identified in families with predominance of glioblastomas	*PTEN* (chromosome 10q)	Subset of families with mutation in *SMAD4 (DRC4)* (chromosome 10q)	*STK11* (chromosome 19p)	*PTEN* (chromosome 10q) in some
Genetic Testing						
Clinical testing of *MLH1* and *MSH2* genes available	Clinical testing of *APC* gene available	Clinical testing of *APC* and *MLH1* genes available	Research testing of *PTEN* gene available	Families being collected for research studies only	Research testing of *STK11* gene available	Research testing of *PTEN* gene available

Colorectal Molecular Subtypes		
CMS1	Predominantly MSI high tumors Tend to be Hypermutated, Methylated and Enriched for BRAF mutations	Right sided tumors Older age at diagnosis Females Intermediate survival Worse survival after relapse
CMS2	High CIN MSS	Left sided tumors Better survival
CMS4	Display proangiogenic properties Poor prognosis- Early relapse and Distant failure	
CMS 3	K RAS and PIK3CA mutations	Intermediate survival

a. **Lynch syndrome I:** Autosomal-dominant inheritance with susceptibility to early onset of colorectal cancer proximal to the splenic flexure in the absence of diffuse polyps

   Lynch syndrome II: Contains most of the features of Lynch I with excess incidence of carcinomas of the endometrium, ovary, kidney, ureter, bladder, bile duct and small bowel and of lymphoma

b. Epidermoid cysts, fibromas, desmoids, dental and osseous abnormalities, intraperitoneal and retroperitoneal fibrosis, ampullary carcinoma, and tumors in other glandular structures. Follow with ophthalmoscopy for associated congenital hypertrophy of the retinal pigment epithelium

c. Hyperpigmentation, alopecia and nail dystrophy

d. Prophylactic colectomy should be considered if 5 to 10 adenomatous polyps are present or if polyps recur

e. Total colectomy with pouch reconstruction. NSAIDS decrease number and size of polyps

Disease	Histology	Distribution of Polyps	Malignant Potential	Associated Manifestations	Age for First FOB Test (years)	Age for First Colonoscopy (years)	Surgery
Discrete polyps and CC	Few AP	Colon	High	None	≥45	≥45	Same as for general population
Hereditary discrete common polyps and CC	AP	Proximal colon	High	Lynch I[a]	30-35	35	Same as for general population
HNPCC	AP →AC	Proximal colon	High	Lynch II[a]	None (ES)	20	Subtotal colectomy
Familial CC	AP	Proximal colon; may be distal	High	None	30-35	35	Same as for general population
FAP and Turcot syndrome	Scattered AP →AC	Colon	High	Central nervous system tumors	None (ES)	Teens	Prophylactic subtotal colectomy
FAP and Oldfield syndrome	Scattered AP →AC	Colon	High	Skin tumors	None (ES)	Teens	Prophylactic subtotal colectomy
FAP and Gardner syndrome	Scattered AP →AC	Usually colon; also stomach and SB	High	See Footnote[b]	None (ES)	Teens	Prophylactic subtotal colectomy
Peutz-Jeghers Syndrome	Hamartomas	Stomach, SB, colon, and ovary	Low	Buccal and cutaneous pigmentation	≥45	≥45	None
Generalized GI juvenile polyposis	JP	Stomach, SB and colon	Low	None	None	≥45	None
Juvenile polyposis coli of infancy	JP	Stomach, SB and colon	None	Protein-losing enteropathy	None	No special indications	None
Cronkhite-Canada syndrome	JP	Stomach, SB and colon	None	Protein-losing enteropathy[c]	None	No special indications	None

CHAPTER 7

COLORECTAL CANCER

- More than 90% of cases diagnosed older than 50 years
- 80% CRC occur sporadically–Most common
- Rectal cancers–More commen in men
- More common in African Americans

RISK FACTORS

- Diet high in Animal fat and Low fiber has lead to carcinogenesis
- Diet high in Saturated or Polyunsaturated fats increase risk of CRC
- ***Diet high in Oleic acid (Olive oil, Coconut oil, Fish oil)–Doesn't increase risk***
- High fiber diet–Protective
- Alcohol
- Calcium, Selenium, Vitamin D, Regular aspirin usage and Plant phenols decrease CRC risk
- Vitamin A, C and E, Carotenoids–Doesn't appear to decrease risk of ployp formation
- **Oral Bisphosphonate**–Associated with Reduced CRC risk (At least 1 year)
- **Tobacco**
  - Associated with increased incidence and mortality of CRC
  - Association is greater with rectal cancers

Obesity and Sedentary life style increase cancer related mortality

Inflammatory bowel disease
• *Patients with long standing colitis from IBD are at increased risk of CRC* • *Duration and Extent of colitis correlate with risk* • *Presence of PSC and Family history of CRC increases risk*
Cancer in these patients is inversely proportional to age of Onset and directly proportional to Extent of colon involvement and Duration of active disease

Cigarette smoking is associated with increased risk of colonic adenoma (>35 years)

- Ureterosigmoidoscopy also increases risk of both adenoma and carcinoma
- Acromegaly also increases risk of CRC
- Pelvic RT increases risk of rectal carcinoma
- About 15% of all colorectal cancers occur in patients with history of colorectal cancer in first-degree relatives
- ***Exposure to asbestos (Brake mechanics) increases incidence of colorectal cancer to 1.5 to 2 times that of average population***

POLYPS

Screen relevant neoplasia: Polyps >1cm, High grade dysplasia and Villous histology

Neoplastic Polyps

- Occurs in 25% of population who is older than 50 years age
- ***Risk of malignancy is related to both Size and Type of Polyp***
- Polyp >1cm→ 2.5 to 4 fold increased risk of cancer
- Multiple polyps→ 5 to 7 fold increased risk of cancer
  - *Tubular adenoma–Malignancy in 5% of cases*
  - *Villous adenoma–Malignancy in 40% of cases*
- Rectal sessile polyps–Transanal resection
- Colectomy–Reserved for patients in which colonoscopic removal is impossible (Large flat lesions/invasive cancer is confirmed)

Hyperplastic polyps

- Usually small (< 5mm)–Not considered premalignant
- Large hyperplastic polyps (>2 cm) may have ***slight risk of malignancy***
- Hyperplastic polyposis–Associated with increased risk of CRC (Multiple large hyperplastic polyps that occur in young adults).

Serrated Polyps

- Treated like adenomatous polyps

Inflammatory polyps (Pseudopolyps)

- Most commonly occurs in context of IBD but may also occur after amoebic colitis, Ischemic colitis and Schistosomal colitis
- ***Not premalignant***
- Extensive polyposis especially in patients with severe colitis

Hamartomatous Polyps (Juvenile Polyps)

- ***Not premalignant***
- Characteristic polyps of childhood
- **Bleeding**–common symptom
- Associated with PTEN mutations

Incidence of Synchronous adenoma with 1 known adenoma–40-50%

Familial Juvenile Polyposis	***Autosomal dominant*** Hundreds of polyps in colon and rectum Annual screening begins between 10 and 12 years If rectum spared–Total abdominal colectomy with Ileorectal anastomosis If rectum involved–Total proctocolectomy **JPS**–*Increased risk of both GI and Extraintestinal cancers, Predominantly hamartomas, Malignant potential of at least 10% in patients with multiple juvenile polyps* Associated with SMAD 4 mutation (50%) ***If rectum is diffusely involved–Restorative proctocolectomy with ileorectal anastomosis***
Peutz Jeghers syndrome	Polyposis of small intestine Melanin spots often on buccal mucosa and lips ***STK 11 germline defect–Chromosome 19p*** Not thought to be significant risk factor for malignancy ***2-10% risk of cancers of intestinal tract, breast, ovary, cervix, fallopian tubes, thyroid, lung, gallbladder, bile ducts, pancreas and testis***

Contd.

Contd.

	Surgery–Reserved for Obstruction/Bleeding, Polyps develop adenomatous features Polyp >1.5 cm→ ***Endoscopically every 2 years***
Cronkite Canada syndrome	GI polyposis Association with Alopecia, Cutaneous Pigmentation, Atrophy of finger and toe nails Diarrhea–Predominant symptom Most patients die of disease **Surgery**–Obstruction
Cowden syndrome	**Autosomal dominant** Hamartomas of all 3 embryonal cell layers Facial trichilemmomas, Ca Breast, Thyroid disease

Fecal Occult Blood Testing

- Known to reduce colorectal cancer mortality by 33% and metastatic disease by 50%
- Decreases both incidence and mortality of CRC
- Detect human globin–More sensitive and specific
- Positive FOBT should be followed by Colonoscopy

Flexible Sigmoidoscopy

- 60-70% reduction in mortality from CRC

Colonoscopy

- Most accurate and most complete method for examining large bowel

Air Contrast Barium Enema

- Highly sensitive for polyps >1cm diameter ***(90% sensitivity)***
- Accuracy is greatest in proximal colon

CT Colonography (Virtual Colonoscopy)

- Highly accurate tool for screening
- In case of obstruction or colonoscopy can't be completed
- Radiographs of the abdomen often reveal characteristic annular, constricting lesions ("apple-core" or "napkin-ring").

Recommended colorectal cancer screening guidelines for asymptomatic average-risk individuals

Beginning at Age 50, All Patients Should Have One of the Screening Options Listed Below

Test	**Frequency**
FOBT (every 3 years) plus flexible sigmoidoscopy (every 5 years)	Ongoing
Fecal occult blood test (gFOBT) or fecal immunochemical test (FIT)	Every years
Colonoscopy[a]	Every 10 years
Flexible sigmoidoscopy[b]	Every 5 years
Double-contrast barium enema[b]	Every 5 years
CT colonography (virtual colonoscopy)[b]	Every 5 years

Advantages and disadvantages of screening modalities for asymptomatic individuals

	Advantages	**Disadvantages**
Fecal occult blood testing	Ease of use and noninvasive Low cost Good sensitivity with repeat testing	May not detect most polyps Low specificity Colonoscopy required for positive result Poor compliance with serial testing

Contd.

Contd.

Sigmoidoscopy	Examines colon most at risk Very sensitive for polyp detection in left colon Does not require full bowel preparation (enemas only)	Invasive Uncomfortable Slight risk of perforation or bleeding May miss proximal lesions Colonoscopy required if polyp identified
Colonoscopy	Examines entire colon High sensitive and specific Therapeutic	Most invasive Uncomfortable and requires sedation Requires bowel preparation Risk of perforation or bleeding Costly
Double-contrast barium enema	Examine entire colon Good sensitivity for polyps >1 cm Examines entire colon	Requires bowel preparation Less sensitivity for polyps <1 cm May miss lesions in the sigmoid colon Colonoscopy required for positive result
Computed tomography colonography (virtual colonoscopy)	Noinvasive Sensitivity may be as good as colonoscopy	Requires bowel preparation Insensitive for small polyps Minimal experience and data Colonoscopy required for positive result

Screening guidelines for colorectal cancer

Population	Initial Age	Recommended Screening Test
Average risk	50 years	Annual FOBT or Flexible sigmoidoscopy every 5 years or Annual FOBT and the flexible sigmoidoscopy every 5 years or Air-contrast barium enema every 5 years or Colonoscopy every 10 years
Adenomatous polyps	50 years	Colonoscopy at first detection; then colonoscopy in 3 years If no further polyps, colonoscopy every 5 years If polyps, colonoscopy every 3 years Annual colonoscopy for > 5 adenomas
Colorectal cancer	At diagnosis	Pretreatment colonoscopy; then at 12 months after curative resection; then colonoscopy after 3 years; then colonoscopy every 5 years, if no new lesions
Ulcerative colitis, Crohn's colitis	At diagnosis; then after 8 years for pancolitis, after 15 years for left-sided colitis	Colonoscopy with multiple biopsies every 1-2 years
FAP	10-12 years	Annual flexible sigmoidoscopy Upper endoscopy every 1-3 after polyps appear
Attenuated FAP	20 years	Annual flexible sigmoidoscopy Upper endoscopy every 1-3 years after polyps appear
HNPCC	20-25 years	Colonoscopy every 1-2 years Endometrial aspiration biopsy every 1-2 years
Familial colorectal cancer first-degree relative	40 years or 10 years before the age of the youngest affected relative	Colonoscopy every 5 years Increase frequency if multiple family members are affected, especially before 5 years

- About half of all carcinomas and large adenomas have associated point mutations, most often in *K-RAS* gene
- Allelic deletions of 17p–are demonstrated in three-fourths of all colorectal carcinomas, and deletions of 5q–are demonstrated in more than one-third of colonic carcinoma and large adenomas

SPREAD

- Most common form of spread–Regional LN involvement
- Bulky and circumferential tumor– Colonic Obstruction

- ***Likelihood of nodal metastasis increases with tumor size, LVI, poorly differentiated histology and depth of Invasion***
- T stage (Depth of Invasion)–Single most significant predictor of LN spread
- ***Number of lymph nodes with metastasis correlates with presence of distant disease and inversely with survival***
- 4/more LN are associated with poor prognosis
- Upper rectum–Inferior mesenteric nodes
- Lower rectum–Lymph nodes along iddle rectal vessels
- Most common site of distant metastasis–Liver
- ***Risk of Hepatic metastasis increases with increase in tumor size and grade***

CLINICAL FEATURES

- Classic first symptoms–Change in bowel habits and rectal bleeding

Left sided–Obstruction

- *Bowel changes for left sided colon and rectal cancers*

Staging	
T1	Tumors invade into but not through the submucosa
T2	Tumors invade into but not through the muscularis propria
T3	Tumors invade through the muscularis propria into the subserosa or into non-peritonealized pericolic or perirectal tissue
T4	T4a–Tumors perforate visceral peritoneum T4b–Tumors invade adherent to other structures or organs macroscopically
N1a	Tumors with metastasis in 1 regional LN
N1b	Tumors with metastasis in two or three nearby LNs
N1c	Presence of tumor deposits found in the subserosa, mesentery, or nonperitonealized pericolic or perirectal/mesorectal tissues (but not in the LNs themselves)
N2a	Metastasis in four to six regional LNs
N2b	Involvement of greater than seven nodes
M1a	Spread of tumor to one distant organ or set of distant LNs
M1b	Spread has occurred to more than one distant organ or sets of LNs or peritoneum
M1c	Metastasis to the peritoneal surface if identified alone or with other site or organ metastasis

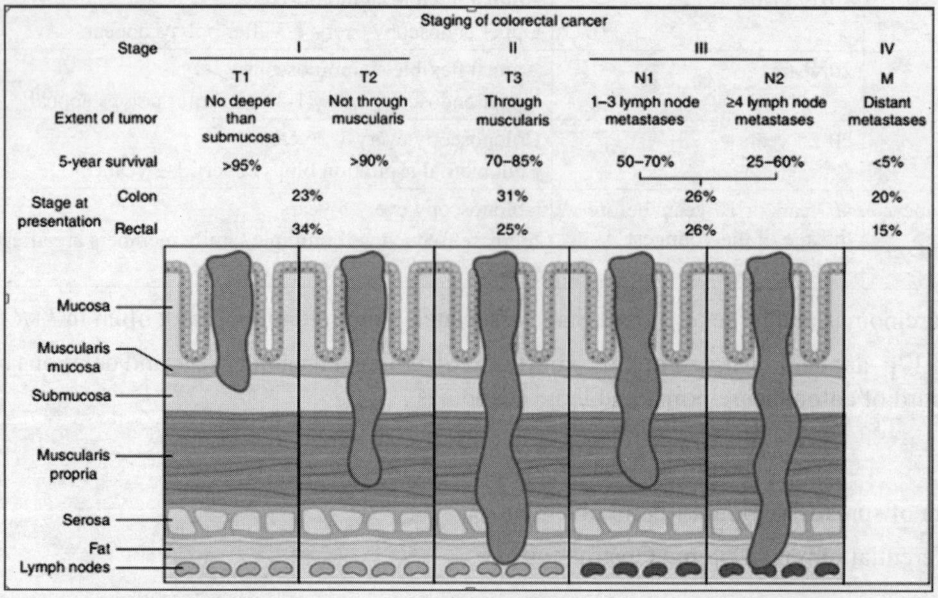

TNM Staging							
	N0	N1	N2a	N2b	M1a	M1b	M1c
Tis	0	-	-	-	IVA	IVB	IVC
T1	0	IIIA	IIIA	IIIB			
T2	I	IIIA	IIIB	IIIB			
T3	IIA	IIIB	IIIB	IIIC			
T4a	IIB	IIIB	IIIC	IIIC			
T4b	IIC	IIIC	IIIC	IIIC			

T1 to T2 N0→ *Stage I,* **T3 to T4 N0→** *Stage II,* **N+→** *Stage III,* **M+→** *Stage IV*

Modified Duke's criteria

- *A–Confined to mucosa*
- *B1– Partially penetrating muscularis propria*
- *B2– Completely penetrating muscularis propria*
- *C1– Spread to 1-4 Lymph nodes*
- *C2– Spread to >4 Lymph nodes*
- *D– Distant metastasis*

Management of Colon Cancer

- Synchronous disease is present in 5% of patients
- ***Field defect***–Presence of synchronous cancers/adenomas or strong family history of colorectal neoplasms suggest that entire colon is at risk for Carcinoma
- ***Second primary cancer***–Metachronous cancers identified during follow up studies
- ***Minimum of 12 LN for adequate staging***

Stage 0:

- No risk of LN metastasis
- Polyps–Excised completely
- Most pedunculated polyps and Many sessile polyps-Completely removed endoscopically
- Polyp can't be removed entirely– ***Segmental colectomy***

Stage I (Malignant polyp):

- Inavsive carcinoma arising in sessile polyp extends into submucosa–Usually treated by Segmental colectomy
- Polyp with poorly differentiated histology or tumor within 1mm resection margin increases risk of local recurrence and metastatic spread

Stage II:

- **Cured with surgical resection**
- Adjuvant chemotherapy–Young and High risk histologic tumors

Stage III:

- Lymph node involvement– Local and Distant recurrence
- **FOLFOX** reduces recurrences and improve survival in this patients
- MSI high Stage III don't benefit from 5FU based therapy–CRYTSAL Trial

Management of Rectal Cancer

- Non-circumferential, benign villous adenoma of rectum–***Transanal excision***
- ***Fulguration***–Reserved for extremely high-risk patients with limited life span who can't tolerate more radical surgery
- ***Upper rectal or mesorectal resections***–*Partial mesorectal excision of at least 5 cm distal to tumor appears adequate*
- ***Extensive pelvic involvement***–*Pelvic exenteration*
- USG–Depth of tumor
- MRI–Mesorectal involvement
- ***When radial margin is threatened/involved–Neoadjuvant chemoradiation***

Stage 0:

- Villous adenoma with high grade dysplasia– Local excision
- 1cm margin should be obtained

Stage I:

- Low risk–Radical resection
- High risk or refused radical resection– Transanal excision +/- Neo adjuvant/ Adjuvant Chemoradiation (Unfavourable histology, Distal third rectum

Stage II:

- Larger rectal tumors if located in distal rectum– More likely to recur locally
- Bulky tumors, Tumor involving adjacent organs and Very low rectal tumors–More extensive surgery

Stage III:

- Neoadjuvant chemoradiation followed by restaging
- If no metastasis proceed with Radical resection

Contd.

Stage IV:	Stage IV:
• Isolated resectable metastasis– Metastatectomy • Most common site of metastasis– LIVER • 15% will have metastasis limited to liver • 20% are potentially curative • All patients should undergo Adjuvant chemotherapy • 20% will have lung metastasis • 1-2% are potentially resectable • Majority are treated by Palliation	• Asymptomatic–CRT • Symptomatic–Palliative

Colon Cancer

- ***Subtotal colectomy with Ileoproctostomy:*** Potentially curable colon cancer with adenoma scattered in colon/Patients with personal history of prior CRC/Family history of CRC in 1st degree relatives
- Excision of a tumor in the right colon should include the right branch of the middle colic artery as well as entire ileocolic and right colic artery
- Excision of a tumor at hepatic or splenic flexure should include the entire distribution of middle colic artery
- ***Obstructing tumors in right colon***–Managed by primary resection and anastomosis
- ***Obstructing tumors in left colon***–Managed with initial decompression (proximal colostomy) or stent insertion followed by resection of tumor and deferred closure of colostomy.
- ***Obstructing Descending/Sigmoid Colon***–Hartmann surgery
- ***Obstructing Rectal obstruction***–Loop colostomy followed by neoadjuvant CRT with resection of primary later
- **Perforated colon cancer**–Initial excision of primary tumor and a proximal colostomy, followed later by reanastomosis and closure of the colostomy
- ***Polypectomy****→Showed Muscularis mucosae involvement/Penetration→ Surgical intervention.*

Presence of specific chromosomal aberrations, particularly mutation in b-raf gene in tumor cells appears to predict for higher risk for metastatic spread.

1. ***Right hemicolectomy***–Cecum, Ascending colon and Hepatic flexure (Resect atleast 6 cm terminal ileum upto transverse colon)
2. ***Extended right hemicolectomy with Ileo Descending Anastomosis***–Transverse colon lesions
3. ***Transverse colectomy***–Resection of transverse colon (Middle colic artery)
4. ***Left hemicolectomy with colorectal anastomosis***–Descending colon lesions
5. ***Sigmoidectomy/High Anterior resection***–Sigmoid carcinoma

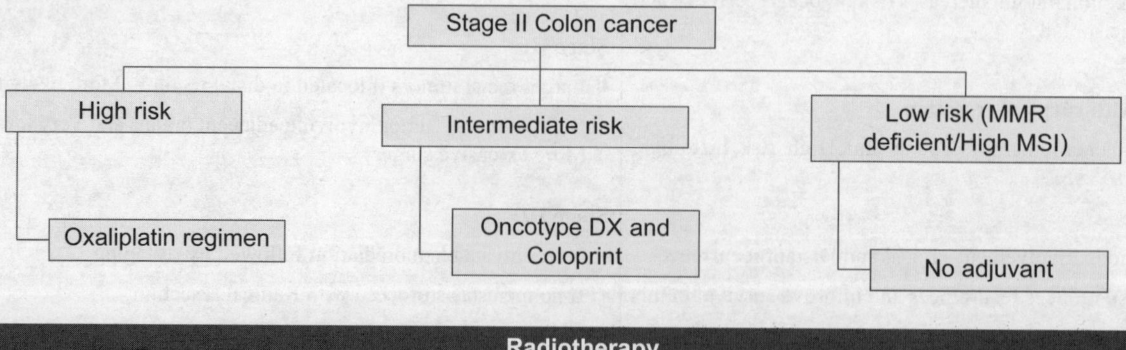

Radiotherapy
• Palliative in Colonic cancer
• Preop and Post op therapy in Rectal cancer–Downstage tumor

Contd.

Contd.

Chemotherapy

- **First line chemotherapy**–5FU + leucovirin, Capecitabine, FOLFIRI/XELIRI, FOLFOX/XELOX

  FOLFOX→No response → FOLFIRI
- Trifluridine/Tipiracil–FDA approved Oral thrapy for Metastatic CRC
- ***Stage III→ FOLFOX/XELOX***
- ***Stage III with pre existing Sensory neuropathy→ FU/LV***
- Best validated High risk factors for stage II to consider adjuvant CT is T4 Stage and <12 lymph nodes retrieved.

Second-line chemotherapy

	FU/leuc	FOLFOX	FOLFIRI	Capecitabine
Nausea/vomiting	+	+	+	+
Diarrhoea	+++	++	+++	++
Mucositis	+++	+	+	+
Myelosuppression	++	+	+++	+
Alopecia	–	–	+	–
Hand-foot syndrome	+	–	++	+++

Rectal Cancer

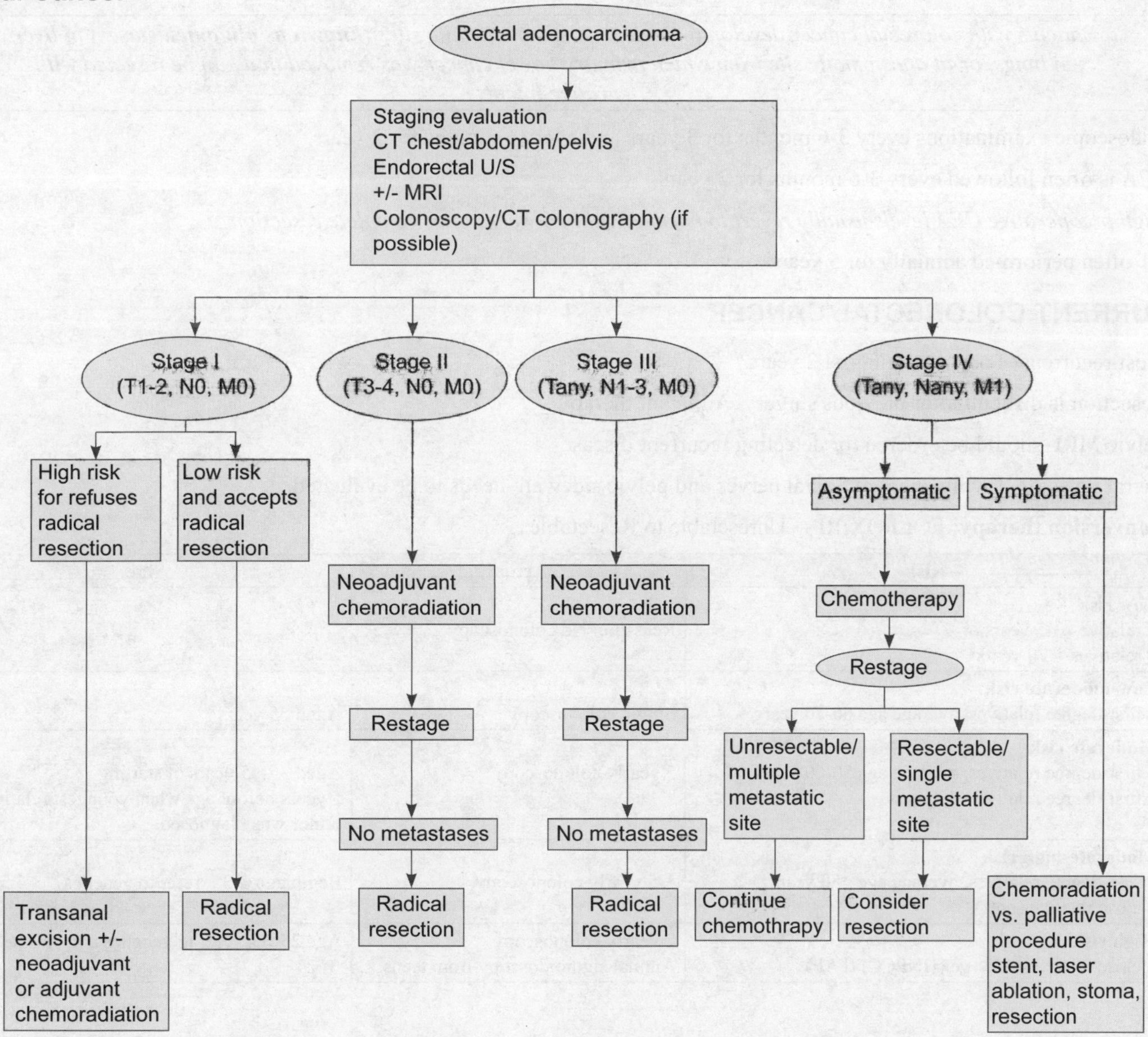

Surgery

- **For Rectal cancers**–Proximal 5 cm and Distal 2 cm margin is adequate
- TME include Resection of entire rectum along with sleeve of surrounding tissue contained within mesorectal fascia ***(From level of sacral promontory to Levator ani muscles)***
- 5% of rectal cancers are removed by non radical transanal surgery
- **Local excision**–Small, low volume, well differentiated cancers on posterior wall *<4 cm, Involving <40% of circumference, <6 cm from anal verge, T1, G1/G2, No Lymphatic or Vascular invasion*
- **Middle and Upper rectum**–Anterior resection of rectum
- **Lower rectum**–APR, Transanal excision, Coloanal anastomosis, Transsphincteric and parasacral approaches, Primary RT
- Best treatment plan for Stage III/Stage II *few cases*→ Chemoradiation followed by Surgery followed by Adjuvant Chemotherapy
- Rectal cancers have a higher incidence of lung metastasis

Follow up and Surveillance

- Colonoscopy should be performed within 1 year after diagnosis of original cancer
- If study is normal colonoscopy should be repeated every 3 to 5 years thereafter

> *Patients with colorectal cancer develop a single or a few metastatic sites* ***(known as oligometastases)*** *in liver, in lungs, or at anastomotic site from which primary bowel cancer was removed that can be resected with curative intent.*

- Endoscopic examinations every 3-6 months for 3 years and every 6 months for 2 years
- CEA is often followed every 3-6 months for 2 years
- *High preoperative CEA levels usually revert to normal within 6 weeks after complete resection*
- CT often performed annually for 5 years

RECURRENT COLORECTAL CANCER

- Most recurrences occur within first 2 years
- Resection is difficult after previous surgery–Adjuvant therapy
- Pelvic MRI–should be ordered for detecting recurrent disease
- Sacral invasion, Involvement of Sacral nerves and pelvic sidewall–needs to be evaluated
- **Conversion therapy:** FOLFOXIRI→ Unresctable to Resectable

Risk	Action	Age
Low risk 1 relative > 45 years or 2 relatives > 70 years	Reassure: No colonoscopy	
Low-moderate risk 2 first-degree relatives, average age 60-70 years	Single colonoscopy	Aged 55 years
Moderate risk 2 first-degree relatives, average age 50-60 years 1 first-degree relative <45 years	5 yearly colonoscopy	Aged 35-65 years of starting 5 years before age when youngest relative's tumor was diagnosed
Moderate-high risk 2 first-degree relatives, average age <50 years 3 close relative (not AC)	3-5 yearly colonoscopy	Begin age 3-35; refer to genetics
High risk 3 close relatives AC +ve (HNPCC) (FAP)	2 yearly colonoscopy Annual sigmoidoscopy from teens	Age 25-65; refer to genetics and counselling

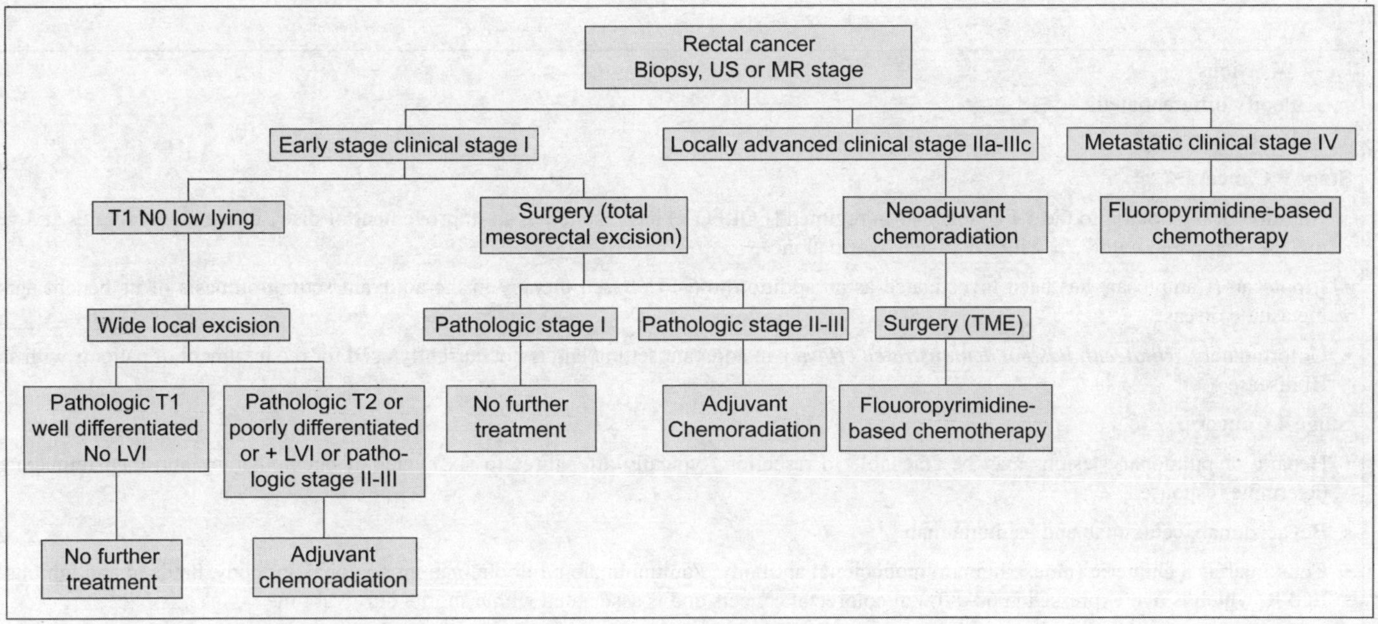

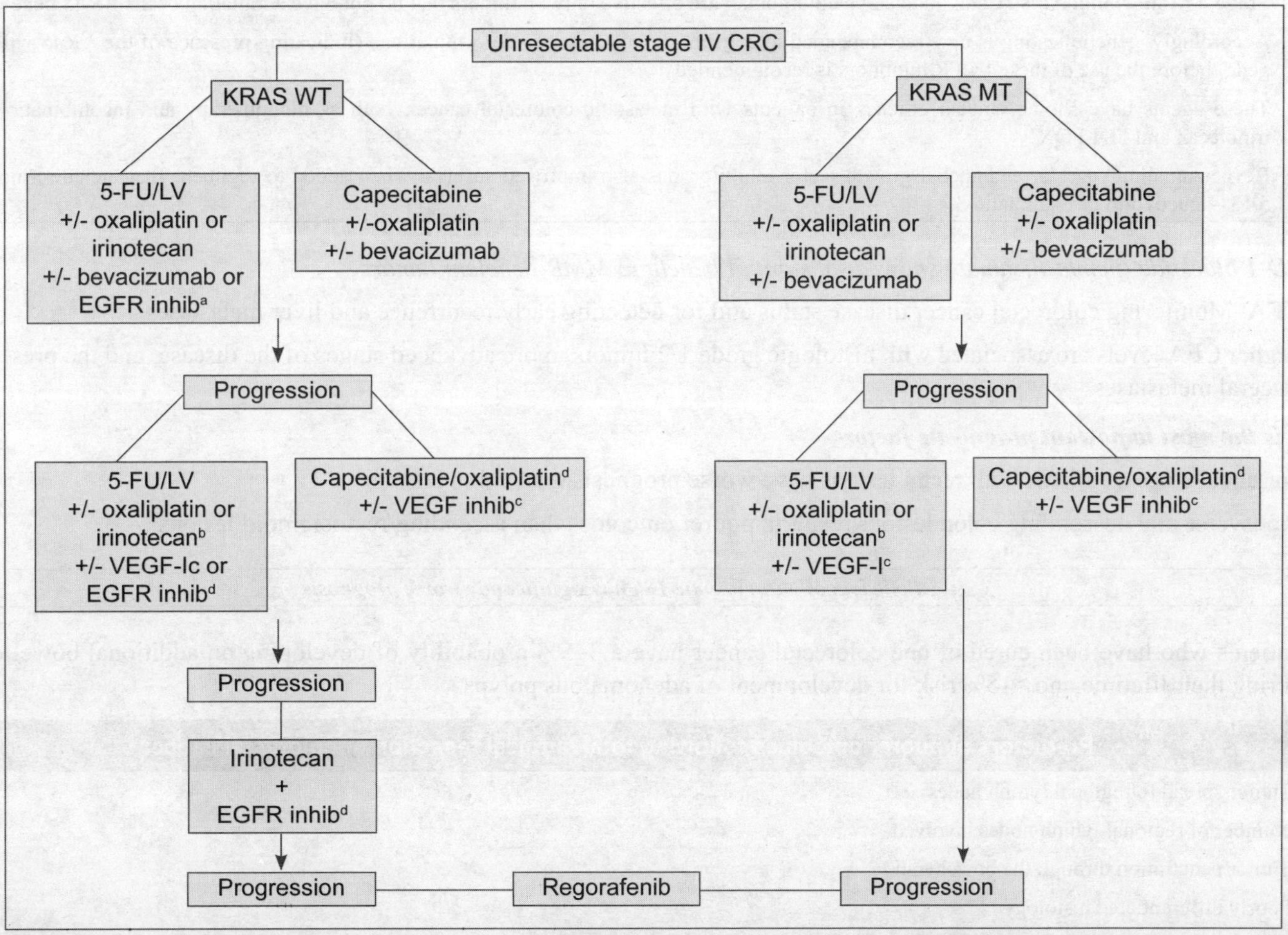

Summary of Colorectalcancer Treatment

Stage 1 Cancers: No adjuvant Chemotherapy given

Stage 2 Cancers: No need of adjuvant chemotherapy except in cases below**

- Adjuvant chemotherapy with 5-FU–Leucovorin is given for following one poor risk factor
  - <12 nodes removed

Contd.

Contd.

- T4 lesions
- Poorly differentiated
- Perforation cases

Stage 3 Cancers:

- Addition of oxaliplatin to the 5-FU–leucovorin regimen (FOLFOX) has resulted in an improvement of disease-free survival rates at 3 years to 78% (compared with 73% with 5-FU–leucovorin alone)
- Irinotecan (Camptosar) has been investigated as an addition to 5-FU–based therapy in the adjuvant setting on basis of its benefit against metastatic disease
- Unfortunately, ***irinotecan has not demonstrated efficacy*** in adjuvant setting and is not currently used for the treatment of patients with stage III disease

Stage 4 Cancers:

- Hepatic or pulmonary lesions may be amenable to resection, typically after three to six cycles of chemotherapy and then reimaging to determine response
- Bevacizumab, cetuximab and panitumumab
- Cetuximab is a chimeric (mouse-human) monoclonal antibody; Panitumumab a fully human monoclonal antibody, binds to and inhibits the EGFR, which is overexpressed in 60–80% of colorectal cancers and is associated with a shorter survival time
- **Stage 4 Monoclonal Ab's**– Cetuximab and panitumumab are effective only on tumors that do not have a mutation of the *KRAS* gene
- Accordingly, genetic testing is now recommended to confirm the absence of *KRAS* mutations (indicating presence of the *KRAS* wild-type gene) before the use of these EGFR inhibitors is recommended
- These agents have shown clinical efficacy in patients with metastatic colorectal cancer, both as monotherapy and incombination with irinotecan and FOLFOX
- Bevacizumab, a vascular endothelial growth factor inhibitor, has also improved survival when added to regimens that include irinotecan, 5-FU- leucovorin or oxaliplatin

- *PD-1 blockade (pembrolizumab) showed substantial benefit in MMR-deficient tumors*
- **CEA**–Monitoring colorectal cancer disease status and for detecting early recurrence and liver metastases
- Higher CEA levels are associated with histologic grade 1/2 tumors, more advanced stages of the disease, and the presence of visceral metastases

Stage is the most important prognostic factor

- **For equal stages, patients with rectal lesions have worse prognosis than colon lesions**
- **Transverse and descending colon lesions result in poorer outcomes than ascending/rectosigmoid lesions**

Allelic loss of chromosome 18q has significantly worse prognosis

- Patients who have been cured of one colorectal cancer have a 3–5% probability of developing an additional bowel cancer during their lifetime and >15% risk for development of adenomatous polyps.

Predictors of poorer outcomes following total surgical resection of colorectal cancer
Tumor spread to regional lymph nodes
Number of regional lymph nodes involved
Tumor penetration through the bowel wall
Poorly differentiated histology
Perforation
Tumor adherence to adjacent organs
Venous invasion
Preoperative elevation of CEA titer (>5 ng/mL)
Specific chromosomal deletion (e.g., mutation in the *b-raf* gene)
Right-sided location of primary tumor

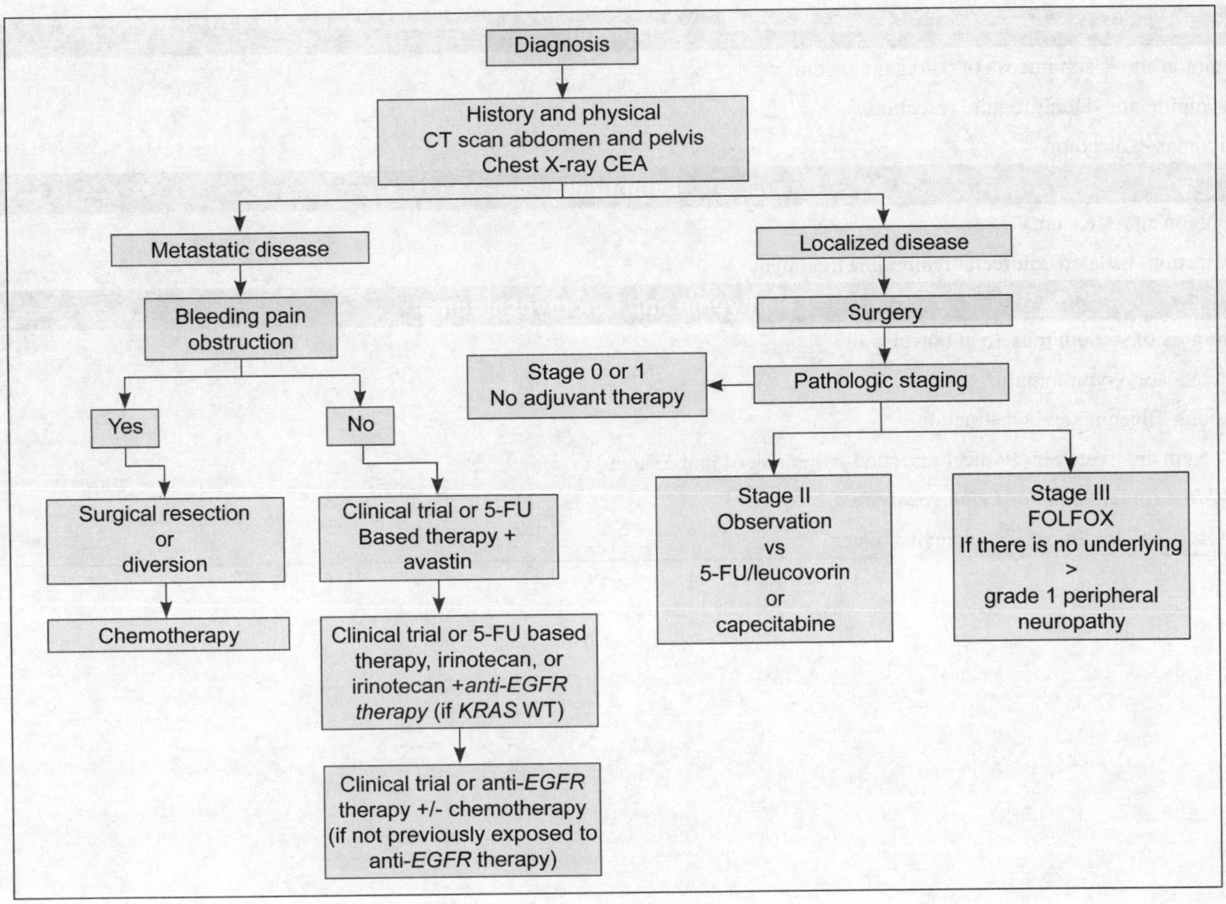
Diagnosis
History and physical
CT scan abdomen and pelvis
Chest X-ray CEA
Metastatic disease
Localized disease
Bleeding pain obstruction
Surgery
Stage 0 or 1
No adjuvant therapy
Pathologic staging
Yes
No
Surgical resection or diversion
Clinical trial or 5-FU Based therapy + avastin
Stage II
Observation
vs
5-FU/leucovorin
or
capecitabine
Stage III
FOLFOX
If there is no underlying
>
grade 1 peripheral neuropathy
Chemotherapy
Clinical trial or 5-FU based therapy, irinotecan, or irinotecan +anti-EGFR therapy (if KRAS WT)
Clinical trial or anti-EGFR therapy +/- chemotherapy (if not previously exposed to anti-EGFR therapy)

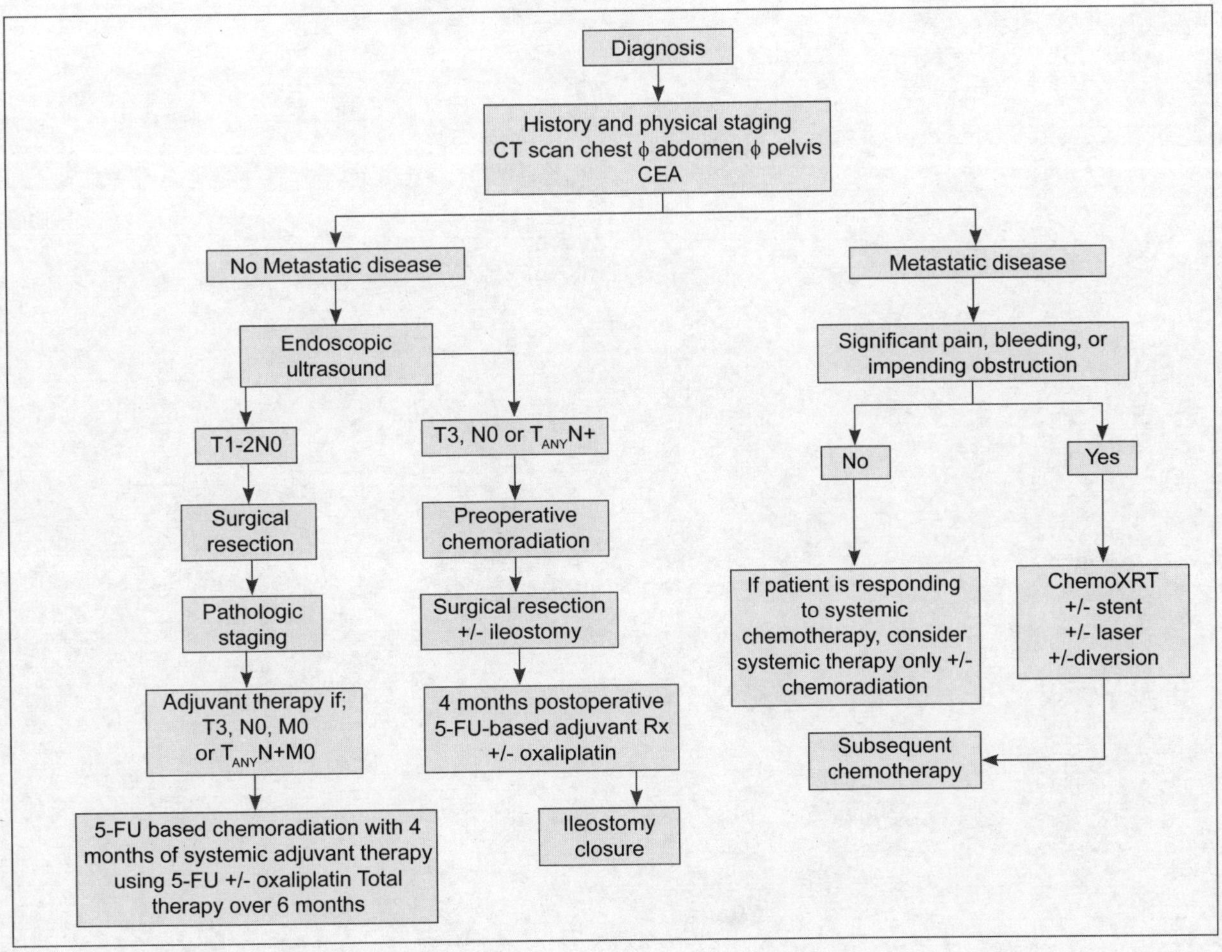
Diagnosis
History and physical staging
CT scan chest ϕ abdomen ϕ pelvis
CEA
No Metastatic disease
Metastatic disease
Endoscopic ultrasound
Significant pain, bleeding, or impending obstruction
T1-2N0
T3, N0 or T ANY N+
No
Yes
Surgical resection
Preoperative chemoradiation
Pathologic staging
Surgical resection +/- ileostomy
If patient is responding to systemic chemotherapy, consider systemic therapy only +/- chemoradiation
ChemoXRT
+/- stent
+/- laser
+/-diversion
Adjuvant therapy if;
T3, N0, M0
or T ANY N+M0
4 months postoperative 5-FU-based adjuvant Rx +/- oxaliplatin
Subsequent chemotherapy
Ileostomy closure
5-FU based chemoradiation with 4 months of systemic adjuvant therapy using 5-FU +/- oxaliplatin Total therapy over 6 months

Lipoma
• Most common site is submucosa of colon and rectum • Small asymptomatic–Don't require resection • Larger lipomas–Colectomy
Lymphoma
• Most common site–Ceacum • Bowel resection–Isolated colorectal lymphoma treatment
Leiomyoma and Leiomyosarcoma
• Benign tumors of smooth muscle of bowel wall • Most patients are Asymptomatic • Large lesions–Bleeding and Obstruction • Lesions >5 cm are treated by Radical resection (High risk of malignancy) • ***Rectum–Most common site of Leiomyosarcoma*** • Radical resection–Treatment for leiomyosarcoma

CHAPTER 8

APPENDICEAL TUMORS

I. CARCINOIDS

- Carcinoid tumors are the most common tumor primary in the appendix
- 0.3% to 0.9% of appendectomy specimens
- ***Size is the best predictor of malignant behavior and metastatic potential***

Treatment:

- Carcinoids <1 cm are typically benign→ Appendectomy
- Patients with carcinoids >2 cm, with involvement of the base/with extension to mesoappendix→right hemicolectomy with regional lymphadenectomy
- For lesions between 1-2 cm in size→careful consideration of the individual tumor characteristics as metastases

II. ADENOCARCINOMA

- Accounts 0.08% to 0.1% of all appendectomies

Treatment:

- Right hemicolectomy with regional lymphadenectomy
- Adjuvant Chemotherapy: 5-fluorouracil, leucovorin and oxaliplatin (FOLFOX)
- FOLFOX is used in neoadjuvant setting in patients with mucinous adenocarcinoma before cytoreductive (debulking) surgery.

III. MUCINOUS TUMORS

- Not frankly malignant
- If ruptured, can result in intraperitoneal spread and the development of pseudomyxoma peritonei (PMP)
- Pseudomyxoma peritonei is a consequence of perforation and direct peritoneal seeding from appendiceal contents
- Avoid rupture if mucocele or mucinous neoplasm is suspected on preoperative imaging or diagnosed intraoperatively
- **Treatment of PMP – Cytoreductive surgery combined with IPHC**

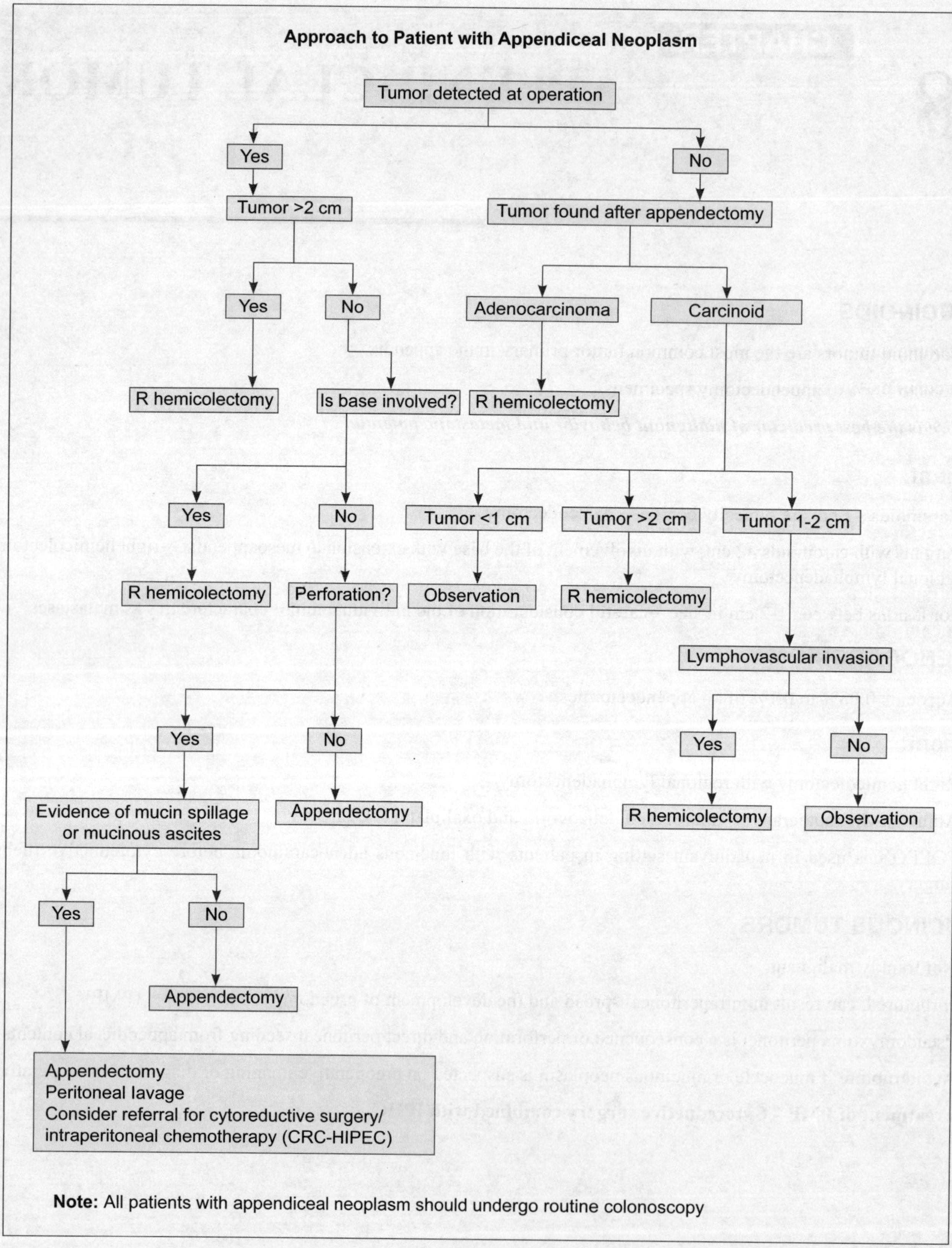
Approach to Patient with Appendiceal Neoplasm
Tumor detected at operation
Yes
No
Tumor >2 cm
Tumor found after appendectomy
Yes
No
Adenocarcinoma
Carcinoid
R hemicolectomy
Is base involved?
R hemicolectomy
Yes
No
Tumor <1 cm
Tumor >2 cm
Tumor 1-2 cm
R hemicolectomy
Perforation?
Observation
R hemicolectomy
Lymphovascular invasion
Yes
No
Yes
No
Evidence of mucin spillage or mucinous ascites
Appendectomy
R hemicolectomy
Observation
Yes
No
Appendectomy
Appendectomy
Peritoneal lavage
Consider referral for cytoreductive surgery/ intraperitoneal chemotherapy (CRC-HIPEC)
Note: All patients with appendiceal neoplasm should undergo routine colonoscopy

CHAPTER 9

TUMORS OF ANAL CANAL AND MARGIN

ANAL CANAL

- Most common type of tumor–SCC
- Most common site of metastasis–Lung
- CRT is most common mode of treatment
- If any residue after CRT treat by APR
- Most common site of LN Metastasis–Inguinal LN
- **Risk factors**–HPV, HIV, Immunosuppression, Smoking, Anal receptive intercourse, Chronic Inflammation and History of Vulvar or Cervical cancer in females
- **Precursor lesion:** Anal Intraepithelial neoplasia
- **Most common symptom**–Bleeding PR
- **Investigation of choice for Anal canal tumors**–Proctoscopy and Biopsy
- **Overall 5 years survival**–66%

Malignant melanoma of anal canal
• Radioresistant and Chemoresistant • Age→50-60 years • Most common in females • Only surgery–WLE • Recurrence is common

ANAL MARGIN

- Late metastasis and Rare tumors
- Malignant ulcers→ Local excision
- Local staging→ MRI

AIN	AIS
• HPV 6,11→ Warts, AIN • HPV 16, 18→ >75% Carcinoma • 10% of AIN3 progress to Carcinoma • 80% of Anal cancer biopsies– AIN3	• Unifocal • Local excision

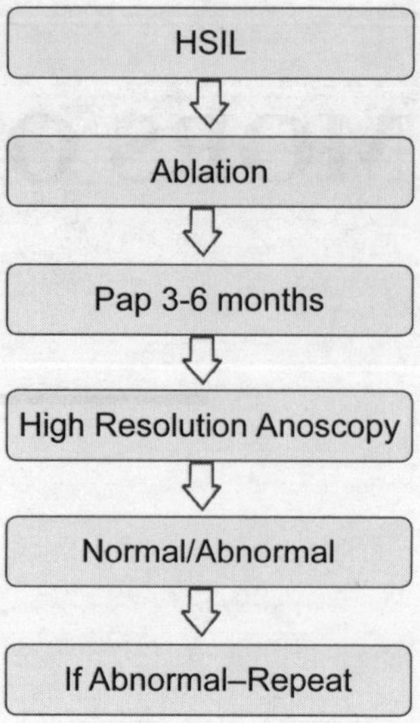

Paget's Disease

- Older age group (7th decade)
- 30-45% associated with invasive carcinoma
- Limited/Non-invasive–WLE+ VY Advancement flap
- Invasive–APR

Verrucous Carcinoma

- Giant condyloma acuminatum
- Buschke Lowenstein tumor
- Slow growing
- Poor prognosis
- WLE

Cancers	Anal Margin	Anal Canal
Squamous cell carcinoma	Small T1→WLE >T1, N+, Advanced→CRT+APR	T1 within 5 cm→ WLE >T1, N+→ CRT **(Nigro regimen)**
Verrucous carcinoma	**WLE**–Poor prognosis	–
Basal cell carcinoma	**WLE**	–
Paget's disease	Invasive–APR Non-invasive–WLE	–
Adenocarcinoma	–	CRT+APR
Melanoma	–	WLE

PART ONE: GI ONCOLOGY - II

CHAPTER 10 LIVER TUMORS

- Right liver typically comprises 2/3rd of total liver volume

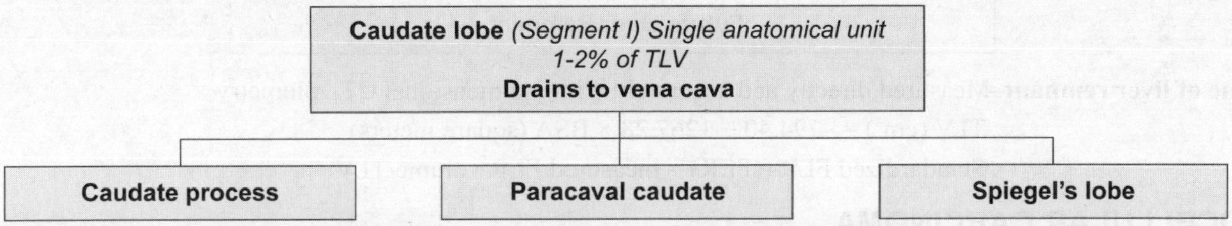

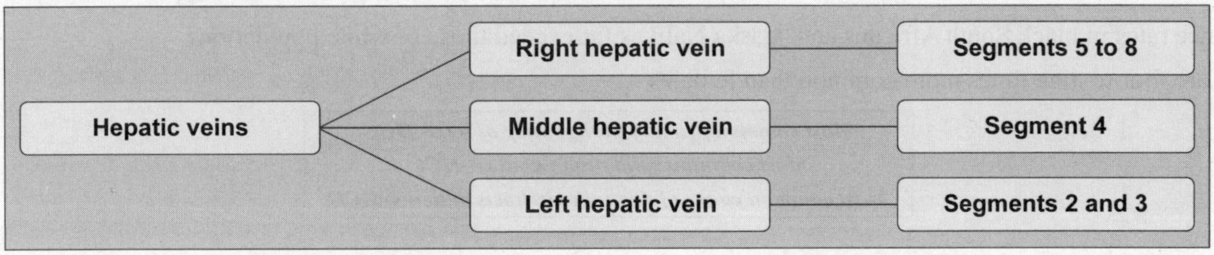

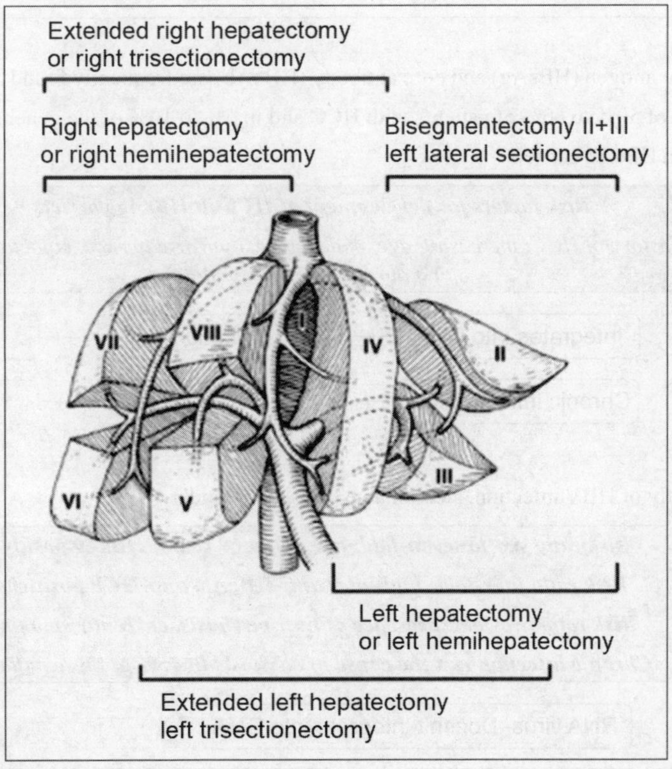

- For patients with tumor-related cholestasis or marked underlying liver disease, a 40% liver remnant is necessary to avoid cholestasis, fluid retention and liver failure

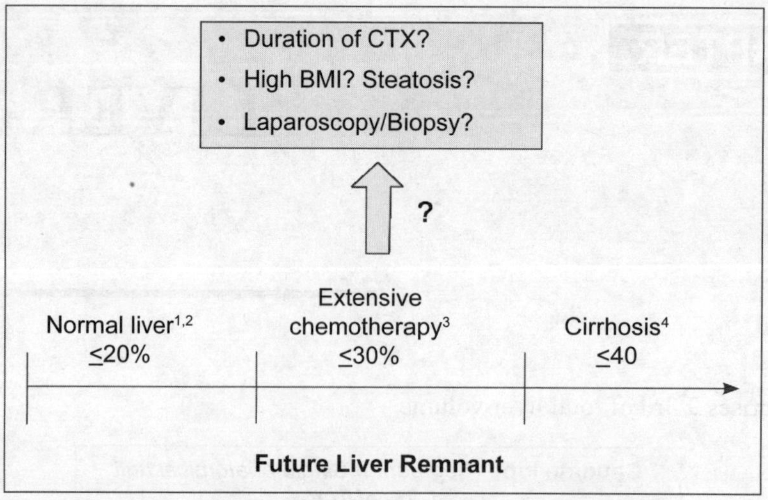

- **Volume of liver remnant**–Measured directly and accurately with 3 dimensional CT volumetry

  TLV (cm^3) = –794.40 + 1267.28 × BSA (square meters)

  Standardized FLR (sFLR) = measured FLR volume/TLV

HEPATOCELLULAR CARCINOMA

- Incidence rates in black South Africans and Alaska Natives far exceed those of white populations
- Males are four to nine times more common than females

> ***Most common primary malignancy of liver–HCC***
> ***Most common solid organ cancer–HCC***
> ***Most common cause of death in cirrhosis patients–HCC***

ETIOLOGY

HEPATITIS B:

- High titers of hepatitis B surface antigen (HBsAg) and core antibody (HBcAb) are frequently found in patients with HCC
- HBsAg was found in the serum of 50% to 60% of patients with HCC and in 5% to 10% of the general population
- HCC is increased by 140-fold in HBsAg carriers

> ***Risk factors for development of HCC in HBsAg carriers***
> *Presence of cirrhosis, family history of HCC, increasing age, male sex, Asian/African race, cofactors (alcohol, aflatoxin and smoking) and duration of carrier state*

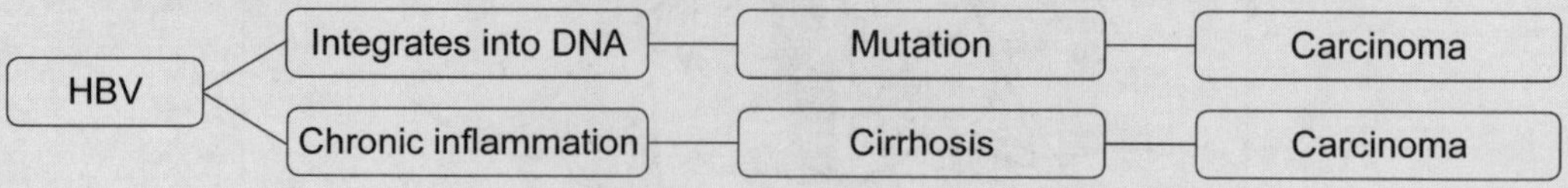

HEPATITIS C:

- HCV infection acts independently of HBV infection, alcohol abuse, age and gender

> ***Risk ratio six- to seven-fold: age, 60 to 69 years; HBsAg positive***
> ***Risk ratio four-fold: high-titer anti-HBcAb, anti-HCV positivity***
> ***Risk ratio two-fold: presence of liver cirrhosis, currently smoking***
> ***Chronic infection was the cause of cirrhosis in 45% of these patients***

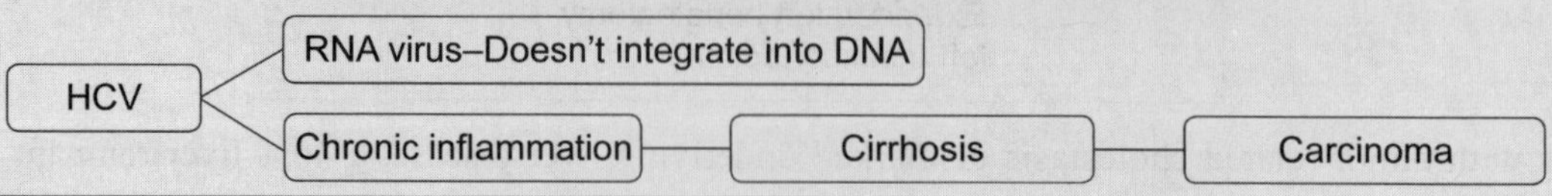

Contd.

Contd.

CIRRHOSIS:

- 60% to 90% of HBsAg-positive subjects have associated cirrhosis
- 20% to 40% of patients with cirrhosis have HCC.

Clear association between alcohol-induced cirrhosis and HCC exists; Associations between alcohol and HCC in absence of cirrhosis is not clear

AFLATOXINS:

- Produced by Aspergillus flavus / Aspergillus parasiticus
- Aflatoxin B1–Hepatocarcinogen

Amount of exposure is correlated with increased HCC risk in humans

SEX HORMONES:

- Risk for liver cell adenomas and HCC is increased in women who have used oral contraceptives for 8 or more years

Observed in people with a history of anabolic steroid use

SMOKING, ALCOHOL. DIABETES AND INSULIN INTAKE

- Cigarette smoking, heavy alcohol consumption and diabetes mellitus, especially with insulin administration, appear to be significant risk factors for HCC
- Alcohol-related cirrhosis is clearly a risk factor

NASH:

Accounts for approximately 10% of all risk factors for HCC

Alpha 1-antitrypsin deficiency, tyrosinemia, and hemochromatosis and Budd chiari syndrome–Increased risk

Phlebotomy therapy can deplete hepatic iron and induce regression of hepatic fibrosis but does not prevent the development of HCC in hemochromatosis

Clonorchiasis, vinyl chloride exposure and administration of thorium dioxide/ methotrexate are also associated with HCC development

MUTATIONS: p53 mutations reported in half of HCC patients

Positive family history have a 150% increased risk of HCC

Radiation exposure–Account for 1% of HCCs

Conditions Associated with Human Hepatocellular Carcinoma

Condition	Risk
Cirrhosis	
Hepatitis B virus	High
Hepatitis C virus	High
Alcohol	High
Autoimmune chronic active hepatitis	High
Cryptogenic cirrhosis	High
Cirrhosis due to nonalcoholic fatty liver disease	High
Primary billiary cirrhosis	High
Hereditary hemochromatosis	High
A1-Antitrypsin deficiency	High
Wilson's disease	Low
Metabolic Diseases (without Cirrhosis)	
Hereditary tyrosinemia	High
A1-Antitrypsin deficiency	Moderate
Ataxia telangictasia	Moderate
Types 1 and 3 glycogen storage disease	Moderate
Galactosemia	Moderate
Citrullinemia	Moderate

Contd.

Contd.

Hereditary hemorrhagic telangiectasia	Moderate
Porphyria cutanea tardis	Moderate
Crotic aciduria	Moderate
Alagille syndrome (congenital cholestatic syndrome)	Moderate
Environment	
Thorotrast	Moderate
Androgenic steroids	Moderate
Cigarette smoking	Low to Moderate
Aflatoxin	Moderate

Pathology–Types

- **GROSS:** Hanging type, Pushing type, Infiltrative type, Multifocal type
- **GROWTH PATTERN:** Massive, Nodular, Diffuse
- **MICROSCOPIC:** Trabecular, solid or tubular
- Sclerosing or fibrosing form–Associated with hypercalcemia

Most HCCs associated with cirrhosis show an expansile growth pattern with fibrous capsule and intra-tumoral septae

Non-cirrhotic livers don't usually have capsule and are generally larger at presentation

Haemorrhage and necrosis are commonly seen within HCC's

Spread	
• *Limited within liver in only 20% cases*	• *Lung metastasis in 35% cases*
• *Invades portal vein in 35% cases*	• *Abdominal LN metastasis occurs in 20% cases*
• *Invades hepatic vein in 15% cases*	• *Thoracic or cervical LN metastasis occurs in 5% cases*
• *Invades contiguous abdominal organs in 15% cases*	• *Vertebrae involved in 5% cases*
• *Invades vena cava and right atrium in 5% cases*	• *Kidney or adrenal involved in 5% cases*
Most patients die from hepatic failure	
Frequently spreads by local extension to diaphragm and adjacent organs and into portal and hepatic veins.	

PARANEOPLASTIC SYNDROMES

Fever, Erythrocytosis, Hypercholesterolemia, Gynecomastia, Hypercalcemia, Hypoglycemia, and Virilization (precocious puberty)

"Most common paraneoplastic syndrome–HYPERCHOLESTEROLEMIA

Clinical Features

- Pain in right subcostal area–***Most common complaint***
- **Others:** Fatigue, Anorexia, Weight loss and Unexplained fever

Hemorrhage into peritoneal cavity-often seen in HCC and may be fatal

- *Sudden deterioration in patient with known liver disease or +ve HbsAg or hepatitis C serology should raise the suspicion of HCC*
- **Ominous prognostic sign**–Ascites/Upper abdominal mass
- Physical findings–Hepatomegaly, Splenomegaly, Ascites , Fever, Jaundice, Hepatic bruit and Cachexia
- Osteolytic bone lesions cause pain as a result of pathological fractures and nerve compression, whilst lung metastases lead to dyspnoea, cough and haemoptysis.

INVESTIGATIONS

- Raised serum bilirubin, LDH and Lowered serum albumin–***Associated with poor survival***

- Serum GGT–II was positive in 90% of patients with HCC–***Valuable for detection of small/subclinical HCC***
- Liver biopsy–Diagnosis
- Indocyanine green clearance is used to provide a functional assessment of the liver and is the basis of determining suitability for resection
- PVE is used to increase volume of FLR prior to resection in patients with Child-Pugh grade A cirrhosis
- If the ICG clearance is <10%, then PVe is indicated if the FLr is ≤40%. For an ICG clearance of 10–15%, then PVE is indicated for an FLr of ≤50%

ICG is not indicated for an ICG clearance of >20%

Serum Markers:

- AFP is often elevated in patients with HCC but can also be elevated in patients with benign chronic liver disease
- Used for monitoring of patients for recurrence
- AFP is increased in 50-90% of all patients with HCC, with levels >400 ng/mL usually found in patients with large or rapidly growing tumors
- AFP >200 ng/mL in association with characteristic imaging findings is nearly 100% sensitive for HCC

AFP–L3 is highly specific for HCC

- **Liver cirrhosis and no HCC**–AFP range from 30 to 460 ng/mL
- **HCC**–AFP concentrations may range from 30 to 7,000 ng/mL
- Serum ferritin levels are also frequently elevated in patients with HCC

AFP	***>20 ng/mL→ Sensitive to predict HCC***
	>400 ng/mL→ Specific for HCC

Ultrasound:

- **HCC**–Usually well circumscribed, hyperechogenic and associated with diffuse distortion of normal hepatic parenchyma
- **Metastasis**–Usually hyperechogenic
- Screening in high risk patients
- Can diagnose early stage HCC

CT:

- **HCC**–Low attenuation isodense with normal parenchyma on CT
- **Metastasis**–Low attenuation with mucin producing tumors of ovary, pancreas, colon and stomach and sarcomas
- HCCs, hepatic adenomas and neuroendocrine tumors–***Arterial phase enhancement***
- Enhancement during portal dominant phase reveals ***hypovascular tumors*** like metastatic adenocarcinoma or cholangiocarcinoma

CECT:

- Enhancement in arterial phase with early wash out of contrast in venous phase
- Definitive diagnosis and treatment planning
- Hypervascularity, Peritoneal metastasis, Vascular involvement, Nodal metastasis, Thrombus in portal/hepatic venous system, Biliary involvement

Selective hepatic, celiac and superior mesenteric angiography

- Confirm portal vein involvement, define arterial supply and identify vascular lesions that are as small as 3 mm in diameter

Diagnostic Laproscopy

- Patients most likely to benefit from DL–Large or ruptured tumors, advanced cirrhosis, or indeterminate nodules in the FLR

AJCC Staging	
T1a	Solitary tumor less than or equal to 2 cm
T1b	Solitary tumor >2 cm without vascular invasion

Contd.

Contd.

T2	Solitary tumor >2 cm with vascular invasion, Multiple tumors none > 5 cm
T3	Multiple tumors atleast one > 5 cm
T4	Single tumor or multiple tumors of any size involving major branch of portal vein/hepatic vein or Tumor with direct invasion of adjacent organs other than gallbladder or with perforation of visceral peritoneum
N1	Regional lymph node metastasis

	N0	**N1**
T1a	IA	IVA
T1b	IB	
T2	II	
T3	IIIA	
T4	IIIB	
M1	IVB	
F0	**Fibrosis score 0-4 (No to moderate fibrosis)**	
F1	**Fibrosis score 5-6 (Severe fibrosis/Cirrhosis)**	

- Presence of severe fibrosis of underlying liver has a negative impact on overall survival

Different Staging Systems	
Okuda Staging	
Factors representing advanced disease - Tumor size > 50% of liver - Ascites - Albumin < 3 g/dL - Bilirubin > 3 mg/dL	
Stage I	No factors present
Stage II	1-2 factors
Stage III	3-4 factors

Child-Turcotte-Pugh Score			
Measurements	Score		
	1	2	3
Encephalopathy	None	Mild	Moderate
Ascites	None	Sight	Moderate
Bilirubin (ml/dL)	1-2	2-3	> 3
Albumin (mg/dL)	> 3.5	2.8-3.5	< 2.8
PT (seconds prolonged)	< 4	4-6	> 6

French Classification				
Weight	0	1	2	3
Kamofsky Index (%)	≥ 80			< 80
Serum bilirubin (μmol/L)	< 50			≥ 50
Serum alkaline phosphatase (ULN)	< 2		> 2	
Serum alpha-fetoprotein (μg/L)	< 35		≥ 35	
Portal obstruction (ultrasonography)	No	Yes		
ULN upper limit of normal				

Japan Integrated Staging (JLS) Scoring System				
Variables	**Scores**			
	0	**1**	**2**	**3**
Child-Pugh stage	A	B	C	
TNM stage by LCSGJ	I	II	III	IV
LCSGJ, Liver Cancer Study Group of Japan				

Model for End Stage Liver Disease (MELD) Score

MELD = $3.78 \times \log_e$ serum billirubin (mg/dL) +
$11.20 \times \log_e$ INR +
$9.57 \times \log_e$ serum creatinine (mg/dL) +
6.43 (constant for liver disease etiology)

Cancer of Liver Italian Program (CLIP) Scoring System			
Variables	**Scores**		
	0	**1**	**2**
Child-Pugh stage	A	B	C
Tumor morphology	Uninodular and extension ≤ 50%	Multinodular and extension ≤ 50%	Massive or extension > 50%
AFP (mg/dL)	< 400	≥ 400	
Portal vein thrombosis	No	Yes	

Weight of Six Prognostic Factors in Chinese University Prognostic Index (CUPI)	
Variable	**Weight**
TNM Stage	
• I and II	-3
• IIa and IIb	-1
• IVa and IVb (reference)	0
Asymptomatic disease on presentation	-4
Ascites	3
AFP ≥ 500 mg/dL	2
Total bilirubin (μmol/L)	
• < 34 (reference)	0
• 34-51	3
• ≥ 52	4
Alkaline phosphatase ≥ 200 IU/L	3
CUPI Stages: Score ≤ 1 (Low risk); 2-7 (Intermediate risk); ≥ 8 (High risk)	

BCLC Staging:

Barcelona Clinic Liver Cancer (BCLC) Staging Classification				
Stage	**PST**	**Tumor Status**		**Liver Function Studies**
		Tumor Stage	**Okuda Stage**	
Stage A: Early HCC				
A1	0	Single	I	No Portal hypertension and normal bilirubin
A2	0	Single	I	Portal hypertension and normal bilirubin
A3	0	Single	I	Portal hypertension and abnormal bilirubin

Contd.

Contd.

A4	0	3 tumors < 3 cm	I-II	Child-Pugh A-B
Stage B: Intermediate HCC	0	Large multinodular	I-II	Child-Pugh A-B
Stage C: Advanced HCC	1-2*	Vascular invasion or extrahepatic spread	I-II	Child-Pugh A-B
Stage D: End-Stage HCC	3-41↑	Any	III	Child-Pugh C
PST, Performance Status Test: A and B, All criteria should be fulfilled; *, Stage C, at least one criteria; PST 1-2 or vascular invasion/ extrahepatic spread; ↑, Stage D, at least one criteria: PST3-4 or Okuda Stage III/Child-Pugh C				

- ***Patients with normal liver function or Child A cirrhosis*–**Good candidates for major or minor resection
- Minor resection may be considered among patients with Child's B cirrhosis
- Patients with HCC in Child's C cirrhosis–considered for OLT if Milan criteria are met
- **Major cause of mortality of HCC–Tumor relates liver failure (Secondary to Biliary obstruction/Vascular compromise)**
- Radiation therapy is therefore most beneficial for patients with unresectable tumors in the hilum or adjacent to main PV or inferior vena cava (IVC) who cannot undergo local ablative therapies
- Mazzaferro *et al.* evaluated patients with Child's B or C cirrhosis and either single tumor ≤5 cm or three tumors ≤3 cm in maximum diameter underwent liver transplantation

Liver Transplatation Criteria		
Milan's Criteria	**UCSF Criteria**	**Silva *et al.***
Single tumor ≤ 5 cm	Single tumor ≤ 6.5 cm	
Or upto 3 tumors ≤ 3 cm	Or upto 3 tumors ≤ 4.5 cm and total sum is ≤ 8 cm	Up to 3 tumors ≤ 5 cm, and total sum is ≤ 10 cm
All three criteria Lists		
No vascular invasion		
No regional nodal/distant metastasis		

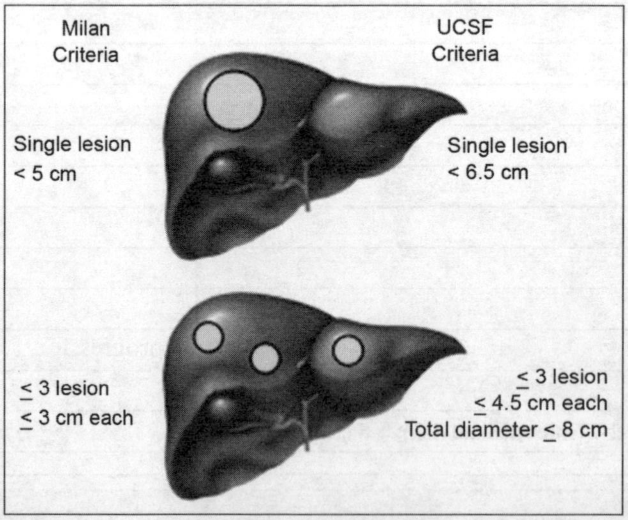

Complications of liver transplantation	
Graft-specific	
Parenchyma	Early—1° non-function, acute rejection, ischaemia-reperfusion injury, chronic rejection Late—Chronic rejection, disease recurrence (HCC or associated liver disease)
Biliary	Bile leak, anastomotic stricture, ascending cholangitis
Hepatic artery/portal vein	Thrombosis, stenosis Systemic immunosuppression Infection—Local or systemic Drug-related toxicity—Cardiovascular, renal, neurological, bone Post-transplant malignancies

Treatment Options for Hepatocellular Carcinoma
• Surgery – Partial hepatectomy – Liver transplantation
• Local ablative therapies – Cryosurgery – Microwave ablation – Ethanol injection – Acetic acid injection – Radiofrequency ablation
• Regional therapies: Hepatic artery transcatheter treatments – Transarterial chemotherapy – Transarterial embolization – Transarterial chemoembolization – Transarterial utrrium-90 Hipiodol – Proton or carbon ion therapy – Conformal radiation therapy – Stereotactic radiation therapy – Palliative low-dose radiation therapy
• Systemic therapies – Chemotherapy – Targeted therapy (sorafenib)* – Immunotherapy – Hormonal therapy
• Supportive care

TREATMENT

- ***Local Ablation***–Who can't undergo resection or bridge to transplantation
- ***Percutaneous ethanol injection/Radiofrequency ablation***–Effective for tumors <2 cm

  Major vessels exert a cooling effect due to the 'heat sink' effect which may reduce efficacy of RFA
- ***Cryotherapy***–Large tumors less suitable to percutaneous approach

TACE–(More than 80% of blood supply is through Hepatic artery)

Treatment of unresectable HCC not suitable for local ablation

Patients awaiting OLT to reduce rate of drop out because of local tumor progression

Best candidate–*Unresectable lesions without vascular invasion/Extrahepatic spread and preserved liver function (Child-Pugh A/B cirrhosis)*

Absolute contraindications: *Complete absence of hepatopetal blood flow (portal vein thrombosis), encephalopathy, biliary obstruction and Child-Pugh C cirrhosis*

RADIATION: Radiosensitive tumor (Extremely radiosensitive organ)

(Normal liver can only tolerate about 20 Gy)

Major drawbacks with RT: *Poor radiation tolerance of normal liver and difficulty with tumor localization*

Selective internal irradiation: *Iodine-131-labeled lipiodol/Yttrium-90- tagged glass microspheres are delivered selectively to the tumor via hepatic artery*

SBRT–*Most applicable to patients with relatively small HCCs who are either inoperable or who refuse operation*

Algorithm:

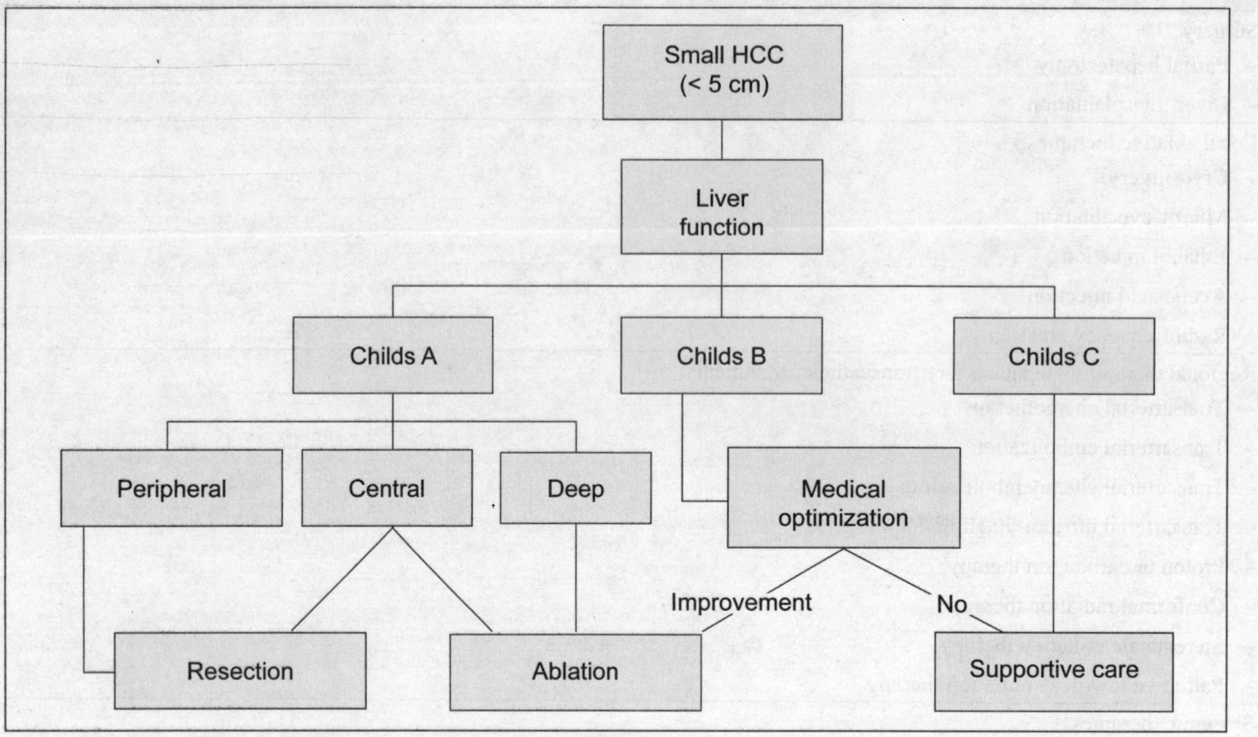

Small HCC
(< 5 cm)
Liver function
Childs A
Childs B
Childs C
Peripheral
Central
Deep
Medical optimization
Improvement
No
Resection
Ablation
Supportive care

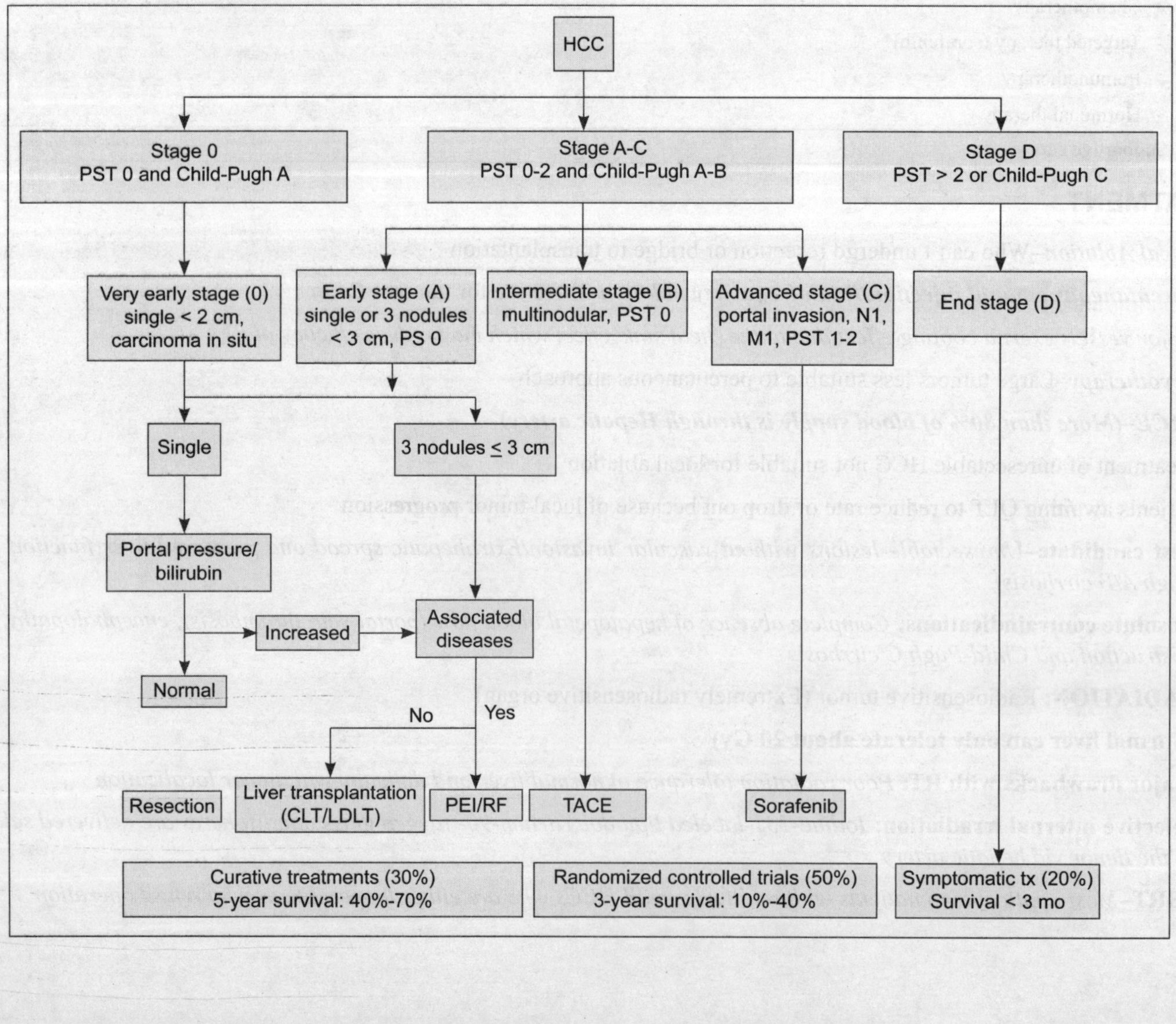

HCC
Stage 0
PST 0 and Child-Pugh A
Stage A-C
PST 0-2 and Child-Pugh A-B
Stage D
PST > 2 or Child-Pugh C
Very early stage (0)
single < 2 cm,
carcinoma in situ
Early stage (A)
single or 3 nodules
< 3 cm, PS 0
Intermediate stage (B)
multinodular, PST 0
Advanced stage (C)
portal invasion, N1,
M1, PST 1-2
End stage (D)
Single
3 nodules ≤ 3 cm
Portal pressure/
bilirubin
Increased
Associated
diseases
Normal
No
Yes
Resection
Liver transplantation
(CLT/LDLT)
PEI/RF
TACE
Sorafenib
Curative treatments (30%)
5-year survival: 40%-70%
Randomized controlled trials (50%)
3-year survival: 10%-40%
Symptomatic tx (20%)
Survival < 3 mo

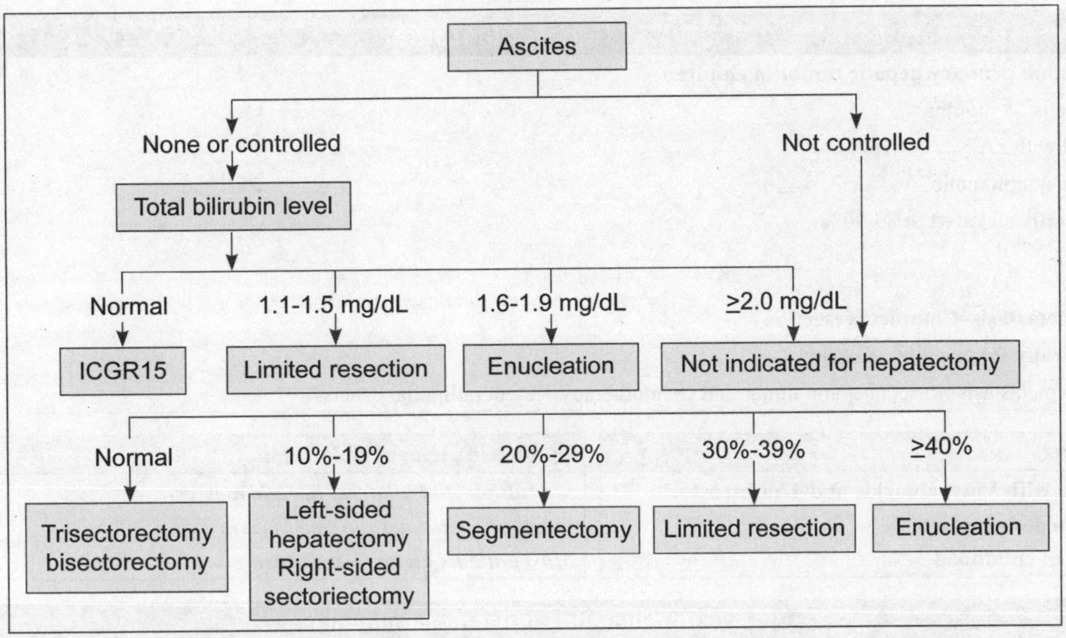

Only 10% HCCs are resectable with solitary/unilobar hepatic lesions at time of diagnosis.

Unresectable
Bilobar or four segment hepatic parenchymal involvement, portal vein thrombus and vena caval involvement with tumor or tumor thrombus.

PROGNOSTIC FACTORS

- No. of liver lesions and presence of vascular involvement are the most significant prognostic determinants in patients with disease limited to liver
- ***Patients with resected HCC, liver is site of disease recurrence in 90% of cases***
- Jaundice–Poor prognostic sign

Factor	**5 years survival**
Number	Solitary→ 45% Multiple→ 15-25%
Size	Small tumors→ 40-45% Large (>5 cm)→ 10%
Patients without cirrhosis with tumors located in left lobe of liver or in right inferior segments (anteriorly or posteriorly) have best prognosis	
All patients with gross tumor thrombi involving portal vein/hepatic vein die within 3 years 5 years survival rate for patients with no vascular involvement of any kind is 30%	
5 years survival rate for patients undergoing curative resection is 55% ***5 years survival rate for patients undergoing noncurative resections is 5%***	
Hepatic lobectomy	5-year survival rate–85%
Subsegmentectomy	5-year survival rate–50%
Wedge enucleation	5-year survival rate–20%

Fibrolamellar HCC

- Fibrolamellar HCC occurs in a much **younger age group** (peak incidence, 3rd decade)
- Can be differentiated from standard HCC as they stain for CK7 and CD68

Usually not associated with cirrhosis or viral hepatitis
Affects males and females equally
Much higher percentage (>15%) with fibrolamellar HCC presents with positive LN

- ***Resection–1st line of therapy***
- For those patients in whom the tumor is thought to be unresectable, liver transplantation provides an effective alternative.
  Total hepatectomy with orthotopic liver transplantation–*Unresectable nonmetastatic fibrolamellar HCC, intrahepatic bile duct cancers, or hemangiosarcoma*

Hepatoblastoma

- **Most common primary hepatic tumor in children**
- Median age is 18 months
- Associated with FAP
- Generally asymptomatic
- **AFP is usually elevated in 85-90%**

Treatment:

- **Without metastasis–Complete resection**
- **Chemotherapy followed by surgery**
- Pulmonary metastasis–Resect hepatic tumor and chemotherapy/Resect pulmonary mets

Angiosarcoma

- **Associated with Vinyl chloride and Thorotrast**
- **Multiple hepatic metastasis**

Can be seen in childhood

Epitheloid Hemangioblastoma

- ***Multiple and bilateral hepatic masses***
- *Extrahepatic metastasis is seen in 25%*

Most patients die of liver failure

Intrahepatic Cholangiocarcinoma

- Most of these tumors involve biliary confluence
- 2nd most common primary hepatic neoplasm

Risk Factors:

PSC, Choledochal cysts, Hepatolithiasis, RPC, HBV, HCV, NASH, Cirrhosis and Diabetes

- Right upper abdominal pain and weight loss–clinical feature
- **AFP levels–Normal**
- CA19–9 and CEA are elevated
- Diagnosis of exclusion
- CT: Focal hepatic mass with peripheral dilatation
- Intrahepatic Metastasis, LN Metastasis, growth along biliary tree often encountered
- **Tretament:** Complete resection is the treatment if choice
- **Poor Outcome:** Multifocality, LN Metastasis, Vascular invasion and Positive margins
- **Chemotherapy is ineffective**

Liver Metastasis

Most common cause of metastasis is Colorectal cancer
Multiple liver secondaries–Gallbladder
Calcified liver secondaries–Colon and Ovary

- Neuroendocrine tumors, Wilms tumor and RCC have 5-year survival rates of 40-70% have been reported after resection

Hepatic resection may also provide excellent palliation in selected patients with hormone secreting neuroendocrine tumors

- 80% of the patients will have malignancies that are amenable to surgical cure
- Approximately 20% of resected cancers will recur within 5 years
- Slowly increasing CEA level usually indicates local or regional recurrence
- Rapidly increasing CEA level suggests hepatic metastases

Overall 75-90% of patients with hepatic CRC metastases have an increased CEA level

- **CT**–Assessment of extrahepatic structures, accurately provides for liver volumetry, accurate localization of tumors within liver, and accurate lesion detection

Multiphase, thin-cut, spiral, hepatic CT is modality of choice

- **MRI**–Useful in patients with metastases poorly visualized on CT and in patients with a significant degree of underlying steatosis
- Consider size, number and location of lesions, colorectal liver metastases are considered resectable if all of disease can be completely resected with negative margin and an adequate FLR remains

Complete radiographic response cannot be equated with a complete pathologic response

Contd.

Contd.

- Preoperative systemic chemotherapy can reduce size and volume of tumors such that all tumor sites can be resected safely and provide long-term survival

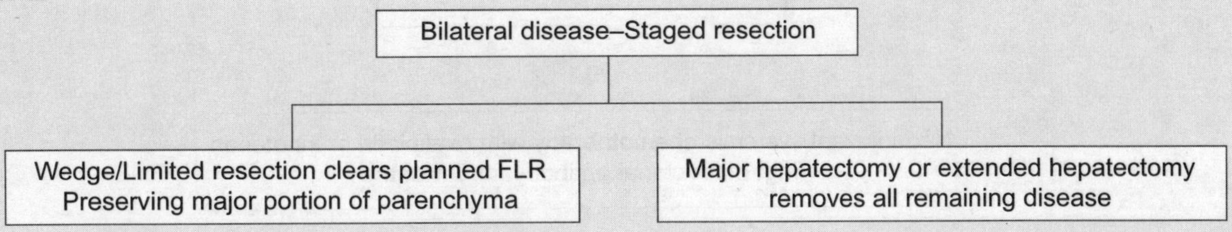

- Solitary, small, peripherally located lesions in healthy, hemodynamically stable patient that can be excised adequately by nonanatomical resection or segmentectomy may be resected at same time as the primary tumor

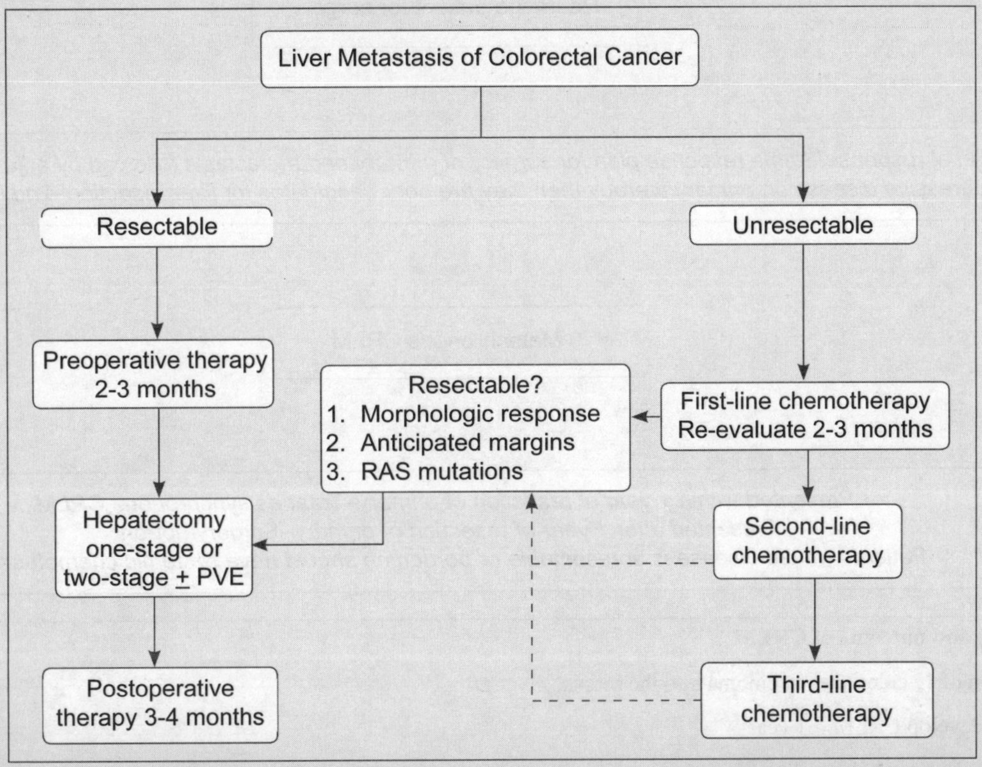

Colorectal Liver Metastasis

- Develop in 50% of patients with colorectal cancer
- Male predominance
- Adenocarcinomas and represent stage IV colorectal cancer
- Frequently in the right side of the liver

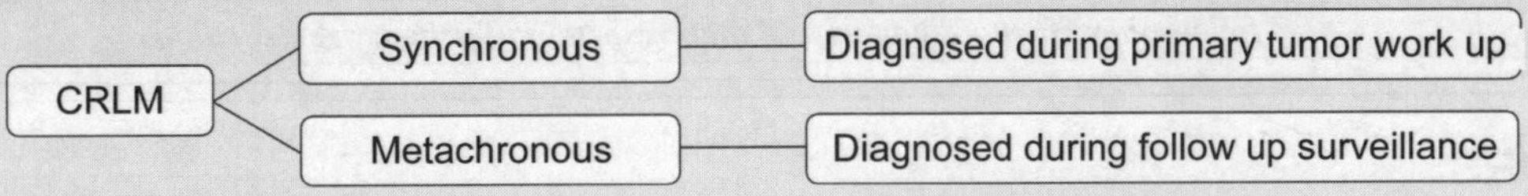

- CEA and CA 19-9 are used to monitor disease recurrence, following resection of primary lesions and CRLM
- Resection is the treatment of choice for resectable CRLM
- 1mm margin is considered R0
- Presence of extra-hepatic disease is no longer considered an absolute contraindication to liver resection
- *If patient is receiving chemotherapy/neoadjuvant therapy is planned, then surgery should be performed after an interval of 6–8 weeks because of risk of associated chemotherapy-related parenchymal damage (sinusoidal obstruction syndrome with oxaliplatin, and steatosis/ steatohepatitis with irinotecan)*

Contd.

Contd.

Synchronous CRLM

↓

Neoadjuvant systemic chemotherapy with oxaliplatin or irinotecan with monoclonal antibody for 3 months

↓

Re image patient for surgery

↓

If partial response/Stable response plan for surgery of primary and metastasis followed by adjuvant therapy
If progressive disease on primary therapy then they are poor candidates for liver resection–2nd line treatment

↓

Metachronous CRLM

↓

Presented within 1 year of resection of primary–Treat as synchronous CRLM
Presented after 1 year of resection of primary–Surgery upfront
Patients whose disease is unresectable or borderline should have systemic chemotherapy

Fong score and outcome of CRLM

- Extension of 1° colorectal carcinoma into the serosa
- Time to develop CRLM > 1 year
- Number of lesions > 1
- Size of largest CRLM > 5 cm
- CEA > 200 mg/mL

Each factor is scored 0 or 1, with a median survival of 74 months reported for patients scoring 0, and 14 months for those with five risk factors

Synchronous liver metastases and rectal cancer–most often treated with neoadjuvant chemotherapy and liver resection, followed by chemoradiation and then resection of primary rectal cancer

BENIGN TUMORS

Hepatic Adenoma:	FNH:
• Low malignant potential–5% (Risk greatest for adenomas >5 cm in size) • Occur mostly in women who use OCP • ***Most are solitary*** • Smooth, encapsulated masses and don't contain kupffer cells • ***Hemoperitoneum occurs in 25% cases***	• No malignant potential • Female-to-male ratio of 2:1 • No clear relation with OCP • Nodular and contain kupffer cells • Symptoms–Rarely

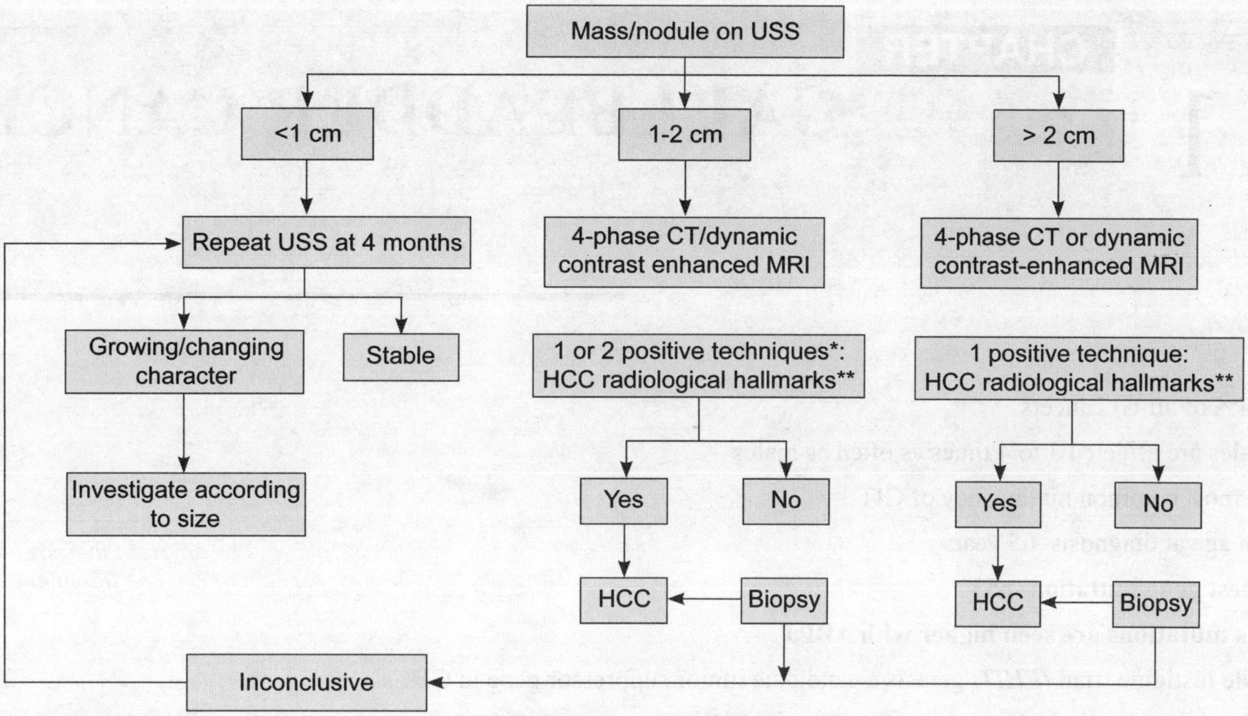

- Metavir F3 [Metavir is a scoring system for hepatic histology that grades fibrosis from 0 to 4 with higher numbers indicating more fibrosis]—or cirrhosis, particularly if associated with HCV genotype 1b
- *PNPLA3* polymorphism is strongly associated with fatty and alcoholic chronic liver diseases and HCC occurrence
- Finally, infection with adeno-associated virus 2 is associated with HCC in individuals without cirrhosis

MOLECULAR ABERRATIONS COMMON IN HCC

Mutations	
Telomere stability	TERT promoter
P53/cell cycle control	TP53
	ATM
	RB1
Wnt/β-cetenin signaling	CTNNB1
	AXIN1
Chromatin remodeling	ARID1A
	ARID2
	KMT2A
	KMT2C
Ras/PI3K/MTOR pathway	RPS6KA3
	TSC1/TSC2
Oxidative stress	NFE2L2
	KEAP1
High-Level Focal Amplifications	
VEGF signaling	VEGFA
FGF signaling	FGF19
Cell-cycle control	CCND1
Target with Homozygeous Deletion	
TP53/cell-cycle control	CDKN2A
	TP53
	RB1
Wnt/β-cetenin/signaling	AXIN1

- HCV infection and alcohol abuse have been associated with *CTNNB1* mutations
- *TP53* mutations are the most frequent alterations with a specific hotspot of mutation (R249S) in patients with aflatoxin B1 exposure

CHAPTER 11 GALLBLADDER CANCER

- 2 to 4% of all GI cancers
- Females are affected 3 to 4 times as often as males
- Fifth most common malignancy of GIT
- Mean age at diagnosis–65 years
- **Earliest gene mutation–p53**
- **K ras mutations are seen higher with ABPJ**
- Fragile histidine triad *(FHIT)* gene is a candidate tumor suppressor gene in GBCs
- GBC tumors may harbor human epidermal growth factor receptor 2 (HER2)/neu alterations in up to 19% of cases
- Gallbladder has thin mucosal wall, narrow lamina propria, and only single muscle layer
- Node-bearing adipose tissue posterior to head of the pancreas and portal vein may be involved early, whereas drainage to the hilum does not occur

Etiology
Cholelithiasis: • Cholelithiasis is present in 75-90% of gallbladder carcinoma • GBC is 7 times more common in patients with gallstones than those without stones • 0.5 to 3% of patients with gallstones develop gallbladder cancer • Patients with larger stones (>3 cm in diameter) have 10 times greater risk (80% risk) of cancer than patients with small stones (<1 cm) • Duration of gallstone disease, patient age, size of gallstones, and possible carcinogenic effects of gallstones, such as from the chemical composition or bacteria within the stones
Type of stone doesn't correlate with increase in incidence of cancer
Risk of malignancy correlates with length of time gallstones have been present
• Patients with symptomatic gallstones have higher risk compared to those of asymptomatic **Other Factors:** • Cholecystoenteric fistulas, Anomalous pancreaticobiliary junction (20%), Chemical carcinogens (Azotoulene, Nitrosamines), IBD, Familial predisposition, Chronic salmonella carrier status and Mirizzi syndrome • ***Patients with APBJ get cancer at a younger age than patients with sporadic GBC. Children with APBJ frequently have epithelial hyperplasia of the gallbladder*** • Obesity (66%), DM, Drugs like ***Methyldopa, Estrogens and Isoniazid***–Increased risk • Polyps >1 cm have greatest malignancy potential and therefore an indication for cholecystectomy. • Polyps more than 3 in number or adenomatous polyps–High risk • Malignant polyps are typically seen in patients **>50 years and Single >1cm** in diameter. • Porcelian gallbladder increases risk of gallbladder cancer by 10-60% (Sabiston <10%, Schwartz >20%, Devita–25%) Prophylactic cholecystectomy–Porcelian GB and ABPBJ

Contd.

Contd.

- Typhoid carriers may also suffer chronic inflammation of the gallbladder and have a sixfold higher risk of GBC
  Stippled, mucosal calcifications appear to be associated with higher risk than diffuse intramural calcifications
- ***Ulcerative colitis*** increases risk for extrahepatic biliary cancer by 5-10 times (15% of these cancers occur in the gallbladder)
- ***PSC***– Associated with an increased risk of GBC and gallbladder polyps
- ***Malignancy in PSC***–Associated with 20-fold increased risk, Early age, multifocal and advanced age–Poor Prognosis. (If associated with IBD–Highest risk)
- Gardener syndrome, NF-1 and HNPCC–Associated with increased risk
- ***Helicobacter bilis and Helicobacter pylori*** have demonstrated to increase the risk of carcinoma by about sixfold.
- Elevated body mass index has been associated with GBC
- Obesity increases risk of cancer by 66%

Rubber industry employees have a higher incidence and earlier onset of GBC
Cholesterol polyps and Adenomyomatosis–No risk

PATHOLOGY

Most common type–Adenocarcinoma (85%)
Most common site–Fundus of gallbladder (60%)

- Slow-growing tumor that arises from fundus in 60% of cases
- Appears firm with a thickened wall
- ***Acalculous carcinoma is more common in women***
- Draining lymph nodal basin for gallbladder cancer–Hepatoduodenal ligament

Papillary adenocarcinoma subtype characteristically grows intraluminally and spreads intraductally-
Less aggressive tumor and carries a better prognosis (<10%)

SPREAD

- Lymph nodes (35%) Adjacent organs (55%)
- Direct invasion of adjacent liver (60%)
- Peritoneal cavity after bile spillage (25%) Distant visceral organs (30%)
- Implanted in biopsy/ laparoscopic port sites

- Only common extra-abdominal site of metastasis is the lung

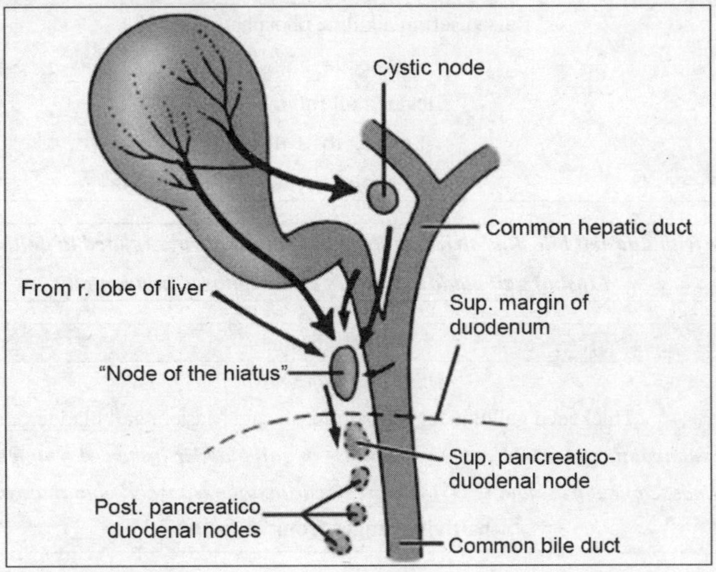

Miyazaki Concept

- No retrograde lymphatic flow in GB
- Direct flow from cystic node to interaortocaval node

*Gall bladder differs from intestines in lack of muscularis mucosa and submucosa, Lymphatics are present in subserosal layer only–**Therefore cancers invading but not growing through muscular layer have minimal risk of nodal disease***

Only 25% have tumors limited to the gallbladder

35% have loco-regional disease

40% have metastatic disease

PRESENTATION

- **Acute cholecystitis**
  Less advanced carcinoma
  High resectability
  Longer survival
- **Chronic cholecystitis**
- **Malignant symptoms**
  Jaundice, weight loss, generalized weakness, anorexia, persistent right upper quadrant pain
- **Benign non-biliary manifestations**
  GI Bleed/Obstruction

Most common site of distant extra-abdominal metastasis is lung

Most common presentation of Gallbladder cancer–Chronic Cholecystitis

Most common symptom of Gallbladder cancer–Abdominal pain

Cystic duct node is usual initial site of regional lymphatic spread

- Right upper quadrant mass/Hepatomegaly and constitutional symptoms suggest GBC

40% of patients with elevated alkaline phosphatase and without bilirubin levels are resectable

- CEA and CA19-9 may be elevated in patients with gallbladder carcinoma
- CA 19-9 is elevated in 80% of cases ***(CA19-9 are also increased in cholelithiasis, xanthogranulomatous cholecystitis and jaundice which are associated with carcinoma)***
- CEA–Specific for Gallbladder cancer but lacks sensitivity
- Invasion of the liver either by direct extension or via draining veins that empty into segments IV and V is seen in >50% of patients
- Courvoisier's law states that if gallbladder is enlarged and if patient has painless jaundice. Cause is unlikely to be gallstones

Lab Diagnosis
Raised serum alkaline phosphatase–65%
Anemia–55%
Elevated bilirubin–40%
Leukocytosis–40%
Leukemoid reaction–1%

Jaundice with mid-left bile duct stricture (type 0)–Almost always related to gallbladder cancer

Most of gall bladder cancers are diagnosed incidentally

Investigations
USG *(20% diagnostic)*
Thickened gallbladder, Cholelithiasis and Mass in gall bladder
Irregularly shaped lesion in subhepatic space, Heterogeneous mass in gall bladder lumen, Asymmetrically thickened gallbladder wall
Endoscopic ultrasound (EUS) is more accurate than transabdominal ultrasound
Sensitivity ranges from 70 to 100%

Triple phase CECT–Diagnostic in 50% of patients Contrast-enhanced CT or MRI will help determine resectability and determines local extent of disease with portal vein/hepatic artery invasion, lymphadenopathy and distant metastases Poor method for nodal spread ***Confirmation of diagnosis–CECT***
PTC–Abnormal in 80% of patients
ERCP–Abnormal in 75% of patients ***MRCP is preferred to ERCP and PTC*** ***Most accurate technique to define staging and vascular and biliary tract invasion–MRCP***
Laparoscopy–Detects resectability
PET CT*–Good means of assessing Metastasis, lymphadenopathy and residual disease in gallbladder, staging incidentally discovered carcinoma prior to radical surgery*

Nevin Staging System for Gallbladder Cancer

Stage	Description
I	Intramucosal only
II	Extends to muscularis
III	Extends through serosa
IV	Transmural involvement and cystic lymph nodes are involved
V	Direct extension to liver or distant metastases

Staging

T1	T1a–Invades Lamina propria T1b–Invades Muscular layer *(Watershed area for Gallbladder cancer management)*
T2	T2a–Invades Perimuscular connective tissue on peritoneal side without serosal involvement T2b–Invades Perimuscular connective tissue on hepatic side with no extension into liver
T3	Perforates serosa (visceral peritoneum) and/or directly invades liver or adjacent organ like stomach, duodenum, colon, pancreas, omentum or extrahepatic bile ducts
T4	Invades main portal vein/hepatic artery or invades two/more extrahepatic organs/structures
N1	1-3 Regional lymph nodes
N2	4/more Regional lymph nodes

<table>
<tr><th></th><th>N0</th><th>N1</th><th>N2</th><th>M1</th></tr>
<tr><td>T1</td><td>I</td><td rowspan="4">IIIB</td><td rowspan="5" colspan="2">IVB</td></tr>
<tr><td>T2a</td><td>IIa</td></tr>
<tr><td>T2b</td><td>IIb</td></tr>
<tr><td>T3</td><td>IIIA</td></tr>
<tr><td>T4</td><td colspan="2">IVA</td></tr>
</table>

Management

T1a	Simple cholecystectomy Cystic duct margin –ve→ Cholecystectomy enough If cystic duct margin +ve→ Bile duct excision and regional lymphadenectomy
T1b/T2, Stage II	Extended cholecystectomy ***(4 and 5 segments of liver along with lymphadenectomy)***
Advanced	Radical surgery ***(Extended right hepatectomy–Segments 4,5,6,7 and 8)***

- **Contraindications to surgery**–Distant metastases, Extensive involvement of porta hepatis causing jaundice, Significant Ascites and Encasement/Occlusion of major vessels
- Absolute contraindications to surgery include distant metastases, vascular involvement, or nodal spread beyond the hepatoduodenal ligament

Direct involvement of adjacent organs is not an absolute contraindication

- RT–No added benefit in adjuvant scenario–*EBRT at dose of 45 Gy can reduce the tumor size in 20% to 70% of cases and relieves jaundice in up to 80% of patients*
- 5 FU based regimen–Most commonly used
- Response rate of locally advanced gallbladder cancer to 5-FU regimens is 12%
- Metastatic disease–Gemcitabine and Cisplatin
- Most common site of metastasis–Liver

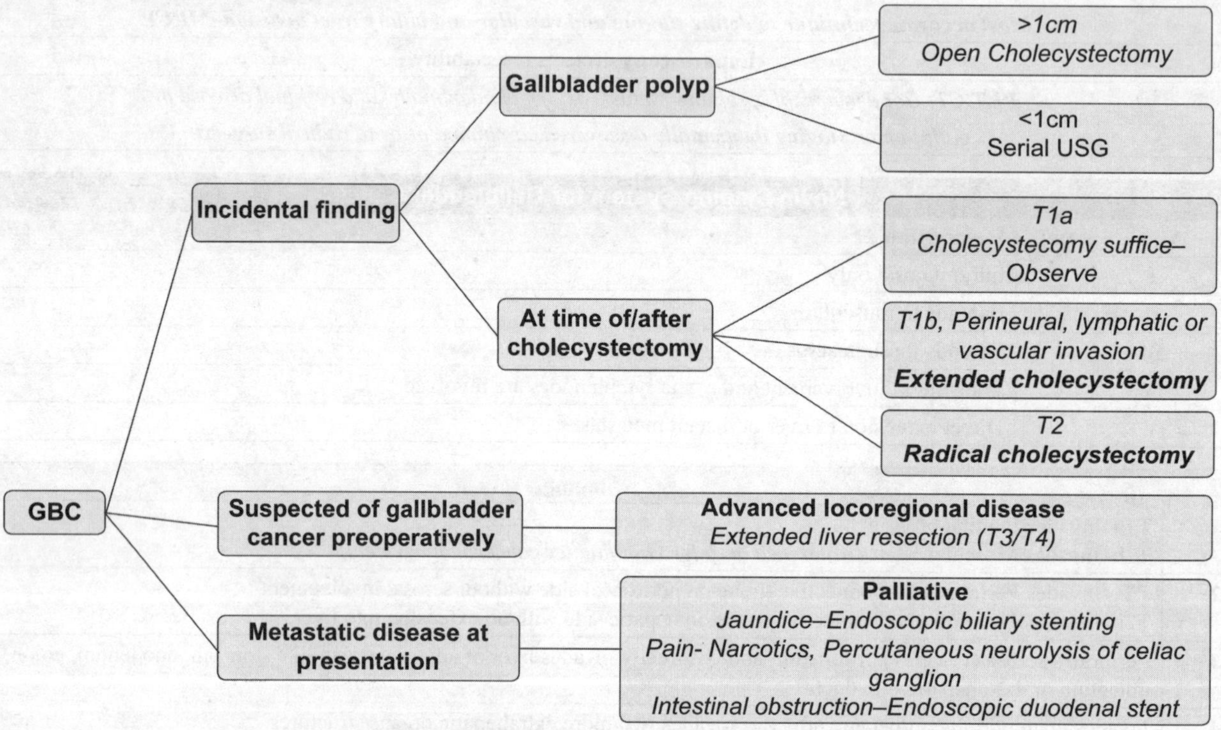

Survival

Survival of patients diagnosed with gallbladder cancer is dependent on stage of disease at presentation

Overall median survival–6 months

Overall 5 years survival rate–5%

- Patients with ***T1a lesions,*** limited to mucosa and lamina propria–***Excellent prognosis***
- Complete resection of ***T1b lesions*** to negative margins–***Excellent prognosis***
- Survival of patients with ***T2 lesions*** depends on nodal status
- Median survival of patients with metastatic disease at presentation–13 months

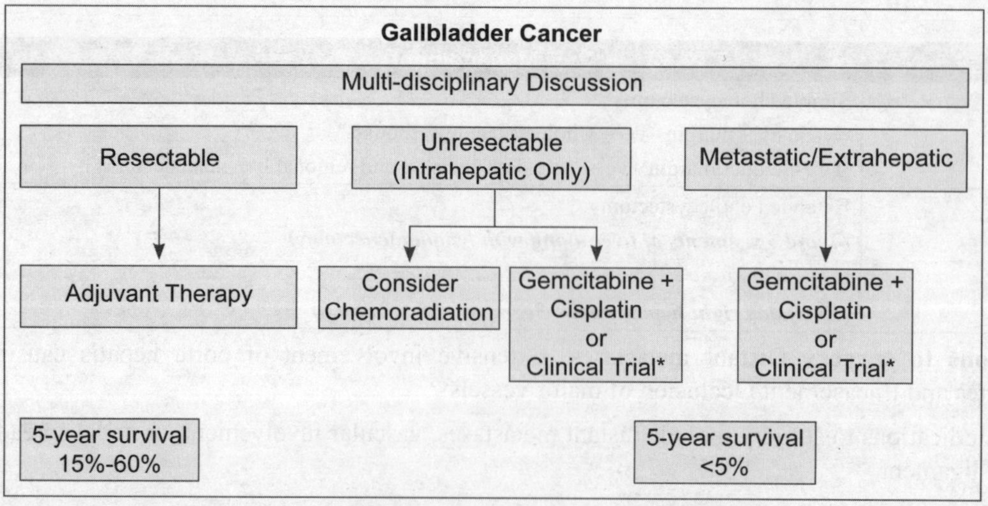

Median survival and 5 year survival			
I	II	III	IV
20 months 60-100%	7 months 10-20%	4 months 5%	2 months 0%

- There are no proven effective options for adjuvant radiation or chemotherapy for patient with gallbladder cancer
- Recurrence after resection most commonly occurs in liver/celiac/retropancreatic nodes
- Open approach is preferred to laparoscopic approach (Ideal for carcinoma gallbladder)
- **Most common cause of death**–Secondary to Biliary sepsis or liver failure
- **Spillage of bile during laparoscopic cholecystectomy**–30% in non-malignant and 50% in carcinoma GB
- Survival of patients with GBC is related to stage and histologic type of cancer
- Survival is worse for tumors on hepatic side of the gallbladder
- Plane of simple cholecystectomy–Between muscularis of gallbladder and cystic plate (Fibrous lining that occupies space between GB and Liver)

CHAPTER 12 CHOLANGIOCARCINOMA

- **More than 2/3rd of cancers are located at Hepatic bifurcation**
- Most patients have advanced disease at the time of diagnosis
- Most patients with unresectable disease die within 1 year of diagnosis
- **Male : Female ratio= 1.3 : 1**
- Average age of presentation→ 50-70 years

ETIOLOGY

- **Primary sclerosing cholangitis**–Most common association (20-fold increased risk)–Multifocal disease and not amenable to resection (5-10% of PSC patients)
- Up to 50% of patients with PSC with CCA have this diagnosed within a year of their initial diagnosis with PSC
- PSC is a clear risk factor for iCCA and pCCA development

> ***PSC with its autoimmune mutifocal strictures of intrahepatic and extrahepatic biliary tree carries increased risk of cholangiocarcinoma***

- **Recurrent pyogenic cholangitis**–Characterized by primary bile duct stone formation with infections and carries risk of cholangiocarcinoma
- **Choledochal cysts and Caroli disease**–*Of patients with choledochal cysts, 10% to 20% will develop CCA if left untreated or managed with surgical drainage alone. Early excision of choledochal cyst has been proposed to reduce the risk of CCA*
- Chronic long-term Ulcerative colitis
- Crohn's disease
- Polycystic kidney disease
- Cystic fibrosis
- **Hepatolithiasis**–*Cancers may develop even after stone removal, potentially related to stasis and cholangitis related to fibrosis induced by stone disease*
- Biliary enteric anastomosis and Biliary papillomatosis

> Clonorchis (Liver flukes)–Induce DNA Mutations and Associated with Intrahepatic stones and Elevated nitrates
> ***Degree of infestation as measured by stool egg count is related to the risk for CCA***

- Chronic typhoid carriers
- Oriental cholangiohepatitis
- Dietary nitrosamines, Thorotrast and Dioxin exposure, OC Pills and Cigarette smoking
- Asbestosis
- **HBV and HCV**–Risk factor for Intrahepatic cholangiocarcinoma
- **Lynch II Syndrome**
- Previous biliary enteric anastomosis
- **Isoniazid**–Increases risk of cholangiocarcinoma
- Congenital hepatic fibrosis

PATHOLOGY

- Most common type–Adenocarcinoma
- Most common morphological subtype–Sclerosing (Perihilar and Distal)
- Intrahepatic cholangiocarcinoma–Mostly nodular
- Most common site–Perihilar location (2/3rd)–**KLATSKIN TUMORS** (65%)
- Most common genetic mutation in Perihilar cholangiocarcinoma–K RAS
- Most common genetic mutation in Intrahepatic cholangiocarcinoma–FGFR2 fusions
- HER 2/neu alterations occur largely in gallbladder and dCCA
- ***Liver flukes-associated CCA have higher incidence of TP53 and SMAD4 mutations***

> *FGFR2 fusions and IDH1/2 mutations only occur in iCCA, whereas ERBB2 amplifications, APOBEC-associated mutation signatures and PKA fusions occur in eCCA*

- Spoardic cases–Tend to occur at bifurcation
- **Sclerosing**–Tend to occur in proximal bile ducts- Periductal fibrosis in concentric pattern and circumferential duct occlusion
- **Nodular**–Firm mass based in duct wall can be seen growing into duct lumen
- **Papillary**–Better prognosis (Less periductal fibrosis)
- **Tend to extend in submucosal route and associated with perineural invasion**
- Nodal involvement is observed frequently (~50% of patients)

> *Perihilar bile duct, the duct located topologically between the right side of the umbilical portion of the left portal vein and the left side of the origin of the right posterior portal vein*

Bismuth Corlette Classification	
Type 1	Common hepatic duct
Type 2	Bifurcation without involvement of secondary intrahepatic ducts
Type 3a	Extend into right secondary intrahepatic duct
Type 3b	Extend into left secondary intrahepatic duct
Type 4	Involves both right and left secondary intrahepatic ducts

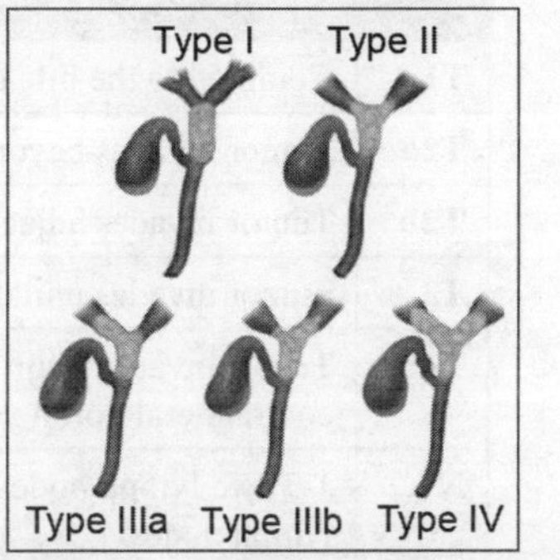

Blumgart Classification of Hilar Cholangiocarcinoma	
Type 1	Tumor involves biliary confluence with **unilateral involvement** upto 2nd order biliary radicles. No portal vein involvement in liver atrophy
Type 2	Tumor involves biliary confluence with **unilateral involvement** upto 2nd order biliary radicles. ***Ipsilateral portal vein involvement or Ipsilateral liver atrophy***
Type 3	Tumor involves biliary confluence with **bilateral involvement** upto 2nd order biliary radicles or Unilateral involvement upto secondary biliary radicles with ***C/L Portal vein involvement*** or Unilateral extension to secondary biliary radicles with ***C/L Liver atrophy*** or Main/Bilateral portal vein involvement

> ***Any patient who has a perihilar stricture, without evidence of ductal disease elsewhere in biliary tree suggestive of PSC, and who has not had previous biliary surgery that might have resulted in stricture, is considered to have pCCA***

- Most perihilar cholangiocarcinomas are infiltrating tumors, in which cancer cells are likely to extend in **subepithelial layer** rather than in the epithelial layer
- Histologically, direct and lymphatic invasion are common routes for invasion to the ductal wall, evoking reactive fibrosis–Cause rigidity, narrowing, tapering and obstruction of duct on cholangiogram
- ***Border of these findings on cholangiograms correspond to leading edge of cancer infiltration***
- ***Superficial spreading cholangiocarcinoma*** is defined as cholangiocarcinoma with a noninvasive cancer extension >2 cm,

characterized by papillary/expansile tumor configuration, length of superficial spread averages 54 mm suggesting that this tumor often requires extensive resection to obtain a negative ductal margin

- ***Diffusely infiltrating cholangiocarcinoma defined*** as a cholangiocarcinoma with an extensive infiltration from the hilar bile duct down to the lower bile duct. A cholangiogram shows that this type has a wide range of irregular biliary strictures
- *Multiplicity* seems to be a characteristic feature of biliary neoplasms
- ***Criteria for multiplicity: No direct continuity between the two tumors, a growth pattern typical of a primary tumor and clear histologic differences between the two tumors***
- Proposed three criteria for multiplicity: No direct continuity between 2 tumors, growth pattern typical of primary tumor and clear histologic differences between 2 tumors

CLINICAL FEATURES

- **Most common clinical presentation**–Painless Jaundice
- Cholangitis–Presenting symptom in 10% of patients
- Except for Jaundice, Physical examination is usually normal in cholangiocarcinoma
- Tumor marker that aids in diagnosis of cholangiocarcinoma most commonly is CA 19-9 (Serum level >129 U/ml)→ Sensitivity= 79% and Specificity= 98%
- ***CA 19-9 levels above 100 U/mL were found to be 89% sensitive and 86% specific for diagnosis of malignancy in patients with PSC***
- CA 19-9 has also been defined as a poor prognostic factor in CCA
- **Constant pain on presentation suggests more advanced disease**

AJCC Staging of Perihilar CCA	
T1	Confined to the bile duct, with extension up to the muscle layer or fibrous tissue
T2a	Tumor invades beyond the wall of the bile duct to surrounding adipose tissue
T2b	Tumor invades adjacent hepatic parenchyma
T3	Tumor invades unilateral branches of the portal vein or hepatic artery
T4	Tumor invades main portal vein or its branches bilaterally, or common hepatic artery, or unilateral second-order biliary radicals with contralateral portal vein or hepatic artery involvement
N1	1-3 +ve lymph nodes typically involving the hilar, cystic duct, CBD, hepatic artery, posterior pancreaticoduodenal, and portal vein lymph nodes
N2	Four or more positive lymph nodes from the sites described for N1
M1	Distant metastasis

	T1	T2	T3	T4
N0	I	II	IIIA	IIIB
N1	IIIC			
N2	IVA			
M1	IVB			

INVESTIGATIONS

- Perihilar location–Dilated Intrahepatic biliary tree and Gallbladder along with extrahepatic biliary tree is normal or collapsed distal to tumor
- Distal location–Dilated extra and intrahepatic bile ducts and gallbladder

USG/CT–Portal vein patency–Can establish level of obstruction but difficult to visualize tumor itself
PTC–Proximal extent of tumor ***(Most important in determining resectability)***
ERCP–Distal extent of tumor

MDCT

- In assessing value of MDCT, ***portal vein invasion*** is defined as absence of a visible hypoattenuated layer between portal bifurcation and adjacent tumor on an Multiplanar image reformation

Perihilar cholangiocarcinoma with Preoperative MDCT is used to assess for

- Distant metastasis
- Nodal metastasis
- Bismuth classification
- Vascular invasion with or without lobar atrophy
- Morphologic subtype
- Biliovascular anatomy
- Liver volume of each sector

Cholangiograms precisely delineate segmental anatomy of intrahepatic bile duct, tumor configuration, and the extent of the tumor border

- ***Biliary tract imaging (cholangiography) with cytology is used to establish diagnosis***
- Mucobilia on ERCP is an uncommon finding that is highly suggestive of papillary CCA

TREATMENT

- ***Surgical excision***–Potentially curative treatment
- ***Best surgical excision is possible with <10% of cases***
- *Surgical exploration*–No signs of metastasis or Locally Unresectable disease

*More than 1/2 who are explored are found to have peritoneal implants, nodal or hepatic metastasis or locally advanced disease–makes resection impossible (Biliary decompression and Chole*cystectomy)

- **Location and Local extent of tumor dictates extent of resection in curative resection**

Length of microscopic invasive and noninvasive cancers is limited to within 1 cm and 2 cm, respectively in 90% of cases of cholangiocarcinomas

This observation clearly guides the optimal resection line of the bile duct so that 1 cm and 2 cm tumor-free margins are recommended for the eradication of invasive and noninvasive cancer cells, respectively

PREOP BILIARY DRAINAGE

- Increases rates of infectious complications of resection
- Generally useful for those with Preop Bilirubinemia (>10 mg/dL) and those with prolonged interval between presentation and resection

PTBD is performed as a second-line procedure only when

- ENBD cannot be placed
- Total liver drainage is necessary for prolonged cholestasis
- Segmental cholangitis of the undrained lobe occurs; or
- ENBD tube is dislodged or kinked repeatedly

Indications for PVE are summarized as follows

- Future liver remnant (FLR) 25% or less in normal liver
- PVE is indicated when estimated FLR is approximately <40% in case of Perihilar cholangiocarcinoma
- Scheduled concomitant extrahepatic surgery or complex hepatectomy; and
- Any major hepatectomy in patients with an underlying chronic disease or an injured liver (resulting from chemotherapy, major steatosis, or cholestasis).

Recommended site for puncture in PVE is Right anterior portal vein*–Because PVE is indicated in patients who are scheduled to undergo right hemihepatectomy or right or left trisectionectomy, right anterior sector is always resected*

Type 1/2 Perihilar tumors with no signs of vascular involvement	Local tumor excision with portal lymphadenectomy, cholecystectomy, CBD excision and Bilateral Roux en Y hepatico jejunostomies
Type 3a/3b	Right/Left hepatic lobectomy added Excision of caudate lobe is required because of direct extension into caudate biliary radicals/ parenchyma
Unresectable perihilar cholangiocarcinoma	Roux en Y cholangiojejunostomy to segment 2/3 bile ducts or to right hepatic duct is done.
Distal bile duct tumors ***Often resectable***	Pylorus preserving pancreatoduodenctomy (Whipple procedure)
Distal bile duct Unresectable	Roux en Y hepaticojejunostomy, Cholecystectomy and GJ

- Liver transplantation is a viable option for the treatment of early stage, unresectable pCCA in highly selected patients.
- Presence of extrahepatic nodal disease or metastases is a contraindication to transplant

If tumors identified unresectable on diagnostic evaluation–***Non operative biliary decompression is performed***
• *Proximal tumors–Percutaneous placement of expandable metal stents or drainage catheters*
• *Distal bile duct tumors–Endoscopic placement*

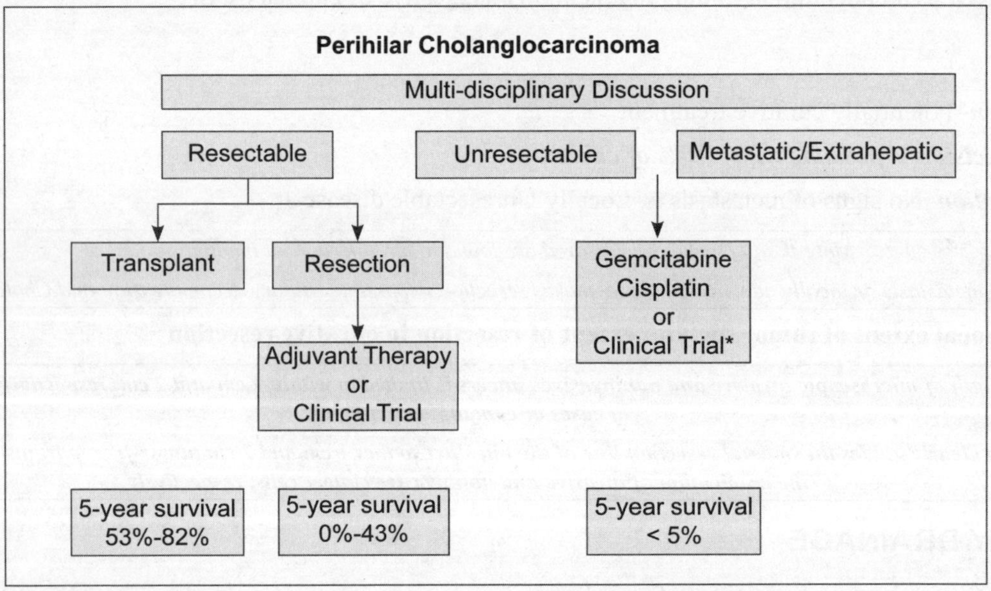

- All procedures include resection of caudate lobe, allowing for complete removal of hilar bile duct
- Proximal duct is resected at ***right side of umbilical portion of the left portal vein in right hemihepatectomy,*** whereas it is ***resected at the left side of the umbilical portion in right trisectionectomy.*** Ductal length is longer in latter than in the former by width of umbilical portion, which measures approximately 10 mm
- Proximal duct is resected at the level of the ***right portal vein in left hemihepatectomy,*** whereas it is resected at the level of ***right posterior portal vein in left trisectionectomy***–Ductal length is longer in the latter than in the former by width of the right anterior portal vein, typically measuring approximately 7 mm

Proximal duct	Resected at right side of umbilical portion of left portal vein in ***right hemihepatectomy***
	Resected at the left side of the umbilical portion in ***right trisectionectomy***
	Resected at the level of right portal vein in ***left hemihepatectomy***
	Resected at the level of right posterior portal vein in ***left trisectionectomy***

Contraindications to Surgery
Bilateral intrahepatic metastases, Any extrahepatic disease, Bilateral hepatic lobar artery or biliary radicals involvement, Significant Ascites, and Encasement of main portal vein
Unilobar vascular structures involvement is managed by resection of primary and affected lobe in continuity

- Overall median survival of perihilar carcinoma is between 5 and 8 months
- 90% die within 1 year
- Overall median survival of distal carcinoma is 32 to 38 months
- Overall 5 year survival rate for resectable perihilar cholangiocarcinoma→ 10-30%
- Overall 5 year survival rate for resectable perihilar cholangiocarcinoma→ 30-50%
- Most common cause of death–Hepatic failure and Cholangitis
- ***Risk factors for recurrence–Positive margins and LN + tumors***
- Therapy for recurrent disease–Palliation (No surgery)
- Most common site of metastasis–Lung
- Survival rate for patients with a positive ductal margin with noninvasive carcinoma was comparable to that of patients with a negative ductal margin, ***which was significantly better than that for patients with a positive ductal margin with invasive carcinoma (BLUMGART)***

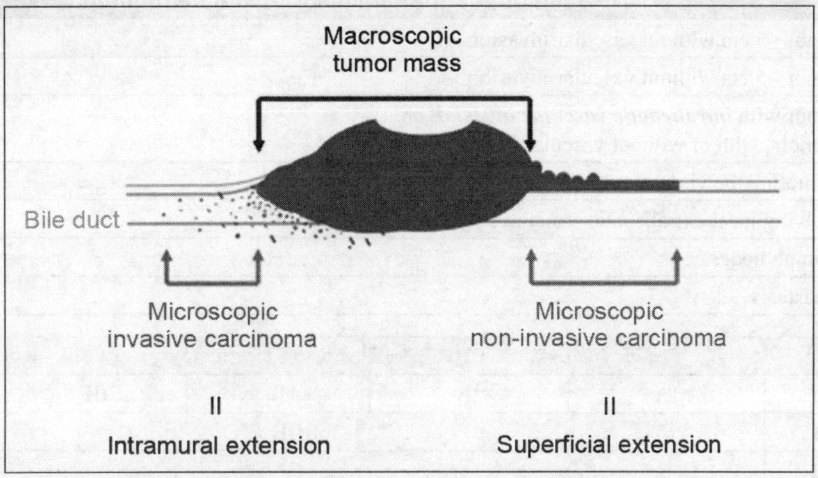

Most common benign neoplasm from glandular epithelium of bile duct–Papilloma
Most common site of papilloma–Periampullary
Most common symptom of papilloma–Jaundice

- Hepatobiliary resection for perihilar cholangiocarcinoma is known to be associated with a high morbidity and mortality, resulting from impaired liver function with cholestasis and cholangitis; reported surgical mortality rate remains high, approximately 10%
- ***Right-sided hepatectomy*** is suitable for ***nodular or flat tumors*** that display an ***infiltrating nature in advancing margin,*** whereas limited surgery, including resection of S1, S1+4, or bile duct resection alone is acceptable for papillary tumors, provided that surgical margin is negative
- ***dCCAs are far less common than pCCAs and have better treatment outcomes***

Intrahepatic Cholangiocarcinoma
• Most of these tumors involve biliary confluence
• *iCCAs arise from intrahepatic bile ducts beyond 2nd order ductal system within liver*
• 2nd most common primary hepatic neoplasm
Risk Factors
PSC, Choledochal cysts, Hepatolithiasis, RPC, HBV, HCV, NASH, Cirrhosis and Diabetes
• Right upper abdominal pain and weight loss–clinical feature
• Jaundice occurs late with iCCAs and usually indicates extensive disease
• **AFP levels–normal**
• CA19-9 and CEA are elevated
• Diagnosis of exclusion

Contd.

Contd.

- CT: Focal hepatic mass with peripheral dilatation
- On CT scan, the lesion is usually of low attenuation with only mild enhancement seen with contrast

Characteristic imaging features of iCCAs that may be helpful in distinguishing these tumors from HCCs are slow uptake of contrast, particularly in highly desmoplastic tumors and peripheral rim of enhancement

- On a T1-weighted MRI, iCCAs are usually of low intensity but may have high intensity on T2-weighted images
- Intrahepatic Metastasis, LN Metastasis, growth along biliary tree often encountered
- Mucin production, fibrosis between acini of tumor tissue, and a more overtly glandular pattern are the main differentiating characteristics from HCC
- ***IDH1 and IDH2*–More commonly identified genetic mutations in iCCA**
- NKG2D Polymorphisms are possible risk factors for Cholangiocarcinoma

AJCC Staging of Intrahepatic Cholangiocarcinoma	
T1a	Solitary tumor ≤5 cm without vascular invasion
T1b	Solitary tumor >5 cm without vascular invasion
T2	Solitary tumor with ***intrahepatic vascular invasion or*** Multiple tumors, with or without vascular invasion
T3	Tumor perforating the visceral peritoneum
T4	Tumor involving local extrahepatic structures by direct invasion
N1	Regional lymph nodes
M1	Distant metastasis

	T1a	**T1b**	**T2**	**T3**	**T4**
N0	IA	IB	II	III	IV
N1	IIIB				
M1	IV				

- **Treatment**: Complete resection is the treatment if choice
- **Chemotherapy is ineffective**
- **Poor Outcome:** Multifocality, LN Metastasis, Vascular invasion and Positive margins
- Intrahepatic metastases tend to occur as multiple satellites, and although their presence impacts prognosis, they should not definitively preclude resectability
- Comorbidities, such as presence of underlying advanced cirrhosis with portal HTN may preclude surgical resection
- Extrahepatic spread also of course precludes resection and portends a poor prognosis
- Median survival after surgical resection is approximately 36 months
- 5 years survival rate with curative R0 resection is approximately 60%

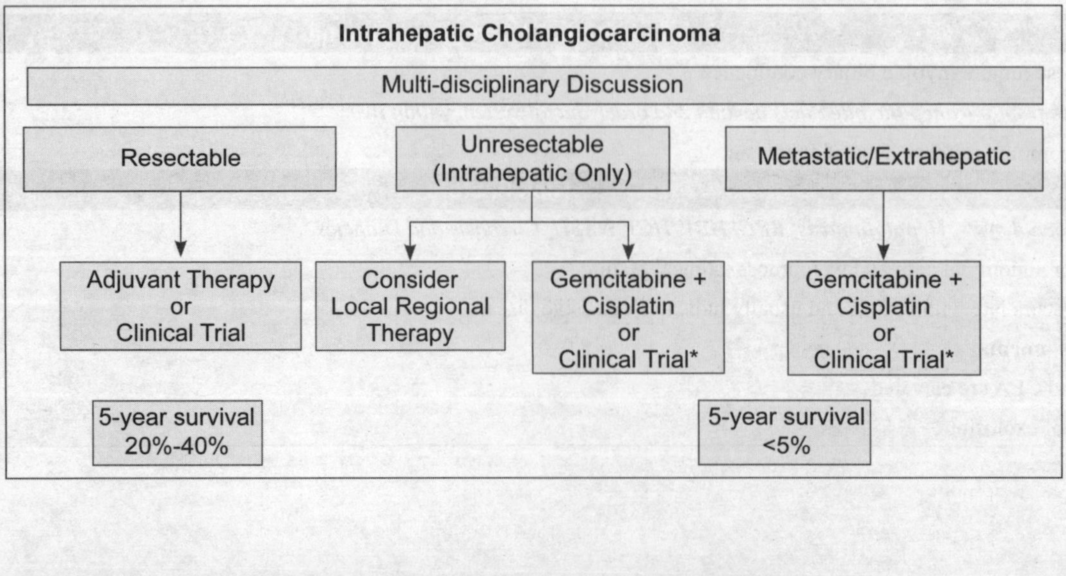

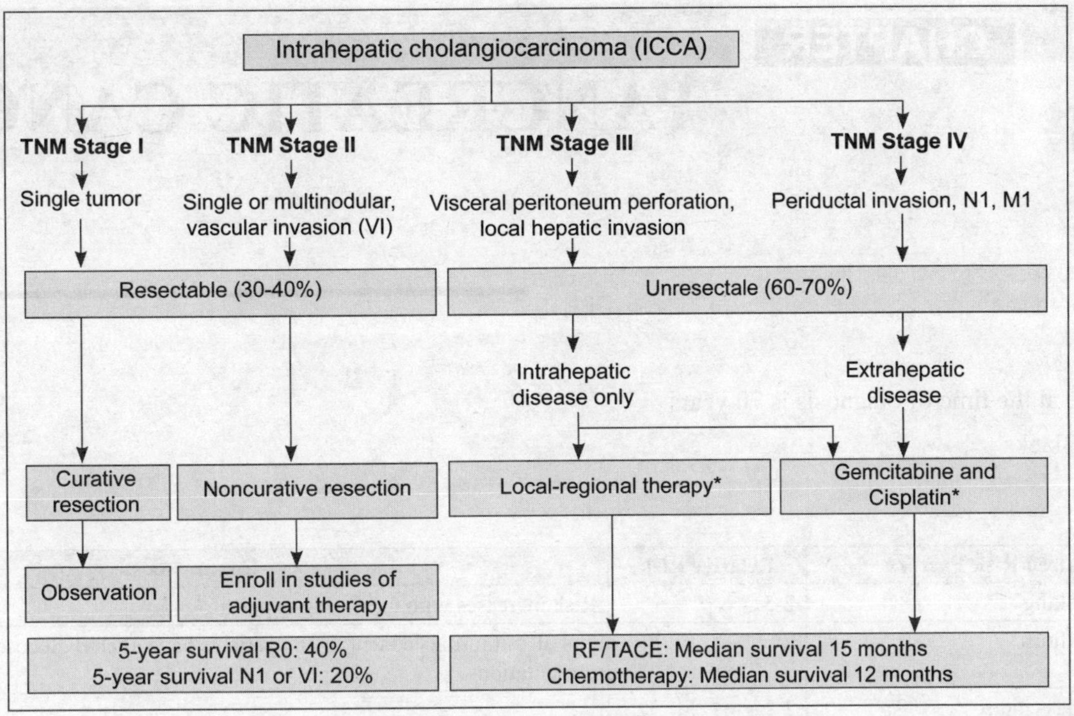

- **Prodige trial**–To receive either gemcitabine plus oxaliplatin (GEMOX) or surveillance following an R0 or R1 resection of a localized cancer
- ***Gemcitabine in combination with cisplatin was established as standard of care for first-line therapy patients with advanced biliary cancers***

CHAPTER 13

PANCREATIC CANCERS

- Median Age at the time of diagnosis is 70 years
- Males and Blacks

ETIOLOGY

Acquired Risk Factors	Relative Risk	Comments
Tobacco smoking	2-5	Risk increases with increasing exposure
Diabetes mellitus	2	Not all authorities concur; many patients have altered glucose metabolism on presentation
High body mass index	2	
Chronic pancreatitis	13-18	Not all authorities concur with this degree of increased risk
Inherited Disorders	**Relative Risk**	**Known Defects**
Hereditary pancreatitis	10-53	PRSS1
FAMMM syndrome	22	P16INK/CDKN2
HNPCC	8	MLH1, MSH2, MSH6
Peutz-Jeghers syndrome	13-30	LBK1/STK11
Familial adenomatous polyposis	4-5	APC
Li-Fraumeni syndrome	?	p53
Familial breast and ovarian cancer	3-5	DNA repair pathways, BRCA2

- **Smoking:** Risk increases with duration and amount of smoking (1.5 times)–***Associated with nitrosamines***
- High intake of fat, meat–Increased risk
- Intake of fresh fruits and vegetables–Protective
- **Partial gastrectomy**–2 to 5 times higher risk of pancreatic cancer (15 to 20 years later)
- **Long term duodenogastric reflux**–Increased risk of pancreatic cancer *(rise in CCK)*
- **Cholecystectomy**–Increases risk of pancreatic cancer *(rise in CCK)*
- **DIABETES**–*Early manifestation of pancreatic cancer/predisposing factor*
- **Chronic pancreatitis**–Associated with 5 to 15 fold increase in risk for pancreatic cancer
- **Hereditary pancreatitis**–50-70 fold increased risk
- Exposure to 2-naphthylamine, benzidine and gasoline derivatives–***5 fold increased risk***
- Prolonged exposure to ***DDT and derivatives***–Increase risk of pancreatic cancer
- **Higher in low socioeconomic patients**
- **Idiopathic DVT**–Associated with mucinous carcinoma development
- **Tonsillectomy**–Protective factor against development of pancreatic cancer (Not confirmed).
- **Familial pancreatic cancer**–5% risk of pancreatic cancer (Germ line mutation of BRCA2)–Autosomal dominant with reduced pentrance
- **Two 1st degree relatives with cancer**–18 to 57 fold increased risk

GENETIC ABNORMALITIES

- Mutant *c-K-RAS* genes have been found in approximately 95% of all human pancreatic carcinoma and metastases
- *BRCA1/2, PALB2 and ATM* genes→ 15-20% of cases
- DPC4 Mutation–Metastatic and Pan I3

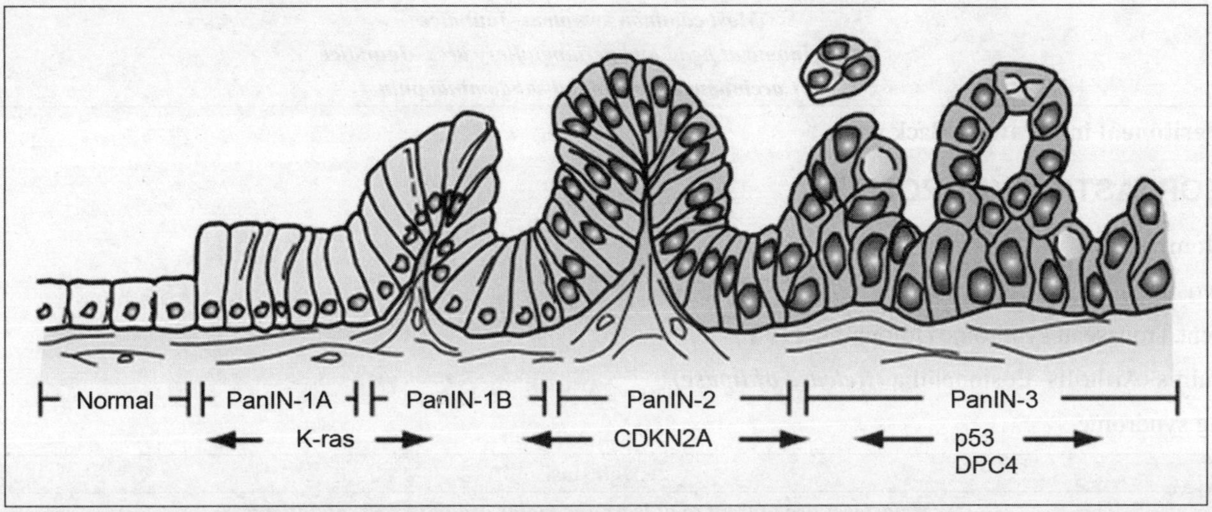

Hereditary Risk Factors Associated with Development of Pancreatic Cancer		
Gene	**Associated Syndrome**	**Clinical Significance**
PRSS1	Familial pancreatitis	Mutation result in chronic pancreatitis and 40% lifetime risk of PDAC
STK11	Peutz-Jeghers syndrome	Mutation result in >100-fold increase in risk of PDAC
CDKN2A	Familial atypical mole and multiple melanoma syndrome	Mutation leads to increased risk of melanoma and >40-fold increase in risk of PDAC
CFTR	Cystic fibrosis	Thick secretions result in chronic pancreatitis and 30-fold increase in risk of PDAC
BRCA2	Hereditary breast and ovarian cancer	Mutation results in elevated risk of breast and ovarian cancer and 10-fold increase in risk of PDAC
MLH1	Lynch syndrome	Mismatch repair gene mutation leads to increased risk of colon cancer and eighthold increase in risk of PDAC
APC	Familial adenomatous polyposis	Mutation result in polyposis coli and colon cancer with four-fold increase in risk of PDAC

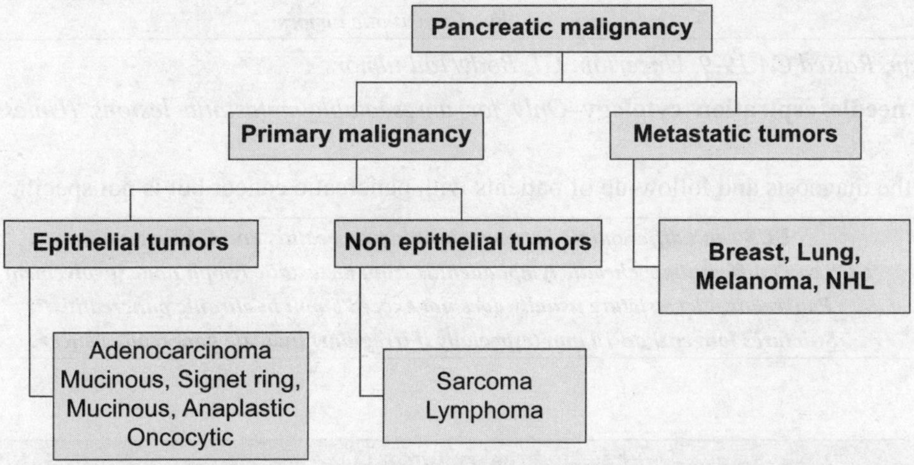

Most common type–Adenocarcinoma

Most common site–Head of pancreas (>85%)

- **Anaplastic carcinoma**–Usually involves body and tail

- **Pure epidermoid carcinoma**–*Usually associated with Hypercalcemia*
- **Periampullary carcinoma**–*Best prognosis*

SYMPTOMS

Most common initial symptom–Jaundice and Abdominal pain
Most common symptom–Jaundice
Carcinoma at head and periampullary area–Jaundice
Carcinoma body and tail–Abdominal pain

- **Retroperitoneal infiltration**–Back pain

PARANEOPLASTIC SYNDROMES

- Dermatomyositis
- Polymyositis
- Recurrent Trousseau syndrome (Idiopathic DVT)
- Panniculitis–Arthritis–Eosinophilia ***(Release of lipase)***
- Cushing syndrome

Metastasis
Metastases are present to at least one major organ in 65% of patients
Liver–45%, Lungs–30%, and Bones–3%

INVESTIGATIONS

- 1st Investigation of choice–**USG** (Detects as small as 2 cm lesion, Hepatic metastasis, Extrapancreatic spread)
- USG shows dilated duct→ Proceed to CECT

Investigation of choice–CECT/MDCT
Most sensitive investigation–ERCP

- **CECT**–Retroperitoneal lymphadenopathy and Invasion *(Atleast 2 cm diameter for detection)*

  Dynamic CECT with continuous infusion–Best for assessing tumor size and Extension
- **ERCP**–Palliation and Biopsy (Obstructed/Encased pancreatic duct >95%)
- **EUS**–T and N Staging, Vasculature, Hepatic metastasis and Extrapacreatic spread <2 cm

EUS is more accurate than standard ultrasound, CT and ERCP for diagnosis, staging and predicting resectability of pancreatic tumors

- **Laparoscopy**– *>3 cm, Raised CA 19-9, Uncertain CT, Body/Tail tumors*
- **Percutaneous fine needle aspiration cytology**–*Only for unresectable/metastatic lesions (Unless Palliative surgery is planned)*
- CA 19-9 is used for the diagnosis and follow-up of patients with pancreatic cancer but is not specific for pancreatic cancer

EUS can't differentiate between chronic pancreatitis and CA Pancreas
EUS can't differentiate chronic lymphadenitis from metastatic lymph node involvement
Pancreatic duct stricture usually does not exceed 5 mm in chronic pancreatitis;
Strictures longer than 10 mm (especially if irregular) indicate pancreatic cancer

TNM STAGING

Primary Tumor (T)	
TX	Primary tumor cannot be assessed
T0	No evidence of primary tumor

Contd.

Contd.

Tis	Carcinoma in situ*
T1	Tumor limited to the pancreas, 2 cm or smaller in greatest dimension
T2	Tumor limited to the pancreas, more than 2 cm in greatest dimension
T3	Tumor extends beyond the pancreas but without involvement of the celiac axis or superior mesenteric artery
T4	Tumor involves the celiac axis or superior mesenteric artery (unresectable primary tomor)
Regional Lymph Nodes (N)	
NX	Regional lymph nodes cannot be assessed
N0	No regional lymph node metastasis
N1	Regional lymph node metastasis
Distant Metastasis (M)	
M0	No distant metastasis
M1	Distant metastasis

Stage	TNM
I	*T1/T2*
II	*T3/N1*
III	*T4*
IV	*M+*

Resectable	T1, T2, T3 (within or just into peripancreatic tissue) No celiac axis/SMA involvement No evidence of Portal vein–SMV axis involvement No evidence of metastasis
Borderline resectable	SMV–Portal vein abutment (<180° of vein is in contact with tumor) SMV–Portal vein encasement (>180° of vein is in contact with tumor) SMV–Portal vein reconstructible short segment occlusion SMA <180° Abutment Reconstructible Abutment/Encasement/Occlusion of Hepatic artery or GDA No SMA, Celiac artery Involvement
Unresectable	T4 (Involves SMA, Celiac artery Stage IV tumor

TREATMENT

Tumors of **head** of the pancreas	**Pylorus preserving pancreaticoduodenectomy or Longmire-Traverso procedure** is preferred
Tumors of **body and tail** of the pancreas	**Distal pancreatectomy** and **en-bloc splenetomy**

- Most complication of pancreaticoduodenectomy is delayed gastric emptying
- Most cause of death following pancreaticoduodenectomy is cardiopulmonary complications
- Most important predictor of post-operative survival is R0 resection
- Most important margin in pancreaticoduodenectomy is retroperitoneal or uncinate margin

Palliative Therapy for Pancreatic Cancer	
Biliary obstruction	• **ERCP** with **metal stent placement (Best)** • Roux-en-Y hepaticojejunostomy
Gastric outlet obstruction	• **Endoscopic stenting (Preferred)** • Double bypass (Roux-en-Y hepaticojejunostomy + gastrojejunostomy)
Pain	• **NSAID** or **opiates** • **Celiac nerve block**

- At the time of presentation 85% of ductal adenocarcinoma are unsuitable for resection
- Standard resection for pancreatic head or Ampullary tumor: pylorus preserving pancreaticoduodenectomy (PPPD or Whipple's procedure)
- Tumors of the body and tail: Distal Pancreatectomy with splenectomy
- Multifocal tumor (main duct IPMN or body and tail too friable for anastomosis): Total Pancreatectomy

Contraindications to surgical resection
• Hepatic metastases • Peritoneal metastases • LN metastasis distant from pancreatic head • Encasement of **superior mesenteric artery, hepatic or Coeliac artery**

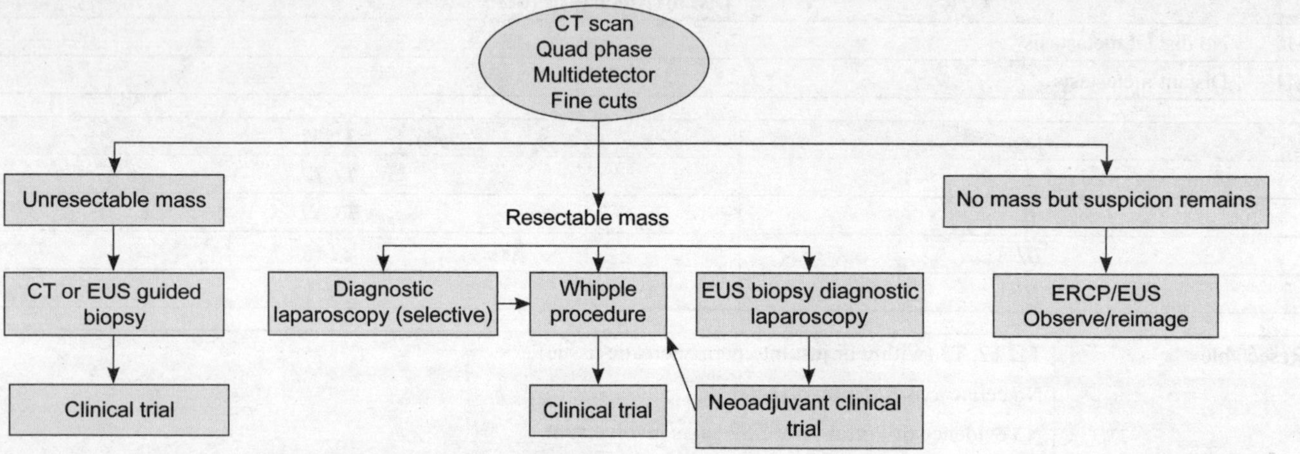

Steps of Standard Pancreaticoduodenctomy:

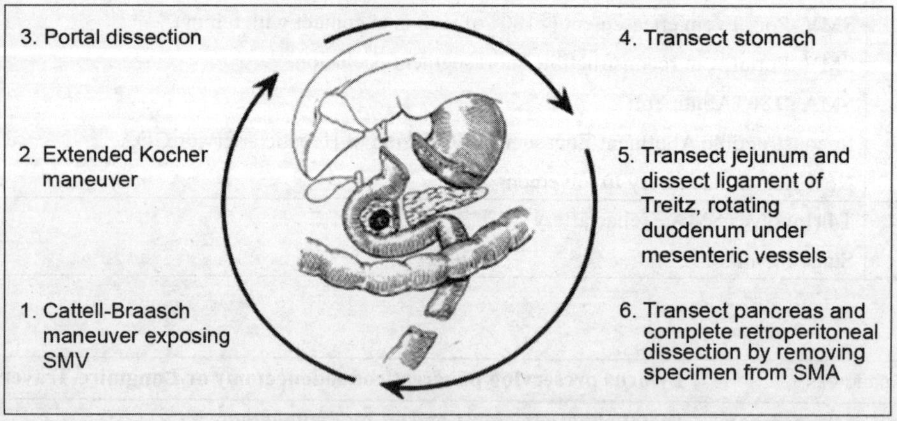

Reconstruction After Pancreaticoduodenectomy:

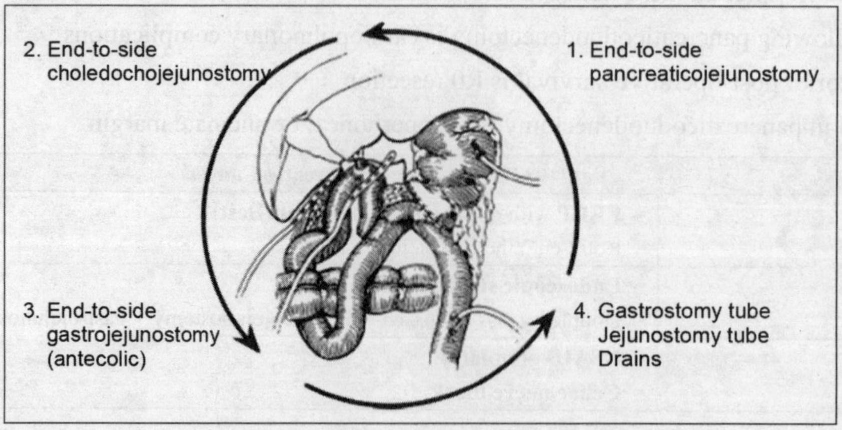

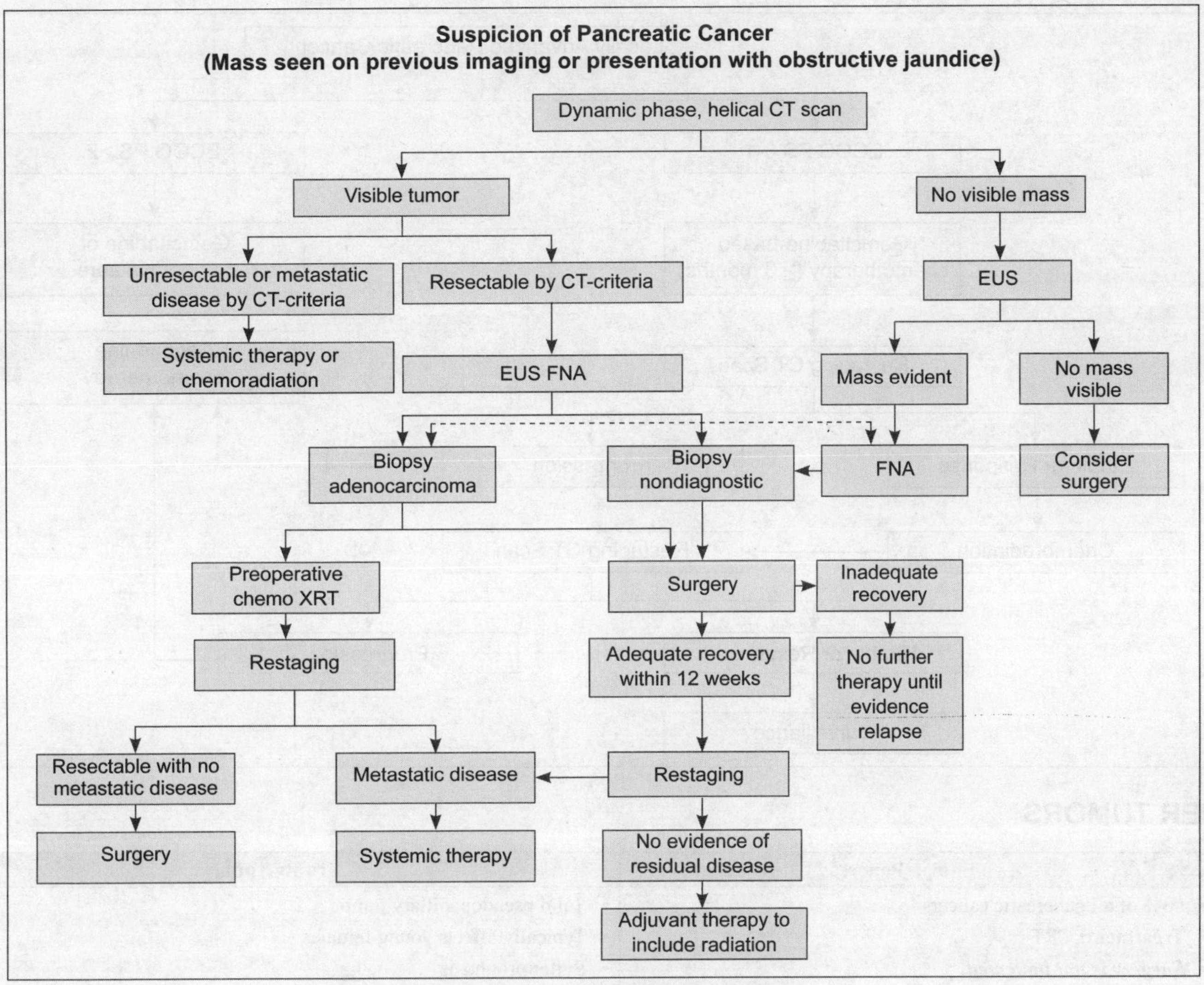
Suspicion of Pancreatic Cancer
(Mass seen on previous imaging or presentation with obstructive jaundice)
Dynamic phase, helical CT scan
Visible tumor
No visible mass
Unresectable or metastatic disease by CT-criteria
Resectable by CT-criteria
EUS
Systemic therapy or chemoradiation
EUS FNA
Mass evident
No mass visible
Biopsy adenocarcinoma
Biopsy nondiagnostic
FNA
Consider surgery
Preoperative chemo XRT
Surgery
Inadequate recovery
Restaging
Adequate recovery within 12 weeks
No further therapy until evidence relapse
Resectable with no metastatic disease
Metastatic disease
Restaging
Surgery
Systemic therapy
No evidence of residual disease
Adjuvant therapy to include radiation

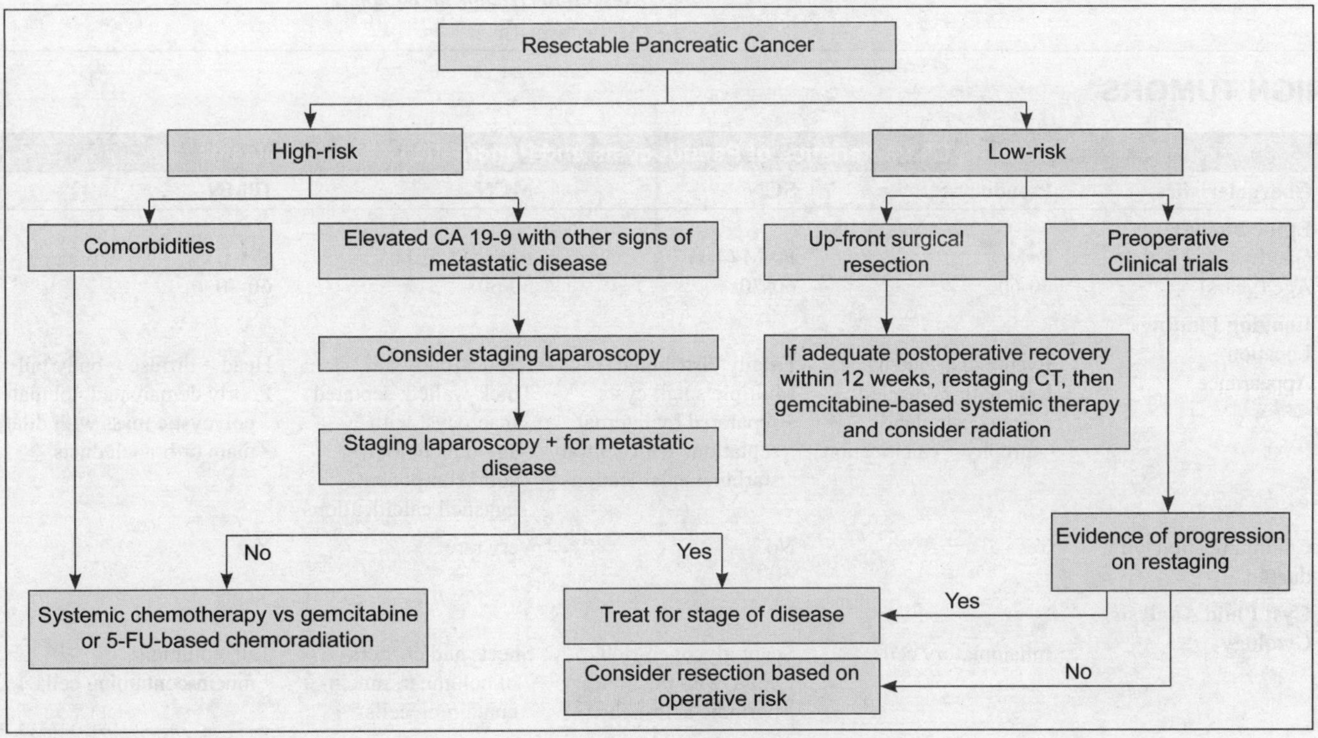
Resectable Pancreatic Cancer
High-risk
Low-risk
Comorbidities
Elevated CA 19-9 with other signs of metastatic disease
Up-front surgical resection
Preoperative Clinical trials
Consider staging laparoscopy
If adequate postoperative recovery within 12 weeks, restaging CT, then gemcitabine-based systemic therapy and consider radiation
Staging laparoscopy + for metastatic disease
No
Yes
Evidence of progression on restaging
Systemic chemotherapy vs gemcitabine or 5-FU-based chemoradiation
Treat for stage of disease
Yes
Consider resection based on operative risk
No

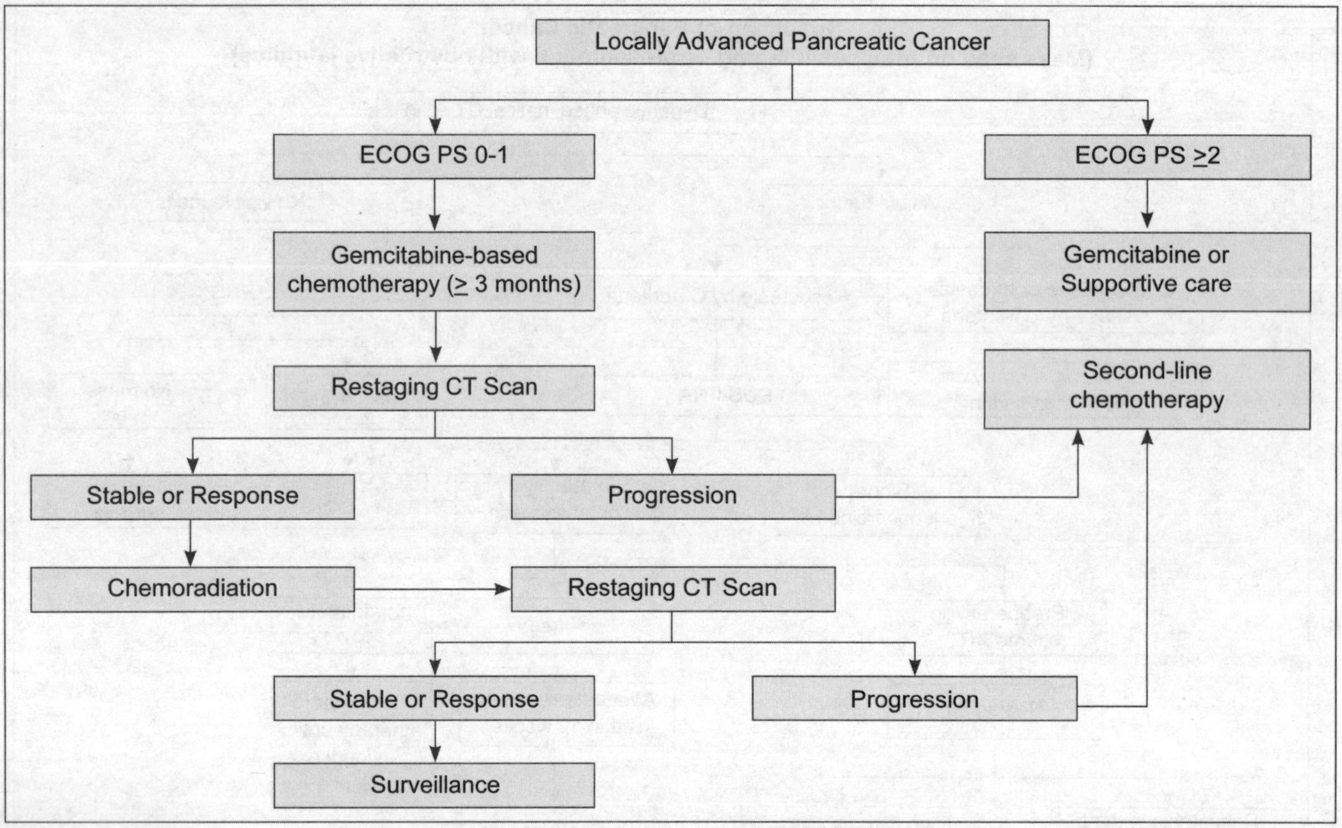

OTHER TUMORS

Lymphoma Pancreas	Frantz Tumor
• <3% of all pancreatic cancers • **Treatment:** CRT • ***Surgery is not indicated***	• Solid pseudopapillary tumor • Typically affects young females • Better prognosis • **Resection**–*Treatment of choice* • **Metastasis**–Liver

BENIGN TUMORS

Defining Characteristics of Pseudocysts and Pancreatic Cystic Neoplasms				
Characteristics	**Pseudocyst**	**SCN**	**MCN**	**IPMN**
Epidemiology				
Gender	F=M	F≫M (4:1)	F ≫M (10:1)	F=M
Age (years)	40-60	60-70	50-60	60-70
Imaging Findings				
Location	Evenly distributed	Evenly distributed	Head ≪ body/tail	Head > diffuse > body/tail
Appearance	Round, thick-walled large cyst; gland atrophy ± calcification	Multiple small cysts separated by internal septations with central starburst calcifications	Thick-walled, septated macrocyst with smooth contour, ± solid component, eggshell calcifications	Poorly demarcated, lobulated, polycystic mass with dilation of main or branch ducts
Communication with ducts	Yes	No	Very rare	Yes
Cyst Fluid Analysis				
Cytology	Inflammatory cells	Scant glycogen-rich cells, with positive periodic acid-Schiff	Sheets and clusters of columnar, mucin-containing cells	Tall, columnar, mucin-containing cells

Contd.

Contd.

Mucin stain	Negative	Negative	Positive	Positive
Amylase	Very high	Low	Low	High
CEA	Low	Low	High	High

SCN	MCN	IPMN
Older women Multiple small cysts **HEAD** Sunburst appearance *>4 cm, Rapid growth→ Resect*	Perimenopausal women Multilocular cyst **BODY/TAIL** *20% history of Pancreatitis* Egg shell, Mural nodule and Large size→ Increased risk of malignancy Pancreatectomy–Treatment of choice	Older men MD-IPMN: Multifocal and Malignant **HEAD** MD–IPMN: 30-50% risk BD–IPMN: 10-15% MD-IPMN→ Total pancreatectomy

A Summary of Worrisome and High-Risk Features of Intraductal Papillary Mucinous Neoplasm

Worrisome Features	High-Risk Features
Main duct 5-9 mm Nonenhancing mural nodule Thickened, enhancing cyst wall BD-IPMN size >3 cm Abrupt caliber charge in main duct with upstream atrophy Lymphadenopathy Pancreatitis	Main duct >1 cm Enhancing solid component Jaundice

MANAGEMENT OF SUSPECTED BD-IPMN

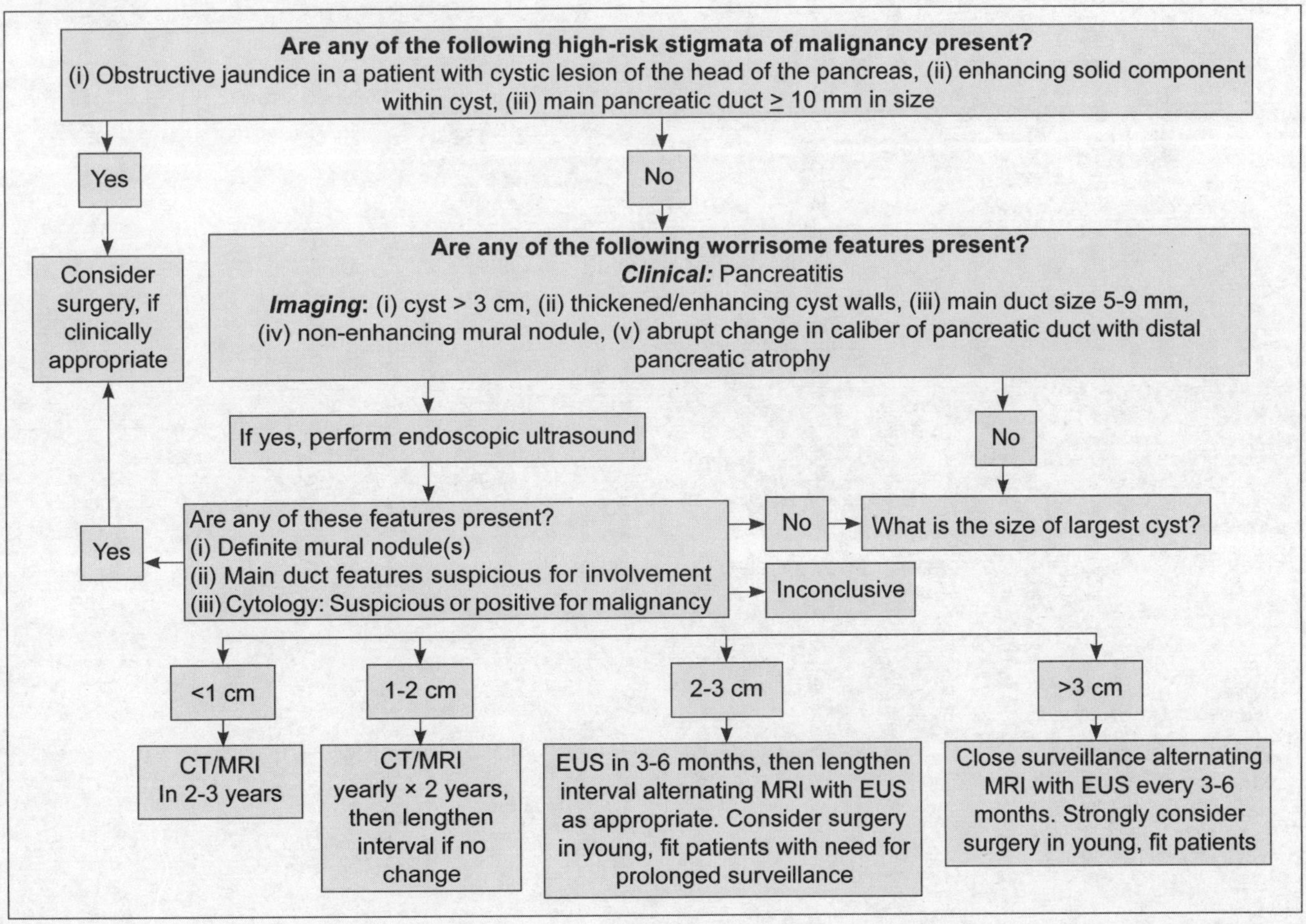

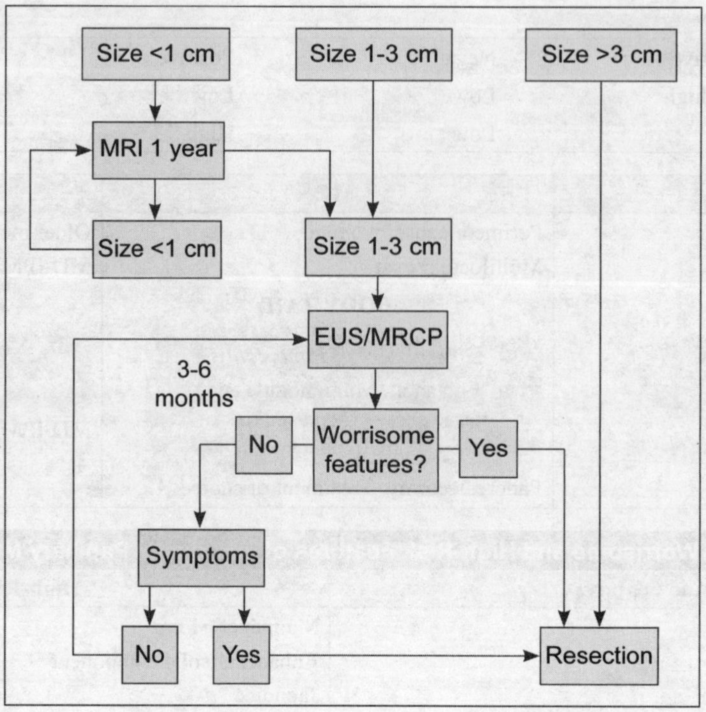
Size <1 cm
Size 1-3 cm
Size >3 cm
MRI 1 year
Size <1 cm
Size 1-3 cm
EUS/MRCP
3-6
months
No
Worrisome
features?
Yes
Symptoms
No
Yes
Resection

PART ONE: GENITOURINARY ONCOLOGY

CHAPTER

14 RENAL CELL CARCINOMA

INTERNIST'S TUMOR, GRAWITZ TUMOR, HYPERNEPHROMA, RENAL ADENOCARCINOMA

One Liners

- Most common type is conventional/clear cell carcinoma
- ***Bilateral RCC***–VHL syndrome
- **Stage is the important prognostic factor**
- Most common symptom is hematuria (painless hematuria)
- Most common paraneoplastic syndrome is raised ESR
- Stauffer's syndrome–Non metastatic hepatic dysfunction
- Carcinoma in chronic dialysis associated cystic disease patients is papillary renal cell carcinoma
- ***Chromophobe Carcinoma***–Best prognosis
- ***Oncocytoma***–Stellate scar/spoke wheel pattern
- ***Plant cell appearance***–Chromophobe carcinoma
- Most common site of distant metastasis–***Lungs***
- 85% of all renal parenchymal tumors
- Constitutes approximately 4% of all adult malignancies

Facts

- More in African Americans
- Males are affected twice as often as females
- 5th to 6th decade
- Median age at diagnosis–**64 years**

Risk Factors

- Smoking
- Obesity
- Hypertension, Diabetes
- Occupational exposure–Cadmium, Asbestosis, Gasoline
- Diuretic use
- Acquired cystic disease of kidney
- Chronic analgesic usage
- Sporadic and VHL–Loss of chromosome region 3p
- Hereditary RCC–Tends to occur at an early age, Bilateral and Multifocal (5%)
- Family history–2 fold

VHL is characterized by cerebellar hemangioblastoma, retinal angiomata, bilateral clear cell RCC (35-45% of RCC–Multiple and Bilateral) and islet cell tumors of pancreas

Hereditary Papillary RCC

- Type 1: Autosomal dominant syndrome → MET (Chromosome 7)–Non random duplication of aberrent chromosome 7 ***(Trisomy 7)***
- Type 2: Hereditary leiomyomatosis → Mutations of ***Fumarate hydratase*** enzyme–Cutaneous and Uterine leiomyoma + Papillary RCC ***(Aggressive clinical course)***–Chromosome 1

Birt-Hogg-Dubé syndrome–Bilateral multifocal tumors with both ***chromophobe RCC and oncocytoma*** histology along with cutaneous fibrofolliculomas, pulmonary cysts and spontaneous pneumothorax–Chromosome 17p11 encodes folliculin protein

Succinate dehydrogenase–SDHB germ line mutations (Pheochromocytoma + Paraganglioma)

Tuberous sclerosis–Angiomyolipoma, Clear cell and Papillary RCC

- RCC is also associated with polycystic kidney disease, tuberous sclerosis, and acquired renal cystic disease
- Bilateral in 2% of sporadic cases

70% of sporadic cases of clear cell RCC are associated with inactivating mutations of both copies of VHL (Overexpression of HIF 1 and VEGF)

PATHOLOGY

- Most common type of histology–Clear cell carcinoma (75-85%)
- Most RCC originate in Proximal tubular cells of kidney
- **Multifocal**–6.5 to 10% (Papillary variety)
- Tumor cells are rich in glycogen and lipid–Clear cell appearance on microscopically and has characteristic yellow appearance grossly
- Chromophobe carcinoma arises from intercalated cells of Collecting system (4%)
- Translocation RCC–Chromosomal translocation in TFE3 (pediatric)
- Collecting duct RCC–Originate in collecting duct

Medullary RCC

Associated with Sickle cell trait characterized by aggressive clinical course

- ***Oncocytoma****–Benign tumor with no malignant potential (7%), originates from collecting ducts*
- All RCC have high grade spindle cells

CLINICAL FEATURES

- ***Gross or Microscopic hematuria***–Most common presenting symptom (50%)
- ***30% Asymptomatic***
- ***Classic triad***–Hematuria, Abdominal mass and flank pain (<10%)
- ***Weight loss***–Presenting feature in <15% of patients
- ***Sudden onset varicocele***–Invasion into renal vein or IVC (Left or right respectively)
- Bone pain and CNS abnormalities–Metastasis
- Lower extremity edema–Advanced disease
- Fever, Plethora, Hypercalcemia symptoms or Anemia–***Presenting features***
- Risk of metastases at presentation and Risk of renal mass being RCC at presentation–Strongly associated with tumor size

Spread
• Direct invasion through renal capsule into perinephric and adjacent structures • Direct invasion into renal vein

Paraneoplastic Syndromes
Erythrocytosis (1-5%):
VHL inactivation is associated with impaired degradation of hypoxia induced transcription factors and increased production of EPO (Independent of oxygen levels)

Contd.

Contd.

Hypercalcemia (15%):
Associated with overproduction of PTHrP
Associated with widespread bony lytic lesions
Fever (10-20%):
Often intermittent with night sweats, anorexia, fatigue and unintentional weight loss
Stauffer's syndrome (15%):
Fever, Leukopenia and areas of hepatic necrosis ***(Non-metastatic Liver dysfunction)–Reversible***
Alkaline phosphatase and Transaminase levels are elevated, Deranged PT, INR and Hypoalbuminemia
Secondary to tumor related cytokine production–Overproduction of GM-CSF and IL-6 by tumor
Hypertension (40%):
Associated with renin production by tumor
Alleviated by tumor removal
Hyperglobulinemia: Result in raised ESR
Amyloidosis: Occurs in 3-5% of patients
Thrombocytosis: Associated with poor prognosis

Investigations

- CT will define tumor mass–***Preferred imaging modality***
- 1st line investigation of hematuria–**USG**
- In case of thrombus involvement of vena cava or renal vein–MRI/CT with 3 dimensional reconstruction–***Extent of tumor thrombus***
- Mass suggests RCC, metastatic work up consisting of Chest X-ray, CT, Liver function tests should be performed
- Patient has increased alkaline phosphatase and bone pain→Bone scan is usually required
- **MRI Brain**–Brain metastasis
- **Cannon ball like lesions**–Round large multiple metastatic deposits of lung

Features Suggestive of Malignancy

- Size >7 cm
- No interface between tumor and renal parenchyma
- Amputation of collecting duct
- Involved perinephric fat and adjacent structures
- Lymphadenopathy and distant metastasis
- Calcification

Robson Staging

Stage	Description	5 year survival
I	Confined to kidney	50-60%
II	Extends into peri renal fat but confined to Gerota's fascia	4-20%
III	Involves Renal vein/IVC/Lymph node involved	20-50%
IV	Adjacent organs/Metastastic disease	0-20%

TNM Staging

T1	Tumor 7 cm or less in greatest dimension, limited to the kidney
	T1a Tumor 4 cm or less *T1b Tumor more than 4 cm but not more than 7 cm*
T2	Tumor more than 7 cm in greatest dimension, limited to kidney
	T2a Tumor >7 cm but not more than 10 cm *T2b Tumor >10 cm, limited to kidney*

Contd.

Contd.

T3	Tumor extends into major veins or perinephric tissues but not into ipsilateral adrenal gland and not beyond Gerota fascia
	*T3a Tumor grossly extends into **renal vein/its segmental (muscle containing) branches**, or tumor invades **perirenal and/or renal sinus fat but not beyond Gerota fascia*** *T3b Tumor grossly extends into vena cava **below diaphragm*** *T3c Tumor grossly extends into vena cava **above diaphragm** or invades **wall of vena cava***
T4	Tumor invades **beyond Gerota fascia** (including contiguous extension into I/L adrenal gland)

<table>
<tr><th></th><th>T1</th><th>T2</th><th>T3</th><th>T4</th></tr>
<tr><td>N0</td><td>I</td><td>II</td><td>III</td><td rowspan="2">IV</td></tr>
<tr><td>N1</td><td colspan="3">III</td></tr>
<tr><td>M1</td><td colspan="4">IV</td></tr>
</table>

MANAGEMENT OF CLEAR CELL CARCINOMA

Localized Tumor–Surgery

Partial Nephrectomy

- *T1a tumor*
- *T1b tumor with need to preserve renal parenchyma*
- *Partial nephrectomy is indicated for bilateral tumor involvement, renal insufficiency, solitary kidney, and hereditary RCC such as VHL*
- *Partial nephrectomy constitutes standard of care for patients with **localized renal tumors <4 cm***
- ***Tumor recurrence after partial nephrectomy–0 to 6%***

Radical Nephrectomy

- Kidney, Ipsilateral adrenal gland, Surrounding Gerota fascia and regional lymph nodes are all resected en bloc
- Indicated for Large locally advanced tumors ***(More than 7 cm limited to kidney)***

Observation

***Small (<4cm) tumors**- Poor surgical candidates/Limited life expectancy*

- *Laparoscopic radical nephrectomy, performed for **<10 cm***
- ***Gold standard** for treatment of patients with localized/locally advanced RCC that is not amenable to nephron-sparing approaches*

***Cryotherapy and radiofrequency ablation**–Treat **small (<4 cm)** renal masses*

- ***Less than 5 cm involving lower pole of kidney–Spare adrenal gland***
- ***<10% of synchronous adrenal metastasis***

Approach

- Modified flank, midline, or subcostal (chevron) incision
- Large upper-pole tumors may be approached through thoracoabdominal incision
- Adrenalectomy is generally not indicated if adrenal gland is not involved with malignancy on imaging or intraoperatively

Nodal Disease

***10% of patients**–regional lymphatic metastases without distant disease*

Incidence of occult nodal involvement is 3% to 5%

- Patients with papillary histology and node metastases that undergo aggressive surgical resection can enjoy an extended progression free and overall survival, in contrast to patients with nodal metastases from clear cell histology
- NCCN guidelines recommend regional lymph node dissection for patients with palpable disease or enlarged nodes identified on preoperative imaging

15% to 20% of RCCs invade Renal vein
8% to 15% invade IVC
50% are localized
25% are locally advanced
40-50% develop metastasis

Mayo classification of vena caval involvement
Level 0: Thrombus is within the renal vein only
Level I: Thrombus extending into IVC but not more than 2 cm above renal vein (Renal)
Level II: Thrombus extends into IVC to >2 cm above renal vein but not to hepatic vein (Infrahepatic)
Level III: Thrombus extending into IVC to above hepatic vein but not to diaphragm (Intrahepatic)
Level IV: Thrombus extending into supradiaphragmatic IVC/right atrium

METASTATIC RCC

- Median survival for patients with metastatic RCC is 12 months
- ***Most common site of distant metastasis–Lungs> Lymph nodes***
- Presence of nodal metastases in setting of distant metastatic disease portends ***worse prognosis and a decreased likelihood of responding to systemic therapy***

Solitary lung metastases *Associated with better survival rate than metastases to other organ sites*
Multiple metastases/multiple sites of metastases *Significantly worse prognosis and usually approached with systemic therapy*
Metastatectomy *Single metastatic lesion and Solitary recurrence > 2 years after definitive nephrectomy*
Cytoreductive nephrectomy *Palliation of intractable hematuria and pain associated with RCC*

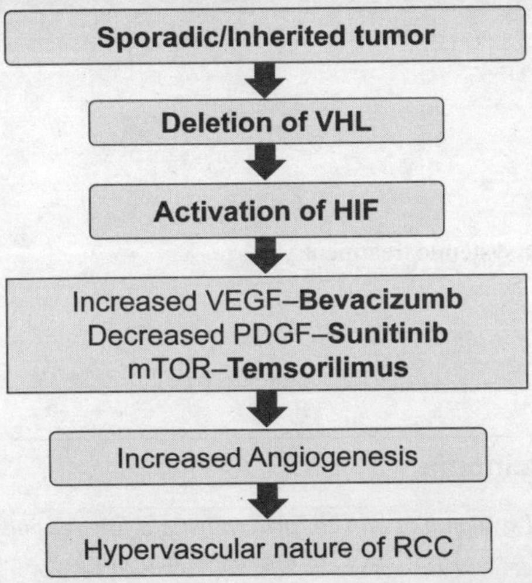

Targeted Therapy
• **Sunitinib**–VEGF TKI is used in 1st line therapy for good to intermediate prognosis renal clear cell carcinoma (Improves Objective response rate, PFS and OS)
• **Sorafenib**–Improved PFS, not ORR and OS
• **Bevacizumab**–Improved OS
• **Pazopanib**–Improved PFS compared to placebo, No improvement in PFS and OS compared to sunitinib
• **Axitinib**–Improved PFS compared to sorafenib
• **Cabozantinib**–Improved PFS
• **Everolimus**–*Worsened PFS compared to sunitinib, Improved disease free survival compared to placebo*
• **Temsirolimus**–*Improved median OS and Prolonged disease free survival compared to INF alpha*
• ***Single agent temsirolimus***–*Reasonable 1st line option for patients with poor prognosis RCC*

Immunotherapy

- IL-2 remains a therapeutic option in selected patients with favorable prognosis–response rate of 15% to 20% in good-risk patients
- **IFN-α** as a single agent has modest antitumor activity in setting of RCC, with a response rate of approximately 15%

Radiotherapy

Palliative radiotherapy is appropriate for: Painful or bleeding primary tumor and non-resectable metastatic disease, e.g., bone, brain, soft tissue

Prognostic Factors

- **Pathologic stage**–Most important prognostic factor
- Tumor >10 cm Size→Associated with poor prognosis
- Renal vein/Vena cava involvement→Associated with poor prognosis
- Sarcomatoid and Unclassified patterns of RCC–Poor prognosis
- Non diploid tumors→Poor prognosis

Leibovich prognostic score runs from 0 to 11 and is based on the tumor's stage, grade, size, involvement of lymph nodes and presence of tumor necrosis histologically

Most widely used grading system for RCC

Fuhrman system (Based on nuclear and nucleolar morphology) 1-4

Short Survival Times

- High LDH levels (>1.5 times upper limit of normal)
- High corrected blood calcium (>10 mg/dl)
- Anemia (Less than lower limit of normal)
- Cancer spread to 2/more distant sites
- Less than a year from diagnosis to need for systemic treatment
- Poor performance status *(KPS<80)*
- Absence of prior nephrectomy

Management of Non-Clear Cell Carcinoma

Currently no standard systemic options of proven benefit for treatment of patients with advanced RCC of non-clear histology

Most common cause of death from kidney cancer–Clear cell carcinoma

RENAL CYSTS

Simple cyst/Fatty tumor → No further follow up is indicated

Hyperechoic lesion on imaging → Follow up

Bosnaik cyst types 3 and 4 are managed as Renal cancers

Hereditary syndromes associated with renal cell carcinoma					
Syndrome	**Gene (position)**	**Protein**	**Incidence of developing a kidney tumor (%)**	**Median age at diagnosis (years)**	**Other phenotypic features**
Clear cell/renal cell carcinoma*					
von Hippel Lindau disease	VHL (3p25-26)	pVHL	25-45	40	Hemangioblastoma Pancreatic neuroendocrine tumors Pheochromocytoma Renal cysts Pancreatic cysts Ovary cystadenoma Epididymal cystadenoma
BAP1 mutant disease (also known as tumor predisposition disease)	BAP1 (3p21)	BRCA-associated Protein	No data	No data	Breast cancer Uveal melanoma Mesothelioma Other cutaneous melanocytic tumors
SDH-associated kidney cancer	SDHB (1p35), SDHC (1q23) and SDHD (11q23)	Succinate dehydrogenase subunits B, C and D	5-15	30	Paraganglioma Carotid body tumors Pheochromocytoma Gastrointestinal stromal tumor
Papillary renal cell carcinoma					
Hereditary leiomyomatosis and renal cell cancer	FH (1q42)	Fumarate hydratase	2-21	46	Uterine leiomyosarcomas Breast cancer Bladder cancer Cutaneous leiomyomas Uterine leiomyomas
Hereditary papillary kidney cancer	MET (7q31)	Hepatocyte growth factor receptor	No data	<60	No additional features
Multiple tumor types					
Birt-Hogg-Dub syndrome	FLCN (17p11.2)	Folliculin	34	50	Fibroclicuttomas and inchaciscomas Pulmonary cysts Pneumothorax
Tuberous sclerosis complex	TSC[1] (9q34) and TSC[2] (16p13)	Hamarain and tuberin	2-4	30	Subependymal giant cell astrocytomas Angiomyolipomas Renal cysts Facial angiofibroma Ungual and periungual fibromas Hypomelanotic macule Forehead plaque Cardiac rhabdomycomas Connective tissue naevus

Contd.

Contd.

Cowden syndrome (also known as multiple hamartoma syndrome)	PTEN (10q23)	Phosphatase and tensin homologue	34	40	Breast cancer Endometrial cancer Thyroid cancer Prostate cancer Macrocephaly Intestinal hamartomatous polyps Benign skin tumors (multiple Trichilemmomas, papillomatous papules and acral keratoses) Dysplastic gangliocytoma of the Cerebellum
Hyperparathyoidism jaw tumor syndrome	MRPT[2](1q31)	Parafibromin	No data	No data	Parathyroid carcinomas Uterine carcinomas Renal cysts and hamartomas Hyperparathyroidism Parathyroid gland tumors Jaw fibromas

Non-clear-cell renal cell carcinomas

Tumor type	Subtype	Cytogenatic alterations	Genes mutated	Gross appearance	Histological features*
Papillary	Type	Gains of 7, 8q, 12q, 16p, 17 and 20 Loss of 9p	MET	Mixed cystic or solid consistency Often whitish in colour and may show hemorrhage and necrosis Frequently with a well-demarcated pseudocapsule	Single layer of cuboid tumor cells Thin, basophillic papilliae with scant pale cytoplasm and low nuclear grade Concentric lamellated calcifications (psamomma bodies) Foamy macrophage infiltration
	Type 2	Gains of 8q Loss of 1p and 9p	CDKN2A SETD2 NRF2		Heterogeneous, thick papillae and eosinophilic cytoplasm, high nuclear grade and pseudostratification Concentric lamellated calcifications Foamy macrophage infiltration
Chromophobe	Classic	Loss of chromosomes 1, 2, 6, 10, 13, 17 and 21	TP53 PTEN	Large, well-circumscribed grey to tan-brown coloured tumors Occasional central scar	Tumor cells with prominent membrane and pale cytoplasm Voluminuous cytoplasm (cytoplasmic accumulation of acid mucopolysaccharides
	Eosinophilic				Large tumor cells with fine eosinophillic granules Distinct cell borders Voluminous cytoplasm
MiT family translocation	NA	Recurrent translocations involving Xp11.23 (TFE3) or 6p21 (TFEB)	TFE3 TFEB	Yellowish tissue Often studded by hemorrhage and necrosis	Papillary or nested architecture Abundant clear or eosinophilic cytoplasm

Contd.

Contd.

Collecting duct	NA	Losses at 8p, 16p, 1p and 9p Gains at 13q	Unknown	Partially cystic White-grey appearance Often exhibit invasion into the renal sinus	Tubulopapillary pattern Often with cells taking columnar pattern with hobnail appearance Presence of mucinous material Desmoplastic stroma
Medullary	NA	Poorly described, but thought to be normal karyotype	SMARCB1	Tan or white appearance Poorly defined capsule Extensive haemorrhage and necrosis	Poorly differentiated, eosinophillic cells Inflammatory infiltrative cells Sheet-like or reticular pattern is common
Oncocytoma	NA	Loss of chromosome 1 and Y chromosome CCND1 rearrangement	Mitochondrial genes (COX1, COX2, MTND4 and MTCYB)	Mahogany colour Circumscribed Occasional central scar Rarely with necrosis	Polygonal cells with abundant eosinophillic cytoplasm Uniform, round nuclei

CHAPTER 15 BLADDER CARCINOMA

One Liners
• Most common type of bladder carcinoma is ***Transitional bladder carcinoma (90-95%)***
• Most common predisposing factor for carcinoma bladder–***Tobacco smoking***
• Lower incidence in African Americans compared to whites
• Intravesical valrubicin is FDA approved drug for BCG refractory patients who refuse/intolerant of cystectomy
• Disease recurs after 2 consecutive induction courses then plan for radical cystectomy
• Schistosomia hematobium infection Chronic inflammation with indwelling catheters and bladder diverticula predisposes to SCC
• Persistent urachus and bladder exstrophy predisposes to adenocarcinoma
• Definitive diagnosis of bladder cancer is by cystoscopy and biopsy
• Most common symptom of bladder cancer is gross painless hematuria
• **TURBT** is the primary tumor staging surgery
• ***Staging is most important prognostic factor for progression and overall survival***
• ***Tumor grade is key prognostic factor for Non-muscle invasive tumors***
• Early BCG administration after TURBT results in BCG sepsis
• Advanced/metastatic disease treatment of choice is MVAC/GC regimen
• Intravesical therapy for low risk disease stage Ta, T1 and Tis is using thiotepa, mitomycin-C, doxorubicin, Epirubicin
• For high risk disease stage Ta, T1 and Tis, Intravesical BCG therapy is given
• For recurrent/persistent tumors, 2nd induction of dose of intravesical BCG given at 3 months follow up

ETIOLOGY

Transitional cell carcinoma	Squamous cell carcinoma
• Tobbcco smoking–most common	• Bladder diverticular
• 2-naphylamine, 4-aminobiphenyl	• Bladder diverticular
• Aromatic amines–dyes, paints, solvents, leather dust, inks combustion products, rubber, textile	• Schistosomia hematobium infection
• Schistosomia hematobium infection	• Chronic inflammation with indwelling catheters
• Pelvic irradiation	• Urinary stones
• ACROLEIN–Metabolite of cyclophosphamide	
• Drugs–Phenacetin and chlomphazine	

- ***Smoking increase risk by 2 to 6 fold***
- Heavy smokers are more likely to have high grade tumor and muscle invasive disease
- Pelvic RT increases bladder cancer by 4 fold
- BALKAN NEPHROPATHY–Increases risk of bladder cancer
- **HNPCC**–*Predominantly MSH2*→ Increases life time risk of urothelial cancer of ureter and renal pelvis
- **Pioglitazone**–Increases risk of bladder cancer

- **Aristocholic acid** *(Found in Chinese herbal remedies)→ Associated with urothelial carcinoma particularly upper tract tumors*
- ***Most common chromosomal abnormality–Loss of chromosome 9***
- ***Most common site of TCC–Bladder***

TYPES

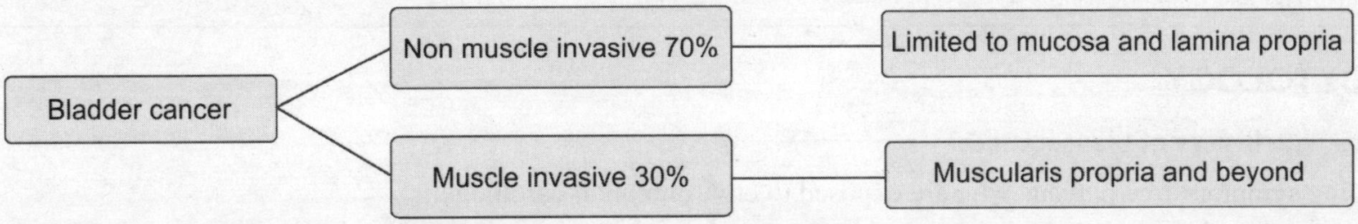

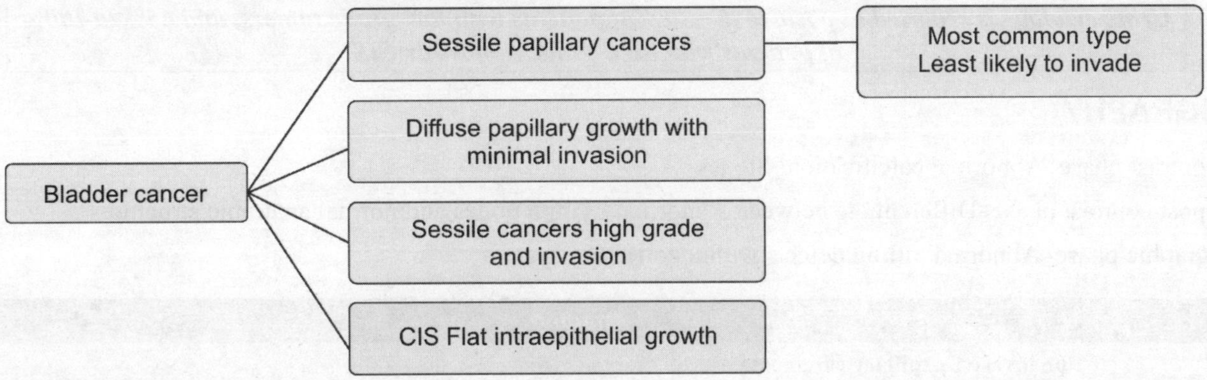

- Most common type of bladder cancer–Transitional cell carcinoma
- ***Carcinoma in situ*** an aggressive form of NMIBC is composed of flat, high-grade urothelial carcinoma limited to the mucosal layer
- ***80% of untreated CIS develop invasive bladder cancer within 10 years after diagnosis***

WHO Classification
• Urothelial carcinoma (91%)
• Squamous cell carcinoma (7%)
• Adenocarcinoma (2%)
• Other variants of urothelial carcinoma (<1%)

Up to 20% of urothelial carcinomas contain areas of squamous differentiation

Up to 7% contain areas of adenomatous differentiation

CLINICAL FEATURES

- 80% present with Gross or microscopic hematuria–Painless and intermittent
- 20% complain of urinary frequency, urgency, dysuria and Strangury (Particularly CIS)
- Uremia by ureteral compression and liver failure–Causes of death

INVESTIGATIONS

- Investigation of choice for diagnosis–***Cystoscopy and Biopsy***
- ***Imaging modality of choice for upper urinary tract- CT urography***
- ***Cystoscopy***–Any gross/microscopic hematuria and normal urinary tract imaging
  Unexplained or chronic lower urinary tract symptoms
  Urinary cytology that is suspicious for cancer
  History of bladder cancer

Grade 3 pT1 and muscle invasive–Staging with chest X-ray and either CT/MRI abdomen and pelvis
• Tumor extent in bladder and extravesical extension to adjacent fat/organs • Pelvic and Para aortic lymphadenopathy • Ureteric obstruction • Bone, Liver and Lung Metastasis

URINE CYTOLOGY

- Patients with history of bladder cancer
- Screening symptom free patients who are exposed to environmental carcinogens
- Evaluating patients with chronic irritative bladder symptoms before cystoscopy is done

Urine cytology is reported as positive in ~30% of patients with low-grade tumors, and 65% to 100% of patients with high-grade tumors or CIS

CT UROGRAPHY

- Non contrast phase–Abnormal calcification/ Stones
- Early post contrast phase–Differentiate between Abnormal Lymph nodes and normal anatomic structures
- Pyelographic phase–Abnormal filling defects within collecting system

Staging	
Ta	**Non invasive papillary carcinoma**
Tis	**CIS (Flat tumor)**
T1	**Invades subepithelial connective tissue**
T2	**Invades muscle** ***T2a–Invades superficial muscularis propria (Inner half)*** ***T2b–Invades deep muscularis propria (Outer half)***
T3	**Invades perivesical tissue** *T3a–Microscopically* *T3b–Macroscopically (Extravesical mass)*
T4	**T4a–Invades prostate stroma, seminal vesicle, uterus and vagina** **T4b–Invades pelvic wall/Abdominal wall**
N1	*Metastasis in Single regional lymph node in true pelvis*
N2	*Metastasis in Multiple regional lymph nodes in true pelvis*
N3	*Metastasis in common iliac node*
M1	Distant metastasis

	T1	T2a T2b	T3a T3b T4a	T4b
N0	I	II	III	IV
N1 **N2** **N3** **M1**	IV			

70% of bladder cancers are NMIBC (Tis, Ta, T1)

70% of NMIBC are Ta, 20% are T1

10% of bladder cancers are Tis/CIS

MANAGEMENT

Non Muscle Invasive

- **TURBT-** Standard treatment for Ta and T1 tumors and visible stage Tis
- Patients with apparently NMIBC at the time of TURBT should receive a single dose of intravesical mitomycin C within 6 hours of resection, if no bladder perforation is evident

Single dose intravesical mitomycin C–decreases risk of bladder cancer recurrence by 40%

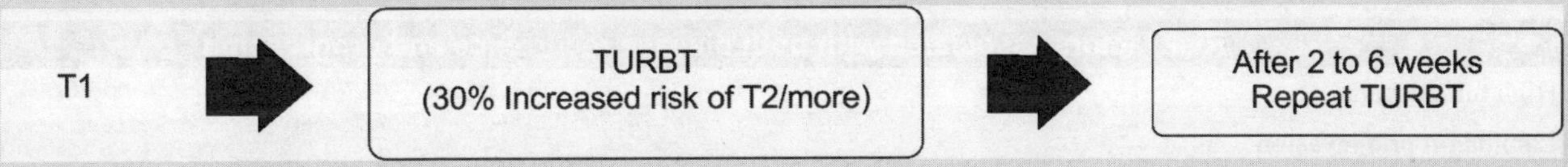

Adjuvant intravesical therapy

- NMIBC with high risk of recurrence and progression including CIS, high-grade Ta or T1 lesions, multifocal and recurrent tumors and rarely residual disease

Most commonly used chemotherapy agen–Mitomycin C
Most widely used intravesical agent in NMIBC–BCG (High grade)

- BCG is typically started 4 to 6 weeks after TURBT
- BCG Started too soon after TURBT ***(before urothelial healing occurs)*** results in BCG sepsis
- Intravesical treatment weekly for 6 weeks, followed by a series of maintenance treatments administered over 12 to 36 months
- *BCG is the treatment of choice for patients who have never received intravesical therapy*

BCG has been shown to eliminate CIS in 80% of patients at 5 year follow-up, reduce tumor recurrence rate for patients with T1 disease to 30% at 4 years and eliminate residual tumor in up to 59% of patients

- **Cystectomy**–Recur within 1 year in spite of ***2 induction courses*** of BCG therapy or BCG maintenance
- **T1 high-grade cancer**–High rate of progression and high risk of death–***Early radical cystectomy (before developing muscle invasion)***

Intravesical valrubicin is FDA approved for BCG-refractory patients who refuse or are intolerant of cystectomy

Muscle Invasive

- Usually primary and solitary tumor
- At dome of bladder
- Doesn't associate with CIS
- Ideal treatment–Partial cystectomy with 2 cm margin
- Primary EBRT→ 65-70 Gy (Surgery not willing/Medically contraindicated)–***Worsened results compared to surgery***

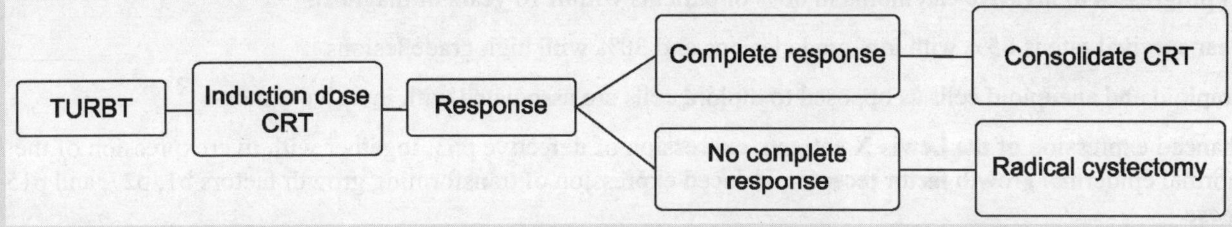

Partial Cystectomy (Segmental resection)

- Solitary
- Localized to the bladder dome
- CIS ruled out with multiple random biopsies
- Able to be removed with a 2-cm margin of healthy tissue
- Patients with adenocarcinomas are best suited for partial cystectomy

Radical Cystectomy
• Muscle invasive tumors
• CIS not responsive to intravesical therapy
• Superficial low-grade tumors that are diffuse, multiple and frequently recurring and becoming difficult to control with recurrent TURBT and intravesical therapy
• High-grade tumors not responsive to intravesical therapy

Risk factors associated with both disease recurrence and progression
• High tumor grade
• Lamina propria invasion
• Tumor diameter >3 cm
• Vascular or lymphatic invasion
• Multiplicity
• Expression of either epidermal growth factor or TGF alpha

Metastatic Disease
• Constitute 5% of tumors
• Cisplatin–Greatest activity against Urothelial carcinoma bladder
• Response rate→10-30%
• Gemcitabine and cisplatin has no significant difference in survival compared to M-VAC

	Radical surgery	Radical RT
Favour	Complete pathological staging Best local and locoregional control Best survival rates	Bladder conservation Option for salvage cystectomy Feasible in patients with extravesical extension and significant comorbidities
Against	Major pelvic surgery Not feasible–Comorbidities and frailty Loss of bladder and sexual function	Poor results in multifocal disease and Tis Normal tissue damage, radiation cystitis and enteritis Worsen urinary symptoms

PROGNOSTIC FACTORS

- Squamous cancers and adenocarcinomas have poorer prognosis than TCC
- **Invasion** of muscle, lymphatics, or perivesical fat is associated with poor prognosis
- **CIS** progresses to invasive carcinoma in 80% of patients within 10 years of diagnosis
- 5-year survival rate is 85% with low-grade lesions and 30% with high grade lesions
- Tetraploid and aneuploid cells as opposed to diploid cells are associated with invasive tumors
- Enhanced expression of the Lewis X antigen; expression of defective p53, together with overexpression of the *Rb* gene and abnormal epidermal growth factor receptor; reduced expression of transforming growth factors b1, p27, and p15–***Aggressive disease***
- Large superficial lesions are more likely to recur
- **Multifocality** is associated with an increased recurrence risk

Stage is most important prognostic factor for bladder cancer
Tumor grade is key prognostic factor in non muscle invasive tumor with potential risk of recurrence and progression

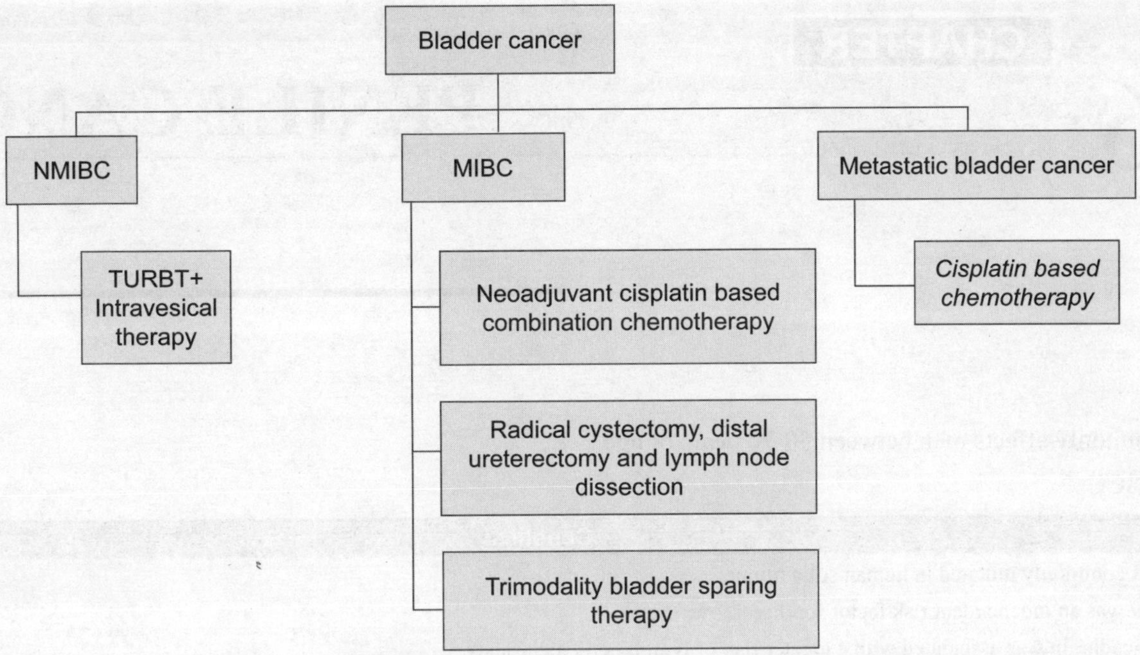

Trimodality therapy*–TURBT, RT and Chemotherapy*

Follow Up	
Superficial low grade cancer	Treated by intravesical chemotherapy→Cystoscopy at 3 months intervals
Cystectomy done	Every 3 months for first 2 years, every 6 months for the next 3 years and yearly thereafter
Ileal conduit/Continent diversion	Urethral washing for cytology is advisable periodically to diagnose local recurrence in urethra
Severe urothelial dysplasia	Urine cytology repeated every 2 to 3 months and cystoscopy with random biopsies every 3 to 6 months

Prevention
Folate-enriched diet has been associated with a decreased risk for bladder cancer
Discourage from smoking
Chemotherapy/Immunotherapy–Used for treatment and prevention of recurrence of superficial TCC

CHAPTER 16 PENILE CANCER

- Most commonly affects men between 50-70 years of age
- 95% are SCC

Genetics

- TP53 is commonly mutated in human solid tumors
- MMP-9 was an independent risk factor for disease recurrence
- Low E-cadherin was associated with a greater risk of lymph node metastasis
- EGFR is overexpressed in majority of penile cancer cases
- EGFR is a useful target for therapy in metastatic penile cancer

ETIOLOGY

- Most common etiology–Poor local hygiene
- Sexually transmitted diseases are not a causative factor
- Circumcision appears to be preventative
- Phimosis–found in 25% to 75% of penile carcinoma patients
- Increased risk with cigarette smoking and immunosuppression
- HIV infection may predispose affected patients to rapid development of SCC from preexisting condyloma infection
- Smegma–Carcinogen
- Smoking–Risk factor

HPV

Factors associated with higher rates of infection with HPV include presence of foreskin, increasing numbers of sexual partners, lack of condom use and smoking

HPV 6, 11 and 42 to 44→Gross condylomata and Low grade dysplasia
HPV 16, 18, 31, 33, 35 and 39→ Malignant disease

Muslims have an intermediate risk for penile cancer. Muslim boys are circumcised at puberty. But disease is almost nonexistent in Jewish men

Premalignant Lesions

CIS–10% risk

- **Erythroplasia of Queyrat**
  - **Glans or prepuce**
    Flat, solitary and reddened; or are velvety plaques and may progress to invasive cancer in 10% of patients
    Development of ulceration may be a sign of progression
- **Bowen disease**
  - **Penile shaft**
    Small eczematoid, dull red plaque with associated crusting and oozing anywhere on penis

Contd.

Contd.

Leukoplakia
- Nonspecific plaques of leukoplakia on glans are almost always associated with SCC
- Lesions of leukoplakia are often adjacent to squamous cell carcinoma lesions

Giant Penile Condyloma (Buschke-Löwenstein Tumor)
- Grossly resembles a cauliflower-like squamous cell cancer and may have foci of cancer
- Surgical excision is mandatory

Others–Cutaneous horn, Condyloma, Kaposi sarcoma, Buschke Lowenstein tumor, Bowenoid papules and Balanitis xerotica obliterans.

HISTOLOGY

- SCC usually well differentiated, constitutes nearly all penile cancers
- Squamous carcinoma of the penis may demonstrate variable degrees of keratin formation
- Usually reveals an exophytic mass
- 50% arise on the glans

CLINICAL FEATURES

- **Most common symptom–Foul smelling discharge**
- Squamous penile cancer usually starts on the glans or coronal sulcus
- As the disease progresses, the corpora cavernosa are invaded
- Urethra is usually spared until late in the disease course
- Earliest lesion of penile carcinoma is described by patients as nonhealing sore, often with an associated foul-smelling discharge
- Many patients have a long history of a painless mass
- Urinary tract symptoms like pain and hematuria are signs of locally advanced disease

Spread

Lymphatic Supply
- Rich lymphatic drainage results in metastases to inguinal nodes (only 1/3rd of palpable nodes are involved with tumor by histology) followed by pelvic nodes and then retroperitoneal nodes
- Approximately 25% of patients with palpable lymph nodes will have bilateral metastases
- For patients at highest risk of lymph node metastases based on features in the primary tumor, surgical staging can be performed by complete bilateral inguinal lymph node dissection, which may also be curative in cases of small-volume metastases

Earliest route of dissemination from penis–metastasis to regional femoral and iliac nodes

Positive p53 immunostain is an independent predictor of lymph node metastasis

Prepuce and Glans→Superficial inguinal nodes

Glans→ Deep inguinal nodes mainly

Early Nodal Metastasis

Flat and Ulcerative growth

>75% of shaft length involved

>5 cm

CABANA Node–Sentinel node for Carcinoma penis

Hypercalcemia without bone metastasis: Correlates with volume of disease and resolves after LN removal (Aggressive saline)

Spread to distant site most commonly occurs to LUNG

Penetration of buck's fascia and tunica albuginea→Vascular invasion

Most common sign of metastatic penile cancer–Priapism

JACKSON STAGING

I – Glans, Prepuce or both

II – Extend to shaft of penis

III – Inguinal node metastasis (Operable)

IV – Adjacent structures (Inoperable inguinal metastasis/Distant metastasis)

Staging	
T1	**Invades subepithelial connective tissue** **T1a**–*without LVI and not poorly differentiated* **T1b**–*with LVI/poorly differentiated*
T2	**Tumor invades corpus spongiosum with or without invasion of the urethra**
T3	**Tumor invades corpus cavernosum with or without invasion of the urethra**
T4	**Tumor invades other adjacent structures**
N1	Palpable mobile unilateral inguinal lymph node
N2	Palpable mobile multiple or bilateral inguinal lymph nodes
N3	Fixed inguinal nodal mass or pelvic lymphadenopathy unilateral/bilateral

	T1a	T1b	T2	T3	T4
N0	I	IIA		IIB	IV
N1	IIIA				
N2	IIIB				
N3	IV				
M1					

STAGE 0

Tis *Carcinoma in situ,*

Ta *Non invasive verrucous carcinoma*

Paraneoplastic Syndromes
Hypercalcemia may develop with no evidence of bony metastasis (20% of patients)

INVESTIGATIONS

- CT has often been the imaging modality chosen in penile cancer to examine the inguinal and pelvic areas as well as to rule out more distant metastases
- Soft tissue planes in CA Penis–Best delineated by MRI

Management

Surgery:

Young Operation–Partial amputation with bilateral Inguinal LN dissection

Piersey Gold Operation–Scrotum removed+ Total penectomy

- ***Partial penectomy is sufficient therapy if there is a 2-cm tumor-free margin***

Partial or total penectomy should be considered in tumors of size 4 cm or more, grade 3 lesions, and those invading deeply into glans, urethra, or corpora cavernosa

- Total penectomy is necessary when you cannot leave at least 2 cm of penile stump
- Circumcision–Younger patients, Tumor confined to prepuce (Recurrence–high)
- **Deeply penetrating and proximal tumors**→ Total penectomy with formation of perineal urethrostomy
- Palpable inguinal lymph nodes should be evaluated with biopsy

A biopsy is not necessary if lymph node sampling is already planned

- Dynamic sentinel node biopsy involves intraoperative lymphatic mapping and sampling one or more nodes where primary tumor is expected to spread

Contd.

Contd.

- Pelvic lymph node dissection remains the standard of care for penile cancer patients following definitive treatment of inguinal lymph node metastases

Inguinal lymph node dissection used to evaluate most frequent site of metastasis

Radical lymphadenectomy is routinely performed in patients with stage T3 tumors

Chemotherapy	Radiotherapy
• **Premalignant lesions**–Topical therapy 5FU or imiquimod cream, Laser therapy • VBM regimen or Cisplatin and 5FU ***(Adjunct to surgery/RT→ T3 and T4 tumors)*** • Response rates of advanced cancer to drugs is as high as 50%	• ***Younger patients–EBRT/Interstitial brachytherapy*** (Avoids penectomy) • *Small primary stage I lesion (<3 cm in diameter)* • ***Results of RT is same as partial amputation***

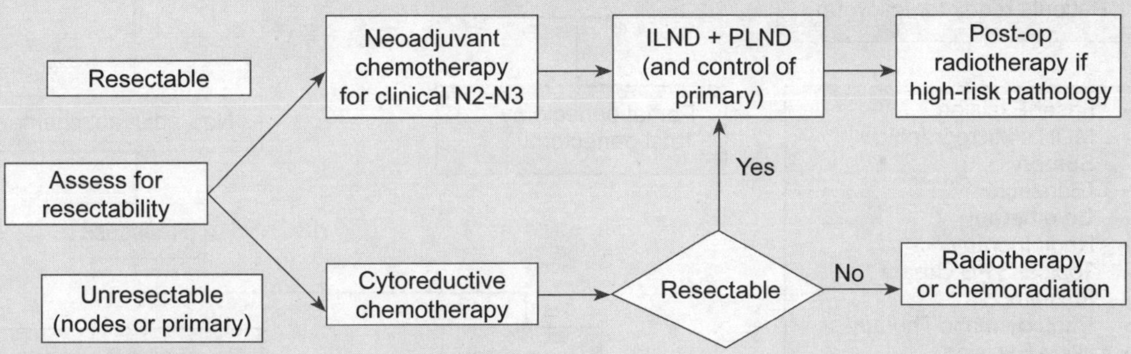

- Tis–Topical fluorouracil, laser therapy, cryotherapy, local excision
- T1–Excision or radiotherapy
- Advanced disease or local recurrence often requires at least partial amputation of penis
- Inoperable disease may be treated with chemotherapy and radiotherapy

PROGNOSTIC FACTORS

- Tumor grade, lymphovascular invasion, and perineural invasion appear to be the most important pathologic prognostic factors for nodal spread and mortality
- Strongest prognostic factor for survival–Nodal metastasis

Poor Prognostic Features
• Endophytic and high-grade lesions
• Shaft invasion and involvement of draining lymph nodes, especially at iliac level or higher
• Of patients with clinical stage Tis, Ta, or T1 (Jackson stage I or II) tumors, 10% have inguinal node involvement proven by surgery

- Lymphovascular invasion in primary tumor has significant prognostic importance
- Metastatic penile cancer is characterized by a relentlessly progressive course, causing death for the majority of untreated patients within 2 years

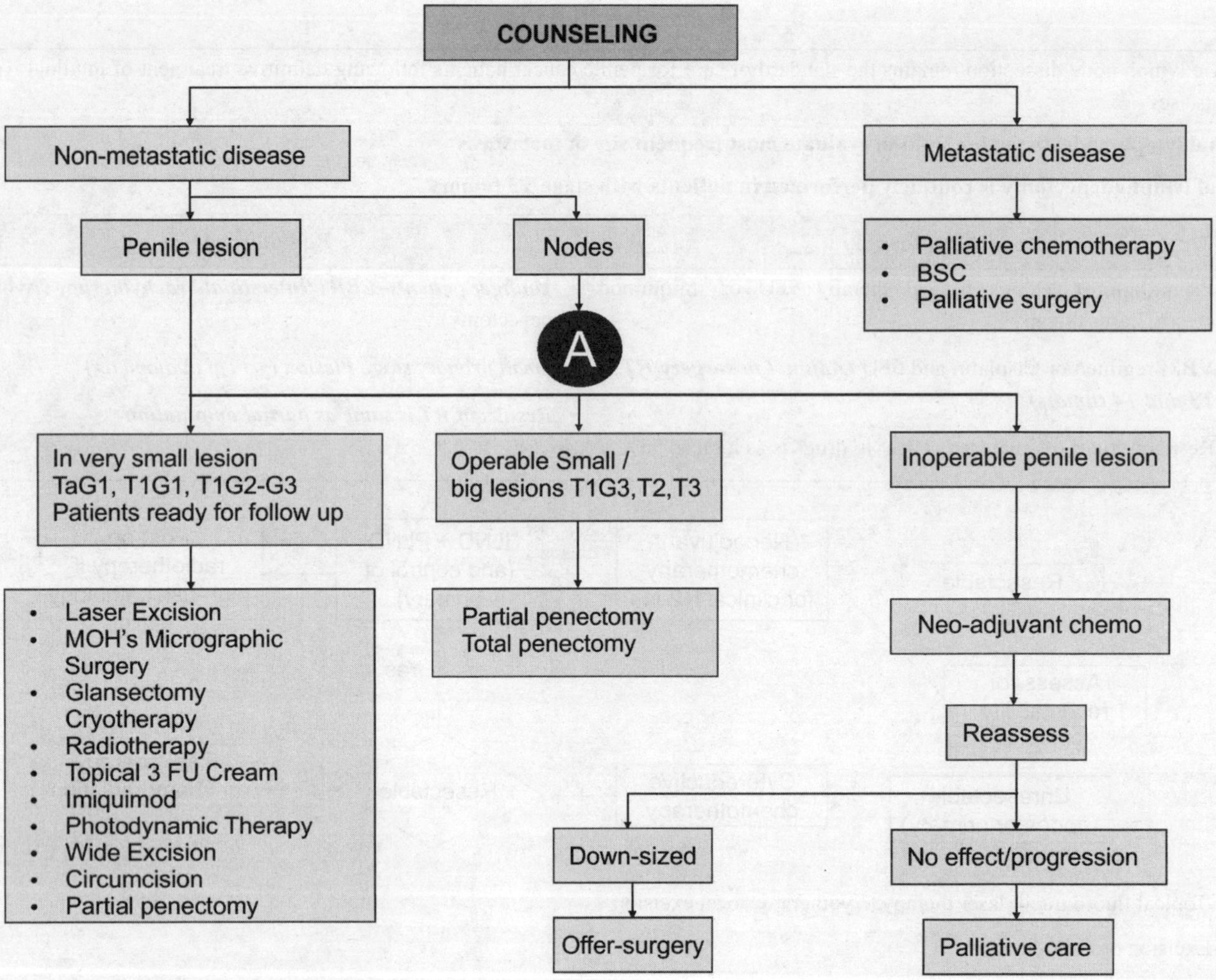
COUNSELING
Non-metastatic disease
Metastatic disease
Penile lesion
Nodes
A
• Palliative chemotherapy
• BSC
• Palliative surgery
In very small lesion
TaG1, T1G1, T1G2-G3
Patients ready for follow up
Operable Small /
big lesions T1G3,T2,T3
Inoperable penile lesion
• Laser Excision
• MOH's Micrographic Surgery
• Glansectomy Cryotherapy
• Radiotherapy
• Topical 3 FU Cream
• Imiquimod
• Photodynamic Therapy
• Wide Excision
• Circumcision
• Partial penectomy
Partial penectomy
Total penectomy
Neo-adjuvant chemo
Reassess
Down-sized
No effect/progression
Offer-surgery
Palliative care

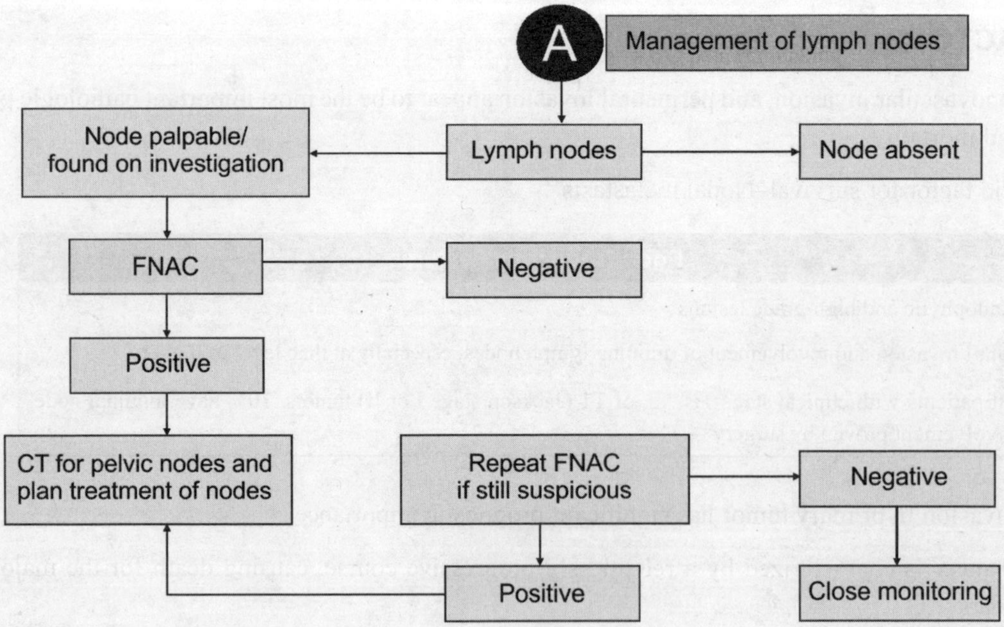
A
Management of lymph nodes
Node palpable/
found on investigation
Lymph nodes
Node absent
FNAC
Negative
Positive
CT for pelvic nodes and
plan treatment of nodes
Repeat FNAC
if still suspicious
Negative
Positive
Close monitoring

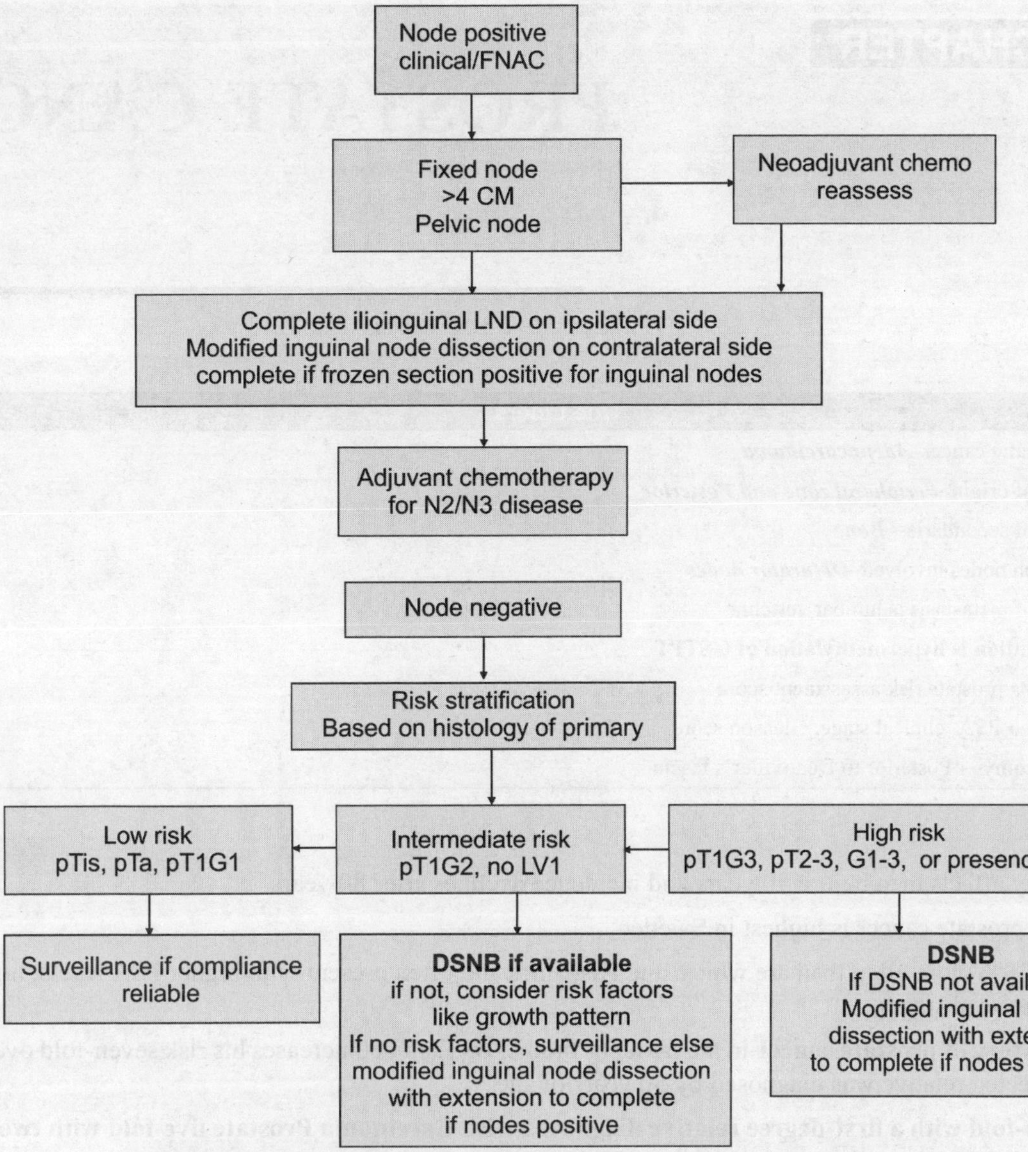

Tis, Ta, T1→ Local surgery→ Follow up for 2 years for inguinal nodes
(Glans→ Inguinal block dissection)
T2,T3→ Local surgery+ Inguinal LN dissection
Any T, N1-3→ Local surgery+ Bilateral inguinal LN dissection
Any T Any N M1/T4→ Only palliative

- Most common flap to Reconstruct penis–Radial forearm free flap
- Most common muscle used to cover femoral vessels after inguinal LN dissection–SARTORIUS
- Most common cause of death in CA Penis–Erosion of femoral vessels

- **Most common mode of penis involvement in Metastatic disease–Corporal involvement**
- **Usg/MRI–Best for cavernosal involvement**

SARCOMA

- Proximal shaft lesions–Malignant
- Distal shaft lesions–Benign
- ***Hemangiopericytoma–Most common***

CHAPTER 17 PROSTATE CANCER

One Liners

- Most common prostatic cancer–***Adenocarcinoma***
- Most common site of origin–***Peripheral zone and Posterior***
- Most common site of secondaries–***Bone***
- Most common lymph nodes involved–***Obturator nodes***
- Most common site of metastasis is lumbar vertebra
- **Most common mutation is hypermethylation of GSTP1**
- CAPRA→Carcinoma prostate risk assessment score
- ***PARTIN TABLES*** → PSA, clinical stage, Gleason score
- **Plane of Prostatectomy**→ Posterior to Denoviller's fascia

ETIOLOGY

- Prostate cancer rarely affects men before 40 years and incidence declines after 80 years
- Risk for developing prostate cancer is highest in Sweden
- Blacks are afflicted 30% more often than are whites and Hispanics and often present with higher PSA levels, higher Gleason scores, and more advanced stages
- **Positive familial history of prostate cancer** in the father or brother of a subject increases his risk seven-fold over the general population if the affected relative was diagnosed by 50 years of age
- **(Risk increases two-fold with a first-degree relative diagnosed with Carcinoma Prostate five-fold with two first-degree relatives)**
- Relative risk declines to 4-fold if diagnosis of first-degree relative was made after 70 years

African-American men are more likely to be diagnosed with advanced disease and have greater than two-fold risk of death from the disease

Consumption of red meat and animal fat has been associated with Carcinoma Prostate

Eating cruciferous vegetables, soy products and lycopene-containing tomato products-protective

Molecular Biology of Prostate Cancer

- Shortened CAG trinucleotide repeat length
- CYP 3A4 polymorphisms
- AMACR upregulation
- Loss of NKX-3-1
- Absence of GSTP1
- Overexpressed PMSA
- Vitamin D polymorphisms
- Reduced E cadherin expression

Contd.

Contd.

- PTEN Mutation
- RB1 and P53 mutation
- LOH for p27

Role of BRCA Mutations In Prostate Cancer

BRCA mutations are associated with increased risk of prostate cancer

- **BRCA 2 mutations** → Associated with 5 fold increased risk and associated with a higher Gleason score and poorer prognosis
- **BRCA1 mutations**→ Associated with 2 fold increased risk and Younger age of diagnosis (< 65 years)

Prostate Cancer Prevention Trial

- Finasteride to block conversion of testosterone to its more active form dihydrotestosterone
- Finasteride prevented formation of new prostate cancers, its use was associated with more frequent diagnosis of high-grade cancers than in control group

Increased intake of vitamin A, Decreased intake of vitamin D
Increased intake of animal fats (Alpha linolenic acid)
Occupational exposure to cadmium, Obesity

Paraneoplastic Syndromes *(Sign of advanced disease)*

DIC, TTP, Primary fibrinolysis and Neuromuscular abnormalities

- Multifocal and frequently (70%) arises from peripheral zone of prostate
- Locally invades along nerve sheaths and metastasizes through lymphatic chains
- Prostate tumors can ***secrete growth factors*** creating new lymphatic vessels in a process known as lymphoangiogenesis

Bone–Most common site of prostate cancer metastases (Osteoblastic)
Pelvis and Lower lumbar vertebrae

PSA–Prostate Specific Antigen

- Used as a screening test: **Serine protease, glycoprotein, liquefaction of semen**
- 15% of patients with nodular hyperplasia have raised PSA
- **After prostate biopsy, PSA is reported to be elevated 6-8 weeks**
- **PSA can be elevated in BPH, Prostatitis, Breast and parotid cancers**

PSA>20 ng/ml
PSA velocity >0.75
PSA density >0.15

Age Specific PSA Levels
40-50 years→ <2.5
50-60 years→ <3.5
60-70 years→ <4.5
70-80 years→ <6.5

- Decreased ratio of free PSA/total PSA associated with probability of CA prostate.
- **PSA<10 ng/ml→Low risk of periprostatic spread and metastasis**
  PSA>10 ng/ml→ >50% patients have capsular penetration
  PSA>50 ng/ml→Metastasis

- **TRUS Guided True cut biopsy:** Hypoechoic appearance on TRUS
- Atleast 12 systemic biopsies cores–*Prostatic biopsies*
- ***MRI with High tesla***→ *Accurate in staging of local disease (eMRI)*

T1a– <5% of resected and well differentiated (TURP)
T1b– >5% of resected (TURP)
T1c– Following PSA Screening
T2a– <One half and Suspicious nodule involving 1 lobe
T2b– More than one half and Suspicious nodule involving 1 lobes
T2c– Suspicious nodule involving both lobes
T3a– Capsule Breached
T3b– Seminal vesicle
T4– Rectum and Pelvis
M1a– Non regional lymph nodes
M1b– Bone
M1c– Other site with or without bone disease

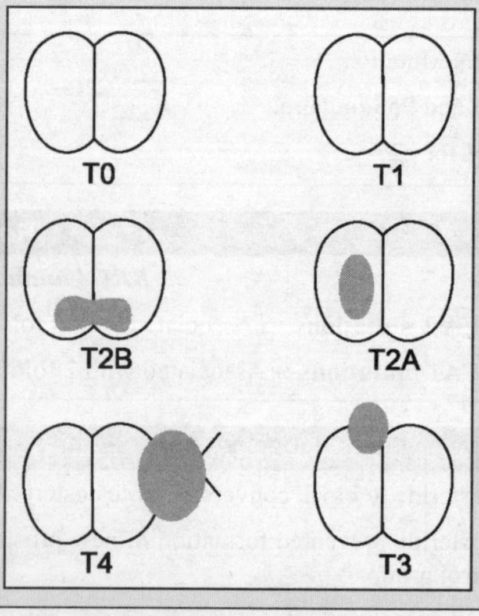

Group	T	N	M	PSA	Gleason
I	T1a-T2a	N0	M0	<10	≤6
	T2a	N0	M0	<10	≤6
	T1a-T2a	N0	M0	X	X
IIA	T1a-c	N0	M0	< 20	7
	T1a-c	N0	M0	≥10 <20	≤6
	T2a	N0	M0	< 20	≤7
	T2b	N0	M0	< 20	≤7
	T2b	N0	M0	X	X
IIB	T2c	N0	M0	Any	Any
	T1-T2	N0	M0	≥ 20	Any
	T1-T2	N0	M0	Any	≥ 8
III	T3a-T3b	N0	M0	Any	Any
IV	T4	N0	M0	Any	Any
	Any T	N1	M0	Any	Any
	Any T	Any N	M1	Any	Any

HIGH RISK PATIENTS

- Confluent with pelvic side wall on DRE
- High Gleason score
- PSA >20 ng/ml

High tumor grades are more frequently associated with LN and Distant metastases

PREVENTION

- Guidelines recommend that PSA screening and DRE begin at age of 50 years
- Screening at the age of 45 should be considered in African American men and in men with positive family history

Management
• **Stage T1-T2:** Watchful waiting, active surveillance, radical prostatectomy and RT

Contd.

Contd.

Management of Localized Prostatic Cancer

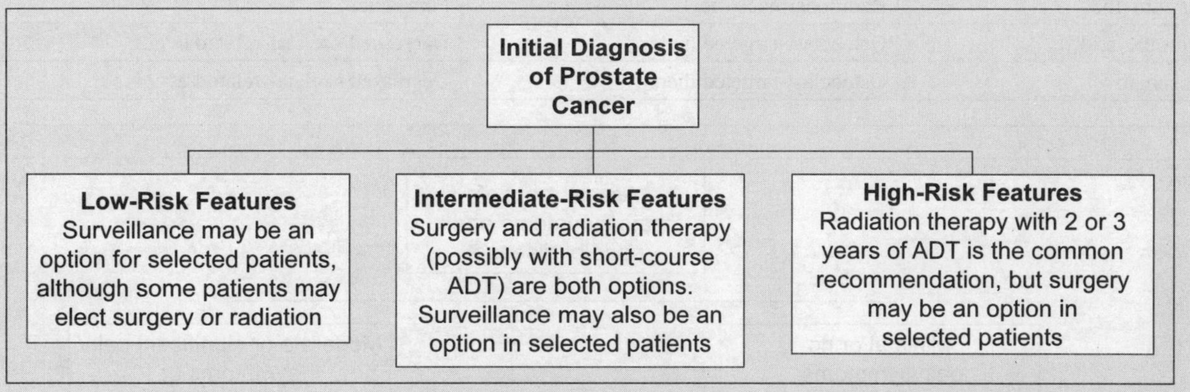

- **Stage T3:** Clinical T3 disease without evidence of distant spread can be cured with surgery
- **Localised (-ve Bone scan and MRI)**→ Radical prostatectomy=Radical RT (Life expectancy more than 10 years)
- **Locally advanced (T3)** → Radiotherapy and Androgen ablation
- Low grade Low volume disease→ I^{125}/Pd^{103}
- **Enzalutamide**→ 2nd generation Androgen receptor blocker
- **Degarelix**→ LHRH Antagonist

Management of Locally Advanced Prostate Cancer

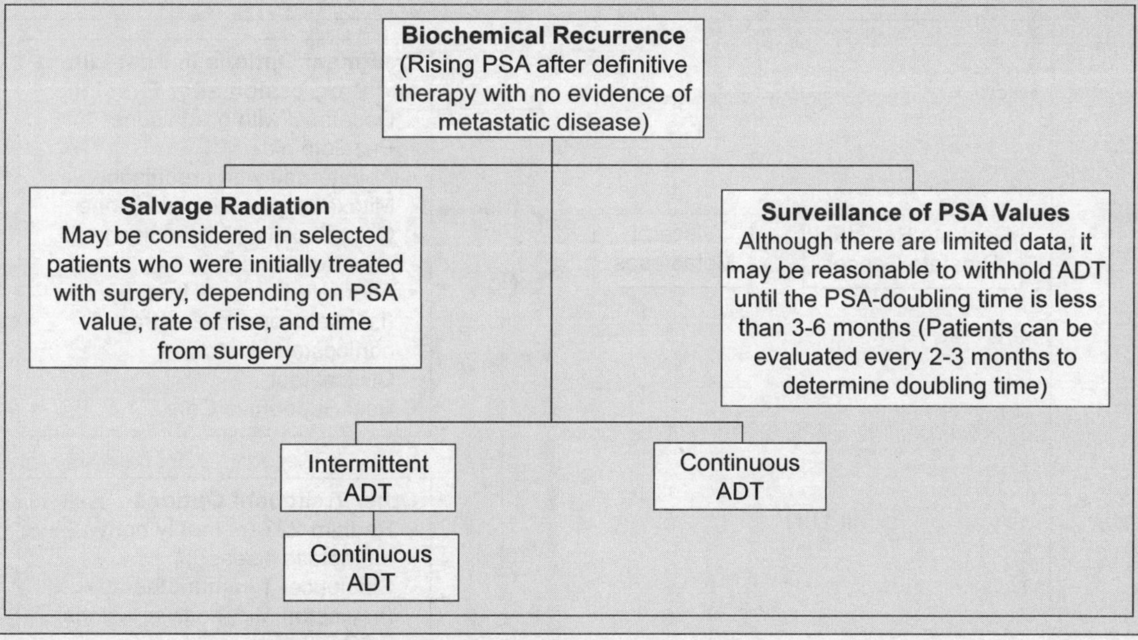

METASTATIC CASTRATION RESISTANT PROSTATE CANCER

Agent	Class	Clinical Benefit
Docetaxel	Chemotherapy	Improved progression-free and overall survival
Cabazitaxel	Chemotherapy	Improved progression-free and overall survival
Mitoxantrone	Chemotherapy	Pain relief
Sipuleucel-T	Immunotherapy	Improved overall survival
Abiraterone acetate	Androgen biosynthesis inhibitor	Improved progression-free and overall survival
Enzalutamide	Androgen-receptor-signaling inhibitor	Improved progression-free and overall survival

Contd.

Contd.

Strontium-89	Radiopharmaceutical	Pain relief
Samarium-153	Radiopharmaceutical	Pain relief
Zoledronic acid	Osteoclast-targeted therapy	Decreased skeletal-related events
Denosumab	Osteoclast-targeted therapy	Decreased skeletal-related events

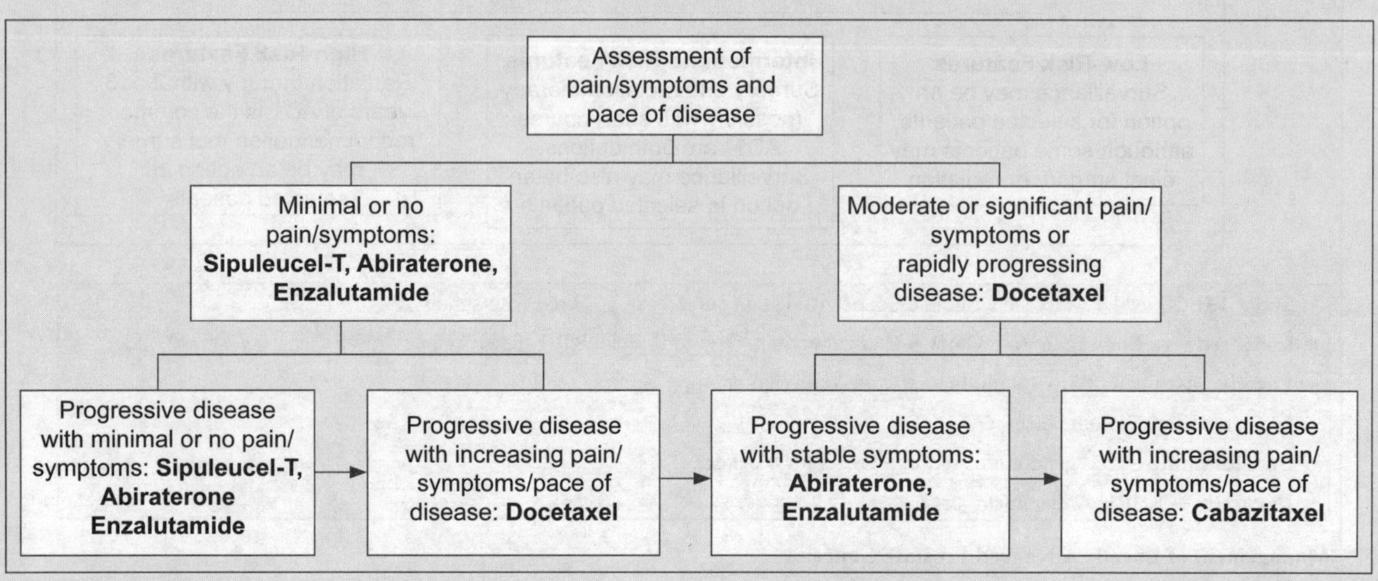

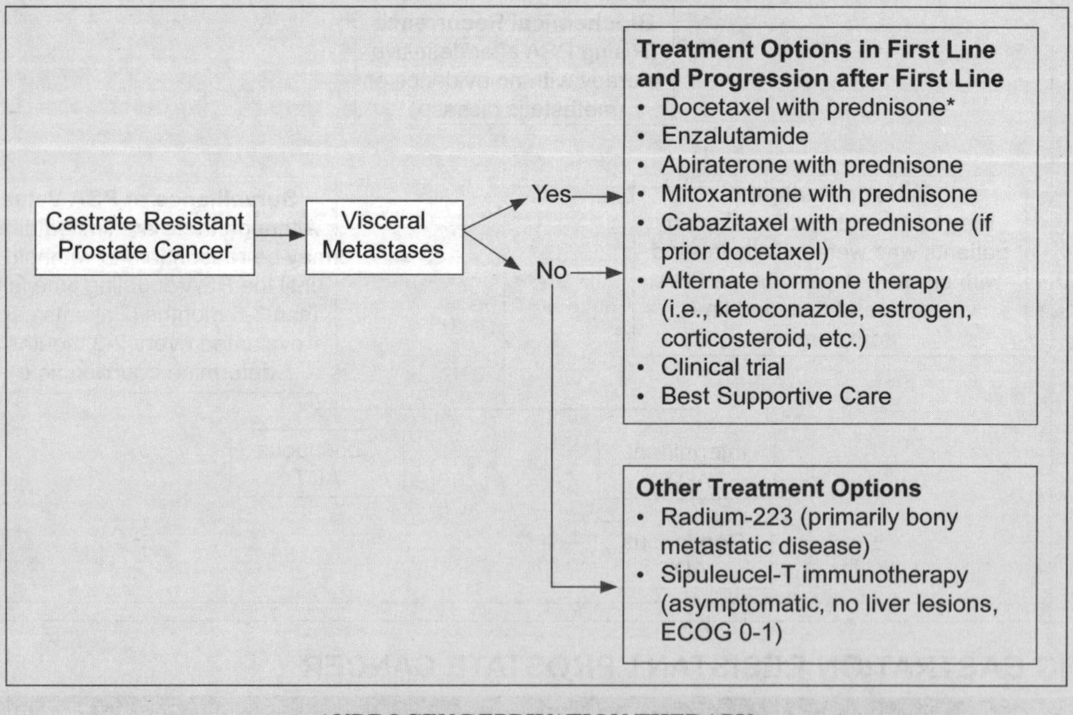

ANDROGEN DEPRIVATION THERAPY

Class	Agents	Mechanism of Action
GnRH against	Leuprolide acetate goserelin	Downregulation of GnRH receptors
GnRH antagonist	Degarelix	Inhibition of GnRH receptors
Estrogen	Diethylstilbestrol	Suppression of pituitary luteinizing hormone production

Contd.

Contd.

Poor Prognosis
Seminal vesicles–*Poor prognosis*
Tumor grade strongly affects prognosis
Extension of tumor beyond prostate capsule–Associated with worse prognosis
Perineural invasion is generally predictor of extraprostatic extension at time of prostatectomy–Associated with higher grade disease, large tumor volume and seminal vesicle invasion
Rapid PSA rise *(high PSA velocity) and short PSA doubling time→ Associated with poor prognosis*
Oncotype Dx and Decipher are clinically useful for prognostication on a molecular level

CHAPTER 18 TESTICULAR CANCERS

- Ninety–five percent of these tumors are of germ cell origin
- Seminoma–4th decade
- Non seminoma–3rd decade
- Most common tumor in Young men–NSGCT
- 90-95% are of GCT
- Lymphoma→ 3 to 7%
- **Risk factors:** *History of testicular enlargement, History of contralateral tumor and Klinefelter's syndrome*

Choriocarcinomas tend to occur between 24 and 28 years of age, embryonal carcinomas from 26 to 34 years of age, seminomas from 32 to 42 years of age, and lymphomas and spermatocytic seminomas after the age of 50 years

Most well-known etiologic factor in development of testicular cancer is cryptorchidism

- CIS is a precursor of testicular germ cell cancer
- Total of 5% to 6% of men with unilateral germ cell tumor have CIS in contralateral testis, and germ cell tumor will develop in 50% of these men
- High risk of CIS are individuals with intersex, cryptorchidism, infertility, or an extragonadal germ cell tumor

Clinical Presentation

- Testicular cancer typically presents as painless testicular mass and/or enlargement
- Advanced disease can present as back pain, flank pain, or with systemic symptoms
- **Leydig cell**–Masculinises, **Sertoli cell**–Feminises

10% of Leydig and Sertoli cell tumors are malignant

Spread

Scrotal skin involvement–Inguinal lymph node affected

Seminoma metastasizes by lymphatics

All teratoma can metastasize

PATHOGENESIS OF GERM CELL TUMORS

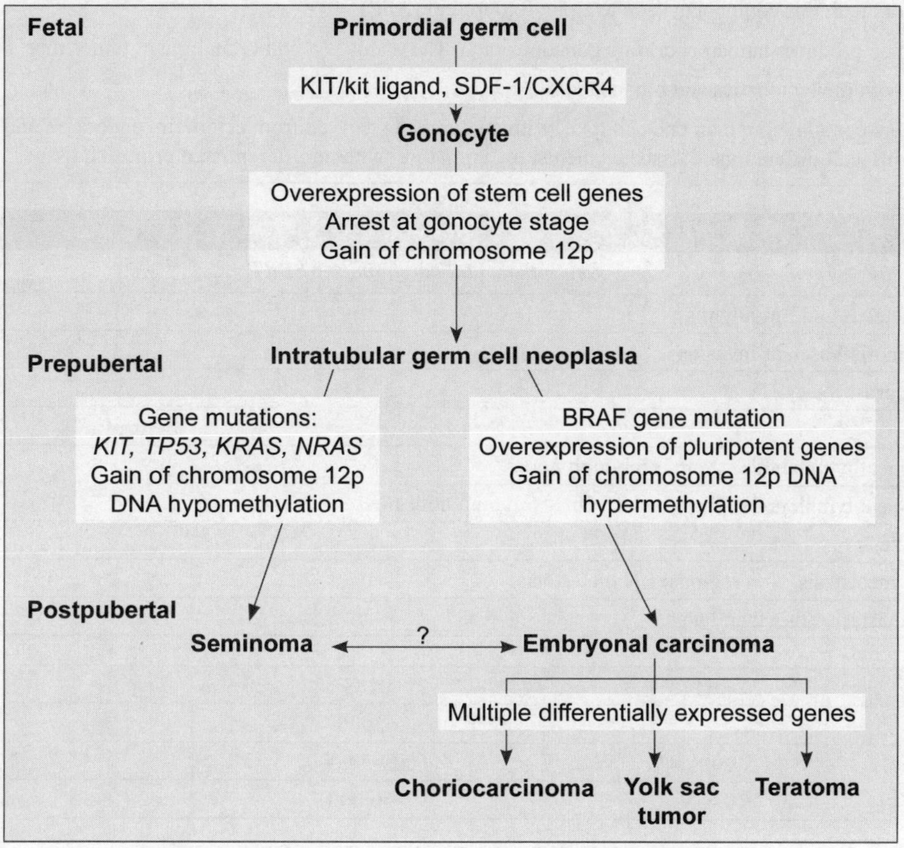

DIAGNOSIS

- Any solid testicular mass is considered a testicular tumor until proven otherwise
- Patients with testicular enlargement that is believed to be inflammatory in nature (epididymo-orchitis) must be re-examined after infection has been treated to rule out the presence of an occult testicular mass
- Before or after radical orchiectomy, staging CT chest, abdomen, and pelvis as well as postorchiectomy serum tumor markers (obtained at least 4 weeks after surgery) should be obtained in all patients for risk stratification to direct subsequent treatment
- **Chest radiograph**–*Obtained in patients with a low risk of thoracic metastasis such as those with normal postorchiectomy tumor markers and normal CT of abdomen/pelvis*
- **Testicular tumors in children are usually Anaplastic teratoma (<3 years)→ FATAL**
- *5% of NSGCT have Gynecomastia*
- *Prepubertal Interstitial Tumors→ Androgens (Sexual precocity, Deep male voice, Suprapubic hair and Prominent Genitalia)*
- *Postpubertal Interstitial Tumors→ Feminizing (Gynecomastia, Azoospermia, Loss of libido and Erectile dysfunction)*
- Diagnosis of Testicular tumor is confirmed by USG
- **USG**–Mandatory in all cases of suspected testicular tumor
- **Interstitial**–*80% Benign, Organ sparing surgery (Larger→ ORCHIDECTOMY)*

Embryonal carcinoma: Highly malignant tumors that occasionally invade cord structures

Yolk sac tumor: Tumors with this component secrete alpha fetoprotein (AFP)

Choriocarcinoma: Often produces human chorionic gonadotropin (hCG). This is a highly malignant tumor that metastasises early via both the lymphatics and bloodstream

Teratoma: These tumors contain more than one cell type, with components derived from ectoderm, endoderm and mesoderm. Tumors may range from 'mature' with well-differentiated tissue elements, to 'immature' with undifferentiated primitive tissues. All can metastasise

Staging	
Tis– Intraductal carcinoma→ EBRT	
T1	Confined to testis and Epididymis
T2	Tunica vaginalis/Vascular invasion
T3	Spermatic cord
T4	Scrotum
N1	Retroperitoneal lymph node <2 cm, <6 lymph nodes
N2	Retroperitoneal lymph node >2 cm and <5 cm, >6 lymph nodes
N3	>5 cm in size
M1a	Pulmonary metastasis, Non regional LN metastasis
M1b	Visceral metastasis other than lungs

	LDH	hCG	AFP
S1	<1.5 × N	<5000	<1000
S2	1.5-10 × N	5000-50,000	1000-10,000
S3	>10 × N	>50,000	>10,000

	T1	T2	T3	T4
N0	IA	IB	IB	IB
N1	IIA			
N2	IIB			
N3	IIC			
M1	III S2/S3			

International Consensus Risk Classification for Germ Cell Tumors		
Prognosis	**Nonseminoma**	**Seminoma**
Good	Testis/retroperitoneal primary. No nonpulmonary visceral metastases. AFP <1,000 mg/mL; HCG <5,000 international units/L (1,000 mg/mL); LDH <1.5 × ULN (56% of all nonseminomas)	Any primary site. No nonpulmonary visceral metastases. Normal AFP, any concentration of HCG; any concentration of LDH (90% of all seminomas)
Intermediate	Testis/retroperitoneal primary. No nonpulmonary visceral metastases. AFP ≥1,000 and ≤ 10,000 ng/mL or HCG ≥ 5,000 milli-international units/ milliliter (mIU/mL) and ≤ 50,000 international units/L or LDH = 1.5 × NL and ≥ 10 × NL (28% of all nonseminomas)	Any primary site. No nonpulmonary visceral metastases. Normal AFP; any concentration of HCG; any concentration of LDH (10% of all seminomas)
Poor	Mediastinal primary or nonpulmonary visceral metastases or AFP > 10,000 ng/mL or HCG >50,000 international units/L (10,000 ng/mL) or LDH >10 × ULN (16% of all nonseminomas)	No patients classified as poor prognosis

SEMINOMA

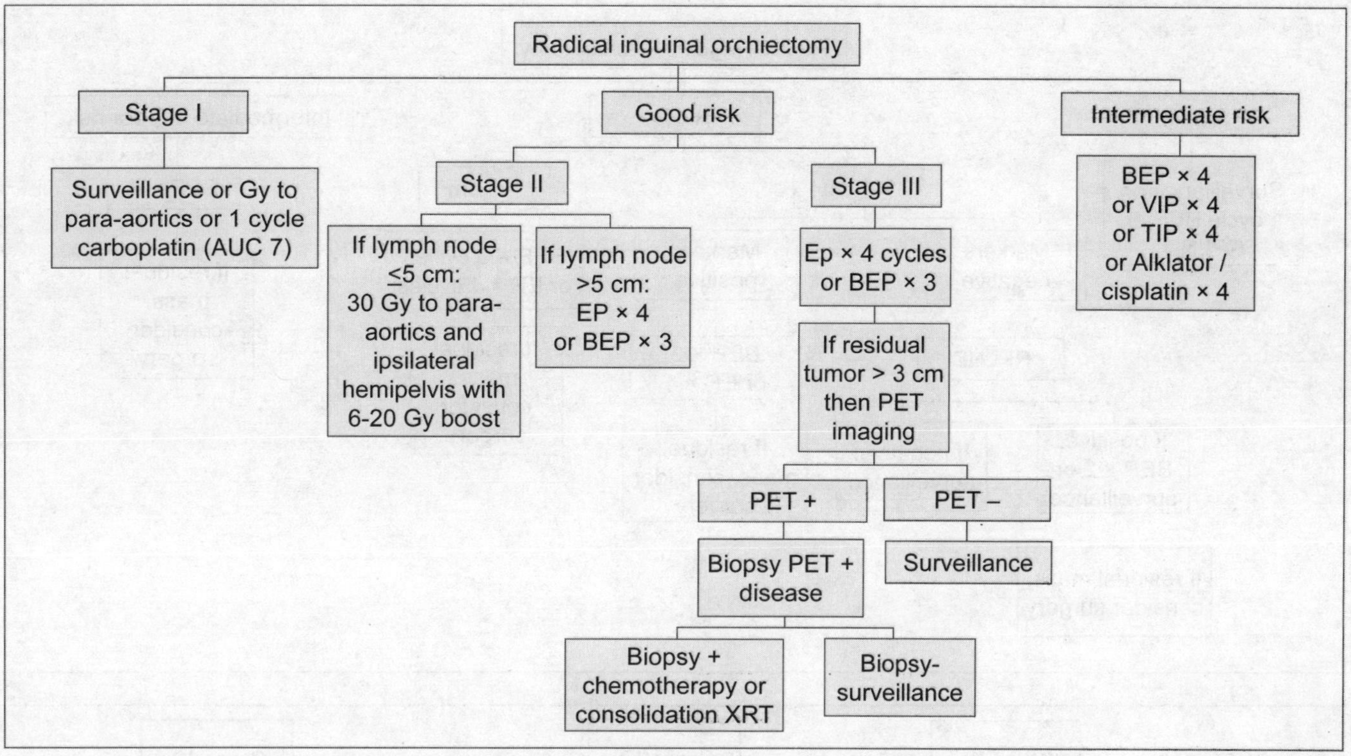
Radical inguinal orchiectomy
Stage I
Good risk
Intermediate risk
Surveillance or Gy to para-aortics or 1 cycle carboplatin (AUC 7)
Stage II
Stage III
BEP × 4 or VIP × 4 or TIP × 4 or Alklator / cisplatin × 4
If lymph node ≤5 cm: 30 Gy to para-aortics and ipsilateral hemipelvis with 6-20 Gy boost
If lymph node >5 cm: EP × 4 or BEP × 3
Ep × 4 cycles or BEP × 3
If residual tumor > 3 cm then PET imaging
PET +
PET –
Biopsy PET + disease
Surveillance
Biopsy + chemotherapy or consolidation XRT
Biopsy-surveillance

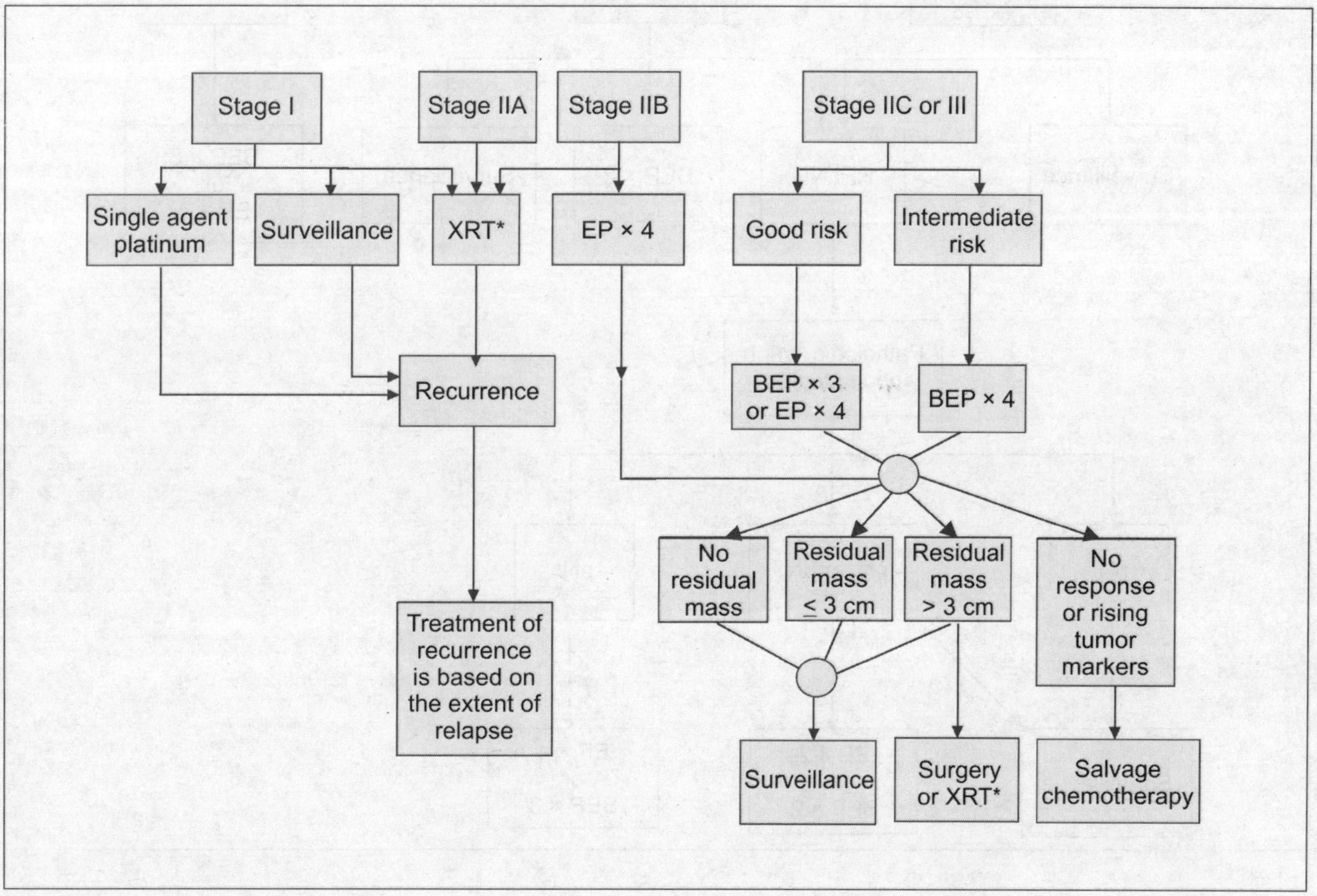
Stage I
Stage IIA
Stage IIB
Stage IIC or III
Single agent platinum
Surveillance
XRT*
EP × 4
Good risk
Intermediate risk
Recurrence
BEP × 3 or EP × 4
BEP × 4
No residual mass
Residual mass ≤ 3 cm
Residual mass > 3 cm
No response or rising tumor markers
Treatment of recurrence is based on the extent of relapse
Surveillance
Surgery or XRT*
Salvage chemotherapy

NON SEMINOMA

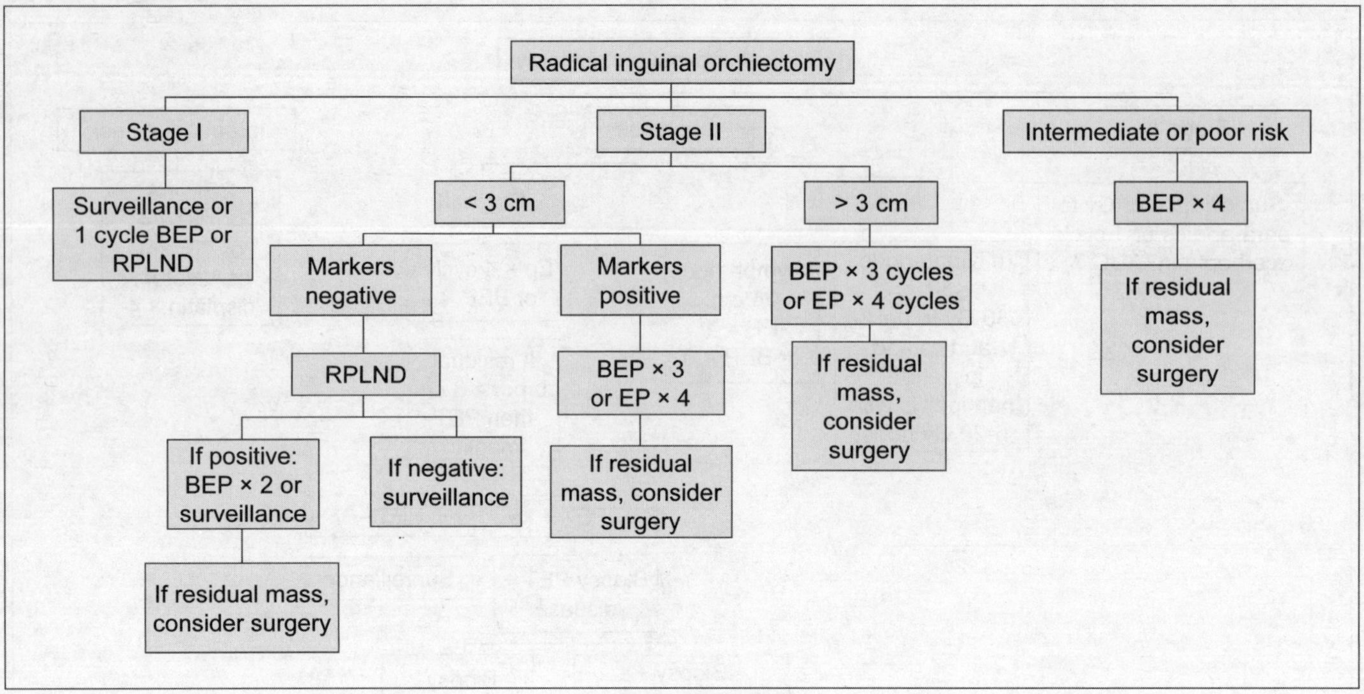

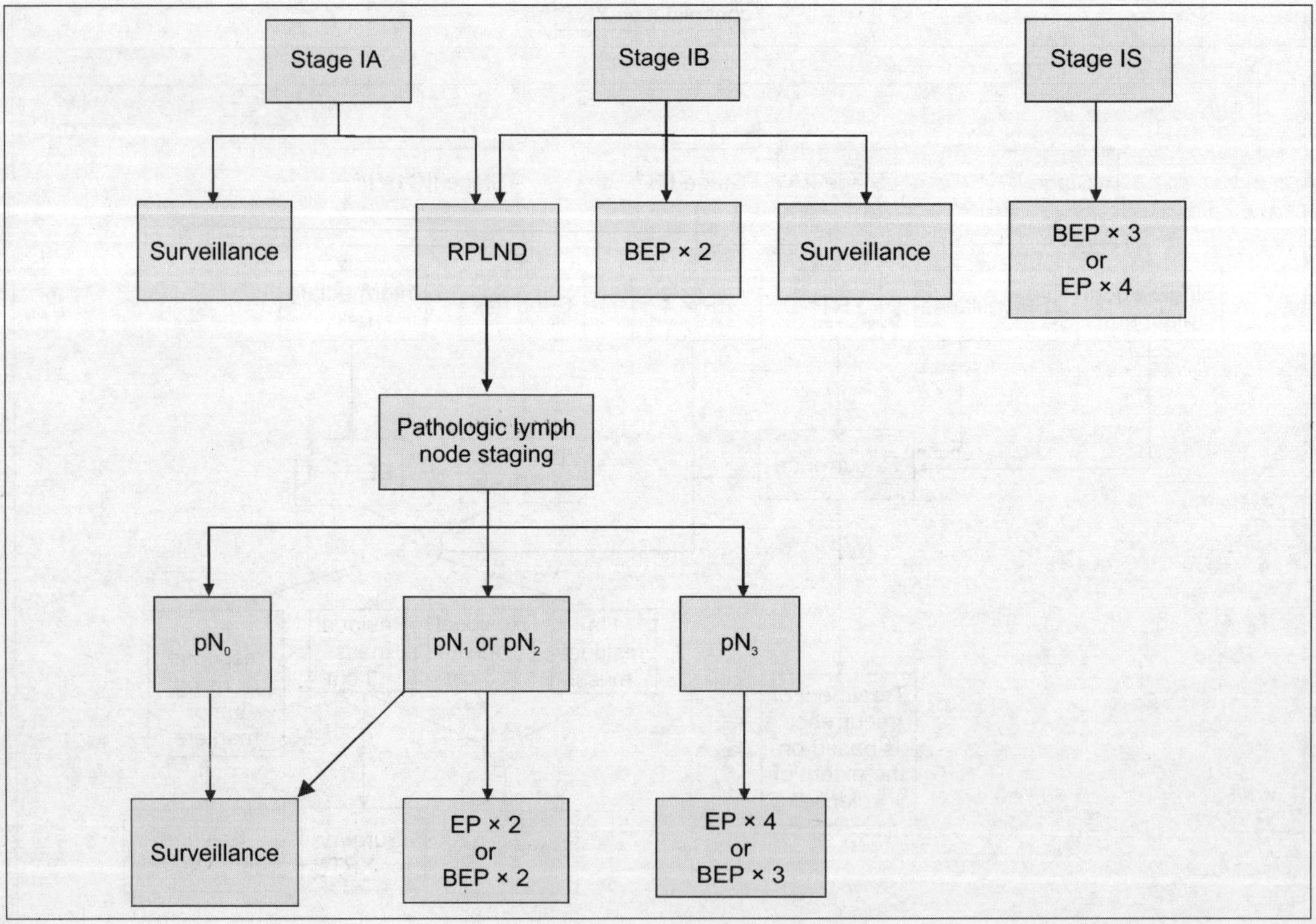

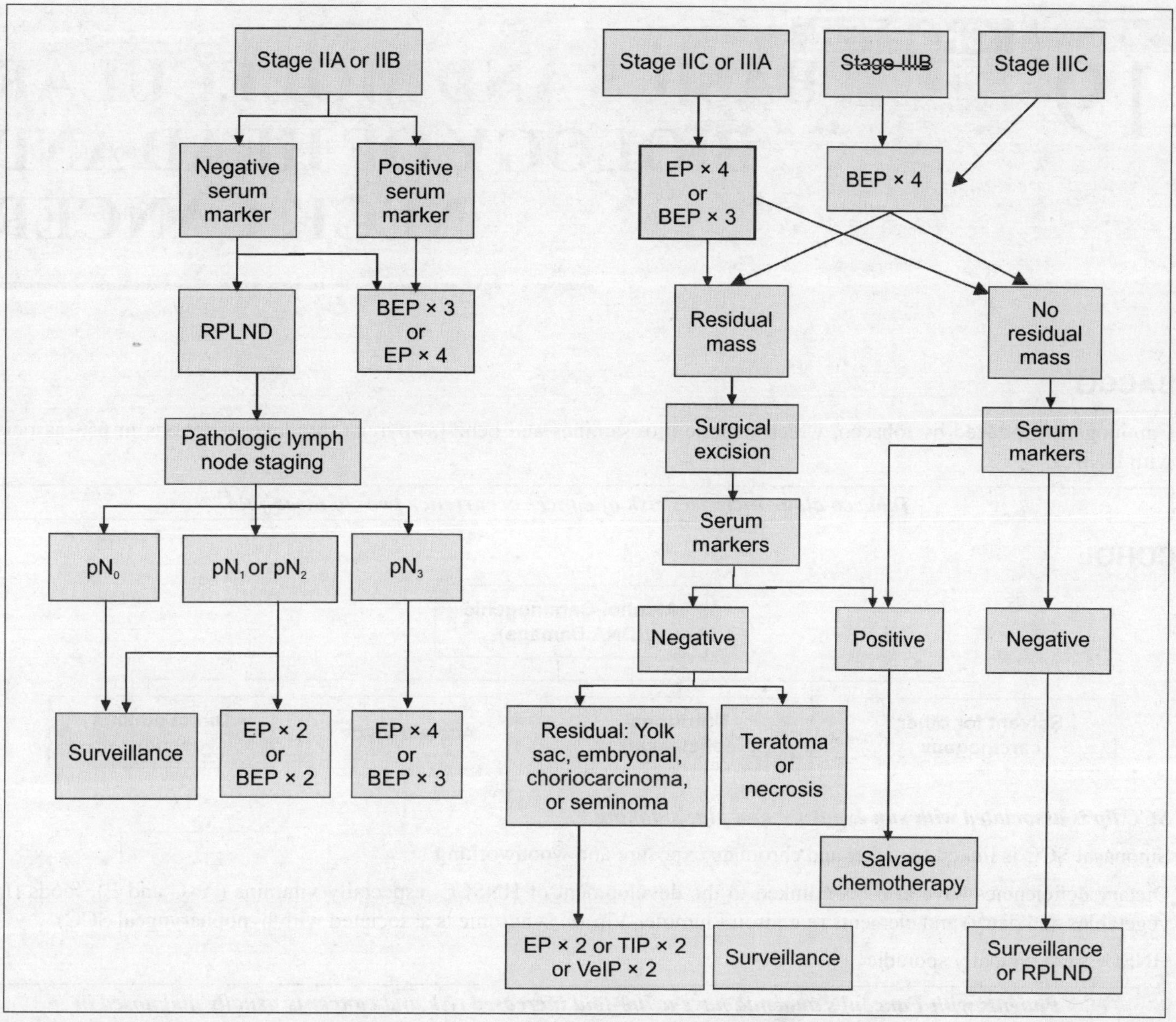
Stage IIA or IIB
Negative serum marker
Positive serum marker
RPLND
BEP × 3 or EP × 4
Pathologic lymph node staging
pN_0
pN_1 or pN_2
pN_3
Surveillance
EP × 2 or BEP × 2
EP × 4 or BEP × 3
Stage IIC or IIIA
Stage IIIB
Stage IIIC
EP × 4 or BEP × 3
BEP × 4
Residual mass
No residual mass
Surgical excision
Serum markers
Serum markers
Negative
Positive
Negative
Residual: Yolk sac, embryonal, choriocarcinoma, or seminoma
Teratoma or necrosis
Salvage chemotherapy
EP × 2 or TIP × 2 or VeIP × 2
Surveillance
Surveillance or RPLND

PART ONE: HEAD AND NECK ONCOLOGY

CHAPTER 19

BASICS AND MOLECULAR BIOLOGY OF HEAD AND NECK CANCER

TOBACCO

- Carcinogens produced by tobacco, which include nitrosamines and benz-(a)-pyrene, produce mutations in p53 associated with HNSCC

Tobacco alone increases risk of cancer occurrence two- to three-fold

ALCOHOL

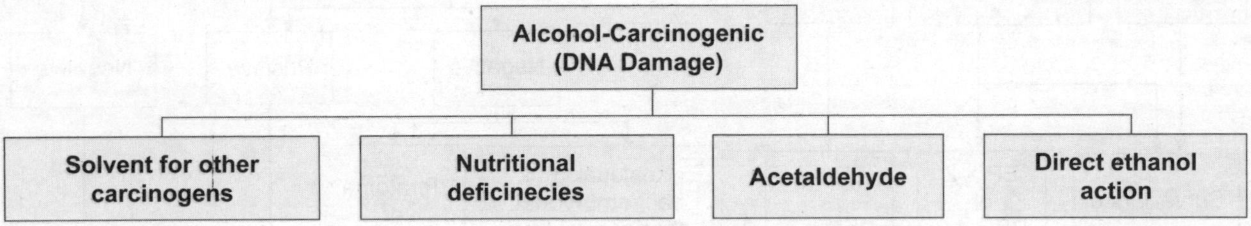

- ***SCC lip is associated with sun exposure and pipe smoking***
- Sinonasal SCC is linked to nickel and chromate exposure and woodworking
- Dietary deficiencies have also been linked to the development of HNSCC, especially vitamins (A, C and E), foods (fruit, vegetables and dairy) and elements (e.g., iron Plummer-Vinson syndrome is associated with hypopharyngeal SCC)
- HNSCCs are typically sporadic

Patients with Fanconi's anaemia have a 700-fold increased risk and cancer is usually diagnosed in 3rd decade

HPV

- In HPV16 infection the E6 and E7 viral oncoproteins cause inactivation of tumor suppressor molecules pRb and p53

Genetics
High levels of EGFR
Associated with poor outcome–Poor Progression free survival and Overall survival

- Tobacco extract induces EGFR phosphorylation in oral cancers

Cancer cells often overexpress NF kB
Cancer cells often express NF-kB that act for proliferation of cells
Activation of NF-kB suppress apoptosis promotes chemoresistance and tumor development

p53 impair ability of cells to repair and undergo apoptosis in response to DNA damage

Most Important Points
• ***LOH of 9p21 seen in 70–80% of HNSCC***
• Loss of pRb causes uncontrolled cell proliferation
• Loss of p53 mediated response to DNA damage leads to genomic stability and reactivation of telomerase driving cell immortality

Markers	Cancer
S100, MelanA, HMB45 and Sox10	Melanoma
CD45, CD79a and CD3	Lymphoma
Cytokeratins 5, 6, 14 Nuclear stained Proteins p40 and p63	Poorly differentiated SCC

Criteria Distinguishes Specific Cellular Proteins For Therapeutic Targeting:

Cellular proteins

- ***Differential expressivity/ Activity of therapeutic target***
- ***Poor clinical outcome associated with the therapeutic target***
- ***Preclinical inhibitor studies demonstrate antitumor effects***

Verrucous Carcinoma

- Well differentiated carcinoma of oral cavity
- Warty, exophytic lesion that arises from a broad base
- Superficial spreading growth
- Lacks significant cellular atypia and is characterized by blunt incursions and an expansile advancing margin

Spindle Cell Carcinoma (Sarcomatoid Carcinoma)

- Typically occurs in upper respiratory tract
- ***Elderly males***
- Previous radiation is a risk factor
- Usually bi-phasic lesion with areas of SCC, and/or high-grade dysplasia, associated with bizarre spindle cell and/or giant cell proliferation of sarcomatoid appearance

Papillary SCC

- Typically affects larynx and hypopharynx
- Lacks typical surface keratinization

Adenosquamous Carcinoma

- Aggressive with poor prognosis
- Affects males in the sixth or seventh decade
- Typically affects larynx and hypopharynx

Basaloid SCC

- High-grade aggressive variant of SCC
- Typically found in middle-aged male patients
- Affects Oropharynx, Larynx and Hypopharynx
- Infiltrating and deeply invasive and presents a typical basaloid appearance
- Cystic degeneration with central comedonecrosis is often a feature

Most Common Site

- Most common site of lip cancer–Lower lip (Vermilion border)
- Most common site of oral cavity–Tongue (Lateral border) [Gingivobuccal sulcus]
- Most common site of Oropharyngeal cancer–Tonsillar region

Contd.

Contd.

• Most common site of Hypopharyngeal cancer–Pyriform sinus • Most common site of laryngeal cancer–Free border on inner surface of true vocal cord • Most common site of nasopharyngeal cancer–Fossa of rosenmuller • Most common site of nasal and sinus cancer–Maxillary antrum • Most common site of Salivary tumor–Parotid

Markers of improved prognosis	Markers of worsened prognosis
p16 overexpression in oropharyngeal carcinoma Low p53/Bcl-xL expression in oropharyngeal carcinoma	Increased EGFR expression in oropharyngeal carcinoma BRAF mutations in PTC and malignant melanoma net/PTC rearrangement in PTC Loss of heterozygosity in p53, p16, E-cadherin, and pRB in hypopharyngeal cancers p53 overexpression in laryngeal carcinoma p21, p53 and pRB alteration in HPV-negative tonsil cancers

Subset of papillary thyroid carcinomas possesses mutated BRAFV600V gene
Presence of BRAF mutation→*Marker for extrathyroidal extension, more aggressive histology and more advanced clinical stage of disease*
BRAF mutations are also seen in malignant melanoma, where they have been correlated with an increased risk of death and significant reduction in survival time

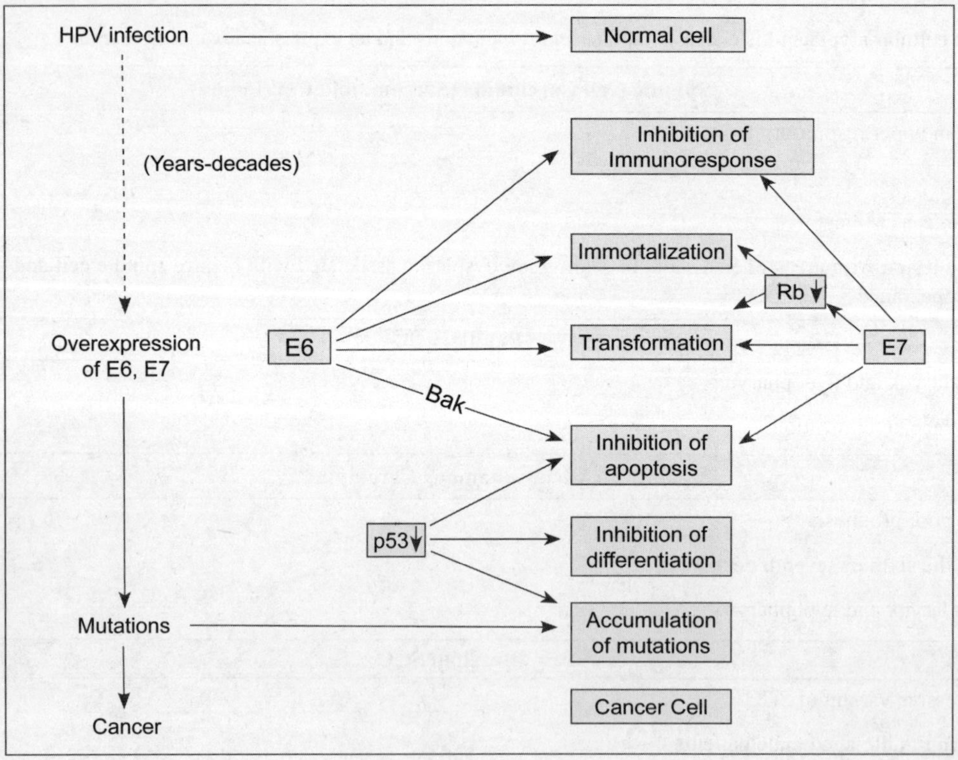

CHAPTER 20 STAGING

ORAL CAVITY

- Tis Carcinoma in situ
- T1 Tumor 2 cm or less in greatest dimension and 5 mm or less depth of invasion

T2
Tumor 2 cm or less in greatest dimension and more than 5 mm but not >10 mm depth of invasion
or
Tumor more than 2 cm but not >4 cm in greatest dimension and depth of invasion not >10 mm

- T3 Tumor more than 4 cm in greatest dimension or more than 10 mm depth of invasion
- T4a *(Lip)* Tumor invades through cortical bone, inferior alveolar nerve, floor of mouth, or skin (of chin/nose)
- T4a *(Oral cavity)* Tumor invades through the cortical bone of the mandible or maxillary sinus, or invades the skin of the face
- T4b *(Lip and oral cavity)* Tumor invades **masticator space,** pterygoid plates, or skull base, or encases ICA

OROPHARYNX

- T1 Tumor **2 cm or less in greatest dimension**
- T2 Tumor more than 2 cm but not more than 4 cm in greatest dimension
- T3 Tumor more than 4 cm in greatest dimension or extension to lingual surface of epiglottis
- T4a Tumor invades any of the following:
  - **Deep/extrinsic muscle of tongue (genioglossus, hyoglossus, palatoglossus and styloglossus), medial pterygoid, hard palate, or mandible, larynx**
- T4b Tumor invades any of the following:
  - **Lateral pterygoid muscle, lateral nasopharynx, skull base; or encases carotid artery, pterygoid plates**

HYPOPHARYNX

- T1 Tumor limited to one subsite of hypopharynx (2 cm or less in greatest dimension)
- T2 Tumor invades **more than one subsite** of hypopharynx or an adjacent site, or measures more than 2 cm but not more than 4 cm in greatest dimension, *without* fixation of hemilarynx
- T3 Tumor >4 cm in greatest dimension, or ***with fixation of hemilarynx or extension to esophagus***
- T4a Tumor invades any of following: Thyroid/cricoid cartilage, hyoid bone, Thyroid gland, **oesophagus,** central compartment soft tissue
- T4b Tumor invades prevertebral fascia, encases carotid artery, or invades mediastinal structures

Nodal Staging
• NX Regional lymph nodes cannot be assessed
• N0 No regional lymph node metastasis

Contd.

Contd.

- N1 Metastasis in a single ipsilateral lymph node, **3 cm or less** in greatest dimension without extranodal extension
- N2a Metastasis in a single ipsilateral lymph node, more than 3 cm but not more than 6 cm in greatest dimension without extranodal extension
- N2b Metastasis in multiple ipsilateral lymph nodes, none more than 6 cm in greatest dimension, without extranodal extension
- N2c Metastasis in bilateral or contralateral lymph nodes, none more than 6 cm in greatest dimension, without extranodal extension
- N3a Metastasis in lymph node more than 6 cm in greatest dimension without extranodal extension
- **N3b Metastasis in a single or multiple lymph nodes with clinical extranodal extension**

NASOPHARYNX

- T1 Tumor confined to nasopharynx, or extends to oropharynx and/or nasal cavity without parapharyngeal involvement
- T2 Tumor with **extension to parapharyngeal space and/or infiltration of the medial pterygoid, lateral pterygoid, and/or prevertebral muscles**
- T3 **Tumor invades bony structures of skull base cervical vertebra, pterygoid structures, and/or paranasal sinuses**
- T4 Tumor with intracranial extension and/or involvement of cranial nerves, hypopharynx, orbit, parotid gland and/or infiltration beyond the lateral surface of the lateral pterygoid muscle.

Oropharynx p-16 Positive

- NX Regional lymph nodes cannot be assessed
- N0 No regional lymph node metastasis
- N1 Unilateral metastasis, in lymph node(s), all 6 cm or less in greatest dimension
- N2 Contralateral/bilateral metastasis in lymph nodes, all 6 cm/less in greatest dimension
- N3 Metastasis in lymph node(s) greater than 6 cm in dimension

Nasopharynx

- NX Regional lymph nodes cannot be assessed
- N0 No regional lymph node metastasis
- N1 Unilateral metastasis, in cervical lymph node(s), and/or unilateral/bilateral metastasis in retropharyngeal lymph nodes, 6 cm or less in greatest dimension, above caudal border of cricoid cartilage
- N2 Bilateral metastasis in cervical lymph node(s), 6 cm or less in greatest dimension, above caudal border of cricoid cartilage
- N3 Metastasis in cervical lymph node(s) greater than 6 cm in dimension and/or extension below caudal border of cricoid cartilage

Supraglottis
• T1 Tumor limited to one subsite of supraglottis with normal vocal cord mobility
• T2 Tumor invades mucosa of > one adjacent subsite of supraglottis or glottis or region outside supraglottis (e.g., **mucosa of base of tongue, vallecula, medial wall of piriform sinus)** without fixation of larynx
• T3 Tumor limited to **larynx with vocal cord fixation** and/or invades any of the following: postcricoid area, pre epiglottic space, paraglottic space, and/or inner cortex thyroid cartilage
• T4a Tumor invades through the thyroid cartilage and/or invades tissues beyond larynx, e.g., trachea, soft tissues of neck including deep/extrinsic muscle of tongue **(genioglossus, hyoglossus, palatoglossus and styloglossus),** strap muscles, thyroid, or oesophagus
• T4b Tumor invades prevertebral space, encases carotid artery, or mediastinal structures

Glottis
• T1 Tumor limited to vocal cord(s) (may involve anterior or posterior commissure) with normal mobility
• T1a Tumor limited to one vocal cord
• T1b Tumor involves both vocal cords
• T2 Tumor extends to supraglottis and/or subglottis, and/or with impaired vocal cord mobility

Contd.

Contd.

• T3 Tumor limited to larynx with vocal cord fixation and/or invades paraglottic space and/or inner cortex of the thyroid cartilage
• T4a Tumor invades through the outer cortex of the thyroid cartilage, and/or invades tissues beyond the larynx, e.g., trachea, soft tissues of neck including deep/extrinsic muscle of tongue **(genioglossus, hyoglossus, palatoglossus and styloglossus), strap muscles,** thyroid, oesophagus
• T4b Tumor invades prevertebral space, encases carotid artery, or mediastinal structures
Subglottis
• T1 Tumor limited to subglottis
• T2 Tumor extends to vocal cord(s) with normal or impaired mobility
• T3 Tumor limited to larynx with vocal cord fixation
• T4a Tumor invades cricoid or thyroid cartilage and/or invades tissues beyond larynx, e.g., trachea, soft tissues of neck including deep/extrinsic muscle of tongue (genioglossus, hyoglossus, palatoglossus and styloglossus), strap muscles, thyroid, oesophagus
• T4b Tumor invades prevertebral space, encases carotid artery, or mediastinal structures

CHAPTER 21

ORAL CAVITY

ANATOMY

- Oral cavity starts at mucocutaneous junction of lips (vermilion border) extending posteriorly to junction of hard and soft palate superiorly, anterior fauces laterally and junction of anterior two-thirds and posterior third of tongue inferiorly
- ***Oral cavity is lined by stratified squamous epithelium of varying degrees of keratinization***

More than 90% of lesions are SCC

- Mean age of transformation of oral dysplastic lesions to malignancy–4.3 years

Pathological features of oral squamous cell papillomas

Subtype	Squamous cell papilloma or verruca vulgaris	Condyloma acuminatum	Multifocal epithelial hyperplasia (Heck's disease)
HPV status	• Approximately half are associated with HPV infection • Squamous cell papilloma HPV 6 and 11 • Verruca vulgaris HPV 2, 4, 40 and 57	• Associated with HPV 6 and 11 • Transmission is venereal or autoinoculation and there is an association with genital condyloma	• HPV 13 and 32 • Disease of children, adolescents and young adults
Macroscopic appearance	Wart-like exophytic lesion	Dome-shaped expophytic nodules, which are usually larger than squamous cell papillomas	Multiple clusters or patches of soft, plaque-like lesions

ORAL CANCERS

- Oral cancer is more common in males, who usually present in the 6th and 7th decade
- Tobacco and alcohol consumption are the major aetiological factors in development of oral cancer

AJCC Staging

Tis Carcinoma in situ

T1 Tumor 2 cm or less in greatest dimension and **5 mm or less depth of invasion**

T2

Tumor 2 cm or less in greatest dimension and more than 5 mm but not >10 mm depth of invasion

Or

Tumor more than 2 cm but not >4 cm in greatest dimension and depth of invasion not >10 mm

T3 Tumor more than 4 cm in greatest dimension or more than 10 mm depth of invasion

T4a *(Lip)*Tumor invades through cortical bone, inferior alveolar nerve, floor of mouth, or skin (of chin/nose)

T4a *(Oral cavity)* Tumor invades through the cortical bone of the mandible or maxillary sinus, or invades the skin of the face

T4b *(Lip and oral cavity)* Tumor invades **masticator space,** pterygoid plates, or skull base, or encases ICA

Contd.

Contd.

Nodal Staging
N0 No regional lymph node metastasis
N1 Metastasis in a single ipsilateral lymph node, **3 cm or less** in greatest dimension without extranodal extension
N2a Metastasis in a single ipsilateral lymph node, more than 3 cm but not more than 6 cm in greatest dimension without extranodal extension
N2b Metastasis in multiple ipsilateral lymph nodes, none more than 6 cm in greatest dimension, without extranodal extension
N2c Metastasis in bilateral or contralateral lymph nodes, none more than 6 cm in greatest dimension, without extranodal extension
N3a Metastasis in lymph node more than 6 cm in greatest dimension without extranodal extension
N3b Metastasis in a single or multiple lymph nodes with clinical extranodal extension

<table>
<tr><th></th><th>T1</th><th>T2</th><th>T3</th><th>T4a</th><th>T4b</th></tr>
<tr><td>N0</td><td>I</td><td>II</td><td>III</td><td rowspan="3">IVA</td><td rowspan="4">IVB</td></tr>
<tr><td>N1</td><td colspan="3">III</td></tr>
<tr><td>N2</td><td colspan="3">IVA</td></tr>
<tr><td>N3</td><td colspan="4">IVB</td></tr>
<tr><td>M1</td><td colspan="5">IVC</td></tr>
</table>

1. Lip Cancer

- Most common site- Lower lip vermilion border
- **Most common type–SCC**
- Usually well differentiated

Lymphatic Drainage
• Upper lip–Submandibular nodes
• Lower lip–Submental, Submandibular and Subdigastric nodes

- *Risk of metastasis to regional LN increases with poorly differentiated, large tumor size*
- *Extension of tumor to lateral commissures (5-10%)*

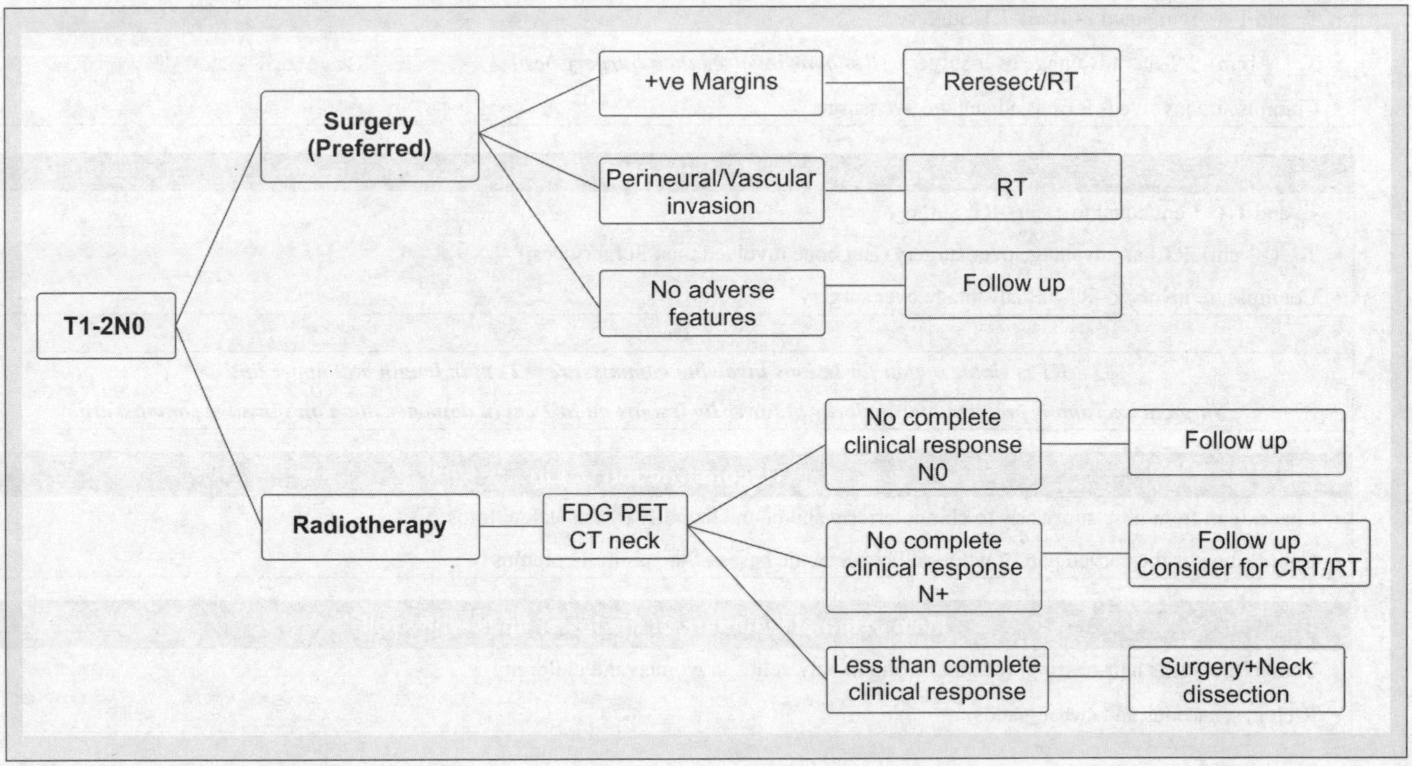

Contd.

Contd.

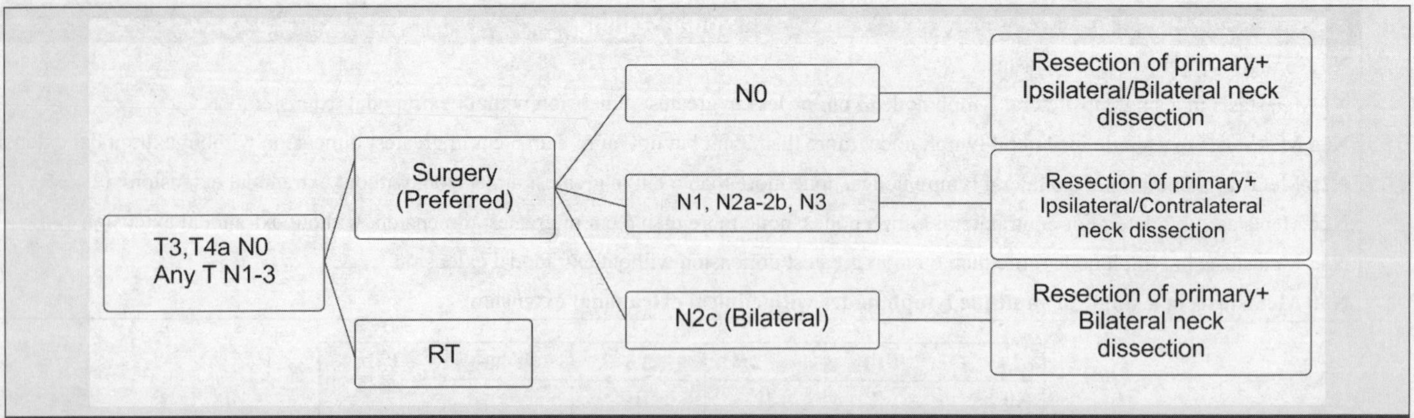

After Resection

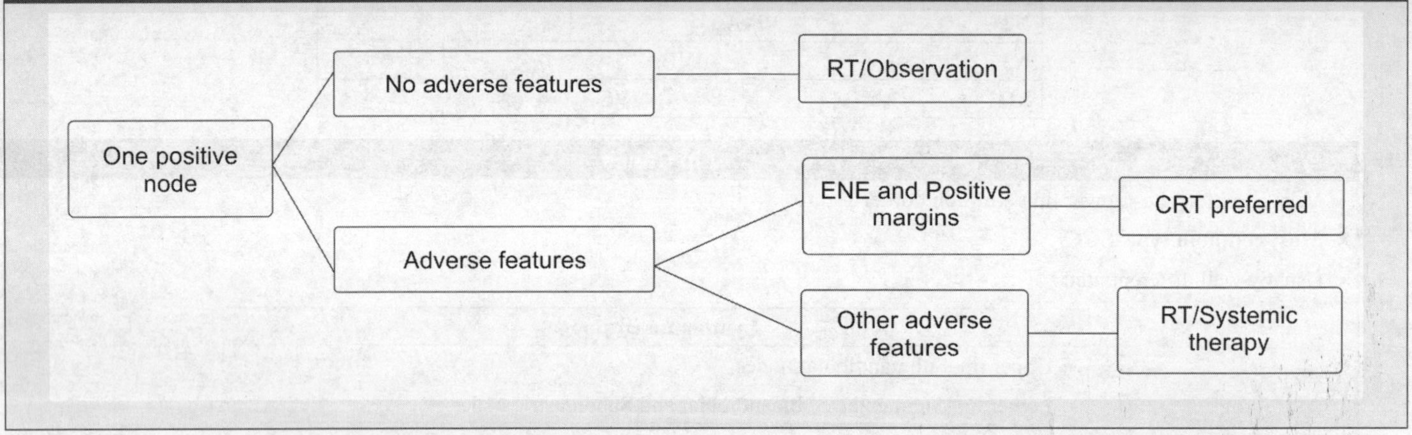

Treatment of Lip Cancer

- Leukoplakia, Severe dysplasia and Limited CIS–Vermilionectomy/Lip shave
- T_{is} and T_1 (<1cm/equal to 1cm)–RT/Surgery
- T_{1-4} (>1cm)- RT has advantage over surgery. ***(But bone involved then Surgery best)***
- Commissure involved- RT has advantage over surgery

Jatin Shah

- T_{is} and T_1 (<1 cm/equal to 1 cm)–RT/Surgery
- T_{1-4} (>1 cm)–RT has advantage over surgery (But bone involved then Surgery best)
- Commissure involved–RT has advantage over surgery

Devita

RT is viable option for lesions involving commissure, >2 cm in length and upper lip

Surgical excision is preferred for majority of lower lip lesions up to 2 cm in diameter that don't involve commissure

Reconstruction of Lip

- Lips extend from nose superiorly to chin inferiorly and bound laterally by nasolabial folds
- Cupid's bow is the curved part of white roll between the bases of the philtral columns

Main external landmark of the lower lip is white roll

- Skin of the lips is hair-bearing, with hair being mostly vellus in women and children
- Rich in sebaceous and sweat glands

Groups of Perioral Musculature

Groups of perioral musculature

- **I — Attached to modiolus**: Orbicularis oris, Buccinator, Levator anguli oris, Depressor anguli oris, Zygomaticus major and Risorius
- **II — Insert into upper lip**: Levator labii superioris, Alaeque nasi abd Zygomaticus minor
- **III — Insert into lower lip**: Depressor labii inferioris, Mentalis and Platysma

Vermilion

Extends from white roll to wet dry border which transforms into mucosa

Vermilion is lined by stratified squamous epithelium

Contains no glands and is dryer and duller in appearance than mucosa

Mucosa is non-keratinized epithelium

- **Paired orbicularis oris**–Sphincter muscles of lips→ Oral competence
- Orbicularis muscles are innervated by buccal branches of the facial nerve
- **Mentalis**–Primary Elevators of lower lip (Lower lip in correct position at rest)–***Large trapezoid muscle***–Innervated by marginal mandibular of 7th nerve

Depressors

- ***Depressor anguli oris and depressor labii inferioris***–Innervated by marginal mandibular branch of 7th nerve
- ***Platysma***–Cervical branches of facial nerve

Elevators

- Levator labii superioris, Zygomaticus major and minor, Levator anguli oris
- Innervated by zygomatic and buccal branches of the facial nerve

Sensory supply	**Infraorbital nerve**–Enters face through infraorbital foramen and provides sensation to nasal sidewall, nasal ala and upper lip **Mental nerve**–Mental nerve exits the mandible between first and second premolar teeth and provides sensation to the lower lip
Arterial supply	Superior and Inferior labial artery
Venous supply	Labial veins can drain into anterior facial veins, transverse cervical veins, superficial temporal veins and the submental veins
Lymphatic supply	**Upper lip**–Submandibular nodes **Commissure**–Periparotid nodes **Lower lip**–I/L submandibular nodes (Midline–submental nodes)

- BCC tend to occur in upper lip and SCC in sun-exposed lower lip
- More common in elderly
- Traumatic lip defects usually occur in young, healthy patients

Principles of Lip Reconstruction

- Preserve nerve supply to reconstructed lip
- Muscle-carrying lip vermilion should also be preserved

Contd.

Contd.

- Lip tissue should preferentially be used to reconstruct lip
- Muscles of the lip should be correctly orientated
- Lip defect is too large to be reconstructed by remaining lip tissue–cheeks
- Insufficient local tissue–free-tissue transfer, should only be performed

Vermilion	**Small defects**–Closed directly • **Lateral superficial defects**–Vermilion flaps/Mucosal and tongue flaps
• ***Vermilion flaps are best suited for defects close to white roll and include vermilion advancement flaps or vermilion 'switch' flaps from opposite lip*** • ***Mucosal advancement flaps–useful for total vermilionectomy defects, broad defects remote from vermilion border*** • ***Tongue flaps–Mucosa is insufficient–best reserved for lateral vermilion defects***	
Upper lip	**Central defects involving <1/2 distance between philtral columns→** Repair primarily or wedge resection **Superficial defects and >1/2 central lip without crossing philtrum→** Full-thickness skin graft **Central defect >1/2 upper lip→** Abbe-Sabattini flap **Abbe-Sabattini flap→** *Lateral lip defects >1/3rd and doesn't involve oral commissure.* **Superficial lateral defects <1/2 width of lateral lip→**Wedge resection **Upper lip defect** <1/2 → Wedge excision 1/2-2/3 → Peri Alar Crescentic, Reverse Karapandzic free flap, Abbe-Estlander >2/3 → Burrow Diffenbach **Defect >1/2 width of lateral lip→** Local flap from cheek **Defects upto 1/3rd in width→** Closed directly **Defects of upper lip >50%** →Larger lip switch flap combination with bilateral perialar crescentic excision and advancement ***(Schuchardt B/L medial advancement flap)***
Lower lip	**Superficial defects lower lip**–Best treated by full thickness wedge excision and primary closure **Karapandzic Technique** • ***Best method*** to reconstruct lower lip defects can't be directly closed–**Karapandzic technique** (both lateral and central lower lip defects) • Supplied by facial artery branches • ***Preserves sensory and motor nerves to lip segment*** **Johanson's Step Technique:** Only applied to lower lip defects ***Defects of lower lip not involving commissure can be reconstructed by Abbe Sabattini flap from upper lip*** ***Defects close to commissure can be reconstructed in single stage by Estlander flap*** **Freeman Modification of Bernard Von Burrow Technique** • **Bernard-von Burow procedure** reconstructs lower lip by medially advancing cheeks (Width of triangular excision is equal to width of defect) • Freeman modification of the Bernard-von Burrow operation is probably the ***best current cheek advancement technique***

Contd.

Contd.

- ***Bilateral cheek advancements can be used for total lower lip reconstruction***

Bandoneon Technique

- Mucomusculocutaneous flap from lower lip can be stretched like 'bandoneon' and advanced to reconstruct lower lip defects up to 2/3rd in width

Steeple Flap

- Island flap of full-thickness tissue from cheek–used for vermilion reconstruction
- For total lower lip reconstruction, bilateral steeple flaps can be used

Microvascular Reconstruction

- A folded free flap like radial forearm flap is best option

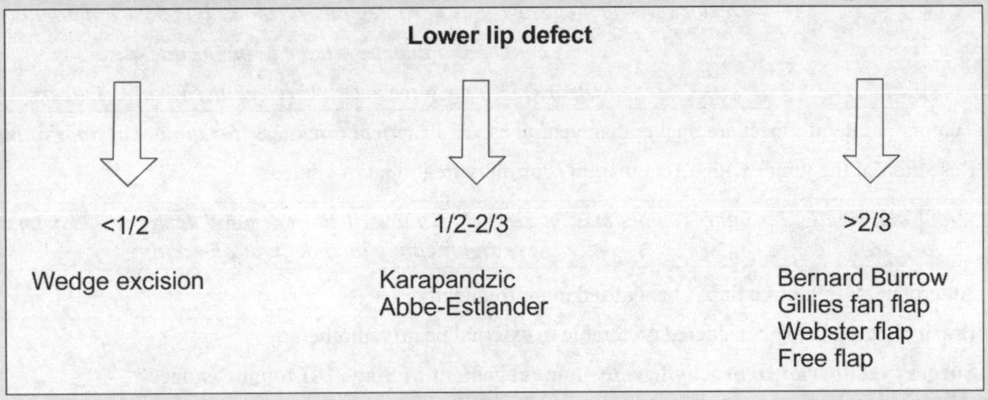

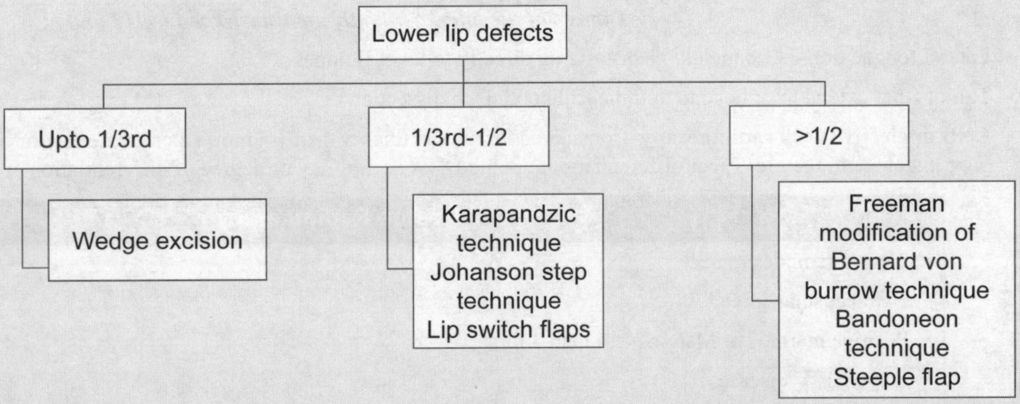

2. Tongue Carcinoma

- Freely mobile anterior two-thirds of the tongue
- Demarcated from base of tongue by circumvallate papillae posteriorly

Ventral and lateral surfaces–Non keratinized stratified squamous epithelium

Dorsum and tip of tongue–Keratinized epithelium

Motor supply	Hypoglossal nerve Palatoglossus–Vagus nerve
Sensory supply	**Lingual nerve**–Sensation of tongue **Sensation of oral tongue**–Fibers of facial nerve that run with lingual nerve
Lymphatic drainage	**Lateral borders of tongue**–I/L cervical nodes Midline, tip and base of tongue–Bilateral
Blood supply	**Lingual artery**

Contd.

Contd.

Most common site–Middle third lateral aspect

- More frequent in males and 6th–8th decade
- 90% occur >40 years age
- Up to 70% report significant tobacco and alcohol use
- ***Lesions of the oral tongue are more likely to be symptomatic***
- Majority of patients with cancer of the ***oral tongue*** present with ***stage I/II disease***
- Cancers of ***base of the tongue*** that are ***usually stage III/IV*** at presentation

> ***Clinically positive cervical lymphadenopathy at presentation is in region of 21–34%***
>
> ***Occult cervical metastasis has been demonstrated in up to 53% of patients with tongue cancer and may be related to tumor thickness***
>
> ***Up to 4.5% may have occult cervical disease in C/L neck***

- Tumors of lateral aspect are thicker than ventral aspect–'***Critical thickness' for tumors of floor of mouth is less than other oral sites***
- Resection of the tumor with a 1cm margin is primary treatment of choice

> ***T1 and small T2 primary tumors may be excised with a vertical wedge and defect closed primarily, if defect does not extend to significantly include floor of mouth***

- Anterolateral thigh free flap is being used more frequently
- Brachytherapy being considered preferable to external beam radiotherapy
- **Surgery is superior to brachytherapy in management of Stage I/II tongue cancer**

Tumors of the tongue initially metastasize to levels I and II

- Lateral tongue tumors frequently metastasizing directly to level II nodes
- Tumors that extend to or beyond midline–Bilateral neck dissection
- **END or elective neck radiotherapy**–Considered for tumors thicker than 3-4 mm, T2 or greater in dimension and T1 tumors that demonstrate poor histological features (poor differentiation, double DNA aneuploidy or degree of differentiation at advancing front).

Postop Radiotherapy

- 2 or more nodes in neck
- Extracapsular spread
- Positive margins or Margins less than 3 mm
- Stage III/IV disease
- ***Tumor thicker than 9-10 mm in absence of other features***
- ***Perineural spread***

- **Recurrence rates for oral tongue carcinoma are 10–50% usually being locoregional**
- Factors that influence local recurrence include tumor thickness and presence of perineural spread
- Younger than 40 years–More likely to develop locoregional failure
- **Metachronous second tumors–Seen in nearly 10% of patients who had tongue cancer**
- Tumor thickness, presence of perineural invasion, cervical metastasis or dysplasia at resection margins have all been demonstrated to influence prognosis

3. **Buccal Mucosa**

- Buccal mucosa is the mucosal lining of the inner surface of the cheek
- Area extends from oral commissure anteriorly to retromolar trigone posteriorly
- Junction between buccal mucosa and retromolar trigone is an arbitrary line drawn from maxillary tuberosity to the distobuccal aspect of mandibular third molar

Lining Mucosa of buccal mucosa is Non keratinizing stratified squamous epithelium

- Mucosa is firmly attached to the underlying buccinator muscle

Contd.

Contd.

- Parotid duct pierces the buccinator muscle to enter the oral cavity adjacent to the first maxillary molar tooth.

Sensory supply	Buccal branch of the mandibular division of trigeminal nerve
Lymphatic drainage	Ipsilateral facial and submandibular nodes to deep cervical chain

- Betel quid is main etiologic factor for submucosal fibrosis
- Strong association with smoking and alcohol consumption, Chewing tobacco, smokeless tobacco
- Pre existing leukoplakia is more common

Male : Female = 4 : 1

- Occurs over 40 years of age

Oral submucous fibrosis and lichen planus may involve buccal mucosa, both being considered premalignant conditions

- **Clinical features**–Intraoral mass, Trismus, Ulceration and Pain
- 40% or more presenting with Stage III/IV disease
- Palpable lymphadenopathy on presentation may be as high as 57% for T3/4 lesions
- Occult nodal metastasis may be present in 26% of those clinically N0 at presentation
- Most patients will require MRI/CT imaging, augmented with ultrasound scan if necessary to help in assessment of depth of primary and cervical lymphadenopathy
- **T1/T2**–Resected perorally down to buccinator
- **T3/T4**–Facial access incisions and bony resection of maxilla and/or mandible

Primary tumor should be resected with 1 cm margin and upto 2 cm if skin is involved

- Small T1 tumors may be resected and reconstructed by primary closure
- Microvascular free flap reconstruction with a radial-free forearm flap or anterolateral thigh flap restores thickness of cheek and if external skin is involved flaps can be bi-paddled to provide reconstruction of mucosal and skin surfaces
- ***T4 tumors–Segmental resection of mandible with composite free flap reconstruction***
- Reconstruction with radial-free forearm flap–better post-operative mouth opening

Regional spread of buccal carcinoma is usually to ipsilateral level I and II lymph nodes

- Patients with palpable lymphadenopathy or pathological nodes on imaging should have a comprehensive neck dissection, although if pathological nodes are only located in level Ia, level I–III SND may be considered

Tumors greater than T2, are poorly differentiated, have a poor lymphocytic response or thicker than 5 mm are more likely to demonstrate cervical metastases–Elective neck dissection

Postop Radiotherapy

- 2 or more nodes in the neck
- Extracapsular spread
- Positive margins or Margins less than 3 mm
- Stage III/IV disease

- Recurrence rates for buccal carcinoma are 26–80% usually occurring within 2 years
- Factors that influence recurrence include tumor thickness, histological margins less than 3 mm and tumor differentiation

Distant failure is more common than regional failure

Factors that potentially influence survival include regional metastasis, ECS, tumor thickness >5–6 mm skin involvement, histological margins <2 mm stage and recurrent disease

4. Floor of Mouth Carcinoma

- Mucosal lining of anterior and lateral floor of the mouth
- Bound anteriorly and laterally by attached mucoperiosteum of mandibular alveolus

Contd.

Contd.

Lateral floor of mouth is bound posteriorly by anterior tonsillar pillars
Medially floor of mouth merges with ventral and lateral aspects of tongue
Lined by Stratified non keratinizing squamous epithelium

- Submandibular ducts enter mouth anteriorly either side of lingual frenum

Sensory supply	Lingual branch of mandibular division of trigeminal nerve
Lymphatic drainage	**Lateral floor of mouth**–Ipsilateral submandibular nodes
	Anterior floor of mouth–Submental nodes

- Occurs more frequently in men
- Age at diagnosis usually being in 6th–7th decade

Leukoplakia of floor of mouth–Considered a premalignant condition with an annual transformation rate of 1–2.9%
Approximately 50% present with advanced disease
Tumor up to 28.6% of patients may have B/L nodal involvement
Cervical lymphadenopathy is present in 17–45% of patients on presentation upto 22% of those clinically N0 at presentation having occult metastasis
Surgical resection with a 1cm margin is preferred treatment modality

- Early extension of floor of mouth tumors into tongue or mandible is demonstrated by requirement of rim or segmental resection of the mandible
- ***Smaller resections at least 3 mm length of duct proximal to orifice*** should be taken to ensure surgical clearance of carcinoma or dysplasia that may extend along duct

Radial free-forearm flap is ideal reconstructive option for Floor of mouth defects–Edentulous mandible
Fibula osteocutaneous flap provides superior reconstruction if segmental resection–Dentate patient

Regional spread of disease in floor of mouth carcinomas–usually due to I/L level I to III lymph nodes

- Towards midline–Bilateral neck dissection
- Lesions that are ***T2 or greater*** should have ***I–III/IV selective neck dissection*** although ENDs have been advocated for T1 lesions

Tumor thickness >4 mm should be considered for END, since risk of occult metastasis >20%

Postop Radiotherapy

- 2 or more nodes in the neck
- Extracapsular spread
- Positive margins or Margins less than 3 mm
- Stage III/IV disease

- Recurrence rates for floor-of-mouth carcinoma are 26–55% usually within first 2 years
- Factors that influence recurrence include tumor size, thickness, histological margins and advanced nodal disease
- ***Overall 5-year survival for floor-of-mouth carcinoma is 52–76%***

5. **Retromolar Carcinoma**

- Triangular area of mucosa that overlies ascending ramus of the mandible
- Base of the triangle is in region of mandibular 3rd molar inferiorly, the apex being adjacent to the maxillary tuberosity superiorly
- Area is bound by buccal mucosa laterally and the anterior tonsillar pillar medially

Lined by non keratinizing stratified squamous epithelium	
Sensory supply	Buccal branch of mandibular division of 5th nerve
Lymphatic drainage	Ipsilateral submandibular and deep cervical nodes

Contd.

Contd.

- *6-7% of carcinoma arise from this site*
- Males and elderly individuals
- Strong association with smoking and alcohol
- Symptoms–Pain, Trismus, Otalgia or lingual parathesia

RETROMOLAR TRIGONE

Buccal mucosa	Oropharynx	Masticator space	Maxilla/Mandible
84%	14%	22%	12-34%

- Posterior maxilla is more frequently involved than mandible
- Tumor extension to masticator space or lower pterygoid–**T4b**
- Usually advanced stage (III/IV)

Spread to regional lymph nodes occurs in 26–56% of patients at presentation 8–15% having occult cervical node involvement

- CT has been demonstrated to have a high specificity, but low sensitivity for predicting mandibular bone invasion of retromolar carcinomas
- MRI is considered imaging modality of choice for retromolar tumors due to its ability to ***accurately stage disease and*** demonstrate ***accurately anatomical relationships*** of tumor
- ***Surgical resection with pre/post-operative radiotherapy or chemoradiotherapy*** dependant on stage of tumor and histological findings–***Treatment of choice***

Resection should be achieved with a 1cm margin in all planes. Small tumors of the retromolar trigone may be resected via a transoral route

- Extensive tumors extending into the masticator space may require a cervicofacial incision, parotidectomy, +/– zygomatic osteotomy and preservation of the facial nerve for access, or an anterior approach including maxillectomy
- A posterior marginal mandibulectomy (including coronoid) conducted via a visor or lip split soft-tissue flap is oncologically safe in patients with no history of previous RT and no radiological signs of cortical bone involvement

Large soft tissue defects–Segmental resection is warranted

- Segmental resection ideally with free-tissue transfer→fibula, scapula or DCIA flaps.
- Scapula flap is versatile in thin individuals and able to reconstruct these extensive defects.
- ***An END (levels I–III/IV) is indicated for any tumor bigger than T1***
- **Post op radiotherapy**–Advanced tumors (Bone invasion and Nodal metastasis)

Lymphatic supply	
N0	Levels I and II
N+	Levels III–V

Local and/or regional recurrence may occur in 20–37%

Frequently presents as Stage III/IV disease with extension into adjacent sites

6. **Maxillary Alveolus and Hard Palate**

- Maxillary alveolus merges laterally with buccal mucosa and lips at gingival sulcus and medially with the hard palate

Osseous alveolar process is lined by stratified squamous epithelium

- Alveolar process extends to the upper end of pterygopalatine arches posteriorly
- Hard palate lies within horseshoe shape of maxillary alveolus merging imperceptively with alveolar mucosa

33% of palatal tumors are derived from salivary epithelium

Contd.

Contd.

- Posteriorly hard palate merges with soft palate at posterior edge of the palatine bone

Sensory supply	Trigeminal nerve branches Nasopalatine nerve–Anterior hard palate Greater palatine nerves–Posterior hard palate
Lymphatic drainage	Ipsilateral cervical nodes through submandibular nodes Posteriorly located tumors–Retropharyngeal nodes

- Carcinoma of hard palate→ Only 1–3% of oral cancers
- Squamous cell carcinoma of maxillary alveolus→3.5–6.5% of oral cancers

Palatal carcinoma is particularly associated with reverse smoking

- 6th–7th decade and females
- Pain, ulceration, loose teeth or poorly fitting dentures.
- Symptoms of advanced disease–Infraorbital parathesia, trismus or nasal obstruction

Most patients present with Stage I or II disease
Extension of tumor through pterygoid plates into the masticator space may render tumor inoperable

- Approximately 8% of patients with carcinoma of hard palate or maxillary alveolus present with cervical lymphadenopathy
- ***27% having occult metastasis***
- **Small tumors**–Per orally
- **Larger tumors**–Upper cheek flap or midfacial degloving to augment access

Superior alveolar ridge lesions–*Inferior or Infrastructure maxillectomy is required*

- An ipsilateral coronoidectomy should be conducted to minimize impingement of the coronoid on the prosthesis or flap reconstruction
- *Small maxillectomy defects–Local flaps like buccal fat pad, temporalis flaps or facial artery musculomucosal flaps*
- *Large defects may require soft tissue or composite free tissue transfer*

Cervical Metastasis

- 35% of patients with hard palate/maxillary alveolar carcinomas an elective I–III neck dissection is appropriate for lesions of T2 size or greater
- **Post op radiotherapy**–T3 or greater disease, positive margins, perineural or perivascular invasion or multiple cervical nodes, particularly ECS

Locoregional control of hard palate and alveolar tumors is in region of 40–45%
(following initial therapy)

- Salvage of local recurrence–**33%**
- Regional recurrence–**71%**
- 5-year absolute survival for hard palate carcinoma–**57%**
- 5-year survival for alveolar carcinoma–**49%**
- Tumor stage and presence of cervical metastasis influence long-term survival

7. Mandibular Alveolus

- Osseous alveolar process of mandible supports dentition and covered by muco periosteum
- Mandibular alveolus merges laterally with the buccal mucosa/lips at gingival sulcus and medially with floor of mouth
- Alveolar process extends to retromolar trigones posteriorly

Sensory supply	Mandibular division of 5th nerve
Lymphatic drainage	Ipsilateral submental and submandibular nodes Midline–Bilateral supply

- Squamous cell carcinoma of the mandibular alveolus→7.5–17.5% of oral cancers

Mandibular alveolar carcinoma is 3 times more common than maxillary alveolar carcinoma

- 7th decade and males

Most common presenting symptom is pain (54–86% of patients)

- Labial parasthesia–presenting feature in upto 14%
- Majority of lesions of the mandibular alveolus are located posterior to the canines, extension to floor of mouth or buccal mucosa being common
- **Cervical lymphadenopathy**→ 24–32% of patients at presentation, usually to levels I and II
- 15% of patients having occult metastasis

Up to 94% of patients have evidence of bone involvement clinically

- ***Small alveolar carcinomas*** with ***no clinical evidence of significant bone involvement*** may be resected via per oral approach with a ***marginal mandibulectomy,*** aiming for a 1cm soft tissue and bony margin

Segmental resection should be considered for tumors abutting mandible previously exposed to radiotherapy, large soft tissue tumors adjacent to the mandible, involvement of inferior dental nerve or intraosseous tumors

- Small, lateral mandibular defects may be reconstructed with reconstruction plate and soft-tissue flap only
- Central defects or larger lateral defects should be reconstructed with vascularized bone to minimize risk of complications

H, C, L, o, m, s classification system accurately describes mandibular surgical defects

Regional Spread

- Mandibular alveolar tumors is usually to Ipsilateral level I–III nodes
- END is indicated in tumors T2 in size or greater or any tumor with demonstrable bone invasion, clearance of levels I–III being adequate
- Lesions overlying the symphysis are thought to be associated with a higher risk of cervical metastasis and may require bilateral neck dissections

PORT: Positive margins (soft tissue/bone), multiple positive nodes or ECS

- ***Higher recurrence rates- Associated with increasing T stage and positive resection margins***
- Overall 5-year survival for lower alveolus carcinoma is 50–60%
- Increasing T stage and particularly tumors > 3 cm, bone involvement (cortical/cancellous), positive resection margins are associated with decreased prognosis

Management of Mandible

- Invasive tumors demonstrate fingers or islands of tumor advancing deeply into bone with no obvious osteoclastic activity
- Erosive tumors have a broad advancing front with osteoclast activity and connective tissue between the tumor and bone, although as depth of invasion increases they may become more invasive in character
- ***Large, deeply invading tumors are more likely to demonstrate an invasive pattern of spread and involve mandible***
- Primarily size and extent of tumor that dictates the pattern of spread once in bone
- Tumors demonstrating an invasive pattern of spread are more likely to give rise to cervical metastasis with extracapsular extension–***Indication of more aggressive nature***

Plain X-rays do not detect initial invasion until 30% demineralization has occurred, giving rise to reduced sensitivity

Contd.

Contd.

- Axial MRI views with T1 and Short-TI Inversion Recovery fat suppression are very sensitive for imaging the primary site of oral cancer with an adequate specificity
- ***SPECT being demonstrated upto 100% sensitivity in determining bone invasion***
- ***Rim resection/marginal mandibulectomy***–Considered for T1/2 tumors with early invasion (< 5 mm) and adequate bone height of the mandible (dependent on pre-operative imaging, clinical examination and periosteal stripping)
- Marginal resections in retromolar region may include coronoid process

If the depth of mandible following rim resection is less than 10 mm then consideration should be given to converting the resection to segmental resection

Segmental mandibular resection and composite reconstruction

Extensive mandibular invasion/deeply invading soft-tissue tumors that abut whole depth of mandible

Presence of bone involvement rather than depth of bone invasion is main determining factor of long-term prognosis

- Rim resection of the mandible maintains bony continuity and hence is usually associated with an excellent functional and cosmetic outcome

CHAPTER 22 SINONASAL MALIGNANCIES

ANATOMY

- Mucosa of nasal cavity is derived from Ectoderm
- Vestibule lined by stratified squamous epithelium, Superior part of nasal cavity–Olfactory epithelium. Rest of nasal cavity–Pseudostratified ciliated columnar epithelium

GENERAL POINTS

- Average delay between the First symptom and diagnosis is approximately 6 months
- Sinonasal malignancies have an incidence of 0.5–1 per 100000 per year
- Account for 0.2–0.8% of all malignancies – **<1% of all neoplasms**
- <3% of upper aerodigestive tract neoplasms
- Most develop in the fifth and sixth decades of life
- **Incidence in men is twice that of women**
- **OAN and Malignant melanoma–Most common in men**

ETIOLOGY

- Biologically active compounds in wood dust impair mucociliary clearance and predispose to carcinogenesis
- Workers exposed to hard wood have a 70 times increased incidence of sinonasal adenocarcinoma, particularly of the ethmoid sinuses
- ***Hardwood exposure increases the risk of developing adenocarcinoma, soft wood exposure is more commonly associated with squamous cell carcinoma (SCC)***
- African mahogany appears to be the most carcinogenic
- Sinonasal adenocarcinoma that develops in wood-workers has a better prognosis than other nasal adenocarcinomas
- ***Exposure to nickel, which increases risk of developing sinonasal SCC 250-fold. Interval between exposure to nickel and development of the tumor can be prolonged***
- Smoking is also thought to play a role in the development of these tumors in a synergistic fashion with wood dust
- Chemicals linked to sinonasal malignancy include chromium, polycyclic hydrocarbons, aflatoxin, mustard gas and thorotrast (thorium dioxide used in paints for watch dials)
- Radiation, viral and genetic causes have also been proposed
- ***Schnederian Papilloma–Risk of SCC is 14.6% (Locally destructive)***
- Papilloma–May result from HPV infection with squamous variants from vestibule of nose

Site
• Most common site is maxillary sinus (55%)
• Nasal cavity (35%), ethmoid sinuses (9%) and frontal and sphenoid sinuses (1%)

SPREAD

Local Invasion

- Ethmoid and maxillary sinuses are intimately related to the orbit
- Olfactory nerves act as tumors that spread intracranially

Patterns of local spread						
Primary site	**Anteriorly**	**Posteriorly**	**Medially**	**Laterally**	**Superiorly**	**Inferiorly**
Frontal sinus	Skin	Anterior cranial tossa, frontal lobes				Ethmoid sinus, nasal cavity
Ethmoid sinus	Skin	Sphenoid, nasopharynx, clivus, pituitary gland	Nasal cavities, cribriform plate	Orbit	Anterior cranial fossa, frontal lobes	Nasal cavity
Maxillary sinus	Cheek, skin	Pterygopalatine fossa, infratemporal fossa, temporal bone, middle cranial fossa	Nasal cavity	Cheek, skin	Orbit	Palate
Sphenoid sinus	Ethmoid sinuses	Clivus, pituitary gland, posterior cranial fossa		Middle cranial fossa, cavernous sinus	Pituitary gland, hypothalamus	Nasopharynx
Nasal cavities	Skin	Sphenoid sinus, nasopharynx		Maxillary sinuses	Anterior cranial fossa, frontal lobes	Palate

Lymphatic Drainage

- Lymphatics of the anteroinferior part of the nasal cavity and skin of nasal vestibule drain via anterior pathway to first eschelon facial, parotid and submandibular lymph nodes
- Remainder of nose and paranasal sinuses drain through a posterior pathway which runs anterior to Eustachian tube to first eschelon nodes in the retropharyngeal space and then onwards to **upper deep cervical chain**
- Around 10% of patients present with nodal disease–marker of locally-advanced disease
- **Submandibular and jugulodigastric nodes are the most commonly involved**

Distant Metastasis

- Seen in 20% of patients with adenocarcinomas in contrast to just 10% of those with SCCs
- Most common sites for metastases are bone, brain, liver, lung and skin
- **Presence of distant metastases is associated with a poor prognosis**

TNM classification	
Maxillary Sinus	
Stage	**Description**
T1	Tumor limited to the antral mucosa with no erosion of bone
T2	Tumor causing bone erosion or destruction, except for the posterior antral wall, including extension into the hard palate and/or middle meatus
T3	Tumor invades any of the following: Bone of the posterior wall of the maxillary sinus, subcutaneous tissues, skin, floor or medial wall of the orbit, infratemporal fossa, pterygold plates, ethmoid sinus
T4a	Tumor invades any of the following: Anterior orbital contents, skin of cheek, pterygoid plates, infratemporal fossa, cribriform plate, sphenoid or frontal sinuses
T4b	Tumor invades any of the following: Orbital apex, dura, brain, middle cranial fossa, cranial nerves other than the maxillary division of V2, nasopharynx or clivus
Ethmoid Sinus	
T1	Tumor confined to ethmoid with or without bone erosion

Contd.

Contd.

T2	Tumor extends into the nasal cavity
T3	Tumor extends into the anterior orbit and/or maxillary sinus
T4a	Tumor invades any of the following: Anterior orbital contents, skin of the nose or cheek, minimal anterior intracranial extension, pterygoid plates, sphenoid or frontal sinuses
T4b	Tumor invades any of the following: Orbital apex, dura, brain, middle cranial fossa, cranial nerves other than V2, nasopharynx or clivus
Nasal Cavity[a]	
T1	Tumor involves one subsite
T2	Tumor involves two subsites or ethmoid
T3	Tumor extends into the Anterior orbit and/or maxillary sinus
T4a	Tumor invades any of the following: anterior orbital contents, skin of the nose or cheek, minimal anterior intracranial extension, pterygoid plates, sphenoid or frontal sinuses
T4b	Tumor invades any of the following: Orbital apex, dura, brain, middle cranial fossa, cranial nerves other than V2, nasopharynx or clivus
[a]Within the nose, four subsites are recognized, namely septum, floor, lateral wall and vestibule.	

<table>
<tr><th></th><th>T1</th><th>T2</th><th>T3</th><th>T4a</th><th>T4b</th></tr>
<tr><td>N0</td><td>I</td><td>II</td><td>III</td><td rowspan="2">IVA</td><td rowspan="4">IVB</td></tr>
<tr><td>N1</td><td>III</td><td>III</td><td>III</td></tr>
<tr><td>N2</td><td colspan="4">IVA</td></tr>
<tr><td>N3</td><td colspan="4">IVB</td></tr>
</table>

SQUAMOUS CELL CARCINOMA

- SCC is most common sinonasal malignancy
- Highest incidence is in **seventh decade** of life
- **Male preponderance**
- Most SCCs arise from **lateral wall of the nasal cavity** with 50% developing on turbinates
- *Two thirds of septal SCCs are found anteriorly in region of mucocutaneous junction*
- Transformation of Schneiderian papilloma occurs to SCC
- Approximately 85% of SCCs are well differentiated tumors
- Papillary and exophytic histological patterns are also recognized

ADENOCARCINOMA

- *Accounts for 9% of sinonasal malignancies*
- **Male predilection**
- **Affect sixth and seventh decades**
- **Found in the upper nasal cavity and ethmoid sinuses**
- Slow growth rate and rarely metastasize
- ***Intestinal variety is most often associated with wood work-induced tumors***
- Sessile and mucoid adenocarcinomas have the worst prognosis
- Papillary adenocarcinomas are least aggressive form

ADENOID CYSTIC CARCINOMA

- Less than 5% of sinonasal malignancies are ACCs
- Tend to grow slowly

- Early perineurial and vascular spread
- Maxillary sinus is the most commonly affected site
- Patients usually present with long history of facial pain

OLFACTORY NEUROBLASTOMA (AESTHESIONEUROBLASTOMA)

- Arises from ***basal cells*** within the olfactory neuroepithelium
- Less than 5% of all sinonasal malignancies
- *Bimodal distribution with peaks at 20 and 50 years of age*
- More common in women
- Capable of causing paraneoplastic syndromes by secreting peptides
- ***Patients with OAN causing Cushing's syndrome, inappropriate antidiuretic hormone secretion or hypertension produced by vasoactive peptides***
- Typically expresses neuroendocrine markers (neurone specific enolase, synaptophysin and chromogranin) and is negative for keratins
- *Hyams et al. developed a four-point histological grading system for OAN based on such features as the degree of differentiation, the tumor architecture, mitotic index, nuclear polymorphism, fibrillary nature of matrix and tumor necrosis*

Hyams' grading classification of olfactory neuroblastoma

Histological Feature	Grade I	Grade II	Grade III	Grade IV
Architecture	Lobular	Lobular	May be lobular	May be lobuar
Mitoses	Absent	Present	Prominent	Marked
Nuclear pleomorphism	Absent	Present	Prominent	Marked
Neurofibrillary matrix	Prominent	Present	May be present	Absent
Rosettes	Homer-Wright rosettes	Homer-Wight rosettes	Flexner-Wintersteiner rosettes	Flexner-Wintersteiner rosettes
Necrosis	Absent	Absent	Present	Prominent

- **Up to 25% of OAN invade the dura and anterior cranial fossa**
- In 5% of patients metastases to cervical nodes are evident at the time of presentation
- Distant metastases are already present in around 7% of patients

Kadish staging system (with Morita's modification)

Stage	Characteristic
A	Limited to nasal cavity
B	Involving nasal cavity and sinuses
C	Extension beyond nasal and paranasal sinuses cavities
D	Tumor with metastasis to cervical nodes or distant sites

Dulguerov staging system

Stage	
T_1	Tumor involving the nasal cavity or paranasal sinuses (excluding the sphenoid sinus) sparing the most superior ethmoidal cells
T_2	Tumor involving the nasal cavity or paranasal sinuses (including the sphenoid sinus) with extension to or erosion of the cribriform plate

Contd.

Contd.

T_3	Tumor extending into the orbit or protruding into the anterior cranial fossa without dural invasion
T_4	Tumor involving the brain
N_0	No cervical lymph node metastases
N_1	Any form of cervical lymph node metastases
M_0	No metastases
M_1	Any distant metastases

SINONASAL UNDIFFERENTIATED CARCINOMA

- Known as anaplastic carcinoma
- Can be hard to distinguish from high-grade OAN
- It is a highly aggressive and invasive tumor commonly containing areas of necrosis but, paradoxically, often produces few symptoms despite its extensive nature
- ***Typically SNUC is negative for Epstein-Barr virus, helping to distinguish it from WHO Type 3 nasopharyngeal carcinoma***

MELANOMA

- **Accounts for 3.6% of all sinonasal malignancies**
- More common in women than men and tends to affect elderly
- Upto 1/3rd are amelanotic

Nasal cavity and septum are usual sites of origin

- Immunohistochemistry shows positivity for S100 and HMB-45
- Sinonasal melanoma metastasizes less frequently to regional cervical lymph nodes than melanoma that develops elsewhere, but more often to the lungs and brain

HAEMANGIOPERICYTOMA

- Rare neoplasms that develop from pericytes within outer capillary wall
- Account for less than 5% of all sarcomas
- 20% of all head and neck haemangiopericytomas develop in **nasal cavity or sinuses**
- **Associated with steroid therapy, coincidental trauma, hypertension and pregnancy**
- Haemangiopericytomas rarely metastasize
- Complete surgical excision is necessary as they are **relatively radioresistant**
- 10–60% recurrence rate

Clinical Presentation

- Progressive unilateral stuffiness and blockage
- Sinus outflow obstruction
- Bleeding or spot nasal secretions
- Distortion of nose
- Maxillary sinus carcinomas cause facial pain
- Erosion of the medial wall is associated with epistaxis and epiphora
- Spread of a tumor superiorly into the orbit gives rise to proptosis and diplopia
- Destruction of posterior wall and spread into pterygopalatine and infratemporal fossae results in progressive trismus as well as maxillary and mandibular trigeminal nerve deficits

IMAGING

- CT gives accurate detail of bone erosion and potential involvement of the skull base
- Gadolinum enhanced MR imaging provides tumor detail that can include flow voids suggesting intense vascularity, detects dural or cerebral infiltration and give an accurate assessment of orbital invasion
- **FDG positron emission tomography/CT is not usually necessary for staging primary tumor** but may be helpful in excluding distant disease, for example in melanoma, or in identifying a primary site if there is concern that disease is metastatic in nature

BIOPSY

- Helps in tissue diagnosis
- Care should be taken while attempting on vascular neoplasms

TREATMENT

- Patients who present early with T1 maxillary tumors may be cured with surgery alone but **majority of patients will require combination therapy**
- *Multimodality therapy (surgery, radiotherapy and chemotherapy) has generally been demonstrated to be most effective approach in treatment of SCC and SNUC*
- Post-operative radiotherapy should start within 6 weeks of surgery with 60–65 Gy delivered over 30 fractions
- Patients with advanced malignant melanoma may have a significant reduction in local symptoms with debulking surgery and post-operative radiotherapy
- **OAN is treated with a combination of surgery and postoperative radiotherapy**
- ***No role for chemotherapy in the initial treatment of mucosal melanoma, the mainstay of which is surgical resection followed by radiotherapy***
- Topical application of 5-fluorouracil has been used for adenocarcinoma of the ethmoid sinus
- **Involvement of facial skin is likewise not contraindication to treatment–best excised and repaired with either a rotation flap or free flap**

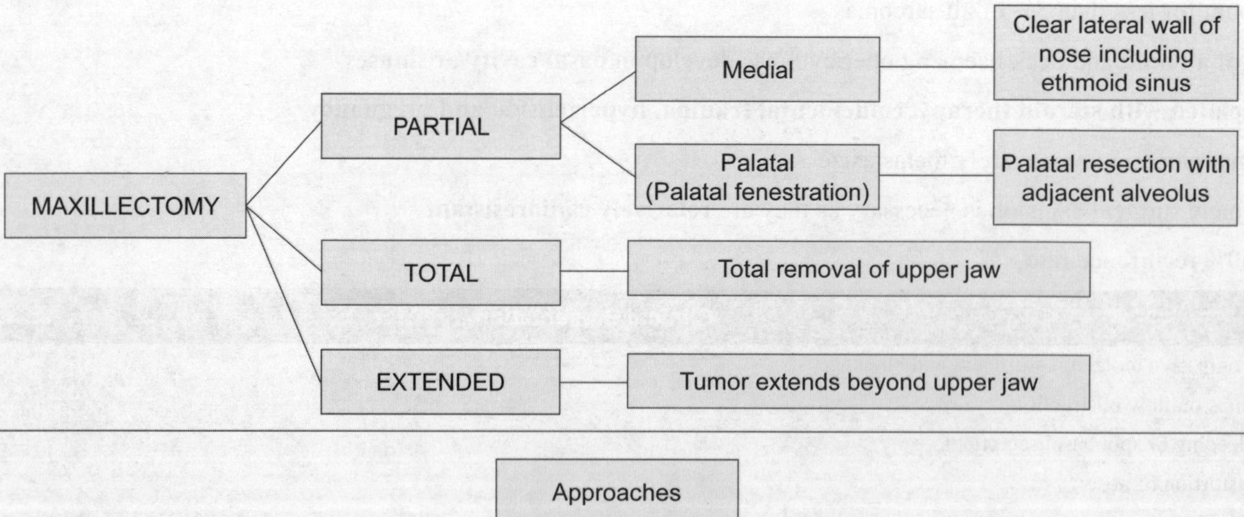

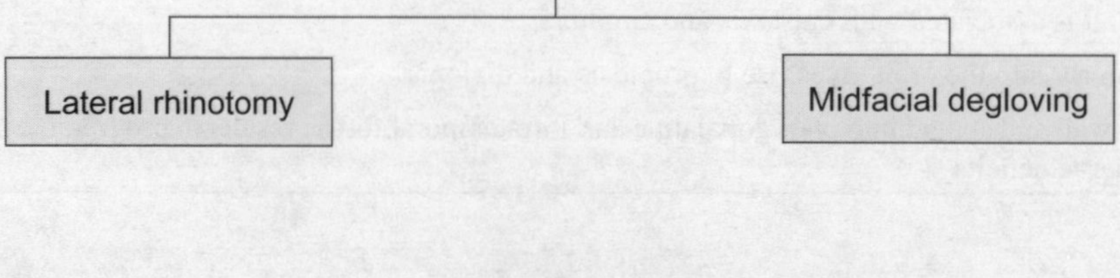

- Maxilla is best exposed by the Weber–Fergusson incision

CHEESMAN AND REDDY CLASSIFICATION

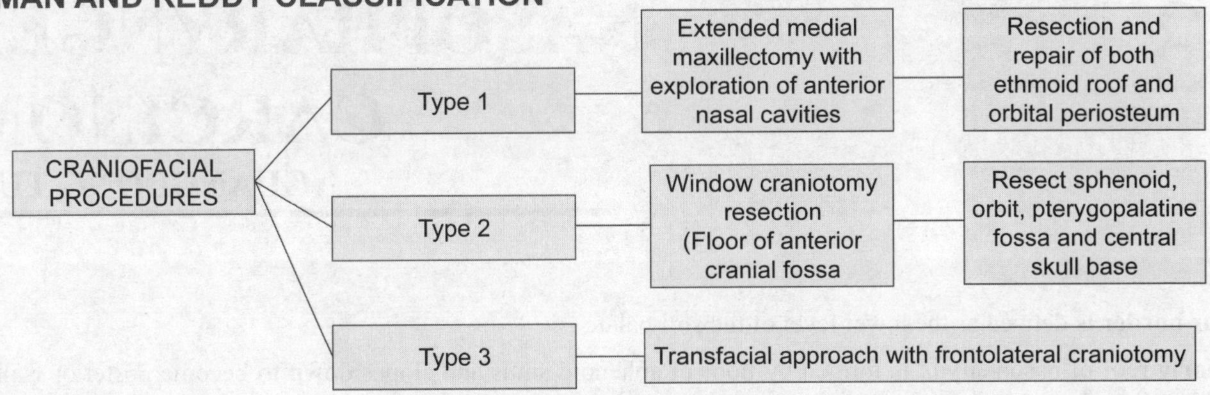

- If there is obvious involvement of the orbital periosteum then exenteration is generally indicated
- Orbital resections leave an obvious cosmetic deformity but titanium implants have revolutionized construction and retention of facial prostheses–**Radiotherapy is not a contraindication to their use**
- Low defects not involving the orbital adnexae can often be successfully treated with dental obturators
- For more extensive maxillary defects a free flap is required
- **Nasomaxillary defects usually require bone to augment loss of nasal bones**
- **Orbitomaxillary cases can be managed with local or soft-tissue free flaps**
- **Unresectable lesions**–Neoadjuvant chemotherapy/CRT

PROGNOSIS

- ***Overall prognosis of sinonasal malignancy is directly related to degree of local control***

Anatomical factors: Location	
Nasal cavity	77
Maxillary sinus	62
Ethmoid sinus	48
Above Ohngren's line	Worse prognosis
Pathological factors: Histological type	
OAN	88
Adenocarcinoma	68
SCC	51
Undifferentiated carcinoma	44
Mucosal melanoma	18
Tumor stage	
T_1	91
T_2	64
T_3	72
T_4	49

- ***Chemoradiotherapy followed by surgery is done for SNUC and advanced ethmoidal SCC***
- Contraindications to aggressive treatment are spread to sphenoid sinus, middle cranial fossa, optic chiasma, cavernous sinus or prevertebral fascia, as well as presence of distant intracranial or systemic metastases

5 Year Survival
• *Best for Olfactory neuroblastoma (>70%)*
• *Worst for Undifferentiated carcinoma (20-40%) and Mucosal melanoma (10-30%)*

CHAPTER 23

NASOPHARYNGEAL CARCINOMA

GUANGDONG TUMOR

- **Inferior border** is defined as the lower level of the soft palate
- **Superiorly** roof of nasopharynx is formed by floor of sphenoid sinus and slopes down to become posterior wall, which is formed by clivus bone

Recess extends posterolaterally on both sides of posterior wall of nasopharynx to form lateral recess of nasopharynx known as fossa of Rosenmüller

- Nasopharynx is covered with pseudostratified squamous epithelium
- Second layer is muscular layer formed by the superior constrictor muscles
- ***Outermost layer of nasopharyngeal wall is pharyngobasilar fascia***
- At upper part of the clivus and roof of nasopharynx, superior constrictor is absent
- Except for the pterygoid plates in the anterior part of the lateral nasopharynx, lateral walls of nasopharynx are devoid of bone
- **1st echelon of lymphatic drainage is retropharyngeal lymph nodes (nodes of Rouvière)**
- Internal carotid artery is located posterolateral to fossa of Rosenmuller and is wrapped by carotid sheath
- **South china–Highest incidence**
- Male to female ratio= 3:1
- Peak age group–50-55 years
- Migrants from high-risk populations who settle in low incidence areas, like Southern Chinese emigrants to North America, have higher incidences than the native population though the incidence reduces in later generations
- Migrants from low incidence areas do not experience an increased risk of NPC even when they emigrate to high incidence areas, like Indian emigrants in Singapore
- ***Caucasian populations have lowest risk***
- **10% has familial clustering**

HLA A2, B14 and B46 are associated with increased risk of NPC while HLA A11, B13 and B22 are associated with lower risk of NPC

- A genome wide association study showed that genes at the 6p21 locus within the HLA region are strongly associated with NPC

Individual HLA subtypes associated with NPC may have impaired immune response to EBV infection and clearance of the virus from epithelium

- ***MDM2 and TP53 and cell-migration gene MMP2 have been shown to be associated with NPC***
- Childhood consumption of salted fish increased incidence of NPC in early adulthood
- Carcinogenic effect of these preserved foods may be due to high nitrosamine content
- Smoking increases risk of NPC development and this risk increase is seen in both low and high incidence populations
- Genetic susceptibility may confer increased risk of a latent EBV infection, while environmental and dietary risk factors may transform the normal nasopharynx epithelium to premalignant stage, supporting the EBV genome in transformed nasopharynx epithelium

WHO Classification:

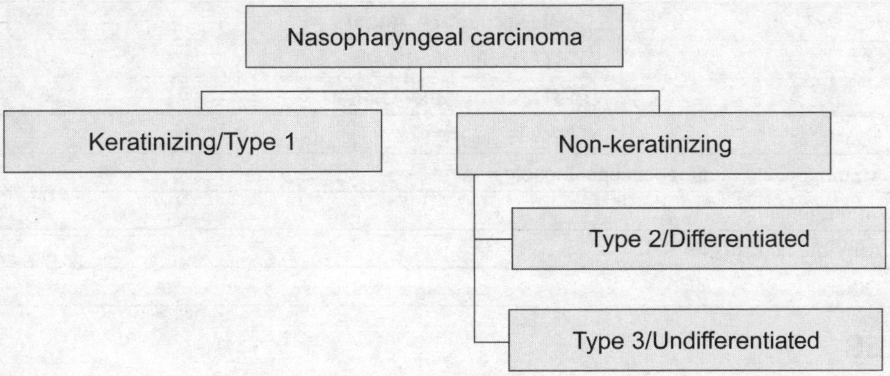

- Immunostaining for EBV in cancer cells can help to differentiate between NPC and different types of head and neck cancer
- Immunostaining for EBV virus encoded small ribonucleic acid (EBER) is commonly used to detect the presence of EBV inside cancer cells
- ***Malignant fibrosarcomas and osteosarcomas are most common form of radiation-induced sarcomas in nasopharynx in NPC patients treated with radiotherapy***–Well differentiated with absent EBV

WHO classification of tumors of the nasopharynx	
I. Epithelial Tumors	
A. Benign	**B. Malignant**
1. Papilloma	1. Nasopharyngeal carcinoma
2. Pleomorphic adenoma	2. Adenocarcinoma
3. Oncocytoma	3. Papillary adenocarcinoma
4. Basal cell adenoma	4. Mucoepidermoid carcinoma
5. Ectopic pituitary adenoma	5. Adenoid cystic carcinoma
	6. Polymorphous low-grade adenocarcinoma
II. Soft Tissue Tumors	
A. Benign	**B. Malignant**
1. Angiofibrama	1. Fibrosarcoma
2. Haemangioma	2. Rhabdomyosarcoma
3. Haemangiopericytoma	3. Angiosarcoma
4. Neurilemmoma	4. Kapoosi's sarcoma
5. Neurofibroma	5. Malignant haemangiopericytoma
6. Paraganglioma	6. Malignant nerve sheath tumor
	7. Synovial sarcoma
III. Tumors of Bone and Cartilage	
IV. Malignant lymphomas	
1. Non-Hodgkin lymphoma	
2. Extramedullary plasmacytoma	
3. Midline malignant reticulosis	
4. Histocytic lymphoma	
5. Hodgkin disease	
V. Miscellaneous tumors	
A. Benign	**B. Malignant**
1. Meningioma	1. Malignant melanoma
2. Craniopharyngioma	2. Chordoma
3. Teratoma	3. Malignant germ cell tumors

Contd.

Contd.

VI. Secondary Tumors
VII. Unclassified Tumors
VIII. Tumor-like Lesions
1. Cysts
2. Meningocoele/meningoencephalocoele
3. Granulomas
4. Amyloid deposits
5. Others

CLINICAL FEATURES

- 50% of the patients have suffered from nasal symptoms
- Most common symptoms are blood stained nasal discharge or post-nasal drip
- Cacosmia or a smell of blood due to bleeding from tumor
- Between 30% and 40% of NPC patients suffer from ear symptom
- An enlarging upper neck mass is the most common symptom
- ***Upto 70% of patients with NPC have enlarged neck lymph nodes on presentation***
- ***One third of patients have bilateral enlarged neck lymph nodes***
- Most frequently involved nodes are level II (upper jugular) and upper level V (apex of posterior triangle)
- ***Isolated enlarged supraclavicular lymph node is almost never a lymph node metastasis from NPC***
- Headache is most common neurological symptom and is present in up to 20% of patients
- ***Involvement of CNIII and CNIV are indicative of cavernous sinus invasion by tumor***
- ***Around 1% of NPC patients develop dermatomvositis as a para-neoplastic syndrome***
- Dermatomyositis can develop concurrently with NPC, late after diagnosis of NPC or months before NPC is clinically and symptomatically apparent
- PET scan can help differentiate between a lung primary and a distant metastasis
- Easy contact bleeding on nasopharyngoscopy is a sign of NPC
- Biopsy under general anaesthesia may be required if multiple deep biopsies are needed to rule in or rule out diagnosis of NPC

AJCC tage classification for NPC			
Primary tumor (T)		**Regional lymph nodes**	
Tx	Primary tumor cannot be assessed	**N1**	Unilateral metastasis, in cervical lymph node(s) and/or unilateral or bilateral metastasis in retropharyngeal lymph nodes, 6 cm or less, above the caudal border of cricoid cartilage
T1	Tumor confined to nasopharynx, or extends to oropharynx and/or nasal cavity without parapharyngeal space involvement	**N2**	Bilateral metastasis in cervical lymph node(s), 6 cm or less above the caudal border of cricoid cartilage
T2	Tumor with extension to parapharyngeal space and/or infiltration of the medial pterygoid, lateral pterygoid, and/or prevertebral muscles	**N3**	Metastasis in cervical lymph node(s) greater than 6 cm in dimension and/or extension below the caudal border of cricoid cartilage
T3	Tumor invades bony structures of skull base cervical vertebra, pterygoid structures, and/or paranasal sinuses		
T4	Tumor with intracranial extension and/or involvement of cranial nerves, hypopharynx, orbit, parotid gland and/or infiltration beyond the lateral surface of the lateral pterygoid muscle		

Contd.

Contd.

Metastatic disease (M)			
M0	No distant metastasis		
M1	Distant metastasis present		

	T1	T2	T3	T4
N0	I	II	III	IV
N1	II			
N2	III			
N3	IV			

INVESTIGATIONS

- Patients with metastatic neck lymph nodes with an unknown primary, persistently raised tumor markers and normal nasopharynx on endoscopy or inconclusive biopsy results will be candidates for GA
- ***Gold standard investigation in diagnosis of NPC is BIOPSY***
- Serum EBV IgG titre signies prior infection by the virus and elevated serum EBV IgM titre indicates recent infection
- **EBV IgA VCA is sensitive but not specific for NPC while EBV IgA EA is specific but not sensitive for detecting NPC**
- Serology has weak correlation with the stage of disease, unable to react the tumor response to therapy and does not show increasing titre in recurrent disease
- **More advanced stage NPC will have a higher tumor load and larger cancer cell turnover**
- Plasma EBV DNA levels can have a prognostic implication–***A high level of EBV DNA before treatment correlates with larger tumor load and more advanced stage of cancer***
- ***Plasma EBV DNA levels rapidly decrease to undetectable or very low levels within 1–2 weeks after completion of treatment***
- Persistently elevated plasma EBV DNA titre after treatment may signify **persistent loco-regional disease or development of distant metastasis** and has been used as a justification for adjuvant chemotherapy
- An initial drop of plasma EBV DNA levels after treatment and a later progressive rise in level may represent tumor recurrence
- Nasopharyngeal brushing for EBV DNA has high sensitivity and specificity of 98.9% and 99.3 respectively

IMAGING

- **MRI is preferred imaging modality for NPC staging and treatment because of its superior soft tissue resolution.**
- MRI can better delineate parapharyngeal extension of tumor, perineural spread and marrow infiltration and can also differentiate between tumor infiltration from retained secretions in the paranasal sinuses, and can define better the limits of the optic chiasma, optic nerves and brainstem
- MRI is more useful than CT in monitoring disease after treatment and imaging recurrent diseases
- Ultrasound combined with fine-needle aspiration cytology can achieve a very high sensitivity and specificity for detection nodal metastasis in NPC
- PET-CT is very useful in assessing residual and recurrent disease after treatment
- PET-CT detects both loco-regional failures and distant failures and is especially recommended in patients with a rising trend of EBV DNA titre after treatment

TREATMENT

- Non-keratinizing subtype of NPC is a very radiosensitive tumor
- Radiotherapy is the mainstay of treatment for primary NPC and surgical treatment is reserved for salvage of radiation failures

- **Stage I and low-risk stage II NPC**–Radical RT alone (Early stage disease)
- **Stage II disease with higher tumor load and stage III, IV disease**–Combination chemotherapy and radiotherapy

- **Gross tumor volume:** GTV includes both primary in NP and for involved neck nodes
- **Clinical target volume:** CTV includes the GTV and covers for subclinical disease spread around NP and neck
  - CTV1 includes GTVs with margin and requires radiation dose of around 70 Gy
  - CTV2 include CTV1 with margin plus areas at risk of microscopic involvement, including entire NP, retropharyngeal nodal regions, skull base, clivus, pterygoid fossae, parapharyngeal space, sphenoid sinus, and posterior part of nasal cavity/maxillary sinuses that includes pterygopalatine fossae atleast 60 Gy
  - A lower dose, 54–60 Gy, may be given for prophylactic irradiation of uninvolved nodal regions
- **Planning target volume:** PTV includes the CTV with a margin to allow for possible errors in daily positioning and treatment of patient during radiotherapy

- In a course of IMRT with 33 fractions over 6.5 weeks, CTV1 may be treated to 70 Gy at 2.12 Gy / fraction while CTV2 can be treated to 66 Gy at 1.82 Gy / fraction
- IMRT has local control rates of over 90%

Pivot Trial
Pivotal Intergroup study 0099 established concurrent cisplatin during RT followed by adjuvant cisplatin and fluorouracil as the standard of care for advanced NPC

- MAC-NPC showed a survival benefit with use of chemotherapy in addition to RT in treatment of NPC
- Distant metastases become the dominant pattern of disease failure in RT patients
- Taxanes and gemcitabine have been found to be useful in treatment of recurrent or metastatic NPC
- Patients with a nasopharyngeal biopsy showing tumor cells at 8 weeks after RT will continue to undergo complete regression by 12 weeks, suggesting that disease should only be considered persistent if biopsy is positive at 12 weeks after radiotherapy
- Most failures occur within 2 years of treatment
- Patients who have persistently enlarged neck lymph nodes 3 months after completion of radiotherapy should be considered to have persistent nodal diseases and offered salvage treatment
- Nasopharyngectomy, is only reserved for salvaging radiation failures
- Tumors that show internal carotid artery encasement, extensive skull base infiltration or intracranial extension are not suitable for salvage surgery
- Transpalatal Approach is extensively used for salvaging NPC local failures
- Radial neck dissection is considered as standard of care for management of nodal failures

- **Transpalatal approach – inferior approach**
- **Transcervico-mandibulo-palatal approach – inferolateral approach**
- **Midfacial degloving approach – anterior approach**
- **Maxillary swing approach – anterolateral approach**
- **Facial translocation approach – anterolateral approach**
- **Lateral skull base approach – lateral approach**

- Spinal accessory nodes are frequently involved in NPC metastasis and together with the high risk of extracapsular spread
- Traditional first-line chemotherapy for metastatic NPC is a combination of cisplatin and 5-fluorouracil and medial overall survival is around 12 months

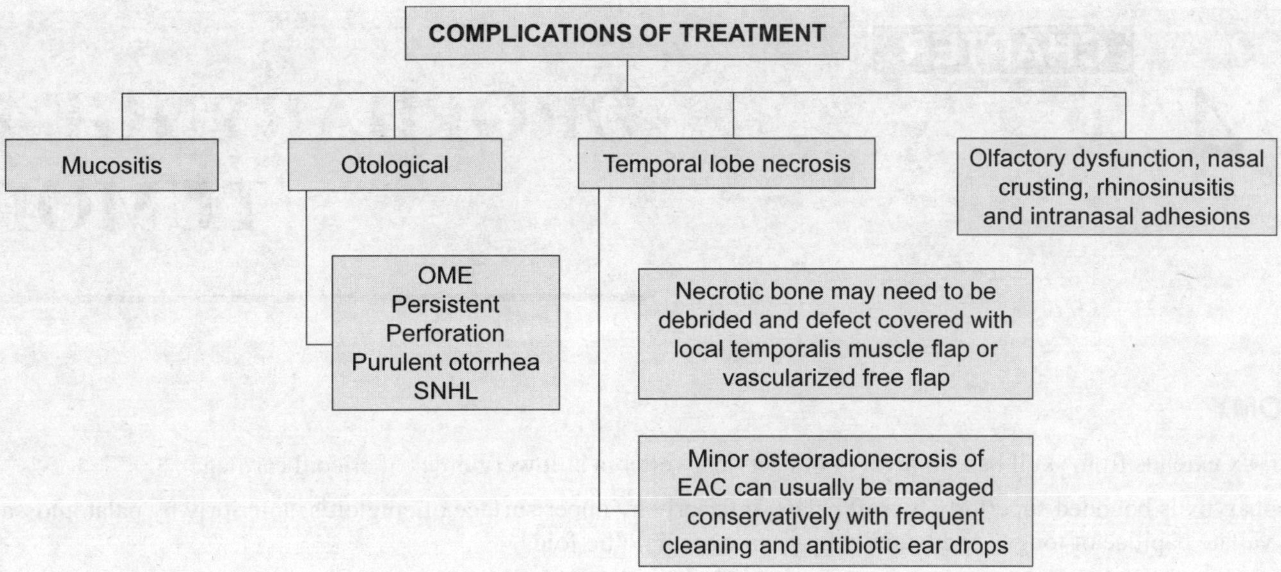

- **Incidence of late complications is around 30%**
- Late dysphagia can affect up to 50% of head and neck cancer patients treated with concurrent chemoradiation and this increase in late dysphagia is also seen in NPC patients
- Radiation-induced malignancies mostly develop beyond 5 years after radiotherapy and occur in around 0.3–3% of patients (rare thyroid malignancy)
- Radiation-induced sarcomas are often of the fibrosarcoma or osteosarcoma subtype and usually occur in patients who have received a high dose of radiation
- Curative resection with clear margins is still the best treatment for radiation-induced malignancies
- **Internal carotid artery aneurysm is a rare life threatening complication after radiotherapy for NPC**–Treatment includes prompt airway control followed by endovascular stenting of internal carotid artery to exclude the aneurysm or ligation of affected internal carotid artery with vascular bypass

CHAPTER 24

OROPHARYNGEAL TUMORS

ANATOMY

- Pharynx extends from skull base to level of 6th cervical vertebra at lower border of cricoid cartilage
- Oropharynx is bounded superiorly by soft palate, inferiorly by upper surface of epiglottis, anteriorly by palatoglossal arches and vallate papillae of tongue and laterally by pharyngoepiglottic folds
- Section of posterior pharyngeal wall included in the oropharynx lies anterior to the vertebral bodies of C2 and C3 and extends from a horizontal line drawn through the hard palate cranially to a horizontal line drawn through the hyoid bone caudally

HISTOLOGY

- Oropharynx is lined with stratified squamous epithelium predominantly non-keratinizing
- Numerous mucous secreting cells as well as minor salivary glands which are most concentrated on oral surface of the soft palate

TUMORS OF OROPHARYNX

- Papillomas are the most common benign tumor of oropharynx

MALIGNANT TUMORS

- **SCC is the most common malignancy presenting in oropharynx**
- Tonsil represent **60%** of all OPSCC tumors
- Base of tongue make up **30%** of all OPSCC tumors
- **Oral surface of soft palate make up 10% of OPSCC.** Soft palate OPSCC presents as a painful ulcerative lesion. Relatively small primary tumors with bilateral cervical lymphadenopathy. More likely to be HPV +ve. Typically behave in a more aggressive fashion with poorer outcomes
- Posterior pharyngeal wall tumors–more likely to be HPV– and typically present late, widespread submucosal spread in all directions
- ***Tumor Fixation as consequence of deep spread to involve prevertebral fascia is a very poor prognostic sign***

LYMPHOMA

- Almost exclusively non-Hodgkin lymphomas
- Arise in lymphoid tissue of the palatine tonsil or BOT
- Usually younger patients (45–55 years)

MINOR SALIVARY GLAND TUMORS

- 6% of all head and neck malignancies
- Hard and soft palate are most common sites for Minor salivary gland cancers
- Surgical resection with adequate surgical margins is primary treatment of choice

- Surgical approach used for Minor salivary gland tumors of oropharynx will **depend on site and size of the mass and the likely functional deficit following resection**
- **Therapeutic neck dissection**→ Clinical or Radiological evidence of **N+**
- **Elective neck dissection** for patients with no evidence of N+ → **Advanced stage or high-grade tumors** (mucoepidermoid carcinoma and adenocarcinoma)

- T3 or T4 tumors, close or involved resection margins, high-grade, perineural/perivascular invasion and N+ disease–**Post op RT**
- ***Inoperable disease, or who refuse surgery→ Primary RT***

Role of HPV in Oropharyngeal Malignancies

- Non-enveloped and circular double-stranded DNA genome
- HPV specifically genotype 16 is independent, risk factor for OPSCC
- ***Increased 8-fold in sexually active individuals***
- Increased with the number of lifetime sexual partners (vaginal or oral) and with recent sexual activity with highest prevalence (>20%) seen in patients reporting >20 lifetime sexual partners

6-20% Oral SCC
20-30% Larynx, NP, PNS
90% Oropharyngeal–HPV+ve

- Usually affects tonsils and BOT
- **Men > Women**
- **Whites > Blacks**
- High socio economic status
- Improved performance and less comorbidities
- Younger, Non-keratinizing, well differentiated, basaloid type with central necrosis

More likely non-smokers
Less commonly heavy alcohol use
More likely Marijuana use

- Increased radiosensitivity
- No tobacco exposure
- Reduced field cancerization and 2nd primary tumors
- **Small primary and Advanced nodal stage**
- HPV E6 and E7 is strongly associated with diagnosis of OPSCC
- ***pRb exerts its influence in late G1***
- EGFR, P53, Surviving is inversely proportional to survival
- ***Advanced primary and nodal stage is associated with reduced salvage and increased distant failure***
- **HPV OPSCC can also present with Cystic nodal metastasis**
- EGFR→ >90% HNSCC
- Low EGFR and High p16→ Surrogate markers for HPV +ve

Low risk	HPV+, <10 Pack years, **N0/N2a** (Platinum CRT)
Intermediate risk	HPV+, >10 Pack years, **N2b/N3**
	HPV-, <10 Pack years, **T2/T3**
High risk	HPV-, <10 Pack years, **T4**
	HPV-, >10 Pack years, **Any stage**

- **HPV-16 DNA** is found in ~50% of oral rinses provided by patients with diagnosed OPSCC and patients with OPSCC are 12 times more likely than patients without OPSCC to have an oral HPV infection, a risk which increases 15-fold when HPV-16 infection alone is considered
- Tobacco use is associated with an increased risk of HPV+OPSCC and Oral HPV infection
- Majority of patients presenting with HPV+OPSCC are still current or past smokers

Contd.

Contd.

HPV-SCCs are typically moderately differentiated and keratinizing tumors arising from dysplastic epithelium

HPV-associated tumors are non-keratinizing, display poorly differentiated predominantly basaloid morphology, are not associated with surface dysplasia but are associated with a high level of tumor infiltrating lymphocytes (TILs)

E1 and E2 are regulatory genes, controlling transcription of the remaining genes

E5–7 are involved in host-cell transformation, and are therefore potentially oncogenic

L1 and L2 are structural proteins necessary for the formation of the viral capsids

- Proteasomal degradation of tumor suppressor protein RB as a consequence of binding by HPV oncoprotein E7 in association with the cullin 2 ubiquitin ligase complex
- Interaction between E7 and p27 resulting in inhibition of cell-cycle arrest
- Interaction between E7 and p21 resulting in inhibition of cell-cycle arrest
- Proteasomal degradation of p53 TSP as a consequence of binding by HPV oncoprotein E6 in association with the ubiquitin ligase E6AP
- Increased expression of p16INK4A as a result of loss of E2F repression which in turn results from RB degradation
- E6 and E6AP degradation of NFX1 resulting in loss of repression of hTERT and consequent reduction in telomere erosion thereby contributing to development of cellular immortality

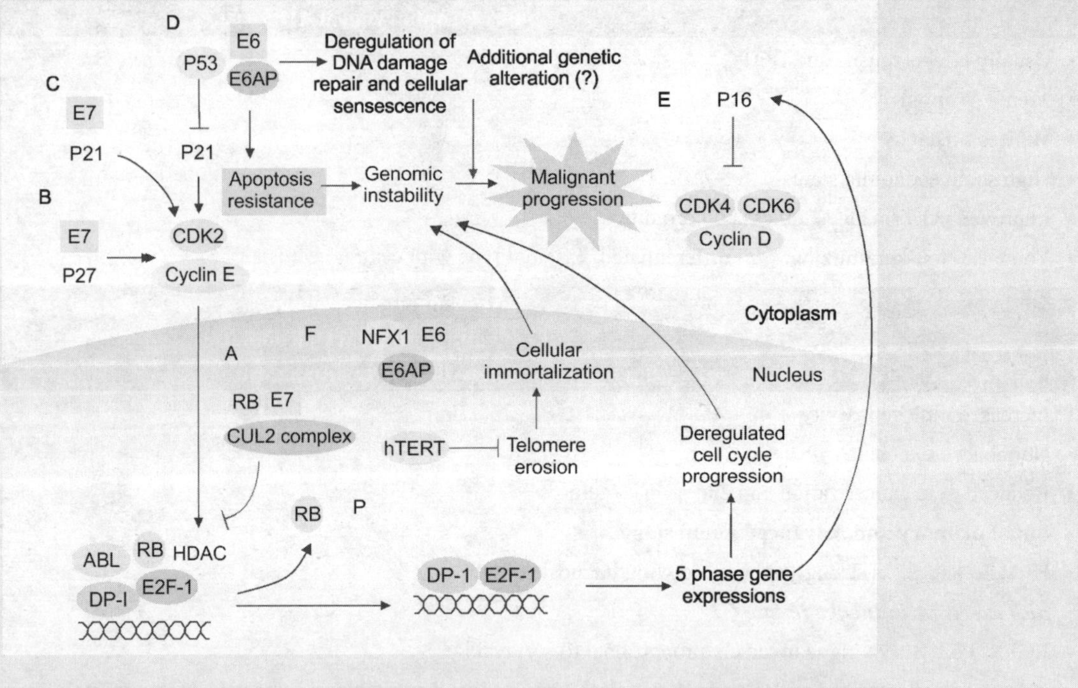

- **Direct detection of E6 and E7 Transcription–Quantitative Reverse transcription PCR→** Current gold standard assay for determining HPV biological activity
- Surrogate marker most often used to detect HPV induced transformation in oropharynx is overexpression of p16INK4a using immunohistochemistry

IN SITU HYBRIDIZATION

- A positive test result is confirmed by the presence of a blue dot under light microscopy
- Allows localization of the HPV DNA to host cell nucleus
- Punctate staining pattern is suggestive of HPV DNA integration

HPV associated SCCHN p16INK4a is typically intact

- P16 overexpression correlates well with clinical outcome and has low specificity for HPV infection

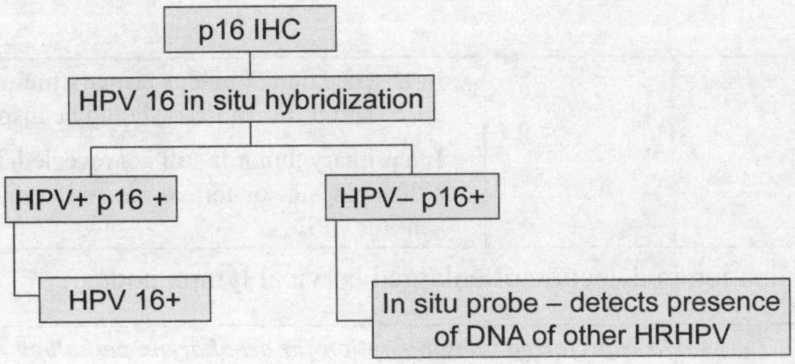

CLINICAL PRESENTATION

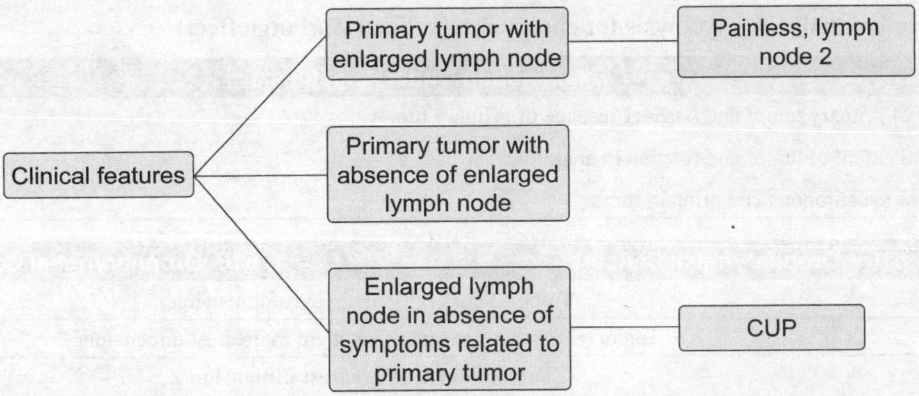

- HPV+OPSCC typically presents with a small primary tumor with multiple, enlarged, cystic cervical lymph nodes with a high prevalence of extracapsular spread
- HPV-OPSCC presents as a more typical head and neck cancer with larger primary tumors and relatively lower tumor burden in cervical lymph nodes

- Ulcerative lesions may be relatively small, present initially with sensation of sore throat with odynophagia
- Larger lesions particularly of the BOT, posterior pharyngeal wall and tonsil may present with continuous pain exacerbated on swallowing and associated with referred otalgia and even dysphagia

Clinically Evident Primary tumor and Enlarged Cervical Node	**USG both sides of neck→ USG guided FNAC** CT/MRI neck CT/PET CT thorax and abdomen (Absence of lung and liver disease) Examination under anesthesia (Upper aerodigestive tract) and Biopsy
Clinically Evident Primary tumor and Absence of Enlarged Cervical Node	CT/MRI neck CT/PET CT thorax and abdomen (Absence of lung and liver disease) Examination under anesthesia (Upper aerodigestive tract) and Biopsy
Clinically occult primary with clinically N+ (CUP)	• **USG both sides of neck→ USG guided FNAC** • HPV testing of FNAC Specimen • CT/MRI neck–absence of obvious primary tumor on clinical examination • CT/PET CT thorax and abdomen (Absence of lung and liver disease) • Examination under anesthesia (UADT) and Biopsy ↓ • MRI/CT head and neck doesn't delineate likely primary tumor, **Whole body PET-CT scan** is investigation of choice as has greater sensitivity for detecting primary tumor site • **PET CT fails→ EUA to examine BOT and Tonsil**

Contd.

Contd.

	• In absence of an obvious primary tumor of tonsil or BOT, ipsilateral post nasal space and piriform fossa should be inspected • If a primary tumor is still not revealed, atleast I/L tonsil should be removed and either biopsies or formal mucosectomy of I/L BOT should be performed and sent for HPE

- USS is more sensitive than palpation in detection of enlarged cervical lymph nodes

MRI is preferred imaging option for oropharynx pathology

- PET-CT has a relatively low specificity with a high false-positive rate
- Cancer cells rely preferentially on glycolysis for energy production (Warburg effect)

Examination Under Anesthesia
• Diagnostic biopsy of primary tumor and Assess Presence of primary tumor • Assess locoregional extent of tumor and relation to anatomical structures • Exclude presence of synchronous 2nd primary tumor

<table>
<tr><th></th><th>p16 + Oropharyngeal Cancers</th><th>p16- Oropharyngeal Cancers</th></tr>
<tr><td>T1</td><td colspan="2">Tumor 2 cm or less in greatest dimension</td></tr>
<tr><td>T2</td><td colspan="2">Tumor >2 cm but not more than 4 cm in greatest dimension</td></tr>
<tr><td>T3</td><td colspan="2">Tumor >4 cm in greatest dimension
OR
Extension to lingual surface of epiglottis</td></tr>
<tr><td>T4</td><td>Tumor invades Larynx, Deep extrinsic tongue muscles, Medial pterygoid, Mandible and Hard palate
Lateral pterygoid, Pterygoid plates, Lateral nasopharynx, Skull base, Encases carotid</td><td>T4a: Larynx, deep extrinsic muscles of tongue, medial pterygoid, mandible and hard palate
T4b: Lateral pterygoid, pterygoid plates, lateral nasopharynx, skull base; or encases the carotid artery</td></tr>
</table>

<table>
<tr><th colspan="2">Clinical N Stage for HPV P16+ Oropharyngeal Cancer</th></tr>
<tr><td>N0</td><td>No regional lymph nodes metastases</td></tr>
<tr><td>N1</td><td>1/more I/L lymph nodes none larger than 6 cm</td></tr>
<tr><td>N2</td><td>C/L or B/L lymph nodes none larger than 6 cm</td></tr>
<tr><td>N3</td><td>Lymph nodes > 6 cm</td></tr>
<tr><td>pN1</td><td>Metastasis in 4 or fewer lymph nodes</td></tr>
<tr><td>pN2</td><td>Metastasis in more than 4 lymph nodes</td></tr>
</table>

<table>
<tr><th colspan="6">Staging of HPV P16+ Oropharyngeal Cancer</th></tr>
<tr><td></td><td>N0</td><td>N1</td><td>N2</td><td>N3</td><td>M1</td></tr>
<tr><td>T1/T2</td><td colspan="2">I</td><td>II</td><td rowspan="2">III</td><td rowspan="3">IV</td></tr>
<tr><td>T3</td><td colspan="3">II</td></tr>
<tr><td>T4</td><td colspan="4">III</td></tr>
</table>

- **T1-T2 N0:** Radical radiotherapy or transoral surgery and neck dissection (with post-operative (chemo) radiotherapy if there are adverse pathological features on histology)

Early stage T1-T2 N0-N1 OPSCC can be effectively treated with RT alone
Advanced T and/or N stage (stage III/IV) OPSCC, CRT is standard of care

- **Other stages:** Primary CRT or surgery and adjuvant (chemo) radiotherapy
- **GORTEC 94-01** study demonstrated a ≥ 20% 3 - and 5-year survival benefit for addition of chemotherapy to RT, albeit in the setting of low overall survival figures

- ***Cisplatin: Weekly low dose–better compliance and Low toxicity***
- ***If cisplatin contraindicated–Carboplatin***
- ***If platinum resistant then concurrent cetuximab***

- Radical RT may be given alone for patients with advanced disease who are not fit for concurrent treatment, particularly if >70 years of age when the benefits of concurrent chemotherapy and cetuximab are reduced
- IC/NACT had a relatively more pronounced effect on distant metastasis rate than concurrent CRT

Gross tumor volume (GTV): Primary tumor (GTVp) and involved lymph nodes (GTVn)
CTV1 includes a 1 cm isotropic margin around primary and nodal GTVs and whole of involved nodal level in neck
CTV2 (Intermediate dose CTV): An optional volume which may include the whole involved nodal level in neck (if not included in CTV1) and/or an additional isotropic margin around CTV1
CTV3 (Prophylactic dose CTV): Includes 'at risk' nodal levels. For node –ve OPSCC, this typically includes levels II–IVa. For node +ve OPSCC, this typically includes levels Ib–V(b or c)
Planning target volume (PTV): A margin (typically 3–5 mm) that is automatically added by the planning system to ensure the CTV is adequately covered on every day of treatment
Organs at risk, including the spinal cord, brainstem, parotid glands and swallowing related structures are also outlined and also given a planning margin called **Planning risk volume (PRV)**

- Key late toxicity affecting QOL is swallowing dysfunction
- ***CRT increases the risk of late toxicity***
- Minimum dose of 57.6 Gy to the primary site with up to 63 Gy to areas of ECS
- Prophylactic treatment for microscopic disease was established by study showing that dose of 50 Gy in 25 fractions was sufficient to control microscopic disease in > 90% of cases

Indications for Port/CRT

- **Primary tumor factors:** Close (1–5 mm) or positive (<1 mm) margins, T3–4 stage, perineural and/or LVSI
- **Nodal factors:** ECS of nodal disease and/or N2-N3 nodal stage

Transoral Surgery

- Most tonsil tumors considered amenable to TLM are T2 in size

TORS

- Extension to the parapharyngeal space and pterygoid musculature are relative contraindications to procedure. ***Retropharyngeal location of ICA is also a contraindication for this procedure***
- Tumor extending across midline of tongue base is a contraindication for the procedure
- Increasing age (>55 years) and extent of TORS resection predicted need for gastrostomy tube and high T stage (pT3/pT4) predicted need for permanent tube feeding
- Patients with T3-4 OPSCCs, which are not transorally resectable, should undergo primary CRT as the standard of care

MANAGEMENT OF NECK

- Prevalence of micrometastatic nodal disease in OPSCC patients presenting without clinical/radiological evidence of nodal disease is estimated to be 10-30%→ ***Elective Neck Dissection***
- Risk of PCF is extremely small, especially if lymph node level I is not dissected
- TORS planned for primary resection then the neck dissection to be carried out as a staged procedure some 2 weeks prior to the primary resection. This is primarily recommended as a strategy to reduce the rate of pharyngocutaneous fistula (PCF)

Lateralized Tumor
Tumor confined to the tonsillar fossa/lateral pharyngeal wall extending onto or into adjacent BOT and/or soft palate by <1 cm and with >1 cm clearance from midline
Non-Lateralized Tumor
Tonsillar/lateral pharyngeal wall tumor that involves adjacent BOT and/or soft palate by ≥1 cm or with ≤ 1 cm clearance from midline

- PD-1 blockade may have a discriminatory advantage in patients with HPV+OPSCC in the recurrent / metastatic setting.

PATHOS TRAIL

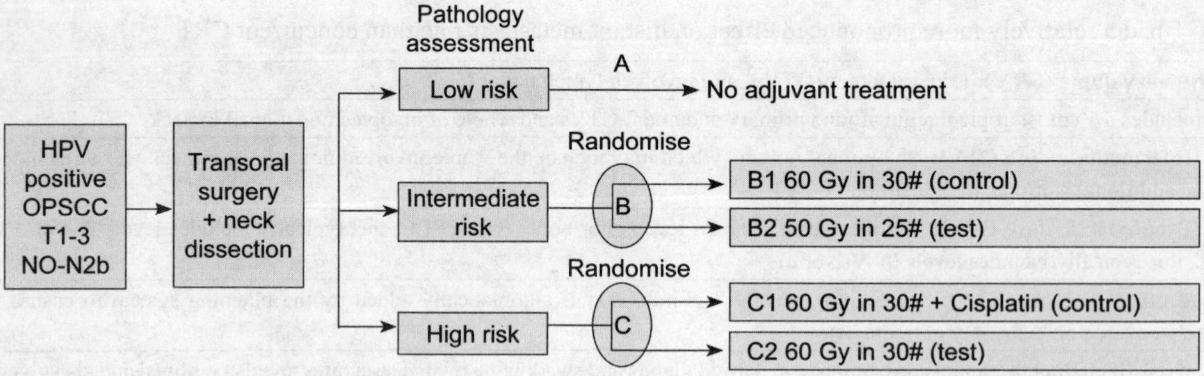

CHAPTER 25

HYPOPHARYNGEAL TUMORS

- Also called as Laryngopharynx
- Extending from the hyoid bone to lower margin of the cricoid cartilage
- Lies below and behind base of tongue and larynx
- Less than 0.5% of all cancers and 3–5% of head and neck cancers
- ***More than 50 years of age***
- Most common site of origin–Pyriform sinus

Post cricoid cancers are predominant in females

- Most common cancer is SCC

PYRIFORM SINUS

- Funnel shaped lateral channel on either side of larynx beginning at level of pharyngoepiglottic fold
- ***Laterally bound by thyrohyoid membrane and medially by aryepiglottic fold***

Pyriform Apex

- Junction of medial and lateral walls, deep and inferior within pyriform sinus
- **Laterally**–Thyroid cartilage
- **Medially**–Cricoid cartilage
- **Inferior** to Paraglottic space
- Pyriform apex tumors lie close proximity to cricoid cartilage. So they should be removed for oncological considerations
- Tumors from the pyriform apex can also escape via cricothyroid membrane early on beyond the laryngeal framework and need careful evaluation

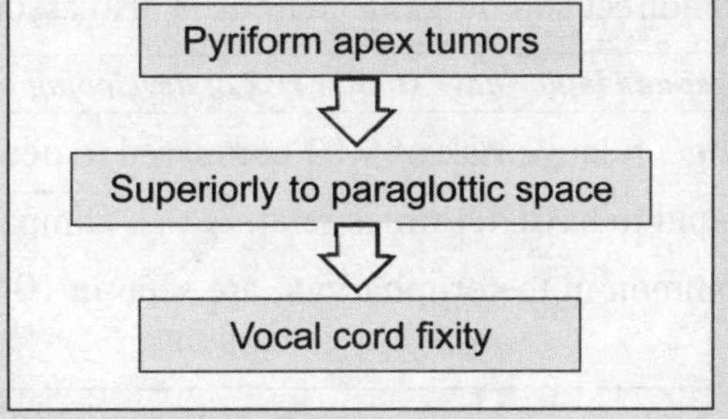

POST CRICOID

- Lies behind larynx and is located below level of the arytenoid cartilages and extends to inferior border of the cricoid cartilage
- Continues below into cricopharynx which lies at upper end of oesophagus

Often involve cricoarytenoid joints causing vocal cord fixity and/or aspiration

POSTERIOR PHARYNGEAL WALL

- Part of the hypopharynx between the lateral walls of pyriform sinuses extend from the hyoid above to the level of the arytenoids below
- Separated from the prevertebral muscles by prevertebral fascia

HISTOLOGY

Layers of hypopharynx

- Non-keratinized stratified squamous epithelium
- Pharyngobasilar fascia
- Muscular layer
- Buccopharyngeal fascia

> ***Blood supply***
> *Superior thyroid arteries along with collaterals from lingual and ascending pharyngeal vessels*

- Motor and sensory supply is provided by pharyngeal plexus, formed by branches of glossopharyngeal and vagus nerves

> ***Vagus nerve via Arnolds nerve provides sensory innervation of external auditory canal and is responsible for referred otalgia in hypopharyngeal cancers***

LYMPHATIC SUPPLY

- Pyriform sinuses drain to deep cervical chain – Jugulodigastric and Jugulo-omohyoid
- Pyriform sinus apex as well as postcricoid area drain into the paratracheal nodes
- Posterior pharyngeal wall drains into retropharyngeal nodes

ETIOLOGY

- Predominantly associated with tobacco and alcohol usage
- Air-cured tobacco is associated with a higher risk than Flue-cured one of developing laryngopharyngeal cancer

> ***Early initiation of smoking and increase in number of cigarettes consumed per day increases cancer risk***

- Smoking cessation is important as it decreases risk of developing head and neck cancers
- Alcohol consumption with direct and indirect carcinogenic actions is also associated with hypopharyngeal cancers

> ***Wine, beer and liquor have similar risk of developing head neck cancers***

- Heavy drinkers (> 4 drinks/day) having a relative risk of 9.03 compared to occasional or non-drinkers
- Consuming dark liquors have been found to have 4.4 times relative risk compared to light liquors
- HPV related cancers, though more common in the oropharynx, are seen in 10.9% of hypopharyngeal cancers with pyriform fossa having the highest association

> ***Lower BMI (< 18.5) is associated with a greater risk of developing hypopharyngeal cancers***

- Meat and fried food intake seem to increase risk of developing hypopharyngeal cancers
- ***Construction workers, potters, butchers, barbers and those exposed to formalin fumes, coal dust, steel dust, iron compounds and fumes are at a higher risk of developing hypopharyngeal carcinoma***

> ***p53 overexpression was seen in 66% of hypopharyngeal tumors***

- Cyclin D1 overexpression correlates with advanced clinical stage, tumor extension and relapse prediction after primary radiotherapy and survival

- **Ki-67**→marker of cell proliferation, is indicative of poor survival

> ***Cyclin D1 has independent prognostic value for cancer-specific survival***

- Hypopharyngeal cancers–moderately or poorly differentiated tumors especially in pyriform sinus

Local Spread

- Pyriform sinus
  - Lateral wall of pyriform sinus
    - Invades thyroid cartilage
  - Medial wall of pyriform sinus
    - Extend anteromedially into paraglottic space
      - Impaired vocal cord movement
  - Apex of pyriform sinus
    - Paraglottic spread and Vocal cord fixity
    - Escape through cricothyroid membrane and involves thyroid gland

- Post cricoid
  - Cricoid and tracheal cartilages
    - Airway obstruction
  - Posterior cricoarytenoid and cricoarytenoid joint
    - Vocal cord fixity and Aspiration
  - Exolaryngeal spread through Cricothyroid membrane to involve thyroid gland
  - Anterolateral spread from predominantly submucous infiltrative postcricoid cancer may present with swelling in region of thyroid and may be misdiagnosed as goitre
  - Inferiorly to Esophagus

- Posterior pharyngeal wall tumors
  - Invades prevertebral fascia
  - Superiorly to base of tonsil
  - Laterally to oropharyngeal wall
  - Inferiorly to postcricoid and cervical esophagus

Regional Spread

- Highest propensity for early lymph nodal metastases

Upto 70% of patients may have lymph nodal metastases

- High incidence of occult nodal metastases
- Level VI metastases are more common in lesions involving post-cricoid or pyriform sinus apex
- Retropharyngeal nodes can be involved in posterior pharyngeal wall cancers

> ***Patients have unilateral clinically positive neck disease, the incidence of contralateral occult lymph node metastases is at least 50%***

- Bilateral occult lymph node metastases in patients with clinically negative neck are most frequently associated with cancers of the pyriform sinus
- Cinically positive neck disease, more than 20% have involvement of the lower nodal stations (level IV and V)

Distant Spread
• Among all head and neck cancers, ***hypopharyngeal primaries*** have highest incidence of distant metastases at presentation (17–24%) and during follow-up, with more than 50% of failures due to distant metastases
• Pulmonary metastases are most common metastases

CLINICAL FEATURES

- ***Usually detected late and Elderly males***
- ***Earliest symptom–mild nonspecific throat discomfort***
- Dysphagia to solid food may be an early presentation in post-cricoid cancers, but is generally seen late in pyriform cancers
    - ***Significant weight loss is especially seen in post-cricoid area and oesophageal tumors***
    - ***Hoarseness of voice may be a late presentation in pyriform and post-cricoid cancers while 'hot potato' speech signifies involvement of the base of the tongue***
    - Loss of laryngeal crepitus ***(Trotter's sign)*** and restriction of neck extension may imply involvement of prevertebral fascia
- Pooling of saliva may obscure the growth especially in pyriform cancers–***JACKSON SIGN***

INVESTIGATIONS

- Barium oesophagogram is an effective screening tool for hypopharyngeal cancers and synchronous cancers in oesophagus
- CT imaging has higher sensitivity for defining T stage of primary tumor (size of tumor, relationship to critical deep structures)

Cartilage Invasion
• MRI is more sensitive than CT
• First imaging of choice–CECT
• Chest X-ray–Screening for distant metastasis
• CT chest–All patients with advanced stage tumors and/or bulky neck disease

- FDG PET/ CECT is a useful imaging modality in assessment of laryngeal and hypopharyngeal cancers, especially in postradiation residual/recurrent disease

Primary tumor	
T1	Tumor limited to one subsite of hypopharynx and/or 2 cm or less in greatest dimension
T2	Tumor invades more than one subsite of hypopharynx or an adjacent site, or measures more than 2 cm but not more than 4 cm in greatest dimension without fixation of hemilarynx
T3	Tumor more than 4 cm in greatest dimension or with fixation of hemilarynx or extension to oesophagus
T4a	Moderately advanced local disease Tumor invades thyroid/cricoid cartilage, hyoid bone, thyroid gland, or central compartment soft tissue (includes prelaryngeal strap muscles)
T4b	Very advanced local disease Tumor invades prevertebral fascia, encases carotid artery, or involves mediastinal structures

Regional lymph nodes (N)	
N0	No regional lymph node metastasis
N1	Metastasis in a single ipsilateral lymph node, 3 cm or less in greatest dimension without extranodal extesion
N2a	Metastasis in a single ipsilateral lymph node, more than 3 cm but not more than 6 cm in gratest dimension without extranodal extension
N2b	Multiple ipsilateral lymph nodes, none more than 6 cm in greatest dimension without extranodal extension
N2c	Bilateral or contralateral lymph nodes, none more than 6 cm in greatest dimension without extranodal extension
N3a	Metastasis in a lymph node, more than 6cm in greatest dimension without extranodal extension
N3b	Metastasis in a single or multiple lymph nodes with clinical extranodal extension*

<table>
<tr><th></th><th>T1</th><th>T2</th><th>T3</th><th>T4a</th><th>T4b</th></tr>
<tr><td>N0</td><td>I</td><td>II</td><td>III</td><td rowspan="3">IVA</td><td rowspan="4">IVB</td></tr>
<tr><td>N1</td><td colspan="3">III</td></tr>
<tr><td>N2</td><td colspan="3">IVA</td></tr>
<tr><td>N3</td><td colspan="4">IVB</td></tr>
<tr><td>M1</td><td colspan="5">IVC</td></tr>
<tr><td colspan="6">Presence of skin involvement or soft tissue invasion with deep fixation / tethering to underlying muscle or adjacent structures or clinical signs of nerve involvement is classified as clinical extranodal extension
Midline nodes are considered ipsilateral nodes</td></tr>
</table>

- ***Squamous cell cancers are biologically more aggressive in hypopharynx due to its rich vascularity and lack of barriers to the spread of tumor***
- Uniquely have substantial submucosal spread well beyond mucosal limits of tumor and are seen up to 20 mm
- Submucosal spread–60% ***(Most commonly inferior)***

Hypopharynx is rich in lymphatics with a high incidence of metastasis to jugular paratracheal and retropharyngeal group of lymph nodes even in early stages of disease which may result in nodal disease as primary manifestation in 65% to 80% and occult metastasis in 30% to 40% of N0 necks

- *More than 75% of patients present in advanced stages III and IV*

Early Hypopharyngeal Cancers

- Treatment of T1 and T2 hypopharyngeal cancers can be with either radiation therapy or conservation surgery
- ***Tumors involving pyriform apex/post-cricoid area and those with poor pulmonary function should not be considered as candidates for partial pharyngolaryngectomy***

Laryngeal conservation surgery–Early hypopharyngeal lesions

Conventional external approach
- Tumors <4 cm (T1–T2)
- Pyriform apex and post-cricoid mucosa free of disease
- Mobile vocal cords
- No erosion of the thyroid cartilage
- No paraglottic spread

Transoral approach
- Tumors less than 4 cm (T1–T2)
- Pyriform apex and post-cricoid mucosa free of disease
- Good exposure
- Mobile vocal cords

CONTRAINDICATIONS
- Oral submucous fibrosis
- Full thickness involvement of pharyngeal muscles
- Thyroid cartilage involvement
- Base tongue and arytenoid involvement
- Cervical oesophagus involvement

Partial Pharyngectomy

- Tumor arises on pharyngeal component of hypopharynx and spares medial wall of pyriform sinus and apex

Partial Pharyngolaryngectomy

- Tumor arises on medial wall of pyriform sinus and extends onto supraglottic structures of larynx
- Partial pharyngectomy can be either an extended supraglottic partial laryngectomy or supracricoid hemilaryngo-pharyngectomy

Resection of the hemilarynx above level of the cricoid and medial aspect of pyriform sinus and ipsilateral supraglottic structures

Transoral Approach

Translaser microsurgery–Elderly and COPD patients also

Transoral robotic surgery (TORS)–Da Vinci robotic system

Transoral videoendoscopic surgery (TOVS)

Advantages of Transoral Over Open Approach

Avoid disruption of laryngeal skeleton and soft tissues, Avoid tracheostomy, Preservation of innervations, Prevention of Oro-cervical fistula formation

Reconstruction

- Pharyngeal defect is reconstructed with either pectoralis myocutaneous flap or free flap usually radial forearm flap
- Incidence of distant metastasis increases as local control rates improve
- Survival is better in patients with T1 disease, those with good surgical margins and in those receiving post-operative radiation
- **Level VI metastasis** confirmed by histopathological analysis, close ***(<5 mm)*** histologic margins, advanced nodal stage and posterior pharyngeal wall tumors were significant independent factors associated with poor disease-specific survival

Management of Neck

- Patients with pT1N0 tumors are either followed up with wait and watch policy for neck with regular US every 2–3 months in the first 2 years, then every 6 months or undergo ipsilateral selective neck dissection of levels II, III and IV

Adjuvant Radiotherapy

- Positive margins, where re-resection is not suitable and for metastatic neck node disease

- 5-year local control rates of 90% for T1 cancers and 80% for T2 lesions with radiotherapy
- Synchronous or metachronous cancers developed in 56.5%
- Early hypopharyngeal cancers tend to have a good prognosis with RT

ADVANCED HYPOPHARYNGEAL CANCERS

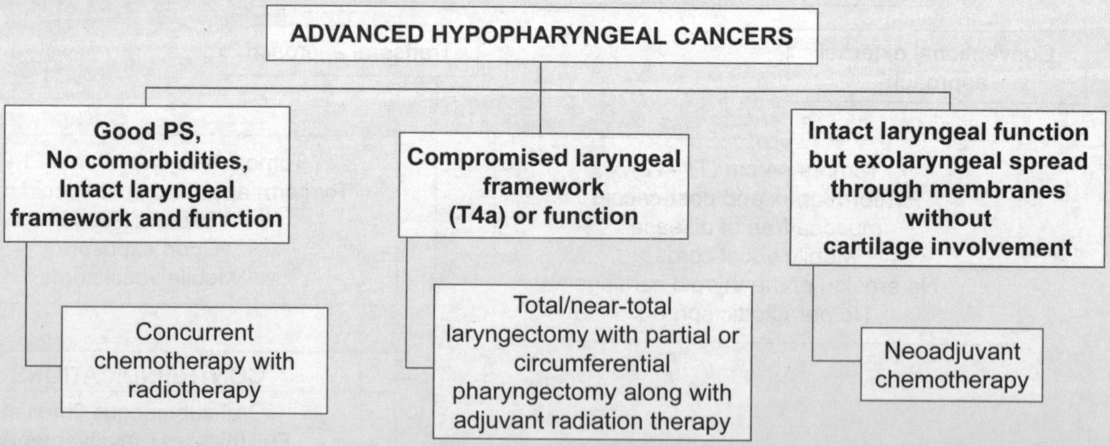

Surgery for Advanced Hypopharyngeal Cancer

Indications	Contraindications
Good general condition Compromised laryngeal function Involved laryngeal framework Salvage surgery following radiation or concurrent chemoradiation	**Poor general condition** **Disease extension:** Involvement of root neck, Prevertebral involvement presents with inability to extend the neck and absence of laryngeal crackle, Superior extension into oropharynx, Lateral extension involving carotid artery **Metastatic disease**

Contd,

Contd.

Near Total Laryngectomy with Partial Pharyngectomy

- **Indications:** Advanced but lateralized hypopharyngeal cancers where ***lesion does not involve post-cricoid mucosa or the interarytenoid region;*** contralateral vocal cord and arytenoid can be preserved and used to form a biological shunt between trachea and neopharynx
- NTLP offers preservation of excellent lung powered speech and may be suitable in almost 20% of advanced, operable, pyriform cancers

Contraindications

- ***Interarytenoid or post-cricoid involvement,*** which makes preservation of contralateral arytenoids oncologically unsafe
- ***Mucosal involvement of more than one-third length of the contralateral cord.*** This does not allow preservation of sufficient laryngeal remnant for shunt formation
- ***Prior radiation therapy is a relative contraindication*** especially if tissues are oedematous

Total laryngectomy with partial pharyngeal resection	Hypopharyngeal lesions involving the inter-arytenoid and post-cricoid mucosa
Total laryngectomy with circumferential pharyngeal resection	Hypopharyngeal lesions involving the postcricoid mucosa where there is no option of preserving any pharyngeal mucosa
Total laryngo-pharyngo-oesophagectomy	Post-cricoid/Hypopharyngeal lesions extending beyond cricopharynx

MANAGEMENT OF NECK

- **Manifest nodes (N1-N3)**
  - Bilateral neck dissection (Level 2-5)
- **Advanced primary (T3/T4)**
  - Bilateral neck dissection (Level 2-4)

Reconstruction

- If the width is <3 cm unstretched or remnant pharynx is not pliant and oedematous a reconstruction should be considered
  - ***Propulsion of the bolus with pharyngeal muscle approximation is more effective***
  - ***Amount of bolus swallowed is better with only mucosal closure***

RECONSTRUCTION OF PHARYNX

- **Partial pharyngeal defects**
  - **Radial artery free flap**
  - **Anterolateral thigh flap**
- **Circumferential defects**
  - **Free jejunal graft**
  - **Free anterolateral thigh–** *High success*
  - **Free radial forearm flap**
- **Gastric pull up**
  - **Following TLPE**
  - Reliable, single-stage vascularized reconstruction with anastomosis in neck, minimizing risk of stricture, fistula and post-operative mediastinitis

Rate of pharyngeal stenosis following NTLP/TLP– 10%

- ***With a remnant pharyngeal mucosa, speech restoration with tracheo-oesophageal prosthesis is successful in >90% of patients***
- Morbidity of surgical treatment in hypopharyngeal cancers is related to the integrity of the neopharynx
- ***Salivary leaks occur more commonly in patients who undergo primary pharyngeal closure for hypopharyngeal cancer surgery compared to those for laryngeal cancers and may be related to remnant pharyngeal width***

- ***Pharyngeal leak rates are higher in post-irradiated patients (50%)***

Contd.

Contd.

Adjuvant Therapy

Advanced primary cancer (T3/T4), close- or positive-cut margins, presence of perineural invasion (PNI), lymphovascular embolii (LVE), extension/invasion to adjacent structures like cartilage, muscle, soft tissues, multiple nodal involvement and finally the presence of extracapsular extension (ECS) in the nodes

Non Surgical Management of Advanced Hypopharyngeal Cancers

- Concomitant chemotherapy was found to be better than induction chemotherapy
- ***Non-surgical treatment is used in resectable advanced hypopharyngeal malignancies for organ preservation and when medical comorbidities preclude surgery***
- Chemoradiation is generally accepted as gold standard of treatment in advanced laryngeal cancers without frank cartilage erosion

Induction Chemotherapy

- ***When induction chemotherapy is used in conjunction with concurrent chemoradiation in HNSCC, the treatment is referred as sequential chemoradiation***
- Drug delivery is better in untreated well-vascularized tumor, and eradication of micrometastatic disease may be achieved because of high response rate and better tolerance to induction chemotherapy in treatment-naive HNSCC patients

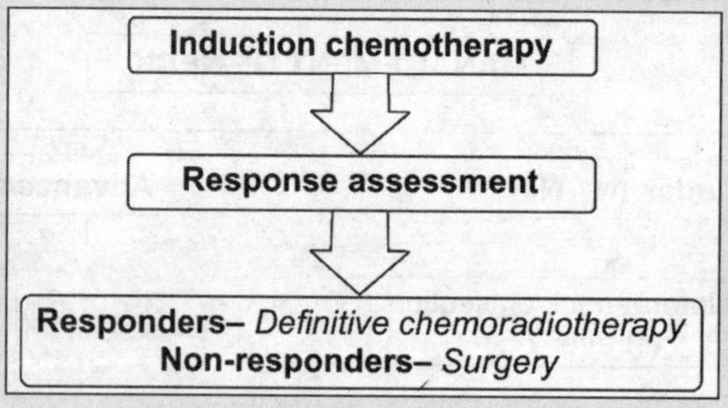

Salvage Therapy

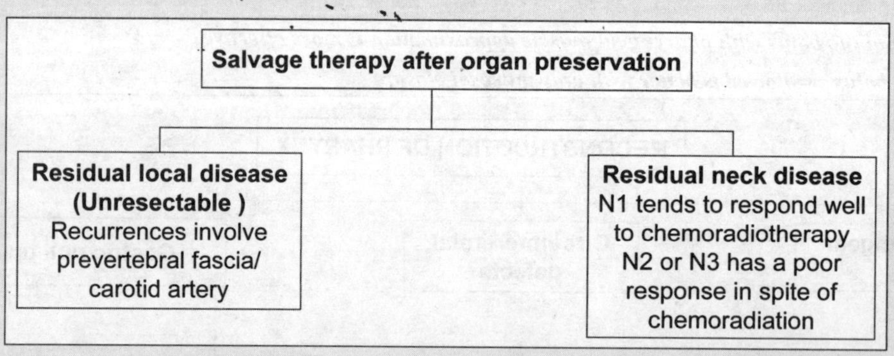

- Control rates after primary radiotherapy/chemoradiation are low, with around 30–50% of patients having residual/ local recurrences, when salvageable, surgery for most cases would be a laryngopharyngectomy with pharyngeal reconstruction
- ***Salvage laryngopharyngectomies have an increased rate of complications especially pharyngocutaneous fistulae 50%***
- Palpable or radiologically obvious remnant neck node–salvage neck dissection is done

Management of Recurrent and Metastatic Disease

Palliative radiation–Local pain and bleeding

Palliative chemotherapy–Good PS and Disseminated disease

- Single-agent cisplatin has been shown to improve overall survival in head and neck cancer patients
- Patients with poor PS should be offered best supportive care and pain medications

FOLLOW UP

- Bimonthly for first 2 years, Quarterly for third year and Biannually for fourth year
- From fifth year annual checkup–2nd primary cancers
- ***Patients should be monitored for second primary cancers in the upper aerodigestive tract which are seen in up to 50% of patients***
- Risk of new cancer development increases by 1% annually

> ***PET-CT scan should be done between 10 and 12 weeks for optimum benefit following radiation in those treated with organ preservation***

- Negative predictive value of PET-CT is above 95% and is an important indicator of disease control

> ***Chance of synchronous tumors is 15%***

> ***Surgery with adjuvant therapy still remains the gold standard in management of advanced hypopharyngeal cancers***
>
> ***Overall 5-year, tumor-specific survival is less than 30%, although the survival of treated patients rises to 50%***

CHAPTER 26

LARYNGEAL TUMORS

- Most common after the age of 60 and less common under 40
- Majority of tumors occurring in Caucasian patients

ETIOLOGY

- ***Smoking remains most common etiological factor for cancers of larynx***
- Alcohol an independent risk factor for developing laryngeal cancer in absence of smoking
- Risk of developing laryngeal cancer is highest in current smokers and increases with number of cigarettes smoked

There is reduction in relative risk of developing laryngeal cancer after stopping smoking and drinking with risk reduction reaching level of never smokers after approximately 20 years

- HPV has linked association with laryngeal cancers
- Asbestos, polycyclic aromatic hydrocarbons, wood dust, coal dust and cement dust are associated with laryngeal tumors

Fanconi anaemia and congenital dyskeratosis are also associated with a higher risk of developing laryngeal tumors

PATHOLOGY

- Most common type of laryngeal cancer–SCC
- Important factors including the type, size and grade of the primary carcinoma, the pattern of invasion and proximity of carcinoma to resection margins

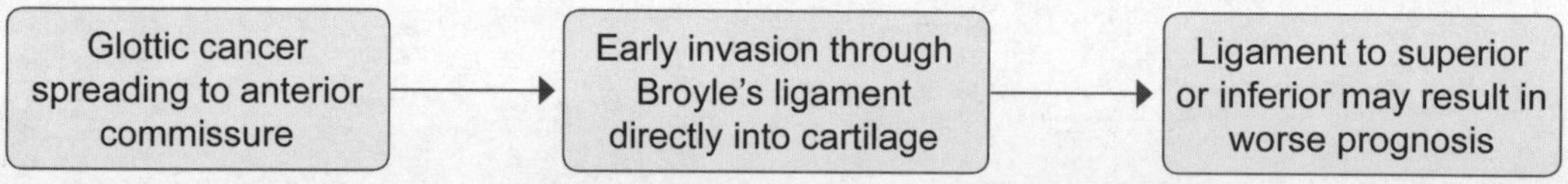

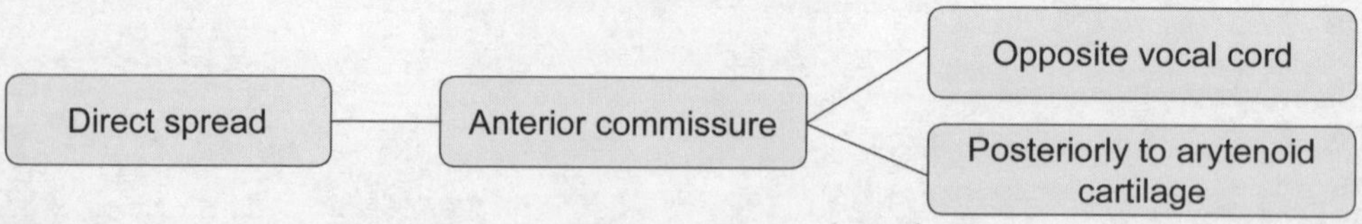

LYMPHATIC SPREAD

Macroscopic lymph node metastasis by disease stage:
<5% (T1), 7% (T2), 14% (T3) and 33% (T4)
'Delphian' node (midline anterior metastatic node or Poirier's pre-laryngeal ganglia node→
Associated with T3 or T4 tumors with significant subglottic extension

- Supraglottic cancers tend to remain locally confined (even with pre-epiglottic or nodal spread) to their subsite until relatively late–***Supraglottic laryngectomy is often a viable option even for bulky tumors***

Approximately 50% of supraglottic cancers spread to glottic region

- 'Suprahyoid supraglottic' carcinomas tend to invade pre-epiglottic space and deep muscles of tongue and spread mucosally into ***piriform fossae*** rather than into paraglottic space

Spread of laryngeal carcinoma		
Primary site		**Look for involvement of**
Supraglottis	Epiglottis	Pre-epiglottic space
	Epiglottic petiole	Anterior commissure
	Intralaryngeal	Paraglottic space
	Mucosa, false cords	
	All	Vocal fold
		Laryngeal cartilage
Glottis	Anterior cord	Anterior commissure/contralateral cord
	Posterior cord	Thyroid cartilage and cricothyoid membrane
	All	Arytenoid cartilage/cricoarytenoid joint/posterior commissure Paraglottic space
		Supraglottic/subglottic spread
Subglottis		Trachea
		Thyroid gland
		Cervical oesophagus

Supraglottic carcinoma has a positive nodal rate of over 60%

- Subglottic carcinoma tends to extend caudally and circumferentially–***50% invade cricoid and 75% have already extended outside larynx by time of diagnosis***
- Due to propensity for inferior extension, nodal dissection for subglottic cancer should include the paratracheal/mediastinal nodes
- Trachea has ***highest density of immunologically active cells*** suggesting that mucosal immunosurveillance may be a crucial factor in defence against airway mutagenesis

Patients with primary subglottic tumors and disease extension into the subglottis have a significantly higher relative risk of thyroid gland invasion

Paraneoplastic Phenomenon:

Peripheral neuropathy and rashes

- **Marginal zone**–Suprahyoid epiglottis and AE folds ***(More aggressive)***

Supraglottis

- T1 Tumor limited to one subsite of supraglottis with normal vocal cord mobility
- T2 Tumor invades mucosa of >one adjacent subsite of supraglottis or glottis or region outside supraglottis (e.g., **mucosa of base of tongue, vallecula, medial wall of piriform sinus**) without fixation of larynx
- T3 Tumor limited to **larynx with vocal cord fixation** and/or invades any of the following: postcricoid area, pre epiglottic space, paraglottic space, and/or inner cortex thyroid cartilage
- T4a Tumor invades through the thyroid cartilage and/or invades tissues beyond larynx, e.g., trachea, soft tissues of neck including deep/extrinsic muscle of tongue **(genioglossus, hyoglossus, palatoglossus and styloglossus),** strap muscles, thyroid, or oesophagus
- T4b Tumor invades prevertebral space, encases carotid artery, or mediastinal structures

Glottis

- T1 Tumor limited to vocal cord(s) (may involve anterior or posterior commissure) with normal mobility
- T1a Tumor limited to one vocal cord
- T1b Tumor involves both vocal cords
- T2 Tumor extends to supraglottis and/or subglottis, and/or with impaired vocal cord mobility
- T3 Tumor limited to larynx with vocal cord fixation and/or invades paraglottic space and/or inner cortex of the thyroid cartilage

Contd.

Contd.

• T4a Tumor invades through the outer cortex of the thyroid cartilage, and/or invades tissues beyond the larynx, e.g., trachea, soft tissues of neck including deep/extrinsic muscle of tongue **(genioglossus, hyoglossus, palatoglossus and styloglossus), strap muscles,** thyroid, oesophagus
• T4b Tumor invades prevertebral space, encases carotid artery, or mediastinal structures

Subglottis
• T1 Tumor limited to subglottis
• T2 Tumor extends to vocal cord(s) with normal or impaired mobility
• T3 Tumor limited to larynx with vocal cord fixation
• T4a Tumor invades cricoid or thyroid cartilage and/or invades tissues beyond larynx, e.g., trachea, soft tissues of neck including deep/extrinsic muscle of tongue (genioglossus, hyoglossus, palatoglossus and styloglossus), strap muscles, thyroid, oesophagus
• T4b Tumor invades prevertebral space, encases carotid artery, or mediastinal structures

GLOTTIC CANCER

- With increasing lesion size, maximum phonation time decreases and with onset of cord-fixation, breathiness may be superimposed with aspiration
- Advanced lesions may lead to airway obstruction causing progressive dyspnoea and stridor

Haemoptysis is usually associated with larger tumors

- Neck nodes are rarely presenting complaint; if present, they signify deep invasion and extension into supraglottis
- Conus elasticus is a strong barrier for lateral extension of cancer from glottis and subglottis and this also accounts for less lymphatic drainage

SUPRAGLOTTIC CANCER

- As tumor bulk increases, phonation is altered, patient presents with a 'hot potato' voice
- If tumors extend to the cords, then hoarseness occurs
- Extension laterally may cause referred otalgia, odynophagia and true dysphagia further

SUBGLOTTIC CANCER

- **Early symptoms**–Feeling of 'globus' or foreign body sensation in the throat
- Any involvement of the glottis or recurrent laryngeal nerves results in hoarseness
- Diplophonia may occur with a shortened maximum phonation time in paralysis

Circumferential progression leads to progressive dyspnoea and stridor, with markedly shortened maximum phonation times and rapid vocal fatigue

EVALUATION

- Larynx is best assessed using flexible nasal laryngoscope in OPD
- ***Laryngeal dysplasia***–Commonly seen in glottis, can be seen virtually anywhere in larynx
- ***MRI scans have higher sensitivity than CT scans in assessing cartilage invasion***

Laryngeal Dysplasia (Laryngeal intraepithelial neoplasia)
• **Ljubljana Classication:** Squamous Intraepithelial Lesion: Low grade SILs and High grade SILs
Malignant transformation rates are between 11% and 25%
• No gold standard in the tool used to resect LD lesion–cold steel or laser resection is recommended over monopolar cautery
• If laser excision is contemplated, CO_2 laser is recommended owing to laser properties enabling minimal penetration thus reducing collateral damage

Contd.

Contd.

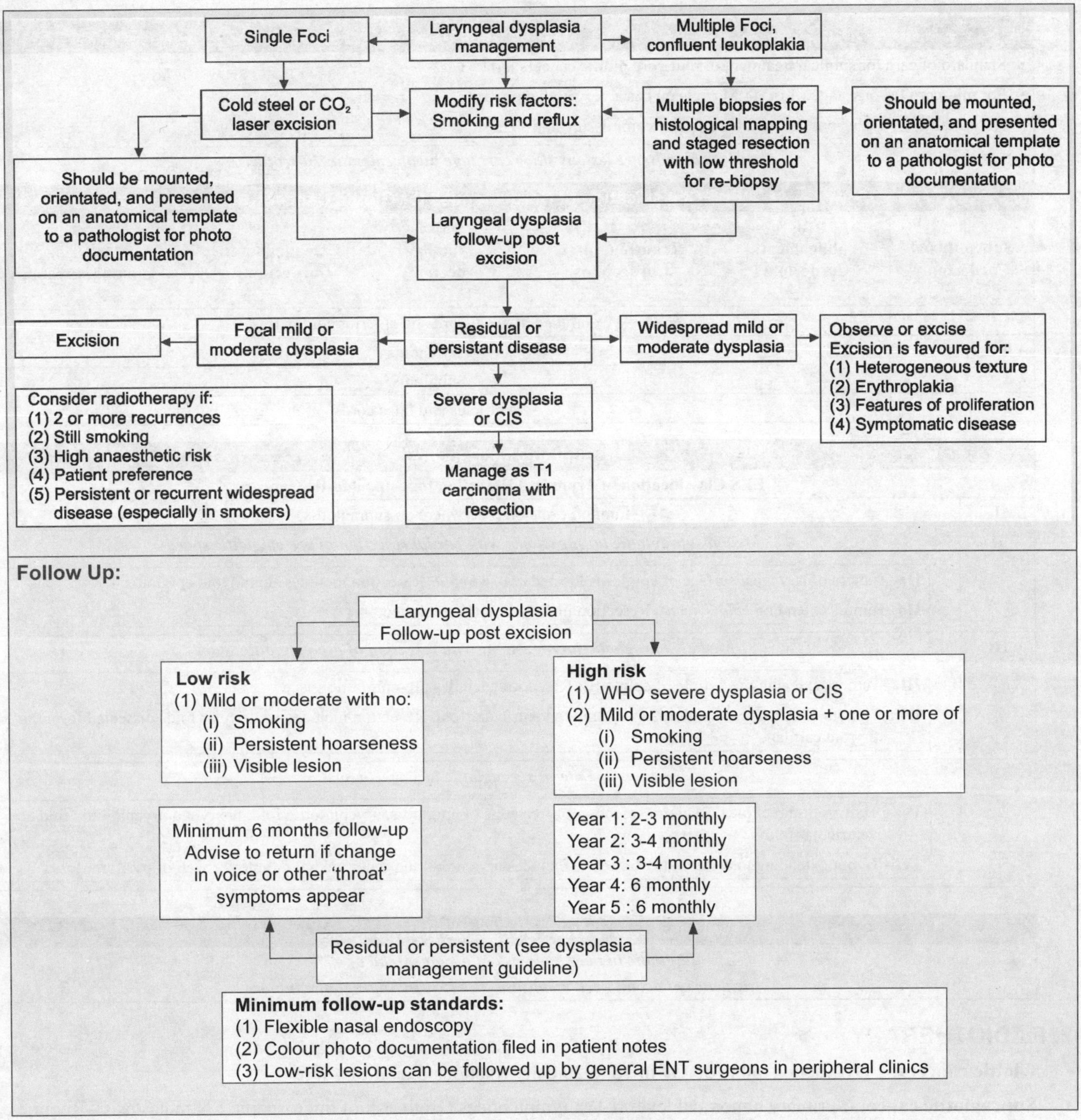

MANAGEMENT OF EARLY STAGE LARYNGEAL CANCERS

- **Laser**–More breathy and wide glottal gap
- **RT**–Less hoarseness related inconvenience 2 years after treatment

> ***Mid cord lesions are largely excised by TLM***
> ***Larger lesions especially when impact on voice is considered to be greater are treated by RT***

1. TRANSLASER MICROSURGERY

Glottic Cancers

- Standard of care for surgical treatment of mid-cord glottic cancers is TLM
- For mid-cord lesions staged T1a, TLM excision has a very high cure rate
- Not suitable for T1 lesions that involve anterior commissure and T2 lesions

Anterior commissure lesions show cartilage involvement in 20% of cases

ELS Classification of Cordectomies for Glottic Cancers

I Subepithelial Cordectomy	II Subligamental Cordectomy	III Transmuscular Cordectomy	IV Total Cordectomy	V Extended total Cordectomy	VI Anterior Commissurectomy

Va	Contralateral vocal cord and anterior commissure
Vb	Arytenoids
Vc	Subglottis
Vd	Ventricles and false cords

Supraglottic Cancers

ELS Classification of Transoral Resection for Supraglottic Cancers

I	Limited excision (Anywhere on supraglottis)
II	***Medial supraglottic laryngectomy with partial resection of pre epiglottic space***
	IIa–Tumors of laryngeal surface of epiglottis located ***above hyoid:*** Resection includes suprahyoid epiglottis **IIb**–Tumors extending *below hyoid:* Resection includes a total epiglottectomy
III	***Medial supraglottic laryngectomy with resection of pre-epiglottic space***
	IIIa–Tumors extending to petiole of epiglottis: Resection includes pre-epiglottic space **IIIb**–Tumors of infrahyoid epiglottis extending to ventricular fold: Resection includes ventricular folds dissected from the thyroid cartilage
IV	***Lateral supraglottic laryngectomy***
	IVa– Tumors of three folds' Region: Resection of free edge of epiglottis, aryepiglottic fold, pharyngo-aryepiglottic fold and ventricular fold **IVb**–Tumor extending to arytenoids: Resection includes arytenoids and inner/medial or anterior wall of pyriform fossa

Neck Management

T2 glottic tumors have risk of occult spread of ~7%

Incidence of occult neck metastases is >15% in Supraglottic tumors

2. RADIOTHERAPY

- **Glottic cancers:** 2 Gy/fraction–50 to 55 Gy in 16 to 20 daily fractions over 3 to 4 weeks
- **Supraglottic cancers:** Primary tumor and level II-IVa lymph nodes (High risk of microscopic LN metastasis)–Regime of 65 Gy in 30 fractions over 6 weeks is used

Recommended treatments for early glottis cancer

T stage	1st choice	2nd choice	3rd choice
T1a	TLM	RT	OPL
T1b	RT or TLM*	OPL	-
T2a	RT or TLM*	OPL	-
T2b	(C) RT	TLM	OPL

Recommended treatments for early supraglottic cancer		
T stage	**1st choice**	**2nd choice**
T1	RT or TLM/TORS*	OPL
T2	RT or TLM/TORS*	OPL

Management of T3 Laryngeal Cancers

Veterans Affairs Study

- Compared induction chemotherapy followed by radiation to Total laryngectomy

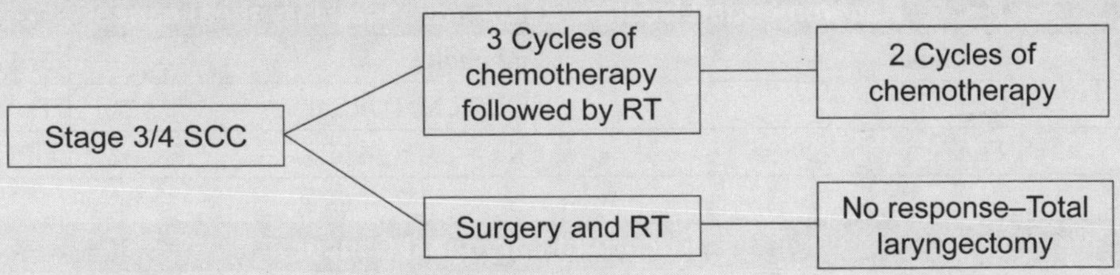

- **Non-surgical treatment**–Valid option for stage III and IV laryngeal tumors
- High proportion of supraglottic tumors and Majority are T3
- Patients who eventually needed a laryngectomy in non-surgical arm had ***glottic tumors, fixed vocal cords, gross cartilage involvement and stage IV/T4 cancers***
- Landmark VA study showed that in patients responding to induction chemotherapy, laryngeal preservation rate was 64% at 2 years with similar survival rates at 2 years (68%) compared to surgery followed by RT
- Salvage laryngectomy rates were significantly lower for T3 compared to T4 disease (29% vs 56%)
- A higher proportion of patients with glottic cancer (those with fixed cord) compared to supraglottic cancer underwent salvage laryngectomy

No improvement in survival following primary surgery
Primary surgery for T3 tumors offers best chance for locoregioal control

RTOG 91-11 (AIIMS SS 2016)

- Higher rates of grade 3 toxicities in chemotherapy arms
- ***Arm 2 has High rate of larynx preserved:*** Higher proportion of patients who received CRT had an intact larynx after RT compared to ICRT or RT

Rate of locoregional control was significantly better with CRT

- Addition of chemotherapy concurrently to RT enhanced chances of laryngeal preservation significantly
- Overall survival did not differ in all 3 groups

Surgical therapy leads to better survival outcomes than non-surgical therapy for patients with advanced laryngeal cancer

- A dysfunctional larynx where airway is compromised, or where the tumor bulk causes significant dysphagia needing tube feeding are circumstances where organ preservation strategies should not be considered, even if tumor stage and extent makes it suitable

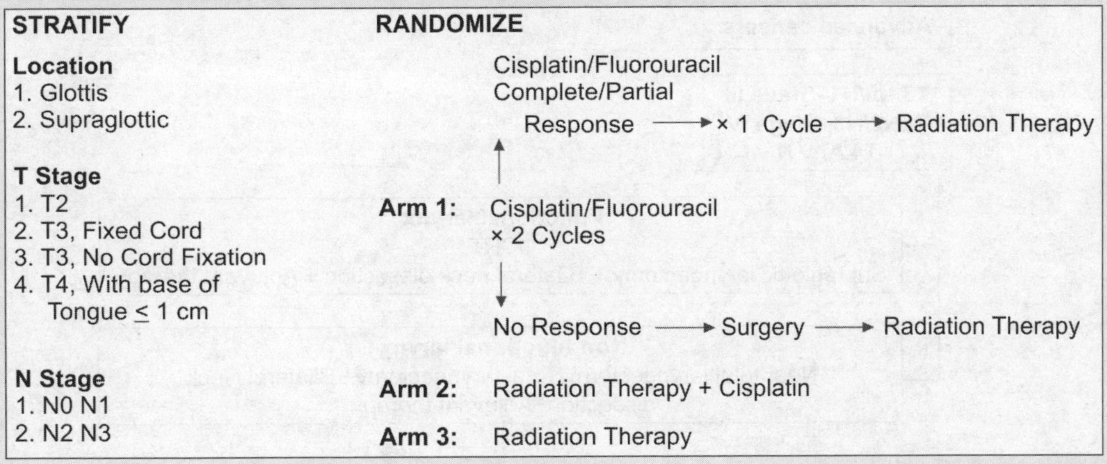

Primary non-surgical treatment with concurrent CRT remains preferred treatment option in patients with

Good performance status, minimal or no comorbidity, disease is limited to confines of larynx with no cartilage invasion, functioning larynx with no airway compromise to achieve best possible outcome of organ and function preservation

Total laryngectomy is a bona de treatment for T3 laryngeal disease, especially in patients who have laryngopharyngeal dysfunction or a fixed cord

Post-operative RT to tumor bed and/or neck in patients at risk of locoregional recurrence can improve locoregional control and survival

- **Risk factors:** pT4 tumors, close or involved resection margins, involved node >3 cm, multiple positive nodes, ECS, perineural invasion and vascular invasion

Recommended treatments for advanced laryngeal cancer

T stage	1st choice	2nd choice	3rd choice
T3	CRT	OPL/TLM/TORS*#	TL*#
T4a	TL#	CRT	OPL/TLM*#

Recurrent Laryngeal Cancer

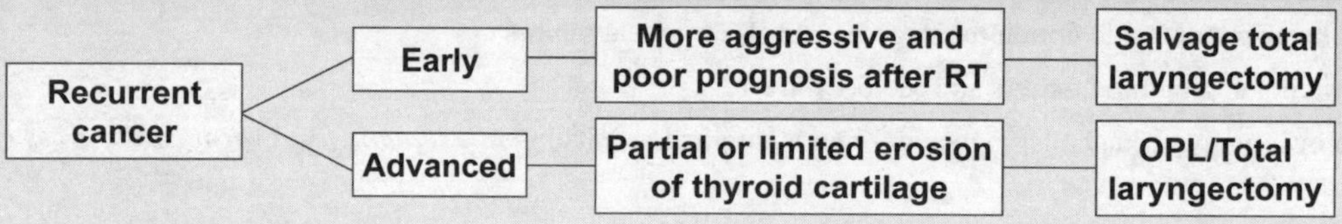

- For more advanced laryngeal tumor recurrences (rT3–4), recommendation was for elective neck dissection (bilateral for supraglottic cancers), particularly if previous radiation fields did not include the lateral neck

SUPRAGLOTTIC CANCERS

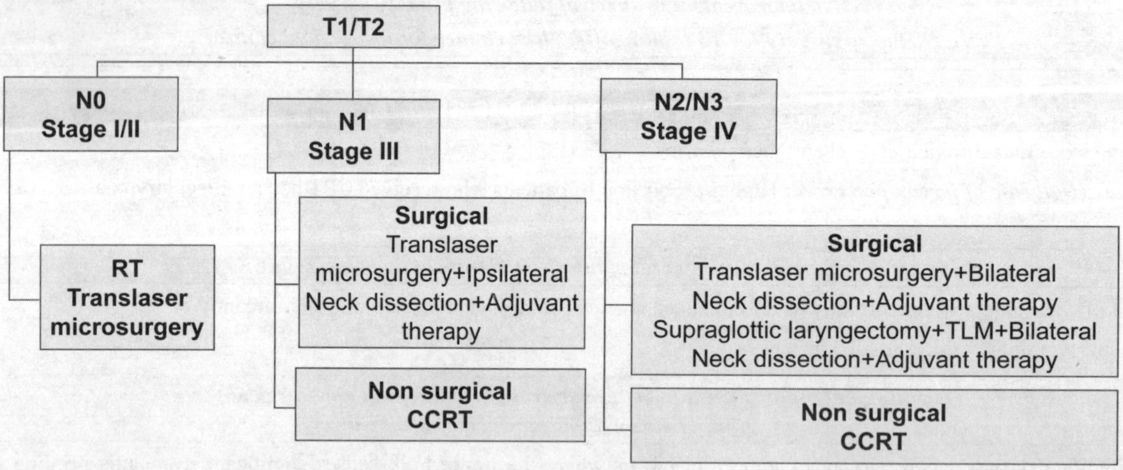

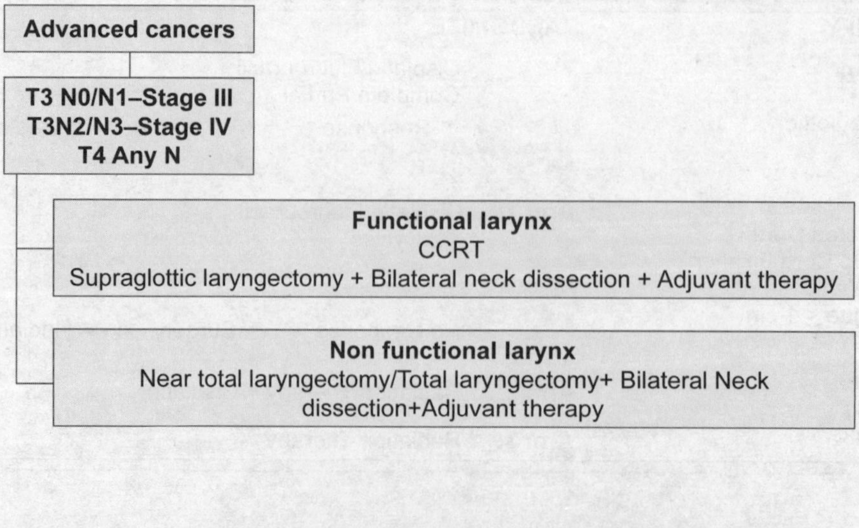

GLOTTIC CANCERS

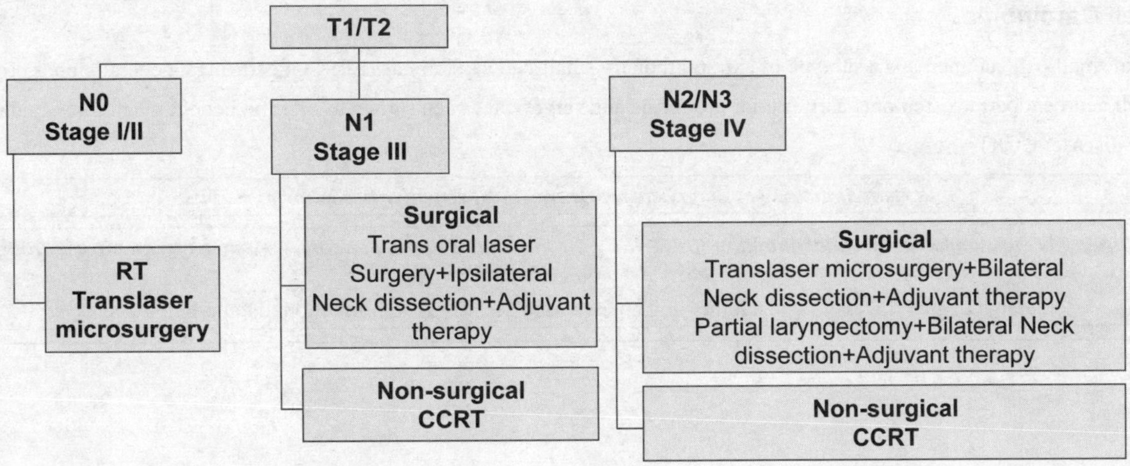

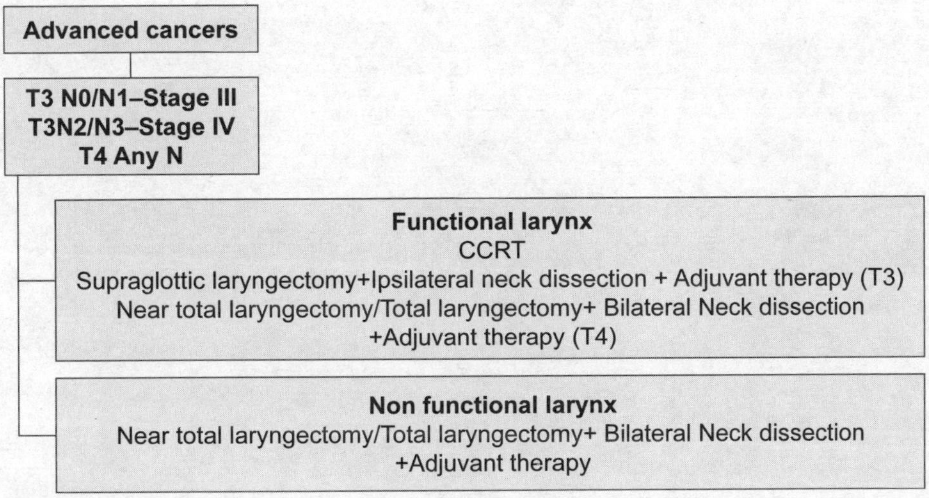

SUBGLOTTIC CANCERS

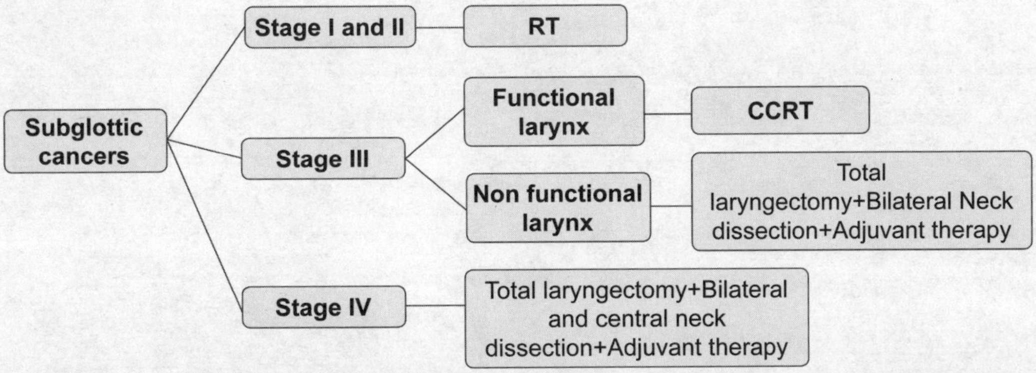

Rare Cancers

- Neuroendocrine tumors are most common nonsquamous tumors of the larynx
- Surgery is the mainstay of treatment for typical and atypical carcinoid
- Atypical carcinoid is considered more aggressive and therefore elective neck dissection is advocated, and adjuvant CRT should be considered

Contd.

Contd.

Small Cell Carcinoma

- Laryngeal small-cell carcinoma is a subtype of extrapulmonary small-cell carcinomas (EPSCC) carrying a generally poor prognosis
- Small cell neuroendocrine carcinoma carries poor prognosis and surgery has been shown to offer no benefit when compared to CRT alone
- **Limited disease:** CCRT= Surgery

Extent of disease at diagnosis represents most sensitive predictor of survival

Surgery is most important treatment option for HNSCC in Fanconi Anemia patients, who merit frequent screening for early detection of malignancies

High degree of genomic instability and an increased sensitivity to bifunctionally alkylating agents

CHAPTER 27

REHABILITATION OF VOICE

- Laryngectomy is carried out conserving as much pharyngeal mucosa as possible, particularly over postcricoid region, piriform fossae and valleculae

> ***For hypopharyngeal tumors mucosa of uninvolved piriform fossa is carefully preserved to minimize need for flap reconstruction***

- ***Ideally transverse, unstretched mucosal width of at least 6 cm at narrowest point is necessary to enable adequate swallowing and effortless tracheo-oesophageal speech***

CRICOPHARYNGEAL MYOTOMY

- Avoid hypertonicity and spasm of these muscles during attempted phonation, and to allow expansion of upper oesophagus providing an air 'reservoir' below pharyngo-oesophageal (PE) segment

TRACHEOESOPHAGEAL PUNCTURE

- Puncture is positioned midline about 10–15 mm below cut edge-posterior tracheal wall

PHARYNGEAL CLOSURE

- **Pharyngeal defect**–Closed using an interrupted/continuous absorbable mucosal suture
- A horizontal closure is considered to produce a wider pharynx above the PE segment and may improve resonance for speech
- An alternative technique is the 'T' closure
- 'Tonic' PE segment at the optimal site in the pharynx with a good reservoir below it and a wide resonating pharyngeal segment above

> ***If the muscles or PE segment wall are hypotonic (e.g., after total pharyngolaryngectomy and reconstruction or if thyropharyngeus is not repaired) voice will be weak because there is minimal or absent muscle in the wall to create a PE segment.***
>
> ***Half Muscle closure technique****–Reduce spasm of pharyngoeophageal segment.*

REPAIR OF SUPRAHYOID MUSCLES

- Suture suprahyoid muscles to thyropharyngeus
- Strengthens mucosa above repair–Avoid pseudoepiglottis and Anterior pouch
- Reattach middle constrictor and other suprahyoid muscles
- Trachea should not be respected too low and sutured to medial margins of sternocleidomastoid

POST OP CARE

- If phonation begins too early, excess pressure during voicing can lead to suture line breakdown

Comparison of speech production before and after laryngectomy			
Physical requirements	**Normal laryngeal voice production**	**Oesophageal speech production**	**Surgical voice production**
Initiator	Moving column of air from the lungs	Moving column of air from the oesophagus	Moving column of air from the lungs
Vibrator	Vocal cords	Vibratory/pharyngo-oesophageal (PE) segment	Vibratory/pharyngo-oesophageal (PE) segment
Resonators	Resonating cavities: nose, mouth, pharynx	Resonating cavities: Nose, mouth, pharynx	Resonating cavities: Nose, mouth pharynx

HYPOTONIC (Too Loose)	Swallow is functional Voice quality is low, weak, whispery and often wet
HYPERTONIC (Too Tight)	Swallowing requires increased pressure Voice is high pitched, effortful and difficult or impossible to maintain

Hypotonicity is managed using digital pressure against outside of neck, artificially increasing tone
Hypertonicity–Open myotomy/Chemical neurectomy
Less severe hypertonicity is managed with a low opening pressure prosthesis

- ***Candida albicans*** interferes with prosthesis valve mechanism causing leakage and aspiration or increasing air flow resistance such that prosthesis becomes non-functional
- **Granulation Tissue:** Small areas can be cauterized using a silver nitrate stick but larger areas require surgical removal
- ***Candida*** interfering with prosthesis valving function is ***most common cause of prosthesis central leakage–aspiration and increases risk of chest infections***

Reasons for peripheral leakage include
• An oversized prosthesis pistoning within the TEP, suctioning the bolus through
• A thinned/weakened party wall (below 8 mm), associated with a wider diameter prosthesis *in situ* often in patients with concurrent comorbidity (e.g. diabetes)

Prevention
• Minimizing trauma by avoiding dilation of TEP and reducing number of changes
• When changing prosthesis, one option is to cut ***in situ*** prosthesis in half, removing anterior portion and allowing posterior portion to pass out through patient
• Hand-load the prosthesis into a smaller gel cap for placement

CHAPTER 28

CARCINOMA OF UNKNOWN PRIMARY (CUP)

- ***Accounts for only up to 5% of patients with head and neck malignancy***
- Presence of clinically overt metastatic disease in absence of a clinically or radiologically obvious primary tumor
- ***Most common primary histological type–SCC (50-80%)***

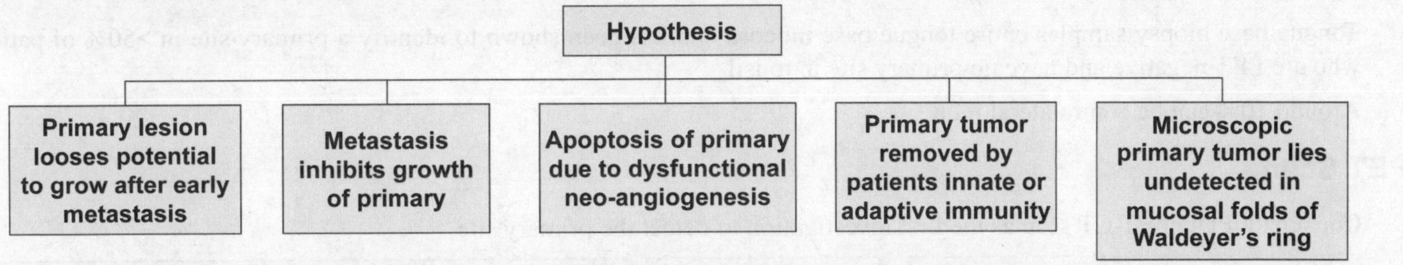

Most common presentation is Painless unilateral neck mass

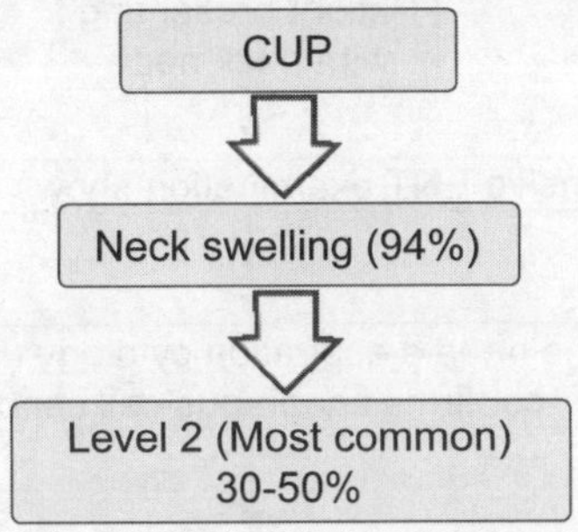

- Usually affects male of age 55-65 years
- Alcohol and tobacco usage–NPC
- Multiple sex partners and Orogenital sex–Oropharyngeal cancer
- Bilateral in <10%
- Usually presents as N2
- Most common presentation of CUP in the head and neck is in context of human papillomavirus (HPV)-associated oropharynx (HPV+OPSCC) carcinoma
- Site of node is an indicator of the primary site

Level I nodes are almost never seen with nasopharyngeal primaries and level V nodes never with laryngeal cancer

EVALUATION

FNAC

- ***First important step in diagnosis is FNAC***
- *Sensitivity–83 to 97% and Specificity–91-100%*

- Repeat FNAC if needed→Core biopsy/Open biopsy

Narrow Band Imaging

- Modification of the standard white light endoscope in which white light is transmitted through optical filters absorbing all but two wavelengths; ***one band centred at 415 nm and another at 540 nm***
- Former wavelength penetrates superficial mucosa and highlights ***submucosal capillaries as brown colour*** while latter penetrates through submucosal layer and identifies ***prominent vessels as cyan in colour***
- SCCs arising from upper aerodigestive tract mucosa are accompanied by neo-angiogenesis
- ***NBI identifies neoplastic tissue at an earlier stage than conventional endoscopy***

Bilateral Tonsillectomy

- Bilateral tonsillectomy should be employed as primary resides in contralateral tonsil in up to 10% of cases

Tongue Base Biopsy

- Tongue base biopsy samples entire tongue base mucosa and has been shown to identify a primary site in >50% of patients who are PET negative and have no primary site in tonsil
- Around 10% can be contralateral foci

PET Scan

- Consider a FDG PET-CT scan as the first investigation to detect the primary site

All patients over age of 35 years with lateral cystic masses must be presumed to have cancer until proven otherwise

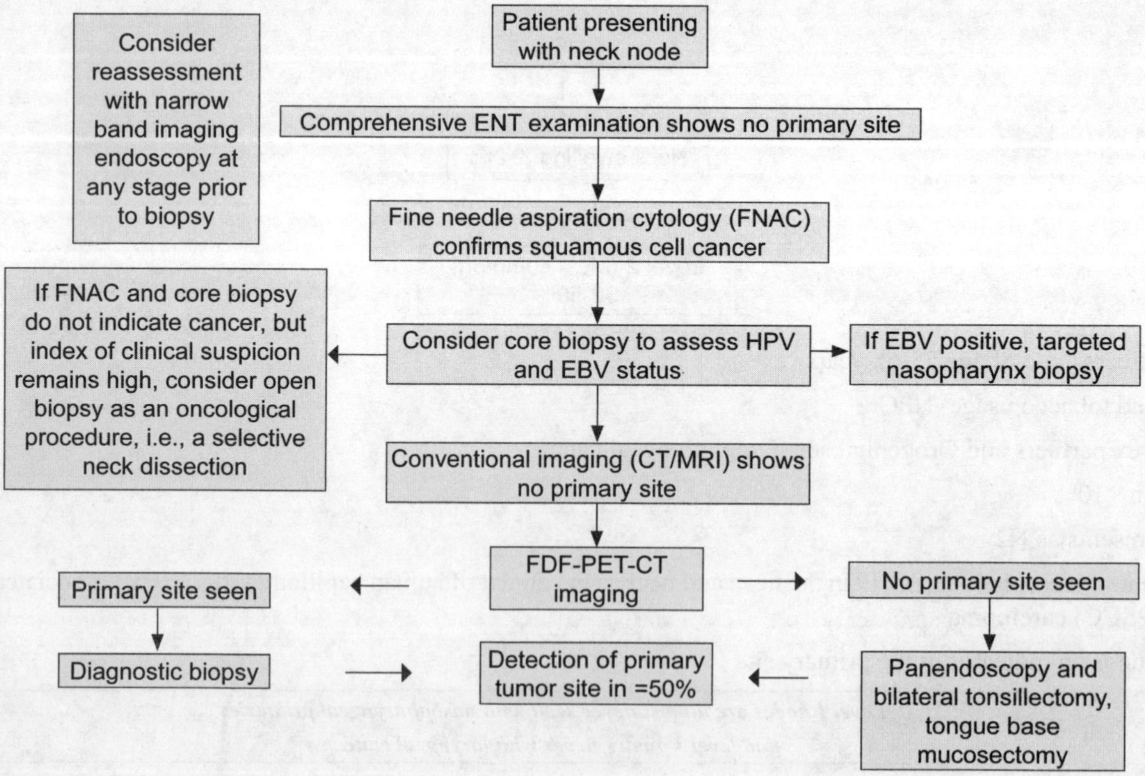

TREATMENT

- **Early disease**–Single-modality therapy→Neck dissection alone/Radiotherapy alone
- **Advanced cases**–Combined modality therapy
- **CRT**–N3, ECS, Resection margins +ve

Primary surgical management of neck is preferred to RT in patients with operable disease

Post-operative selective or total mucosal radiotherapy is indicated for most patients with advanced operable disease
Total mucosal irradiation has demonstrated a reduction in primary site recurrence without any improvement in overall survival

For total mucosal irradiation, a dose of 50 Gy in 25 daily fractions, five fractions per week is sufficient for control of occult primary disease

Selective neck dissection has been suggested as a valid option for patients with N2a and N2b disease as the risk of metastases in levels I and V has proven to be rare in patients with CUP unless they present with N3 neck disease

cT0N1M0 without ENE found on histopathological/radiological studies	Single modality treatment either with selective neck dissection or involved field radiotherapy alone
pT1N0M0 with ENE	Post-operative RT if ENE is identified
T0N2M0 AND T0N3M0	Primary CRT followed by PET-CT guided surveillance or combined modality treatment including neck dissection followed by RT or CRT

Stage	Surgery	Radiotherapy	Chemotherapy
T0N 1 M0 (No ECS)	SND or MRND	No unless for mucosal sites	No
T0N 1 M0 (ECS)	SND or MRND	Yes to neck	Should be considered
T0N 2 M0	SND or MRND	Yes–ipsilateral but contralateral should be considered	Should be considered
T0N 3 M0	MRND or RND	Yes–ipsilateral but contralateral should be considered	Should be considered

Overall 5-year survival for all stages of HNSCC with unknown primary site would be in range of 52% and 75%

FAILURE

- If EBRT is used, disease recurrence is usually in neck and in form of distant metastasis
- FDG-PET-CT scan is probably best method of detection and diagnosis of recurrences
- ***Distant metastasis usually occurs within a year of completion of treatment–most commonly to Lung***
- Recurrence in primary→ 0 to 66% (Treated by surgery alone)

Nodal stage is the most important risk factor for local recurrence

CHAPTER 29

BENIGN SALIVARY GLAND TUMORS

- 80% within the parotid gland, and 10% within the submandibular and minor salivary glands respectively
- ***Around 75% of salivary gland tumors are benign***
- Peak incidence in sixth decade
- Female preponderance, with exception of Warthin's tumors ***(more common in males)***

Frequency of epithelia salivary gland tumors and malignancy analyzed by site		
Site	**Benign vs malignant (%)**	
	Eveson and Cawson	**Bradley and McGurk**
Parotid	85	91
Submandibular	64	75
Sublingual	14	0
Minor glands	54	60

- Radiation has possible association with Warthin's tumor
- Malignancy is relatively more likely in younger patients and in submandibular tumors (40% malignant)
- If FNAC is non-diagnostic/false negative and tumor is then found to be malignant, imaging performed preop will help to stage tumor and plan further treatment if necessary
- If FNAC is non-diagnostic, imaging may assist in diagnosis and plan urgency of resection

MRI/CT (Axial images)
• Tumors that are large (e.g. > 3 cm) • Deep lobe/parapharyngeal space involvement • Suspicion of malignancy
MR is generally preferred because it gives better definition of tumor–normal salivary gland interface

- Irregular capsule, or extracapsular invasion, hypervascularity and imaging features consistent with necrosis–Imaging features of malignancy
- ***Ultrasound is primary and initial imaging modality for benign tumors***

PLEOMORPHIC ADENOMA

- Almost mucoid nature of many pleomorphic adenomas makes them extremely fragile so that they can rupture at operation
- *Approximately 50% of all salivary gland tumors, 65% of parotid tumors and 40% of intra-oral minor salivary gland tumors*

Pleomorphic adenomas are derived from intercalated duct and myoepithelial cells ***Only 0.15% of pleomorphic adenomas have features of malignant change***
Pleomorphic adenomas of the submandibular gland are treated with excision of the gland ***Pleomorphic adenomas of the minor oral salivary glands is treated by wide local excision***

- Deep lobe tumors generally require total conservative parotidectomy
- ***Overall recurrence rates of pleomorphic adenomas–2%***
- MR scan is the imaging of choice–both to characterize the identified recurrence(s) and detect further foci

- Radiotherapy is effective in reducing further recurrence of pleomorphic adenoma
- ***Much higher chance of malignant change within recurrent tumors, about 3%***

Risk of Malignant Transformation
• Older patient age • Male patient • Long duration of tumor • Multiple recurrences • Deep lobe parotid location

Arguments in favour for extracapsular dissection and partial parotidectomy with cuff in the surgical treatment of parotid pleomorphic adenoma	
Extracapsular dissection	**Partial parotidectomy with cuff or superficial parotidectomy**
Recurrence rates are the same in this method as in superficial parotidectomy	On histopathology, the tumor capsule is incomplete and tumor cells extend through into adjacent tissue. Therefore, a cuff of tissue is necessary to achieve microscopic clearance and reduce chance of recurrence
Less cosmetic deformity	If the histology demonstrates an unexpected malignancy then clearance may still be adequate (if a low-grade tumor)
Lower incidence of Frey's syndrome There is no possible cuff in the tumor adjacent to one significant facial nerve branch in most cases	Dissecting close on the capsule may cause rupture (although when this does happen, it tends to be when dissecting capsule off facial nerve branch (i.e., no scope for a cuff here anyway)
If revision surgery is required (e.g., malignant on histopathology) than the tissue planes used to dissect and identify the main facial nerve and some branches are virginal	

WARTHIN'S TUMOR

- Accounts for 20% of benign parotid tumors

Seventh decade and Men ***Strong association between the development of Warthin's tumors and smoking***

- Racial association in that it is ***comparatively rare in afrocaribbeans***
- Arises from salivary duct inclusions within intra parotid lymph nodes
- Treatment of Warthin's tumor is generally through surgical excision
- ***May undergo rapid expansion possibly caused by cystic change***
- Most tumors are managed through a partial superficial partotidectomy
- Older age group–Observation
- ***Synchronous or metachronous tumors are more frequently associated with Warthin's tumors than any other salivary tumor***

MYOEPITHELIOMA

- Myoepithelial cells are a prominent component of pleomorphic adenomas
- No apparent predominance in either sex and all salivary glands can be affected
- ***Average age at presentation is 40 years***

ONCOCYTOMA (OXYPHILIC ADENOMA)

- Predominantly tumors of middle age–***7th decade/ 8th decade***
- ***Parotid gland are most frequent site***
- Slow growing and may rarely be bilateral
- ***Benign and excision is curative***

SURGERY OF PAROTID GLAND

- Permanent facial palsy is in the region of 1–2%
- Area of sensory loss generally decreases in first 12 months post-operatively
- Stump neuroma presents as very localized tender nodule just anterior to superior part of sternomastoid muscle
- Can be managed by simple local excision and burying of the fresh nerve end in muscle
- Mobile lesions in the parotid tail are most suitable for ECD, or smaller tumors fairly supercial within the superficial lobe
- Inflammatory lesions, large tumors and those extending into the deep lobe are unsuitable for ECD, as are those where malignancy is suspected

First Bite Syndrome
• Intense pain in the parotid gland when just about to eat and it quickly passes after beginning to eat occurs as a result of sympathetic denervation of remaining parotid tissue
• **Treatment:** Botulinum toxin into parotid gland can be effective as can high dose Gabapentin/Pregabalin. ***Generally self-limiting***

SUBMANDIBULAR SURGERY

1. **Damage to the marginal branch of the facial nerve:** Incidence as a permanent complication is around 2–3%
2. **Lingual and hypoglossal nerve damage:** It is more likely to be sustained when gland is removed for chronic sialadenitis than tumor. Incidence as a complication is around <1%
3. **Marginal mandibular nerve:** It enters neck **1cm in front of the angle of mandible,** loops over the facial artery and vein 2 cm below lower border of body of mandible before sweeping superiorly to the angle of the mouth

Protection of mandibular branch of facial nerve

- Facial vessels can be transected at a low level on surface of submandibular gland and reflected superiorly
  - Nerve lies lateral to facial vessels, can then be lifted out of operative field by traction on transected end of vessels
- Capsule of gland can be opened at level of hyoid bone and dissection continued beneath it

Long Term Follow Up
• Incomplete resection (as distinct from completely excised but with incomplete capsule)
• Tumor rupture/spillage at operation
• Complications that need management
• Recurrent disease

CHAPTER 30 MALIGNANT SALIVARY GLAND TUMORS

- Minor salivary glands are unencapsulated seromucinous glands distributed throughout the entire upper aerodigestive tract, numbering between 500 and 1000, with the majority (<90%) being located in oral cavity and oropharynx
- ***0.5% of all malignancies***
- ***Epithelial tumors account for majority (95%) of malignant salivary gland tumors***
- Up to 70% arise in the parotid gland and typically 1–3% of all head and neck carcinomas are reported to be parotid carcinomas
- **Atomic bomb**–increased incidence of both benign (Warthin's tumor and pleomorphic adenoma) and malignant (mucoepidermoid carcinoma) salivary gland tumors
- ***Incidence of Warthin's tumor is doubled and multicentric in smokers***

Epstein Barr Virus–Bilateral Warthin's tumors and undifferentiated parotid carcinoma
CMV– Mucoepidermoid carcinoma

- ***Inverse relationship exists between diet rich in PUFA and salivary cancers***
- Increased risk of salivary cancer in workers involved with livestock feed processing, possibly related to naturally occurring mycotoxins produced by ***Aspergillus***

Chromosomal translocations in salivary gland tumors

Salivary tumor	Fusion oncogene	Diagnostic utility
Pleomorphic adenoma	PLAG-1 fused to CTNNB 1, TCEA 1 or others	*PLAG-1* abnormality in 30% of tumors
Mucoepidermoid carcinoma	CRTC 1-MAML 2 (>80%) CRTC 3-MAML2 (<10%)	Present in low and intermediate grade tumors
Adenoid cystic carcinoma	MYB-NF IB MYBL 1-NFIB	Present 80-90% of tumors
Secretory carcinoma	ETV 6-NTRK3	Defines the entity

- ***Secretory carcinoma***–Low grade salivary gland carcinoma defined by a translocation (12;15)(p13;q25) leading to formation of an ETV6-NTRK3 fusion oncogene

HISTOLOGY

- Major glands have a true excretory ductal system
- Minor salivary glands are composed of unencapsulated acini with a short or absent ductal system
- ***Serous acinus cells predominate in parotid and submandibular gland***
- Mucous acinus cells are main source of saliva in sublingual and submandibular glands and only source of saliva in minor salivary glands
- Tumors originating from the intercalated duct reserve cells are adenocarcinoma not otherwise specified (ACNOS), acinic cell carcinoma **(AcCC)**, adenoid cystic carcinoma **(AdCC), mixed malignant tumor** and **oncocytic tumors)**
- Tumors that originate from the excretory duct reserve cells are mucoepidermoid carcinoma **(MEC)**, squamous cell carcinoma **(SCC)** and salivary duct carcinoma **(SDC)**

- ***'Multicellular theory'*** favours a transformation of the entire ducto-acinar unit and requires various 'differentiated' cells to become 'de-differentiated', deranged in their growth pattern, resulting in microscopically different components in various types of salivary gland tumors
- ***'Reserve cell theory'*** states that both normal salivary gland unit and the different tumor types are result of differentiation of undifferentiated pluripotent precursor cells, and tumor cells originate from a problem in normal differentiation process

- 1% of parotid tumors arise in accessory parotid gland (along the Stensen duct)
- A diagnosis of a ***malignancy*** is suggested by ***rapid increase in size, pain, associated cervical lymphadenopathy, fixation of salivary mass to deep structures or facial skin or presence of VII nerve dysfunction***

44% has pain, 25% have VII Nerve paresis or paralysis

- Incidence of parotid carcinoma has been estimated to be ***as high as 6%*** in patients presenting with LMN VII Nerve paralysis where no aetiology has been identified after initial MRI scans
- Paresis has been slow in onset, progressive in nature, shows no evidence of recovery, affects only isolated branches of the VII Nerve and if facial tics are present

Imaging is strongly advised when tumor mobility is impaired, tumor >4 cm, VII Nerve is clinically involved and there are palpable cervical nodes

- ***MRI is superior to CT*** in evaluating parotid tumors and allows better demonstration of retromandibular parotid, stylomastoid foramen area, VIIN invasion and perineural extension
- Diffusion weighted MRI is considered to have superior diagnostic efficacy in identifying malignancy based on a specific diffusion pattern

Warthin's tumors and pleomorphic adenomas demonstrate an increased FDG uptake

MUCOEPIDERMOID CARCINOMA

- ***Mucoepidermoid carcinoma is most common malignant salivary gland neoplasm***
- More frequently in female patients
- Major risk factor for development is previous therapeutic radiation exposure with a latent period of 7–32 years

Grading system for mucoepidermoid carcinoma

Parameter	**Point value**	
Intracystic component < 20%	2	
Neural invasion	2	
Necrosis	3	
Mitoses (>4 per 10 HPF)	3	
Anaplasia	4	
Grade	**Total score**	**Overall survival (10 years)**
Low	0-4	90%
Intermediate	5-6	70%
High	7-14	25%

ACINIC CELL CARCINOMA

- Accounts for 7–17.5% of all malignant salivary gland neoplasms
- Approximately 80% arise from parotid gland
- Male preponderance and usually present in third decade of life
- Usually rounded, well circumscribed and can be encapsulated
- Recurrent tumors tend to be less well demarcated and can appear multinodular
- Reactive lymphoid tissue is characteristic of acinic cell carcinoma and may mimic lymph node involvement
- ***Demonstrate zymogen granules in serous acinar cells***

Growth patterns of acinic cell carcinoa	
Growth pattern	**Features**
Solid	Cells aggregate into sheets forming lobules or nodules
Microcystic	The tumor has a sieve-like appearance due to the presence of microcysts
Papillary-cystic	The tumor contains prominent cysts with intraluminal papillary projections
Follicular	Contain multiple variable-sized cysts loosely resembling thyroid parenchyma

ADENOCARCINOMA NOT OTHERWISE SPECIFIED

- More common in women
- Frequently seen in the fifth to eighth decade ***(mean age of diagnosis of 58 years)***
- ***Sixty per cent occur in major salivary glands, usually parotid***

Adenocarcinoma not otherwise specified
- Degree of gland formation, cellular pleomorphism and mitotic count
  - Low grade: Easily identifiable gland and duct-like structures. Single cell type with small nucleoli, abundant cytoplasm, distinct cell borders and little nuclear pleomorphism with few mitoses
  - Intermediate grade: Easily identified gland and duct-like structures. *Greater nuclear pleomorphism with more mitoses*
  - High grade: Solid, with areas of haemorrhage and necrosis Gland and duct-like structures are much sparser

ADENOID CYSTIC CARCINOMA

- 10–12% of all malignant salivary gland tumors
- ***Most common malignant tumor of submandibular gland***
- 5% of parotid neoplasms and 30–50% of minor salivary gland neoplasms
- No sex predilection
- Usually seen in patients in 40s to 60 years
- Poorly circumscribed solid white tumor

> ***Tubular pattern represents the most differentiated form of AdCC***
> ***Cribriform pattern is most common pattern***
> ***Solid pattern is the least common type***

- Overall pattern resembles 'Swiss cheese'

> ***High-grade (solid) AdCC is an aggressive, destructive malignancy***

GRADES
- **I** — **Mostly tubular with some cribriform elements**
- **II** — **Entirely cribriform or cribriform/tubular with <30% solid component**
- **III** — **Any tumor with >30% solid growth**

CARCINOMA EX PLEOMORPHIC ADENOMA

- Approximately 12% of all salivary gland malignancies and 6.2% of all pleomorphic adenomas
- Arises from within a pre-existing PSA or at the site of a previous pleomorphic adenoma

Risk factors for malignant transformation of a pleomorphic adenoma
• Older age (mean, 61 years)
• Male sex
• Prolonged duration of tumor
• Multiple recurrences

8th Edition (2017) UICC TNM classification and stage regrouping for major salivary gland malignancies	
T	**Primary Tumor**
Tx	Primary tumor cannot be assessed
T0	No evidence of primary tumor
T1	Tumor 2 cm or less, without extraparenchymal extension*
T2	Tumor > 2-4 cm, without extraparenchymal extension
T3	Tumor >4-6 cm, and/or extraparenchymal extension
T4a	Tumor invades skin, mandible, ear canal and/or VIIh nerve involvement
T4b	Tumor invades base of skull and/or pterygoid plates and/or encases carotid artery
N	**Regional Lymph Nodes**
N1	Metastasis in a single ipsilateral node, 3 cm or less in greatest dimension, without extranodal extension
N2a	Single ipsilateral node > 3-6 cm, without extranodal extension
N2b	Multiple ipsilateral nodes < 6 cm
N2c	Bilateral or contralateral nodes < 6 cm
N3a	Node(s) > 6 cm, without extranodal extension
N3b	Single or multiple nodes, with extranodal extension**
M	**Distant Metastasis**
M0	No distant metastasis
M1	Distant metastasis

	T1	T2	T3	T4a	T4b
N0	I	II	III	IVA	IVB
N1	III				
N2	IVA				
N3	IVB				
M1	IVC				

Superficial lobe of parotid contains lymph nodes that serve as primary echelon nodes for Anterolateral scalp, Lateral face and Auricular cutaneous malignancies → Superficial parotidectomy is included in treatment of malignancies of these regions (Regional metastasis)

- **Elective neck dissection**→ High grade lesions, Major nerve invasion and Intraparotid lymph node metastasis
- **Radiotherapy**→ High grade cancers, Advanced locoregional disease

CHAPTER

31 PARAPHARYNGEAL TUMORS

- Only 0.5% of all head and neck masses

ANATOMY

Pterygomaxillary space, pharyngomaxillary space, pterygopharyngeal space and lateral pharyngeal space

- Inverted pyramidal-shaped potential space
- Its base lies superiorly at ***skull base***
- This area includes jugular and hypoglossal canal and the foramen lacerum
- Its apex lies inferiorly at the ***greater cornu of the hyoid bone***

Anterior leading edge is pterygomandibular raphe

- Medial surface–***distensible*** and comprises superior pharyngeal constrictor muscle, the buccopharyngeal membrane and the pharynx
- Lateral surface–***relatively immobile,*** comprises medial pterygoid muscle, ramus of the mandible, and deep lobe of parotid gland, and below level of mandible, lateral aspect is bordered by fascia of posterior belly of digastric muscle
- ***Posterior surface is part of prevertebral fascia, bordered by carotid sheath posterolaterally and the retropharyngeal space posteromedially***

Fascia
• Parapharyngeal space is divided into two parts by fascial condensation called aponeurosis of Zuckerkandl and Testut–***fascia joining styloid process to TVP divides parapharyngeal space into pre-styloid and post-styloid compartments***
• Condensation of cervical fascia forms a band that extends from near apex of styloid process of temporal bone to angle and posterior border of mandible

- Stylomandibular ligament, lying posteriorly and posterior border of mandible, lying anteriorly, form stylomandibular tunnel.
- ***Tunnel is deep relation of deep lobe of parotid gland***
- **Salivary gland tumors–82%** benign and 18% malignant–***Most common tumors are of salivary gland origin, accounting for 45% of all lesions–Pleomorphic adenoma***

Malignant salivary gland tumors
• Parotidectomy with sparing of facial nerve dependent on pre-operative nerve function with a transcervical approach

- **Neurogenic lesions** accounted for 41% of lesions in parapharyngeal space–***52% were paragangliomas and Malignant lesions account for 5%***
- Miscellaneous lesions account for 12%–***Internal carotid artery aneurysms, branchial cleft cysts, haemangiomas and meningiomas***
- ***Metastatic lesions account for 3% of lesions and 2% of lesions are of lymphoid origin***

PARAGANGLIOMA

- 30% of these tumors are believed to have a genetic origin related to the *Succinyl Dehydrogense (SDH)* gene locus

- 10% of paragangliomas are multicentric
- 3% may be secretory
- ***Usual indications–Suspected malignancy as evidenced by multiple lesions, erosion of adjacent bone or involvement of adjacent cranial nerves or associated regional lymphadenopathy***
- Surgery is also indicated if increasing tumor size causes pressure effects on surrounding vascular and neurological structures
- Displacement of angle between the internal and external carotid arteries–***'Lyre' sign***
- Characteristic imaging features including demonstration of vascularity called ***'salt and pepper' appearance***

SCHWANNOMA

- Between 30 and 70 years of age
- Benign neurogenic tumors
- Considered to originate from either Schwann cells/Fibroblasts supporting nerve
- Vagus nerve–Origin of 50% of parapharyngeal schwannomas–***Dysphagia and Hoarseness***
- Schwannomas are characterized by slow and asymptomatic growth
- Usually fusiform along long axis of nerve or round
- Transcervical or transoral biopsy of parapharyngeal space schwannomas is usually associated with unique pain not usually reported by patients undergoing Fine needle aspiration biopsy and may be complicated by hemorrhage, infection and rarely cranial nerve injury

> ***Most common metastases to parapharyngeal space is from NPC–30% of cases***

- Nodes may also be involved in tonsil and tongue base cancers and maxillary sinus cancer
- Benign tumors of parapharyngeal space have ***low levels of recurrence*** with a 5 year PFS rates of 93%. Malignant tumors of parapharyngeal space have 5 year PFS rate of 61%
- ***Usually asymptomatic oropharyngeal masses***–At least 3 cm before they become apparent and present as a neck mass

> ***Most common presentation of parapharyngeal mass- Asymptomatic neck mass with blunting of mandibular angle or inferior displacement of submandibular gland***

IMAGING

- Parapharyngeal space appears as a small triangular space on axial imaging with an image density or signal consistent with fat

> ***Presence of a fat plane between parotid and lesion differentiates truly parapharyngeal space lesion from an extension of deep lobe parotid lesion through stylomandibular tunnel into parapharyngeal space***
>
> ***Lesion arising in pre-styloid space may have a rim of parapharyngeal fat anteromedially, but*** *displaces parapharyngeal fat and internal carotid artery posterolaterally*
>
> ***A lesion in post-styloid compartment will displace*** *parapharyngeal fat and internal carotid artery anteromedially*
>
> *On MRI,* ***Congenital*** *cysts appear as T1-weighted hypointense and T2-weighted hyperintense lesions with peripheral enhancement on post-contrast study and low attenuation on CT scan*

Schwannomas
• Fusiform, sharply circumscribed masses seen on CT as soft-tissue density masses with few cystic areas within
• Uniform enhancement on post-contrast study
• On MRI heterogeneously hyperintense on T2-weighted images and isointense to hypointense on T1-weighted images

TREATMENT

- Lesions of parapharyngeal space are predominantly treated by surgery
- ***Adjuvant radiotherapy is reserved for malignant lesions or recurrent benign lesions with high risk of recidivism and considered a high surgical risk or unresectable lesions***

- **Chemotherapy:** Rhabdomyosarcoma, Positive margin status, Tumor histology, Perineural and Lympho-vascular spread

Choice of surgical technique is dependent on tumor size, its relationship to parotid gland and skull base and if tumor is malignant

TRANSCERVICAL APPROACH

- *Ideal for small benign tumors independent of deep lobe of the parotid gland*

TRANSCERVICAL-TRANSPAROTID APPROACH

- Suited for lesions arising from the deep lobe of the parotid gland, for vascular tumors (as it allows access to vessels in the neck) and for resection of malignant lesions

MANDIBULOTOMY

- Excision of ***infiltrating malignancy and multifocal recurrent benign tumors***
- Better visual access to superior aspect of parapharyngeal space and skull base

TORS
Ideal indications for TORS parapharyngeal space resection are benign salivary gland tumors occurring in pre-styloid compartment, displacing carotid artery posteriorly and laterally
• An absolute contraindication is tumor adherent or involving carotid artery

COMPLICATIONS

- Vagus–Most common to be injured in about 13% of carotid body tumors resection
- ***First bite syndrome:*** Loss of sympathetic supply to the parotid gland with subsequent increased sensitivity of myoepithelial cells to parasympathetic innervation

CHAPTER 32

TEMPORAL BONE TUMORS

Classification of tumors of the temporal bone						
Cutaneous neoplasms	**Glandular neoplasms**	**Vascular/ haematological**	**Paraganglions**	**Bone**	**Neural**	**Developmental and congenital**
Squamous cell papilloma and carcinoma	Ceruminous adenoma and adenocarcinoma	Haemangioma	Glomus tympanicum	Osteoma	V, VII, VIII, IX, X, schwannoma	Chordoma
Basal cell papilloma and carcinoma	Pleomorphic adenoma	Haemangiopericytoma	Glomus jugulare	Secondary tumurs	Meningioma	Demoid
Malignant melanoma	Adenoid cystic carcinoma	Leukaemia	Glomus vagale	Rhabdomyosarcoma		Teratoma
	Middle ear adenoma	Lymphoma		Chondrosarcoma		Choriostoma
	Endolymphatic sac tumors	Plasmacytoma		Ewing sarcoma		
		Langerhans cell histocytosis		Osteogenic sarcoma		

CERUMINOUS ADENOMA

- ***Well-differentiated tumors derived from ceruminous glands***
- Inner layer–Cuboidal/Coloumnar, Outer layer–Myoepithelial
- ***Wide excision–Local recurrence common, RT has no role***

CERUMINOUS ADENOCARCINOMA

- ***Surgical resection with post-operative radiotherapy–Appropriate therapy***

ADENOID CYSTIC CARCINOMA

- Local tissue destruction
- Perineural and perivascular invasion
- Tends to metastasize to lymph nodes
- ***Best management-***Aggressive surgical resection followed by RT

Bone invasion, perineural spread and tumor extension outside the external auditory canal are considered indicators of poor prognosis

SCHWANNOMA

- ***Most common neoplasm affecting temporal bone-Vestibular Schwannoma***
- NF2 gene is inactivated in 67% of Schwannomas
- Schwannomas are strongly S100-positive; neurofibromas tend to be weakly positive and also contain neurofilament positive fibres

NEUROENDOCRINE TUMORS OF MIDDLE EAR

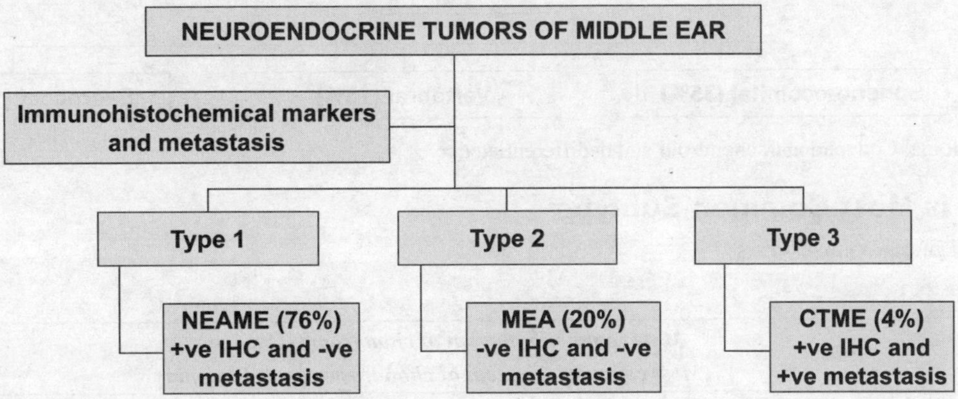

- ***Wide surgical resection is generally recommended***
- Hearing can often be preserved
- Radiotherapy does not have a role to play in the treatment

Endolymphatic SAC Tumors

- **Heffner tumor, Low grade adenocarcinoma of endolymphatic sac origin and Aggressive papillary middle ear tumor**
- ***Progressive unilateral, sensorineural hearing loss is most prominent feature***
- On microscopy, tumors demonstrate a papillary ultrastructure, composed of cuboidal/low columnar cells
- ***Growth and spread to cerebellopontine angle and posterior fossa is most commonly seen***
- Associated with vHL (3p)–***female-to-male ratio of 2:1 for VHL disease***
- An excellent prognosis (survival and hearing preservation) with early surgical resection
- Radiation therapy may be considered when surgical treatment is not an option or as a palliative measure following partial tumor removal

INVERTED PAPILLOMA

- HPV–implicated in inverted papilloma of middle ear
- Surgery is mainstay of treatment

Patients with evidence of carcinoma- Radical resection with post-operative radiotherapy

HEMANGIOMA

- Most common site–***Geniculate ganglion***
- May regress spontaneously, others continue to grow and are locally destructive
- Surgical excision is the treatment of choice

HEMANGIOPERICYTOMA

- 15–25% of haemangiopericytomas develop in the head and neck
- Fifty percent are malignant
- Treatment is by wide surgical excision
- Radioresistant

OSTEOMA

- Most common site of origin in temporal bone–Mastoid (20% middle ear)

Chordoma

- ***Arises from dendritic processes at the cephalic end of primitive notochord***
- LOH 1p36 is implicated, Loss of 1p36 is associated with sporadic chordoma

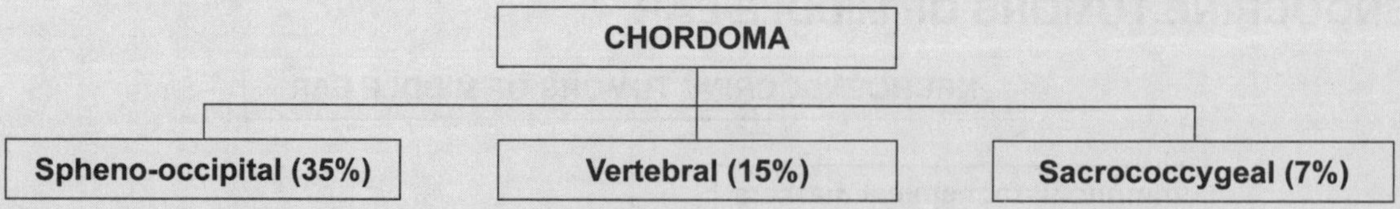

- Types of chordoma: Conventional, chondroid and dedifferentiated

Chondroid is Most Common Subtype

- Mean age if diagnosis–35 to 45 years
- Male : Female= 2 : 1

Most common symptom of chondroma–Headache
Most common symptom of chondrosarcoma–Diplopia

- Surgical removal of chordoma is mainstay of treatment
- Successful resection depends on the degree of spread of the tumor and degree of involvement of vital structures, such as the carotid artery and the brain
- Proton beam therapy is now considered gold standard radiotherapy modality

Lack of 1p36 LOH, or the presence of TNFRSF8 expression–associated with a better prognosis

Chondrosarcoma

- Arise from chondrocytes that persist as embryonal cell rests at or about foramen lacerum

Hyaline and myxoid types are more common and are referred to as 'conventional' chondrosarcoma

- Mean age at presentation is in fourth decade and male : female ratio is approximately equal
- Chondrosarcoma has a much better overall prognosis than that of chordoma

Surgical resection is the mainstay of treatment
Complete removal is not always possible but adjunctive radiation therapy, particularly proton beam is used

SECONDARY TUMORS OF TEMPORAL BONE

Haematological malignancies have significant propensity to spread to temporal bone
Most common site of origin of secondary temporal bone tumors–BREAST
Most common symptom at presentation is hearing loss
Petrous apex is the most common site

- Development of unilateral hearing loss in a patient who has had a previous malignancy may indicate a secondary tumor in the temporal bone

Rhabdomyosarcoma

- Extremely aggressive tumor of striated muscle origin
- ***Most common soft tissue tumor of childhood***
- ***Most common symptom of Rhabdomyosarcoma–Mass in ear region***

Langerhans Cell Histiocytosis

- Proliferation of histiocytes share characteristic langerhans cells–**HISTIOCYTOSIS X**
- Presence of inclusion bodies in cytoplasm–**BIRBECK GRANULES**

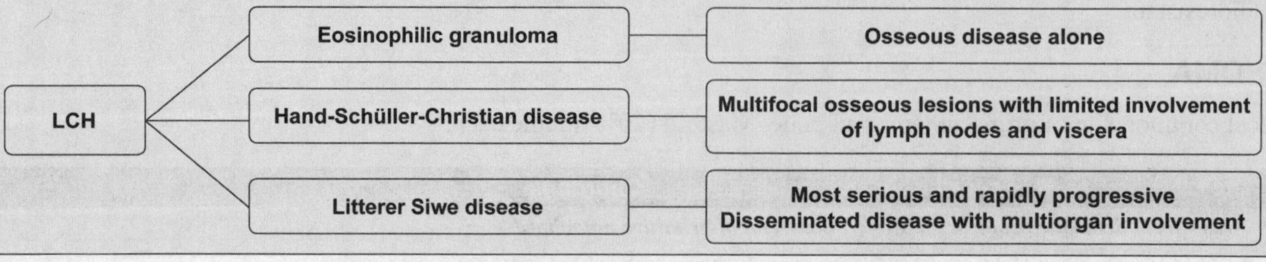

Contd.

Contd.

- Thirty per cent of patients with temporal bone involvement have bilateral involvement

Characteristic radiological appearance of temporal bone is 'punched out' or lytic appearance

- Age at presentation of less than 2 years with organ dysfunction is an indicator of a much poorer prognosis

Disseminated disease is rapidly fatal

TEMPORAL BONE CARCINOMAS

- <1% of all head and neck malignancies
- ***Most common involved part–Auricle***
- ***Males***–More commonly involved
- ***Sun exposure***–Important risk factor
- Most common histologic cancer–***SCC***
- Most common tumor staging for Temporal bone carcinoma–***Pittsbugh staging***

ETIOLOGY AND RISK FACTORS

- **Genetics:** NF2 (22q), Hereditary paraganglioma (11q), vHL (3p)
- **Ionizing radiation**–Latency period before symptoms detected ranged from 5 to 30 years

Cahan established criteria for radiation induced sarcoma in bone

Lustig Criteria

- Second neoplasm must develop in the irradiated field
- A latent period of at least several years must elapse between radiation exposure and development of a second primary
- Previous condition must show histological, radiographic and microscopic evidence of neoplasia
- Second tumor must be of a different histological type from that previously irradiated

- **UV light:** Most common type of primary cancer in the EAC is SCC
- **CSOM:** Cellular trauma must be a contributory factor
- **HPV:** HPV 16/18 at both tissue and molecular levels in patients with carcinoma of middle ear and associated chronic otitis media
- Exposure to ultraviolet light–risk factor for SCC that originates in EAC

CLINICAL FEATURES

- Otalgia, otorrhoea, hearing loss and vertigo are main features
- ***Alarming features***–Facial palsy or bleeding
- Invasion of blood vessels of EAC gives rise to bloody otorrhoea
- Trismus
- Hemifacial spasm or progressive facial weakness
- Lower cranial nerve palsies (IX, X, XI and XII)
- Headache and localized pain
- Cervical metastases

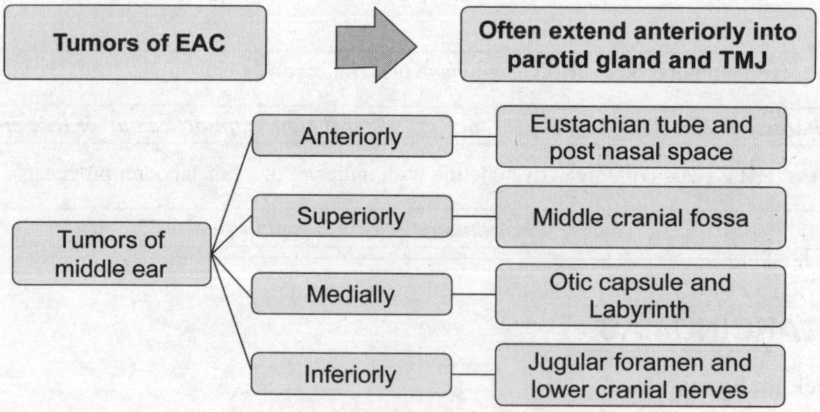

- Stell and McCormick proposed system for staging Carcinoma of External and Middle ear
- Arriaga have also proposed system for staging Tumors of External auditory canal
- First echelon lymph nodes are often within parotid gland and these drain into pre-auricular nodes en route to the jugulodigastric and deep cervical chain of lymph nodes

Presence of metastatic lymph nodes in the neck are a poor prognostic indicator–neck dissection does not improve survival

INVESTIGATION

An endophytic or exophytic mass within the EAC is likely to be malignant and is a strong indication for an urgent biopsy

- Staging CT chest and neck is done
- CT pelvis is not needed unless adenocarcinoma, lymphoma and melanoma

University of Pittsburgh staging system for squamous cell carcinoma of the temporal bone	
T Status	
T1:	Tumor limited to the external auditory canal without bony erosion or evidence of soft-tissue extension
T2:	Tumor with limited external auditory canal bony erosion (not full thickness) or radiographic finding consistent with limited (<0.5 cm) soft-tissue involvement
T3:	Tumor eroding the osseous external auditory canal (full thickness) with limited (<0.5 cm) soft-tissue involvement, or tumor involving middle ear and/or mastoid or patients presenting with facial paralysis
T4:	Tumor eroding the cochlea, petrous apex, medial wall of the middle ear, carotid canal, jugular foramen or dura or with extensive (> 0.5 cm) soft-tissue involvement
N Status	
Lymph Node involvement is a poor prognostic sign and places the patient in an advanced stage (i.e., T1 N1 (Stage III) and T2, 3, 4 N1 [Stage IV])	
M Status	
M1 disease is stage IV and is considered a very poor prognostic sign	

Modified Pittsburgh staging system		
Stage		**Description**
T Classification	T1	Limited to the EAC without bony erosion or evidence of soft tissue involvement
	T2	Limited to the EAC with bone erosion (not full thickness) or limited soft tissue involvement (< 0.5 cm)
	T3	Erosion through the osseous EAC (full thickness) with limited soft tissue involvement (< 0.5 cm), or tumor involvement in the middle ear and/or mastoid
	T4	Erosion of the cochlea, petrous apex, medial wall of the middle ear, carotid canal, jugular foramen, or dura; with extensive soft tissue involvement (>0.5 cm, such as involvement of the TMJ or styloid process); or ***evidence of facial paresis***

Contd.

Contd.

N Classification	N0	No regional nodes involved
	N1	Single metastatic regional node < 3 cm in size
	N2a	Single ipsilateral metastatic node 3-6 cm in size
	N2b	Multiple ipsilateral metastatic lymph nodes
	N2c	Contratateral metastatic lymph node
	N3	Metastatic lymph node > 6 cm in size

–	T1	T2	T3	T4
N0	I	II	III	IV
N1	IV			
N2				
N3				

- Surgery preferred treatment for SCC and BCC
- Small lesions–***WLE***
- Large lesions–***Partial/Total auriculectomy***
- Early EAC lesions–***Sleeve resection***
- Large tumors with medial extension or bony erosion–***Lateral temporal bone resection***
- Most extensive tumors–Subtotal temporal bone resection

Lesions elsewhere involving temporal bone–Auriculectomy and Lateral temporal bone resection

- Overall survival is 20-30% at 5 years
- Cancers of outer ear– >90% Survival. Middle ear extension–30%

SURGICAL ASPECTS OF TEMPORAL BONE CARCINOMA ***En bloc resection with post-operative radiotherapy is current treatment of choice***

Tumors lateral to tympanic membrane ***(T1 and T2)*** can be resected adequately by a ***lateral temporal bone resection***
• Aggressive nature of this disease, pinna is only preserved if a wide soft tissue margin (>1cm) exists between the lateral aspect of the tumor and the external auditory meatus
Anterior border of the malignancy is the posterior limit of TMJ

An ***extended temporal bone resection*** is required when invasion extends medial to TM or into the mastoid ***(T3/T4 disease)***
• Margins of resection are the ICA anteriorly, middle fossa dura superiorly, sigmoid sinus and posterior fossa dura posteriorly, petrous apex medially and jugular bulb inferiorly

RECONSTRUCTION

- Free tissue transfer is routinely used to reconstruct pyramidal defect that typically remains following ablative surgery
- Anterolateral thigh flap is a common choice as it provides skin and fascial covering and can be taken with muscle if more bulk is required
- Thigh donor site provides access for fascia lata if required for static slings for simultaneous facial palsy reconstruction

SURVIVAL

- Early stage tumors generally have favorable outcome with most reporting an 80–100% survival rate
- Malignant invasive disease may sometimes be limited to the adventitia and as a consequence the tumor can be dissected clear without need for ligation and division of the artery

PART ONE: NEURO-ONCOLOGY

CHAPTER

33 NEURO-ONCOLOGY

Most Common
• Most common primary intracranial malignancy–GBM
• Most common malignancy of brain–Metastasis
• Most common tumor of brain in children–Juvenile astrocytoma
• Most common posterior fossa tumor in children–Cerebellar astrocytoma
• Most common malignant posterior fossa tumor in children–Medulloblastoma
• Most common brain stem tumor–Pontine glioma
• Most common symptom of brain tumor–Headache
• Most common sign of brain tumor–Hemiparesis
• **Most common Primary intracranial tumor–MENINGIOMA**
• Most common site of Primary CNS lymphoma–Frontal lobe
• Most common site of Oligodendroglioma–Frontal lobe
• Most active agent against CNS lymphoma–Methotrexate
• Highly radiosensitive brain tumor–Medulloblastoma
• **Most common site of pineal meningioma–VELUM**
• Most common site of medulloblastoma in children–VERMIS, Adults–Cerbellar hemisphere
• Most common site of metastasis of medulloblastoma–Subarachnoid space
• Most important prognostic factor of medulloblastoma–Disseminated disease
• Most common site of meningioma–Parasagittal
• Most common site of choroid plexus Tumors–4th ventricle
• Most common benign Non glial brain tumor in children–**CRANIOPHARYNGIOMA**
• Most common site of chondrosarcoma–Petrous apex
• Most common site of Heamgioblastoma–Cerebellar hemisphere (VHL)
• Most common location of Origin of Vestibular schwannoma–Internal auditory canal
• Most common nerve of origin of Vestibular schwannoma–Superior vestibular nerve
• Most common type of Lymphoma of brain–DLBCL
• Most common type of pineal tumor–**GERMINOMA**
• Most common malignant pineal parenchymal tumor–**Pinealoblastoma**
• Most differentiated pineal tumor–**Pineocytoma**
• Most common type of pituitary adenoma–**PROLACTINOMA**
• Most common primary for brain secondaries–Carcinoma Lung > Breast Ca
• High prosensity to metastatise to brain (MULTIPLE)–Malignant melanoma
• Most common metastasis to cause Intratumoral bleed–Malignant melanoma
• Most common Intracerebral metastasis in children–Neuroblastoma
• Most common metastasis to present as cystic lesions–Breast and lung cancers

Contd.

Contd.

- **Most common cancer to cause leptomeningeal metastasis–CA BREAST**
- **Most common orbital tumor in children–DERMOID CYST**
- **Most common bony tumor of orbit–OSTEOMA**
- **Most common sarcoma of orbit–RHABDOMYOSARCOMA**
- **Most common mesenchymal tumor of orbit in adults–Fibrous histiocytoma**
- **Most common benign lacrimal gland tumor–Pleomorphic adenoma**
- **Most common malignant lacrimal gland tumor–Adenoid cystic carcinoma**

Risk Factors

- **VHL–Hemangioblastoma**
- **Tuberous Sclerosis–SEGA**
- **NF1–Optic glioma**
- **NF2–Schwannoma and meningioma**
- **Turcot syndrome–Medulloblastoma**
- **Lynch syndrome–GBM**
- **Gorlin syndrome–Medulloblastoma**
- **Family History**
- **EBV–Primary CNS lymphoma**
- **SPECIAL EDGE: (Proposed not established)**
  - Farmers and petrochemical workers–Primary tumors
  - Radiation–Superficial meningioma
  - CT scan–Increases risk of Intracranial meningioma
  - Cell phones–Glioma/Meningioma
  - Vinyl chloride–Astrocytoma

Chromosomal abnormalities associated with brain tumors

Syndrome	Gene defect	Tumor
Neurofibromatosis type 1	Neurofibromin (Chr 17)	Astrocytomas
Neurofibromatosis type 2	Schwannomin (Chr 22)	Acoustic neuromas (bilateral); meningiomas
Cowden's disease	PETN (Chr 10)	Astrocytomas
Hereditary non-polyposis colorectal cancer	Multiple	Astrocytomas
Li-Fraumeni syndrome	P53 (Chr17)	Astrocytomas

Condition	Inheritance and genetics	Cutaneous manifestations	Eye	Nervous system	Brain tumors
Von Recklinghausen's neurofibromatosis (NF-1)	Autosomal dominant NF-1 gene (encodes neurofibromin that regulates GT Pases in signal transduction	Café au lait macules, axillary, freckles	Lisch nodules (pigmented iris hamartomas)	Neurofibromata	Schwann cell tumors of spinal and cranial nerves, meningiomas ependymomas, optic gliomas
Acoustic neurofibromatosis (NF-2)	Autosomal dominant NF-2 gene (encodes Merlin protein involved in cell adhesion)	Café au lait macules less common than in NF-1	Presenile catarcts	Bilateral acoustic neuromas Neurofibromata	Schwann cell tumors of spinal and cranial nerves, meningiomas, astrocytomas, ependymomas, optic gliomas
Tuberous sclerosis	Autosomal dominant TSC1 gene (encodes hamartin protein) and TSC2 gene (encodes tuberin protein)	Adenoma sebaceum, Shagreen patches, subungual fibromata, café au lait spots		Seizures, mental retardation	Giant cell astrocytoma of the foramen of Munro, gliomas, ependymomas

Contd.

Contd.

Von Hippel-Lindau	Autosomal dominant VHL gene (encodes VHL protein involved in ubiquination)	Skin hamartomas	Retinal angiomas		Cerebellar haemangioblastomas ependymomas phaeochromocytoma

SEX

- Meningioma and Schwannoma–Females
- Glioma and medulloblastoma (others)–Males

SYMPTOMS

Patterns of deficit generally associated with certain tumors	
Tumor location	**Expected deficit**
Pituitary (e.g., pituitary adenoma)	Bitemporal hemianopia; gaze palsies
Cerebellopontine angle (e.g., vestibular schwannoma)	Hearing loss; balance disturbance; tinnitus
Anterior skull base (e.g., olfactory groove meningioma)	Anosmia; ipsilateral optic atrophy; contralateral papilloedema (Foster-Kennedy syndrome)
Occipital (e.g., glioma, metastasis)	Homonymous hemianopia with central sparing
Parietal (dominant hemisphere)	Acalculia; agraphia; left-right disorientation; finger agnosia (Gerstamann syndrome)
Parietal (e.g., glioma)	Sensory inattention; dressing apraxia; astereognosis
Temporal (e.g., glioma)	Memory disturbance; contralateral superior quadrantanopia; dysphasia (dominant hemisphere)
Frontal (e.g., glioma)	Personality changes; gait disturbance; urinary incontinence
Brainstem (e.g., brainstem glioma)	Multiple cranial nerve deficits; long tract signs; nystagmus
Posterior fossa (e.g., medulloblastoma)	Ataxia; hydrocephalus
Parasagittal falx	Progressive spastic weakness Numbness of legs
Olfactory groove	Anosmia Visual loss Papilloedema (Foster-Kennedy syndrome) Frontal lobe syndrome
Sella turcica	Visual field loss
Sphenoid ridge	Cavernous sinus syndrome (medial) Exophthalmos and visual loss (middle) Temporal bone swelling and skull deformity (lateral)
Posterior fossa (foramen magnum tentorium)	Hydrocephalus (tentorium) Galt atacela and cranial neuropathies V, VII, VIII, IX and X (cerebellopontine angle) Suboceipital pain, ipsilateral arm and leg weakness (foramen magnum)

TUMORS

I. Glioma:

- **30% to 50% of all pediatric CNS tumors**
- **IDH Mutation–Better prognosis**
- Hemispheric (10%-15%)
- Midline (10%-15%)
- Optic pathways (5%)

- Favorable prognosis, indolent course, remote risk of malignant transformation
- 40% of GBM has EGFR Amplification

Grading of gliomas by subtype				
	Astrocytoma	**Oligodendroglioma**	**Mixed glioma**	**Ependymoma**
Grade 1	Pilocytoic, giant cell			Subependymoma, myxopapillary ependymoma
Grade 2	Diffuse, pilomyxoid pleomorphic xanthoastrocytoma	Oligodendroglioma	Oligoastrocytoma	Ependymoma
Grade 3	Anaplastic astrocytoma	Anaplastic Oligodendroglioma	Anaplastic oligoastrocytoma	Anaplastic ependymoma

PILOCYTIC ASTROCYTOMA

- **Most common glial tumor**
- Less invasive
- Circumscribed
- 90% BRAF V600 E mutation
- Treatment–Surgery

> - ***Most common feature of Low grade glioma–Low grade seizures***
> - ***Most common feature of subcortical and cortical tumors is seizures***

Tumor	Site
Pilomyxoid astrocytomas	Hypothalamus
Gangliogliomas and pxas	Temporal lobe
Sega	Periventricular
Oligodendrogliomas	Frontal lobe

OPTIC GLIOMA

- 1% of all intracranial tumors
- Unilateral
- Females > males
- **Most common location is the optic pathway (60%)**
- 75% occur in <10 years of age
- **Strong association with NF1**
- >70% of ONG have NF1, 30% of those with NF1 develop optic glioma
- 75% symptomatic in the first decade and 90% asymptomatic before 20

Types

- Pre-chiasmatic optic nerve glioma
- Diffuse chiasmatic glioma
- Dorsal-chiasmatic–hypothalamic glioma

Signs/Symptoms

- Decreased visual function, Acute loss of vision, Proptosis, Strabismus, Disc edema, Vascular compromise-chronic compression of central retinal vein leading to occlusion venous stasis retinopathy optociliary shunt vessels/neovascular glaucoma

MRI

– ONG without NF1 the optic nerve is enlarged in a fusiform manner with a clear-cut margin produced by intact dural sheath
– ONG with NF1 nerve is irregular with kinking and buckling secondary to the mass
– Hypo- to iso on T1 and hyper on T2 Variable contrast enhancement
– Intracranial extension not related to optic anal enlargement

Most common optic nerve GLIOMA is Pilocytic Astrocytoma

- **Most common mutated gene in GBM-p53**
- **Most common type of adult brain tumor–Malignant astrocytoma/GBM**
- **Most common site of oligodendroglioma–Frontal lobe**
- **Fried egg appearance is seen in Oligodendroglioma**

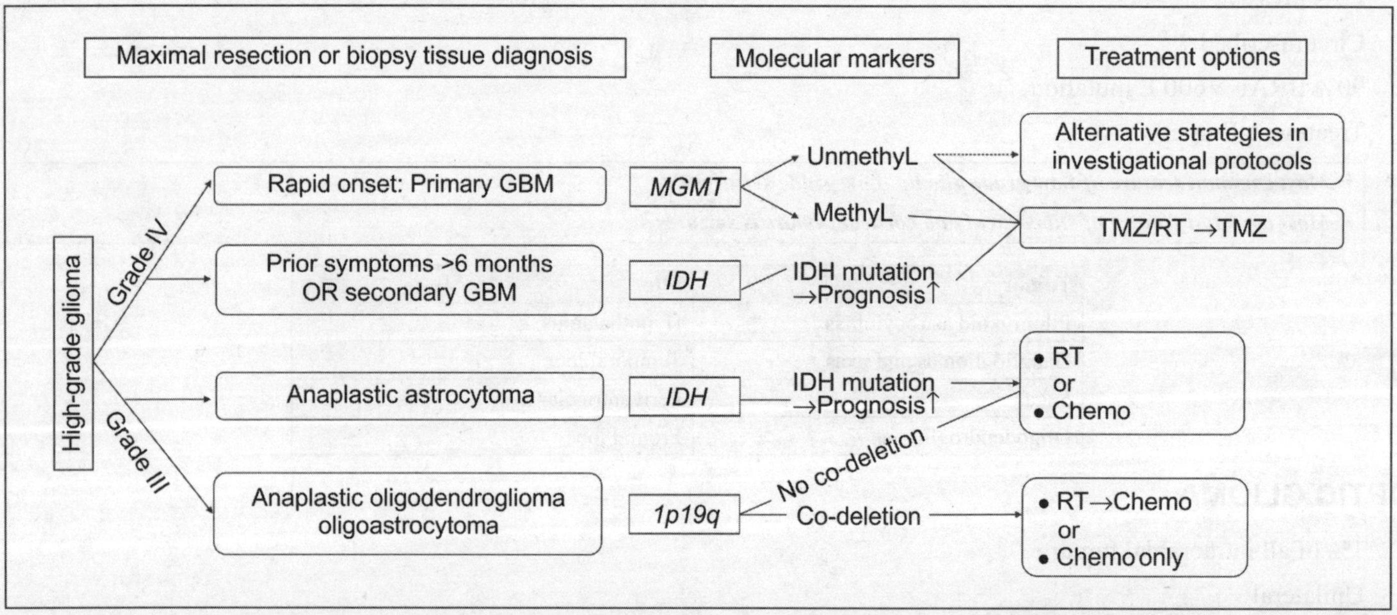

Molecular genetics of gliomas		
Genetic Alteration	**Primary (De Novo) GBM (90%)**	**Secondary GBM (10%)**
IDHI mutation	Absent	> 95% (indicates progression from grade 2 astrocytoma)
LOH 10p	50%	Rare, possibly never
LOH 19q	~5%	~30-50%
LOH 10q	~70%	~70%
PTEN mutation (10q23.3)	25%	Uncommon, <5%
EGFR amplification	~35-45%	Uncommon, 0-6.5%
TP53 mutation	~20-35%	~60-85%

Tumor	5-year survival
Grade I glioma (cerebellar)	90-100%
Grade I glioma (other sites)	50-60%
Grade II (astrocytoma)	16-46%
Grade III (anaplastic astrocytoma)	10-30%
Grade IV (glioblastoma multiforme)	1-10%
Oligodendroglioma	50-80%
Meningioma	70-80%

II. Meningioma

- Most common site is Falx–Parasagittal
- Benign slow growing extra Axial tumor
- Arises from arachnoid cap cells

Risk Factors: NF2–80% sporadic meningioma, CA breast, Radiation, Female sex

- Usually benign (70-80%), 10% Multiple
- Malignant meningioma–Loss of 1p, 10 and 14q
- GLOBULAR/SIEVE calcification
- DURAL TAIL SIGN
- Calvarial hyperosteosis
- **TRAF4–Anterior, NF2–Posterolateral**
- Recurrent KLF4 K409 mutation–WHO 1 meningioma
- Most useful predictor for recurrence is VEGF

Who Grading of Meningioma

WHO grade	Criteria
I	Mitosis < 4/10 HPF
II	Mitosis 4-19/10 HPF or 3 or more of the following five features • Increased cellularity • Uninterrupted patternless or sheet-like growth • Smell cells with a high nuclear/cytoplasmic ratio • Prominent nucleoli • Foci of 'spontaneous' or 'geographic' necrosis
III	Mitosis ≥ 20/10 HPF or exhibiting loss of differentiated features resulting in carcinoma, melanoma, or sarcoma-like appearances

SIMPSON GRADING OF RESECTION

Resection Grade	Definition	Recurrence%
1	GTR of tumor, dural attachments and abnormal bone	9
2	GTR of tumor, coagulation of dural attachments	19
3	GTR of tumor w/o resection or coagulation of dural attachments or extradural extensions (invaded or hyperostotic bone)	29
4	Partial resection of tumor	44
5	Simple decompression (biopsy)	–

Treatment

- Surgical resection, Recurrence rate–1 to 2%
- Inoperable, Incomplete resection WHO GRADE 3–RADIOTHERAPY (54 Gy–Benign, 60 Gy–Malignant)
- **Simpsons grade 0, 1, 2–No radiotherapy given**
- **Optic sheath meningioma–Radiotherapy**

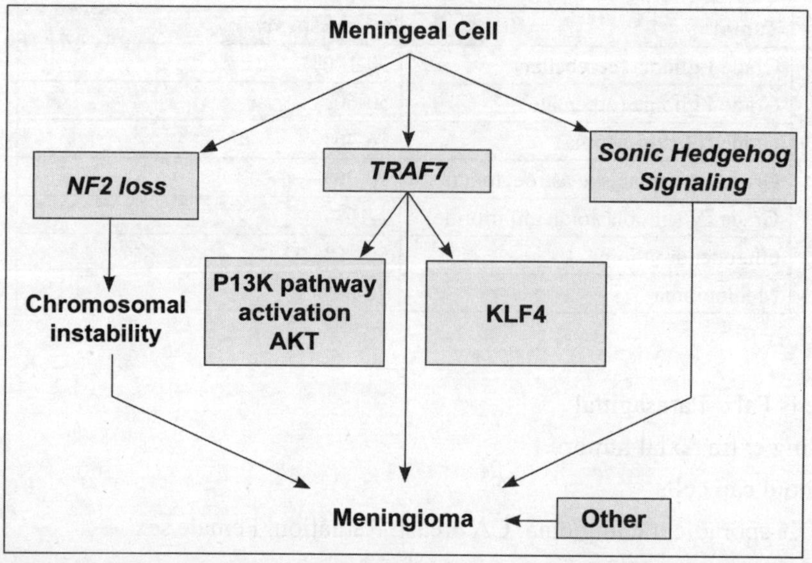

Hakuba modification of bonnal and brotchi classification of parasagittal meningioma	
Type I:	The meningioma is attached to the sole outer layer of the sinus well. The outer dural layer is resected and the site of attachment coagulated, leaving a clean and glistening dural surface
Type II:	The lateral recess is invaded. The intrasinusal fragment is extracted and the dural defect repaired with either a simple running suture or a patch made of autologous aponeurosis (dura mater, periosteum, fascia lata, or, better, fascia temporalis)
Type III:	The ipsilateral lateral wall is invaded. The invaded wall is resected and repaired with a patch
Type IV:	The ipsilateral wall and the roof are both invaded. The invaded walls are resected and the sinus is kept patent with a patch reconstruction
Types V and VI:	The sinus is totally occluded. In Type V, one wall is free of tumor. Although the current theory is to remove the invaded portion of the sinus without reestablishing venous circulation, our preference is to restore this circulation. In tumors of type V, circulation can be restored with a patch after the two invaded walls (or, ipsilateral wall and roof) have been resected and the fragment that occludes the sinus extracted. In tumors of type VI, restoration must be done with a bypass, which can be end-to-side before tumor removal or end-to-end after removal. For meningiomas in the posterior third of the SSS, the torcular or the lateral sinus, a sino-jugular bypass at the neck can be done before sacrifice of the invaded portion

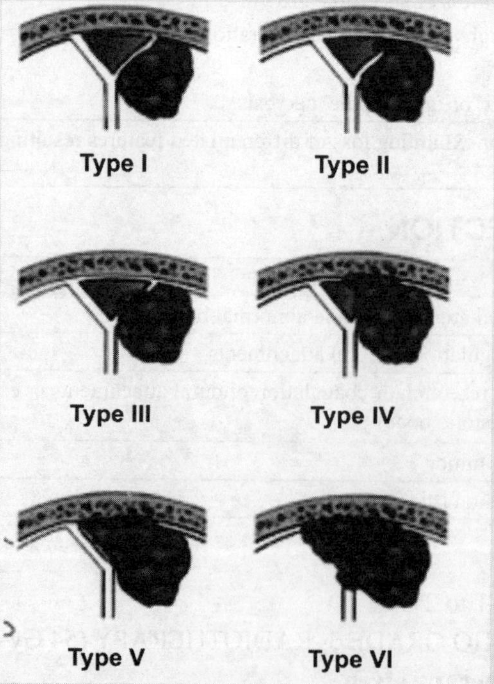

Contd.

Contd.

Anterior Clinoidal Meningioma

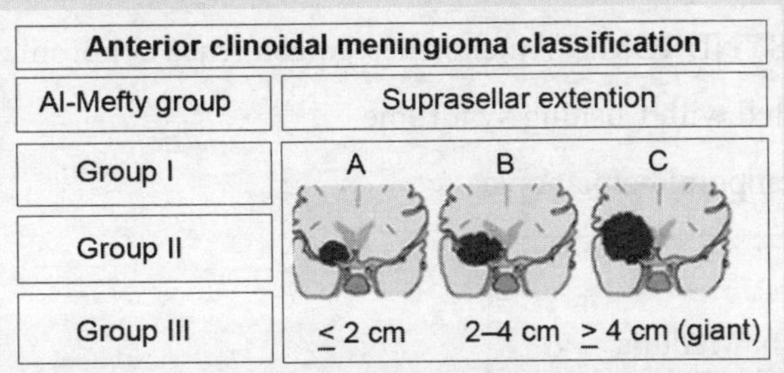

Cavernous Meningioma

- Grade 0: Adenoma does not extend the medial carotid line
- Grade 1: Adenoma extends the medial line, but doesn't reach median line, so-called "intracarotid" line
- Grade 2: Tumor extends beyond the median line, but doesn't extend beyond or tangent to lateral line
- Grade 3: Tumor extends beyond the lateral line
- Grade 4: Tumor totally wraps around the intracavernous carotid artery

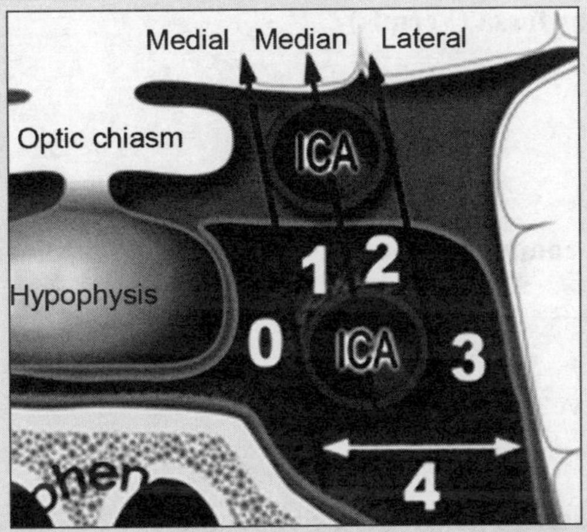

Posterior Fossa Meningioma

Type	Location	Anatomical extension
I	Cerebellar convexity, lateral tentorial	Tentorium, transverse and signmoid sinus
II	CP angle	Petrous ridge, IAC
III	Jugular foramen	Cerebello-medullary angle, internal jugular vein, extracranial
IV	Petro clival	Upper 2/3rd clivus, cavernous sinus, meckles cave, petrous ridge
V	Foramen magnum	Lower 1/3rd clivus and C1, C2 area
VI	Unclassifed	Entire clivus, mid and lower clivus and other types

III. Acoustic Neuroma

- Most are unilateral
- NF2- bilateral
- ***M=F***
- ***50 years***

Most Common Location–Internal Auditory Canal

- Gd enhanced MRI–Investigation of choice

Treatment:

- **Observe**–Small tumors, Old age, Multiple medical comorbidities

IV. Pituitary Tumors

- Anterior pituitary–10%
- FORBES–ALBRIGHT SYNDROME–Amenorrhea galactorrhea syndrome–Hypersecretion of prolactin
- Most commonly associated with Cushing syndrome
- OPTIC CHIASMA–Bitemporal hemianopia

V. Brainstem Glioma

- **Focal**– < 2 cm, Mid brain, Medulla
- **Diffuse–Pons**
- **Cervicomedullary**–Upper cervical cord
- **Dorsal exophytic**–Floor of 4th ventricle

VI. Medulloblastoma

- **Most common PNET**
- **Most common site is Posterior fossa (Vermis)**
- Metastasis occurs to bone

Types:

- **Classical–Most common**
- **Desmoplastic/nodular–Most common variant**
- Anaplastic
- Large cell
- Medulloblastoma with extensive nodularity

Molecular Groups:

- **WNT–Best prognosis–Monosomy 6–TURCOT Syndrome**
- SHH–Desmoplastic–Del PTCH, MYCN and GLI 2 Amplification
- **Group 3–Worst prognosis**
- Group 4–Intermediate prognosis **(*MOST COMMON TYPE)**
- **Posterior fossa/Cerebellar mutism syndrome**–Diminished speech, Emotional liablility, Urinary retention, Decreased respiratory drive, Ataxia, Bulbar dysfunction
- Needs aggressive resection
- Highly radiosensitive
- Most common site of metastasis– Subarachnoid space
- **CT**–Discrete hyperattenuated Verminian mass
- **MRI–Gold standard**

Group	Progenitor Cell	Growth	Prognosis	Characteristic mutations	Structural Events
WNT	Lower Rhombic lip	4th ventricle with dorsal brainstem infiltration	Good	CTNN1(91%) DOX3X SMARCA4, MLL2, TP53	Monosomy 6

Contd.

Contd.

SHH	Cerebellar granule neuron precursors of the external granule layer	Cerebellar hemispheres	Intermediate	PTCH1, SUFU, SMO, TP53, MLL2, DOX3X	Genome Instability, including frequent amplification of MYCN and GLF2, deletion of PTCH1
Group 3	Cerebellar granule neuron precursors of the external granule layer, neural stem cells	–30%, metastatic at diagnosis (47% for infants)	Poor		Genome instability including MYC amplification. MYC/PVT1 fusion somase copy number alterations in TGFB signaling members including amplifications of OTX2
Group 4	Unknown	~30% metastatic at diagnoses (30% for infants)	Intermediate	KDMBA	Genome instability including SNCAP tandem duplication MYCN amplification

Treatment

Surgery + Post op RT whole brain

- Disseminated disease is most important prognostic factor
- Relapsed–High dose chemotherapy and Autologous stem cell rescue
- Age < 3 years, Extent of resection and Disseminated disease are poor prognostic factors
- Anaplastic < 3 years–High risk→ CRANIOSPINAL IRRADIATION

Chang staging system for Medulloblastoma	
T1	Tumor < 3 cm in diameter
T2	Tumor > 3 cm in diameter
T3a	Tumor > 3 cm in diameter with extension into aqueduct of Sylvius or foramen of Luschka
T3b	Tumor > 3 cm in diameter with unequivocal extension into the brainstem
T4	Tumor > 3 cm in diameter with extension up past the aqueduct of Sylvius and/or down past the foramen magnum (i.e., Beyond the posterior fossa)
M0	No evidence of subarachnoid or hematogenous metastasis
M1	Tumor cells found in cerebrospinal fluid
M2	Intracranial tumor beyond primary site
M3	Gross nodular seeding in spinal subarachnoid space
M4	Metastasis outside the cerebrospinal axis (especially to bone marrow, bone)

VII. Ependymoma

- **Most common site in adults–Infratentorial**
- **Most common site in pediatric population–Supratentorial**
- NF2 association present

Origin–Radial glial cells

- **Group A**–Laterally located, Younger, >50% recurrence
- **Group B**–Favourable, Older

Ependymoma subtype characteristics

Anatomical Location	Population	Genomic Characteristic
Supratentorial	Adult	CDKN2A deletion, amplification of $EPHB_2$
Infratentorial, medial	Pediatric	Chr1q gain
Infratentorial, lateral	Young adult	NF2 chr22 loss
Spinal	Adult	NF2 chr 22 loss

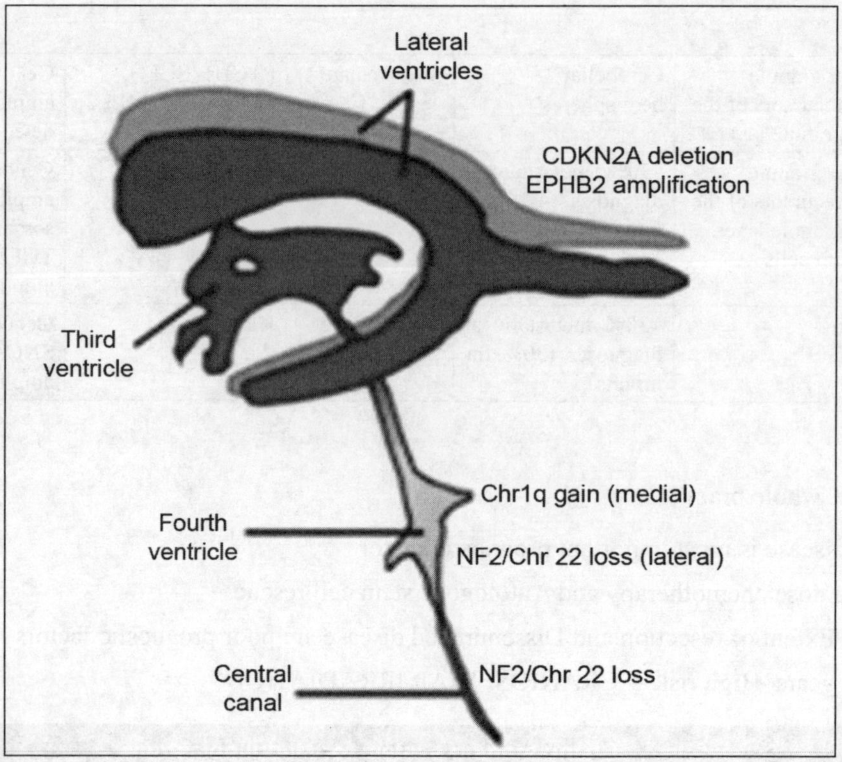

VIII. Lymphoma

Risk Factors–EBV, Immunocompromised, AIDS, Organ transplantation

- **Usually >60 years**
- Deletion of CDKN2A
- **Ring enhancing mass lesion** that disappears after starting steroids is strongly suggestive of lymphoma
- **Periventricular/subcortical white matter**
- **Frontal lobe is most commonly involved**

Ommaya Reservoir: Methotrexate high dose+ Ara-C

- **Surgery is the treatment of choice**

Extra Edge

- 20% of cancers in ages 1 to 4 years and 30% in 5 to 9 years
- 75% of all primary childhood CNS tumors are gliomas
- Supratentorial tumors constitute 31% of pediatric CNS tumors
- **Most common benign peripheral nerve tumor–Solitary NF**
- Operative resection–Pain, Paraesthesia or weakness in nerve distribution
- **Indication For Surgical Resection of Solitary NF:** Large tumor mass, Accelerated growth, Neurologic deficit, Pain
- ***Most malignant peripheral nerve tumor–MPSNT***
- Tumor capable of metastasis to extracranial sites–Medulloblastoma
- Tumor spread along CSF pathway–Ependymoma
- **Bubbly appearance–Orbital lymphangioma**

MISCELLANEOUS

I. Metastasis

- **Most common tumor to metastatize to brain–CA LUNG**

Features

- **Multiple lesions**
- **Grey/white matter lesions**
- **Increased vasogenic edema/Tumor size**

Tissue of origin for brain metastases (approximate)	
Origin	**Percentage**
Lung	40
Breast	15
Melanoma	10
Renal/genitourinary	10
Other/unknown	25

II. Choroid Plexus Tumors

- **Most common site–4th ventricle (adult), Children–lateral ventricle**
- ***Associated with VHL and Li Fraumeni syndrome→ Propensity to carcinoma***
- *Most common presentation–Raised ICT without focal findings*
- **Increased signal on T2W MRI imaging**

WHO Grading

- **1-Choroid plexus papilloma (CPP)**
- **2-Atypical Choroid plexus papilloma (Atypical CPP)**
- **3-Choroid plexus carcinoma (CPC)**
- *Typically choroid plexus papilloma never progress to carcinoma*

Treatment

- Surgical resection (total)–CPP

Choroid Plexus Carcinoma (CPC)

- Adult→ surgery
- Children→ Open biopsy, chemotherapy and surgery

III. Pineal Tumors

- **Most malignant pineal tumor–Germinoma (Extremely malignant)**
- **Most common pineal tumor–Germinoma**
- ***PARINAUD SYNDROME–Paralysis of conjugate upward gaze***
- SYLVIAN AQUEDUCT SYNDROME
- ***Pineal tumor that spreads along ventricular walls/leptomeninges–Germinoma***
- CT–Hyperdense, MRI–Hypointense on T2 W
- Germinoma–Bifocally synchronous involvement of suprasellar and Pineal gland

- **Type 1–S100 +ve, NSE +ve**
- **Type 2–S100 –ve, NSE +ve**

- Treatment of germinoma–RT (40 Gy + 15 Gy boost)
- **Non-germinoma–Radical resection and Cisplatin etoposide chemotherapy**
- ***Disseminated/multiple germinoma–Chemotherapy (craniospinal irradiation)***
- 90% 5 year survival

IV. Chordoma

- Arises from primitive notochord
- Younger women
- ***Extradural, pseudoencapsulated, multilobulated***
- **Physaliferous cells**
- Chondroid chordoma–Cartilage features
- **HYPERINTENSE ON T2 W MRI**
- Dedifferentiated chordoma–High grade/poorly differentiated spindle cell sarcoma
- **TREATMENT: Surgery + RT**

V. Chondrosarcoma

- **Most common site is Petrous apex**
- **Most common site is Temporo-occipital synchondrosis**
- S100 +ve

VI. Craniopharyngioma

- **Most common nonglial brain tumor in children**
- Remnants of Rathke pouch
- Proteinaceous cyst fluid–Oily cellular debris
- **SUPRASELLAR CALCIFICATION–Pathognomonic (30-50%) on CT**

Treatment

- **Surgery–Subfrontal/pterional approach–Treatment of choice**
- Large–Supraorbital craniotomy
- Cystic–SRS, Endoscopic Y90, P32
- Radiosurgery–Optic chiasma, Brainstem, Pituitary fossa

VII. Hemangioblastoma

- **Most common site–VERMIS**
- Sporadic mostly, Associated with VHL (3rd decade)
- **Spinal cord tumors–Post to dentate line (90%)**
- MRI–Solid enhanced nodule with peritumoral cyst
- Uncal herniation–Hemispheric lesion
- Tonsillar herniation–Posterior fossa

Treatment

- VHL–Observe till symptomatic
- Unresectable, recurrent, incompletely excised–RT

SPINAL TUMORS

- Extradural–55%
- Most common extradural tumors–metastatic

- Schwannoma–THORACIC SPINE, Meningioma–FORAMEN MAGNUM
- Most common intramedullary tumor–Ependymoma
- Most common site of metastatic spinal tumors–Thoracic and Lumbar
- Most common source of spine metastasis–Lymphoma
- Most lesions of spinal metastasis–Osteolytic

Extra Dural	Extra Medullary	Intramedullary
Vertebral body, Thoracic spine	Within dura	Spinal cord
Lung metastasis	Meningioma, NF, Schwannoma	Astrocytoma, Ependymoma
Pain along Axial spine and trunk in radicular pattern		Myelopathy Cauda equine syndrome
Treatment: Surgery+RT	**Treatment:** EBRT	**Treatment:** Surgery

- **SURGERY–Failure of RT, Spinal instability, Recurrence after RT, Diagnosis of unknown primary**

- Hemangioma–Vertebral bodies of thoracoabdominal spine
- Most common intradural extramedullary tumor–Benign, slow growing and well circumscribed
- Most Intramedullary tumors in adults–Ependymoma
- **Best prognosis among spinal tumors–Myxopapillary**

SUMMARY

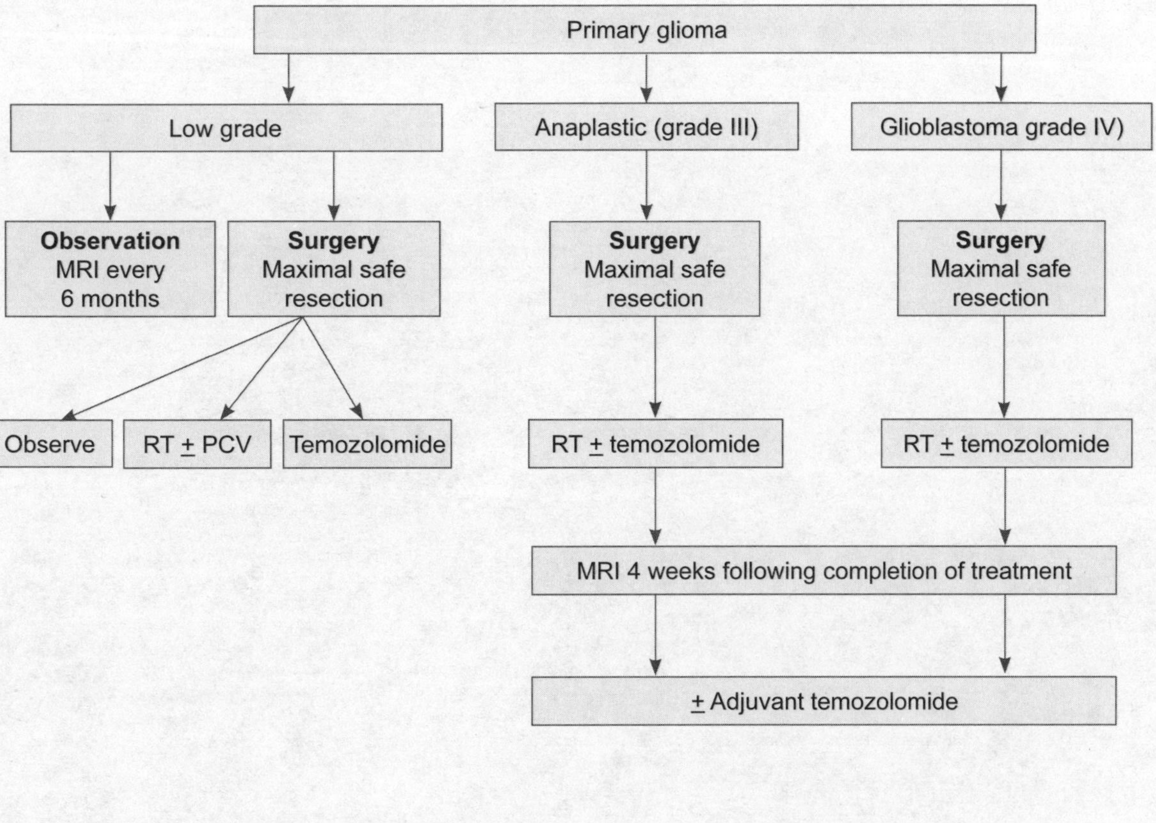

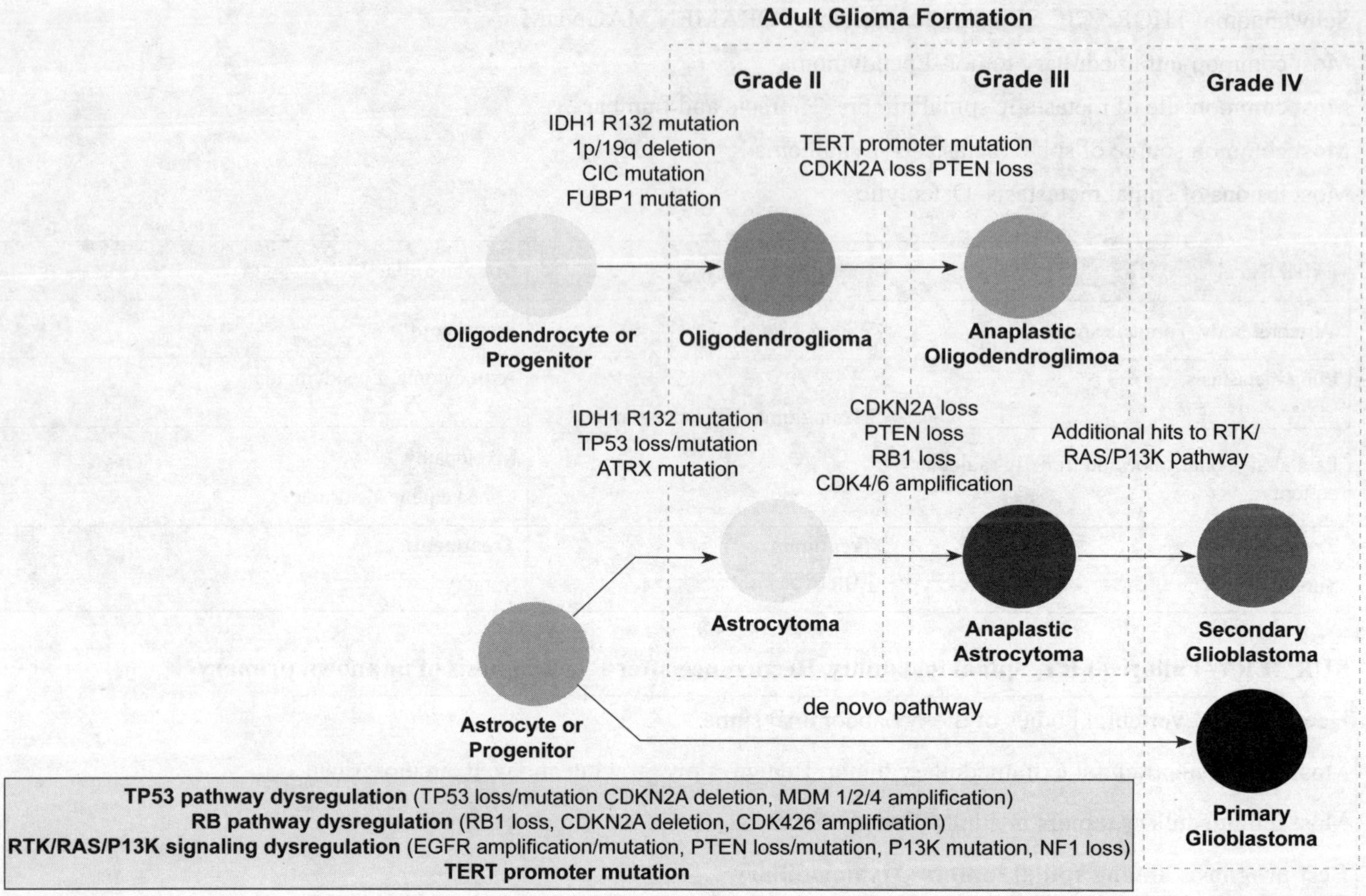
Adult Glioma Formation
Grade II
Grade III
Grade IV
IDH1 R132 mutation
1p/19q deletion
CIC mutation
FUBP1 mutation
TERT promoter mutation
CDKN2A loss PTEN loss
Oligodendrocyte or Progenitor
Oligodendroglioma
Anaplastic Oligodendroglimoa
IDH1 R132 mutation
TP53 loss/mutation
ATRX mutation
CDKN2A loss
PTEN loss
RB1 loss
CDK4/6 amplification
Additional hits to RTK/ RAS/P13K pathway
Astrocytoma
Anaplastic Astrocytoma
Secondary Glioblastoma
Astrocyte or Progenitor
de novo pathway
Primary Glioblastoma
TP53 pathway dysregulation (TP53 loss/mutation CDKN2A deletion, MDM 1/2/4 amplification)
RB pathway dysregulation (RB1 loss, CDKN2A deletion, CDK426 amplification)
RTK/RAS/P13K signaling dysregulation (EGFR amplification/mutation, PTEN loss/mutation, P13K mutation, NF1 loss)
TERT promoter mutation

PART ONE: ENDOCRINE ONCOLOGY

CHAPTER

34 THYROID MALIGNANCIES

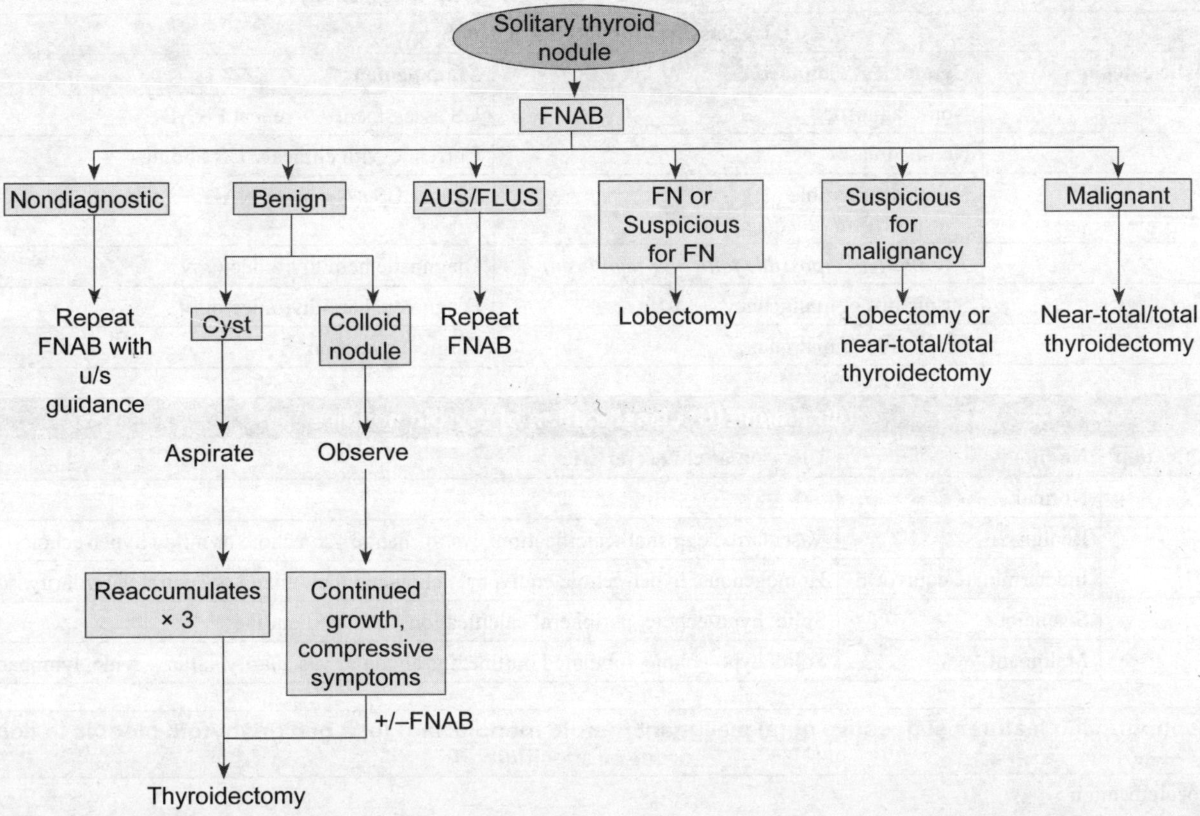

Bathedsa Classification		
Diagnostic Category	**Estimated Risk of Malignancy (%)**	**Usual Management**
Nondiagnostic	1-4	Repeat FNA with ultrasound guidance
Benign	0-3	Clinical follow-up
Atypical cells of undetermined significance (ACUS), follicular lesion of undetermined significance (FLUS)	5-15	Clinical/imaging correlation, repeat FNA for most
Follicular neoplasm or suspicious for a follicular neoplasm	15-30	Surgical lobectomy
• Specify if Hurthle cell type • Suspicious for malignancy • Suspicious for papillary carcinoma • Suspicious for lymphoma • Suspicious for metastatic tumor • Other	60-75	Total thyroidectomy or surgical lobectomy
Malignant	97-99	Total thyroidectomy

Cytological classification of fine-needle aspirates and action required

ATA classification (Bethesda System)

Diagnostic category	Cytological diagnosis	Management
I	Non-diagnostic	Repeat US-guided FNA
II	Benign	Clinical follow-up
III	Atypia/follicular lesion of undertermined significance	Repeat FNA
IV	Suspicious	Surgical hemithyroidectomy
V	Suspicious	Near-total thyroidectomy/surgical hemithyroidectomy
VI	Malignant	Near-total hemithyroidectomy

BTA classification (RCPath Thy System)

Diagnostic category	Cytological diagnosis	Management
Thy 1	Non-diagnostic	US assessment +/– repeat FNAB
Thy 2	Non-neoplastic	Correlate with clinical / US findings
Thy 3	Neoplasm possible *Thy 3a-Atypia (uncategorized)*	Further US +/–repeat FNAB
	Thy 3r-Atypia (possible follicular neoplasm)	Diagnostic hemithyroidectomy
Thy 4	Suspicious of malignancy	Diagnostic hemithyroidectomy
Thy 5	Diagnostic of malignancy	Surgical resection

Ultrasound (U) classification of thyroid nodules

U classification	Nodule type	Ultrasound characteristic
U1	Normal	
U2	Benign	Vascularity, egg shell calcification, cystic change, iso-echoic or mildy hyper-echoic
U3	Indeterminate/equivocal	Homogenous, hyper-echoic equivocal echogenic foci, mixed or central vascularity, solid or halo
U4	Suspicious	Solid, hypo-echoic, peripheral calcification, lobulated outline
U5	Malignant	Solid, hypo-echoic, lobulated outline, intranodular vascularity, taller > wide, lymphadenopathy

Ultrasonographic features suggestive of (a) malignant thyroid module, and (b) a benign thyroid module in decreasing order of specificity

- Microcalcification
  - Irregularity of the border of the nodule
  - Increased blood flow in nodule on colour-flow Doppler
  - Hypoechogenicity
  - Absence of a halo
- Diameter less than 1 cm (those less than 0.5 cm do not require further intervention)
  - Simple cyst with no solid component
  - Comet tail sign, due to colloid content
  - Honeycomb appearance

Clinical features associated with increased risk of malignancy

Age < 20 years
Presence of cervical lymphadenopathy
History of radiation to the head and neck during childhood
Family history of medullary thyroid cancer of MEN types 2A and 2B
Hard fixed nodule
Recent nodule growth
Hoarseness of voice (indicating invasion of recurrent laryngeal nerve)

Malignancy	Relative incidence
Papillary carcinoma	80%
Follicular carcinoma	10%
Poorly differentiated/anaplastic carcinoma	5%
Medullary carcinoma	2.5%
Lymphoma	2.5%

Familial cancer syndromes involving non-medullary thyroid cancer

Syndrome	Gene	Manifestation	Thyroid tumor
Cowden's syndrome	*PTEN*	Intestinal hamartomas, benign and malignant breast tumors	FTC, rarely PTC and Hurthle cell tumors
FAP	*APC*	Colon polyps and cancer, duodenal neoplasms, desmoids	PTC cribriform growth pattern
Werner's syndrome	*WRN*	Adult progeroid syndrome	PTC, FTC, anaplastic cancer
Carney complex type I	*PRKAR1α*	Cutaneous and cardiac myxomas, breast and adrenal tumors	PTC, FTC
McCune-Albright syndrome	*GNASI*	Polyostotic fibrous dysplasia, endocrine abnormalities, café-au-lait spots	PTC clear cell
DICER 1 syndrome		Pleuropulmonary blastoma, cystic nephroma, ovarian sex cord-stromal tumors	Multinodular goiter, thyroid cancer

Clinical and genetic characteristics of familial medullary thyroid cancer syndromes

Syndrome	Characteristic Features
FMTC	MTC
MEN2A	MTC Adrenal medulla (pheochromocytoma) Parathyroid hyperplasia
MEN2A with cutaneous lichen amyloidosis	MEN2A and a pruritic cutaneous lesion located over the upper back
MEN2A or FMTC with Hirschsprung disease	MEN2A or FMTC with Hirschsprung disease
MEN2B	MTC Adrenal medulla (pheochromocytoma) Intestinal and mucosal ganglioneuromatosis Characteristic marfanoid habitus

Clinical and genetic characteristics of familial thyroid follicular cell carcinoma susceptibility syndromes

Syndrome	Chromosome Linkage/ Gene	Characteristics
Papillary thyroid carcinoma with papillary renal neoplasia	1q21	Associate with papillary renal neoplasia Autosomal dominant with partial penetrance
Familial nonmedullary thyroid carcinoma	2q21 and 19p13	Two genetic loci identified Autosomal dominant with partial penetrance
Familial thyroid tumors with cell oxyphilia	19p13.2	Characteristic oxyphilic cells Autosomal dominant with partial penetrance
Familial adenomatous polyposis	5q21-22/*APC*	Papillary thyroid carcinoma with <10 × increased prevalence Colorectal carcinoma, ampullary carcinoma, ampullary carcinoma, hepatoblastoma, medulloblastoma Autosomal dominant

Contd.

Contd.

Cowden disease (multiple hematoma syndrome)	10q23.3/*PTEN*	Follicular and papillary thyroid carcinoma Multiple hamartomas, breast and endometrial cancer Autosomal dominant
Carney complex 1	17q/*PRKAR1A*	Follicular and papillary thyroid carcinoma Skin pigmentation and cardiac, endocrine, cutaneous and neural mydomalous tumors Autosomal dominant

Main genes involved in thyroid oncogenesis: Classification, tumor types and prevalence

Genes	Histologic type	Prevalence	Comments
		Receptor	
TSH	Autonomous follicular adenoma	3%-82%	TSH activation mutation are not oncogenic
TRK	PTC	6%-20%	Tyrosine kinase receptor, somatic mutation absent in benign thyroid neoplasms
RET/PTC	PTC	2.5%-85%, higher with radiation exposune	Tyrosine kinase receptor, somatic mutation Higher prevalence with radiation exposure Possibly associated with more aggressive tumors Five chimeric subtypes have been identified
Met	PTC, FTC	-75% PTC -25% FTC	Tyrosine kinase receptor, somatic mutation Possibly associated with aggressive tumors Overexpressed mostly in PTC and poorly DTC
c-erb-2	PTC	-50% PTC	Tyrosine kinase activity, similar to epidermal growth factor receptor Overexpressed in PTC, but oncogene is not overamplified
		Signal Transduction Proteins	
ras	PTC, FTC, HCC, autonomous follicular adenoma	7%-92% (-30% overall)	Early event in carcinogenesis May be associated with aggressive PTC
BRAF	PTC	40%-50% PTC	*BRAF*^{CODE} most common mutation, may confer worse prognosis
gsp	Autonomous follicular adenoma	7%-28%	Early event in carcinogenesis Similar frequency in benign and malignant thyroid neoplasms Coexisting *ras* and *gsp* mutations in same tumor may be associated with aggressive DTC
		Tumor Suppressor Genes and Nuclear Oncogenes	
PAX8/ PPABγ	FTC	75%	Presence of this fusion oncoprotein may be used to differentiate follicular adenoma from carcinoma
p53	Poorly DTC, ATC	-75%	p53 immunohistochemistry may be predictive of tumor aggressiveness Thought to occur as a late genetic event in thyroid carcinogenesis
PTEN	Benign follicular adenoma, infrequently in DTC	26% of benign, 6% of malignant	Higher rate in benign than malignant tumor questions the presence of strict adenoma-to-carcinoma sequence

Risk factors associated with differentiated thyroid carcinoma
Exposure to ionizing radiation, especially during childhood
Familial adenomatous polyposis (Gardner syndrome)
Carney complex
Werner syndrome
Cowden syndrome (phosphatase and tensin homolog [PTEN]-hamartoma tumor syndrome)
Pendred syndrome
Familial papillary thyroid cancer

Prognostic Risk Classification for Patients With Differentiated Thyroid Carcinoma (AMES or AGES)		
	Low Risk	**High Risk**
Age	≤40 Year	>40 years
Sex	Female	Male
Extent	No local extension, intrathyroidal, no capsular invasion	Capsular invasion, extrathyroidal extension
Metastasis	None	Regional or distant
Size	<2 cm	>4 cm
Grade	Well differentiated	Poorly differentiated

Dynamic risk stratification following treatment for thyroid cancer			
Response	**Criteria**	**Risk stratification**	**Follow-up**
Excellent	*All of the following:* Suppressed and stimulated Tg <1 mcg/l Neck USS without evidence of disease Cross-sectional and/or nuclear medicine imaging negative (if performed)	High	6-monthly for first year Annually thereafter
Indeterminate	*Any of the following:* Suppressed Tg <1 mcg/l and stimulated Tg ≥1 and <10 mcg/l Neck USS with non-specific changes or stable sub-1 cm nodes Cross-sectional and/or nuclear medicine imaging with non-specific changes, not completely normal	Intermediate	More frequently depending on individual need
Incomplete	*Any of the following:* Suppressed Tg ≥1 mcg/l or stimulated Tg ≥10 mcg/l Rising Tg values Persistent or newly identified disease on cross-sectional and/or nuclear medicine imaging	Low	Investigate and more frequently depending on individual need

Prognostic scoring systems for AGES, AMES and MACIS
AGES (Age, Tumor Grade, Tumor Extent, Tumor Size)
Prognostic score = 0.05 × age (if age 40 years and older)
+1 (if grade 2)
+3 (if grade 3 or 4)
+1 (if extrathyroid)
+3 (if distant spread)
+ 0.2 × tumor size (cm maximum diameter)
Survival by AGES score (20 years):
≤3.99 = 99%
4-4.99 = 80%
5-5.99 = 67%
≥6 = 13%
AMES (Age, Metastatic Disease, Extrathyroidal Extension, Size)
Low risk: Younger patients (men 40 years and younger, women 50 years and younger) with no metastases
Older patients (intrathyroid papillary, minor capsular invasion for follicular lesions)

Contd.

Contd.

Primary cancers <5 cm
No distant metastases
High risk: All patients with distant metastases
Extrathyroid papillary, major capsular invasion follicular
Primary cancers ≥5 cm in older patients (men older than 40 years, women older than 50 years)
Survival by AMES risk groups (20 years)
Low risk = 99%
High risk = 61%
MACIS (Metastasis, Patient Age, Completeness of Resection, Local Invasion and Tumor Size)
Score = 3.1 (if age younger than 40 years) or 0.08 × age (if age 40 years and older)
+0.3 × tumor size (cm maximum diameter)
+ 1 (if incompletely resected)
+ 1 (if locally invasive)
+ 3 (if distant spread)
<6 = 99%
6-6.99=89%
7-7.99=56%
≥8=24%

Grading of TSH suppression

Response	TSH suppression (mU/l)
Excellent	0.3-2.0
Indeterminate	0.1-0.5 (for 5-10 years)
Incomplete	<0.1 (indefinitely)

Non-Surgical Management of Differentiated Thyroid Cancer

- *Radioiodine uptake is usually seen in thyroid bed following total or near-total thyroidectomy*
- *^{131}I destruction of this residual tissue is called radioiodine remnant ablation (RRA)*

No Indication for ^{131}I Ablation

- Low risk of recurrence or cancer specific mortality
- Tumor <1cm unifocal/multifocal and on histology classical papillary or follicular variant/follicular minimally invasive without angioinvasion and no capsule invasion

Definite indications for ^{131}I ablation
• *Tumor >4 cm*
• *Any tumor size with gross extrathyroidal extension (pT4)*
• *Distant metastases present*

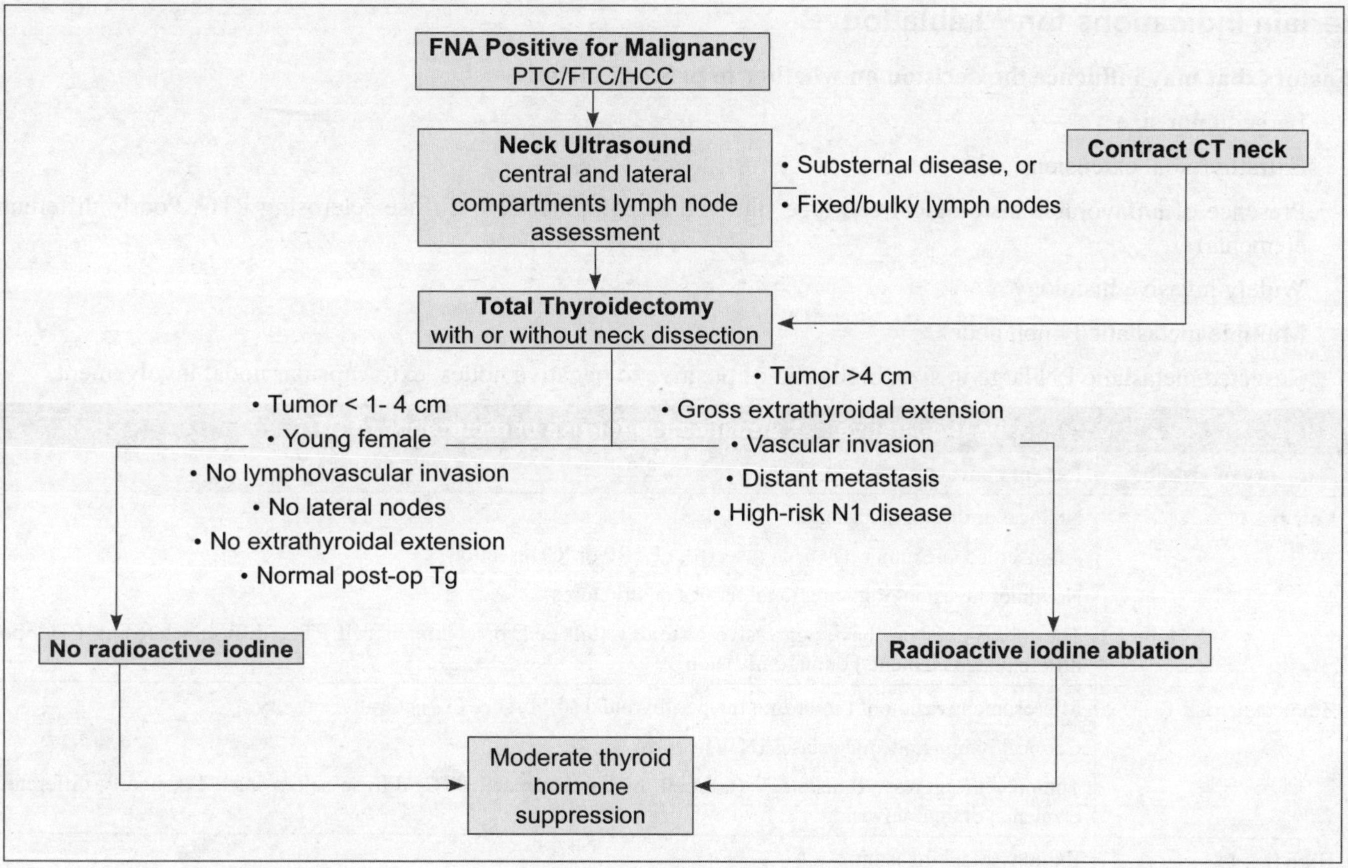
FNA Positive for Malignancy
PTC/FTC/HCC
Neck Ultrasound
central and lateral compartments lymph node assessment
• Substernal disease, or
• Fixed/bulky lymph nodes
Contract CT neck
Total Thyroidectomy
with or without neck dissection
• Tumor < 1- 4 cm
• Young female
• No lymphovascular invasion
• No lateral nodes
• No extrathyroidal extension
• Normal post-op Tg
• Tumor >4 cm
• Gross extrathyroidal extension
• Vascular invasion
• Distant metastasis
• High-risk N1 disease
No radioactive iodine
Radioactive iodine ablation
Moderate thyroid hormone suppression

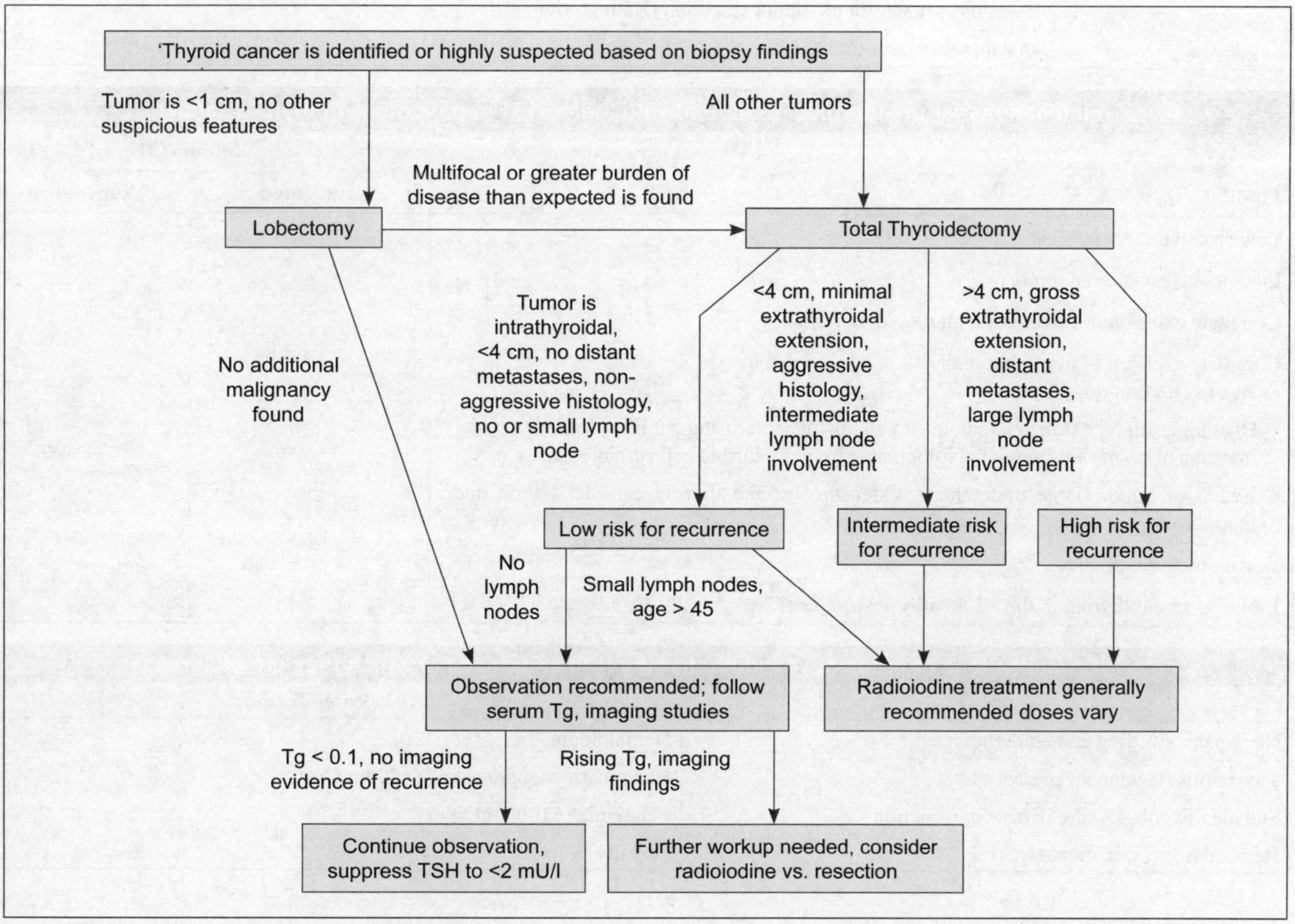
'Thyroid cancer is identified or highly suspected based on biopsy findings
Tumor is <1 cm, no other suspicious features
All other tumors
Multifocal or greater burden of disease than expected is found
Lobectomy
Total Thyroidectomy
No additional malignancy found
Tumor is intrathyroidal, <4 cm, no distant metastases, non-aggressive histology, no or small lymph node
<4 cm, minimal extrathyroidal extension, aggressive histology, intermediate lymph node involvement
>4 cm, gross extrathyroidal extension, distant metastases, large lymph node involvement
Low risk for recurrence
Intermediate risk for recurrence
High risk for recurrence
No lymph nodes
Small lymph nodes, age > 45
Observation recommended; follow serum Tg, imaging studies
Radioiodine treatment generally recommended doses vary
Tg < 0.1, no imaging evidence of recurrence
Rising Tg, imaging findings
Continue observation, suppress TSH to <2 mU/l
Further workup needed, consider radioiodine vs. resection

Uncertain indications for ^{131}I ablation

- **Factors that may influence the decision on whether to proceed include**
  - Large tumor size
  - Extrathyroidal extension
  - Presence of unfavorable histological cell type (tall cell or columnar cell, diffuse sclerosing PTC, Poorly differentiated elements)
  - Widely invasive histology
  - Multiple metastatic lymph nodes
  - Resected metastatic LN large in size, high ratio of positive to negative nodes, extracapsular nodal involvement.

Post-operative risk stratification for risk of recurrence of DTC

Category of risk	Patient characteristics
Low risk	No local or distant metastases All macroscopic tumor has been resected, i.e., R0 or R1 resection No tumor invasion of locoregional tissues or structures The tumor does not have aggressive histology (tall cell, or columnar cell PTC, diffuse sclerosing PTC, poorly differentiated elements) or angioinvasion
Immediate risk	Microsopic invasion of tumor into the perithyroidal soft tissues (T3) at initial surgery Cervical lymph node metastases (N1a or N1b) Tumor with aggressive histology (tall cell, or columnar cell PTC, diffuse sclerosing PTC, poorly differentiated elements) or angioinvasion
High risk	Extrathyroidal invasion Incomplete macroscopic tumor resection (R2 resection) Distant metastases (M1)

Indications for postsurgical treatment with Iodine-131 in patients with thyroid cancer

Finding	Iodine-131	
	Indicated	Not Indicated
Low risk of cancer-specific mortality or relapse		×
Incomplete excision of tumor	×	
Complete excision of tumor but high risk of mortality	×	
Complete excision of tumor but high risk of relapse due to • Age (<16 years or >45 years) • Histologic subtype (tall cell, columnar cell, diffuse sclerosing papillary variants; widely invasive or poorly differentiated follicular subtypes; Hurthle cell carcinomas) • Extent of tumor (large tumor mass, extension beyond thyroid capsule, lymph node metastases	×	
Distant metastases	×	
Elevated serum thyroglobulin >3 months postsurgery	×	

Complications of radioactive iodine therapy (^{131}I) and doses at which they are observed

Acute	Long-Term
Neck pain, swelling and tenderness	Hematologic
Thyroiditis (if remnant present	Bone marrow suppression (>500 mCi)
Sialadenitis (50-450 mCi), taste dysfunction	Leukemia (>1000 mCi)
Hemorrhage (brain metastases)	Fertility

Contd.

Contd.

Cerebral edema (brain metastases, 200 mCi) Vocal cord paralysis Nausea and vomiting (50-450 mCi) Bone marrow suppression (200 mCi)	Ovarian/testicular damage, infertility Increased spontaneous abortion rate Pulmonary fibrosis Chronic sialadenitis, nodules, taste dysfunction Increased risk of cancer Anaplastic thyroid cancer Gastric cancer Hepatocellular cancer Lung cancer Breast cancer (>1000 mCi) Bladder cancer Hypoparathyroidism

Non-Surgical Management of Medullary Thyroid Cancer

- Surgery is the main modality of treatment for this disease and monitoring of serum calcitonin post-operatively
- Calcitonin level of patients, however, remains elevated after surgery and it is frequently difficult to locate the site of residual disease and determine whether it is local or at a distant site
- Blood samples taken for calcitonin must be immediately stored in ice
- CEA is also commonly raised and can similarly be used to monitor progress and response to therapeutic intervention

> *Calcitonin doubling time >2 years was associated with long-term survival*
> *Patients with a doubling time of <6 months all die due medullary thyroid cancer*

Radiotherapy may be indicated in

- Post-operatively, when disease was locally advanced at presentation and macroscopic clearance has not been achieved
- Multiple involved lymph nodes, especially if extracapsular spread is present
- Bulky inoperable tumors
- Palliation of distant metastases (e.g., bone)

> ***For successful remnant ablation to be achieved, the TSH level prior to the isotope administration must be elevated to >25–30 mU/l***

- If liothyronine is commenced (usual dose 20 mcg tds), this should be withdrawn 14 days prior to radioactive iodine treatment
- If levothyroxine is used, it should be substituted with liothyronine starting 28 days prior to radioactive iodine treatment and this is then stopped for the last 14 days prior to treatment

METASTATIC MTC

- Diarrhoea as a result of excess peptide release or symptoms related to excess hormone production
- Often with urgency, wheezing and flushing
- No curative treatment option
- Treatment interventions are therefore usually reserved until patient becomes ***symptomatic and/or develops significant radiological progression with accelerated calcitonin doubling times*** rather than at first presentation of asymptomatic radiologically diagnosed metastases or raised tumor markers
- Diarrhea–Loperamide and Codeine, Octreotide *(Blocking somatostatin receptors can result in a decrease in the amount of peptide and calcitonin released)*

CHAPTER 35 PARATHYROID CARCINOMA

- 1% of Hyperparathyroidism
- Most commonly manifests in the fourth to fifth decades
- Male = Female
- PTCA is often firm, is densely scarred, and obliterates normal tissue planes.
- Associated with MEN1, MEN2A, Familial Hyperparathyroidism and Hyperparathyroidism–Jaw tumor
- History of previous neck irradiation–Risk factor for Parathyroid carcinoma
- Cyclin D1 overexpression (11q13)

HPT-JT (Hyperparathyroidism- Jaw tumor)
• Autosomal dominant
• >10%
• 1q25-32 (HRPT2 gene)
• CDC73 Mutations (Frameshift and Nonsense)
• Parafibromin gene

- **Suspected**–Severe symptoms, Calcium >14 mg/dl, Raises PTH (5 times), Palpable parathyroid/Neck mass
- 15% LN+
- 1.8% Distant metastasis
- 40% Local invasion
- Palpable neck mass is found in 36–52% of patients with parathyroid carcinomas
- Large mass with whitish capsule adherent to adjacent structures
- Definitive diagnosis of Carcinoma Parathyroid–Locoregional invasion and Metastasis
- Hypercalcemia, Normal PTH and Hypocalcemia and Calcium/Creatinine clearance <0.01
- Salt and Pepper skull

Major Criteria
• Capsular and Vascular invasion
• Trabecular/Fibrous stroma invasion
• Mitoses

Parathyroid carcinoma proposed staging system	
Proposed Staging System	
T1	Primary tumor < 3 cm
T2	Primary tumor > 3 cm
T3	Primary tumor of any size with invasion of the surrounding soft tissues (thyroid gland, strap muscles, etc.)
T4	Massive central compartment disease invading trachea and esophagus or recurrence parathyroid cancer

Contd.

Contd.

N0	No regional lymph node metastases
N1	Regional lymph node metastases
M0	No evidence of distant metastases
M1	Evidence of distant metastases
Stage	
I	T1 N0 M0
II	T2 N0 M0
IIIa	T3 N0 M0
IIIb	T3 N0 M0
IIIc	Any T, N1 Mo
IV	Any T, any N, M1

I-T1, II-T2, IIIa-T3, IIIb-T3, IIIc-N+, IV-M+

Treatment

- Surgery is the treatment of choice
- Neck exploration–Enbloc tumor excision and Ipsilateral tumor lobe excision with tracheoesophageal, paratracheal and upper mediastinal nodes
- Avoid capsular rupture

Adjuvant RT

- High risk of local recurrence
- Close/+ve margins
- Invasion to surrounding structures
- Tumor rupture

- Bisphosphonates–Hypercalcemia associated with Parathyroid carcinoma
- Cinacalet hydrochloride–Calcimimetic, Reduces PTH, Binds to CaSR cells on Parathyroid
- Amifostine–Inhibits PTH release
- +ve Margins→Predict recurrence
- Localised recurrent tumors→ Cervical and Mediastinal exploration
- Prophylactic Neck dissection has no improved survival and has increased morbidity
- Most common site of metastasis–Lung
- PTH and Calcium monitoring–Best way for follow up
- Best approach for recurrence–High resolution USG
- Selective venous sampling for PTH→ Attempt to localize site of recurrence
- ***Local recurrence→ Reresection***

Familial hyperparathyroid disorders, genetic characteristics, presentation of hyperparathyroidism and associated features					
Disorder	**Inheritance**	**Gene**	**Chromosome**	**HPT**	**Associated tumors**
MEN1	AD	*MEN1*	11q13	90% penetrance; multiglandular	Pituitary tumor, EPT
MEN2A	AD	*RET*	10q21	20% penetrance; multiglandular/adenoma	MTC, pheochromocytoma
HPT-JT	AD	*HRPT2*	1q21-q32	Cystic parathyroid tumors (15% risk of carcinoma)	Jaw tumor, renal tumor
FIHPT	AD	*HRPT2*	1q21-q32	Adenoma/multiglandular	—
		MEN1	11q13	Adenoma/multiglandular	
ADMH	AD	*CASR*	3q13-21	Multiglandular/adenoma	—
FHH	AD	*CASR*	3q13-21	Mildly hyperplastic	—
NSHPT	AR/AD	*CASR*	3q13-21	Markedly hyperplastic	—

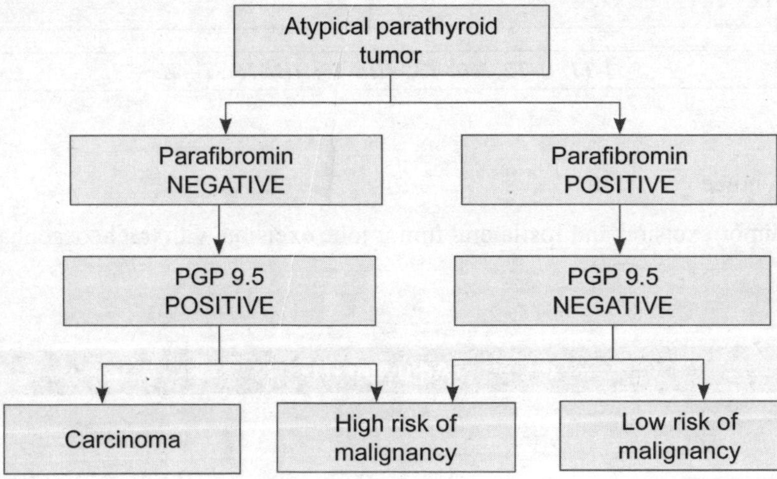

- Immunohistochemical evidence of downregulation of parafibromin has a sensitivity of 67% and specificity of 100% for detecting parathyroid carcinoma and protein gene product 9.5 (PGP 9.5)
- Parafibromin immunohistochemistry may be used with immunohistochemistry for PGP 9.5. This is a protein encoded by ubiquitin carboxyl terminal esterase L1
- Upregulated in parathyroid carcinoma
- Has sensitivity of 78% and specificity of 100%

CHAPTER 36

ADRENOCORTICAL CARCINOMA

- *Slight female preponderance*
- *Associated with Beckwith Wiedemann syndrome, Li fraumeni syndrome and Carney complex*
- Cushing syndrome + Virilization/Feminization + Mineralocorticoid excess–Adrenocortical carcinoma
- FNAC–Only done if mass is suspected to be metastatic from another malignancy
- MRI–IVC involvement
- Investigation of choice–CT Abdomen (>10 to 13 HU and <50% Washout)
- **Malignancy features on Imaging**–Size > 6 cm, Heterogeneity, Irregular borders, Calcification and Necrosis with hemorrhage
- Weiss criteria–3/more of 9 criteria
- Mitotic rate–Important criteria and Indicates malignancy (>5 mitosis/50 HPF)
- Mitotic rate >20/HPF→ High grade Adrenocortical carcinoma

	Macfarlane	Sullivian	Icard	Lee
</= 5 cm	T1	T1	T1	T1
>5 cm	T2	T2	T2	T2
Local invasion	Without involved adjacent organs, Mobile N+	Local invasion with N+	T3	T3 IVC thrombus and Direct extension
Invades adjacent organs, Fixed nodes, Distant metastasis	T4	T4	T4	T4

Adrenocortical Carcinoma (ACC)		
AJCC Stage (Eighth Edition)/ENSAT		
Stage	**TNM**	**Notes**
I	T1 N0 M0	T1: primary tumor ≤5 cm
II	T2 N0 M0	T2: primary tumor >5 cm T3: local invasion (no organ invasion)
III	T1 N1 M0, T2 N1 M0, T3 any N M0, T4 any N M0	T4: invasion of kidney, diaphragm, or any large blood vessels
IV	Any T any N M1	N1: metastasis in regional lymph node(s) M1: distant metastasis

I- T1, II- T2,
III- T1, T2 N1 or III- T3/T4, N0/N1
IV- M+

- Strongest predictor for outcome in Adrenocortical carcinoma–Complete resection
- Most common form of relapse–Local recurrence
- ***Stage 1 to 3*** → En bloc resection + Adjuvant Mitotane

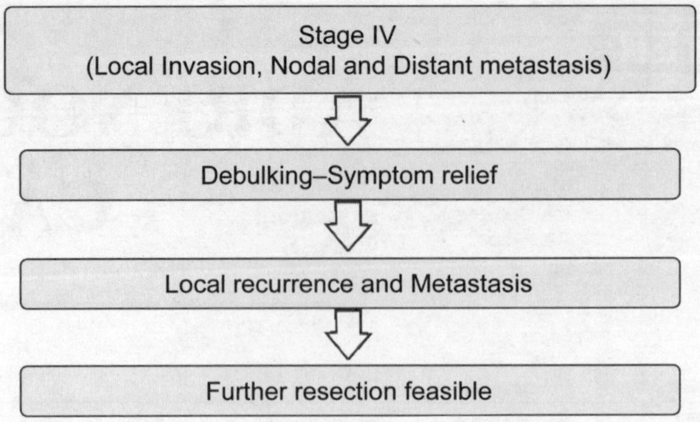

- ***Prophylactic nephrectomy****–Involved renal vein/Capsule*
- ***Celiac axis and SMA root partially encased–***Contraindication for adrenalectomy
- Chemotherapy regimen–Mitotane/Cisplatin+ Etoposide + Doxorubicin
- Most common site of distant metastasis–Lungs
- > 6 cm / < 6 cm suspected of being malignant→ Open adrenalectomy

• Minimally Invasive Adrenalectomy–Benign adrenocortical tumors and PCPGL
Posterior retroperitoneal approach–Not advised (Significant subcutaneous/perinephric fat, Unfavourable, >8 cm)
• Cortical sparing adrenalectomy (Partial)→Familial, Benign and Bilateral tumors (Bilateral PCPGL, VHL and MEN2)

PHEOCHROMOCYTOMA

- *Triad of Pheochromocytoma–Headache, Perspiration and Tachycardia*
- Tuberous sclerosis, Struge Weber syndrome, Familial paraganglioma syndrome, MEN1, NF1 and VHL–Risk for Pheochromocytoma

Hereditary syndromes associated with pheochromocytoma		
Syndrome	**Gene mutation**	**Phenotype**
Multiple endocrine neoplasia type 2A	*RET*	Medullary thyroid cancer, primary hyperparathyroidism
Multiple endocrine neoplasia type 2B	*RET*	Medullary thyroid cancer, marfanoid habitus, mucosal neuromas
Neurofibromatosis type 1 (von Recklinghausen disease)	*NF1*	Neurofibromas, café au lait spots, Lisch nodules (benign iris hamartomas)
von Hippel-Lindau	*VHL*	Retinal angioma, central nervous system hemangioblastoma, renal cell cancer, primitive neuroectodermal tumor, pancreatic and renal cysts
Familial paraganglioma syndrome	*SDHA, SDHB, SDHC, SDHD*	Gastrointestinal stromal tumor *SDHB* may be associated with renal cell cancer
Hereditary pheochromocytoma	*TMEM127*	Possibly other tumors
Hereditary pheochromocytoma	*MAX*	Possibly other tumors
Hereditary pheochromocytoma	*HIF2A*	Familial polycythemia, somatostatinomas

- Associated with Hyperglycemia, Increased gallstones, Polycythemia, Cushing's syndrome, Hypercalcemia
- Most common extra-adrenal site of Pheochromocytoma–Organ of Zuckerkandl (IMA and Aortic bifurcation) > Urinary bladder > Thorax > Renal hilum
- Most common symptom–Sustained paroxysmal hypertension
- Most specific tool for pheochromocytoma–24-hour urinary fractionated metanephrines
- Most sensitive test for pheochromocytoma–Plasma fractionated metanephrines

Cutoff values for biochemical diagnosis of pheochromocytoma					
	Cutoff Value				
Test*	mol	g	Definitions	Sensitivity (%)	Specificity (%)
Plasma free metanephrine	0.3 nmol/liter	59 μg/liter	Paired test, positive result if either or both values are elevated	99	85-89
Plasma free normetanephrine	0.6 nmol/liter	110 μg/liter			
Urinary total metanephrines	6.6 μmol/day	1.3 mg/day		71	99.6
Urinary epinephrine	191 nmol/day	35 μg/day		29	99.6
Urinary norepinephrine	1005 nmol/day	170 μg/day		50	99.6
Urinary dopamine	4571 nmol/day	700 μg/day		8	100
Urinary total metanephrines and catecholamines	-		Grouped test, positive result if any one of the following three urinary values is elevated: total metanephrines, epinephrine, norepinephrine, dopamine	88	99
Urinary vanillylmandelic acid	40 μmol/day	7.9 mg/day		64	95
Clonidine suppression test			Positive result = elevated level after clonidine and fall of <40	96	100
Plasma free normetanephrine	0.61 nmol/l	112 μg/liter			

T2 weighted MRI images can identify chromaffin tissue
T2 weighted adrenal mass/Liver ratio of pheochromocytoma >3

- *Most common site of Metastasis in Malignant Pheochromocytoma–Lung*
- Only criterion absolute for differentiation of malignancy of pheochromocytoma–Presence of secondary tumor in sites where chromaffin cells don't exist
- ***Only criterion adopted by WHO for Malignant PCPGL–Metastasis***

Pheochromocytoma/Paraganglioma (PC/PGL)		
AJCC Stage (Eighth Edition)	TNM	Notes
I	T1 N0 M0	T1: PC < 5 cm in greatest dimension with no organ invasion
II	T2 N0 M0	T2: PC ≥ 5 cm or any PGL of any size, with no organ invasion
III	T1 N1 M0, T2 N1 M0, T3 any N M0	T3: PC of any size with invasion of surrounding tissues
		N1: metastasis in regional lymph node(s)
IV	Any T any N M1	M1: distant metastasis: subtypes exist to denote location of metastases

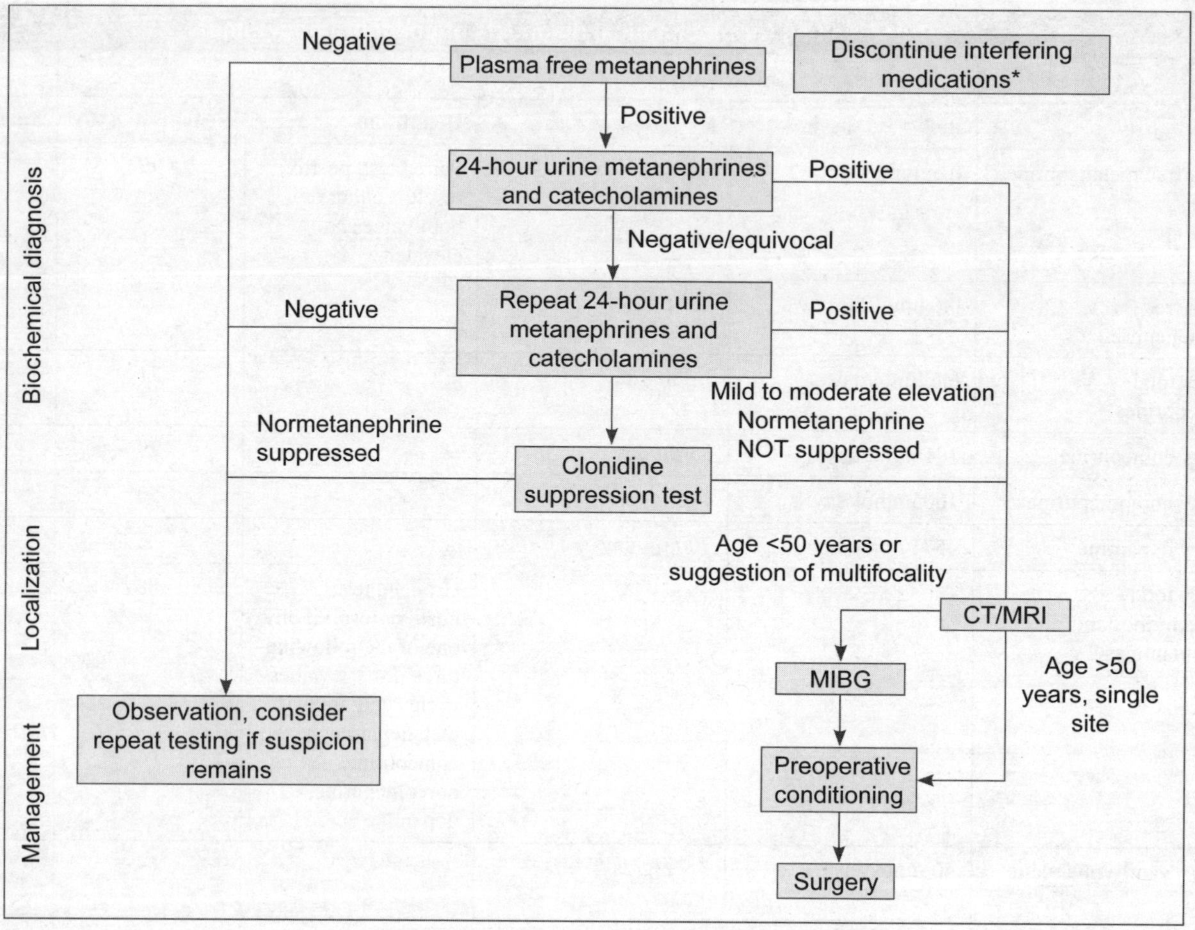

Management of Recurrent/Metastatic Pheochromocytoma

- Familial and Larger, Malignant→50% Recurrence
- Most common site of metastasis in PCPGL–Bones
- Treatment–Palliative
- Debulking and Metastatectomy→ Resectable
- Cyclophosphamide and Dacarbazine→ ***Symptomatic Unresectable***
- Childhood Adrenal tumors

Pheochromocytoma– and paraganglioma–associated familial syndromes		
Gene	**Syndrome**	**Prominent Extra-Adrenal Clinical Features**
VHL	von Hippel-Lindau	Clear cell renal carcinoma, CNS/retinal hemangioblastomas, pancreatic neuroendocrine tumors
RET	Multiple endocrine neoplasia types 2A and 2B	Medullary thyroid carcinoma, primary hyperparathyroidism, marfanoid habitus (MEN2B only)
NF1	Neurofibromatosis type 1	Neurofibromas, schwannomas, gliomas, Lisch nodules, cafe-au-lait spots
SDHB	Pheochromocytoma-paraganglioma syndrome, type 4 (PGL 4)	
SDHD	PGL 1	Renal cell carcinoma, gastrointestinal stromal tumor (GIST), paraganglioma
SDHC	PGL3	
SDHA	PGL 5	GIST, paraganglioma
SDHAF2	PGL2	Head and neck paraganglioma

Contd.

Contd.

TMEM127	Familial pheochromocytoma	Renal cell carcinoma
MAX		Paraganglioma
EPAS1	Polycythemia paraganglioma syndrome	Polycythemia, paraganglioma, somatostatinoma
FH	Leiomyomatosis and renal cell cancer	Cutaneous and uterine leiomyomas, papillary renal cell carcinoma, paraganglioma

Childhood Adrenal Tumors

- **PCPGL:**
  - Males, SDHB and VHL
  - Definitive treatment→ Surgical resection + preop blockade and volume expansion
  - Pregnancy–Associated with PCPGL in 1st 2 trimesters
- **Adrenocortical carcinoma:**
  - Females, >60% of Adrenocortical tumors
  - P53 mutations
  - Early childhood Adrenocortical carcinoma–Virilization

Treatment:
- Early–Surgery
- Advanced–Multimodal treatment

Adrenal Incidentaloma

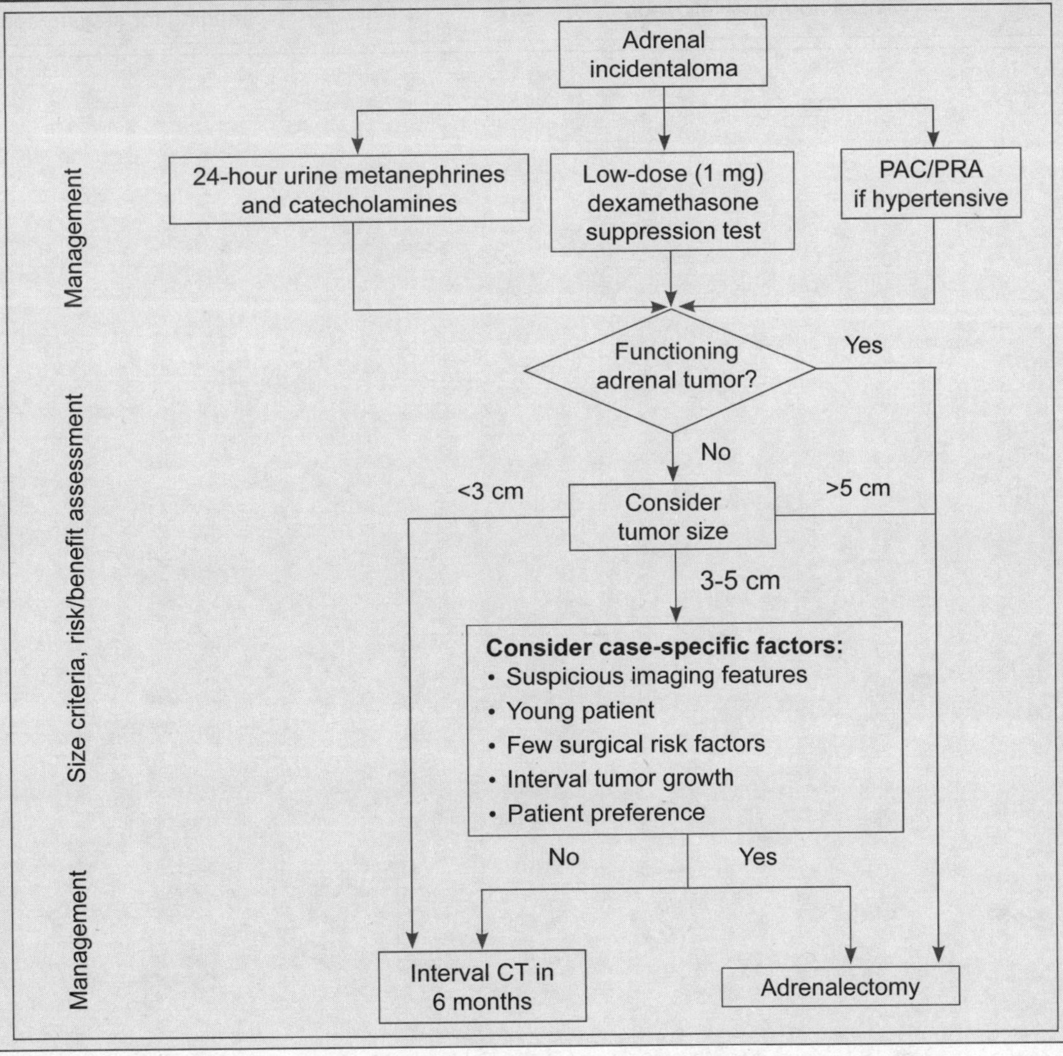

Contd.

Contd.

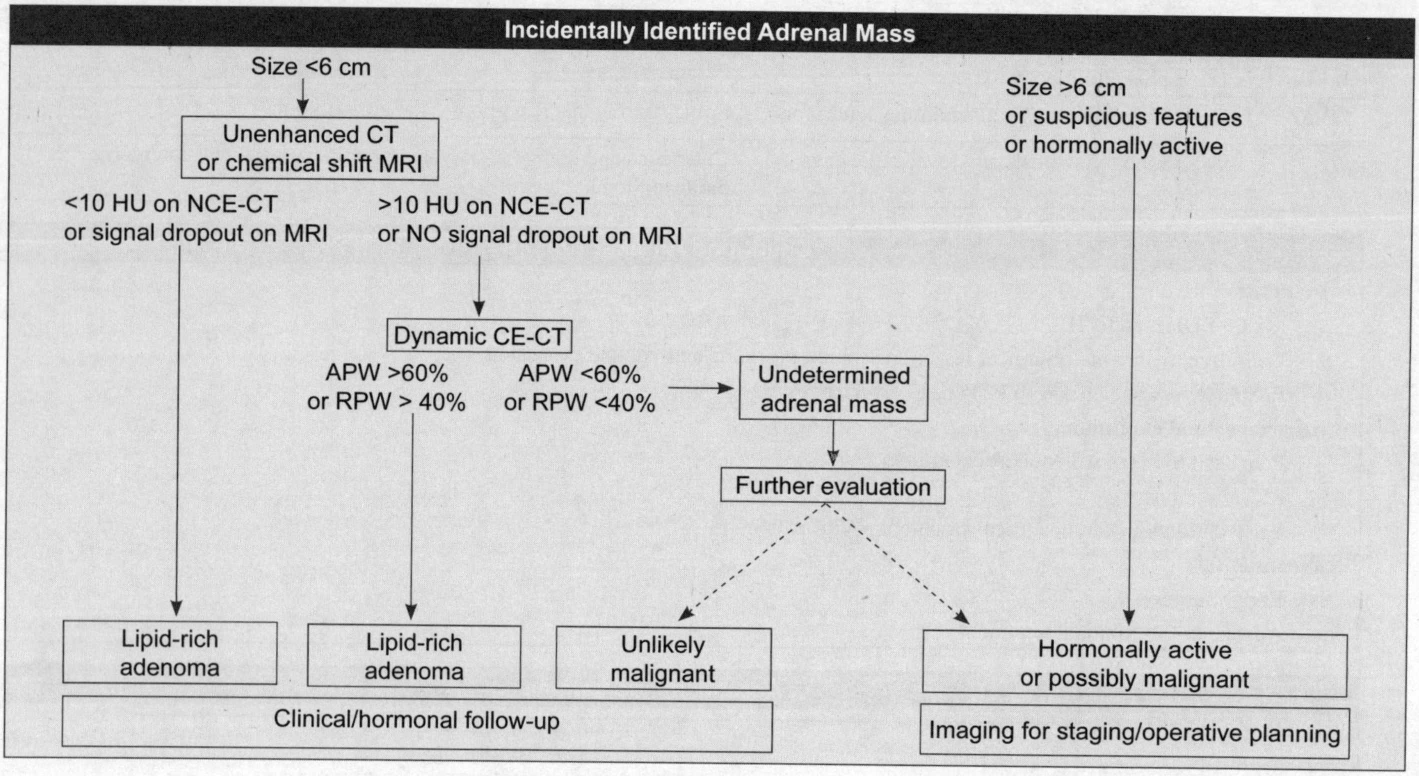

Incidentally Identified Adrenal Mass
Size <6 cm
Unenhanced CT or chemical shift MRI
<10 HU on NCE-CT or signal dropout on MRI
>10 HU on NCE-CT or NO signal dropout on MRI
Dynamic CE-CT
APW >60% or RPW > 40%
APW <60% or RPW <40%
Undetermined adrenal mass
Further evaluation
Size >6 cm or suspicious features or hormonally active
Lipid-rich adenoma
Lipid-rich adenoma
Unlikely malignant
Hormonally active or possibly malignant
Clinical/hormonal follow-up
Imaging for staging/operative planning

CHAPTER 37 MEN SYNDROME

- Autosomal dominant syndromes with variable penetrance
- Younger age than sporadic counterpart
- Arises in multiple organs synchronously/sequentially
- Usually preceded by asymptomatic endocrine hyperplasia
- Often multifocal
- Usually more aggressive

MEN I (Wermer's Syndrome)

- **3 P's–parathyroid, pancreas, pituitary**
- Most common presentation of MEN1 is primary hyperparathyroidism
- 1st clinical manifestation of MEN 1 is primary hyperparathyroidism
- **Subtotal/total parathyroidectomy with cervical thymectomy is the surgical treatment of choice**
- Most common Enteropancreatic tumor in MEN1 is Gastrinoma
- Patients with MEN 1 associated gastrinomas and concomitant PHTP should undergo parathyroidectomy achieving normocalcemia that decreases serum gastrin levels
- **Metastatic pancreatic endocrine tumors–Most frequent cause of death in MEN 1**
- Pancreatic tumors→gastrinomas, insulinomas, glucagonoma, VIPoma, prolactinoma
- Bronchial and thymic, Gastric carcinoid tumors
- Cutaneous tumors include Multiple angiofibromas, Collagenomas and lipomas
- Meningiomas, Ependymomas, Leiomyomas and adrenal cortical tumors are present
- **Angiofibroma and collagenomas are markers for MEN 1 syndrome**
- Pituitary adenomas→Prolactinoma, Acromegaly and ACTH producing adenoma
- Prolactinomas associated with MEN 1 have poorer prognosis than sporadic type
- Mutation of MEN 1 gene which encodes protein **MENIN**
- **Tumor suppressor gene located on gene 11q13**
- Intron 34ss gene codon mutation is seen in VIPomas
- Most aggressive carcinoid arises from thymus gland and have poor prognosis
- **Diagnosis**→Atleast 2/more classic MEN 1 tumors/one of the classic tumors and atleast one close relative with clinical diagnosis of MEN 1
- Most common thyroid malignancy associated with MEN 1 is papillary carcinoma
- **Screening should be done in high risk patients/patients with MEN 1 mutation**

  At age of 8 years–Annual Serum calcium and PTH levels in Primary hyperparathyroidism

  At age of 5 years–Annual Serum prolactin and IGF–1 levels

Yearly serum fasting glucose, Insulin, Gastrin, Chromogranin A, Glucagon and proinsulin→CT/MRI Abdomen every 1-3 years

- Inability to suppress GH levels <5 ng/dl after administering oral glucose is diagnostic of Somatostatinoma

MEN 2A (Sipple Syndrome)

- Associated with RET proto-oncogene mutation (10q11)
- Presents with medullary carcinoma thyroid, pheochromocytoma B/L, **primary hyperparathyroidism-634 mutation (adenoma)**
- Most common tumor in MEN II is Medullary carcinoma thyroid
- Others: **Hirschsprung's disease, lichen planus, amyloidosis**
- Baseline serum calcitonin and CEA levels should be measured 2-3 months following operative intervention and every 6-12 months thereafter, Cervical ultrasound should be performed 6 months after surgical resection
- Prophylactic thyroidectomy is done at <5 years in MEN 2A and <1 year in MEN 2B

MEN 2B/MEN 3

(Williams-Pollock Syndrome, Gorlin Vickers Syndrome, Wagenmann Froboese Syndrome)

- Associated with RET proto-oncogene mutation (10q11)
- Presents with medullary carcinoma thyroid, pheochromocytoma B/L
- **Multiple mucocutaneous ganglioneuromas (Lips, tongue, eyelids) and Marfanoid habitus, Megacolon. Medullated corneal nerve fibres, High arched palate, pes cavus, diverticulae and sugar loaf skull**
- Ectopic ACTH production causes Cushing syndrome
- Most common operative approach in patients with unilateral pheochromocytoma is laproscopic adrenalectomy.
- In Medullary carcinoma associated with MEN 2, Screening should be done at the age of 5 years
- In Medullary carcinoma associated with Familial medullary carcinoma, Screening should be done at the age of 21 years
- MEN 2B with M918T mutation is the most aggressive form of MTC

MEN 4 (MEN X)

- Parathyroid adenoma, Pituitary adenoma, Testicular cancer, Neuroendocrine cervical cancer, Adrenal and renal tumors, Cataracts
- **Gene mutation seen is CDNK1B that encodes p27Kip1**
- **Involves chromosome 12q13**

- Thompson procedure→Distal pancreatectomy, Enucleation of palpable/USG visible tumors in head, lymphadenectomy and duodenotomy to identify occult gastrinomas
- **Familial forms of medullary carcinoma thyroid are always bilateral but sporadic MTC are usually unilateral**
- Parathyroid hyperplasia (Asymmetrically enlarged) associated with MEN 2 is pseudonodular hyperplasia
- Strongest predictor of survival in patients with MTC is stage of the disease at time of thyroidectomy
- Prognosis is excellent in patients with familial medullary carcinoma who have preop calcitonin <150 pg/ml, MTC< 1 cm and no lymph node metastasis
- Reliable indicator for progression of medullary carcinoma thyroid is calcitonin/CEA doubling time
- **Vandetanib and Cabozantinib are FDA approved drugs in MTC to prolong progression free survival**
- Poor prognosis of pNET in MTC is ***high fasting gastrin levels, presence of more than one functional hormonal syndrome, need >3 parathyroid surgical procedures, presence of liver metastasis, aggressive primary tumor growth, large pNET >4 cm, pNET with areas of poor vascular enhancement on CT and serial imaging with evidence for progression***

Affected Organs in Multiple Endocrine Neoplasia Type 1			
Endocrine gland affected	**Frequency (%)**	**Hormone**	**Clinical syndrome**
Parathyroids	90	PTH	pHPT
Pancreas, duodenum (mostly multiple)			
Gastrinoma	50-80	Gastrin	Zollinger-Ellison syndrome
Insulinoma		Insulin	Hypoglycemia syndrome
Non-functioning tumors		PP	-
VIPoma		VIP	Verner-Morrison syndrome
Glucagonoma		Glucagon	Glucagonoma syndrome
Anterio pituitary gland	30-60		
Prolactinoma		Prolactin	Galactorrhea
Non-functioning adenoma		-	Non-specific
Other manifestations			
Adrenals	40-50 Cortisol?	Mostly non-functioning	
NET in lung, thymus, stomach	3-10	-	-
Lipoma	5-10	-	-

Frequency of Diseases in Multiple Endocrine Neoplasia Type 2 Related to Mutation in Different Codons				
Syndrome	**Frequently affected codons in *RET***	**MTC (%)**	**pHPT (%)**	**PCC (%)**
FMTC	533, 630, 768, 844	90-100	-	-
MEN 2A	609, 634, 790, 804	90-100	20-30	10-50
MEN 2B	883, 918	100	-	10-50

Prophyactic Thyroidectomy for Medullary Thyroid cancer Depending on the Site of Mutation of the *RET* Protooncogene in Multiple endocrine Neoplasia TYpe 2 Patients with Normal Calcitonin Levels			
	Risk group		
	High	**Medium**	**Low**
Codon	883, 918, 922	609, 611, 618, 820, 634	768, 790, 791, 804, 891
Thyroidectomy at age (years)	<1	6	<20

CHAPTER 38 PANCREATIC NEUROENDOCRINE TUMORS

Endocrine cells of the pancress and tumor syndromes

Cell Type	% Islet Cell Mass	Location within Islet	Location within Pancreas	Major (Minor) Hormone Secreted	Associated Tumor Syndrome	Diagnostic Hormone Levels
A (alpha)	10%	Peripheral	Evenly distributed	Glucagon (glicentin, TRH, CCK, endorphin, PP, pancreastatin)	Glucagonoma: necrolytic migratory erythema, diabetes, hypoaminoacidemia	Normal= <150 pg/mL
B (beta)	70%	Central	Body/tail	Insulin (TRH, CGRP, amylin, pancreastatin, prolactin)	Insulinoma: hypoglycemia and associated symptoms	>5 μU/mL in the face of hypoglycemia
D	5%*	Evenly distributed	Evenly distributed	Somatostatin (metencephalon)	Somatostatinoma: diabetes, gallstones, steatorrhea	Normal = 10-25 pg/mL
D_2	5%*	Evenly distributed	Evenly distributed	VIP	VIPoma: high-volume secretory diarrhea, hypokalemia, metabolic acidosis, hypochlorhydria	Normal = <200 pg/mL
F	15%	Peripheral	Head and uncinate process	PP	None	NA
EC	<1%	Evenly distributed	Evenly distributed	Substance P. serotonin	None	NA
G	Not present in normal physiologic state	NA	Head, uncinate process, duodenum	Gastrin, ACTH-related peptides	Gastrinoma: Acid hypersecretion, gastric/duodenal ulcers, diarrhea	Normal = <100 pg/ml Suspicious = >100 pg/ml with secretin test, an increase >200 pg/ml diagnostic

Tumor (syndrome)	Incidence (%)	Presentation	Malignancy (%)
Insulinoma	70-80	Weakness, sweating, tremor, tachycardia, anxiety, fatigue, dizziness, disorientation, seizures	<10
Gastrinoma	20-25	Intractable or recurrent peptic ulcer disease (hemorrhage, perforation), complications of peptic ulcer, diarrhea	60-80
Non-functional tumors	30-50	Obstructive jaundice, pancreatitis, epigastric pain, duodenal obstruction, weight loss, fatigue	60-90

Contd.

Contd.

VIPoma	4	Profuse watery diarrhea, hypotension, abdominal pain	80
Glucagonoma	4	Migratory necrolytic skin rash, glossitis, stomatitis, angular cheilitis, diabetes, severe weight loss, diarrhoea	80
Somatostatinoma	<5	Cholelithiasis, diarrhea, neurofibromatosis	50
Carcinoid	<1	Flushing, sweating, diarrhea, oedema	90
ACTHoma	<1	Cushing's syndrome	>90
GRFoma	<1	Acromegaly	30

- Least malignant–Insulinoma
- Most malignant–ACTH oma
- Most common–Insulinoma
- 10-20% of cases associated with MEN 1
- Investigation of choice–MDCT
- Majority are Nonfunctioning

American joint committee on cancer staging for pancreatic neuroendocrine tumors

Primary Tumor (T)			
TX	Tumor cannot be assessed		
T0	No evidence of primary tumor		
Tis	Carcinoma in situ (includes Pan-IN 3)		
T1	Tumor limited to pancreas, ≤ 2 cm in size		
T2	Tumor limited to pancreas, >2 cm in size		
T3	Tumor extends beyond the pancreas but without involvement of the celiac axis or superior mesenteric artery		
Regional Lymph Nodes (N)			
NX	Regional lymph nodes cannot be assessed		
N0	No regional lymph node metastasis		
N1	Regional lymph node metastasis		
Distant Metastasis (M)			
M0	No distant metastasis		
M1	Distant metastasis		
Anatomic Stage			
Stage 0	Tis	N0	M0
Stage IA	T1	N0	M0
Stage IB	T2	N0	M0
Stage IIA	T3	N0	M0
Stage IIB	T1	N1	M0
	T2	N1	M0
	T3	N1	M0
Stage III	T4	Any N	M0
Stage IV	Any T	Any N	M1

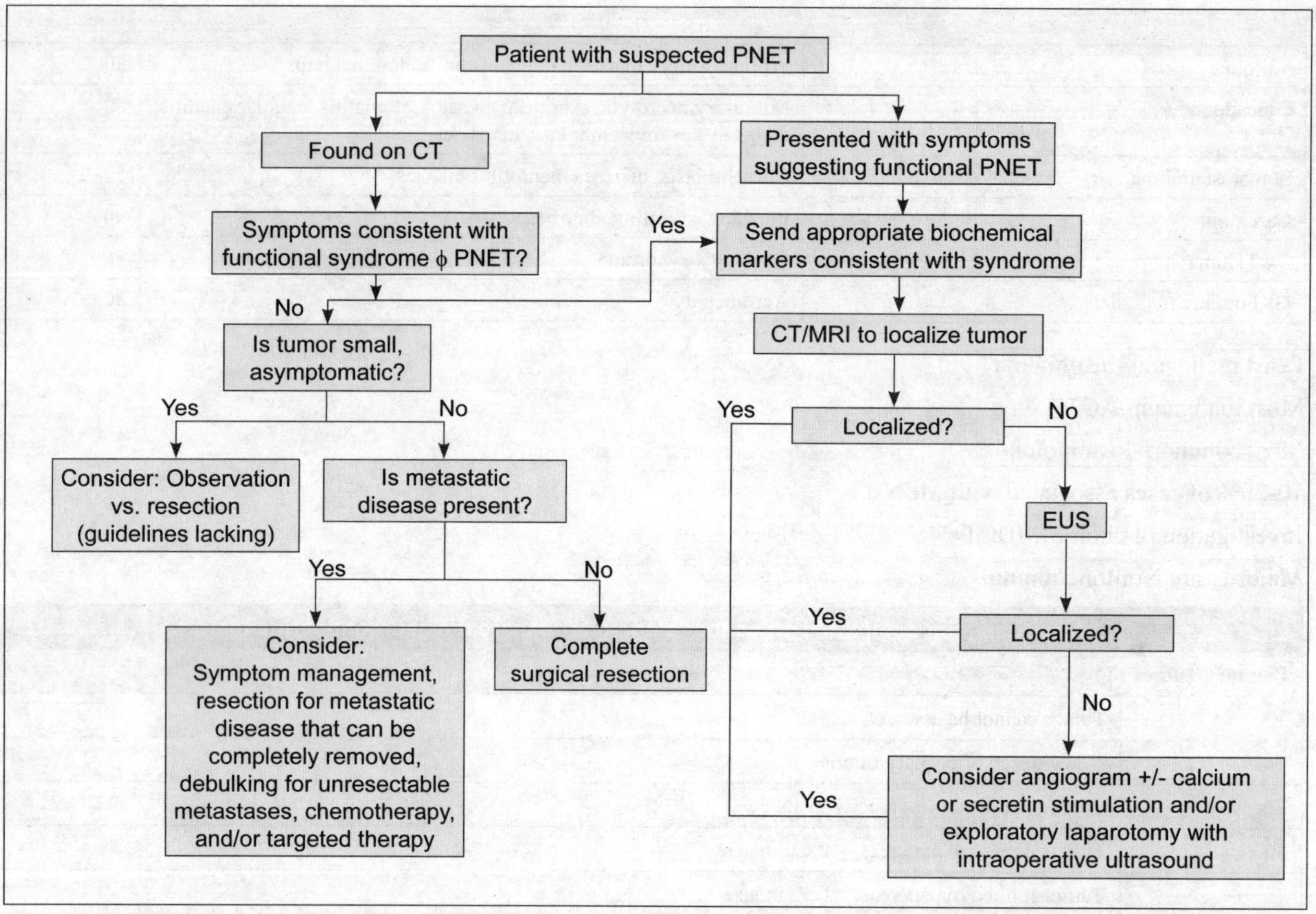

Insulinoma

- 70-80% of tumors
- 4th to 6th decade
- Women
- **Whipple's triad**–Symptoms of Hypoglycemia after fasting/Exercise, Plasma glucose <2.8 mmol/l and Relief of symptoms on intravenous glucose

Head= Body= Tail

- 10% MEN1–Multiple
- 10% Malignant
- Less than 2 cm, No vascular invasion/Metastasis→ Benign

Management:

- Best method of localization–Intraoperative USG
- ***Intra-operative USG→Confirms presence of tumor***
- Surgical treatment of choice–Enucleation
- Body/Tail, >2 cm, close to pancreatic duct→ Distal pancreatectomy
- Diazoxide–Unresectable metastatic, Unwilling/Unable to surgery
- Streptozotocin and Doxorubicin→ Metastatic

ZES/Gastrinoma

- Fulminant stomach ulcer, duodenum and atypical sites
- Recurrent ulceration despite therapy
- Non beta islet cell tumor
- 20%
- Males, 38 years
- Head of pancreas–Sporadic→ WORSE PROGNOSIS
- >60% are malignant
- 70% MEN1
- Involves 1st and 2nd part of duodenum
- ***Abdominal pain–Most common symptom (75%)***
- **Diarrhea** (halted by nasogastric aspiration of gastric secretions is characteristic) and GERD are also common
- 20-40% multiple
- Most common site is the **duodenum** (mostly first part; never in fourth part)

> ***Most common (80%) found in the gastrinoma triangle (Passaro)*** *formed by connecting lines between*
> *– Junction of cystic duct with common bile duct superiorly*
> *– The junction of 2nd and 3rd part of duodenum inferiorly*
> *– The junction between the neck and body of the pancreas medially*

- May be sporadic or associated with MEN 1
- Even malignant sporadic gastrinomas have indolent course
- **Tumors found outside the triangle have worse prognosis**
- Most patients have a typical duodenal ulcer

Factors suggesting gastrinoma

- *Ulcer of unusual nature – refractory/resistant to medical therapy*
- *Unusual number –* ***multiple peptic ulcers***
- *Unusual recurrence – recurrence after vagotomy/antrectomy*
- *Unusual sites – jejunum*
- *Unusual age – young and old*
- *Severe esophagitis*

- **Ulcers in the absence of H.pylori** infection or NSAID ingestion
- Ulcers associated with prominent gastric folds

Diagnosis

- Normal basal serum gastrin level is <120 pg/ml
- Serum gastrin level in ZES is typically 200 to 1000 pg/ml
- Gastric pH < 2 and fasting serum gastrin > 1000 pg/ml – diagnosis of ZES is confirmed
- PPIs have to be discontinued for 1 week before gastrin determination
- Basal acid output is usually >15 mEq/hour
  - Gastric pH<2.5 and Gastrin >1000 pg/ml→ Confirmed
  - 100-500 pg/ml→ Secretin test→ Gastrin >200 pg/ml (GASTRINOMA)
  - BAO/GAO >0.6
  - Secretin test: Rise above 200 pg/ml over the pretreatment value is diagnostic of ZES
  - Localization of tumor for preoperative staging–Somatostatin receptor scintigraphy (SRS) with radio labeled octreotide along with Endoscopic Ultrasound

Contd.

Contd.

Management:

- PPI, Octreotide
- Streptozotocin, 5 FU/Doxorubicin–Metastatic
- **Pancreatic Gastrinoma**–Head of pancreas, Worse prognosis, >1cm, Detected by EUS, Enucleation
- Head or uncinate process: **Enucleation with peripancreatic lymph node dissection**
- Body or tail: **Enucleation or distal resection**
- **Duodenal gastrinomas**:
  - < 5 mm Enucleated with overlying mucosa
  - Larger tumors: Excision with full thickness excision of duodenal wall

Non Functional PET

- Doesn't cause any syndrome
- Large, Unifocal
- 40-50 years
- >5 cm
- Most commonly involves Head
- Worse prognosis
- 70% Malignant
- Raised Chromagranin and Pancreatic Polypeptide
- Most common site of metastasis–Lung

Management

- Curative resection

Somatostatinoma

- Somatostatin-secreting PNET→ Steatorrhea, Diabetes mellitus, Hypochlorhydria and Gallstones
- Inhibition of pancreatic enzyme and hormone secretion by unregulated hypersecretion of somatostatin causes steatorrhea, diabetes, malabsorption, and cholelithiasis resulting from reduced gallbladder emptying
- Usually solitary and 85% are larger than 2 cm
- >60% are found in the pancreas, usually the head
- Typically 50 to 60 years old at time of diagnosis
- In patient with diabetes, gallstones and steatorrhea, with or without finding of pancreatic or duodenal mass on radiographic studies, fasting plasma somatostatin level should be measured
- ***Concentration >160 pg/ml is suggestive of diagnosis***
- ***Associated with Von Recklinghausen disease and Pheochromocytoma***

Glucagonoma

- Glucagonoma syndrome is a rare syndrome, with ***classic presentation of the "4 D's": diabetes, dermatitis, deep vein thrombosis and depression***
- Characterized by severe catabolic state with weight loss, depletion of fat and protein stores, and associated vitamin deficiencies
- Characteristic skin lesion, necrolytic migrating erythema is noted in approximately two thirds of patients and often appears before other symptoms of the syndrome
- Diagnosis of glucagonoma is established by measuring glucagon levels
- Normal fasting glucagon levels are less than 100 pg/ml
- Fasting glucagon level higher than 1000 pg/ ml is considered diagnostic

Carcinoma Pancreas	Non-functioning Pancreatic Endocrine Tumors
<5 cm	>5 cm
Hypodense and No calcifications	Hyperdense and calcification
-	+ve Chromogranin
-	+ve SRS

Comparison of commonly mutated genes in pancreatic neuroendocrine tumor and pancreatic ductal adenocarcinoma

Genes	PNET (%)	PDAC (%)
MEN1	44	0
DAXX, ATRX	43	0
Genes in mTOR pathway	15	0.8
TP53	3	85
KRAS	0	100
CDKN2A	0	25
TGFBR1, SMAD3, SMAD4	0	38

Causes of hypergastrinemia

High Gastric Acid Output	Normal, Low or No Gastric Acid Output
ZES (gastrinoma)	H_2 receptor antagonist therapy
Gastric outlet obstruction	PPI therapy
G cell hyperplasia	Prior acid-reducing procedure
Retained gastric antrum	Atrophic gastritis, pernicious anemia, gastric cancer, vitiligo, achlorhydria, vagotomy, renal failure

CHAPTER 39

CARCINOID TUMORS AND NET

1. **Arises from enterochromaffin cells/kulchitsky cells found in crypts of lieberkuhn**
2. Order of involvement of carcinoids is bronchus > ileum > rectum > appendix
3. Most common system involved in carcinoids is GIT (85%)
4. Life threatening form of carcinoid syndrome is carcinoid crisis
5. Least commonly associated with malignant potential is **Rectum > Lung**
6. Most common GI carcinoids to be associated with carcinoid syndrome is **midgut carcinoids**
7. Carcinoid tumors that have the best prognosis is small bowel carcinoids
8. Foregut carcinoids produce low levels of serotonin
9. **Midgut carcinoids produce high level of serotonin**
10. Hindgut carcinoids rarely produce serotonin, but may produce somatostatin and peptide YY
11. **Ileal carcinoids are more likely to metastatize to liver**
12. Most common site of hindgut carcinoids is Colon
13. Small bowel carcinoids occur most commonly in terminal 60 cm of ileum–**Distal 1/3rd**
14. Most common site of foregut carcinoids is bronchus > stomach
15. Most common site of midgut carcinoids is ileum
16. Pulmonary carcinoids are usually perihilar and ectopic ACTH and GH releasing factor results in Cushing syndrome and acromegaly
17. **Hindgut carcinoids rarely produce carcinoid syndrome but presents with bleeding**
18. **Carcinoid syndrome** is precipitated by alcohol intake, exercise, stress, eating and vigorous palpation of liver while **carcinoid crisis** is precipitated by anesthesia, surgery and chemotherapy
19. Atypical carcinoid syndrome is seen in sporadic foregut carcinoids due to histamine release
20. High levels of Ki-67 associated with decreased survival of carcinoid patients
21. 5-HIAA correlates with tumor burden in carcinoid syndrome
22. **Most common symptom of carcinoid syndrome is flushing**
23. **Appendectomy is treatment of choice in appendiceal tumors <1.5 cms**
24. **Right hemicolectomy with regional lymphadenectomy is treatment of choice in appendiceal tumors >1.5 cms, base involvement, invasion of mesoappendix wall, blood vessels and regional lymph nodes >2 cm**
25. Chromogranin A can be used in detection of functional and nonfunctional tumors
26. Abdominal CT scan is useful for assessing involvement of retroperitoneum and liver metastasis
27. SPOKE WHEEL APPEARANCE–In small bowel carcinoids on CT Scan due to extensive mesenteric fibrosis and calcification
28. Positive immunohistochemical staining for MIB-1 and p53 are associated with metastatic behavior
29. All patients with metastatic carcinoids should receive octreotide therapy preoperatively to prevent carcinoid crisis

30. Carcinoid syndrome is seen in patients with liver metastasis, retroperitoneal disease and carcinoids outside GIT as with bronchial, ovarian or testicular tumors
31. Surgical resection depends upon size of primary lesion and mesenteric lymph node involvement in small bowel carcinoids as they are multicentric and metastasizing
32. Surgical treatment of rectal carcinoids depends on size and depth of invasion
33. For recurrent/metastatic disease, somatostatin analogue is used to reduce tumor burden and carcinoid syndrome
34. **Prophylactic cholecystectomy-patients on long term octreotide therapy**
35. Rectal carcinoids <1 cm→local excision

    Rectal carcinoids 1-2 cm and no LVSI and muscularis propria involvement→Wide local excision

    Rectal carcinoids 1-2 cm with LVSI and muscularis propria involvement→TME

    Rectal carcinoids >2 cms→TME with sphincter preservation (Total mesorectal excision)

    High grade rectal carcinoids→neoadjuvant chemoradiation followed by radical resection
36. **Type 1 gastric carcinoids are most common of all gastric carcinoids**
37. **Type 1→75% of Gastric carcinoids are associated with chronic atrophic gastritis type A (CAGA) and Pernicious Anemia→gastrin increased, reduced acid→EMR is treatment**
38. **Type 2 gastric carcinoids→5-10% associated with ZES (MEN 1), multifocal, higher metastasis→increased gastrin and acid→Total gastrectomy and pancreaticoduodenectomy**
39. **Type 3 gastric carcinoids→15-25%, males, sporadic. Aggressive, ATYPICAL CARCINOID SYNDROME→Surgery and chemotherapy**
40. Small pedunculated gastric carcinoids→endoscopically

    Large gastric carcinoids→wedge resection/partial gastrectomy

    Multiple gastric carcinoids→Total gastrectomy
41. **Bright red patchy flushing is typically seen in gastric NET's due to histamine,** Purple flush involving upper trunk and face <30 min is seen in ileal carcinoids, Deep dusky purple flush over entire body
42. **Most common cardiac lesion in carcinoid disease–Tricuspid regurgitation/Pulmonary stenosis**
43. **Platelet/urine serotonin levels are useful in foregut carcinoids**
44. Indication for surgical intervention in unresectable and metastatic small bowel carcinoids are obstruction and perforation.
45. Everolimus→Improved survival in pancreatic NET
46. Bronchial carcinoids rarely metastatise→surgery is curative
47. Most common symptom of bronchial carcinoid-hemoptysis
48. Most common symptom of small bowel carcinoids-abdominal pain
49. Small bowel, bronchus, pancreas, ovary and testis is associated with malignant carcinoid syndrome
50. Ovary and retroperitoneum NET's bypass the liver causing carcinoid syndrome without hepatic metastasis
51. **Size→Best predictor of malignant and metastatic potential, including lymphovascular invasion**
52. Diarrhea in carcinoid syndrome is episodic, watery and often explosive→5HT
53. Increased N-terminal pro-brain natriuretic peptide (NT pro-BNP) and Chromogranin A has showed worse prognosis
54. Barium studies showed fibrosis of small bowel with multiple filling defects and kinking in small bowel carcinoids
55. CT Scan Small bowel carcinoids→Solid mass with speculated borders and radiating strands within mesenteric fat and kinking of bowel
56. MRI Small bowel carcinoids→Diagnosis of liver metastasis

    Usually low signal intensity on T1 and high signal intensity on T2 weighted images
57. After Gd enhanced contrast, liver metastasis enhances peripherally in hepatic arterial phase and hypointense defects in portal venous phase

58. Most of the NET's have low Ki-67 expression and have low sensitivity of PET-CT
59. Carcinoid tumors produce intense desmoplastic reaction causing mesenteric fibrosis and **parachute intestine** (intestinal obstruction)
60. **LUBARSCH 1st described the carcinoid tumor in 1888**
61. **OBERNDORFER coined the term KARZINOIDE**
62. Most important principle of management of metastatic carcinoids is therapeutic restraint
63. Most life threatening complication of carcinoid syndrome is hypotension mediated by kinins and precipitated by catecholamines
64. Monoamine oxidase inhibitors are contraindicated in carcinoid syndrome as they precipitate symptoms
65. CARCINOID CRISIS→Avoid morphine, succinyl choline and curare

    Preop octreotide 100 mg SC three times daily for 2 weeks, During and after surgery, IV at rate of 50 mcg/h starting before anesthesia and gradually tapered over 1 week postop
66. Ga^{68} DOTATATE PET-CT is clinically useful imaging technique to localize primary tumors in patients with neuroendocrine metastasis of unknown origin as well as to define existence and extent of metastatic disease
67. **CLARINET trial-Lanreotide significantly improved progression free survival among patients with metastatic enteropancreatic NET's of grade 1/2 (Ki-67 marker <10%)**
68. NET's have best prognosis of all small bowel tumors
69. **An elevated level of CgA is an independent predictor of adverse prognosis, probably most useful factor identified**
70. Patients with metastatic NET's determined that tumor uptake is predictive for both survival after Y^{90} DOTA-TOC treatment and occurrence of renal toxicity
71. IFN alpha is used in palliation of diarrhea and flushing→stimulates T cells, Inhibits angiogenesis, Induces cell cycle arrest in G_0 and G_1 phases
72. Pancreatic NET's have mutations in mTOR genes in approximately 15% of cases
73. **Radiofrequency ablation is used for liver metastasis in carcinoids which are centrally located, <3 cms and not near major blood vessels/ducts**
74. TACE is used for patients with diffuse/widely scattered bilateral liver metastasis
75. Negative prognostic factors for liver transplantation in liver metastasis are High hepatic tumor burden, Ki-67 index elevated, Pancreatic primary tumor
76. **Risk factors for development of midgut carcinoids are age, male sex, Increased body mass index and menopausal therapy**
77. In midgut carcinoids, only primary site in which size doesn't correlate with metastasis
78. Overall 5 year survival rate of all patients with GI NET's is 28.5%
79. Thymic carcinoids→Secrete ectopic ACTH, associated with MEN 1 syndrome (25%)
80. **Stage 1 and 2 thymic NET's are treated by radical thymectomy and Stage 3 thymic NET's are treated by Chemotherapy**
81. Bronchial carcinoids are not related to smoking, associated with MEN 1, close to hilum
82. Well differentiated bronchial carcinoids are treated by resection while small cell NET's are treated by chemotherapy
83. Atypical bronchial carcinoids have more uptake of deoxyglucose on PET Scan and Typical carcinoids have more uptake of octreotide
84. Esophageal NET's are most common in distal esophagus just proximal to GEJ
85. Gastrinomas are most common duodenal NET's→proximal duodenum
86. **Esophageal carcinoids with no incidence of lymph node metastasis and tumor amenable to complete resection→Endoscopic mucosal resection**

    Esophageal carcinoids with lymph node metastasis→ open resection

87. **Non ampullary duodenal NET's: <1cm→EMR, >2 cm→surgical excision**
    >3 cm→whipples pancreaticoduodenectomy
88. Periampullary duodenal NET's→local excision/whipples pancreaticoduodenectomy
    Depending on age, size of tumor, relation to ampulla→Secretes Somatostatin
89. Periampullary duodenal NET's are associated with Von Recklinghausen neurofibromatosis
90. **Colonic carcinoids are more common on right side, Ascending/transverse colon**
91. **Midgut carcinoids are most common source of carcinoid syndrome, associated with 2nd primary tumor (colon and breast) and MEN 1**
92. Initial imaging procedure to localize and stage carcinoids-SRS (Identify extraabdominal metastatic disease/primary cant be appreciated on CT scan
93. One of the major determinants of survival→presence of liver metastasis
94. Extensive involvement of small intestine is associated with Higher probability of liver Metastasis
95. Appendiceal carcinoids are more common in females
    Type 3 gastric carcinoids are more common in men
96. Maximum malignant potential is associated with pancreatic carcinoids
97. **SMART BOMBS–Radiolabelled somatostatin analogues that deliver radiation specifically to carcinoid cells**
98. Somatostatin receptor scintigraphy with In^{111} labelled pantreotide has shown higher sensitivity than CT scan
99. Endocardial fibroelastosis is cardiac manifestation of carcinoid syndrome
100. Young age and females are associated with good prognosis
101. Most common site of appendiceal

PART ONE: THORACIC ONCOLOGY (LUNG AND CHEST WALL)

CHAPTER

40 CARCINOMA LUNG

One Liners

- Most common visceral malignancy
- Most common cause of cancer related death in both men and women
- Most common lung cancer is adenocarcinoma
- Most common lung cancer in smokers is squamous cell carcinoma
- Most common lung cancer in non smokers is adenocarcinoma
- Most common lung cancer in males is squamous cell carcinoma
- Most common lung cancer in females is adenocarcinoma
- Most common primary malignant tumor of lung–Bronchogenic carcinoma

Genetics

- Mutations of K-RAS are most commonly seen in NSCLC (90% of adenocarcinoma)
- **In presence of K-RAS mutations patient doesn't respond to TKI therapy**
- Loss of PTEN expression by IHC/RT-PCR seen in 73% of NSCLC
- Mutations of p53 occur in 50% of NSCLC
- 90% of EGFR mutations are Exon 19 deletion/substitution of aminoacid at 858 position in Exon 21
- **MET is associated with adenocarcinoma**

Etiology

SMOKING

- Cigarette smoking is cause of 85% to 90% of lung cancer cases
- 80% of lung cancers are seen in active smokers or stopped smoking recently

Risk for lung cancer in smokers is 30 times greater than in nonsmokers

- Frequency of lung cancers and pack years of smoking are related

Smoking cigars or pipes doubles risk for lung cancer compared with risk in non-smokers

- 60 times more in smokers, Smoking causes chromosomal breakages
- P450 polymorphisms activate pro-carcinogens in smoking
- 95% of small cell lung cancers occur in current/former smokers

Cancers in non-smokers are likely to have EGFR mutations and never K-RAS

- Passive smoking probably increases risk of lung cancer about two-fold
- Proportion of the risk associated with active inhalation is about 20-fold

	Smokers	**Never Smokers/Light Smokers**
Age	Older (>60)	Younger (<60)
Gender	Male > Female	Female < Male
Ethnicity	Caucasian predominant	East Asian > Caucasian

Contd.

Contd.

Histological subtype	All	Adenocarcinoma
Associated mutations/alternations	KRAS, PIK3CA, RB p53	EGFR, EML4-ALK

INDUSTRIAL

- Asbestosis, Arsenic, Chromium, Uranium, Nickel, Vinyl chloride, Ionizing radiation, Radon gas, Uranium miners
- **Asbestosis**–Increased risk of lung cancer. Three times greater risk than smoking alone
- Radon has been associated with up to 6% of lung cancer cases

Lung scars and chronic obstructive pulmonary disease are associated with an increased risk for lung cancer

Precursor Lesions

- Squamous dysplasia and CIS
- Atypical adenomatous hyperplasia
- Adenocarcinoma in situ
- DIPNCH–diffuse idiopathic pulmonary neuroendocrine hyperplasia

- Accounts for 1/3rd of cancer related deaths

Tumors

Squamous Cell Carcinoma	Adenocarcinoma
• Arise from segmental bronchi • Highest frequency of p53 mutation • Bronchial obstruction and post obstruction pneumonia • Keratinization and intercellular bridges are very specific • ***Central location, Cavitating lesion*** • ***Most common paraneoplastic syndrome associated hypercalcemia–PTHrP*** **TYPES** • **Papillary:** Exophytic and papillary • **Clear cell:** Clear cell cytoplasm • **Small cell:** Glanular nuclear chromatin • **Basaloid:** Palisiding nest of cells	• Usually peripheral, Associated with K-ras mutation • Glandular pattern of growth, Cells are positive for mucin and TTF-1 • Arises from previous scars • ***Most common in non-smokers*** • ***Most common in young females***
Sarcomatoid Tumors (<2%)	**Pulmonary Blastoma**
Atleast 10% of sarcomatous features No distinguishing radiologic features Both central and peripheral location **TYPES** • **Pleomorphic** • **Spindle cell** • **Giant cell** • **Pulmonary blastoma**–Women, 4th decade	Primitive, biphasic tumor ***Mainly adults*** Pleuropulmonary variety occurs in pediatric patients
Salivary Gland Neoplasms	**Large Cell Carcinoma**
Mucoepidermoid-segmental and subsegmental bronchi Adenoid cystic-intraluminal and tracheobronchial Epithelial-myoepithelial carcinoma (myoepithelioma)-outer myoepithelial and inner layer	Lacks cytologic features of small cell carcinoma and glandular/squamous differentiation Cells with prominent nucleoli and moderate amount of cytoplasm **Associated with gynaecomastia** **TYPES** • **Lymphoepithelioma**–EBER1 RNA • **Basaloid**–poor prognosis

Contd.

Contd.

	• **Clear cell**–Associated with clear cell carcinoma kidney • **Rhabdoid**–Prominent eosinophilic cytoplasmic globules Large cell neuroendocrine carcinoma is diagnosed by presence of nucleoli with prominent cytoplasm which differentiates it from small cell carcinoma
Bronchoalveolar Carcinoma	**Adenosquamous Carcinoma**
Subtype of adenocarcinoma Histologically tumor is characterized by growth along pre existing structure (Lepidic pattern) with no evidence of stromal,vascular or pleural invasion or alveolar destruction Ultrastructurally they contain mucin secreting bronchiolar cells, clara cells Spreads transbronchially by aerosolisation	At least 10% are squamous and 10% are adenomatous
Cystic Adenoid Carcinomas ("Cylindroma")	
Locally invasive cancers ***Locoregional recurrence is most common,*** but they may also metastasize to other areas of lung and to distant sites	

NEUROENDOCRINE TUMORS

Feature of neuroendocrine lung tumors

	Typical Carcinoid	Atypical Carcinoid	LCNEC	SCIC
NE features	Well differentiated	Well differentiated	Poorly differentiated	Poorly differentiated
Cell size	Intermediate	Intermediate	Large to intermediate	Small to intermediate
Mitotic rate	Low < 2 mitoses/^{2} mm^2	Intermediate 2-10 mitoses/^{2} mm^2	High median 70 mitoses/^{2} mm^2	High median 80 mitoses/^{2} mm^2
NE markers by IHC	+++	++–+++	+–+++	±
Necrosis	–	+ (focal)	+++	+++
KI-67 index	≤ 5%	5-20%	50-100%	80-100%
5-years survival	90-95%	60-70%	10-40%	≤ 5-10%

TYPICAL CARCINOID TUMOR

- WHO cut off <2 mitosis/HPF
- Associated with MEN-1
- But not with tobacco smoking
- CENTRAL TYPE–endobronchial mass pneumonia/hemoptysis
- PERIPHERAL TYPE–subpleural, fusiform cells, airway fibrosis
- **COLLAR BUTTON LESION*****
- 5-15% lymph node metastasis
- 3% are distant metastasis
- **SALT AND PEPPER CHROMATIN******

ATYPICAL CARCINOID TUMOR

- Usually with punctate necrosis
- 2-10 mitosis/HPF
- 40-50% lymph node metastasis
- 20% distant metastasis

Contd.

Contd.

SMALL CELL LUNG CARCINOMA

- **Most common pulmonary neuroendocrine tumor**
- High expression of Bcl-2 in majority of tumors
- Cells are smaller than size of 3 resting lymphocytes
- Small/absent nucleoli
- OAT CELL CARCINOMA
- **AZZOPARDI EFFECT**–Basophilic staining of vascular walls is frequently present
- Central location
- Significant smoking history
- **Nuclear molding is present**
- Presence of neurosecretory granules
- Best response to chemotherapy and radiotherapy
- Most aggressive lung cancer
- Paraneoplastic syndrome–SIADH and Cushing syndrome
- Large central mass with mediastinal extension and widespread metastasis
- SVC SYNDROME, RLN palsy and dysphagia are associated.
- Bcl-2 is positive in 90% of cases
- RB1 muatations are seen in >90% of small cell lung cancers
- Loss of heterozygosity of 9p and 10q (PTEN).
- Also +ve for keratin, EMA and BER-EP4
- Deletions in 3p occur in 90% of small cell lung cancers
- **Ki-67 index→80-100%**
- 75% staining +ve for at least 1 NE marker-NSE, Chromogranin, CD 56
- P53 mutations are most common abnormality in 75-80% of tumors (But Squamous cell carcinomas are associated with majority of p53 mutations)
- **Classical autocrine agent in small cell carcinoma is GRP**
- Elevated levels of IGF-1 are seen in 75% of tumors
- Median survival of untreated cancers–4 to 6 months
- Median survival of metastatic tumors–5 to 9 months

More often central or hilar (95%)

Relapse after radiation therapy (RT) or chemotherapy occurs in the sites initially affected as well as in previously uninvolved sites

Associated paraneoplastic syndromes include ***SIADH-most common,*** hypercoagulable state (common), Ectopic ACTH syndrome and Eaton-Lambert (myasthenic) syndrome

Hypercalcemia occurs rarely in SCLC, even in presence of extensive bony metastases

CLINICAL FEATURES

Signs and Symptoms	Range of Reported Frequencies (%)
Cough	8-75
Weight loss	0-68
Dyspnea	3-60
Chest pain	20-49
Hemoptysis	6-25
Bone pain	6-25
Fever	0-20

Contd.

Contd.

Weakness	0-10
Superior vena cava obstruction	0-4
Dysphagia	0-2
Wheezing	0-2

Symptoms	Weight loss > 10 B
	Focal skeletal pain
	Neurologic symptoms: Headache, syncope, seizures, focal extremity weakness, altered mentation
Signs	Palpable lymphadenopathy (> 1 cm)
	Hoarseness or SVC syndrome
	Bone tenderness
	Hepatomegaly (>13 cm)
	Focal neurologic signs
	Soft tissue mass
Laboratory testing	Hematocrit < 40% in men or < 35% in women
	Elevated alkaline phosphatase, liver function tests

INVESTIGATIONS

Early stage (I/II) and PET mediastinum is –ve→Surgery

If PET +ve→Endobronchial biopsy via EBUS or→ EUS or mediastinoscopy depending on node location

False –ve PET scan→Carcinoids and Lepidic growth adenocarcinoma

MRI–Indicated for evaluating Superior sulcus tumors with concern for neurovascular or spine involvement

PARANEOPLASTIC SYNDROMES

Most common tumor associated with SIADH is small cell lung cancer

Associated with acanthosis nigricans, trousseau syndrome

Most common paraneoplastic neurologic disorder associated with Small cell lung cancer is **SUBACUTE PERIPHERAL SENSORY NEUROPATHY**

SUPERIOR SULCUS SYNDROME

Apical lung tumor causing compression of sympathetic plexus resulting in Horner's syndrome and pain in ulnar nerve distribution

Mostly due to adenocarcinoma

SVC SYNDROME: *Mostly due to small cell cancer lung*

Primary treatment of hyponatremia in small cell carcinoma is chemotherapy

Primary treatment of cushing syndrome in small cell carcinoma is chemotherapy

Syndrome	Presentation/Symptoms	Laboratory Values	Management/Treatment*
SIADH	Gait disturbances falls, headaches, nausea, fatigue, muscle cramps, anorexia, confusion, lethargy, seizures respiratory depression, coma	Hyponatremia Mild = serum sodium 130-134 mmol/l Severe = serum sodium less than 125 mmol/l Increases urine osmolality (> 100 mOsm/Kg) in the context of euvolemic hyponatremia	Fluid restriction (and encourage adequate salt and protein intake) Discontinuation of offending drugs Demeclocycline Vasopression-receptor antagonists Conlvaptan Tolyaptan Hypertonic (3%) saline (if acute onset)

Contd.

Contd.

Cushing syndrome	Muscular weakness, peripheral edema, hypertension, weight gain	Hypokalemia typically less than 3.0 mmol/L Elevated base line serum cortisol greater than 800 nmol/L Normal to elevated midnight serum ACTH (not suppressed with dexamethasone) greater than 100 mg/L	Ketoconazole Octreotide Aminoglutethimide Metyrapone Mitortane Etomidate Miferistone

Syndrome	Clinical Presentation	Associated Antibodies	Additional Diagnostic Studies	Management/Treatment
Limbic Encephalitis (LE)	Mood changes, hallucinations, memory loss, seizures, less commonly hypothalamic symptoms (hyperthermia, somnolence, endocrine dysfunction); onset over days to months	Anti-Hu (ANNA-II) Anti-CRMPS (anti-CV2) Anti-Ma Anti-amphiphysin	EEG epileptic foci in temporal lobe(s); focal or generalized slow activity FDG-PET increased metabolism in temporal lobe(s) MRI hyperintensity in medial temporal lobe(s) CSF plenocytosis, elevated protein, elevated IgG, oligodonal bands	IMG Corticosteroids Plasma exchange Cyctophosphamide Rituximab
Paraneoplastic Cerebellar Degeneration (PCD)	Ataxia, diplopia, dysphagia/dysarthria; prodrome of dizziness, nausea vomiting	Anti-Hu (ANNA-II) Anti-Yo Anti-CRMPS (anti-CV2) Anti-Ma Anti-Tr Anti-Ri Anti-VGCC Anti-mGluRl	FDG-PET increased metabolism (early stage) and then decreased metabolism (late stage) in cerebelium MRI cerebellar atrophy (late stage)	IMG Corticosteroids Plasma exchange Cyclophosphamide Rituximab
Lambert-Eaton Myasthenic Syndrome (LEMS)	Lower extremity proximal muscle weakness, fatigue, diaphragmatic weakness, bulbar symptoms (usually milder than in myasthenia gravis): Later in course autonomic symptoms (ptosis, impotence, dry mouth) in most patients	Anti-VGCC (P/Q type)	EMG low compound muscle action potential amplitude; decremental response with low-rate stimulation but incremental response with high-rate stimulation	3,4-Diaminopyridine (DAP) Guanidline Pyridostigmine Corticosteroids Azathioprine IMG

Contd.

Contd.

Subacute (Peripheral Sensory Neuropathy)	Paresthesia/pain (typically upper extremities before lower) followed by ataxia; multifocal/ asymmetric distribution; all sensory modalities decreased but especially deep sensation/ pseudoathetosis of hands; deep tendon reflexes decreased/ absent; onset over weeks to months.	Anti-Hu (ANNA-1) Anit-CRMPS (anti-CV2) Anti-amphilhysin	NCS reduced/absent sensory nerve action potentials CSF pleocytosis, high IgG, oligoclonal bands	Corticosteroids Cycliphosphamide IMG Plasma exchange
Autonomic Neuropathy	Panautonomic neuropathy, often subacute (weeks) onset, involving sympathetic, parasympathetic, and enteric systems: Orthostatic hypotension, GI dysfuncion, dry eyes/ mouth, bowel/bladder dysfunction, altered pupillary light reflexes, loss of sinus arrhythmia Chronic Gastrointestinal Pseudoobstruction (CGP): Constipation, nausea/vomitting dysphagia, weight loss, abdominal distension	Anti-Hu (ANNA-I) Anti-CV2 (CRMPS) Anti-nAchR Anti-amphiphysin	Abdominal X-ray/ barfum studies/CT GI dilatation but no mechanical obstruction (for CGP) Esophageal manometry achalasia or spasms (for CGP)	For orthostatic hypotension: Water, salt intake Fludrocortisone Midodrine Caffeine For pseudobstruction: Neostigmine

NODAL INVOLVEMENT

4 specimen has shown to be adequate for diagnostic yield for endobronchial tumors

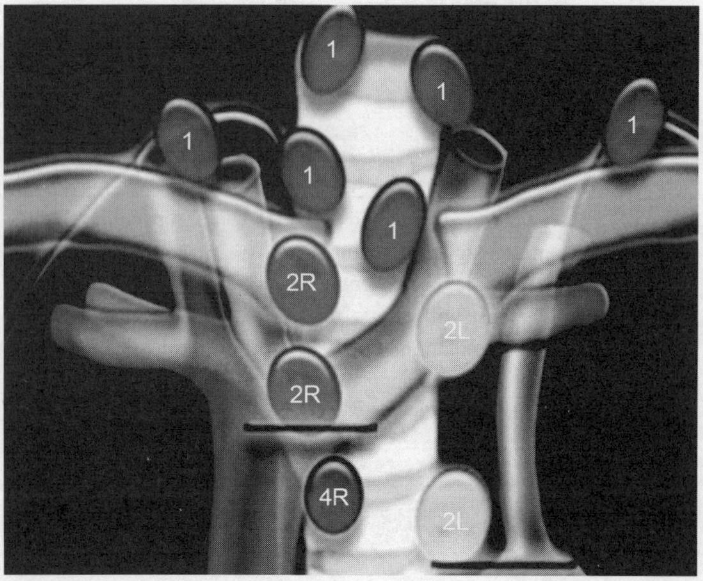

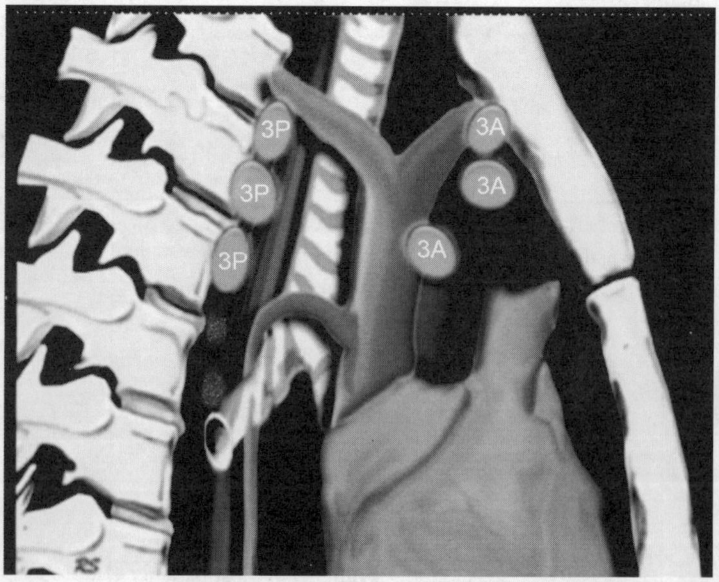

Contd.

Contd.

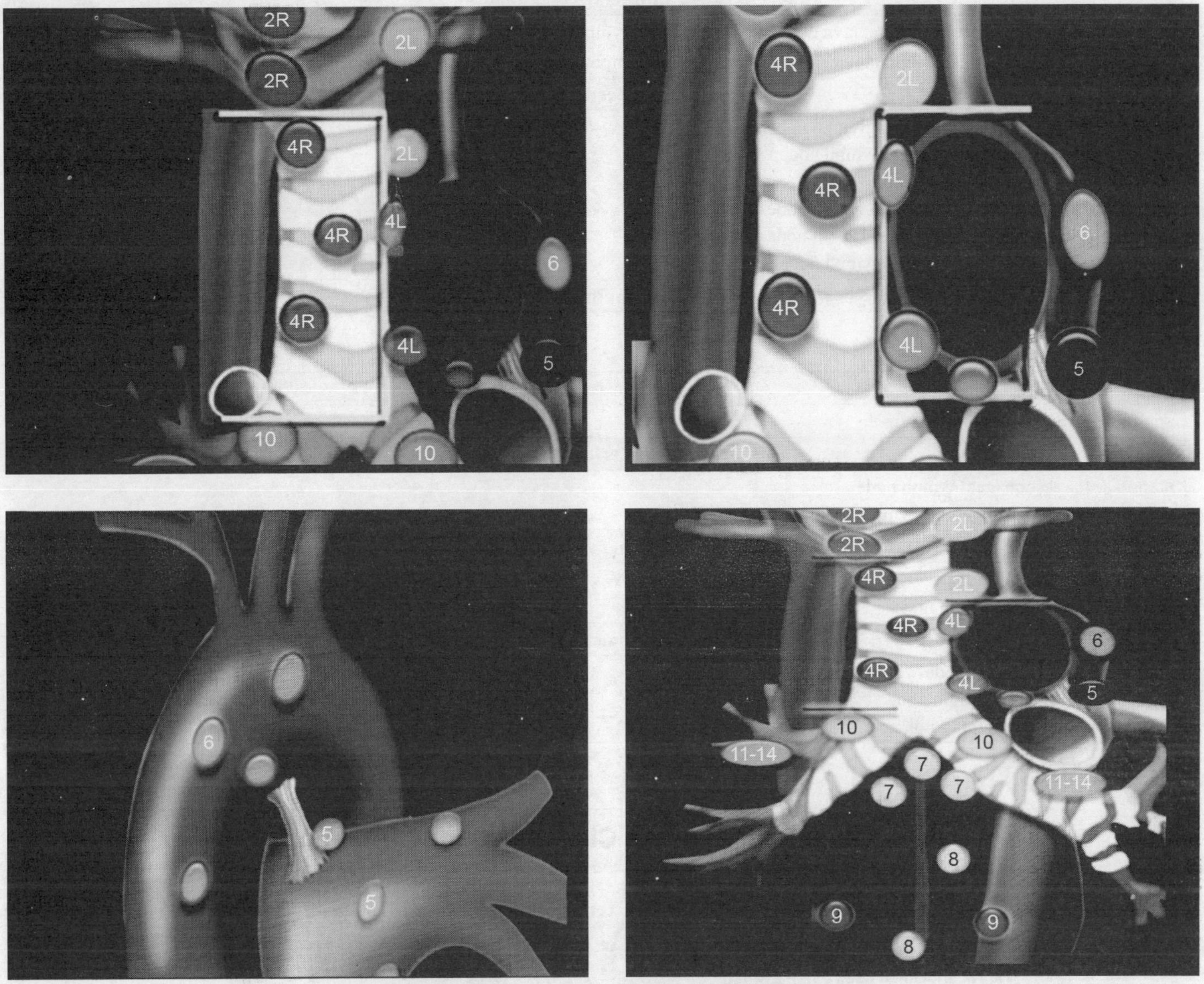
2R
2R
2L
4R
2L
4R
4L
6
4R
4L
5
10
10
4R
2L
4L
4R
6
4R
4L
5
10
6
5
5
2R
2L
2R
4R
2L
4R
4L
6
4R
4L
5
10
11-14
10
7
7
7
11-14
8
9
9
8

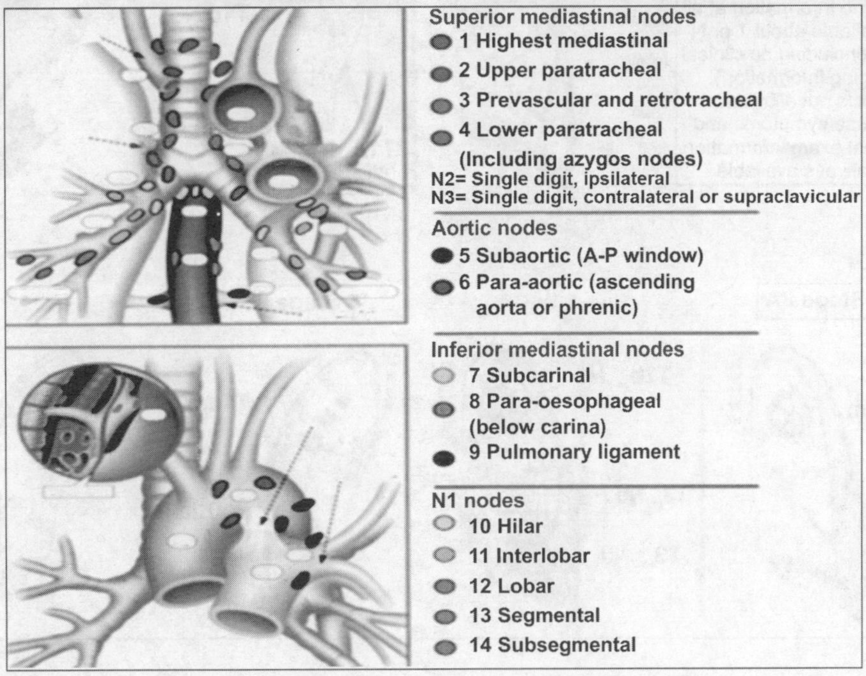
Superior mediastinal nodes
1 Highest mediastinal
2 Upper paratracheal
3 Prevascular and retrotracheal
4 Lower paratracheal
(Including azygos nodes)
N2= Single digit, ipsilateral
N3= Single digit, contralateral or supraclavicular
Aortic nodes
5 Subaortic (A-P window)
6 Para-aortic (ascending
aorta or phrenic)
Inferior mediastinal nodes
7 Subcarinal
8 Para-oesophageal
(below carina)
9 Pulmonary ligament
N1 nodes
10 Hilar
11 Interlobar
12 Lobar
13 Segmental
14 Subsegmental

Supraclavicular zone
Station 1L: Right low cervical, supraclavicular, and sternal notch lymph nodes Station 1L: Left low cervical, supraclavicular and sternal notch lymph nodes
Upper zone (superior mediastinal nodes)
Station 2R: Right upper paratracheal lymph node Station 2L: Left upper paratracheal lymph node Station 3A: Prevascular lymph node Station 4R: Right lower paratracheal lymph node Station 4R: Right lower paratracheal lymph node Station 4L: Left lower paratracheal lymph node
Aortopulmonary zone
Station 5: Subaortic lymph node Station 6: Paraaortic lymph node
Subcarinal zone
Station 7: Subcarinal lymph node
Lower zone (inferior mediastinal nodes)
Station 8: Paraesophageal lymph node Station 9: Pulmonary ligament lymph node
Hilar and Interlober zone (pulmonary nodes)
Station 10: Hilar lymph node Station 11: Interlobar lymph node
Peripheral zone (pulmonary nodes)
Station 12: Lobar lymph node Station 13: Segmental lymph node Station 14: Subsegmental lymph node

AJCC STAGING 8th EDITION

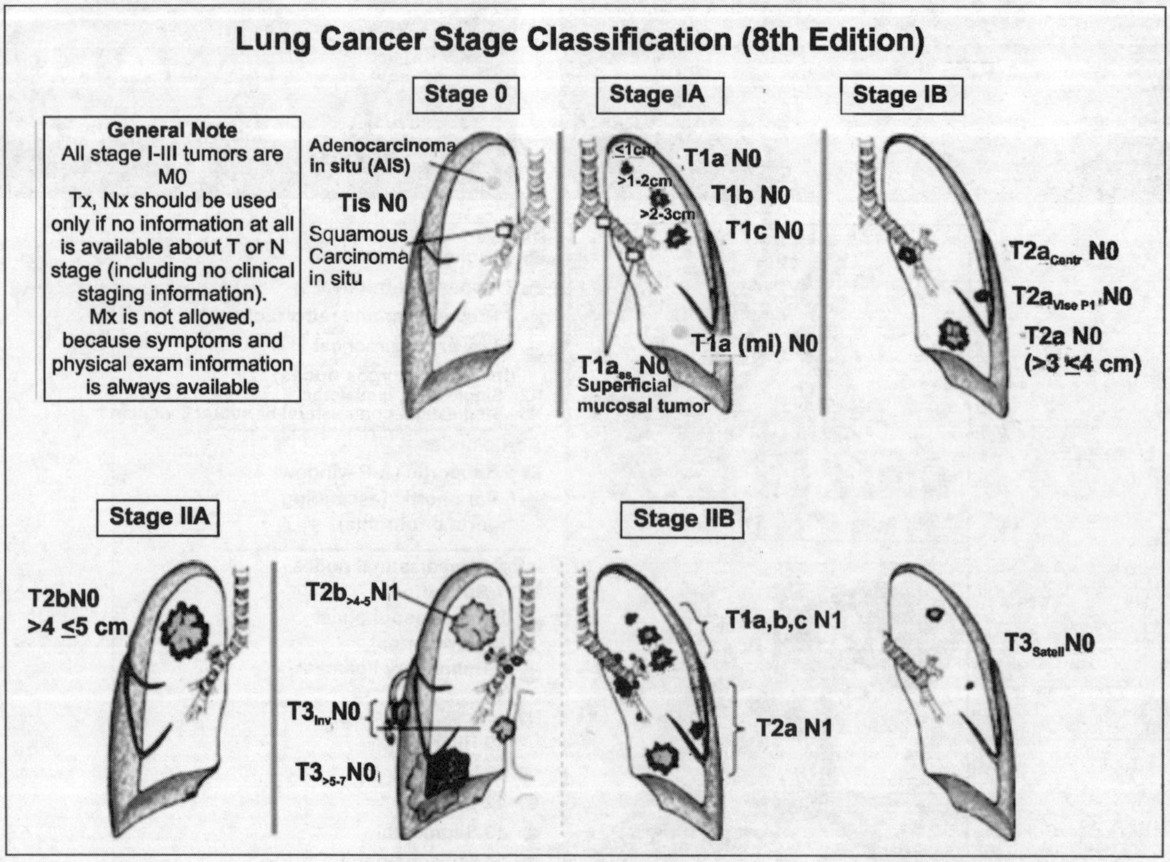

	N0	N1	N2	N3
T1	IA	IIB	IIIA	IIIB
T2a	IB	IIB	IIIA	IIIB
T2b	IIA	IIB	IIIA	IIIB
T3	IIB	IIIA	IIIB	IIIC
T4	IIIA	IIIA	IIIB	IIIC
M1a	IVA	IVA	IVA	IVA
M1b	IVA	IVA	IVA	IVA
M1c	IVB	IVB	IVB	IVB

Pulmonary assessment and Risk for thoracic resection

	Average risk	High risk	Prohibitive risk
ppoFEV1	> 40%	20-40%	<20%
ppoDLCO	>40%	20-40%	<20%
pO_2	>60	45-60	<45
pCO_2	<45	45-60	>60
VO_2 max	>15	10-15	<10

Management

NON SMALL CELL LUNG CANCER:

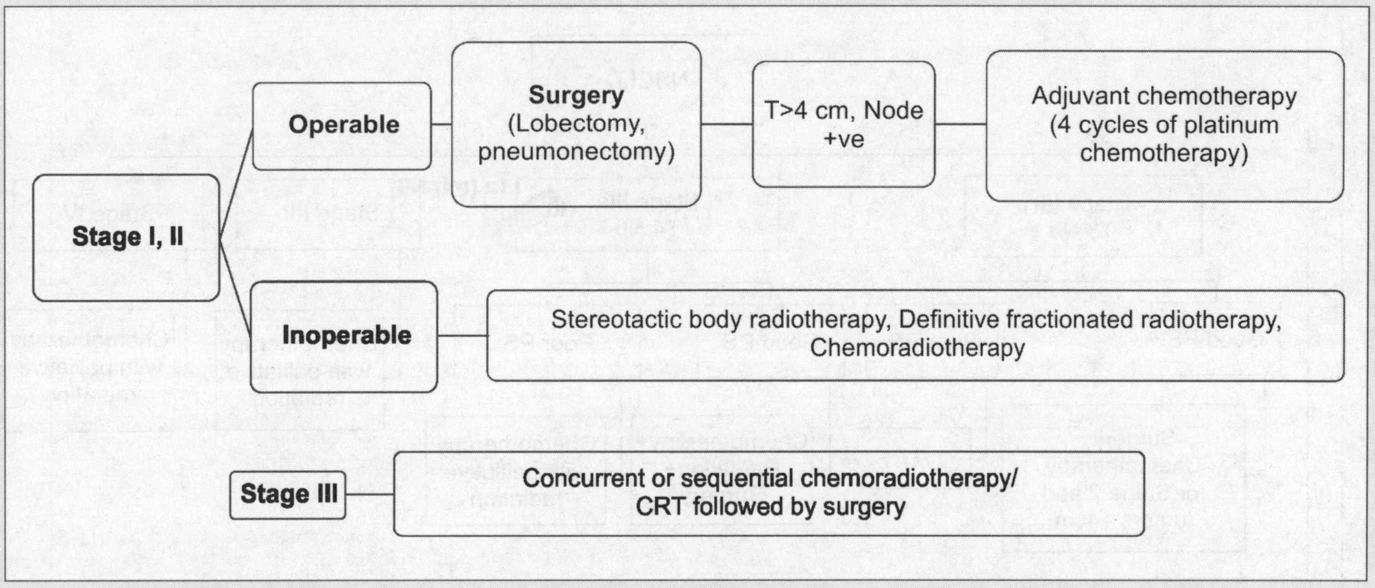

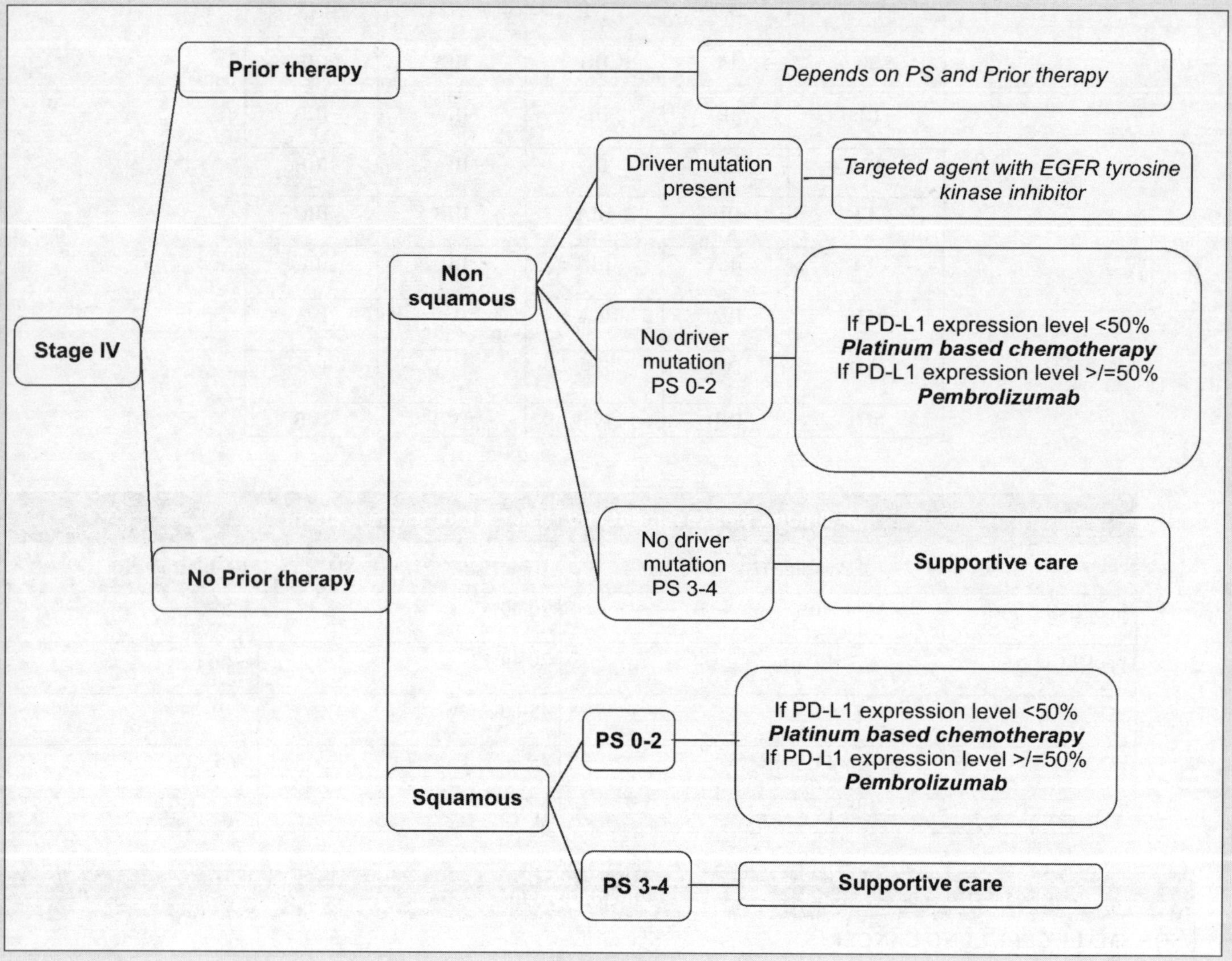
Prior therapy
Depends on PS and Prior therapy
Driver mutation present
Targeted agent with EGFR tyrosine kinase inhibitor
Non squamous
Stage IV
No driver mutation PS 0-2
If PD-L1 expression level <50%
Platinum based chemotherapy
If PD-L1 expression level >/=50%
Pembrolizumab
No driver mutation PS 3-4
Supportive care
No Prior therapy
PS 0-2
If PD-L1 expression level <50%
Platinum based chemotherapy
If PD-L1 expression level >/=50%
Pembrolizumab
Squamous
PS 3-4
Supportive care

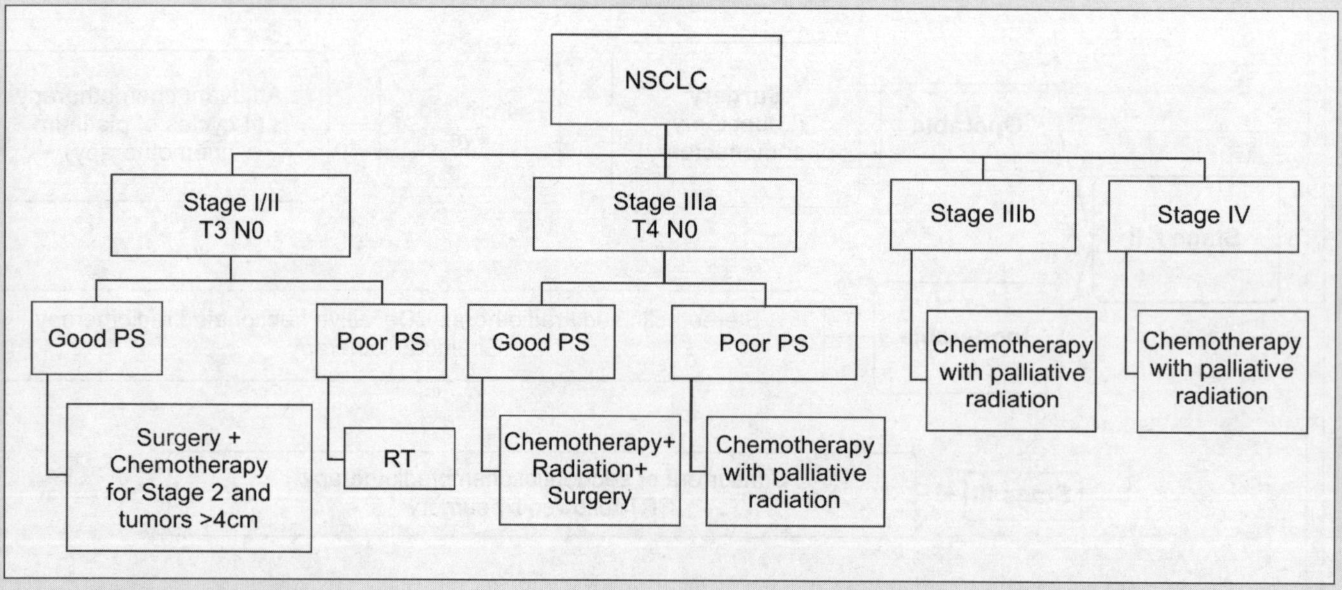
NSCLC
Stage I/II T3 N0
Stage IIIa T4 N0
Stage IIIb
Stage IV
Good PS
Poor PS
Good PS
Poor PS
Chemotherapy with palliative radiation
Chemotherapy with palliative radiation
Surgery + Chemotherapy for Stage 2 and tumors >4cm
RT
Chemotherapy+ Radiation+ Surgery
Chemotherapy with palliative radiation

50-70% present with advanced disease

- Physiologically fit patients with early-stage lesions (stage I or II) are treated with surgery
- Chest wall involvement without nodal spread (T3N0) is considered an early-stage lesion (stage IIb)–Can't tolerate surgery→***Definitive radiation combined with chemotherapy***
- Stage IIIa disease (N2 disease or chest wall with nodal involvement–***Induction chemotherapy***

Mediastinal node–Contraindication to surgery and Mandates Radiation for lung primary

SBRT–Early stage disease with comorbidities

Induction therapy is recommended for all patients with single mediastinal nodal station biopsy–proven stage IIIa disease who are believed to be resection candidates

Unresectable NSCLC

- Distant metastasis (Mets to opposite lung also)
- Persistent pleural effusion with malignant cells
- SVC obstruction

Involvement of following structures:

- Supraclavicular/Neck lymph nodes histologically proven
- Contralateral mediastinal lymph node histologically proven
- Tracheal wall
- RLN
- Mainstem Bronchus <2 cm from carina (Resectable by sleeve technique)

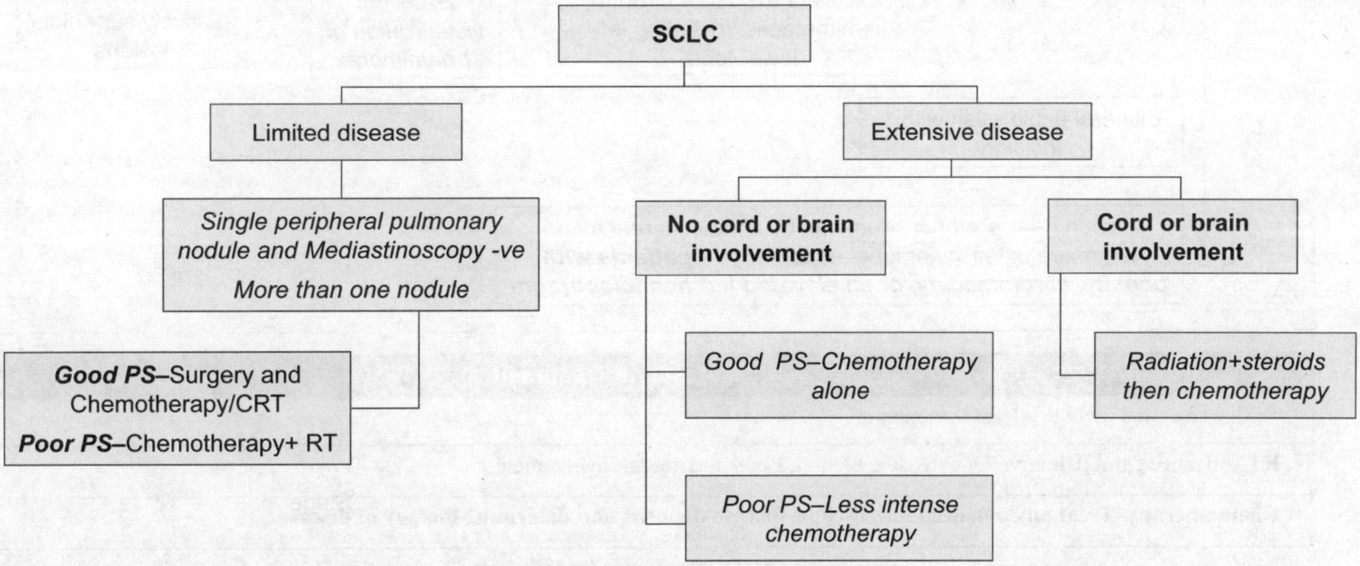

- **Limited disease**–Disease confined to one hemithorax, Ipsilateral or contralateral hilar or mediastinal nodes and Ipsilateral supraclavicular nodes
- **Extended disease**–Spread to contralateral supraclavicular nodes or distant sites like contralateral lung, liver, brain or bone marrow
- **STAGING** of SCLC–Whole body PET–CT and MRI Brain
- SCLC is very sensitive to chemotherapy and more than two-thirds of patients achieve partial response after systemic therapy with multidrug regimens
- ***Thoracic radiation therapy has been shown to improve local control of primary tumor and is often included as part of the treatment for limited SCLC***

- Prophylactic cranial irradiation is given even in absence of brain metastasis–***80% of SCLC patients present with brain metastasis during disease course***

Solitary peripheral pulmonary nodules with no evidence of metastatic disease after evaluation with CT abdomen and chest, MRI brain, PET-CT and mediastinoscopy can be treated with lobectomy postop chemotherapy and prophylactic brain irradiation

METASTASIS TO LUNG

- **Parameters of prognostic significance include:**
  - Resectability
  - Disease free interval
  - Number of metastasis
- **Favourable histology for long term survival**–Sarcoma, Breast, Colon and Genitourinary
- **Unfavourable histology for long term survival**–Melanoma, Stomach, Esophagus and Pancreas

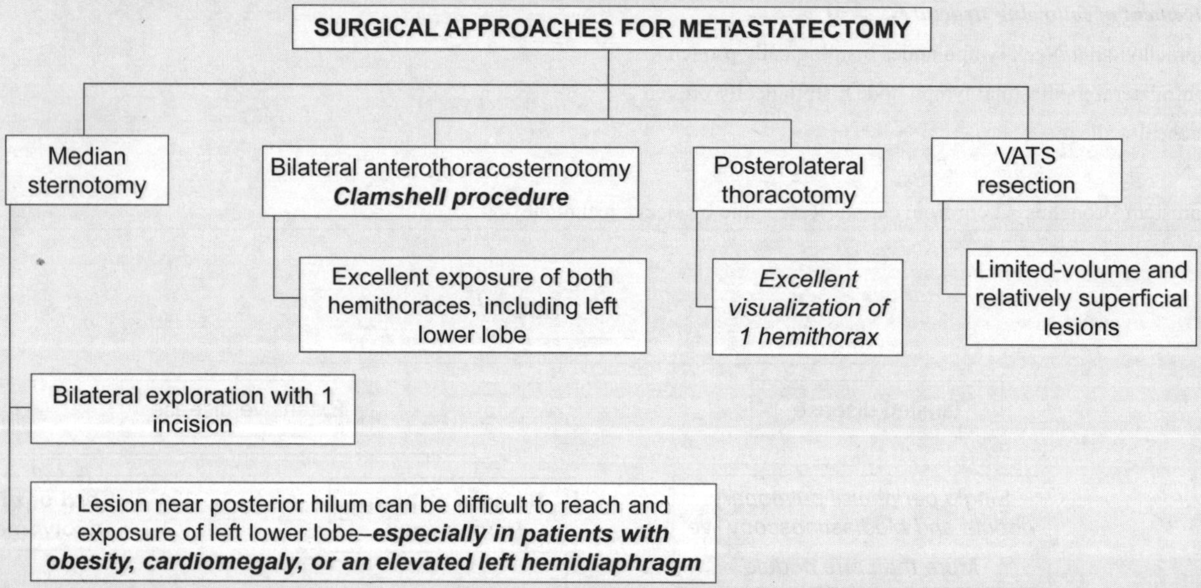

Metastasis Treatment
• Wedge resection include atleast 1cm margin
• **RT**–Advanced and Palliative for extensive Pleural, Bony and neural involvement
• **Chemotherapy–Treat any potential microscopic disease deposits and determine biology of disease**
CT Surveillance for follow up

Gene	Drug
ALK	Crizotinib
EGFR	EGFR TKIs; erlotinib, gefitinib afatinib
	EGFR monoclonal antibodies; cetuximab, matuzumab, necitumumab, panitumumab
MEK	AZD6244
MET	Tivantinib, cabozantinib, foretinib, crizotinib, MetMAb
mTOR	Everolimus
RAF	Sorafenib

TRAILS

- **TRIBUTE TRAIL**–Carboplatin and paclitaxel with erlotinib
- **FLEX TRAIL**–Cisplatin, vinorelbine and cetuximab in advanced EGFR mutation +ve NSCLC
- **LUX-LUNG 1 TRAIL**–Patients with lung adenocarcinoma treated with platinum based regimen and followed by 12 weeks
- **LUX-LUNG 3 TRAIL**–Afatinib efficacy compared with pemtrexed/cisplatin in EGFR mutation +ve stage 3/4 lung adenocarcinoma
- **BATTLE TRAIL**–Sorafenib active against tumors mutated/wild type K-RAS

EML4-ALK FUSION

- Younger patients, never smokers/former smokers
- **Associated with adenocarcinoma**
- **CRIZOTINIB–competitive inhibitor targeted to ATP binding pocket of ALK-TK**

EGFR THERAPY

- **ONCOGENE ADDICTION HYPOTHESIS:** EGFR mutation lung cancers develop in setting in which mutated receptor is constantly transducing high level of antiapoptotic signals, cancer cells are addicted to EGFR Kinase prosurvival signaling. Sudden interruption of TKI's leads to massive cell death
- **ONCOGENE SHOCK HYPOTHESIS:** Pro-apoptotic cells signals are still present in EGFR Mutant lung cancer cells. On TKI therapy antiapoptotic substances decay faster than pro-apoptotic resulting in cell death

RESISTANCE

All patients responding to TKI therapy develop resistance and suffer relapse due to

- **50% are due to secondary mutations-threonine to methionine at T790M**
- **MET overexpression/gene amplification**

JACKMAN'S CRITERIA

- Clinical exposure to TKI
- Benefit from TKI
- Evidence of disease progression by RECIST Criteria
- Lack of exposure to other drugs

Surgical Aspects of Lung Cancer	
Pneumonectomy	Removal of the whole lung Higher mortality (4% to 10%) and morbidity than anatomical lobectomy
Lobectomy	***Perioperative mortality rate 2%*** Complete tumor removal along with the resection of intralobar lymph nodes and lymphatic pathway
Segmentectomies and nonanatomical wedge resections	Predominantly in higher-risk patients with limited pulmonary reserve and tumors <2 cm, who may not tolerate lobectomy
Minimally invasive thoracic surgery	Early stage tumors
Thoracotomy	More advanced disease or complex resections
Workhorse for Lung cancer surgery–Lobectomy	

Mediastinal Lymph Node Dissection

Complete mediastinal lymph node dissection improves accuracy of lung cancer staging, improves indications for subsequent adjuvant therapy and may decrease locoregional recurrence

CHEMOTHERAPY
High PD L1 expression is associated with diminished overall survival and poor tumor differentiation
High PD L1 expression is associated with good response to immunotherapy and suggests
PD L1 as a predictive biomarker
Pembrolizumab is first line approved drug for metastatic lung carcinoma expressing >50%

PROGNOSTIC FACTORS
Bcl2–***Favourable prognostic factor***
TTF1, COX2, EGFR Overexpression, ras, Ki67, HER2, VEGF, Microvascular density, p53, Aneuploidy–***Adverse prognostic factor***

CHAPTER 41 MISCELLANEOUS

I. MESOTHELIOMA

- Mesothelioma develops from the mesothelial cells that line the pleural cavity–localized or diffuse
- Histologic subtypes include epithelial, sarcomatoid, or mixed histology
- ***Epithelial histology has a more favorable prognosis***

Localized

- Solitary fibrous tumor of the pleura, benign mesothelioma.
- Usually well-defined, encapsulated tumor, **not associated with asbestos exposure**
- Typically Presentation–Asymptomatic mass on a chest radiograph
- **Complete surgical resection is the treatment of choice**

Diffuse

- Diffuse malignant pleural mesothelioma–locally aggressive tumor, **associated with asbestos exposure**
- Diagnostic imaging includes CXR, CT and FDG-PET scan to determine the extent of invasion and to evaluate occult metastases, including mediastinal metastases
- Echocardiography is also performed to determine cardiac involvement
- Diagnosis is made with pleural biopsy (thoracentesis or pleural biopsy alone or incisional biopsies via thoracoscopy or open techniques)
- Survival for this disease is poor, ranging from 4 to 12 month
- Treatment–Chemotherapy, Standard and conformal RT and extrapleural pneumonectomy
- Extrapleural pneumonectomy and total pleurectomy are two commonly used surgical procedures

II. MEDIASTINAL TUMORS

A. Neuroendocrine Tumors

- Arise from cells of Kulchitsky located in the thymus
- Occur in men, 40-50 years, Aggressive
- **Most common site is Anterosuperior mediastinum**
- 20% have metastatic spread to mediastinal and cervical lymph nodes, liver, bone, skin and lungs
- More than 50% of thymic neuroendocrine
- Usually Hormonally active-often associated with **Cushing syndrome (ACTH)**
- Less frequently associated with MEN and only rarely associated with carcinoid syndrome (0.6%)

Treatment

- Complete excision
- Irradiation should be used particularly in patients with capsular invasion

B. Thyroid Tumors

- Tumors arise from **heterotopic thyroid tissue**
- Only 1% of all mediastinal masses
- **Occurs most commonly in anterosuperior mediastinum**
- Substernal extension of a cervical goiter is common, totally intrathoracic thyroid tumors are rare
- True intrathoracic thyroid gland derives its blood supply from thoracic vessels
- **Substernal extensions can usually be excised–cervical approach**

C. Parathyroid Tumors

- Occur in the mediastinum in 10% of patient
- **Most often adenomas are found in the anterosuperior mediastinum (80%)** embedded in or near the superior pole of the thymus
- Mediastinal adenoma–excised after a negative exploration of cervical region
- Usually accessible through the **cervical incision**
- **If residual parathyroid in mediastinum→ Mediastinal exploration using a median sternotomy or thoracoscopy is indicated**
- Parathyroid carcinomas are **usually hormonally active,** higher serum calcium levels and manifest more severe symptoms of hyperparathyroidism, **resection is the optimal therapy**

D. Lymphoma

- Mediastinum is frequently involved in lymphoma during the course of disease
- Infrequently the sole site of disease at the time of presentation
- Patients usually have symptoms–chest pain, cough, dyspnea, hoarseness and superior vena cava syndrome are the most common clinical manifestations
- **Symptoms characteristic of Hodgkin lymphoma include chest pain after consumption of alcohol and Pel-Ebstein fever**

Treatment

CHEMOTHERAPY→R-CHOP

- Surgical excision of all disease is rarely possible
- Needle biopsy doesn't provide significant diagnostic material, particularly nodular sclerosing lesions
- Thoracoscopy, mediastinoscopy, or mediastinotomy and rarely thoracotomy/median sternotomy may be necessary to obtain sufficient tissue
- **Staging laparotomy**–Only current indication is for patients with clinically limited disease who opt for limited treatment
- **Lymphoblastic lymphoma represent 60% of cases of mediastinal NHL**
- CT cannot differentiate fibrosis or necrosis from residual tumor
- **FDG-PET:** Noninvasive way to detect active mediastinal disease and predict relapse in **lymphoma, but tissue confirmation is required**
- Transthoracic incisional biopsy under general anesthesia is often needed given the significant fibrosis that remains after therapy

E. Paraganglioma

- *Usually <1% of all mediastinal tumors and less than 2% of all pheochromocytomas*
- Most are found in ***paravertebral sulcus***
- Multiple paragangliomas occur in 10% of patients
- More common in patients with MEN, family history of disease and Carney syndrome
- In patients who had excision of an adrenal pheochromocytoma and continue to have symptoms, a search for extra-adrenal lesion is undertaken
- **Tumor localization**→CT and iodine–^{131} MIBG particularly when the tumors are hormonally active

Treatment

- **Surgical resection is treatment of choice**
- In patients with tumors involving the middle mediastinum, cardiopulmonary bypass done to enable resection
- Preoperative embolization to reduce perioperative bleeding
- Although half of tumors are malignant

- ***Most common mediastinal tumor is neurogenic tumors (Overall)***
- ***Most common anterior mediastinal tumor is thymoma***
- ***Most common middle mediastinal tumor is lymphoma***
- ***Most common middle mediastinal mass is bronchogenic cysts***
- ***Most common posterior mediastinal tumor is neurogenic tumors***
- ***Most common site of tumor in mediastinum is anterosuperior region***
- ***Most common mediastinal mass in children is Neurogenic tumor***

PART ONE: MUSCULOSKELETAL ONCOLOGY

CHAPTER

42 BONE TUMORS

One Liners

- Most common bone tumor–**Metastasis**
- Most common primary tumor in adult–**Chondrosarcoma (Young)**
- Most common primary tumor in Old age–Osteosarcoma (Sabiston)
- Multiple myeloma (Other books)
- Most common tumor to metastasize to bone–Breast
- Most common site of bone metastasis–Spine
- **High risk for Osteosarcoma**–Maffucci syndrome, Olliers disease and Familial Retinoblastoma
- Osteosarcomas account for approximately 60% of malignant bone tumors in the first two decades of life
- Acral/Intracortical metastasis occur mainly from **Carcinoma Lung**
- ***Most common bone tumor of hand–Enchondroma***
- Bone metastasis of Unknown origin–Ca Lung and RCC
- **Transcortical biopsy**–Intraosseous Diaphyseal tumors
- **Metastasis in Diaphysis**–*Intramedullary Nail*
- **Mirel score >/= 8 High risk**→ *Prophylactic fixation*
- **Mirel score <7**→ *RT and Medical treatment*
- **Mirel score indicates risk of Pathological fracture**
- Most prominent cytokine for osteoclastogenesis–RANKL

OVER REVIEW

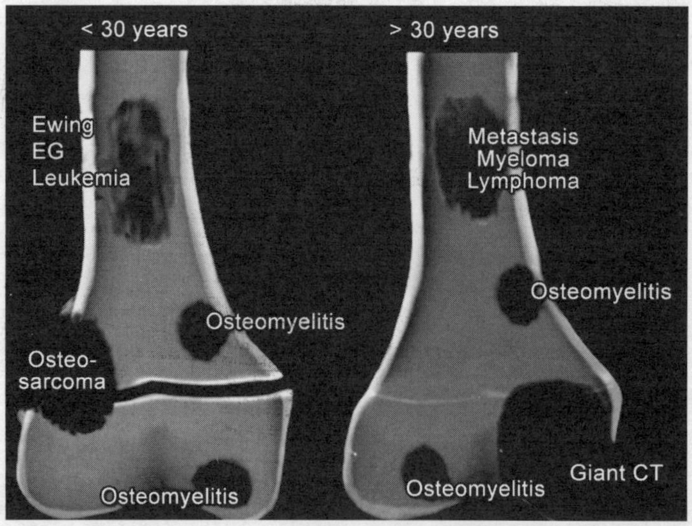

Epiphysis
• Chondroblastoma • Giant Cell Tumor • Clear Cell Chondrosarcoma
Diaphysis
• Ewing's Sarcoma (5-25 Years) • Fibrous Dysplasia (5-30 Years) • Adamantinoma • Histiocytosis (5-30 Years) • Lymphoma (Adult)
Metaphysis
• Osteochondroma • Chondrosarcoma • Osteosarcoma • Fibrosarcoma • Secondaries

GENETICS

Tumor	Cytogenetic Abnormality	Gene Product
Aneurysmal bone cyst	t(16;17)(q22;p13) t(1;17)(p34.3;p13) t(3;17)(q21;p13) t(9;17)(q22;p13) t(17;17)(q21;p13)	*CDH11-USP6* *THRAP3-USP6* *CNBP-USP6* *OMD-USP6* *COL1A1-USP6*
Chondrosarcoma or chondroma		*IDH1 or IDH2* *Point mutation*
Ewing's sarcoma/PNET family	t(11;22)(q24;q12) t(21;22)(q22;q12) t(7;22)(p22;q12) t(2;22)(q33; q12) t(17;22)(q12;q12) inv(22)(q12;q12) t(16;21)(p11;q22)	*EWS1-FLI1* *ESW1-ERG* *ESWR1-ETV1* *EWSR1-FEV* *EWSR1-E1AF* *EWSR1-ZSG* *FUS-ERG*
Fibrous dysplasia	Activating oncogenic mutations	*GNAS1*
Mesenchymal chondrosarcoma	t(8;8)(q13;q21)	*HEY1-NCOA2*
Osteosarcoma, low-grade (parosteal and intramedullary)	12q 14-15 (ring chromosomes, giant marker chromosomes)	Amplification of *CDK4, MDM2, HMGA2, GLI and SAS*
Osteosarcoma		Multiple genetic aberrations

OSTEOBLASTOMA
• More than 2 cm • Aggressive • Low risk of malignancy • SPINE

CHONDROBLASTOMA
• Epiphysis • Children • Knee

- Osteoid osteoma: ***Proximal femur***

CT guided thermocoagulation is used for Osteoid osteoma–Majority resolve spontaneously

GIANT CELL TUMOR

- 20-45 years after physis closed
- Epiphysis of long bones
- Knee
- 1-2% of lung metastasis
- Radical curettage
- **DENOSUMAB**–RANKL mediated

FIBROUS DYSPLASIA

- Shepherd Crook deformity
- Ground glass appearance

Simple Bone Cyst	Aneurysmal Bone Cyst
• Proximal long bones • Fallen fragment sign • Conservative–Steroids and Curettage	• More aggressive • Fluid levels

Enneking Staging	
Benign	**Malignant**
• Latent–Osteochondroma • Active–Osteoid osteoma • Aggressive–GCT	• **Low grade:** Intracompartmental–IA, Extracompartmental–IB • **High grade:** Intracompartmental–IIA, Extracompartmental–IIB • **Any grade:** Metastasis→ III
Majority of malignant tumors are 2B	

- ***Solitary Osteochondroma:*** 1% Malignant
- ***Multiple Osteochondroma:*** 10-30% Malignant
- ***Maffucci syndrome:*** Enchondroma+Angioma (Inevitable–100%)
- ***Ollier's disease:*** 20% malignant risk

Conditions associated with an increased risk of malignant disease in bone and cartilage		
High risk	**Moderate risk**	**Low risk**
Maffucci syndrome (enchondromatosis and angiomas of soft tissue)	Hereditary multiple exostoses	Chronic osteomyelitis
Ollier disease (enchondromatosis)	Polyostotic Paget's disease	Osteonecrosis
Familial retinoblastoma syndrome	Radiation osteitis	Fibrous dysplasia, osteogenesis imperfeta, osteoblastoma and chondroblastoma

Tumor and site		
Diaphyseal	**Metaphyseal**	**Epiphyseal**
Eosinophilic granuloma	Most	Chondroblastoma
Osteoid osteoma		Intra-articular osteoid osteoma
Fibrous dysplasia		Giant cell tumor (physis closed)
Adamantinoma		Clear cell chondrosarcoma
Ewing's sarcoma		

Common diaphyseal bone tumors according to age	
Age and most common diaphyseal tumor	
<10 years	Eosinophilic granuloma
Teenage	Ewing's sarcoma
Adult	Lymphoma
>60 years	Metastasis/myeloma

Classification of surgical resection margins	
Surgical margins	
Inralesional	Resection through the tumor
Marginal	Resection through the reactive zone of the tumor
Wide	Resection outside the reactive zone of the tumor
Radical	Resection of the whole anatomical compartment

1. Osteoid Osteoma

- It is the most common true benign tumor of the bone
- Pathologically, it consists of a *nidus of tangled arrays of partially mineralised osteoid* trabeculae surrounded by dense sclerotic bone
- **Tibia most common bone involved**
- Located in the diaphysis of long bones
- Posterior elements of the vertebrae are a common site
- Presenting complaint is a nagging pain, worst at night, and is relieved by salicylates
- **Diagnosis:** Generally confirmed on X-ray
- The tumor is visible as a zone of sclerosis surrounding a radiolucent nidus, usually less than 1 cm in size
- In some cases, the nidus may not be seen on a plain X-ray because of extensive surrounding sclerosis, and may be detected on a CT scan

Treatment

- Complete excision of the nidus along with the sclerotic bone is done
- Prognosis is good
- It is not a pre-malignant condition

2. Osteochondroma (Cartilage-Capped Exostosis)

- Site–Occurs in metaphysic of long bones. Originates in growth plate
- *Most common site is distal femur followed by proximal tibia and proximal humerus*
- Clinical features–Asymptomatic, firm non tender swelling fixed to the bone around the joint–Most common clinical finding
- Pressure symptoms include bursitis, pressure neuritis, etc
- *X-rays-**pathognomonic**→well-defined exostosis from metaphysic with base coextensive with the present bone*

Complications

- **Bursitis** (Most common)
- **Others:** Pressure neuropathy, and false aneurysm, Fracture of bony stalk due to trauma. Malignant change (Secondary chondrosarcoma)

Treatment

- Not required until symptomatic. Sometimes resolve it
- En block resection preferred, i.e., extraperiosteal resection/with entire cartilaginous cap
- Recurrence rare, caused by failure to remove the cap

3. Chondroma [Enchondroma] (Chondromyxoma)

- Centrally located, also known as cartilaginous hematomas
- Juxtacortical or subperiosteal chondroma–eccentric located
- Site—metaphysis, small tubular bones of hands and feet are most commonly involved, phalanges
- Clinical feature: After pathological fracture and in the absence of fracture pain and swelling
- X-ray-centrally located cystic lesion (loculated or nonloculated). Fibrous septa may be seen interspersing the central cavity. Cortex thinned and expanded
- Stippling or calcification may be present. No reactive bone formation
- Treatment–Curettage and bone grafts. Radical resection for tumor of long bones and pelvis

Multiple enchondromatosis **(Ollier diseases):** caused by failure of normal endochondral ossification, nonfamilial

- Location—epiphysis
- Maffucci syndrome. Enchondromas + cavernous hemangioma + soft-tissue phleboliths
- Malignant change—up to 50%
- Benign (occasionally aggressive) types of bone tumors

4. Giant Cell Tumor

- Benign tumor with malignant potential changes
- Site–epiphysis in skeletally mature and metaphysic in skeletally immature
- Pathology–ragged friable bleeding tissue fitted with various-sized cysts and cavities without periosteal reactions
- Clinical features–Main presentation is swelling with stretched skin without dilated veins and local temperature not raised
- Egg shell crackling is characteristic clinical finding
- X-ray–an eccentric radiolucent area in epiphysis. Soap bubble appearance
- Treatment of choice–en block resection with BG/allograft or prosthesis (2 cm of normal tissue is excised along with the tumor) giant cell variants

5. Chondroblastoma (Codman's Tumor)

- Site-epiphysis
- Most common feature progressive pain
- X-ray–characteristic–rounded, well–demarcated radiolucent area in the epiphysis with eccentric location
- **MOTTLED AREAS OF CALCIFICATION is seen on X-ray**
- Pathology–cancellers bone is destroyed and multiple Calcium deposits are usually found
- Treatment–curettage with Bone grafting

6. Osteoblastoma (Giant Osteoid Osteoma)

- Most common site is spine
- Most common symptom is pain
- Treatment–excision with Bone grafting

7. Nonossifying Fibroma

- X-rays–eccentrically located, multiloculated app, or ridges in bony wall, sclerotic scalloped borders, erosion of cortex, etc.
- T/T–resolve spontaneously

8. Ossifying Fibroma of Long Bones

- Campanacci disease
- Osteofibrous dysplasia

9. Hemangioma of Bone

- Most common vascular bone tumor
- Most common Site is spine, often between T_4 and L_4
- Most common site of Vertebral compression is T_4
- X-ray–characteristic corduroy appearance (coarse vertical trabeculation due to loss of horizontal striations)
- Treatment of choice is radiotherapy

10. Osteosarcoma

- Most common primary malignant tumor of young age
- Pathology–arise from multifocal mesenchymal tissue
- Characteristic is Leg of mutton appearance
- Main symptom pain
- X-ray–pain roentgenograms are the most valuable tools for making the correct diagnosis

Frequently Asked Points

- *Sun burst/sun ray appearance is seen in subperiosteal area. It is due to bone deposition along the vessels*
- *Codman's triangle—reactive bone formation parallel to the bone and triangle in shape*
- *CT scan—best to detect chest metastasis*
- *MRI—best to detect extent*
- *Biopsy—for definitive diagnosis*

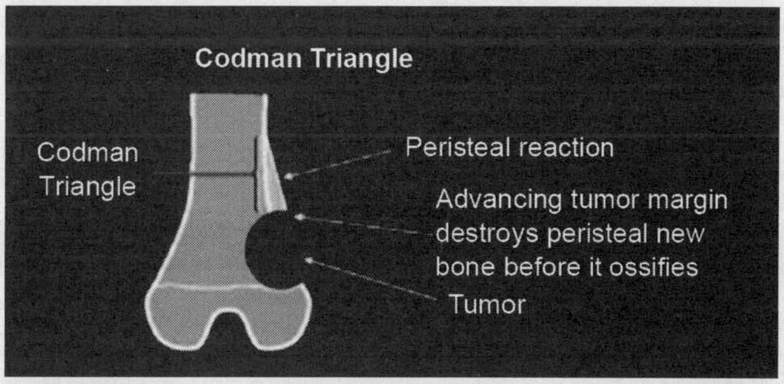

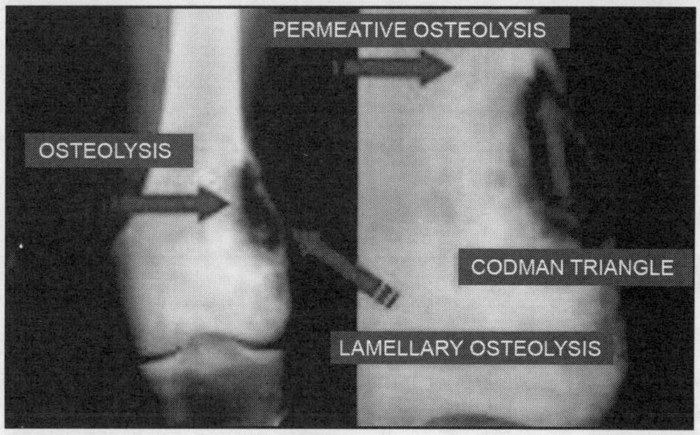

- **SECONDARY OSTEOSARCOMA:** Paget's disease, Osteochondroma, Enchondroma, Fibrous dysplasia, Post irradiation, Bone infarcts, Chronic osteomyelitis, Melorheostosis and Osteogenesis imperfecta

- **SPREAD:** *Lungs are the Most common site of metastasis (80%)*

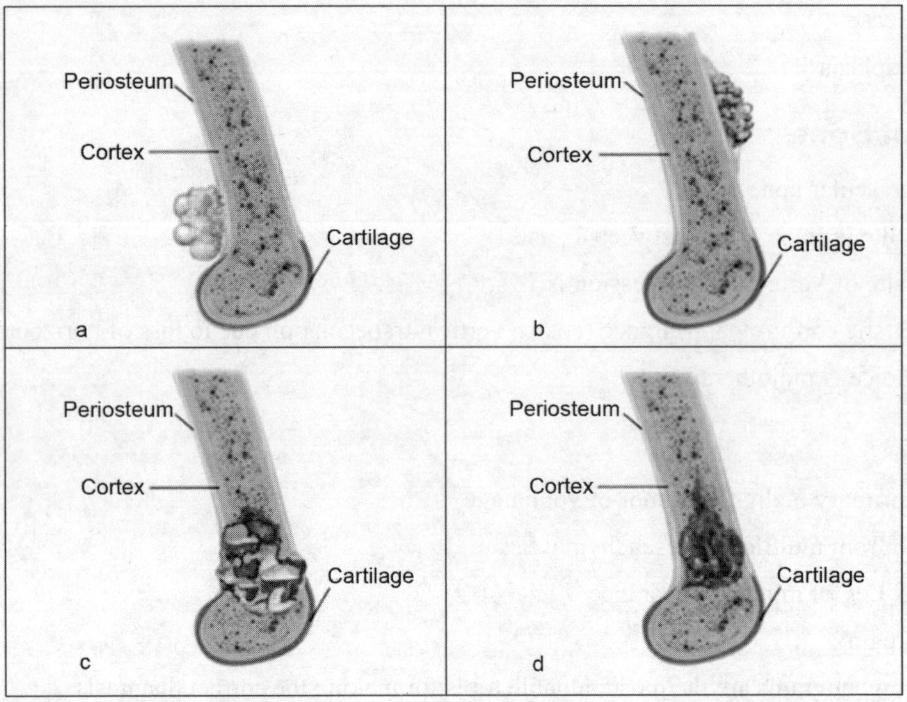

(a) Parosteal osteosarcoma arises from the surface of bone (usually the posterior femur)

(b) Periosteal osteosarcoma arises from the surface with mineralization and a sunburst pattern

(c) Telangiectatic osteosarcoma arises from the metaphysis as a lytic mass

(d) High-grade intramedullary osteosarcoma is the most common primary sarcoma of bone

- Treatment–early and radical ablation is procedure of choice. Generally combined approach is used: first put on chemotherapy and then irradiation, and next is radical ablation
- Pulmonary metastasis–small lesion–chemotherapy
- Large lesion–wide resection or lobotomy after chemotherapy
- Chemotherapy used–adriamycin + blomycin + cyclophosphamide + MTX (methotrexate)

Prognosis of lesion
• Prognosis–Most important factor is extent of disease at the time of diagnosis
• Grade–High grade has bad prognosis
• Size–Larger size with worse prognosis
• Location–Proximal tumor does worse
• Paget's OS–Poor
• Radiation induced–Poor

11. Solitary Lesions of Bone

Features	Giant cell tumor	Simple bone cyst	Aneurysmal bone cyst	Fibrous dysplasia
Age	20-40 years	< 20 years	10-40 years	20-30 years
Common bones	Lower femur, Upper tibia Lower radius	Upper humerus Upper femur	Tibia Humerus	Neck of the femur Tibia

Contd.

Contd.

Location	Epiphysis	Metaphysis	Metaphysis	Metaphysis
X-ray	Soap-bubble appearance, eccentrically placed	Maximum width less than width of the growth plate	Distending lesion, 'ballooning' the bone	Multi-loculated Ground-glass appearance Trabeculations++
Treatment preferred	Excision	Curettage and bone graft	Curettage and bone graft	Curettage and bone graft

	Aneurysmal bone cyst	Unicameral bone cyst
Presentation	Pain, swelling	Pathologic fracture
Location	Distal femur, proximal tibia, pelvis, posterior elements of spine	Proximal humerus, proximal femur
Imaging	Metaphyseal lytic lesion, wider than physis MRI: Fluid-fluid levels	Metaphyseal, lytic lesion, less than width of physis Filling leaf sign
Treatment	Curettage, bone graft	Methylprednisolone Curettage/bone graft (proximal femur)

12. Chondrosarcoma

- Arises from cartilage cells
- Most common site is ilium (pelvis)

Classification

- Primary Chondrosarcoma arises in any that develops in cartilage
- Secondary Chondrosarcoma arise at the site of preexisting benign cartilage lesion

X-rays-Central CS, central radiolucent area with calcification

- Calcification is punctate, popcorn or comma-shaped, cottonwool or bread crumb
- Biopsy–for definitive diagnosis
- Treatment–Primary treatment is wide or radical, resection or amputation

13. Ewing's Sarcoma

- Most common primary malignant tumor in age <10 years
- Most common location is physis of long bone with extension into tibia (Most common site), femur and flat bones
- Pathology–arise from endothelial cells of bone marrow
- Course–exacerbation and remission common
- Most common site of metastasis-lung and lymphatic spread present
- X-ray–characteristic–**onion peel app.**–due to periosteal new bone formation in layers
- **Moth eaten app. or cracked ice app.**–diaphysial lesion with irregular destruction
- *Laboratory investigations–Hb decreased: ESR increased: CRP increased: urine for (VMA) vanilmandelic acid, tissue for glycogens stain PAS+ve*
- Most radiosensitive bone tumor is Ewing's sarcoma
- Best treatment or treatment of choice for Ewing's is radiotherapy

Highlights

Unfavorable Prognostic Features

- Male gender
- Humerus involved
- Pelvis involved
- Distant metastasis (worst prognostic factor)
- Increased age of presentation
- Disease relapse

14. Multiple Myeloma (Plasmacytoma)

- Characterized by the presence of cell resembling plasma cells which replace bone
- Pathology-chiefly within the medullary cavity with eaten-up cortex
- Most common complaint is bone pain

X-Ray Features:

- Multiple punched-out lesions in skull and pelvis
- Wedge collapse of Vertebrae commonly in thoracic spine
- Diffuse osteoporosis
- Diffuse rarefaction of bone when involve vertebrae and pedicles are more commonly involved called pedicle sign (common in secondaries)
- Urine analysis–Bence Jones protein-excretion of light chain in 30% cases
- Serum protein electrophoresis–abnormal spikes in regions of gamma globulins (myeloma spikes): 90% S. globulins increased with A/G ratio reversed with total proteins normal or increased
- Protein electrophoresis: **Monoclonal band**
- Bone biopsy is definitive, diagnostic test

Treatment:

General	Specific
• Anemia: correction • Infection: antibiotics • Renal impairment: hemodialysis • Hypocalcaemia: bisphosphonates	• Chemotherapy is main stay of treatment • Cyclophosphamide (DOC), melphalan, steroids and urethane

15. Chordoma

- Site–5% sacrococcygeal area, 30% at the base of skull
- Sacrococcygeal: Low backache–MOST COMMON SYMPTOM
- Cervical tumor: Headache is most common
- X-ray–A well-circumscribed radiolucent expansile defect in lower sacrum
- **TREATMENT:** Surgical resection with wide margin
- Prognosis–favorable: Male gender, younger age and distal location

16. Adamantinoma (Ameloblastoma)

- Most common Site is Mandible
- Tibia–Most common in appendicle skeleton (85%)
- X-ray–Most common appearance is multiple sharply demarcated radiolucent lesions separated by dense, sclerotic bone (HONEYCOMB APPEARANCE)

The Mirels scoring system for risk of pathological fracture

	Score		
	1	2	3
Site	Upper limb	Lower limb	Peritrochanteric
Pain	Mild	Moderate	Functional
Size	<1/3	1/3-2/3	>2/3
Lesion	Blastic	Mixed	Lytic
Score ≥ 8, high risk of fracture – urgent prophylactic fixation should be considered: Score <8, low risk of fracture – orthopaedic intervention may not be required			

Mirels Scoring System

Score	Site of Lesion	Size of Lesion	Lesion type	Pain
1	Upper limb	> ⅓ cortex	Blastic	Mild
2	Lower limb	⅓–⅔ cortex	Mixed	Moderate
3	Trochanteric	> ⅔ cortex	Lytic	Functional

17. Metastatic Carcinoma

- Most common source–Breast
- Most common site of secondaries is Vertebrae
- Most common site of primary for suspected metastasis with unknown origin is Lung

- Osteolytic lesions more common than osteoblastic lesions

Osteoblastic	Breast prostate
Osteolytic	Kidney, thyroid
Mixed app.	Lung

- Most common route of spread is Hematogenous
- Bone scan is most sensitive to detect silent metastasis
- Treatment of choice is Radiotherapy Co-60 (3000 reds for 3-4 weeks)

CHEMOTHERAPY IN BONE TUMORS

Drug	Mechanism of Action	Toxicity	Tumor
Adriamycin/doxorubicin	Block DNA/RNA synthesis by inhibiting topoisomerase II	Cardiotoxicity	Osteogenic sarcoma

Contd.

Contd.

Cis-platinum	DNA cross-linking, interrupts covalent bonding	Nephrotoxicity, ototoxicity, neurotoxicity	Osteogenic sarcoma
Methotrexate	Inhibits dihydrofolate reductase	Ulcerative stomatitis, leucopenia, cystitis	Osteogenic sarcoma
Ifosfamide	DNA alkylating agent	Nephrotoxicity encephalopathy	Osteogenic sarcoma and Ewing's sarcoma
Vincristine	Vinca alkyloid, disrupts microtubule assembly	Peripheral neuropathy	Ewing's sarcoma
Etoposide	Topoisomerase II inhibitor	Bone marrow suppression	Ewing's sarcoma
Cyclophosphamide	DNA alkylating agent	Myelosuppression, hemorrhagic cystitis	Ewing's sarcoma
Actinomycin	Transcription inhibitor	Bone marrow suppression	Ewing's sarcoma

OSTEOSARCOMA

- ***Distal femur***–Most common site

Risk factors for osteosarcoma
Familial cancer
Secondary osteosarcoma
Li-Fraumeni syndrome
Irradiated bones
Bilateral retinoblastoma (independent of therapy modality)
Loss of tumor-suppressor genes p53 and Rb (retinoblastoma)

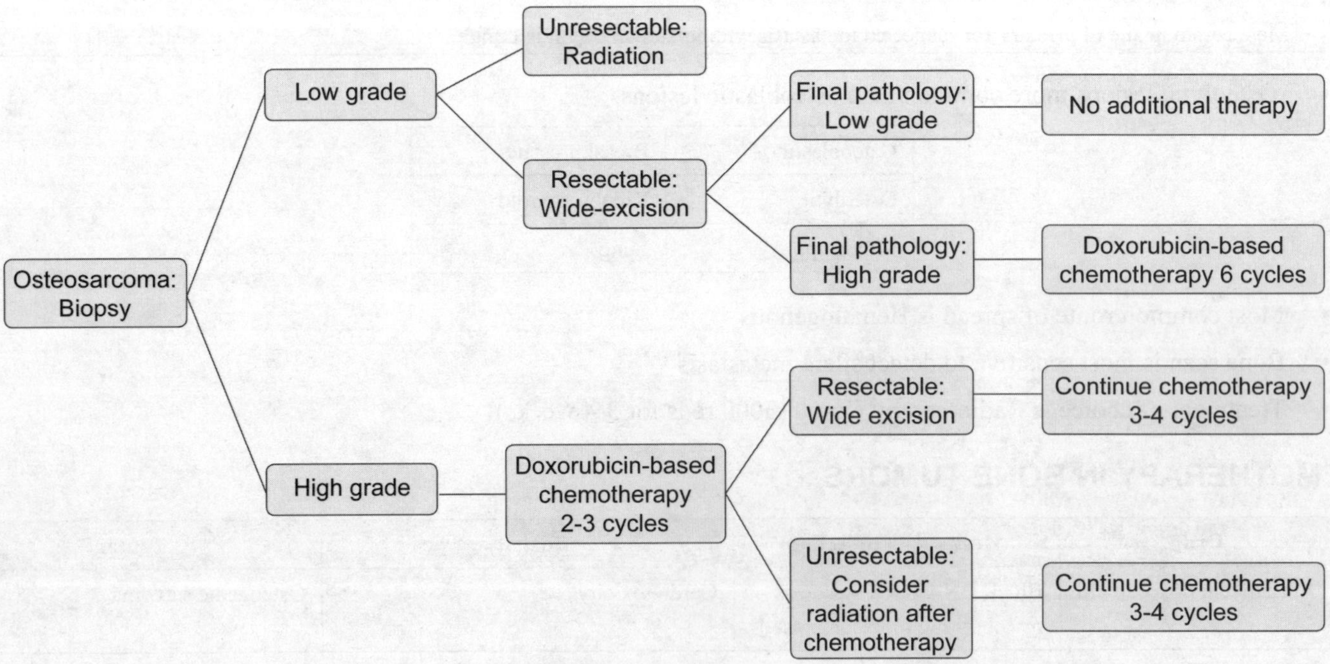

Localized and metastatic types: Preoperative chemotherapy

↓

Standards:

Preoperative chemotherapy: Association of drugs

Options:

- Mechotrexate HD + adriamycin
- Adriamycin + cisplatin
- Mechotrexate HD + cisplatin
- Ifosfamide + cisplatin

Recommendations:

- Inclusion in evaluated protocol
- Adults: FNCLCC, EORTC
- Children: SFOP, protocol comprising methotrexate HD

↓

Metastatic type on initial examination?

- No → Localized osteosarcoma types
  Local treatment
- Yes → Metastatic osteosarcomas
  Local treatment

For administration of methotrexate, the possibility of assaying methotrexate and the possibility of resuscitation with dialysis are required

Localized types: Local treatment for osteosarcoma

↓

Presurgical workup: Reexamination of lesions by same paraclinical examinations

↓

Contraindication to surgery?

- No → **Contraindication to conservative surgery?**
  - No / Yes → Recommendation:
    - Conservative surgery with large exesises and resection of tumor on bloc
    - Resection of biopsy scar
    - Reconstruction by prosthesis or graft if necessary

    → Postoperative chemotherapy
- Yes → Radiation therapy
  Recommendation:
  Photons + neutron therapy

  Recommendation:
  Amputation

  → Postoperative chemotherapy

Metastasized types: Local treatment

↓

Presurgial workup: Reexamination of lesions by same paraclinical examinations

↓

Standard surgery of primary tumor and metastases

Recommendations:

- Conservative surgery with large exercises and resection of tumor en bloc
- Resection of biopsy scar
- Amputation must remain the exception
- Surgery of metastases according to localization

↓

Postoperative chemotherapy

Metastatic types after surgery

↓

Good responder: Grades III and IV according to Huvos grading system of tumor and metastases?

Yes →

Standard:

Postoperative chemotherapy: Same protocol as in preoperative

No →

Standard:

- Postoperative chemotherapy:
- Other drugs effective in osteosarcoma

Options:

If methotrexate and adriamycin in preoperative:

- Ifosfamide + VP16 or
- Ifosfamide + cisplatin

Recommendation:

Protocol evaluated:

- Adults: FNCLCC, EORTC
- Children: SFOP
- Adults and children: Phase 2 trial

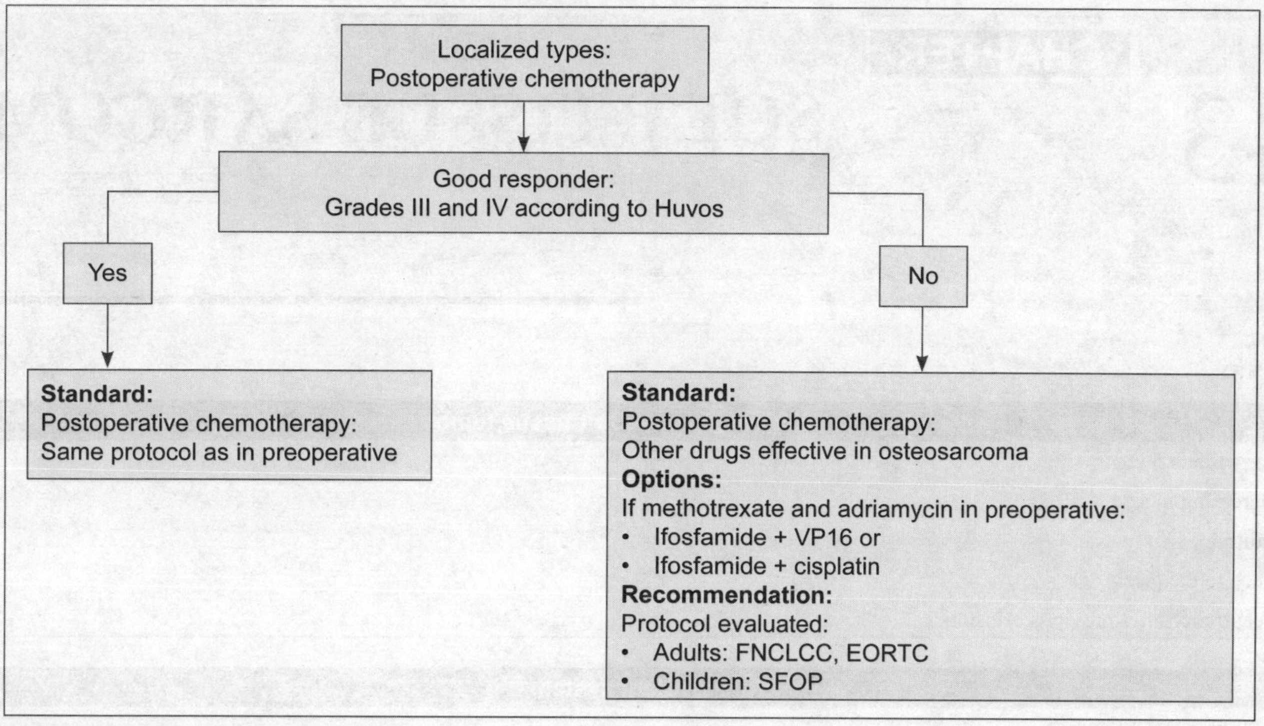

- Limb salvage–Preserved for recurrent tumors
- Most common osteosarcoma–Spontaneous (RB, Li fraumeni syndrome)

EWING'S SARCOMA

- Anemia and associated with raised ESR
- Diaphysis
- EWS-FHR/FLI1
- MIC2/CD99 +
- Moth eaten/Onion skin appearance

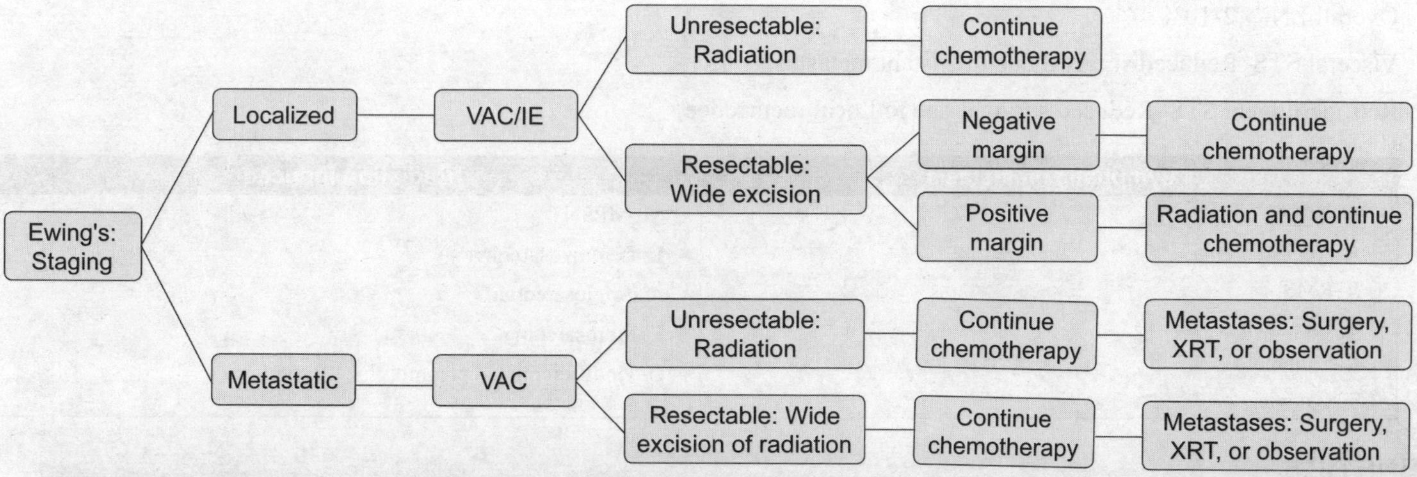

Clinical presentation of osteosarcoma and Ewing Family of Tumors (EFT)		
Tumor site	**Radiographic characteristics**	**Associated signs**
Osteosarcoma		
Metaphyseal bone	Periosteal elevation with new bone formation ("sunburst")	Soft-tissue swelling
EFT		
Diaphyseal/flat bones	Patchy bone destruction ("motheaten") Periosteal lamellation ("onion skin")	Soft-tissue swelling, pleural effusion

CHAPTER 43 SOFT TISSUE SARCOMA

Warning signs–Soft tissue tumor
• Larger than 5 cm • Increasing in size • Painful • Deep to the fascia • Recurrence after previous excision

Trojani system
• T–Tumor differentiation • N–Necrosis • M–Mitotic count

- MRI Spine–Useful for spinal metastasis
- Most useful imaging in determining diagnosis of primary bone tumor–X-ray
- CT Scan–Confirmation and Staging
- JAMSHIDI Neddle–Bone biopsy
- TRUCUT Needle–Soft tissue biopsy
- Overall LN→ 2-10%
- Visceral STS–Reduced survival due to Distant metastasis
- Retroperitoneal STS–Reduced survival due to Local recurrence

Lymphatic metastasis	Radiation induced
• **M**–MFH • **A**–Angiosarcoma • **R**–RMS • **C**–Clear cell • **E**–Epitheloid • **S**–Synovial	• **M**–MPSNT • **L**–Leiomyosarcoma • **A**–Angiosarcoma • **F**–Fibrosarcoma • **U**–Undifferentiated pleomorphic sarcoma

GENETICS

- **NF1**–17p11.2, Neurofibromin, Autosomal dominant, 10% risk of Malignant peripheral nerve sheath tumor (20-50 years), Schwannoma and Glioma
- **Li-Fraumeni syndrome**–P53 muatation, 17p13.1, Breast (Most common), RMS, Undifferentiated pleomorphic sarcoma, Brain tumors, Osteosarcoma and Hematologic cancers
- **FAP**–Sporadic, CTNNB1 mutation, 5q21-22, Desmoids (Intraabdominal)→20%

Cytogenetic abnormalities in sarcomas and the genes involved		
Sarcoma	**Translocation**	**Genes involved**
Ewing's tumors	11;22	*EWS-Fli1*
Liposarcoma (myxoid and round cell)	12;16	*TLS (FUS)-CHOP*
Synovial sarcoma	X;18	*SYT-SSX1 and 2*
Rhabdomyosarcoma (alveolar)	2;13	*PAX3-FKHR*
Clear cell sarcoma	12;22	*EWS-ATF1*

Genetic abnormalities shared by different tumor types	
ETC6-NTRK3/t (12;15)	Infantile fibrosarcoma Acute myeloid leukaemia Secretory carcinoma of the breast
ALK gene fusions	Inflammatory myofibroblastic tumor Large cell anaplastic lymphoma Lung carcinoma
FUS-ERG/t(16;21)	Ewing sarcoma Acute myeloid leukaemia
ASPL-TFE3/t (X;17)	Alveolar soft part sarcoma Subset of paediatric renal cell carcinoma
EWS-ATF1/t(12;22) and ESW-CREB1/t(2;22)	Clear cell sarcoma Angiomatoid fibrous histiocytoma

Tumor	Cytogenetic Abnormality	Gene Product
Alveolar rhabdomyosarcoma	t(2;13) (q35;q) 14) t(1;13)(p36; q14) t(x;2) (q 13;q35)	*PAX3-FOXO1A* *PAX7-FOXO1A* *PAX3-AFX*
Alveolar soft tissue sarcoma	t(X;17) (p11.2;q25)	*ASPL-TFE3*
Clear cell sarcoma	t(12;22) (q13;q12) t(2;22)(q32;q12)	*EWSR1-ATF1* *EWSR1-CREB1*
Congenital fibrosarcoma	t(12;15)(p13;q25)	*ETV6-NTRK3*
Dermatofibrosarcoma protuberans	t(17;22)(q22;q13)	*COL1A1-PDGFB*
Desmoplastic small round cell tumor Epithelioid hemangioendothelioma	t(11;22)(p13;q12) t(1;3) (p36;q25)	*EWSR1-WT1* *WWTR1-CAMTA1*
Endometrial stromal sarcoma	t(7;17)(p15;q11)	*JAZF1-SUZ12*
Gastrointestinal stromal tumor	Activating mutations Overexpression Loss of 14q LOH of 22q Loss of 1p	*KIT, PDGFR, BRAF* *ETV1*
Inflammatory myofibroblastic tumor	t(1;2)(q22-23;p23) t(2;19)(p23;p13.1)	*TPM3-ALK* *TPM4-ALK*
Low-grade fibromyxoid sarcoma	t(7;16)(q32-34;p11) t(11;16)(p11;p11)	*FUS-CREB3L2* *FUS-CREB3L1*
Lipoma	t(3;12)(q27-28, q14-15)	*HMGA2-LPP*
Malignant peripheral nerve sheath tumor	Inactivating	*Deletion of NF1*
Myxoid chondrosarcoma	t(9;22)(q22-31;q11-12) t(9;17)(q22;q11) t(9;15)(q22;q21)	*ESWR1-NR4A3* *TAF15-NR4A3* *TCF12-NR4A3*
Myxoid liposarcoma	t(12;16)(q13;p11) t(12;22)(q13;q12)	*FUS-DDIT3* *EWSR1-DDϕT3* *P1K3CA mutation*
Synovial sarcoma	t(X;18)(p11;q11)	*SS18-SSX1* *SS18-SSX2* *SS18-SSX4*
WDLPS/ALT and DDLPS	12q14-15 (supernumerary ring chromosomes; giant marker chromosomes)	*Amplification of MDM2, CDK4* *HMGA2, SAS, GLI and JUN*
Uterine leiomyosarcoma	t(12;14)(q7-)	

Mutations associated with soft tissue sarcoma				
Syndrome	**Inheritance Pattern**	**Locus**	**Gene**	**Associated Soft-Tissue Sarcomas**
Familial gastrointestinal stromal tumor syndrome	AD	4q12	*KIT*	Gastrointestinal stromal tumor
Familial infiltrative fibromatosis	AD	5q21	*APC*	Desmoid fibromatosis
Li-Fraumeni syndrome	AD	17p13 22q11	*TP53* *CHK2*	Multiple types
Neurofibromatosis type 1 (von Recklinghausen's disease)	AD	17q11	*NF1*	Malignant peripheral nerve sheath tumors
Retinoblastoma	AD	13q14	*RBI*	Multiple types
Rhabdoid predisposition syndrome	AD	22q11	*SNFS/INII*	Malignant rhabdoid tumors
Werner's syndrome	AR	8p11-12	*WRN*	Multiple types

Risk factors			
Factor	**Agent**	**Patient Population**	**Comment**
Radiotherapy	Orthovoltage and megavoltage radiation	Therapeutic radiation patients	Most commonly osteosarcoma; dose-response relationship
Chemotherapy	Alkylating agents: cyclophosphamide, melphalan, procarbazine, nitrosourea and chlorambucil	Pediatric cancer patients	Relative risk of bone sarcoma increased with cumulative drug exposure
Chemical exposure	Phenoxyacetic acids: 2,4-dichlorophenoxyacetic acid (2,4-D); 2,4,5 trichlorophenoxy acetic acid (2,4,5-T); 2 methyl-4 chlorophenoxyacetic acid (MCPA)	Forestry and agricultural workers	Phenoxy herbicide and defoliant exposure
	2,3,7,8-tetrachlorodibenzo-p-dioxin (TCDD); dioxin	Vietnam veterans	No clear link demonstrable for dioxin (Agent Orange)
	Chlorophenols	Sawmill workers	
	Thorotrast	Diagnostic X-ray patients	Hepatic angiosarcoma
	Vinyl chloride	Vinyl chloride workers	Hepatic angiosarcoma
	Arsenic	Vineyard workers	Hepatic angiosarcoma after exposure to arsenical herbicides
Chronic lymphedema		Postsurgery patients Postradiation patients Patients with congenital Lymphadema or filariasis	Stewart-Treves syndrome (lymphangiosarcoma)

The three phases of assessment of lesions		
Phase 1 (within 24 hours)	**Phase 2 (within first week)**	**Phase 3 (at specialist centre)**
History and examination	Bone scan	CT-scan lesion
Bloods	Ultrasound scan abdomen	MRI-scan lesion
Radiograph whole bone	CT-scan chest	Biopsy
Chest radiograph		

Grading of sarcoma
Low Metastatic Potential
Desmoid tumor
Atypical lipomatous tumor/Well-differentiated liposarcoma
Dermatofibroasarcoma protuberans
Hemangiopericytoma
Intermediate Metastatic Potential
Myxoid liposarcoma
Myxofibrosarcoma (previous myxoid malignant fibrous histiocytoma)
Extraskeletal chondrosarcoma
High Metastatic Potential
Undifferentiated pleomorphic sarcoma (previously pleomorphic malignant fibrous histiocytoma)
Liposarcoma (dedifferentiated and pleomorphic)
Leiomyosarcoma
Angiosarcoma
Alveolar soft-part sarcoma
Clear-cell sarcoma
Epithelioid sarcoma
Extraskeletal Ewing sarcoma
Extraskeletal osteosarcoma
Neurogenic sarcoma (malignant schwannoma)
Rhabdomyosarcoma
Synovial sarcoma

RHABDOMYOSARCOMA

- Orbit: Proptosis
- Nasopharynx: Nasal discharge and obstruction
- Basal skull and posterior orbit: Cranial nerve palsies and visual loss
- Parameninges: Headache and meningism
- Vagina or uterus: Vaginal polyp/discharge
- Bladder or prostate: Urinary obstruction
- Male genitals: Paratesticular scrotal mass

Embryonal RMS
Characteristic loss of heterogenicity (LOK) 11p15.5 (IGH-II gene)
Hyperdiploid DNA
Alveolar RMS
Characteristic translocations
PAX3/FKHR t(2,13) (q35;q14)
PAX7/FKHR t(1;13) (p36;q14)
Tetraploid DNA

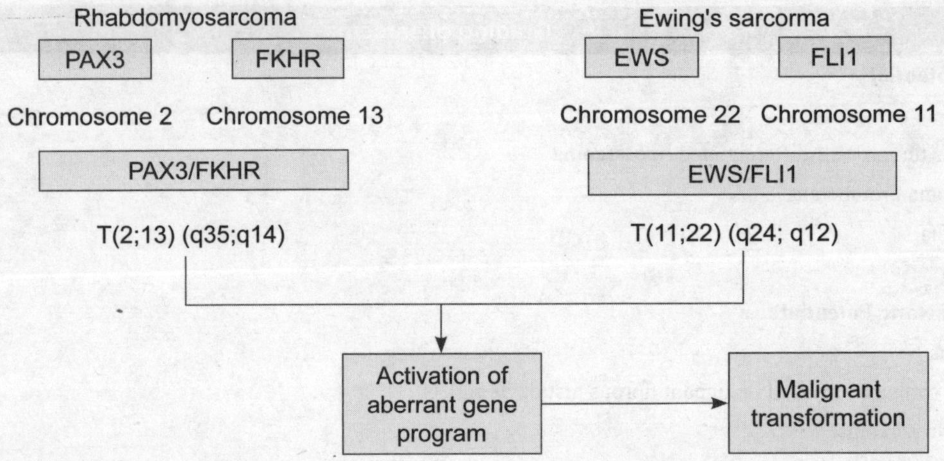

Risks factors for rhabdomyosarcoma in children and adolescents
Genetic
Familial cancer
Germline mutant p53
Congenital abnormalities
Neurofibromatosis type I
Li-Fraumeni syndrome
Parental behaviors
Smoking
Use of recreational drugs
Prenatal consumption of alcohol
Chemical exposure at workplace

Prognostic factors in rhabdomyosarcoma	
Good	**Poor**
Orbit, paratesticular, vagina, extremities	Parameningeal, retroperitoneal
Localized to tissue of origin	Contiguous spread, nodal or metastatic disease
Complete resection feasible	Unresectable
Embryonal histology	Alveolar histology
Infant or child	Adult
Complete response to chemotherapy	Poor response to chemotherapy

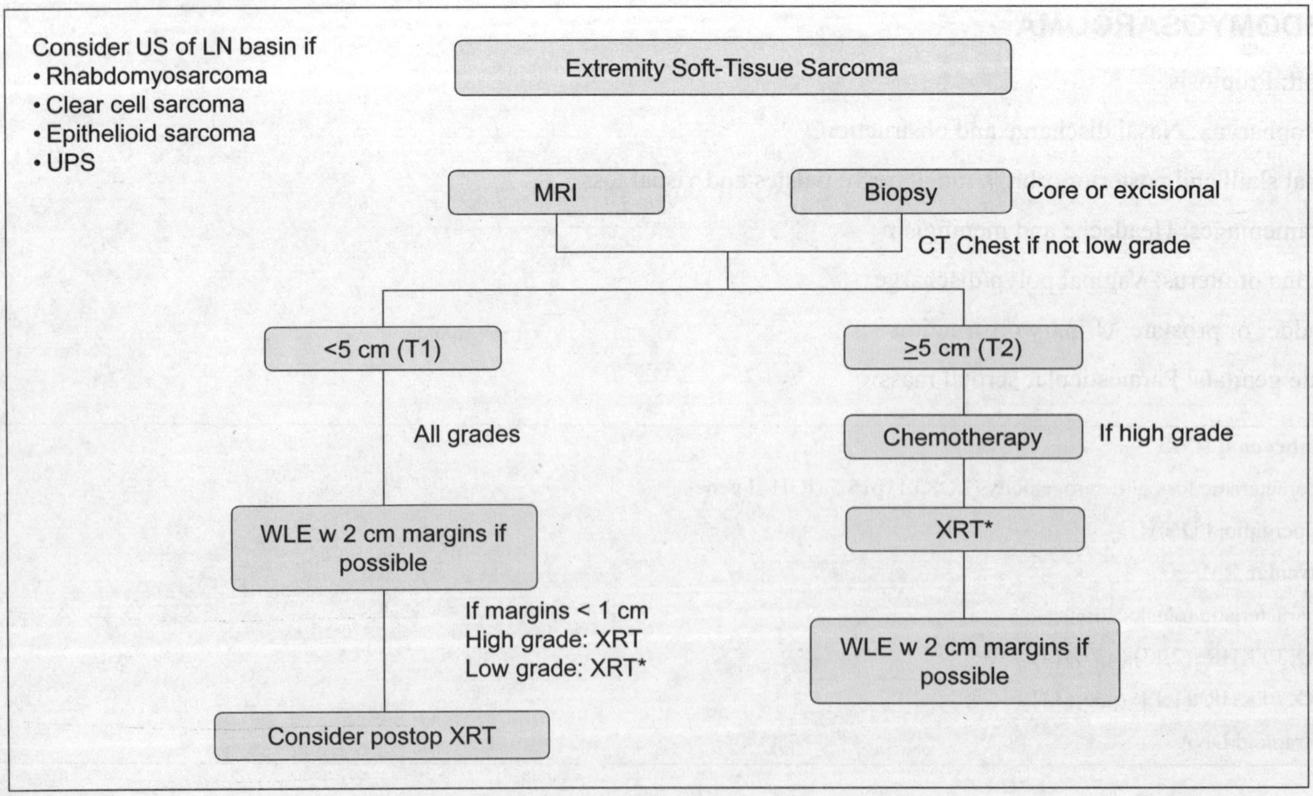

LIPOSARCOMA

- T (12,16) translocation
- Extremity LPS–Surgery (Limb salvage surgery)
- **CT Scan** > 10 cm, >2 mm septa, Non adipose areas, <75% adipose tissue →Indicates Malignancy
- ***Round cell–Worse outcome***

LEIOMYOSARCOMA

- Most common site–Retroperitoneum (Uterus)
- 6th to 7th decade
- Women
- Risk factors–RT, Immunosuppression and EBV
- +ve Desmin, Smooth muscle actin
- ***Most common site in GIT–Rectum***
- ***Most common site for Vascular leiomyosarcoma–Pulmonary artery***
- Resection with –ve margins

RETROPERITONEAL SARCOMA

- 15% STS
- M=F
- 54 years
- Worse prognosis
- Most common–Liposarcoma
- 70% relapse
- Poor prognosis–High grade, Unresectable, Gross residual disease after surgery
- 60-70 Gy–Sarcoma lethal dose
- Metastatic–Anthracyclines

Relative Chemosensitivity	Example
Highly sensitive (chemotherapy standard of care in management)	Ewing's sarcoma family of tumors/PNET Embryonal and alveolar rhabdomyosarcoma
Sensitive to chemotherapy	Synovial sarcoma Small cell sarcoma Myxoid/round cell liposarcoma Uterine leiomyosarcoma
Moderate sensitivity to chemotherapy	Pleomorphic liposarcoma Myxofibrosarcoma Epithelioid sarcoma Pleomorphic rhabdomyosarcoma Leiomyosarcoma Malignant peripheral nerve sheath tumor (MPNST) Angiosarcoma Desmoplastic small round cell tumor (DSRCT)
Insensitive to chemotherapy	Dedifferentiated liposarcoma Clear cell sarcoma Endometrial stromal sarcoma
Chemoresistant (chemotherapy risk clearly outweighs benefit)	Gastrointestional stromal tumor (GIST) Alveolar soft parts sarcoma (ASPS) Extraskeletal myxoid chondrosarcoma

Type	Frequency	Age Distribution	Gender	Common Sites	Radiologic Features	Pathologic Features
Osteosarcoma	45%	10-20 years	M > F	Metaphysis	Sunburst calcifications	Spindle cells, osteoid matrix
MFH	8%	20-80 years	M > F	Long bones	Radiolucent with ill-defined margins	Pleomorphic spindle cells, NO osteoid
Chondrosarcoma	22%	20-80 years	M > F	Pelvis/shoulder girdles	Lobulated appearance	Lobules, chondroid matrix
Ewing/PNET	15%	10-20 years	F > M	Diaphyses	Lytic with soft tissue component	Small round blue cells

Prognostic Factors

Endpoint	Adverse Prognostic Factor
Local recurrence	Age > 50 years Local recurrence at presentation Microscopically positive margin Fibrosarcoma Malignant peripheral nerve tumor
Distant recurrence	Size 5.0-10.0 cm Size > 10.0 cm High-grade Deep location Local recurrence Leiomyosarcoma Other nonliposarcoma histology
Disease-specific survival	Size > 10.0 cm Deep location Local recurrence at presentation Leiomyosarcoma Malignant peripheral nerve tumor Microscopically positive margin Lower-extremity site

IMMUNOHISTOCHEMISTRY

Antibody	Histotype
ALK	Inflammatory myofibroblastic tumor
Beta-catenin	Desmoid fibromatosis
CD 31	Vascular tumors Histiocytes
CD 34	DFSP Solitary fibrous tumor Vascular tumors
CD 99	Ewing's sarcoma Synovial sarcoma
CD 117 (KIT)	Gastrointestinal stromal tumor Metanocytic tumors Seminoma Mast cell disease
Cytokeratin AE1/AE3	Synovial sarcoma Epithelioid sarcoma Desmoplastic small round cell tumor Myoepithelioma

Contd.

Contd.

h-Caldesmon	Leiomyosarcoma
Desmin	Rhabdomyosarcoma Leiomyosarcoma Desmoplastic small round cell tumor Classifying fibromyxoid tumor
DOG1	Gastrointestinal stromal tumor
EMA	Synovial sarcoma Myoeithelial tumors
ERG	Vascular tumors
FVIII-RA	Vascular tumors
FLI-1	Ewing's sarcoma Vascular tumors
GFAP	Glial tumors Neural tumors Myoepithelial tumors
HHSV8	Kaposi sarcoma
HMB45	PE Coma Clear cell sarcoma Metanocytic tumors

Antibody	**Histotype**
INI1 (loss of expression)	Epithelioid sarcoma Myoepithelioma
MDM2	Well-differentiated/differentiated liposarcoma Low-grade central osteosarcoma
Myogenin	Rhabdomyosarcoma
MUC4	Low-grade fibromyxoid sarcoma
Smooth muscle actin	Leiomyosarcoma Myofibroblastic tumors
S100 protein	Neural tumors Myoeithelial tumors Melanocytic tumors Clear cell sarcoma Synovial sarcoma
SOX9	Chondrogenic tumors
TFE3	Alveolar soft part sarcoma PEComa
TLE1	Synovial sarcoma
WT1 (n-terminal)	Desmoplastic small round cell tumor

PART ONE: DERMATO-ONCOLOGY

CHAPTER 44

MELANOMA

One Liners
• Melanocytes are derived from neural crest cells
• Most common histological type of malignant melanoma is superficial spreading type
• Worst prognosis is with nodular melanoma
• Melanoma with equal frequency in blacks and whites- ***Acral lentigenous melanoma***
• Melanoma showing neurotropism–***Desmoplastic (Amelanotic) melanoma***
• FDA approved combination of Trametinib (MEK inhibitor) and Dabrafenib (BRAF inhibitor) for treatment of patients with unresectable/ metastatic melanoma
• Histologically, melanocytic proliferation originating in basal layers of epidermis
• Prognosis depends on Breslow thickness (depth of invasion), Clark level of invasion, No. of inflammatory cells and type of melanoma
Greater the number of lymphocytes in tumor the better the prognosis
• Malignant melanoma arising from lentigo maligna has better prognosis than invasive superficial spreading melanoma

Differences between acquired melanocytic and dysplastic nevi

Acquired Melanocytic Nevus	Dysplastic Nevus
Develops in early childhood through fourth decade	Develops throughout life
<5 mm in diameter, sharp borders, evenly pigmented	6-8 mm in diameter, irregular borders, variegated pigment and topographic asymmetry
Risk for melanoma development increases by 10-fold if more than 100 in number	Risk factor for melanoma development

- Accounts for about 2% of all skin cancers
- Responsible for 80% of deaths
- Before the age of 45, women have a higher risk than men
- After 60 years age, the risk for men is twice as high as for women
- White people have a 2.4% lifetime risk for development of melanoma and African Americans 0.1%
- Melanoma is neoplastic disorder produced by Malignant transformation of normal melanocytes
- Site most commonly associated with melanocytic transformation in the skin, where melanocytes reside at the dermo-epidermal junction (junctional melanocytes)
- Most common site of MM in men: Back and trunk
- Most common site of MM in women: Lower extremity
- Most susceptible individuals: Fair complexion, red or blonde hair, blue eyes and freckles and who tan poorly and sunburn easily, multiple nevi

Arises from
• De novo • Congenital giant pigmented nevus • Lentigo maligna • Nevocellular nevus • Superficial spreading melanoma in situ

RISK FACTORS

- Strongest risk factors for melanoma are family history of melanoma, multiple benign or atypical nevi and previous melanoma
- Others–Immunosuppression, sun sensitivity and exposure to UV radiation

Risk Factor	Features
Personal history of melanoma	9x increased risk of developing a second melanoma (vs general population)
Family history of melanoma	First-degree relatives have a higher risk, and 10% of all melanomas are familial (FAMMM syndrome and dysplastic nevus syndrome)
Total number of nevi	Relative risk of 5 to 17 with presence of > 50 nevi
Congenital nevi	6% lifetime risk with large (>20 cm) congenital nevi
Dysplastic nevi	3- to 20-fold higher risk of developing melanoma than general population
Immunosuppressant	Chronic immune suppressant use, HV infection and organ transplantation
MC 1R variants	Associated with fair skin, red hair and freckles
Exposure to ultraviolet light	Tanning bed use, sunburn

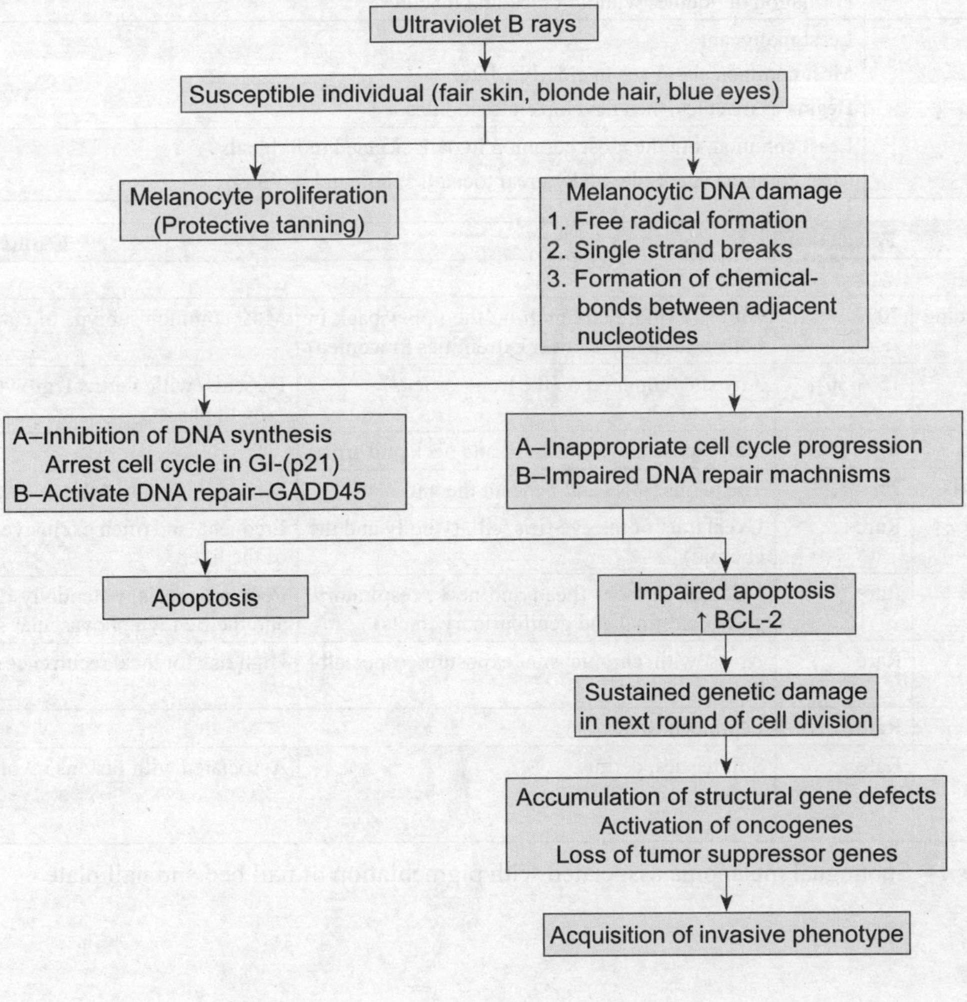

Familial
Approximately 10% of melanomas are familial

High Penetrance Genes
CDKN2A and CDK4, are associated with high-penetrance susceptibility
Mutated CDKN2A–Most prevalent gene in families with melanoma (Located on chromosome 9p21)
CDK4 encodes cyclin-dependent kinase 4
Other High penetrance genes–BAP1, TERT, XP

Low Penetrance Genes
BRCA2, MC1R, MITF E318K, shelterin complex genes (POT1, ACD, TERF2IP)

Familial atypical mole melanoma syndrome

- Familial dysplastic nevus syndrome
- Members suffered from melanoma and had multiple (usually >100) large moles of variable size and color (reddish brown to bright red) with pigmentary leakage
- Autosomal dominant
- Males develop melanoma less frequently at an older age than women

Classification of melanoma

Superficial spreading	Most common type of MM in light skinned individuals Most common site: Torso
Nodular	Most malignant Most common site: Head, neck and trunk Vertical growth phase only Formation of nodules without preceding macules
Lentigo maligna	Least malignant Most common site: Face in elderly whites Begins as macules, then develops into nodules
Acral lentiginous	Least common, but the most common in dark skinned individuals Most common site: Sole, under great toenail, subungual regions

Type	Frequency	Sites	Features
Cutaneous			
• Superfical spreading	70%	Any site (more common on the upper back in both sexes and the lower extremities in women)	Most common subtype of cutaneous melanomas
• Nodular	15%-30%	Any site (common on the trunk or legs)	Presents with vertical growth phase without radial growth phase
• Lentigo maligna	4%-15%	Sun-exposed area (the head and neck and arms)	
• Acral lentiginous	2%-8%	The palms, soles and beneath the nail plate	More common in African Americans and Asians
Uveal	Rare	Uveal tract of the eye (iris, ciliary body and the choroid)	Frequent, and often exclusive, metastatic involvement of the liver
Mucosal	Rare	Mucosal surfaces (head and neck, respiratory, gastrointestinal and genitourinary tracts)	Poor prognosis, potentially due to delayed diagnosis and the rich lymphovascular supply of the mucosa
Desmoplastic	Rare	Areas with chronic sun exposure, especially head and neck	High risk for local recurrence and growth along nerves
Primary CNS	Rare	Leptomeninges	
Melanoma of soft parts (Clear cell sarcoma)	Rare	Soft tissues, dermis	Associated with fusions involving the *EWSRI* gene

- ***Hutchinson's Sign*** – Subungual melanoma associated with pigmentation of nail bed and nail plate

BASED ON ONCOGENIC MUTATIONS

	Mutations			
Melanoma subtype	**BRAF**	**NRAS**	**KIT**	***GNAQ/GNA11***
Cutaneous without CSD	50%	15%-20%	1%-2%	–
Cutaneous with CSD	5%-30%	10%-15%	2%-17%	–
Acral lentiginous	10%-15%	10%-15%	15%-20%	–
Mucosal	5%	5%-10%	15%-20%	–
Uveal	–	–	–	85%

Clark's levels (on the basis of depth of invasion)	
I	Melanoma restricting to Epidermis and appendages
II	Invading papillary dermis without filling it
III	Reaching interface of papillary and reticular dermis
IV	Invading reticular dermis
V	Invading subcutaneous tissue

Breslow's Thickness (Actual measurement of the deepest invasion from the granular layer)	
Stage I	<0.75 mm
Stage II	0.75-1.5 mm
Stage III	1.6-4.0 mm
Stage IV	>4.0 mm

Prognostic Factors (Depends Most Importantly on Staging)

- Depth of invasion (most important lymph node status prognostic factor)
- Satellite lesion
- Presence of ulceration carries worst prognosis
- Distant metastasis
- Regression: Poor prognosis
- Presence of lymphocytes between tumor cells – Good Prognosis

CHARACTERISTIC FEATURES

- Classic appearance of melanoma: ABCD (Asymmetry, Border irregularity, Color variation, Diameter > 6 mm)
- **Most common route of metastasis: Through Lymphatics**
- **Most common site of systemic metastasis: Liver**
- Microsatellites: Discrete tumor nests > 0.05 mm in diameter, separated from main body of tumor by normal dermal collagen or subcutaneous fat
- Microsatellites are associated with increased risk of regional LN metastasis

DIAGNOSIS

- Confirmed by full thickness excisional biopsy
- Incisional biopsy for large lesions and lesions in proximity to important structures (eye, nose, ear)
- HPE; Aggregates and irregular nests of atypical melanocytes in epidermis and dermis

AJCC 8th edition staging			
T Classification		**Thickness**	**Ulceration Status, Thickness Detail**
TX		Thickness cannot be assessed	
T0		No evidence of primary tumor (e.g. unknown or regressed primary)	
		Mission Oncology	
Tis		**Melanoma is situ**	
T1		≤ 1.0 mm	a: <0.8 mm without ulceration b: Ulcerated or 0.8-1.0 mm
T2		1.1-2.0 mm	a: Without ulceration b: With ulceration
T3		2.1-4.0 mm	a: Without ulceration b: With ulceration
T4		>4.0 mm	a: Without ulceration b: With ulceration
N Classification		**No. and Size of Metastatic Nodes**	**In-Transit ϕ Satellite Metastases**
NX		Regional notes not assessed: except for T1, use cN	
N0		None	None
N1	a	1 clinically occult node	None
	b	1 clinically detected node	None
	c	None	Yes
N2	a	2-3 clinically occult nodes	None
	b	2-3 nodes, with ≥ 1 clinically detected	None
	c	1 node (clinically occult or clinically detected)	Yes
N3	a	4 or more clinically occult nodes	None
	b	4 nodes, with ≥ 1 clinically detected; or any matted nodes	None
	c	2 or more nodes (clinically occult or clinically detected) and/or matted nodes	Yes
M Classification		**Site**	**Serum Lactate Dehydrogenase**
M0		No evidence of distant metastasis	
M1a		Distant skin, subcutaneous, soft tissue (including muscle), or nodal metastases	(0) Not elevated (1) Elevated
M1b		Lung metastases	(0) Not elevated (1) Elevated
M1c		Other non-CNS visceral metastases	(0) Not elevated (1) Elevated
M1d		CNS metastasis	(0) Not elevated (1) Elevated

	Tis	T1a	T1b	T2a	T2b	T3a	T3b	T4a	T4b
N0	0	IA	IB	IB	IIA	IIA	IIB	IIB	IIC
N1-3	III								
M1	IV								

Risk of identifying a metastatic deposit in a sentinel lymph node, according to the 1° tumor thickness	
	Risk of metastatic deposit in sentinel node (%)
Breslow depth < 0.75 mm	1
≥0.75 Breslow depth < 1.5 mm	8
≥ 1.50 Breslow depth < 4.0 mm	23
Breslow depth ≥4.0 mm	36

Management

A. Primary:

- Definitive surgical treatment for primary cutaneous melanoma is a wide excision

Tumor Thickness (mm)	Recommended Surgical Margin (cm)
In situ	0.5-1
<1	1
1.01-2	1-2
2.01-4	2
>4	2

- Mohs micrographic surgery may contribute to favorable outcomes, especially on head and neck where extensive subclinical spread is relatively common

Unusual sites

- Subungual melanoma is treated with partial digital amputation
- Plantar melanoma–Wide excision with reconstructive flap procedures (Weight bearing surface)
- **Mucosal melanoma**

  Localised–Craniofacial resection for skull base tumors, radical vulvectomy for vulvar melanomas, or APR for anorectal melanomas

B. Regional Lymph Node Metastasis:

- **Sentinel Lymph node biopsy** can adequately detect lymph node metastasis with decreased morbidity
- SLN is identified by lymphoscintigraphy

Patients who do not have clinically involved regional lymph nodes and whose primary tumor is thicker than >1 mm or thicker than 0.75 mm with high-risk features (ulceration, Clark level IV and V, histologic regression, or high mitotic rate) undergo SLNB

- Only 1% to 2% of patients who have an uninvolved SLN have metastases to non-SLN
- Patients with positive SLNB→ Recommendation is to have elective lymph node dissection
- ***Inguinofemoral lymph nodes are clinically positive/3 or more are involved microscopically or if Cloquet node is positive***–Elective Iliac and Obturator LN dissection is considered

Complications occur more frequently after Inguinal lymphadenectomy than after axillary lymphadenectomy

C. Intransit Metastasis:

- Patients with unresectable in transit metastasis or for whom surgery would not provide a meaningful control of disease should be managed as patients with metastatic disease

ISOLATED LIMB PERFUSION

- **Indication**–Lesion in extremities, Unresectable recurrence, Multiple intransit metastasis
- **Hyperthermic perfusion of Melphalan/L-phenylalanine mustard is used**

Brain Metastasis
• Patients at especially high risk for development of brain metastases are ***males with primary lesions located on mucosal surfaces or on skin of trunk/head and neck, with thick/ulcerated primary lesions, or with acral lentiginous/nodular lesions***
Favorable prognostic factors
Good performance status, Younger age, Absence of extracranial metastases and presence of solitary brain metastasis
• *All patients with a new diagnosis of brain metastasis from melanoma should be evaluated for possible surgical resection or stereotactic irradiation*
Multiple simultaneous metastasis (>5)–*Whole brain radiation therapy*
• Response rate to ipilimumab when used alone or in combination with stereotactic radiosurgery was similar in brain and outside brain in patients who were asymptomatic or minimally symptomatic and who were not on steroids or were on a low dose of steroids • BRAF inhibitors have also activity against brain metastases of V600E BRAF mutated melanomas

Median survival from time of diagnosis of brain metastasis – 4 months

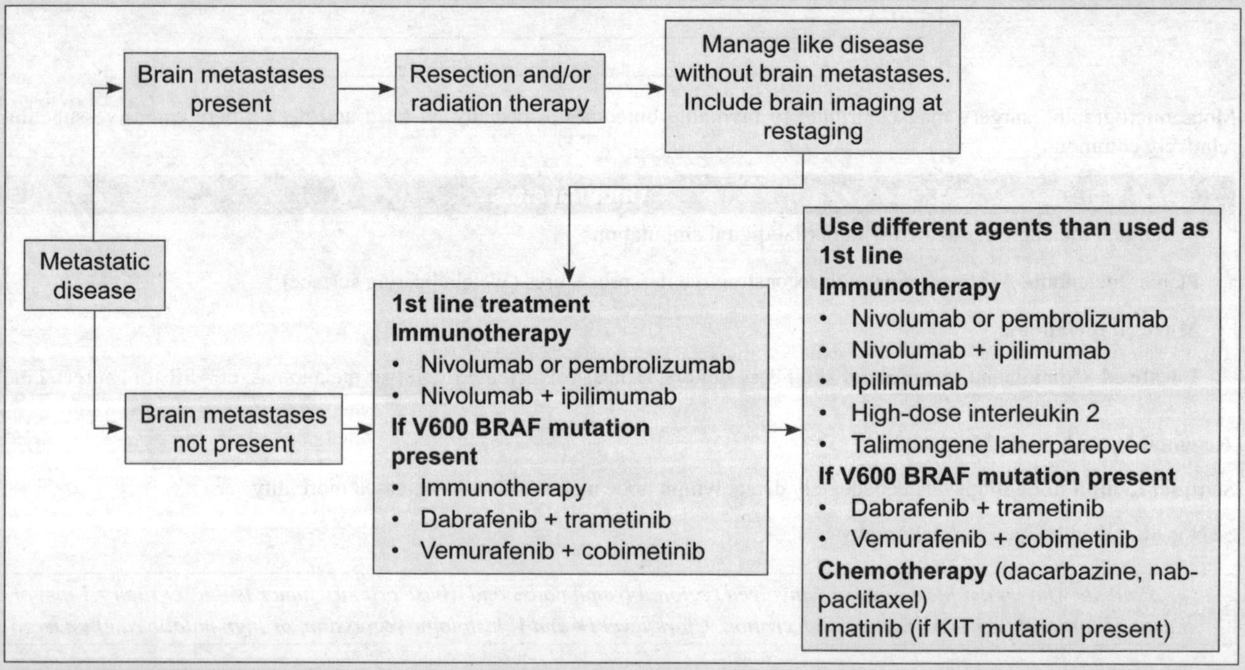

Molecular targeted therapy for Metastatic melanoma

1. **BRAF Inhibitors:**
   - Vemurafenib and Dabrafenib
   - BRAF V600 mutation is seen in about 40-50% of melanoma patients
2. **MEK Inhibitors:**
   - Block MAPK pathway by inhibiting MEK activity (Downstream kinase from BRAF)
   - Trametinib–BRAF mutated melanoma
   - Binimetinib–N RAS mutated melanoma
3. **BRAF and MEK Inhibitor combinations:**
   - Patients with BRAF V600 E mutations can be offered combination therapy
4. **Kit Inhibitors:**
   - Response is better with c-kit mutated melanoma

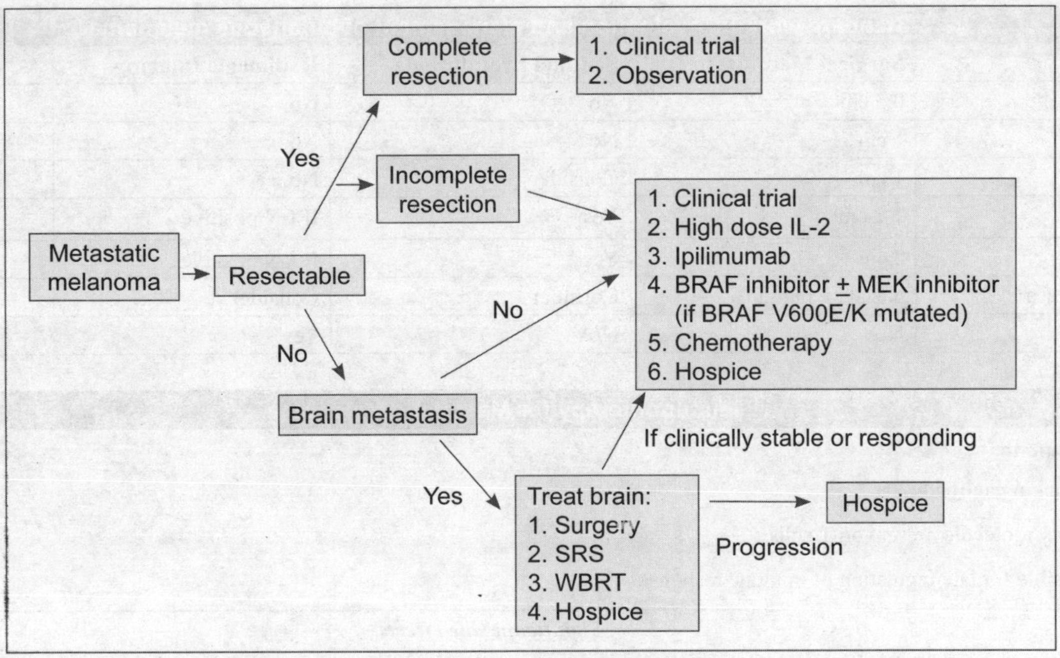
Complete resection
1. Clinical trial
2. Observation
Yes
Incomplete resection
Metastatic melanoma
Resectable
1. Clinical trial
2. High dose IL-2
3. Ipilimumab
4. BRAF inhibitor ± MEK inhibitor (if BRAF V600E/K mutated)
5. Chemotherapy
6. Hospice
No
No
Brain metastasis
If clinically stable or responding
Yes
Treat brain:
1. Surgery
2. SRS
3. WBRT
4. Hospice
Hospice
Progression

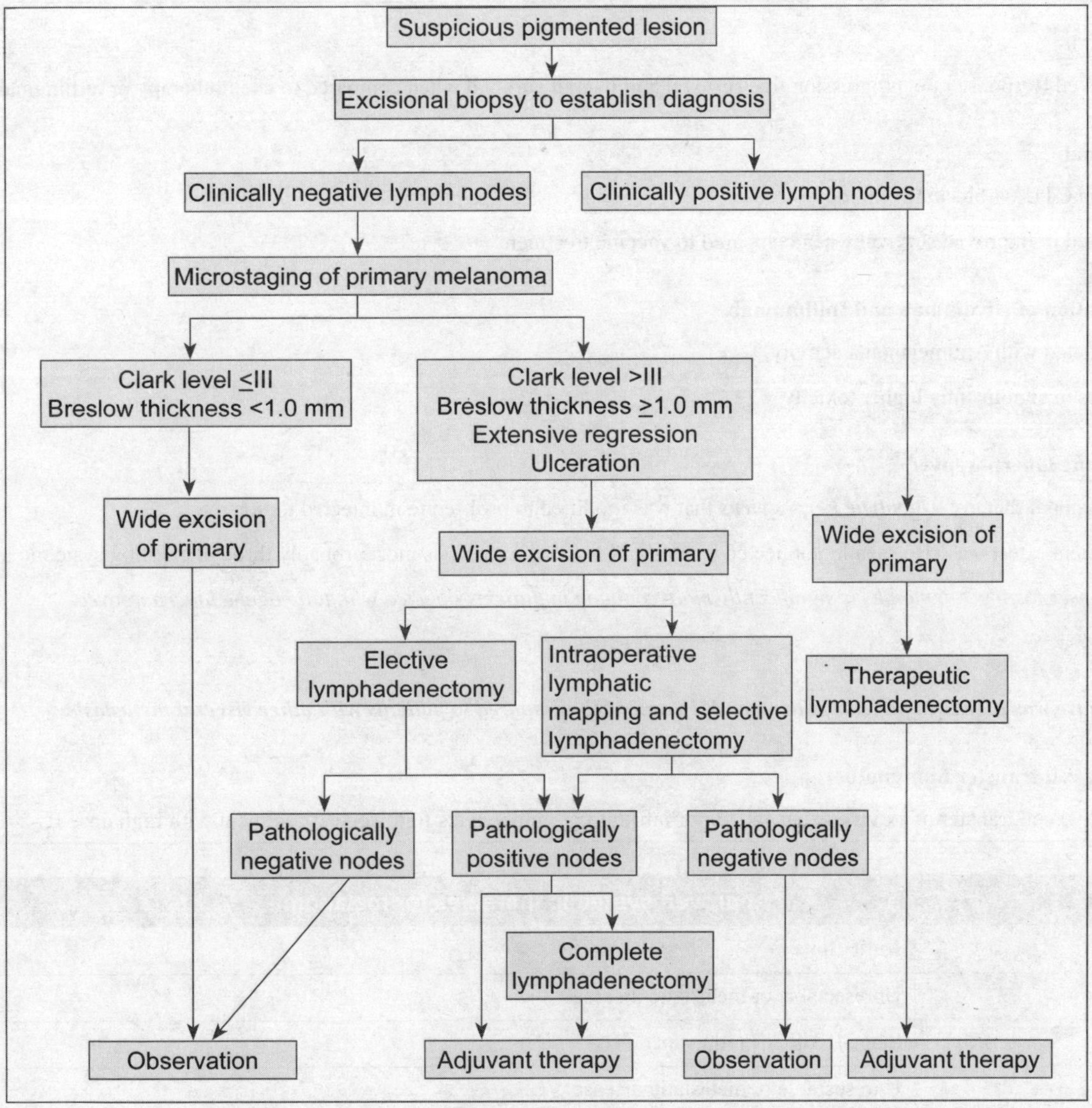
Suspicious pigmented lesion
Excisional biopsy to establish diagnosis
Clinically negative lymph nodes
Clinically positive lymph nodes
Microstaging of primary melanoma
Clark level ≤III
Breslow thickness <1.0 mm
Clark level >III
Breslow thickness ≥1.0 mm
Extensive regression
Ulceration
Wide excision of primary
Wide excision of primary
Wide excision of primary
Elective lymphadenectomy
Intraoperative lymphatic mapping and selective lymphadenectomy
Therapeutic lymphadenectomy
Pathologically negative nodes
Pathologically positive nodes
Pathologically negative nodes
Complete lymphadenectomy
Observation
Adjuvant therapy
Observation
Adjuvant therapy

Standard workup, evaluation and management of cutaneous melanoma				
Melanoma	**Surgical Margins**	**Sentinel Lymph Node**	**Radiologic Imaging**	**Labs**
In situ	0.5 cm	No	No	No
<0.75 mm	1 cm	No	No	No
0.75-1 mm	1 cm	Consider	No	No
1-2 mm	1-2 cm	Yes	If LN positive	No
>2 mm	2 cm	Yes	If LN positive	No
In-transit disease	Negative margin	Consider	Consider	Consider LDH
Stage IV	N/A	N/A	Yes	LDH

Immunotherapy for Metastatic Melanoma

1. Pembrolizumab

- PD1 blocking antibody
- Inhibitory molecule present on T cells
- Responsible for late regulation of immune responses

> ***Significant side effects***
> *Diarrhea, Colitis, Hepatitis, Pneumonitis, Hypo/Hyperthyroidism, Type 1 DM*

2. Nivolumab

- Improved Response rate, progression free survival and overall survival when compared to chemotherapy or ipilimumab

3. Ipilimumab

- Human CTLA 4 blocking antibody
- Resulted in improved survival when compared to vaccine treatment

4. Combination of Nivolumab and Ipilimumab

- Associated with Antimelanoma activity
- Results in significantly higher toxicity

5. Talimogene laherparepvec

- Intralesional therapy–***Oncolytic herpes virus*** that was modified to proliferate in injected tumor
- Treatment effect was also seen in uninjected lesions and visceral metastasis most probably through eliciting systemic immune responses
- *Responses lasting > 6 months is significantly more common in patients injected with talimogene laherparepvec*

6. IL 2

- ***Response was higher in patients with stage M1a and M1b compared to patients with other visceral metastasis***

7. Adoptive cell transfer immunotherapy

- Adoptive cell transfer of ex vivo expanded tumor infiltrating lymphocytes followed by treatment with high dose IL-2

Approved systemic therapies for melanoma	
Agent	**Indication**
Dacarbazine	Unresectable or metastatic disease
Interferon	Stage IIB/IIC/II (adjuvant)
Interleukin-2	Unresectable or metastatic disease

Contd.

Contd.

Pegylated interferon	Stage III (adjuvant)
Ipilimumab	Unresectable or metastatic disease
Vemurafenib	Unresectable or metastatic disease with *BRAF*^{v600} mutation
Dabrafenib	Unresectable or metastatic disease with *BRAF*^{v600} mutation
Trametinib	Unresectable or metastatic disease with *BRAF*^{v600} mutation
Dabrafenib + trametinib	Unresectable or metastatic disease with *BRAF*^{v600} mutation
Pembrolizumab	Unresectable or metastatic disease after ipilimumab (and after *BRAF* inhibitor if *BRAF*^{v600} mutation present)
Nivolumab	Unresectable or metastatic disease after ipilimumab (and after *BRAF* inhibitor if *BRAF*^{v600} mutation present)
Ipilimumab + nivolumab	*BRAF*^{v600} wild-type, unresectable or metastatic disease
Vemurafenib + cobimetinib	Unresectable or metastatic disease with *BRAF*^{v600} mutation

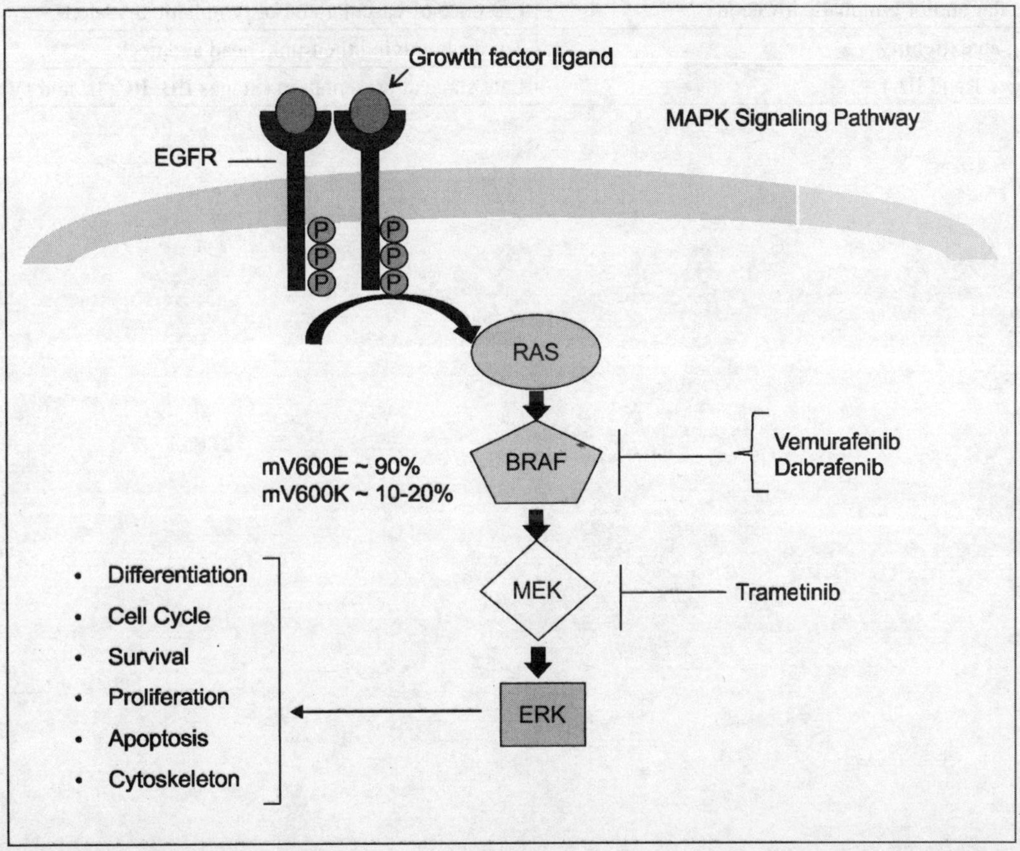

Chemotherapy for metastatic melanoma
Choice for patients whose disease progressed on Immunotherapy and Targeted therapy
1. **Dacarbazine** 2. **Temozolomide** • *Brain metastasis* • Oral analogue of Dacarbazine • Penetrates blood brain barrier • Degraded to MTIC in body • When compared to DTIC–No significant improvement in median survival

Contd.

Contd.

3. **Nab-paclitaxel**
   - Improved Progressive free survival
   - No improvement in OS and Response rate
4. **Other single agents**
   - Platinum containing agents, Nitrosureas, Microtubule toxins and taxanes

Prognostic factors of melanoma	
Good Prognostic Factors	**Poor Prognostic Factors**
Thin tumor (tumor ≤ 1 mm deep)	Thick tumor (tumor >1 mm deep). Nodular tumor
No ulceration of tumor	Tumor ulceration present
No tumor cell mitosis	Tumor mitosis present
Absence of foci of regression and/or tumor satellites in the reticular dermis and subcutaneous fat	Presence of foci of regression and/or tumor satellites in reticular dermis and subcutaneous fat
Absence of vascular and/or lymphatic invasion	Presence of vascular and/or lymphatic invasion
Tumor involving an extremity	Tumor involving the trunk, head and neck
Early stage (stages 1 and IIA)	Late stage at presentation (Stages IIB, IIC, III and IV)

CHAPTER

45 NON MELANOMATOUS SKIN CANCER – SCC AND BCC

Etiology
• BCC is four to five times more common than SCC
Occurs due to intense intermittent UV exposure
• Fair skin, Light eyes, Blond or red hair increase UV Sensitivity
Use of tanning devices increase risk of SCC and BCC in 2 fold
• **PUVA therapy**–8.6 for SCC and low for BCC
• **Long term immunosuppresssion**–100 fold increased risk of SCC and 10 fold increased risk of BCC ***(Overall 3 fold)***
SCC in immunosuppressed patients tend to be behave more aggressively and associated with greater tumor depth, higher risk of recurrence and more frequently associated with perineural or lymphovascular invasion ***Sirolimus reduces incidence and severity of post transplant NMSC***
• Persistent HPV infection may act synergistically with UV exposure to increase risk
Epidermodysplasia verruciformis*–HPV 5 and 8* ***Verrucous carcinoma****–HPV 6 and 11* ***SCC****–HPV 16 and 18* ***Periungual SCC****–HPV 16*
• Exposure to ionizing radiation ***increases risk of NMSC three fold*** and often presents decades after initial exposure (Dose dependent)
• ***Arsenic, tar, soot, tobacco, asphalt and mineral oil have all been associated with an increased risk of SCC***
• SCC can also arise from areas of chronic inflammation and healing such as from scars, burn sites, or ulcers; this type of SCC is also known as a Marjolin ulcer (Discoid lupus)
• Xeroderma pigmentosum, albinism, Muir-Torre syndrome, ***dystrophic epidermolysis bullosa,*** Fanconi anemia, Werner syndrome, nevoid basal cell syndrome, and Li Fraumeni syndrome have an increased incidence of NMSC
• Previous diagnosis of cutaneous carcinoma increases the risk of future NMSCs to as high as 35% at 3 years and 50% at 5 years
• Voriconazole–Antifungal agent facilitate actinic damage
• Nasolabial folds, Floor of nose, Columella, Preauricular regions, Inner and Outer canthus of eye are more aggressive with higher risk of recurrence
Nevoid basal cell syndrome
• Autosomal dominant disorder characterized by development of multiple BCCs
• Often quite small but can number in hundreds on any given skin surface
• Sonic hedgehog signaling pathway ***(PTCH1 gene, chromosome 9q22)*** has significant etiologic role in nevoid BCC syndrome and ***90% of sporadic BCC***
• Macrocephaly, Frontal bossing, Bifid ribs, Bone cysts, Palmar and Plantar pitting, Kyphoscoliosis, Spina bifida, Short metacarpals, Hyperresponsiveness to parathormone and Ovarian fibroma, Calcification of falx cerebri, ***Medulloblastoma***
• Exquisitely sensitive to radiation and should avoid excessive sun exposure and RT
Xeroderma pigmentosum
• Autosomal recessive disease
• Characterized by photophobia, severe sun sensitivity and advanced sun damage

Contd.

Contd.

- Affected individuals have defective DNA excision repair, and when exposed to UV radiation, develop malignancies of the skin and eyes at a rate 1,000 times that of general population
- Aggressive sun protection in the form of full-body sun suits and regular skin examinations are critical for patients with xeroderma pigmentosum
- **De Sanctis Cacchione syndrome**–Severe form (Microcephaly, Mental deficiency, Dwarfism and Failure of gonadal development
- 10% of Nevus sebaceous develop into BCC
- **Actinic keratoses**–Premalignant lesions with potential to develop into SCCs. 60% of cases SCC arises from Actinic Keratosis
- **Keratoacanthoma**–Older, sun-damaged skin and is most commonly found on the neck and face– 3 to 5 mm margins excision recommended

Bazex syndrome

- X linked dominant disorder
- Characterized clinically by follicular atrophoderma, hypotrichosis, hypohidrosis, milia, epidermoid cysts and facial BCCs

Rombo syndrome

- Bazex syndrome with peripheral vasodilation with cyanosis

Basal cell carcinoma

- Malignant transformation of sebaceous cyst results in basal cell carcinoma
- Also called as rodent ulcer
- ***Most common skin cancer (95%)***
- ***Most common on Nose***
- Men > Women
- Elderly/Middle aged and occasionally Younger individuals
- *Arise from hair follicle cells*–Almost exclusively on hair-bearing skin
- ***Occult BCC→ 3% Rhinophyma***
- **Strongest risk factor for BCC**–UV radiation
- Most common histologic subtype is Nodular BCC

> **Higher-risk subtypes**–Sclerosing, infiltrating, micronodular, morpheaform (or desmoplastic) and basosquamous carcinoma- ***Subclinical extension exceeding visible borders of lesion***

- **Nodular**–Pearly pink elevated translucent nodules with central umbilication and **"rolled edges"**. ***Often pigmented.*** Predominantly on face–***Most common type (60%)***
- **Superficial**–Predominantly on limbs and trunk. Slow-growing, scaly pink plaque (30%)–***Trunk***
- **Infiltrative**–***Predominantly head and neck (5%)***–Spiky appearance. Palisiding is characteristically absent
- **Sclerosing/Morpheaform**–Poorly defined indurated/ sclerotic plaque (5-10%), Spreads rapidly–***Secretes collagenase 4*** (Least common/ Most malignant)
- **Basosquamous Carcinoma/Metatypical**–Aggressive tumors with potential to metastasize, though metastatic risk is determined by degree of squamous component
- **Fibroepithelioma of Pinkus**–***Torso and Extremities (1%)***
- **Hyperkeratotic Carcinoma**–Multicentric ulcer and scar tissue or exophytic type or cystic type presenting as blue gray nodule on face or as sessile growth on lower trunk
- **Perineural invasion**–*Most often in recurrent clinically aggressive lesions and periauricular and Malar areas*
- Turban tumor is BCC arising from basal cells of hair follicles and sweat glands
- **RT**–Best suited in older patients with extensive lesions on ear, lower limbs/eyelids
- **Cyclopamin**–Competitive inhibitor of SMO signaling, binding directly to PTCH1 or SMO

Prolonged exposure to arsenic results in Multiple BCC, SCC and Bowen's disease

Contd.

Contd.

Grossly involved disease recurrence–67%

Microscopic/Close margin recurrence–33%

Tricholemmoma

- 10% form BCC life long
- Nevus Sebaceous of Jodassohn
- Congenital hamartoma

- **Death**–Direct extension to blood vessels and Intracranially
- **Margins**–4 mm for superficial and 1cm for Morpheaform/Recurrent BCC
- No apparent precursor lesion
- Develops proportional to initial dose of carcinogen (Not duration)
- Eyelids. Tear ducts and Nasal tip–**X-ray therapy**

Squamous cell carcinoma

- Accounts for 20% of all NMSCs
- SCC is responsible for majority of deaths from NMSC
- Origin–Epidermal Keratinocytes
- Can arise from actinic keratosis or base of cutaneous horn
- Lesions are usually red, poorly defined plaques/nodules with an ulcerated friable surface

Bowen disease/SCC in situ**–***Characterized by rapidly growing, well-demarcated ulcerating tumor in pre-existing scaly, erythematous plaque. Upto 5% of Bowen disease may become invasive*

- Higher metastatic potential than BCC
- Overall 5-year recurrence 8% and metastatic risk 5%
- Tumors of head and neck–***parotid gland*** is a common site for metastases
- Most common site of metastasis–Regional lymph node
- Actinic SCC metastasis–<3%, Non actinic SCC metastasis 35%
- Self healing SCC–Keratoacanthoma and Smith Ferguson syndrome

High risk for SCC

- Size ≥ 20 mm on trunk or extremities
- Size ≥ 10 mm on cheeks, forehead, scalp, neck or pretibia
- Size ≥ 6 mm on central face, eyelids, eyebrows, periorbital nose, lips, chin, mandible, preauricular and postauricular skin/sulci, temple, ear, genitalia, hands and feet; poorly defined borders
- Recurrent tumors
- Immunosuppression
- Tumor in site of previous radiation or inflammation; rapid growth; neurologic symptoms
- Moderate or poor differentiation
- Adenoid, adenosquamous and desmoplastic; depth ≥ 2 mm; perineural/perivascular invasion

3-5% of in situ carcinoma patients develop SCC

10% of Erythroplasia of Quyret patients develop SCC

10-30% of patients with Chronic inflammation and at mucocutaneous junction develop SCC

Keratoacanthoma–20% SCC

Cutaneous horn–10% SCC

Actinic keratosis–20% SCC

- **Marjolin's ulcer**–Chronic scars to SCC–Least malignant lymph node spread

Contd.

Contd.

- **BRAF inhibitors**–Associated with increased risk of SCC
- 2% Overall metastasis
- Local recurrence rate–20%
- High recurrence–Penis, Lips, Ears and Dorsum of hand
- **Worse prognosis**–Extremities
- **Most common skin cancer in darkly pigmented race–SCC**
- **Spindle Cell:** Occurs more commonly at scar site, trauma, or burn; Elongated nuclei arranged in ***swirling pattern, more aggressive form***
- **Adenoid:** ***Pseudoglandular arrangement,*** Commonly located ***periauricular in elderly, more aggressive form***
- **Verrucous:** Warty appearance, ***less aggressive***
- Smith Ferguson syndrome–Self healing SCC (Chromosome 9q)
- **Bowen's disease**–*4 mm margin*
- 4 mm margin→ < 2 cm SCC
- 1 cm margin→ > 2 cm SCC
- **Depth >6 mm→**15% metastasis, **> 2 cm surface lesion**→Worse prognosis

Biopsy

- Biopsy of suspicious pigmented lesions should be limited to punch or excisional biopsy techniques in which the full thickness of the dermis can be evaluated
- Shave biopsy is an excellent technique for superficial lesions/nonpigmented lesions suspicious for BCC or SCC
- Excisional biopsy involves removal of the entire lesion with a margin of clinically clear tissue and is generally used for superficial SCCs or nodular and superficial BCCs

Surgical Techniques

- Complete excision with a margin of clinically normal tissue is associated with 5-year disease-free rates of over 98% for BCC and 92% for SCC

For well-defined, low-risk lesions <2 cm, excision with 4 mm margin around tumor border is expected to definitively treat tumor in 95% of cases

- For high-risk tumors, a larger margin of at least 6 mm is indicated, and European guidelines suggest at least 10 mm margin should be used
- Recurrent BCC is associated with poor cure rate and 10 mm excision margin is recommended
- **Incompletely excised**–Re excise lesion
- Patients with tumors < 2 cm, 2.1 to 3 cm, and >3 cm in diameter, the proportions of patients with a positive SLN were 0%, 15.8% and 30.4%, respectively

Curretage

- *Tumors (<1 cm), primary, low risk, or superficial tumors in non-hair-bearing areas, and as such is not suitable for recurrent or ill-defined tumors*
- Primarily reserved for treatment of precancerous lesions like **AKs and small, superficial, low-risk, primary BCCs or SCCs**

MOH's micrographic surgery

(Chemosurgery-zinc chloride fixative)

Indications:

- Recurrent/incompletely excised BCC/SCC
- Primary BCC/SCC with indistinct borders
- Lesions in high risk areas–eyelids, nose, ear, nasolabial folds, upper lip, vermilion border, columella, periorbital, temples, preauricular and postauricular areas, scalp
- Cosmetically and functionally important areas
- Tumors with aggressive clinical behavior (rapidly growing, >1cm)
- Tumors at site of prior Radiotherapy
- Tumors with aggressive histology (Morpheaform, basosquamous, perineural invasion, periappendiceal, perivascular, adenoidal, multicentric lesions

Contd.

Contd.

Microscopically controlled surgery and tissue section examined under light microscopy • Cure rate of BCC is 97-99% and SCC is about 96% • Mohs micrographic surgery of primary and recurrent NMSC of the head and neck has a cure rate (negative histologic margin) of 97%

Topical Therapies
• **5 FU and Imiquimod**–AKs as well as for superficial BCCs and SCCs in situ
Topical 5-FU is ***not appropriate for nodular BCC and not recommended for SCC*** due to high recurrence rates
• ***Imiquimod therapy is approved for the treatment of AKs and superficial BCC (<2 cm diameter on neck, trunk or extremities)***
Imiquimod therapy should not be used for SCC
• ***Imiquimod can also be used for nodular BCC,*** treatment duration requires 12 weeks and response is lower (76%) compared to > 85% success rate for superficial BCC
Cryosurgery–Small clinically well defined primary tumors

Radiotherapy
• *Recurrent or histologically aggressive tumors particularly those with perineural invasion, high-grade NMSC with perineural involvement or invasion into bone, adjuvant or palliative treatment for lymph node metastases*
Contraindicated in Nevoid BCC, Xeroderma pigmentosum, Epidermodysplasia verruciformis, recurrent or morpheaform lesions

Risk factors for recurrence and metastases in squamous cell carcinoma

	Low-risk feature	High-risk feature
Clinical Factors		
Tumor size	< 2 cm	> 2 cm
Location	Trunk, extremities	Mucosal surfaces, genitalia, mask areas of face including eyelids, periorbital nose, lips, chin, pre- and post-auricular areas, ear and prior burn scars of irradiated areas
Borders	Well defined	Ill defined
Arising from scar, inflammation	No	Yes
Prior radiation	No	Yes
History of immunosuppression	No	Yes
Primary vs. recurrent	Primary	Current
Histology		
Differentiation	Well differentiation	Poorly differentiated
Perineural invasion	No	Yes
Lymphovascular invasion	No	Yes
Depth of invasion	< 2 mm or < Clark level IV	≥ 2 mm or Clark level IV/V
Subtype	—	Bowen disease, desmoplastic SCC, acantholytic SCC, adenosquamous SCC, basosquamous SCC
Excision	Complete	Incomplete
Patients with SCC, most recurrences or metastases will occur within 2 years		

- Vismodegib and Sonidegib–Inactivation of SMO–Locally advanced and metastatic BCC
- Chemoprevention with low-dose oral retinoids is used in prevention of SCC for chronic immunosuppressed patients who have undergone organ transplantation
- **Screening**–Recommended for light skin types, immunosuppression and a family or personal history of skin cancer

CHAPTER 46

OTHER MALIGNANT SKIN CANCERS

MOST FREQUENTLY ASKED TOPICS IN INSTITUTE BASED EXAMS

Merkel cell carcinoma

Neuroendocrine tumor of skin

Trabecular carcinoma skin

Cutaneous APUDomas

- Arises from merkel cells of basal layer of epidermis ***(Mechanoreceptors)***
- ***Most important cause of merkel cell carcinoma is Polyoma virus (80%)***
- **Risk Factors:** Sun exposure, Advanced age and Chronic immunosuppression
- Median age of presentation–**65 years**
- ***Most common site***–Head and neck (30-45%) and Extremities (35%)
- 75% are localized, LN–25% of cases, Distant metastasis–2 to 4%
- Diagnosis–**Biopsy**
- **Treatment: WLE (2-3 cm)**
- Radiosensitive–Unfit for surgery
- Adjuvant Radiation–Incomplete resection/Larger tumor size (>2cm/more)
- N+ → *Lymph node dissection followed by RT*
- Extent of disease is most important prognostic factor
- ***Nodal disease–Decreases overall survival***
- Radiologically demonstrable nodal involvement–Total lymphadenectomy
- Most common site of distant metastasis–Liver > Brain and Lungs
- **Chemotherapy**–Not considered for node –ve disease

  High risk and metastatic disease
- **Stain +ve for NSE and Anticytokeratin antibody CAM 5.2**

Angiosarcoma

(Malignant Heamangioendothelioma, Hemangiosarcoma):

- 2% of sarcomas
- Elderly whites
- **Women, Multifocal**
- **Most common site involved–Head and neck *(Scalp)***

TYPES
Idiopathic–Most common (50-60%)–Head and neck
Stewart Treves syndrome–Lymphedema associated Angiosarcoma
Radiation induced Angiosarcoma
Epitheloid Angiosarcoma

Contd.

Contd.

- Most common mode of spread–Hematogenous
- High grade lesion–***Lung metastasis***
- Post Mastectomy–Stewart Treves syndrome
- **Treatment: Resect+RT**
- **Associated with CD31–FLI 1**
- 5 years survival rate–35%
- **Poor prognosis**→ >5 cm, Epitheloid

DFSP
(Dermatofibrosarcoma Protuberans)

- **Low grade**
- Arise from dermal fibroblasts
- **Most common site**–*TRUNK*
- Associated with PDGF beta
- *90% Associated with t (17,22)/COLA1A1–PDGF Beta translocation*
- Fibrosarcoma–Aggressive and High risk of distant spread
- **Treatment:** WLE (2-4 cm)
- **Recurrence**→ Resection + RT

Extramammary Paget's Disease	Kaposi Sarcoma
• **Most common site involved–*Vulva***	• Associated with HHV 8 and HIV
• **Diagnosis**–Biopsy	• **Treatment:**
• **Treatment:** Excision	Antiretroviral therapy
• **Increased risk** of GI and Genitourinary malignancies	Symptomatic–RT
• **RT**– Reduces recurrence	

CHAPTER 47

MALIGNANT MUCOSAL MELANOMA

- Most common site of mucosal melanoma is head and neck
- Most common site of head and neck mucosal melanoma is sinonasal region
- Most common site in sinonasal region is nasal cavity (80%)
- Anterior portion of nasal septum accounts for most cases of nasal cavity mucosal melanoma
- Maxillary sinus is the most common site involved among paranasal sinus
- **Most common site of laryngeal mucosal melanoma is Supraglottic region**

PART ONE: BREAST CANCER

CHAPTER 48 BREAST CANCER

A. BREAST CANCER

LYMPHATIC SUPPLY

- Level I nodes–Located lateral to the lateral border of the pectoralis minor muscle
- Level II nodes–Located between medial and lateral border of pectoralis minor muscle both anteriorly and posteriorly
- Level III nodes–Located medial to pectoralis minor muscle and include subclavicular nodes

Surgical levels	Anatomical importance
I	Pectoral axillary lymph nodes (anterior) Subscapsular axillary lymph nodes (posterior) Humeral axillary lymph nodes (lateral)
II	Central axillary lymph nodes Some apical axillary lymph nodes Interpectoral lymph nodes (Rotter's)*
III	Apical axillary lymph nodes

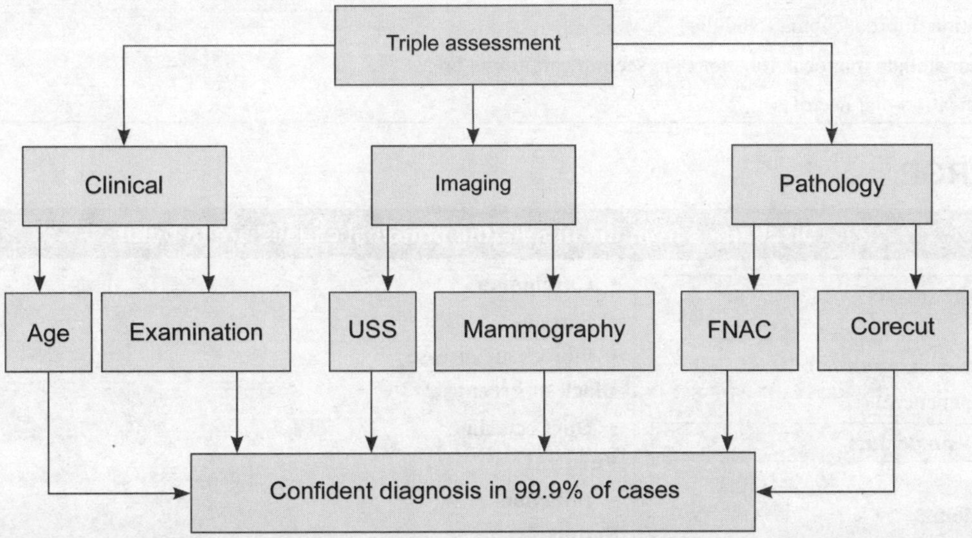

Investigation of a breast lump (after imaging performed) using fine-needle aspiration cytology		
Cystic	Lump disappears; clear fluid (many colours)	Discharge patient
	Residual thickening; blood-stained fluid	Investigate–? core biopsy
Solid	Benign	Offer excision or observe
	Atypical	Investigate– ?core biopsy
	Malignant	Treat for cancer

SENTINEL LYMPH NODE BIOPSY

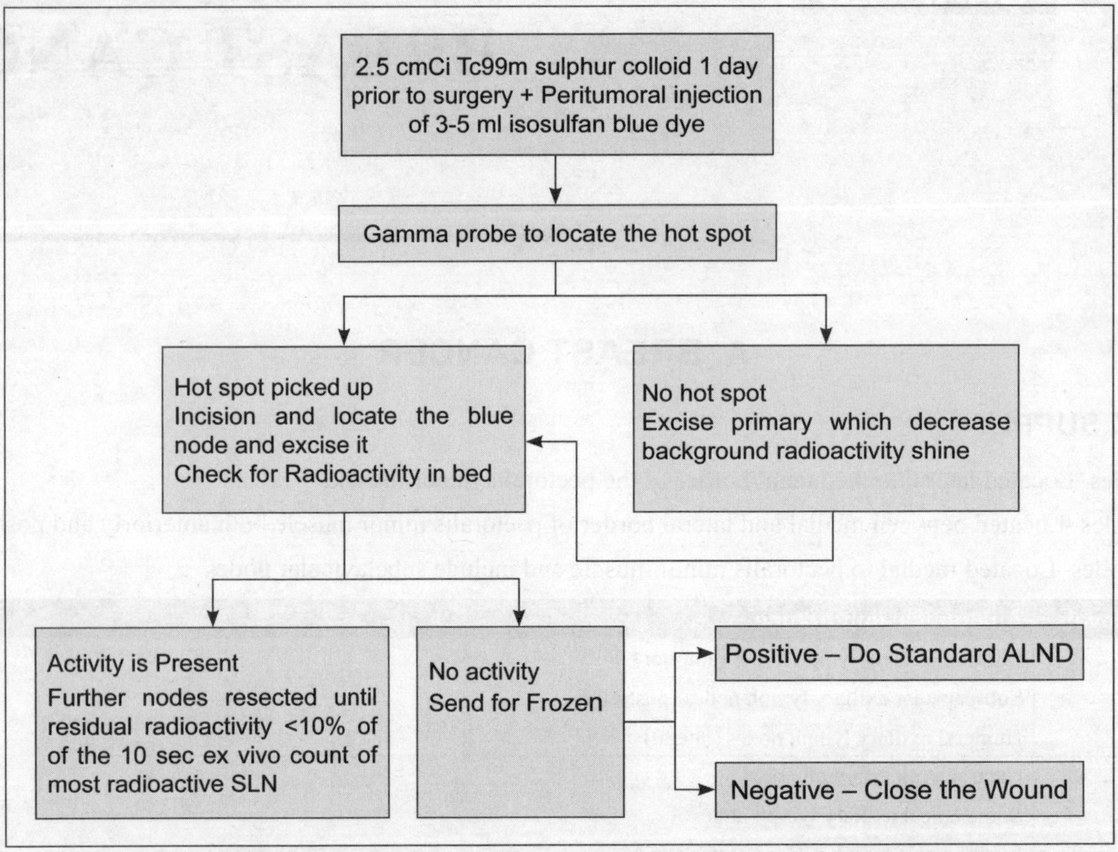

Mammographic findings
• Powdery calcification–Fibrocystic disease • Popcorn calcification–Fibroadenoma (Nodular) • Pleomorphic linear stellate microcalcifications are seen in carcinoma breast • Curvilinear calcification–Fat necrosis

NIPPLE DISCHARGE

Discharges from the nipple (the principal causes are in bold)	
Discharge from the surface • Paget's disease • Skin diseases (aczema, psoriasis) • Rare causes (e.g. chancre) **Discharge from a single duct** **Blood-stained** • **Intraduct papilloma** • **Intraduct carcinoma** • Duct ectasia **Serous (any colour)** • **Fibrocystic disease** • **Duct ectasia** • Carcinoama **Discharge from more than duct** **Blood-stained**	• **Carcinoma** • Ectasia • Fibrocystic disease **Black or green:** • **Duct ectasia** **Purulent** • **Infection** **Serous** • **Fibrocystic disease** • Duct ectasia • Carcinoma **Milk** • **Lactation** • Rare cause (hypothyroidism, pituitary tumor)

	Mutation	Associated Risk
BRCA1	Chromosome 17q	Malignancies of the breast, ovaries, and possibly prostate and colon
BRCA2	Chromosome 13q	Malignancies of the breast (including male), ovaries, prostate, larynx and pancreas
Li-Fraumeni	p53 gene on chromosome 17p	Malignancies of the breast, brain and adrenal glands; soft-tissue sarcomas
Cowden disease	Mutation in the *PTEN* gene on chromosome 10q	Malignancies of the breast, colon, uterus, thyroid, lung and bladder, hamartomatous polyps in GI tract
Peutz-Jeghers	Mutation in the *STK11* gene on chromosome 19p	Malignancies of the breast and pancreas; mucocutaneous melanin deposition, hamartomas of the GI tract

Risk factors for breast cancer in women

- Increasing age
- Family history of breast cancer at a younger age
- Nulliparity
- Early menarche and Late menopause
- **Genetic mutations–BRCA 1 and 2 (85%)**
- Older age at 1st child birth
- Atypical lobular hyperplasia/ductal hyperplasia
- Prior breast biopsies
- Increased mammographic breast density
- Long term postmenopausal estrogen replacement
- Early exposure to ionizing radiation

Relative risk of invasive breast carcinoma based on pathological examination of benign breast tissue (American College of Pathologists Consensus Statement)

No increased risk	Adenosis, sclerosing or florid
	Apocrine metaplasia
	Cysts, macro and/or micro
	Duct ectasia
	Fibroadenoma
	Fibrosis
	Hyperplasia
	Mastitis (inflammation)
	Periductal mastitis
	Squamous metaplasia
Slightly increased risk (1.5-2 times)	Hyperplasia, moderate or florid, solid or papillary
	Papilloma with a fibrovascular core
Moderately increased risk (5 times)	Atypical hyperplasia (ductal or lobular)
Insufficient data to assign a risk	Solitary papilloma of lactiferous sinus
	Radial scar lesion

Likelihood of genetic mutation with family history

No. of family cases <50 years old	*BRCA1* (96)	*BRCA2* (%)
2	4	3
3	17	13
4	41	33
5	55	44

Recommended guidelines for screening
• BSE (Breast self examination) monthly started at age of 18 years
• Clinical breast examination every 3 years starting at age 25 years and annually for women above 40 years age
• Annual mammogram and breast MRI starting at age 25/5 years Earlier than youngest relative based on family history
• Bilateral prophylactic mastectomy could prevent breast cancer in 90 to 100%

TYPES OF CALCIFICATION

Type of Calcification	Description
Typical Benign	
Skin (dermal)	Typical lucent-centered deposits that are pathognomonic. Atypical forms may be confirmed by tangential views to be in the skin
Vascular	Parallel track or linear tubular calcifications that are clearly associated with blood vessels
Coarse or popcorn-like	The classic calcifications produced by an involuting fibroadenoma
Large rod-like	Benign calcification forming continuous rods that occasionally may be branching. They usually are >1 mm in diameter, and may have lucent centers, if calcium surrounds rather than fills an ectatic duct. These are the kinds of calcifications found in secretory disease, "plasma cell mastitis" and duct ectasia
Round	When multiple, they may vary in size. They usually are considered benign, and when small (<1 mm), they often are formed in the acini of lobules. When <0.5 mm, the term "punctate" can be used
Lucent-centered	Benign calcification ranging from <1 mm to ≥1 cm. These deposits have a smooth surface, are round or oval, and have a lucent center. The "wall" that is created is thicker than the "rim" or "eggshell" type of calcifications, included are areas of fat necrosis, calcified debris in ducts, and occasional fibroadenomas
Eggshell or rim	Very thin, benign calcification that appear as calcium deposited on the surface of a sphere. These deposits usually are <1 mm thick when viewed on edge. Although fat necrosis can produce these thin deposits, calcification in the walls of cysts are the most common "rim" calcifications
Milk of calcium	Consistent with sedimented calcifications in cysts. On the craniocaudal image, they often are less evident and appear as fuzzy, round amorphous deposits; on the 90-degree lateral view, they are sharply defined, similunar, crescent-shaped, curvilinear, or linear, defining the dependent portions of cysts
Suture	Calcium deposited on suture material. They are relatively common in the postirradiated breast. They typically are linear or tubular in appearance, and knots often are visible
Dystrophic	Calcifications that usually form in the irradiated breast or in the breast after trauma. Although irregular in shape, they usually are >0.5 mm in size . They often have lucent centers
Punctate	Round or oval, >0.5 mm, with well-defined margins
Intermediate Concern	
Amorphous or indistinct	Often round or flake-shaped calcifications that are so small or hazy that a more specific morphologic classification cannot be determined
Higher Probability of Malignancy	
Pleomorphic or heterogeneous (granular)	Usually more conspicuous than the amorphic forms. They are neither typically benign nor typically malignant irregular calcifications. They vary in size and shape and are usually <0.5 mm in diameter
Fine linear, or fine linear branching (casting)	Thin, irregular calcifications that appear linear, but are discontinuous and <0.5 mm wide. Their appearance suggests filling of the lumen of a duct involved irregularly by breast cancer
Distribution Modifiers	Used as modifiers of the basic morphologic description. These terms describe the arrangement of the calcification. Multiple similar groups may be indicated when there is more than one group of calcifications that are similar in morphology and distribution
Grouped or clustered	Although historically the term "clustered" has connoted suspicion, the term is now used as a neutral distribution modifier and may reflect benign or malignant processes. It is used when multiple calcifications occupy a small volume (<2 mL) of tissue
Linear	Calcification are arrayed in a line that have branch points
Segmental	Worrisome in that their distribution suggests deposits in a duct and its branches, raising the possibility of multifocal breast cancer in a lobe or segment of the breast. Although benign causes of segmental calcifications exist (e.g., secretory disease), this distribution is of greater concern when the morphology of the calcifications is not specifically benign

Contd.

Contd.

Regional	Calcifications scattered in a large volume of breast tissue and not necessarily conforming to a duct distribution. They are likely benign, but are not everywhere in the breast, and do not fit the other, more suspicious categories
Diffuse/scattered	Calcifications that are distributed randomly throughout the breast

GAIL MODEL: *Deals with women's absolute risk of developing breast cancer*

GAIL RISK MODEL→1.66%

- Age
- Age at menarche
- Age at 1st live birth
- No. of previous biopsies
- History of atypical ductal hyperplasia
- No. of 1st degree relatives with breast cancer

Histology

- Most common site is upper outer quadrant
- ***Most common type is infiltrating ductal carcinoma–NOS***
- Best prognosis is seen with Tubular and colloidal
- Worst prognosis is with Infiltrating ductal type
- Earliest metastasis is seen with Infiltrating ductal type
- ***INDIAN FILE PATTERN** is seen with **INFILTRATING LOBULAR CARCINOMA***
- **Nottingham's prognostic index:** SCORE= (0.2*size in cm) + stage of node + tumor grade
- **Inflammatory breast cancer is the most aggressive forms of CA Breast**
- Mucinous and Tubular types have better prognosis
- Triple –ve CA breast had more aggressive clinical course

Association of clinicopathologic features of breast cancer with intrinsic subtype

Intrinsic subtype	Luminal A	Luminal B	*HER2* Enriched	Basal-like
ER/PR expression	Positive–strong	Positive–variable	Positive or negative	Negative
HER2 amplification	Rare	Rare though small percentage positive	Common	Negative
Grade	Low to intermediate	Intermediate to high	Intermediate to high	High
P53 mutation	Rare	Uncommon	Common	Common
Ki67	Low	Intermediate to high	High	High
DNA copy number	Diploid	Aneuploid	Aneuploid; high genomic instability	Aneuploid; high genomic instability
mRNA expression signature	High ER cluster, low proliferation	Lower ER cluster, high proliferation	High *HER2* amplicon, high proliferation	Basal signature, high proliferation

A pragmatic classification of breast cancer

Group	Approximate 5-year survival rate (%)	Example	Treatment
'Very low risk' primary breast cancer	>90	Screen-detected DCIS, tubular or special types	Local
'Low-risk' primary breast cancer	70-90	Node negative with favourable histology	Locoregional with/without systemic
'High-risk' primary breast cancer	<70	Node positive or unfavourable histology	Locoregional with systemic
Locally advanced	<30	Large primary or inflammatory	Primary systemic
Metastatic	–	–	Primary systemic

BIRADS SCORING

Categories	Inference	Remarks
0	Incomplete	Needs additional imaging
I	Negative	No features (Nothing to comment on)
II	Benign	Benign lesions (fibroadenoma, lipoma, cyst, galactocele)
III	Possibly benign	<2% malignant risk
		Noncalcified circumscribed solid mass/focal asymmetry/cluster of punctate calcifications
		Needs follow up for short interval
IV	Suspicious abnormality	Biopsy to be considered
		A,B,C – Low intermediate and moderate risk
		2-95% malignant risk
V	Highly suggestive of malignancy	>95% probability of cancer. Appropriate action should be taken
VI	Known biopsy proven malignancy	

NCCN Guidelines Indicate that Following Needs Genetic Risk Evaluation

- Early age onset breast cancer
- Triple –ve breast cancer
- >2 breast primaries in single individual / 2 different individuals from same side of family
- >1 close blood relative with breast cancer <50 years age
- >2 close blood relative with breast cancer/pancreatic cancer at any age
- Population at increased risk
- Male breast cancer

Role of MRI in Breast Cancer

- BRCA Mutations
- Life time risk of breast cancer exceeds >20%
- Patients with prior radiotherapy who are >25 years age and women with genetic predisposition for breast cancer starting at the age of 25
- Extent of disease in cancer patients–multifocal, multicentric, chest involved, C/L breast, pectoralis involvement
- Response to neoadjuvant chemotherapy
- Axillary adenopathy
- Postlumpectomy for residual disease (+ve margins)
- Inconclusive mammographic findings, USG, Examination

Modified Van Nuys Prognostic Index→

VNPI: 4 to 6→100%, 7 to 9→100%, 10 to 12→97.6% (5 year survival)

Score	1	2	3
Size (mm)	<15	16-40	>41
Margins (mm)	>10	1-9	<1
Age	<61	40-60	<39
Pathology	Non high grade without necrosis	Non high grade with necrosis	High grade with /without necrosis

Classification of breast ductal carcinoma in situ (DCIS)			
Histologic Subtype	Determining Characteristics		DCIS Grade
	Nuclear Grade	Necrosis	
Comedo	High	Extensive	High
Intermediate	Intermediate	Focal or absent	Intermediate
Noncomedo	Low	Absent	Low

Salient characteristics of in situ ductal (DCIS) and lobular (LCIS) carcinoma of the breast		
	LCIS	DCIS
Age (years)	44-47	54-58
Incidence	2%-5%	5%-10%
Clinical signs	None	Mass, pain, nipple discharge
Mammographic signs	None	Microcalcifications
Premenopausal	2/3	1/3
Incidence of synchronous invasive carcinoma	5%	2%-46%
Multicentricity	60%-90%	40%-80%
Bilaterality	50%-70%	10%-20%
Axillary metastasis	1%	1%-2%
Subsequent Carcinomas		
• Incidence	25%-35%	25%-70%
• Laterality	Bilateral	Ipsilateral
• Interval to diagnosis	15-20 years	5-10 years
• Histologic type	Ductal	Ductal

Indications for Surgical Biopsy after Core Needle Biopsy

- Failure to sample calcifications
- Diagnosis of alypical ductal hyperplasia
- Diagnosis of pleomorphic LCIS
- Lack of concordance between imaging findings and histologic diagnosis
- Radical scar or complex sclerosing lesions
- Papillary lesions

American College of Radiology BI-RADS System for Reporting Mammographic Findings as follows:

- **Category 1:** *Negative*
- **Category 2:** *Benign finding*
- **Category 3:** *Probably benign finding.* Short interval follow-up is suggested. The findings have very high probability of being benign, but the radiologist would prefer to establish stability
- **Category 4:** *Suspicious abnormality:* Biopsy should be considered. These are lesions that don't have characteristic findings of breast cancer, but have definite probability of being malignant
- **Category 5:** *Highly suggestive of malignancy*

- In western countries >90% of patients will have localized disease only
- About 5 to 10% of breast cancers are familial/hereditary
- Most common mutations of genes involves are BRCA 1 and BRCA 2

- Mutations of BRCA 1 and 2 involve 45 to 84% life time risk for breast cancer as well as increased risk of contralateral breast cancer
- Mutations of BRCA 1 and 2 involve 11 to 62% life time risk of ovarian cancer
- Positive genetic test indicates that there exists mutation in BRCA 1/2 that has been associated with inherited risk of developing breast cancer
- ***Bilateral salpingo-oophorectomy ideally recommended between age of 35 and 40 years/after completing child bearing. BSO alone reduces breast cancer risk by 50% and ovarian cancer by 95%***
- There is 49% reduction of risk in incidence of invasive breast cancer in high risk patients who took tamoxifen at dose of 20 mg daily for 5 years
- Raloxifene won't decrease the risk of DCIS or LCIS unlike tamoxifen
- Positive HER 2/neu is either IHC 3+/FISH amplified (HER-2/neu to CEP 17) ratio >2 or Average HER-2/neu gene copy number >6 signals/nucleus
- Indices of proliferation include Mitotic index, Ki-67/Sphase
- **Ki-67 is helpful in distinguishing Luminal A versus B in ER/PR +ve lesions**
- PET scan is useful in locally advanced and metastatic breast cancers
- **Most important prognostic factor in Carcinoma Breast is Axillary lymph node involvement**

Modified scarff bloom Richardson grading system assigns score (1 to 3)–Size, Mitosis, Tubule formation
3-5 points→low grade, 6-7 points→intermediate grade and 8-9 points→high grade
Scarff bloom Richardson and Fisher nuclear grading systems are used

- ER and PR +ve tumors have better prognosis and these patients are eligible for endocrine therapy
- HER 2/neu overexpression is poor prognostic factor in CA Breast

Oncotype Dx

- Diagnostic genomic assay based on RT-PCR on paraffin embedded tissue
- Likelihood of cancer recurrence in women with newly diagnosed stage 1 and 2, node –ve, ER +ve CA Breast

Based on expression of panel of 21 genes

- *Low risk→<18→Endocrine therapy*
- *Intermediate risk→18-30→Endocrine+Chemotherapy*
- *High risk→>31→Endocrine+Chemotherapy*

Mammaprint

- Mammaprint is a DNA microassay of 70 genes designed to predict recurrence of early stage breast cancer
- FDA approved Mammaprint for patients <61 years, size <5 cm and lymph node –ve

- ER –ve breast cancers are basal like, claudin low, interferon rich, androgen receptor and Normal like subtypes
- Atypical ductal hyperplasia→Reduces risk of development of invasive breast cancer→Tamoxifen 20 mg for 5 years/Raloxifene 60 mg daily for 5 years (postmenopausal)
- **LCIS is a marker of increased risk of developing invasive breast cancer → Multicentric and bilateral**
- LCIS patients are followed up for Clinical breast examination every 4 to 12 months and annual mammogram/MRI
- Comedocarcinoma is a type of DCIS with poor prognosis
- **Lumpectomy followed by radiation followed by tamoxifen for 5 years is standard treatment option for DCIS**

  Breast conservation treatment is preferred for early invasive breast cancer

Contraindications to BCT
• Prior Radiotherapy to breast/chest wall
• Radiation therapy during pregnancy
• Diffuse suspicious/malignant appearing microcalcifications
• Widespread disease that can't be incorporated by local excision through single incision that achieves –ve margins with satisfactory cosmetic result
• +ve pathologic margins

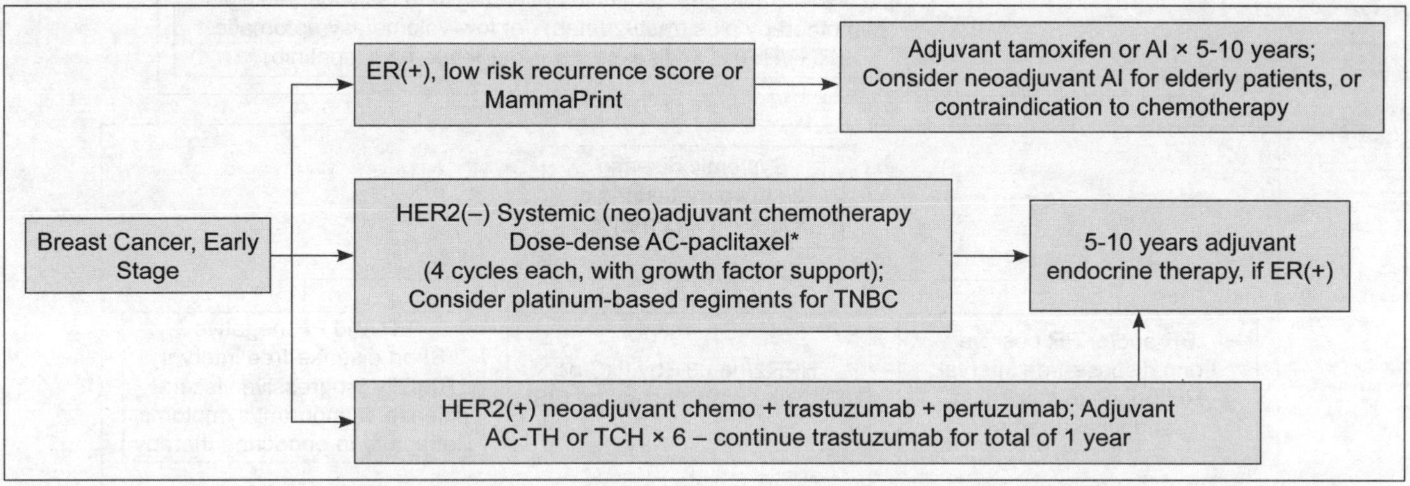

- In developed countries breast cancer is the most commonly diagnosed malignancy and 2nd leading cause of cancer death
- Full field mammography has highest diagnostic accuracy in patients with dense breasts, women under 50 years age, premenopausal and perimenopausal women

Chemotherapy should be considered in following patients
• ER/PR –ve patients
• HER 2/neu +ve patients
• Triple –ve patients
• Node +ve patients
• High risk patients based on Oncotype Dx, Mammaprint or other prognostic classification
• Patients under age of 35 years

ASCO guidelines for indications of post mastectomy RT
a. Patients with T3N1, or stage III tumors
b. Patients with ≥4 positive axillary nodes
c. Positive or close (<1 mm) surgical margins

- APBI→Brachytherapy is used treatment 34 Gy in 10 fractions delivered twice daily
- **Neoadjuvant preoperative chemotherapy→IIB, IIIA, IIIB, IIIC (locally advanced breast cancer) and Inflammatory breast cancer**
- Aromatase inhibitors are approved by FDA for use in **postmenopausal** women with breast cancer as adjuvant chemotherapy agents (Anastrozole 1 mg PO daily for 5 years and Letrozole 2.5 mg PO daily for 5 years
- HER 2/neu Premenopausal women→Tamoxifen 20 mg + Ovarian ablation/suppression with endocrine therapy (Aromatase inhibitors)
- ***LD flap is safer in obese or who have compromised vascular supply due to diabetes/smoking***

Management of Metastatic Breast Cancer

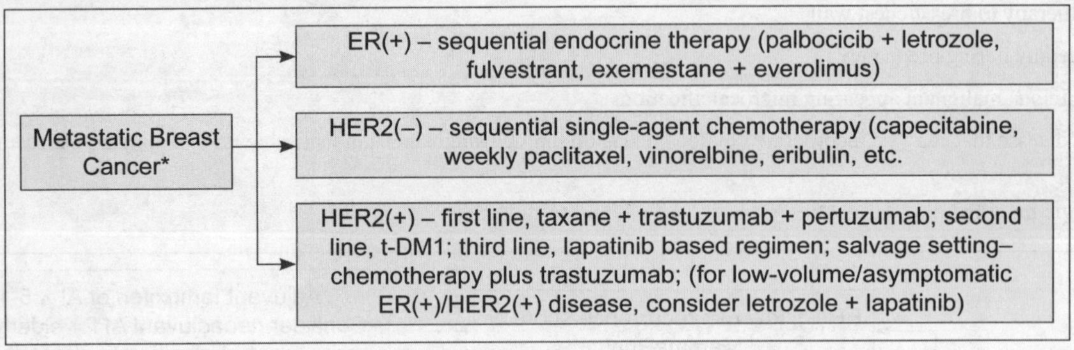

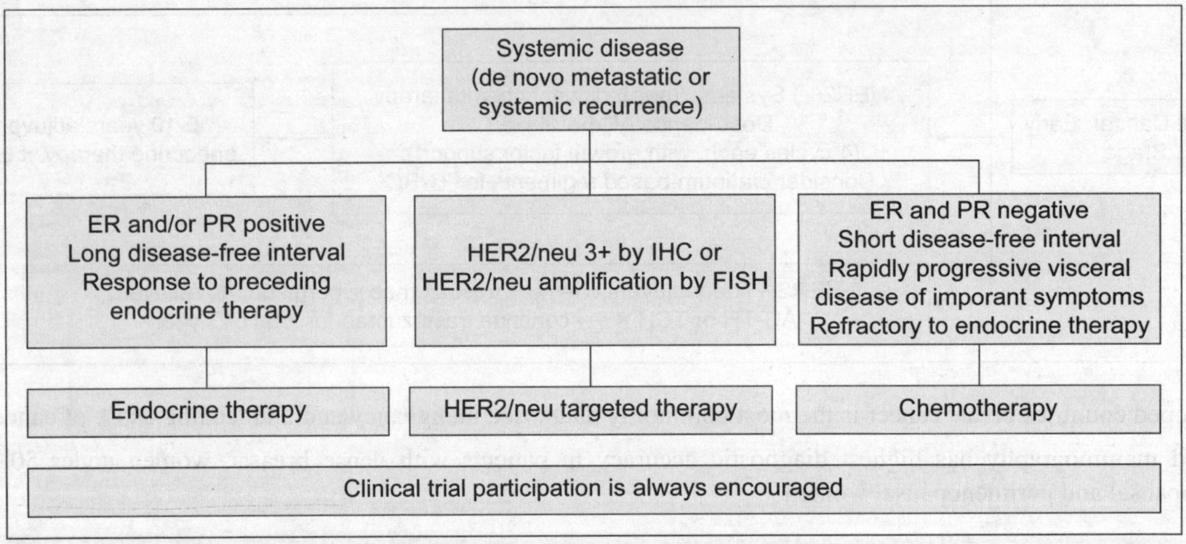

Endocrine Therapies for Metastatic Breast Cancer

- Ovarian suppression/ablation (premenopausal women)
- Selective estrogen receptor modulators (tamoxifen, toremifene)
- Aromatase inhibitors (anastrozole, letrozole, exemestance, postmenopausal women)
- Antiestrogens (fulvestrant; postmenopausal women)
- Progestins (megestrol and medroxyprogesterone)
- Other steroid hormones (high-dose estrogens, androgens; principally of historical interest)

Trials

- **ATAC trial**→Non-significant reduction in contralateral breast cancers in women treated with anastrozole alone compared to tamoxifen
- **BIG 1-98 Trial**→Compared postmenopausal women with early stage breast cancer to those who underwent 5 years of therapy and found that risk of breast cancer recurrence was lower in women in letrozole arm compared to tamoxifen arm
- **MAP.3 Trial**→Role of exemestane in risk reduction setting randomizing women to either exemastane or placebo

Women aged 40 years and older at an average risk of breast cancer should have mammograms every 1-2 years

- **DMIST (Digital mammographic imaging screening Trial)**→Pre/perimenopausal women under the age of 50/Women at any age with dense breasts had accurate detection of breast cancer with digital mammogram
- ACOSOG Z 0011 clinical trial showed no difference in overall survival and disease free survival in doing complete axillary node dissection in patients with clinical T1-T2 invasive breast cancer without palpable adenopathy and pathologic evidence of 1-2 SLN containing metastases
- **TCH and HERA Trial had less cardiac toxicity than compared to anthracycline containing regimen**
- **NeoSphere study design**

Contd.

Contd.

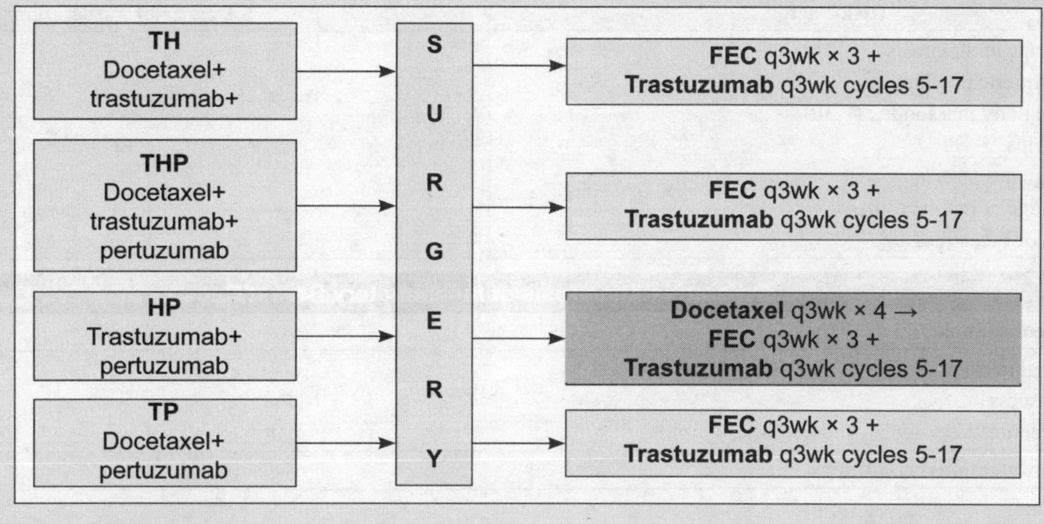

- **TRYPHAENA study design**

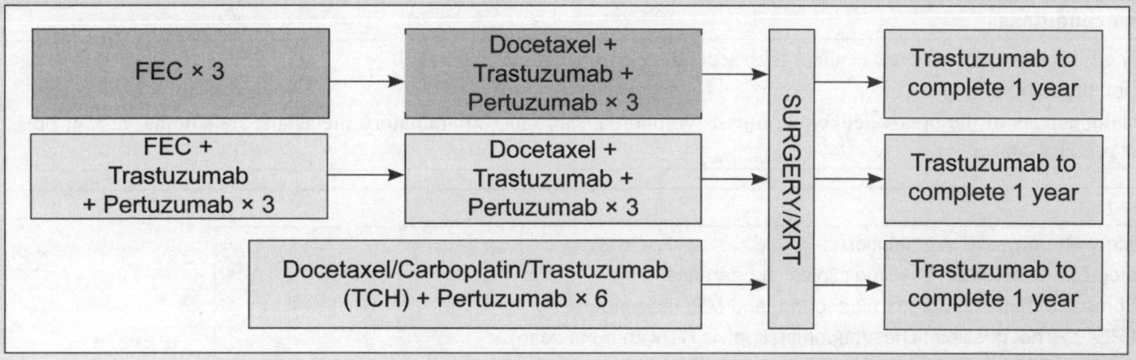

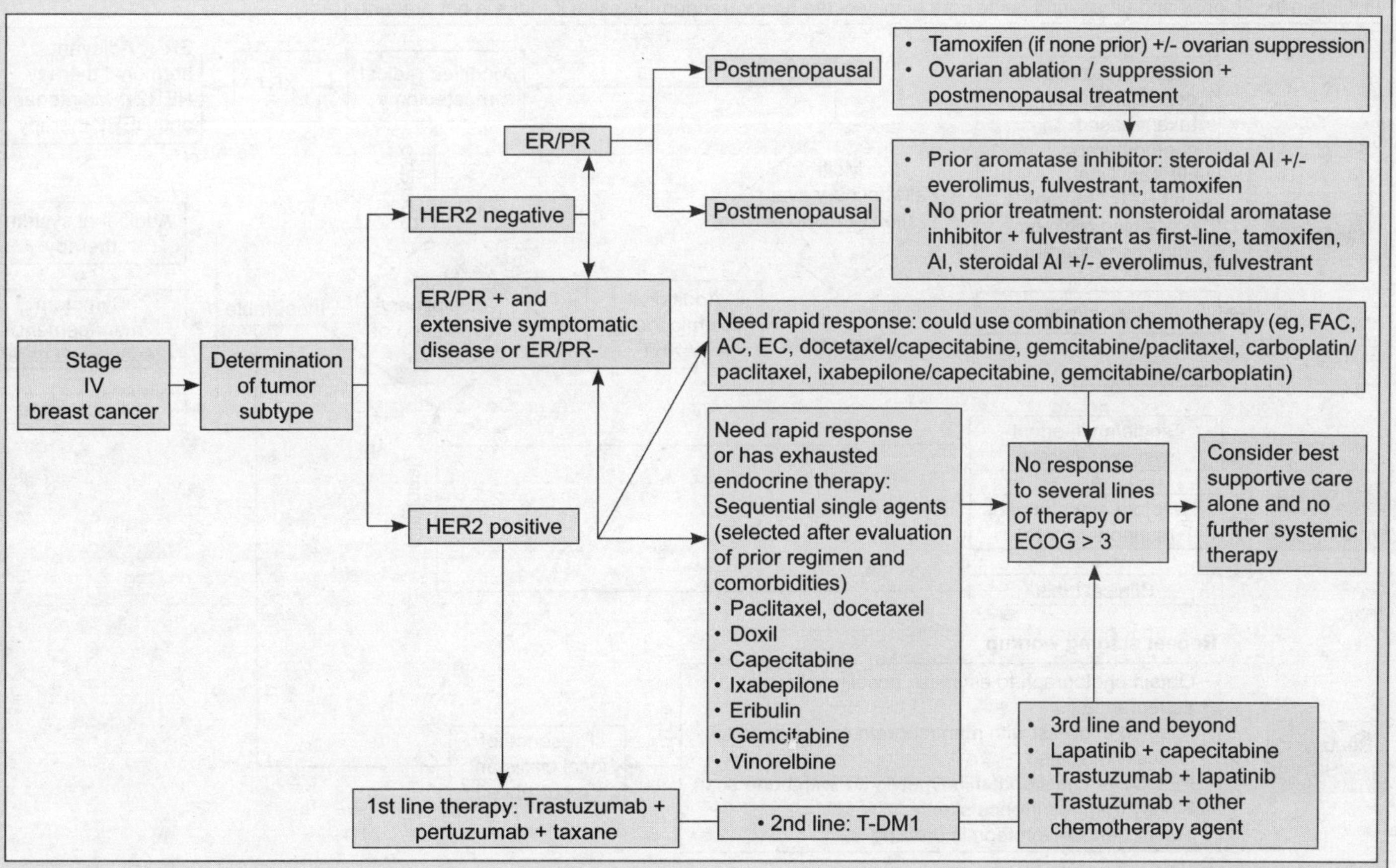

Risk Factors Associated With the Development of Inflammatory Breast Cancer	
Risk Factor	**Degree of Association**
• Younger age at diagnosis	+++
• African American ethnicity	+++
• Increased body mass index (≥ 30)	+++
• North Africa	++
• Ever pregnant	+
• Younger age at live first birth	+
• Duration of breastfeeding	+

Differential Diagnosis of Inflammatory Breast Cancer
Infectious conditions
• Lactational mastitis • Breast abscess • Other infections: erysipelas, tuberculosis, syphilis
Benign (noninfectious) conditions
• Dermatitis • Duct ectasia
Malignant conditions
• Locally advanced neglected breast cancer with secondary erythematous changes • Radiation dermatitis • Rare malignancies of the breast: leukemia, breast lymphoma, sarcoma, inflammatory metastatic melanoma, distant breast metastasis from another primary cancer

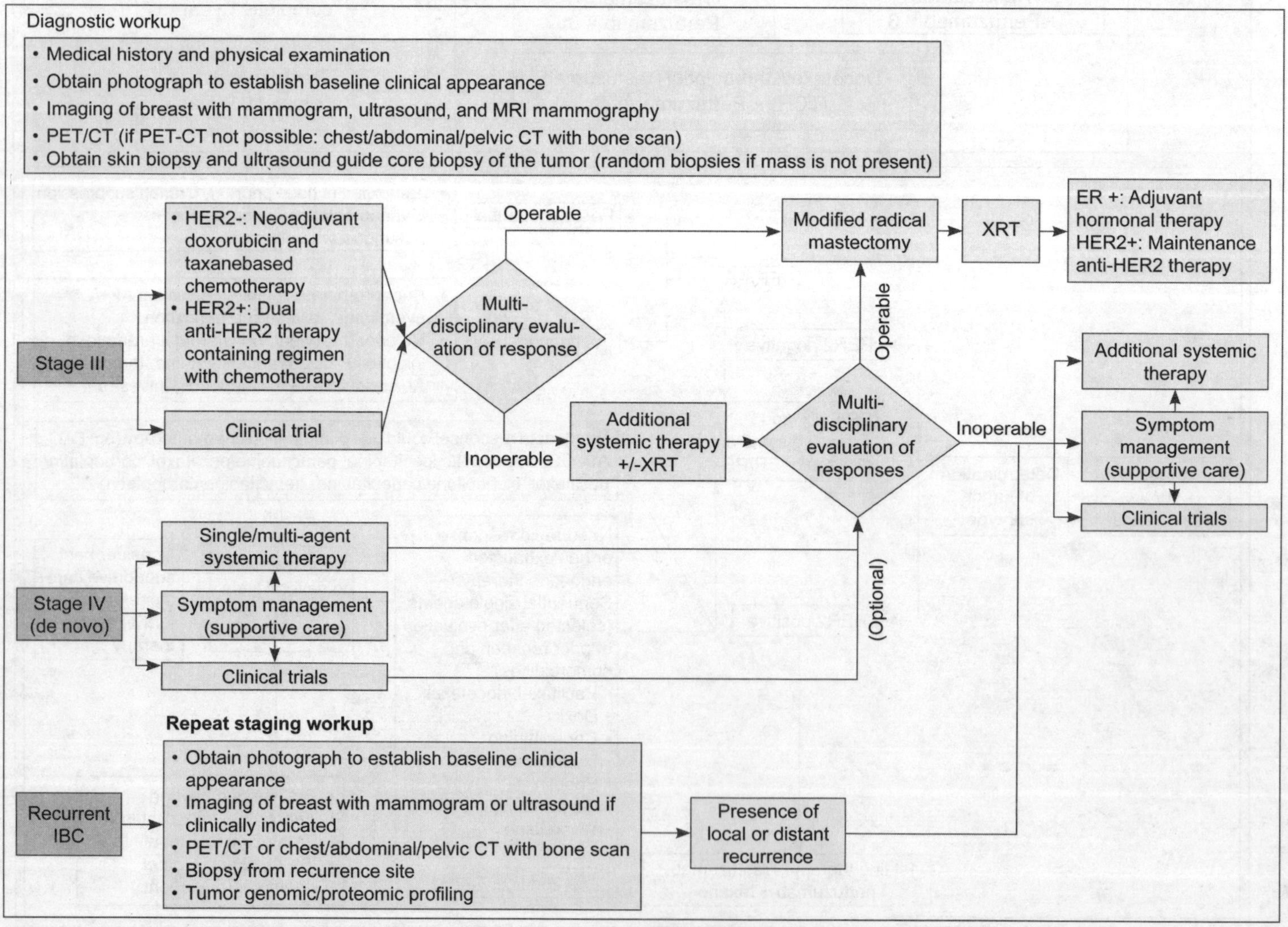

Overview of Adjuvant Treatment Approaches in Breast Cancer		
Tumor *HER* Status	**Tumor Hormone Receptor Status**	
	Positive	**Negative**
HER2 negative/normal	Endocrine therapy ± chemotherapy	Chemotherapy
HER2 positive/overexpressed	Endocrine therapy + chemotherapy + anti-HER2 antibodies	Chemotherapy + anti-HER2 antibodies

INITIAL ENDOCRINE THERAPY OPTIONS

No prior endocrine therapy or over one year since endocrine therapy

- Premenopausal→Anti-estrogen or OFS with endocrine therapy like postmenopausal women
- Postmenopausal→ Aromatase inhibitor or anti-estrogen

Prior endocrine therapy

- Second-line endocrine therapy (see below)

SUBSEQUENT ENDOCRINE THERAPY OPTIONS

Premenopausal patients

- Add OFS and treat like postmenopausal women

Postmenopausal patients

- Nonsteroidal (anastrozole, letrozole) or steroidal (exemestane) aromatase inhibitor

  Note: Men of any age should not receive an aromatase inhibitor without concomitant use of an LH-RH agonist
- Fulvestrant
- Tamoxifen or Toremifene
- Megestrol acetate
- Fluoxymesterone
- Ethinyl estradiol

Indications for Postmastectomy Radiation
Tumor >5 cm
T4 tumor
Involvement of 4 or more axillary lymph nodes
Gross extracapsular nodal disease
Residual disease after mastectomy
Additional Considerations
Involvement of 1 to 3 axillary lymph nodes
Gross multifocality
Extension into the nipple or skin

Breast Cancer Follow-up	
Recommended for Routine Surveillance	
History/physical examination	Every 3-6 months for the first 3 years, every 6-12 months for years 4 to 5 and annually thereafter
Mammography	Annually, beginning no earlier than 6 months after radiation therapy
Breast self-examination	All women should be counseled to perform monthly
Pelvic examination	Annually
Coordination of care	Continuity of care with breast cancer specialist and appropriate other health care providers
Not Recommended for Routine Surveillance	
Routine blood tests	Complete blood cell count and liver function tests are not recommended
Imaging studies	Chest radiograph, bone scans, liver ultrasound, computed tomography scans, fluorodeoxglucose–position emission tomography scans and breast magnetic resonance imaging are not recommended for routine breast cancer surveillance
Tumor markers	Cancer antigen 15-3, cancer antigen 27, 29 and carcinoembryonic antigen are not recommended

Breast Cancer in Pregnancy

- More aggressive and poorly differentiated
- **Breast biopsy is safe in all stages of pregnancy**
- 1 in 3000 pregnancies
- Core needle biopsy is preferred for histologic diagnosis and biomarker analysis
- Ductal carcinoma is the most common type
- Breast ultrasound is highly sensitive and specific in diagnosing breast cancer during pregnancy
- Overall poor outcome is likely related to advanced stage at time of diagnosis
- Mammography is difficult to interpret because of increased breast density
- Lumpectomy and axillary lymph node dissection is done in 3rd trimester and RT can be safely delayed until delivery
- MRM is the treatment of choice in 1st and 2nd trimester
- Breast cancer is most often associated with larger tumor size and lymph node metastasis
- More frequently ER -ve, PR –ve and HER 2 neu +ve
- Clinically node +ve/T3 breast lesions→Ultrasound liver and MRI thoracic and lumbar spine without contrast can be used
- Termination of pregnancy is contraindicated

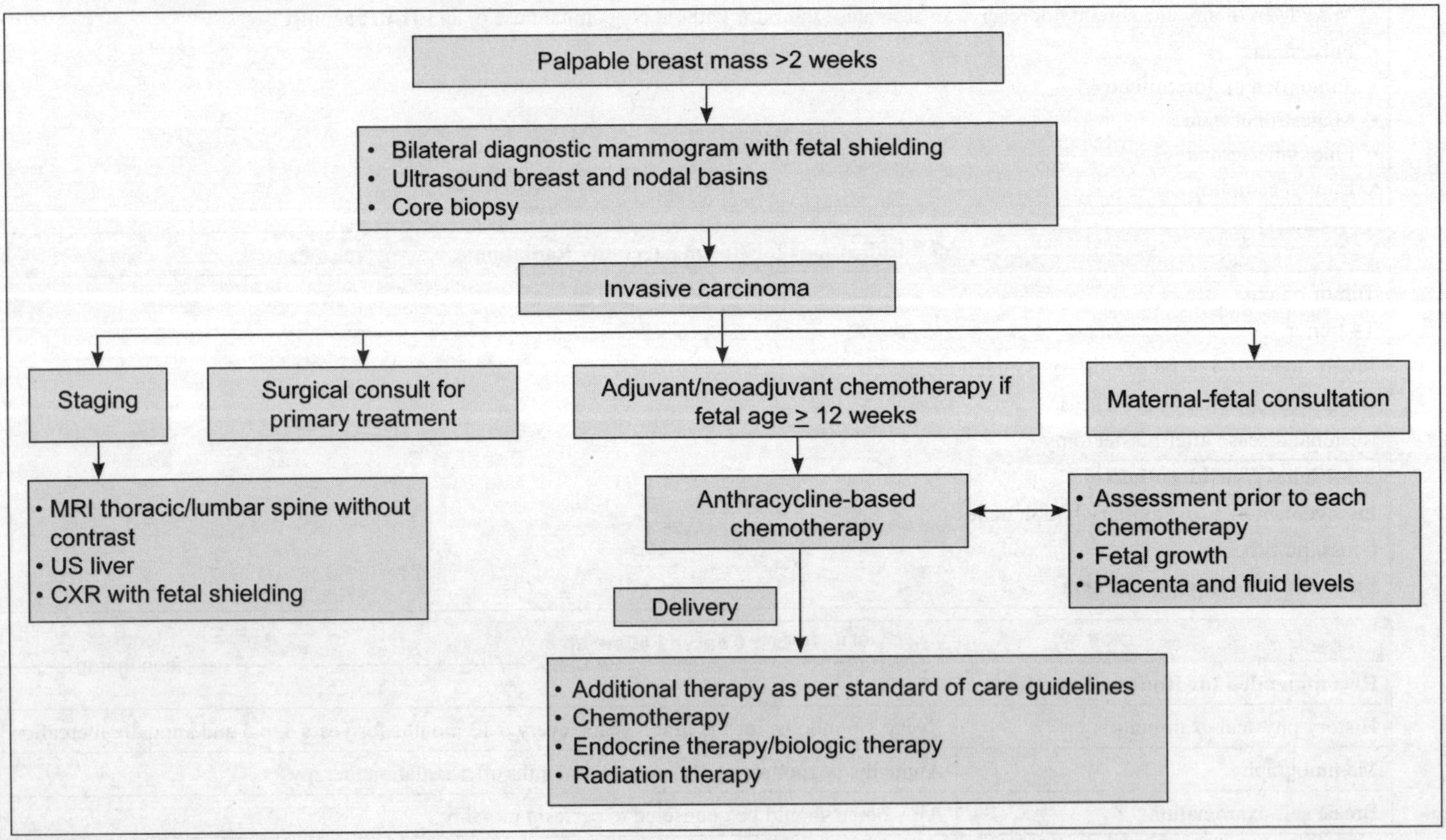

CYSTOSARCOMA PHYLLODES

- Constitute <1% of all breast neoplasms
- About 90% of phyllodes tumors are benign and about 10% are malignant
- Tumors rarely metastasize, they can recur locally
- Surgical resection with ample margins is necessary to optimize local control

ALGORITHMS

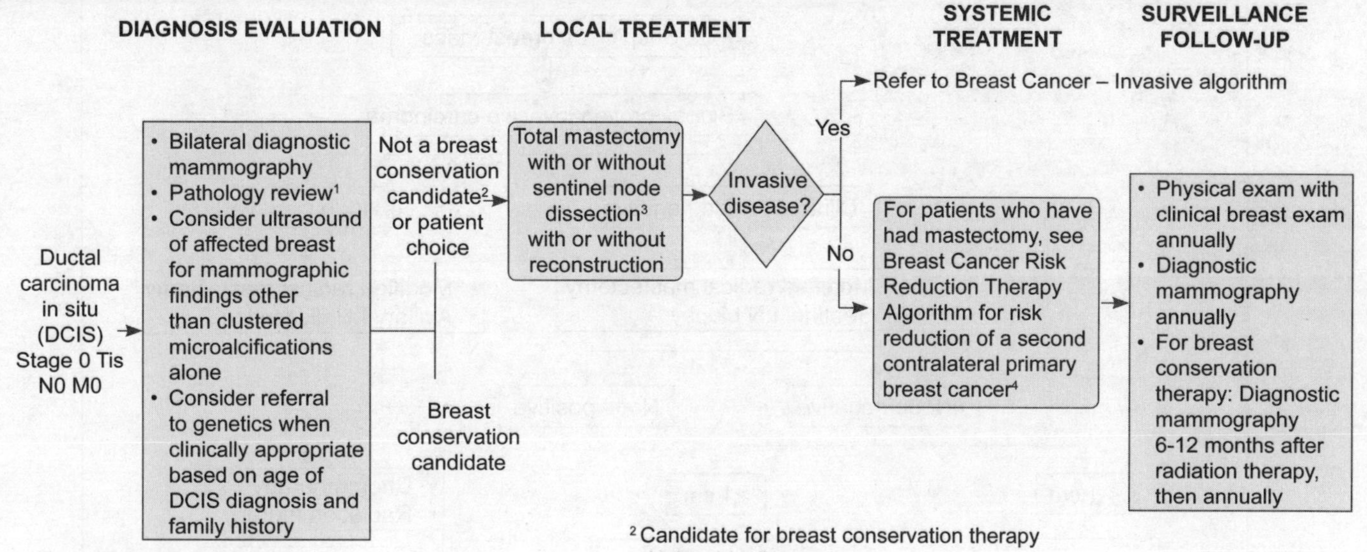

[1] Pathology review to include:
- Tumor size
- Rule out invasive component
- Lymph node status if lymph node surgery performed
- ER/PR status, preferably on the surgical specimen (unless patient is undergoing bilateral mastectomy)
- Margin status
- Nuclear grade
- Histologic type/necrosis

[2] Candidate for breast conservation therapy
- Unicentric disease
- Tumor to breast size ratio allows for acceptable cosmetic result
- Attempt margins greater than or equal to 2 mm
- No evidence of diffuse microcalcifications on mammography
- No contraindication to radiation therapy

[3] DCIS lymph node evaluation not recommended unless patient having total mastectomy which would preclude mapping at a later date if invasive disease noted on final pathology

[4] For estrogen receptor (ER) of progesterone receptor (PR) positive DCIS, Endocrine therapy with tamoxifen for 5 years or aromatise inhibitor (AI) therapy is also an option for postmenopausal patients for risk reduction. See Breast Cancer Risk Reduction Therapy algorithm for risk reduction of a second contralateral primary breast cancer. For patients who underwent bilateral mastectomy, there is 0 indication for risk reduction therapy

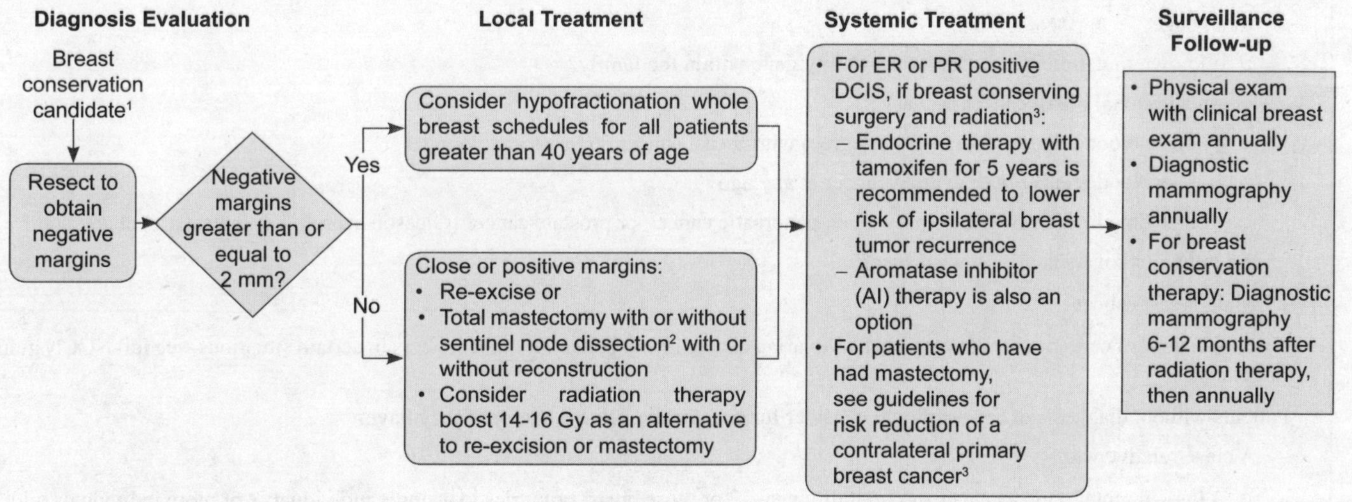

[1] Candidates for breast conservation therapy:
- Unicentric disease
- Tumor to breast size ratio allows for acceptable cosmetic result
- Attempt margins greater than or equal to 2 mm
- No evidence of diffuse microcalcification on mammography
- No contraindication to radiotherapy

[2] DCIS lymph node evaluation not recommended unless patient having total mastectomy which would prelude mapping at a later date if invasive disease noted on final pathology

[3] For ER or PR positive DCIS, if patient undergoes breast conserving surgery and radiation endocrine therapy is recommended to lower risk of ipsilateral breast tumor recurrence. The magnitude of local recurrence risk reduction depends on absolute risk of local recurrence based on factors such as grade and size (molecular profiling impact still is uncertain). Tamoxifen 20 mg daily for 5 mg daily for 5 years is approved to lower ipsilateral breast tumor recurrence after breast conserving surgery and radiation AI therapy (anastrazole 1mg daily for 5 years) has been shown to be equally effective, yet not FDA-approved for this indication. Endocrine therapy can also be considered for ER or PR positive DCIS treated with breast conserving surgery without radiation, but less supportive data exists. For patients undergoing mastectomy, refer to breast cancer prevention guidelines for prevention of a contralateral breast cancer

MALE BREAST CANCER

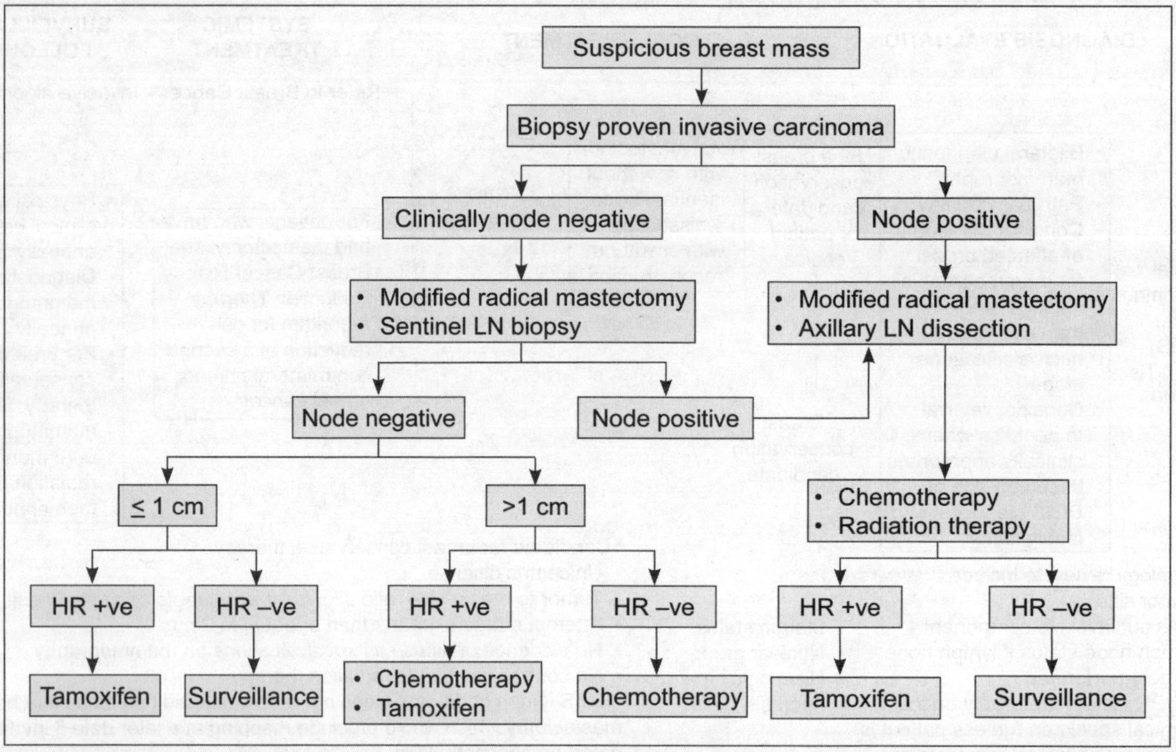

Factors Warranting Further Genetic Risk Evaluation

- Personal diagnosis of DCIS or invasive breast cancer + one or more the following:
  - Diagnosed 50 years and younger
  - Triple-negative breast cancer diagnosed 60 years and younger
  - At any age:
    - A known mutation in a cancer susceptibility gene within the family
    - An additional breast cancer primary
    - ≥1 close blood relative (first to third degree) with breast cancer 50 years and younger
    - ≥ close blood relative with ovarian cancer at any age
    - ≥ close blood relatives with breast cancer, pancreatic cancer, or prostate cancer (Gleason score ≥7 or metastatic) at any age
  - An individual of Ashkenazi Jewish ancestry
  - Male breast cancer
- Personal history of certain other cancers (such as ovarian cancer in any patient or other cancers in certain situations–see full NCCN guidelines for details)
- Patients without diagnosis of cancer should consider further genetic risk evaluation if they have:
  - A close relative with:
    - A known mutation in a cancer susceptibility gene: 2 or more breast primaries in a single individual: 2 or more individuals with breast cancer on the same side of the family with at least one diagnosed at age 50 years or younger; ovarian cancer; male breast cancer
  - A first or second degree relative with cancer at age 45 years or younger
  - A family history of 3 or the following: breast cancer, pancreatic cancer, prostate cancer (Gleason 7 or higher or metastatic), melanoma, sarcoma, adrenal cortical carcinoma, brain tumors, leukemia, diffuse gastric cancer, colon cancer, endometrial cancer, thyroid cancer, kidney cancer, dermatologic manifestations, and/or macrocephaly, or hamartomatous polyps of GI tract

B. BREAST RECONSTRUCTION

- **Lattismus dorsi–work horse flap for U/L defects in thin women with minimal donor sites, small breast women and salvage for failed breast reconstruction**

- **TUG FLAP–Transverse upper gracilis flap→Ascending branch of medial circumflex femoral artery**
- **TAZINI**–1st used lattismus dorsi flap
- TRAM flap is 1st used by **Robbins**
- **CZERNY** attempted breast reconstruction
- "To attempt to close the breast wound more or less regularly by any plastic method is hazardous, and in my opinion, to be vigorously discounted" is by **HALSTED**

One Liners
• Ruben flap is based on deep circumflex iliac artery (NEET SS)
• Best myocutaneous flap for breast reconstruction is TRAM flap (AIIMS SS)
• Best for bilateral reconstruction of breast is Implants (NEET SS)

- **ZONES FOR VASCULAR TERRITORIES OF TRAM FLAP:**
  - Zone 1→Perfusion is best overlying rectus muscle on the side (pedicle) used
  - Zone 2→The region overlying the contralateral rectus muscle
  - Zone 3→Ipsilateral outer region of tissue
  - Zone 4→ Region perfused the least is the farthest from the rectus pedicle

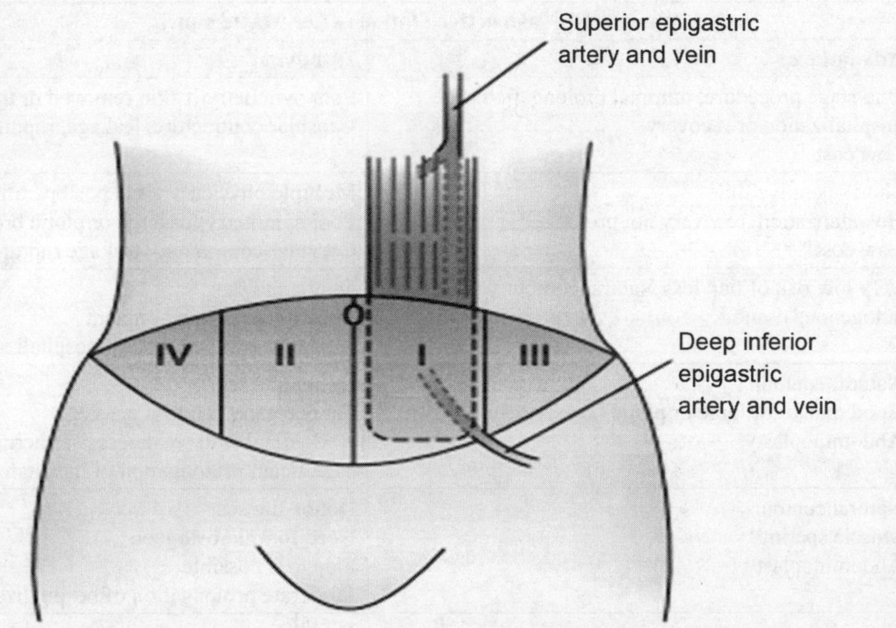

Vascular territories of the abdominal wall provided by a unilateral TRAM flap (as determined by Moon and Taylor). Blood flow is best in zone I, followed by zones II, III and IV

• Ideal time for breast reconstruction is immediately after mastectomy
• Ideal time for creating areola is 4-6 weeks after nipple reconstruction
• Ideal time for nipple reconstruction is 2-3 months after creating breast mound

- Most common complication of implant based reconstruction-capsular contraction
- ***Most common complication of LD flap reconstruction is Seroma***
- **Best investigation for recurrence after breast reconstruction is MRI**
- Contraindications to breast reconstruction include Extreme age, obesity, severe CVS disease, Advanced breast disease
- Reconstruction of breasts with inadequate donor sites is Implants

- Surgical reconstruction should never be done prior to radiation therapy
- Most common method of breast reconstruction now-a-days is silicone implants

Options for Breast Reconstruction	
Autogenous	Thoracoepigastric flap
• Abdominal-based flaps	Lateral thigh flap*
• TRAM	Breast-splitting procedure†
• Single pedicle	Alloplastic
• Double pedicle	• Silicone gel implant
• Free flap*	• Silicone implant with saline fill
• Deep interior epigastric perforator flap*	• Smooth wall
• Upper abdominal horizontal flap	• Textured wall
• Vertical abdominal flap	• Round
• Tubed abdominal flap	• Anatomic shaped
Latissimus dorsi musculocutaneous flap	• Silicone injection†
Gluteal flap*	Combination procedures
• Superiorly based	• Latissimus dorsi flap with implant
• Inferiorly based	• TRAM flap with implant
Rubens flap*	

Common Reconstructive Options after Mastectomy		
Type	**Advamtages**	**Disadvantages**
Implant	One-stage procedure, minimal prolongation of hospitalization or recovery Low cost	Poor symmetry if skin removed or in large ptotic breasts Capsular contracture, leakage, rupture possible
Tissue expander	Short operative time Hospitalization, recovery not prolonged Low cost	Multiple physician visits postoperatively Poor symmetry for large or ptotic breasts Capsular contracture, leakage rupture possible
Latissimus dorsi flap	Very low risk of flap loss Natural contour with autogenous tissue	Donor site scar Usually requires an implant Moderate prolongation of hospitalization and recovery
TRAM flap	Natural contour Good match for large or ptotic breasts Abdominoplasty	Donor site scar Fat necrosis, flap loss possible Abdominal wall weakness plus hernia Significant prolongation of hospitalization and recovery
DIEP flap	Natural contour Muscle sparing Abdominoplasty	Donor site scar Need for microsurgeon Flap loss possible Moderate prolongation of hospitalization and recovery
Superior gluteal artery perforator flap	Natural contour Alternative donor site	Donor site scar Need for microsurgeon Flap loss possible Moderate prolongation of hospitalization and recovery

Implant Reconstruction	
Indications	**Relative Contraindications**
Bilateral reconstruction	Young age (may need implant replaced multiple times)
Patient requesting augmentation in addition to reconstruction	Patient unwilling to adhere to follow-up
Patient not suited for long surgery	Very large breast
Lack of adequate abdominal tissue	Very ptotic breast
Patient unwilling to have additional scars on back or abdomen	Silicon allergy
Small breast mound, with minimal ptosis	Implant fear
	Previous failed implants
	Need for adjuvant radiation therapy

Latissimus Dorsi Reconstruction	
Indications Small breast Minor breast ptosis Abdominal donor site unavailable (e.g., scars, lack of tissue) Salvage of previous breast reconstruction **Relative Contraindications** Planned postoperative radiation therapy Bilateral reconstruction Significant breast ptosis	**Contraindications** Previous lateral thoracotomy Very large breast in patient who does not desire reduction

Transverse Rectus Abdominis Muscle Flap Reconstruction	
Indications Breasts of all sizes Breast ptosis **Relative Contraindications** Smoking Abdominal liposuction Previous abdominal surgery Pulmonary disease Obesity	**Contraindications** Previous abdominoplasty Patient unable to tolerate 4- to 6-week recovery period Patient unable to tolerate longer procedure

PART ONE: PEDIATRIC ONCOLOGY

CHAPTER

49 NEUROBLASTOMA

- 80% before 4 years age
- Adrenal glands involved
- 2/3rd present as Asymptomatic Abdominal Mass
- 60% Retrobulbar metastasis→ Proptosis and Periorbital Ecchymosis
- 3% Opsoclonus/Myoclonus→ Good prognosis (Immune mediated)

CRITERIA

- Unequivocal pathologic diagnosis
- Bone marrow aspirate/Biopsy with Unequivocal tumor cells
- Increased catecholamines

SHIMDA CLASSIFICATION

Degree, Mitosis–Karyorrhexis index, Schwannian stroma

TREATMENT

- Localised→Surgery + RT
- Unresectable→ CT+RT and Surgery
- NACT+Surgery→95% Resection
- Spontaneous Regression is seen with Stage IVS

- ***Hyperdiploidy→ Favourable***
- ***N myc Amplification→ Poor prognosis***

CHAPTER 50

WILM'S TUMOR

- Most common primary malignancy of kidney in children
- 97% → Sporadic
- Heritable→ Bilateral and Early presentation
- 5% → Bilateral
- Left→ 50% and Right→ 45%
- 90% cure rate

GENETICS

- WT1–Tumor suppressor gene, located on chromosome 11, constitutively deleted in patients with WAGR syndrome (Wilms' tumor associated with Aniridia, Genitourinary abnormalities and Mental Retardation)
- WT2–Beckwith–Wiedemann syndrome (WT associated with overgrowth) is also linked with changes in chromosome 11, involving second Wilms' tumor locus
- *WTX* has been identified on X chromosome

CLINICAL FEATURES

- Usually affects 1-5 years of age
- Most common symptom–Asymptomatic Mass
- Others–Pain, Haematuria, Fever, weight loss and Hypertension

Favourable histology (90%)	**Unfavourable histology**
• Classical triphasic histology–epithelial, blastemal and stromal elements are all present • Rhabdomyoblastic differentiation • Monomorphic epithelial variant	• Anaplasia is an unfavourable feature, occasionally observed in triphasic tumors • Major unfavourable histological types are probably distinct cancers • Bone-metastasizing renal tumor of childhood • Malignant rhabdoid tumor

National Wilms' Tumor Study Group staging system:

- Stage I–Tumor confined within the renal capsule and fully resected
- Stage II–Tumor beyond renal capsule, but fully resected; Preop biopsy; ruptured; confined to flank
- Stage III–Tumor outside capsule and incompletely resected; Lymph node involvement at hilum/paraaortic chain
- Stage IV–Haematogenous metastases, e.g., to the lungs, liver, bone, or brain
- Stage V–Bilateral renal tumors

TREATMENT

- Surgical resection is, and almost certainly will remain, the cornerstone treatment for WT

- Only 5% are suitable for partial nephrectomy
- Usually surgery is done by open technique with wide excision, taking care to avoid rupture or spillage of the tumor
- Unilateral–Radical Nephroureterectomy
- Bilateral–Chemotherapy followed by Nephron sparing surgery

Current treatment for WT

Stage	Treatment
I, Low risk	No adjuvant therapy
I, Intermediate risk	Adjuvant vincristine, actinomycin
I, High risk	Adjuvant vincristine, actinomycin, doxorubicin
II, low risk	Vincristine, actinomycin
II-III, Intermediate risk	Vincristine actinomycin, + doxorubicin
II-III, High risk	Cyclophosphamide, doxorubicin, etoposide, carboplatin, and radiotherapy
Metastatic	Neoadjuvant vincristine, actinomycin, doxorubicin, then surgery, then further chemotherapy ± etoposide, carboplatin and radiotherapy

CHAPTER 51

HEPATOBLASTOMA

- **Most common primary hepatic tumor in children**
- Median age is 18 months
- Associated with FAP, Beckwith Wiedemann syndrome, Hemihyperplasia (10%)
- Isosexual precocity→ Penile and Testicular enlargement
- Hemihyperplasia is seen in 10%
- Isosexual precocity–Penile and Testicular enlargement
- Generally Asymptomatic
- Most common symptom–Abdominal Mass
- 2/3rd of Liver tumors–Malignant
- Most often Unifocal
- ***AFP is usually elevated in 85-90%***

Stage	Metastasis	Resection	Cure Rate
I	No	Complete resection	90%
II	No	Microscopic residual, Tumor rupture/spill	90%
III	No	Unresectable/Resected with gross residual, N+	60%
IV	Yes	Unresectable/Resected with gross residual, N+	20%

TREATMENT

- **Without metastasis–Complete resection**
- ***Metastasis–Chemotherapy followed by surgery***
- Pulmonary metastasis–Resect hepatic tumor and chemotherapy/Resect pulmonary metastasis
- ***Survival rate→70% (HCC→25%)***

CHAPTER 52 RETINOBLASTOMA

1. Most common intraocular malignancy of childhood
2. Most common inherited malignancy
3. AD inheritance, **Chromosomal deletion 13q14**
4. Usually multicentric, Mostly unilateral, 30% bilateral
5. **Trilateral retinoblastoma- Bilateral retinoblastoma + midline intracranial tumor (pinealoblastoma)**
6. Microscopy-Flexner wintersteiner rosettes, Homer wright rosettes and flourettes
7. Most common presentation is Leucocoria/Amaurotic cats eye
8. Staging systems are Rees-Ellisworth Classification, COG classification, Chantada *et al.*
9. Most sensitive investigation is CT scan
10. **Most common site of metastasis in retinoblastoma is BONE**
11. **Most common malignancy associated with retinoblastoma is osteosarcoma**
12. Enzyme markers for retinoblastoma are LDH and phosphoglucoisomerase
13. The sparse cytoplasm is located at one side of the cell, suggesting the **appearance of an embryonal retinal cell/nuclear layers of retina**
14. Retinoblastoma is the most frequent malignant ocular tumor in pediatric patients and one of the most curable neoplasms affecting young children, with survival rates exceeding 90%
15. Also called as Glioma retinae
16. Among children with unilateral disease, 10% to 15% have hereditary germ line deletions of chromosome 13, band q14, which contains RB 1 locus
17. Diagnosis of retinoblastoma is based on clinical history (including family history) and results of examination of both eyes under general anesthesia
18. MRI is used to define the extent of the intraocular tumor, to assess vitreal seeding, and to determine the presence and extent of extraocular disease
19. Radionuclide bone scans should be obtained only for patients with extensive ocular involvement, symptoms suggesting the presence of a bone metastasis, and bone marrow involvement
20. **REES ELLISWORTH CLASSIFICATION:**
    (See table on the next page)
21. The eye may be red and painful because of uveitis after spontaneous necrosis of a retinal tumor or from neovascular glaucoma
22. Standard surgical technique is modified to allow excision of longest possible segment of optic nerve in continuity with the globe in advanced unilateral disease
23. **Patients with limited unilateral or bilateral residual or focal recurrent disease may benefit from local surgical modalities, including photocoagulation, cryotherapy, or radioactive plaque brachytherapy**

Staging System for Retinoblastoma	
Group	**Description**
Group1	
A	Solitary tumor, <4 disc diameters in size, at or behind the equator
B	Multiple tumors, 4-10 disc diameters in size, all at or behind the equator
Group II	
A	Solitary tumor, 4-10 disc diameters in size, at or behind equator
B	Multiple tumors, 4-10 disc diameters in size, behind the equator
Group III	
A	Any lesion anterior to the equator
B	Solitary tumors >10 disc diameters behind the equator
Group IV	
A	Multiple tumors, some >10 disc diameters
B	Any lesion extending anteriorly to the ora serrata
Group V	
A	Massive tumors involving more than one-half the retina
B	Vitreous seeding

24. **INDICATIONS FOR ENUCLEATION:**
    a. Retinoblastoma unilateral that completely fills globe or that has damaged and disrupted retina or vitreous so extensively that restoration of useful vision is not possible
    b. Retinoblastoma bilateral in which previously mentioned conditions exist in only 1 eye
    c. Tumor present in the anterior chamber
    d. Painful glaucoma with loss of vision after rubeosis iridis
    e. Extensive b/l retinoblastoma with no potential for restoration of useful vision
    f. Retinoblastoma unresponsive to all other forms of local therapy
    g. Cases with permanent vision loss in which extraocular tumor is suspected
25. Radioactive plaque brachytherapy is more commonly used for salvage in the setting of localized recurrence
26. Tumors 2.5 mm or less in thickness and 4.5 mm or less in diameter are considered appropriate candidates are considered for laser photocoagulation
27. Bilateral retinoblastoma is currently treated with initial chemotherapy, with careful assessment of treatment response by examination under anesthesia after each cycle
28. External beam radiation therapy is indicated for bilateral disease where the eye has advanced disease, has not responded adequately to chemotherapy and local treatments, but has useful vision
29. Proton therapy can potentially decrease dosage to the surrounding bony orbits by more than 60% and avoid significant dosage to the hypothalamus compared with intensity-modulated radiotherapy, with equivalent target coverage
30. Risk of osteosarcomas was higher in patients who received chemotherapy with radiation, compared with radiation alone
31. Local irradiation, after enucleation is recommended for all patients with extension of retinoblastoma into the orbit
32. Presentation with exophthalmos or a palpable mass through the eyelids suggests the presence of orbital extension of the tumor
33. B scan shows cauliflower like mass arising from retina while A scan shows characteristic V-Y pattern
34. **ESSON PROGNOSIS CLASSIFICATION** is used for assessing prognosis of Retinoblastoma
35. **“VITREOUS SEEDING shows Cottage cheese appearance”**

International Classification System for Intraocular Retinoblastoma	
Group	**Description**
Group A	**Very low risk** Eyes with small discrete tumors away from critical structures. All tumors 3 mm or smaller, confined to the retina and located 3 mm from the foveola and 1.5 mm from the optic nerve. No vitreous or subretinal seeding
Group B	**Low risk** Eyes with no vitreous or subretinal seeding and discrete retinal tumor of any size or location. Any retinal tumor not in group A. No vitreous or subretinal seeding. A small cuff of subretinal fluid no more than 5 mm from the base of the tumor is allowed
Group C	**Moderate risk** Eye with focal vitreous or subretinal seeing and discrete retinal tumors of any size or location. Any seeding must be local, fine and limited, Retinal tumors are discrete and of any size and location. Up to one quadrant of subretinal fluid may be present
Group D	**High risk** Eyes with diffuse vitreous or subretinal seeding and/or massive, nondiscrete endophytic and exophytic disease. Eyes with more extensive seeding than group C Intraocular disseminated disease may consist of fine or "greasy" vitreous seeding or avascular mass

PART ONE: MISCELLANEOUS

CHAPTER

53 RADIOTHERAPY

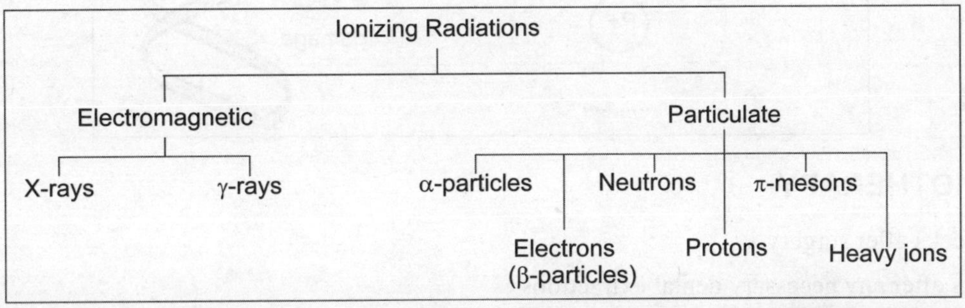

Electrons
• Limited tissue penetration
• Negligible exit dose from beam
• Particularly useful for superficial tumors, e.g., skin, head and neck, breast cancers
• Reduced dose to normal tissues beneath target, e.g., spinal cord, lung
Photons
• Suitable tissue penetration characteristics for the treatment of deep-seated cancers
• Skin sparing
• Beam characteristics facilitate beam matching and crossfire treatment plans

TYPES OF RADIATION

- **Photon:** *Most common form of radiation used (6 megavolts)*
- **Electron:** Superficial penetration ideal for skin
- **Neutron:** High-energy particle and highly toxic–Selectively used for **salivary gland malignancies**
- **Proton:** Low-energy particle with a sharp falloff of dose beyond the target (Bragg peak)–**used for skull base lesions**
- **Carbon ion:** High-energy particle with a sharp Bragg peak

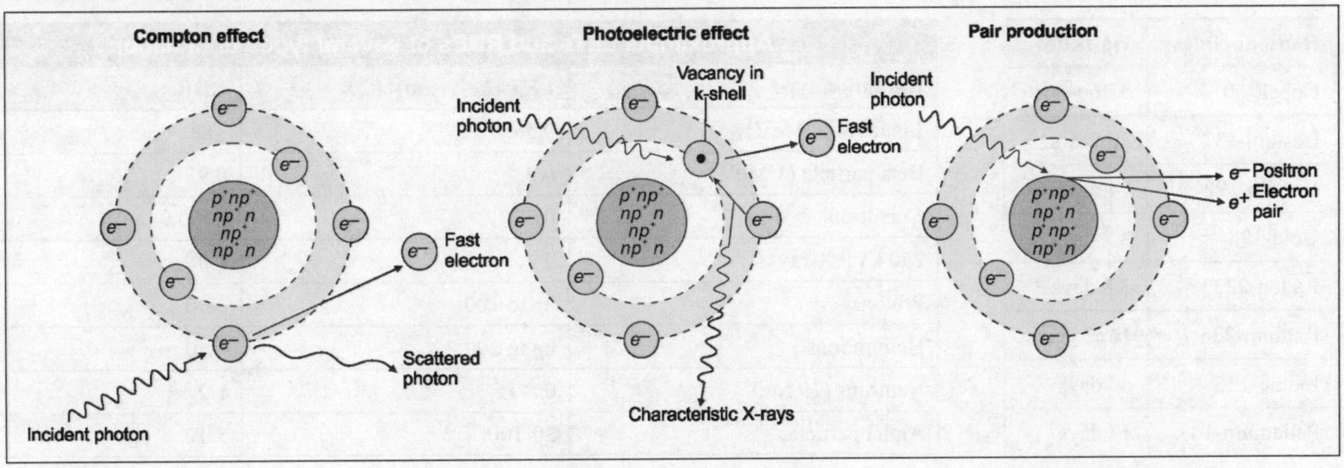

MECHANISM OF RADIOTHERAPY

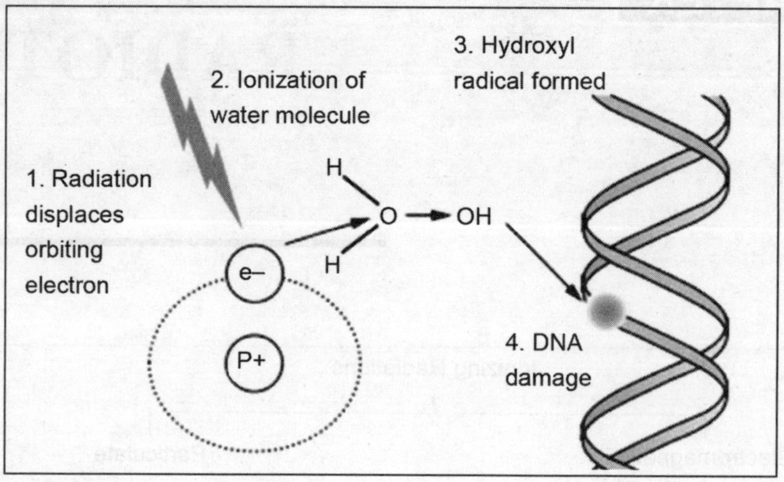

TIMING OF RADIOTHERAPY

- **Adjuvant:** 4-6 weeks after surgery
- **Primary:** 2 weeks after any necessary dental extractions

High risk
• Primary tumor and involved lymph nodes (this includes possible local subclinical infiltration at primary site and at high-risk level lymph nodes. 66 to 70 Gy daily (Monday-Friday in 6 to 7 weeks)
Low to Intermediate risk
• Sites of suspected subclinical spread 44-50 Gy to 54-63 Gy

Interval between EBRT and Brachytherapy should be atleast 1-2 weeks
Interval between high dose radiotherapy fractions should be atleast 6 hours
Preferred gap between surgery and RT is <6 weeks

Brachytherapy
Low dose rate (LDR) brachytherapy (0.4-0.5 Gy per hour):
• Consider LDR boost 20-35 Gy if combined with 50 Gy EBRT or 60-70 Gy over several days if using LDR as sole therapy
High dose rate (HDR) brachytherapy:
• Consider HDR boost 21 Gy at 3 Gy/fraction if combined with 40–50 Gy EBRT or 45–60 Gy at Gy/fraction if using HDR as sole therapy

Radionuclides	Half-life
Cobalt-60	5.26 years
Cesium-137	30 years
Iridium-192	74 days
Gold-198	2.7 days
Radon-222	3.8 days
Radium-226	1622 years
Iodine-125	60 days
Palladium-103	17 days

Approximate LETs and RBEs of several types of radiation

Radiation type	LET (ke V/μm)	RBE
Linac (6-15 MeV)	0.3	-0.8
Beta particle (1 MeV)	0.3	0.9
Cobalt-60	0.3	0.8-0.9
250 kVP X-rays	2	1.0
Protons	up to 100	~1.0
Helium ions	up to 200	~1.0
Neutrons (19 MeV)	0.5-15	1-2
Alpha particles	30-100	5-10

Indications for Postop Radiotherapy

- Advanced-stage disease: pT3, pT4
- Multiple positive nodes
- Positive surgical margins
- Perineural invasion

Salient Features of Altered Fractionation Schemes

Hyperfractionation

- Smaller fraction size (115-120 cGy) compared with conventional fractionation (180-200 cGy)
- BID to TID fractionation
- Larger total dosage (7440-8460 cGy) than conventional fractionation (7000 cGy)
- Similar overall treatment duration as conventional fractionation

Accelerated Fractionation

- Similar fraction size as conventional fractionation (180-200 cGy)
- BID to TID fractionation
- Similar total dosage as conventional fractionation
- Shortened overall treatment duration compared with conventional fractionation

Hypofractionation

- Larger fraction size (600-800 cGy) compared with conventional fractionation (180-200 cGy)
- Fractions delivered several days apart
- Lower total dosage (2100-3200 cGY) than conventional fractionation (7000 cGy)
- Shortened overall treatment duration compared with conventional fractionation

Schematic Representation of Altered Fractionation Protocols

<table>
<tr><th></th><th>Week</th><th>1</th><th>2</th><th>3</th><th>4</th><th></th><th></th><th></th><th>Fx. No.</th><th>Fx. Size</th><th>Total</th></tr>
<tr><td>ACCELERATED</td><td>AM</td><td>|||||</td><td>|||||</td><td>|||||</td><td>|||||</td><td>|*</td><td></td><td></td><td>42</td><td>1.6 Gy</td><td>67.2 Gy</td></tr>
<tr><td>FRACTIONATION*</td><td>PM</td><td>|||||</td><td>|||||</td><td>|||||</td><td>|||||</td><td>|</td><td></td><td></td><td></td><td></td><td></td></tr>
<tr><th></th><th>Week</th><th>1</th><th>2</th><th>3</th><th>4</th><th>5</th><th>6</th><th>7</th><th>Fx. No.</th><th>Fx. Size</th><th>Total</th></tr>
<tr><td>HYPERFRACTIONATION</td><td>AM</td><td>|||||</td><td>|||||</td><td>|||||</td><td>|||||</td><td>|||||</td><td>|||||</td><td>|||||</td><td>70</td><td>1.15 Gy</td><td>80.5 Gy</td></tr>
<tr><td></td><td>PM</td><td>|||||</td><td>|||||</td><td>|||||</td><td>|||||</td><td>|||||</td><td>|||||</td><td>|||||</td><td></td><td></td><td></td></tr>
<tr><th></th><th>Week</th><th>1</th><th>2</th><th>3</th><th>4</th><th>5</th><th>6</th><th>7</th><th>Fx. No.</th><th>Fx. Size</th><th>Total</th></tr>
<tr><td>ACCELERATED</td><td>AM</td><td>|||||</td><td>|||||</td><td>|||||</td><td>|||||</td><td>|||||</td><td>|||||</td><td></td><td>40</td><td>1.8 Gy</td><td>60 Gy</td></tr>
<tr><td>BOOST</td><td>PM</td><td></td><td></td><td></td><td></td><td>|||||</td><td>|||||</td><td></td><td></td><td>1.5 Gy</td><td></td></tr>
</table>

Features of megavoltage X-rays

- High dose delivered at depth through tissue
- Maximum dose below skin surface
- Skin sparing
- Absorbed dose falls off exponentially with depth in tissue
- Sharp 'fall-off ' of dose at beam edge (penumbra)
- Beam shape can be modified by metal blocks or multileaf collimators, now an integral part of modern linear accelerators
- Metal filters or wedges can be used to create a gradient in the dose across the beam
- Treatment from any direction is feasible
- Crossfire technique with 2–4 beams gives higher target dose and relative sparing of adjacent normal tissues

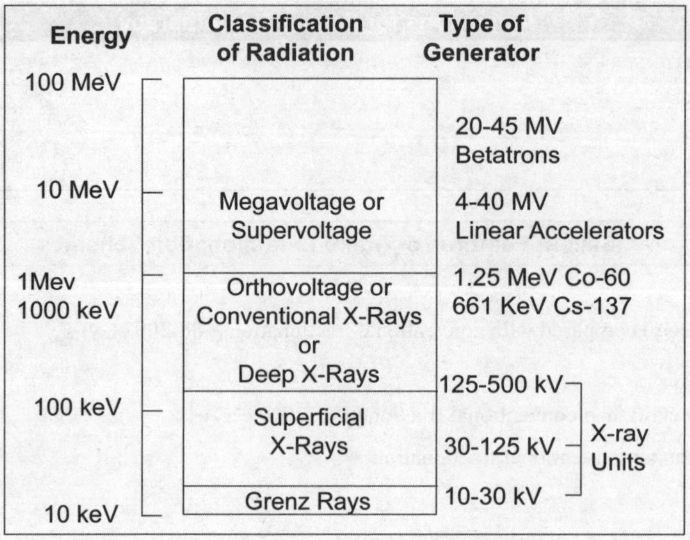

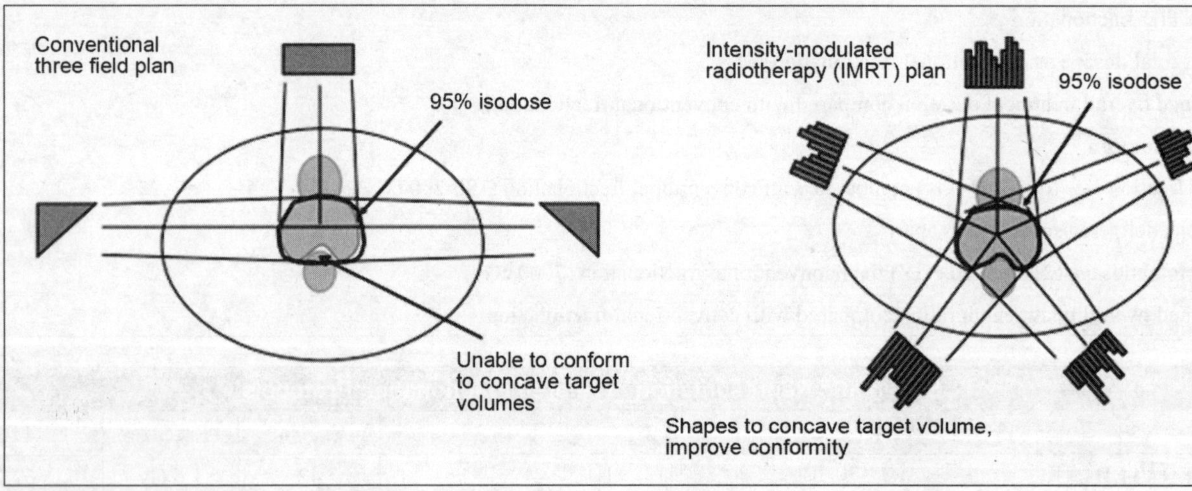

Interaction of anticancer drugs with radiation		
Drug	**In combination with XRT**	**Toxicity**
5FU	Increased cell kill with increased concentration or exposure time	Lower GI, mucous membranes, skin, heart, marrow
Cisplatin	Cell kill enhancement occurs to greater extent in cells sensitive to cisplatin. Concentration dependent enhancement Postradiation enhancement also occurs and may be most important clinically	Skin, mucous membranes, CNS
Mitomycin	Scheduling with XRT unimportant. May work best early on when fraction of hypoxic cells is greatest	Lung, marrow
Adriamycin or Actinomycin	Post-XRT usage may result in recall of radiation reaction	Heart, lung, kidney, skin, esophagus, mucous memb., lower GI
Hydroxyurea	May synchronize cells by inhibiting entry into S from G1	Marrow
Bleomycin	Tumor dependent variation in optimum treatment schedule	Lung
Nitrosourea	Can penetrate CNS	Marrow
Cytoxan	Hemorrhagic cystitis can occur with or without XRT	Marrow, bladder
Vincristine	Peripheral neuropathy may occur with or without XRT	Peripheral nerves
Methotrexate	Often excluded when treating breast cancer patients to avoid excessive skin reactions	CNS, skin

Palliative radiation			
Condition	**Work-up**	**Dose Schedule**	**Acute Side Effects**
Bronchial Obstruction (Lung Collapse)	Bronchoscopy CT Imaging	30 Gy/10 Fractions 20 Gy/5 Fractions	Cough Mild Skin Changes Esophagitis
Brain Metastases	CT/MRI Brain	35 Gy/15 Fractions 30 Gy/10 Fractions	Alopecia Fatigue Skin Erythema
Limited Skeletal Metastases	Bone Scan Skeletal Survey	30 Gy/10 Fractions	Mild Skin Changes Neutropenia
Extensive Skeletal Metastases	Bone Scan Skeletal Survey	Systemic Radiotherapy with Strontium-89/Sumarium-97	Neutropenia Thrombocytopenia Fatigue
Hepatic Metastases	LFT's Abdominal CT/Ultrasound	21-24 Gy/7-8 Fractions	Mild Nausea
Extensive Nodal Enlargement	Physical Exam CT/MRI Imaging	20-30 Gy/10-15 Fractions	Mild Skin Changes
Intraabdominal Carcinomatosis (Ascites)	CT Imaging Ultrasound	30 Gy/15-20 Fractions	Nausea Fatigue
Esophageal Obstruction	Barium Swallow CT Imaging	30-40 Gy/10-15 Fractions	Esophagitis
Obstructive Jaundice (G.G./Pancreas)	CT Imaging Ultrasound	45 Gy/25 Fractions 30 Gy/10 Fractions	Fatigue Nausea

COMPLICATIONS OF RADIATION

1. **Mucositis (World Health Organization scale)**
   - Grade 1: Soreness with erythema
   - Grade 2: Erythema, ulcers and can eat solids
   - Grade 3: Ulcers and liquid diet only
   - Grade 4: Alimentation is not possible

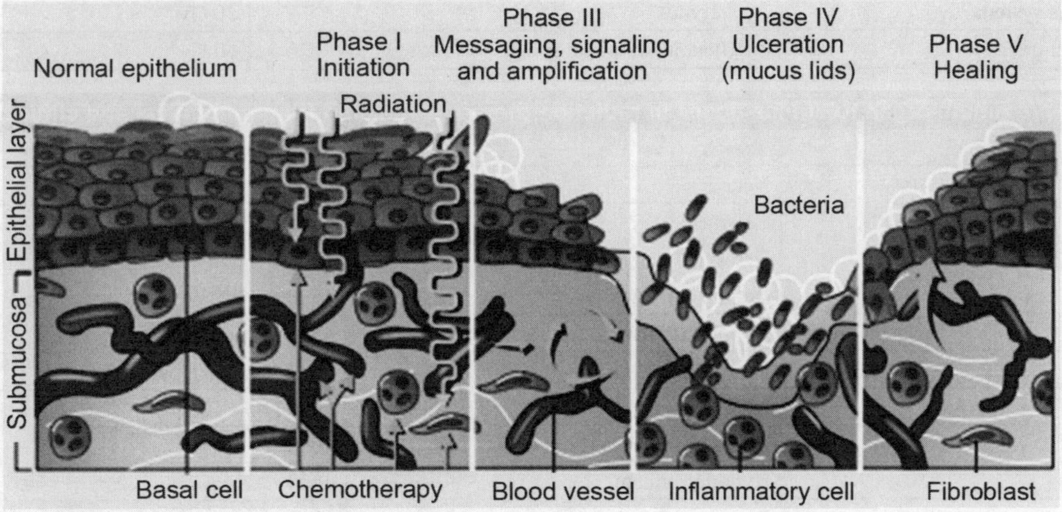

2. **Xerostomia:**
   - **Prevention:** IMRT to spare salivary glands and submandibular gland transfer
   - **Treatment:**
     - Saliva substitutes and mucosal lubricants
     - Stimulation of saliva
     - Sugar-free hard candy or gum
     - Pilocarpine

3. **Osteoradionecrosis:**
   - Mandible, Temporal bone, Maxilla

Acute effects after radical radiotherapy		
Site	**Effect**	**Treatment**
Skin	Erythema leading, if severe, to desquamation	Minimal; avoid irritants, trauma Aqueous or weak hydrocortisone cream
Bowel	Diarrhoea/colic	Low residue diet Codeine or loperamide
Bladder	Frequency/dysuria	Exclude infection
Scalp	Hair loss	Order wig in advance; hair will regrow after palliative but not radical doses
Mouth/pharynx	Mucositis	Avoid irritants and alcohol; treat candidiasis; topical chlorhexidine or benzydamine

Late effects after radical radiotherapy		
Site	**Effect**	**Treatment**
Skin	Fibrosis; telangiectasia; rarely necrosis	Usually none
Bowel	Stricture; perforation; bleeding fistulae	If severe, resection of affected segment
Bladder	Fibrosis causing frequency; haematuria; fistulae	If severe, surgical resection
CNS	Myelitis causing paraplegia; cerebral necrosis	None
Lung	Fibrosis	None

Tissue	Radiation effect	Dosage
Testis	Sterility	0.2 Gy
Eye	Cataract	10 Gy
Lung	Pneumonitis	20 Gy
Kidney	Nephritis	25 Gy
Liver	Hepatitis	30 Gy
Central nervous system	Nervous	50 Gy
Gastrointestinal tract	Ulceration, haemorrhage	60 Gy

Approximate organ tolerance doses in radiation therapy estimated from preclinical and clinical data		
Organ	**Toxicity**	**Tolerance Dose (cGy)***
Brain	Necrosis	6000
Eye	Cataract	600
	Keratitis	5000
	Retinal damage	4500
Pituitary	Hypopituitarism	4500
Spinal cord	Paralysis	5000 (5 cm segment)
Skin	Necrosis	6000 (10 × 10 cm)
Salivary gland	Xerostomia	4000
Thyroid	Hypothyroidism	4500
Lung	Pneumonitis	2000
Heart	Peri-/paracarditis	4500
Esophagus	Stricture	6000
Liver	Hepatitis	3000
Stomach	Ulcer/hemorrhage	5000
Kidney	Nephritis	2000
Rectum	Ulcer/hemorrhage	6000
Ovary	Sterility/menopause	600
Testis	Sterility	200
Bladder	Contracture	6500

Examples of radiation-induced cancers		
Sources of Exposure	**Exposure Circumstances**	**Cancer Types**
Explosions of Nuclear Weapons		
Blast	Atomic bombing survivors in Hiroshima and Nagasaki	Leukemia, breast, lung, thyroid, stomach, colon, multiple myeloma, esophagus, ovary
Fallout	Populations exposed through atmospheric testing, including Marshall Islanders, veterans in the Pacific, general population in Nevada, Utah	Thyroid
Diagnostic Procedures		
X-rays	Children exposed in utero	Leukemia
Thorotrast	Cerebral and limb angiography; of biliary passages	Liver
Fluoroscopic X-ray	Monitoring of lung infections in patients with tuberculosis	Breast
Therapeutic Procedures		
X-ray	Postpartum mastitis	Breast
X-ray	Ankylosing spondylitis	Leukemia, lung, stomach, esophagus
Cobalt-60	Treatment for cancer of the cervix	Leukemia, stomach, rectum, bladder, vagina, female genital, lung, buccal cavity, nasopharynx, esophagus
X-ray	Treatment of benign head and neck conditions	Thyroid, skin, central nervous system
Radium-224	Ankylosing spondylitis, bone tuberculosis	Bone sarcoma
Professional Exposures		
X-ray	Early radiologists	Skin, leukemia
Radon	Uranium, hard-rock miners	Lung cancer
X-ray, γ-rays, neutrons	Nuclear industry	Multiple myeloma
Radium isotopes	Radium dial painters	Bone, head sarcoma

Potential interactions between herbal medicines and conventional drugs		
Herb(s)	**Drug(s)**	**Potential Interaction/Effect(s)**
St. John's wort	Irinotecan, protease inhibitors, other drugs metabolized by cytochrome P-450 Cyclosporine Oral contraceptives	Reduced drug levels
Hawthorn flower, devil's claw, licorice	Digoxin	Alters pharmacodynamics; drug level monitoring is prudent
Licorice	Potassium-sparing diuretics	Affects potassium levels
Kelp	Thyroxine	Iodine content of herb may interfere with thyroid replacement
Kava	Alprazolam Terazosin	Additive sedative effects, coma
Evening primrose oil	Anticonvulsants	Lowered seizure threshold
Feverfew, garlic, ginseng, gingko, ginger, dong quai	Warfarin	Altered bleeding time
Yohimbe bark	Centrally active antihypertensive agents	Yohimbine may antagonize guanabenz and methyldopa through its α_2-adrenoceptor-antagonistic properties
Ginseng	Phenelzine sulfate	Headache, tremulousness, manic episodes
	Estrogens, corticosteroids	Additive effects

CHAPTER 54

ANTICANCER DRUGS

CELL CYCLE

- All normal tissues have the capacity for cellular division and growth
- There are three general types of normal tissue growth: static, expanding and renewing

- **Static population** comprises relatively well-differentiated cells that after initial proliferative activity in the embryonic and neonatal period, rarely undergo cell division. **Typical examples are striated muscle and neurons**
- **Expanding population** of cells is characterized by the capacity to proliferate under special stimuli (tissue injury). Under those circumstances, the normally quiescent tissue (liver or kidney) undergoes a surge of proliferation with regrowth
- **Renewing population** of cells is constantly in a proliferative state. There is constant cell division, a high degree of cell turnover and constant cell loss. This occurs in bone marrow, epidermis, and gastrointestinal mucosa

Gap 1 (G_1) (Synthesis of enzymes and regulatory proteins)	Postmitotic	4-24 hours (variable)
DNA Synthesis (S) and Replication		10-20 hours
Gap 2 (G_2) RNA synthesis Protein synthesis	Premitotic	2-10 hours
Mitosis (M)		0.5-1 hour
G_0 Resting phase		Variable Period

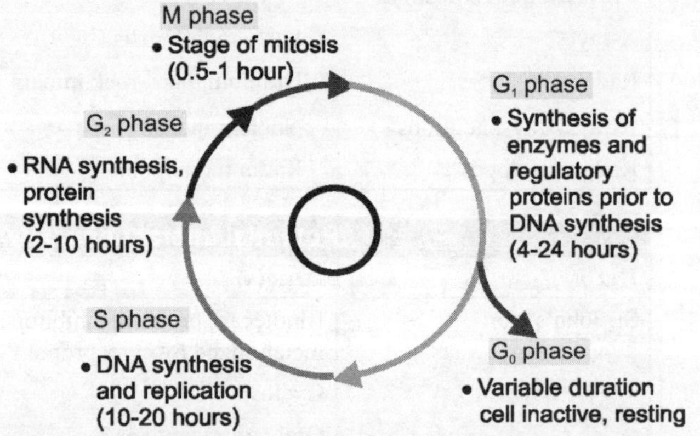

CLASSIFICATION OF CHEMOTHERAPEUTIC AGENTS

Drug Activity in the Cell Cycle		
Cell cycle	**Non-specific**	Cyclophosphamide Cisplatin Carboplatin
Cell cycle	**Specific:** On G_1	Actinomycin D
	On S phase	Methotrexate 5 FU, Doxorubicin
	On G_2	Bleomycin Etoposide
	On M phase	Vinblastine Vincristine Taxanes
	G_0	Nitrosoureas (BCNU, CCNU)

Relationship of chemotherapy agents to intracellular targets and cell-cycle progression			
Classification	**Cell-Cycle Specificity**	**Cellular Targets and Mechanisms**	**Examples**
Inhibition of DNA synthesis and repair	G_1,S	Inhibition of nucleotide synthesis and metabolism. Inhibition of thymidylate synthase, thymidylate phosphorylase, dihydrofolate reductase, ribonucleotide reductase	Antifolates (methotrexate, pemetrexed), nucleoside analogues (6-mercaptopurine, 5-fluorouracil, cytarabine, fludarabine, gemcitabine), hydroxyurea
	S	Stabilization of DNA-topoisomerase II cleavable complex, DNA intercalation, +/- free radical formation	Anthracyclines (doxorubicin, daunomycin, idarubicin, epirubicin), anthracenediones (mitoxantrone), epipodophyllotoxins (etoposide), actinomycin D
	S	Stabilisation of DNA-topoisomerase I cleavable complex	Camptothecins (topotecan, irinotecan)
Alkylating agents and related compounds	G_1, G_2, S	Direct DNA damage, DNA adduct formation, free radical production, strand breakage	Radiation, platinum compounds (cisplatin, carboplatin, oxaliplatin), bleomycin, mitomycin C, nitrogen mustard, nitrosoureas, ecteinascidin
Antimicrotubule reagents	M	Inhibition of tubulin polymerization	Vinca alkaloids (vinristine, vinblastine, vinorelbine), colchicines
		Promotion of tubulin polymerization	Taxanes (paclitaxel, docetaxel), epothilones
		Kinesin spindle proteins	Investigational agents
Cell cycle agents	$G_{1,}$ S, G_2, M	Mitotic checkpoint control, cyclin-dependent kinases (CDK), aurora kinases	Flavopiridol, investigational agents
Signal transduction modulators	$G_{0,}$ G_1, S, G_2	Growth factor sequestration, receptor blockade	Trastuzumab, cetuximab, pertuzumab, aflibercept, bevacizumab
		Inhibition of tyrosine kinase-mediated signal transduction	Erlotinib, gefitinib, desatinib, imatinib, sorafenib, sunitinib, lapatinib
		Modulation of protein kinase C	Bryostatin, enzastaurin
		Inhibition of hormonal pathways	Tamoxifen, raloxifene, anastrazole, letrozole, fulvestrant, megestrol, mifepristone, flutamide, leuprolide
Gene regulation	NA	Gene regulation by inhibition of promoter methylation, DNA methyltransferase, or histone deacetylase	Azacytidine, suberoylanilide hydroxamic acid (vorinostat, belinostat)
Protein modifications	NA	Posttranslational protein modifications, inhibition of farnesylation	Tipifarnib, bisphosphonates
		Inhibition of the proteasome complex and clearance of ubiquinated proteins	Bortezomib

COMBINATION CHEMOTHERAPY

Important factors in the design of drug combinations	
1.	The drugs used must be active as single agents against the particular tumor
2.	The drugs should have different mechanisms of action to minimize emergence of drug resistance
3.	The combination of drugs should have additive or preferably synergistic effects
4.	The drugs chosen should have a different spectrum of toxicity so that they can be used for maximum cell kill at (or near) full doses
5.	The drugs chosen should be administered intermittently so that cell kill is enhanced and prolonged myelosuppression is minimized

Representative agents for development of combination regimens

Agent	Cellular Target	Mechanism of Action	Schedule-Dependent Effects	Patterns of Resistance	Interaction with Platinum
Platinum	DNA	DNA adduct formation	Generally independent of schedule	↑ GSH ↑ DNA repair ↑ Damage tolerance ↓ Accumulation	NA
Paclitaxel	β tubulin	↑ Tubulin aggregation	↑ Heme and mucosal toxicity with prolonged infusion ↑ Efficacy with weekly schedule	↑ MDR 1 (P 170) ↑ Tubulin-β3 isoforms	↓ Platelet toxicity ↑ Neuropathy
Topotecan	Topoisomerase-I	Stabilize DNA-topoisomerase complex	↑ Efficacy with 5-day exposure Sequence-dependent toxicity	↓ Topoisomerase-I ↑ BCRP (ABCG2)	↑ Heme toxicity
Gemcitabine	Ribonucleotide reductase, DNA, nucleotide pool	↓ DNA synthesis ↓ Nucleotide pools Masked chain termination	Saturated uptake and phosphorylation with rapid infusion	↑ Ribonucleotide reductase	↑ Heme toxicity
PEG-liposomal doxorubicin	Topoisomerase-II	↓ DNA synthesis	Prolonged clearance (PEG formulation)	↑ MDR 1 (P 170)	↑ Heme toxicity

RESPONSE ASSESSMENT

RECIST 1.1 Definitions of response

Complete response (CR)	Disappearance of all target lesions
Partial response (PR)	At least a 30% decrease in the sum of the longest diameter (LD) of target lesions, taking as reference the baseline sum LD
Progressive disease (PD)	At least a 20% increase in the sum of the LD of target lesions taking as reference the smallest sum LD recorded since the treatment started or the appearance of one or more new lesions
Stable disease (SD)	Neither sufficient shrinkage to qualify for PR nor sufficient increase to qualify for PD, taking as reference the smallest sum LD since the treatment started

DRUG INTERACTIONS

Drug interactions in cancer chemotherapy

Effect	Caused by	Interaction	Resulting in	Bioavailable Drug
↓ Renal function/excretion	Nephrotoxic antibiotics	*Methotrexate; cisplatin*	↓ Excretion	↑
↓ Hepatic metabolism/biliary excretion	*Vincristine*	*Doxorubicin*	↓ Excretion	↑
↓ Displacement from albumin or plasma proteins	Sulfonamides; salicylates	*Methotrexate; cisplatin*	↓ Binding	↑

Contd.

Contd.

↓ Intestinal absorption	*Neomycin*	*Methotrexate*	↓ Absorption	↓
↓ Direct chemical interaction	*Mannitol*	*Cisplatin*	↑ Excretion	↓
↓ Direct effect on metabolism	*Phenobarbitol* *methotrexate* *5-fluorouracil*	*Cyclophosphamide* *5-fluorouracil* *methotrexate*	↑ Metabolism ↑ Activation ↓ Metabolism	↑

Physiologic and pharmacologic interactions in cancer chemotherapy

Physiologic Condition	Causation	Impact and Examples
Renal insufficiency	Obstruction, chronic kidney disease, hypovolemia, hypotension, nonsteroidals, nephrotoxins (aminoglycosides, cisplatin)	Decreased clearance of methotrexate, carboplatin and other agents
Hepatobiliary dysfunction	Biliary obstruction, hepatitis, cirrhosis	Decreased clearance of doxorubicin, mitoxantrone, vincristine, vinblastine, etoposide, paclitaxel, docetaxel
	Gilbert's syndrome, impaired glucuronidation and polymorphisms (UGTA 1A)	Increased exposure to SN-38 (from irinotecan)
	Decreased microsomal activity	Impaired activation of cyclophosphamide and ifosfamide
Reduced protein binding	Carrier displacement (sulfonamide, salicylates, phenytoin) Reduced carrier proteins (malnutrition)	Increased toxicity, higher free drug levels (methotrexate) Increased toxicity, higher free drug levels (cisplatin, paclitaxel, docetaxel, etoposide, SN-38)
Altered intestinal absorption	Oral antibiotics (neomycin) High-fat meal	Decreased absorption of methotrexate Increased bioavailability of lapatinib Decreased bioavailability of capecitabine
	Grapefruit juice (intestinal CYP3A4 inhibition)	Increased bioavailability (cyclosporine, erythromycin, benzodiazepines)
Decreased metabolism	Caused by allopurinol	Delayed clearance of 6-mercaptopurine
	Dihydropyrimidine dehydrogenase (DPD) deficiency	Lethal toxicity from 5-fluorouracil
Cholinesterase inhibition	Caused by cyclophosphamide	Decreased clearance of succinylcholine
Monoamine oxidase inhibition	Caused by procarbazine	Neurotoxicity and seizures (tricyclic antidepressants and phenothiazines)
MDR-1 competition	Associated with natural products and other substrates, including verapamil, cyclosporine, tamoxifen	Decreased efflux and increased toxicity from natural products (doxorubicin, vincristine, paclitaxel, docetaxel)
CYP2C9 Inhibition	Caused by capecitabine	Increased AUC of warfarin
CYP3A4 Induction	Caused by glucocorticoids, barbiturates, rifampin	Increased activation of cyclophosphamide
Inhibition	Caused by ketoconazole, itraconazole, fluconazole, erythromycin	Decreased metabolism of substrates (potentially significant)
Substrate competition	Caused by cyclophosphamide, ifosfamide, paclitaxel, docetaxel, etoposide, vincristine, vinblastine, tamoxifen, gefitinib	Decreased metabolism of other substrates (usually not clinically significant)

ADVERSE EFFECTS

Chemotherapy induced nausea/vomiting (CINV) risk by agent	
Risk category	**Agents**
High risk (>90%)	Cisplatin Dacarbazine Doxorubicin >60 mg/m^2 Ifosfamide $\geq$2 g/m^2/dose
Moderate risk (31-90%)	Carboplatin Dactinomycin Doxorubicin <60 mg/m^2 Epirubicin $\leq$90 mg/m^2 Ifosfamide <2 g/m^2/dose Irinotecan Melphalan Methotrexate $\geq$ 250 mg/m^2 Oxaliplatin Temozolomide
Low risk (10-30%)	Docetaxel Liposomal doxorubicin Etoposide Fluorouracil Gemcitabine Mitomycin Paclitaxel Pemetrexed Topotecan
Minimal risk (<10%)	Bevacizumab Bleomycin Vinblastine Vincristine Vinorelbine

Severity/grade of chemotherapy-induced diarrhea					
	Grade 1	**Grade 2**	**Grade 3**	**Grade 4**	**Grade 5**
Diarrhea	Increase of <4 stools per day over baseline; mild increase in ostomy output compared to baseline	Increase of 4-6 stools per day over baseline; moderate increase in ostomy output compared to baseline	Increase of >6 stools per day over baseline; incontinence; severe increase in ostomy output compared to baseline; limiting self-care ADL	Life-threatening consequences; urgent intervention indicated	Death

Chemotherapy agents commonly causing peripheral neuropathy			
Drug	**Onset dosage**	**Incidence**	**Notes**
Cisplatin	300 mg/m^2	28-100%	Worsens in combination with taxane May progress after discontinuation
Oxaliplatin	Acute: Any Persistent: 500 mg/m^2	Acute: 65-80% Persistent: 43%	Acute neuropathy, transient and triggered by cold Persistent neuropathy similar to cisplatin
Carboplatin	600-800 mg/m^2	6-42%	Less neurotoxic than other platinums Worsens in combination with taxane

Contd.

Contd.

Paclitaxel	100-1,000 mg/m^2	57-83%	Worsens in combination with platinum Increased incidence with short/frequent infusions
Docetaxel	400 mg/m^2	11-64%	Less severe neurotoxicity compared to paclitaxel Worsens in combination with platinum
Vincristine	Onset: 4 mg/m^2 Motor dysfunction: >6 mg/m^2		May cause autonomic neuropathy Motor neuropathy more common
Altretamine		31%	Generally reversible upon discontinuation

Peripheral neuropathy severity/grading

	Grade 1	Grade 2	Grade 3	Grade 4	Grade 5
Paresthesia	Mild symptoms	Moderate symptoms; limiting instrumental ADL	Severe symptoms; limiting self-care ADL	–	–
Peripheral neuropathy	Asymptomatic; observation; intervention not indicated	Moderate symptoms; limiting instrumental ADL	Severe symptoms; limiting self-care ADL; assistive device indicated	Life-threatening consequences; urgent intervention indicated	Death

Agents commonly used for chemotherapy-induced peripheral neuropathy pain

Drug	Dose	Adverse effects
Duloxetine	Starting: 20-30 mg/day Maximum: 120 mg/day	Nausea, xerostomia, constipation, diarrhea
Gabapentin	Starting: 100-300 mg nightly Maximum: 1,200 mg TID	Somnolence, dizziness, nausea, diarrhea, edema, discoordination
Lidocaine 5% patch	3 Patches daily	Rash
Opioids	Variable	Constipation, nausea, vomiting, sedation, respiratory depression
Pregabalin	Starting: 25-50 mg TID Maximum: 200 mg TID	Dizziness, somnolence, xerostomia, edema, blurred vision, decreased concentration
Tramadol	Starting: 50 mg 1-2/day Maximum: 100 mg q^{6h} or q^{8h} for elderly	Dizziness, constipation, nausea, somnolence, seizure, serotonin syndrome
Tricyclic antidepressants	Variable	Anticholinergic effects, cardiovascular effects dizziness, somnolence

MASCC scoring index for evaluation of febrile neutropenia

Characteristics	Score
Illness extent (choose 1 item below) • No symptoms • Mild symptoms • Moderate symptoms	 5 5 3
No hypotension (SBP ≥90 mm Hg without pressors)	5
No chronic obstructive pulmonary disease	4
Solid tumors (if have hematologic malignancy–no previous fungal infection)	4
No dehydration	3
Outpatient at onset of fever	3
Age <60 years (does not apply for patients <16 years)	2

Type of hypersensitivity reaction of platinums and their characteristics					
Type of hypersensitivity reactions	**Antigen**	**Mediated by**	**Mechanism**	**Involved in platinum hypersensitivity**	**Symptoms related**
1	Soluble antigen	IgE	Mast cell and basophil degranulation	Carboplatin, cisplatin, oxaliplatin (most)	Early onset symptoms; itching, chest pain, rash, anaphylactic reactions
II	Cell- or matrix associated antigen	IgG, IgM	Phagocyte and NK-cell activation	Oxaliplatin	Hemolysis, thrombocytopenia
III	Soluble antigen	IgG	Immune complex, phagocyte and NK- cell activation complement fixation	Oxaliplatin	Chronic urticaria, joint pain, proteinuria
IV	Soluble or cell-associated antigen	T-cell	Macrophage and eosinophil activation, cytotoxicity	Carboplatin, cisplatin	Delayed reactions, hours or even days after infusion

Grading of HSR					
	Grade				
	1	2	3	4	5
Hypersensitivity (allergic reaction)	Transient flushing or rash, drug fever <380°C, intervention not indicated	Intervention or infusion interruption indicated; responds promptly to symptomatic treatment (e.g., antihistamines, NSAIDS, narcotics); prophylactic medications indicated for ≤24 h	Pronlonged (e.g., not rapidly responsive to symptomatic medication and/or brief interruption of infusion); recurrence of symptoms following initial improvement; hospitalization indicated for clinical sequelae (e.g., renal impairment, pulmonary infiltrates)	Life-threatening consequences; urgent intervention indicated	Death
Acute infusion reactions (cytokine release syndrome)	Mild reaction; infusion interruption not indicated; intervention not indicated	Therapy or infusion interruption indicated but responds promptly to symptomatic treatment (e.g., antihihistamines, NSAIDS, narcotics, IV fluids); prophylactic medications indicated for ≤24 h	Prolonged (e.g., not rapidly responsive to symptomatic medication and/or brief interruption of infusion); recurrence of symptoms following initial improvement; hospitalization indicated for clinical sequelae (e.g., renal impairment) pulmonary infiltrates)	Life-threatening consequences; pressor or ventilator support indicated	Death

CTCAE grading of myelosuppression				
Element	**Grade**			
	1	**2**	**3**	**4**
Leukocytes (per mm^3)	LLN to 3,000	< 3,000 to 2,000	<2,000 to 1,000	<1,000
Granulocytes (per mm^3)	LLN to 1,500	<1,500 to 1,000	<1,000 to 500	<500
Hemoglobin (g/dL)	LLN to 10.0	<10.0 to 8.0	<8.0 to 6.5	<6.5
Platelets (per mm^3)	LLN to 75,000	<75,000 to 50,000	<50,000 to 25,000	<25,000

Representative drug dose modifications for hematologic toxicity			
Category (Timing)	**Parameters**	**CTCAE Grade**	**Dose or Schedule Modifications**
Granulocytes (day of therapy)	>1,500/mm^3 <1,500/mm^3	0,1 2,3,4	Full does of all drugs Delay until recovered. If delay >7 days, reduce doses by one level or add G-CSF. If delay >14 days, reduce doses by one level and add G-CSF

Contd.

Contd.

Platelets (day of therapy)	WNL <LLN to 75,000/mm³ <75,000/mm³	0 1 2, 3, 4	Full doses of all drugs Delay until recovered Delay until recovered. If delay > 7 days, reduce doses by one level
Granulocytes (cycle nadir)	>1,000/mm³ <500/mm³ for ≥ 7 days <1,000/mm³ with fever	0, 1, 2 4 3, 4	Full doses of all drugs Reduce doses by one level. If already reduced, add G-CSF for future cycles Add G-CSF for current episode, reduce doses by one level for future cycles. If already reduced, add G-CSF for future cycles.
Platelets (cycle nadir)	≥50,000/mm³ <50,000/mm³ with bleed <25,000/mm³	3 3, 4 4	Full doses of all drugs Reduce doses by one level Reduce doses by one level

I. DRUG RESISTANCE

Specific mechanisms of tumor drug resistance

Resistance Mechanism	Examples	Specific Cellular Target or Effects
Impaired activation	5-Fluorouracil	Reduced levels of thymidylate synthase, thymidylate phosphorylase, or dihydropyrimidine dehydrogenase
	Methotrexate	Reduced intracellular polyglutamation
	Doxorubicin	Low P450 enzymes
	Cyclophosphamide, ifosfamide	Decreased microsomal transformation
	Gemcitabine	Decreased deoxycytidine kinase
Increased drug efflux	Natural products	Increased MDR 1 (P 170)
	Topotecan, mitoxantrone	Increased BCRP (ABCG2)
Increased drug inactivation	Alkylating agents, platinum	Elevated glutathione and other cellular thiols
Accelerated DNA repair	Alkylating agents, platinum, radiation	Induction of DNA repair enzymes
Increased damage tolerance	Alkylating agents, platinum, radiation	Loss of DNA mismatch repair
Transport defects	Melphalan	Reduced carrier-mediated uptake
	Gemcitabine	Decreased nucleoside transporter
	Platinum	Decreased copper transporter-1
Target alterations	Methotrexate	DHFR gene amplification
	Paclitaxel, docetaxel	Increased tubulin-β3 isoforms or mutations
	Hydroxyurea, gemcitabine	Decreased ribonucleotide reductase
	Glucocorticoids	Decreased receptor binding
	Camptothecins	Decreased topoisomerase-I
	Anthracyclines, etoposide	Decreased topoisomerase-II

Site of action in the cell cycle

Portion of Cell Cycle	*Drugs*
G_1	*Actinomycin D*
Early S	*Hydroxyurea, cytosine arabinoside, 5-fluorouracil, methotrexate*
Late S	*Doxorubicin*
G_2	*Bleomycin, etoposide, teniposide, carboplatin, cisplatin, topotecan*
M	*Paclitaxel, vincristine, vinblastine*

Assessment of performance status

Score	Karnofsky Performance Status Scale
100	Normal, no complaints; no evidence of disease
90	Able to carry on normal activity, minor signs or symptoms of disease
80	Normal activity with effort; some signs or symptoms of disease
70	Cares for self but unable to carry on normal activity or do active work

Contd.

Contd.

60	Requires occasional assistance but is able to care for most personal needs
50	Requires considerable assistance and frequent medical care
40	Disabled; requires special care and assistance
30	Severely disabled; hospitalization indicated, although death not imminent
20	Very sick; hospitalization necessary; active support treatment necessary
10	Moribund; fatal process progressing rapidly
0	Dead
Grade	**Gynecologic Oncology Group Performance Status Scale**
1	Fully active, able to carry on all predisease performance without restriction
2	Restricted in physically strenuous activity but ambulatory and able to carry out work of a light or sedentary nature (e.g., light housework, office work)
3	Capable of only limited self-care, confined to bed or chair > 50% of waking hours
4	Completely disabled; cannot carry on any self-care; totally confined to bed or chair
5	Dead

Chemosensitivity	Tumor
Sensitive and curable	Leukaemias Lymphomas Germ cell tumors Childhood tumors
Sensitive and normally incurable (radical palliation) Moderately sensitive (palliation or adjuvant treatments)	Small cell lung cancer Myeloma Breast cancer Colorectal cancer Ovarian cancer Bladder cancer
Low sensitivity (chemotherapy of limited use)	Kidney cancer Melanoma Adult brain tumors Prostate cancer

Carcinogenic drug	Associated tumor
Cytotoxics (especially alkylating agents and topoisomerase II inhibitors)	Acute myeloid leukaemia
Cyclophosphamide Immunosuppression	Bladder cancer Kaposi's sarcoma, post-transplantation lymphoproliferation
Oestrogens (unopposed)	Endometrial cancer
Oestrogens (transplacental)	Vaginal adenocarcinoma
Oral contraceptive pill	Hepatic adenoma
Androgenic anabolic steroids	Hepatocellular carcinoma
Phenacetin	Renal pelvis transitional cell cancer
Chloramphenicol	Acute leukaemia
Phenytoin	Lymphoma, neuroblastoma

Name	Target	Class	Clinical uses
Bevacizumab	VEGF	Monoclonal antibody	Colon cancer and NSCLC
Cetuximab	EGFR	Monoclonal antibody	Colon cancer and head and neck cancer
Dasatinib	BCR/ABL	Small molecule	CML
Erlotinib	EGFR	Small molecule	NSCLC
Gefitinib	EGFR	Small molecule	NSCLC
Imatinib	BCR/ABL	Small molecule	CML and GIST
Lapatinib	EGFR and Her2	Small molecule	Breast cancer
Sorafenib	Multiple target kinases	Small molecule	Kidney cancer and liver cancer
Sunitinib	Multiple target kinases	Small molecule	Kidney cancer and GIST
Trastuzumab	Her2	Monoclonal antibody	Breast cancer

CHAPTER 55 MISCELLANEOUS

ONE LINERS

1. Most common cancer to cause opsoclonus in children–Neuroblastoma
2. Most common cancer to cause opsoclonus in Adults–Ca LUNG
3. Most common cause of subacute cortical cerebellar degeneration is Ca Ovary
4. Most common cancer associated with Guillain Barre syndrome is Hodgkin lymphoma
5. **Most common tumor associated with POEMS Syndrome is Myeloma**
6. Impaired horizontal gaze and Orofacial spasm is associated most commonly with Ca Prostate
7. Life threatening complication of SVC Syndrome is Tracheal obstruction
8. Most common tumor causing spinal cord compression is Ca Lung
9. Most common tumor to metastasize to bones is Ca Breast
10. Most common tumor to metastatize to brain is Ca Lung
11. Ball's disease (Intracranial leucocytosis) is seen in AML
12. Drug most commonly causes Hemolytic uremic syndrome is Mitomycin C
13. Drug most commonly associated with Raynaud's phenomenon is Bleomycin
14. Radiation fibrosis/Pneumonitis occurs if dose is greater than 40 Gy
15. Tumor that causes Non islet cell Hypoglycemia is Soft tissue sarcoma (IGF-2)
16. Most common Paraneoplastic Endocrine syndrome is Hypercalcemia
17. Molecule causing Paraneoplastic thrombocytosis is IL-6
18. Paraneoplastic Eosinophilia is due to IL-5 (Leukemic Lymphoma)
19. Tumor most commonly associated with paraneoplastic neurologic syndrome is Ca Lung
20. Only hormone used as tumor marker is hCG
21. **TUMOR MARKERS:**
    - Rhabdomyosarcoma–Myoglobin
    - Kaposi sarcoma–Factor 8
    - Melanoma–S100 (More specific marker is HMB 45)
    - Lymphoma–CD 45
    - Hodgkin's Lymphoma–Leu M1
    - Carcinoma–Cytokeratin
    - Sarcoma–Desmin
    - Breast–GCDP (Gross cystic fluid protein)

22. **CHROMOSOMAL MARKERS:**
    - t(x,18)→Synovial sarcoma
    - t(11, 22)→Ewing's sarcoma
    - 3p- →Small cell carcinoma lung, RCC
    - 1p- →Neuroblastoma
    - 12p- →GCT
23. Peritoneal carcinomatosis is most commonly caused by Ca Ovary
24. Most sensitive investigation for response to chemotherapy is Angiography
25. X-ray bone shows mottled/punctate/Annular calcification. Most probable diagnosis is Chondrosarcoma
26. **BONE METASTASIS:**

	Osteolytic	**Osteoblastic**
Best investigation	Plain X-ray	Bone scan
Calcium	Hyper	Hypo (If extensive)
Urine hydroxyl proline	+	–
Increased Alk. phosphatase	–	+

27. Most common symptom of bone metastasis is Bone pain
28. Damecles syndrome→ fear of cancer relapse
29. **HIGH FAT DIET:**
    - Carcinoma Breast
    - Carcinoma Colon
    - Carcinoma Prostate
    - Carcinoma Endometrium
30. Cigarette smoke acts as both **initiator and promoter** of carcinogenesis→ **COMPLETE CARCINOGEN**
31. Familial cancer syndromes are usually inherited as Autosomal Dominant (Not all)
32. DNA repair abnormalities are usually inherited as Autosomal Recessive (Not all)
33. Most common malignancy associated with Li Fraumeni syndrome is Ca Breast
34. Gaurdian of Genome is P53
35. Gaurdian of G2 check point is P53
36. Most common genetic alteration in human cancer is P53
37. Most treatment failure and death are caused by Metastatic dissemination
38. Most common cause of death in Epidermolysis Bullosa is SCC
39. Most common prophylactic surgery is removal of premalignant skin lesions
40. A 10 cm tumor mass has 10^{12} tumor cells
41. MEGAVOLTAGE THERAPY–Deep lesions
42. ORTHOVOLTAGE THERAPY–Superficial lesion
43. Electron beam therapy–Superficial tumors (Skin cancers)
44. **RADIATION TOLERANCE:**
    - Brain–60 Gy
    - Heart–45 Gy
    - Intestine–45 to 50 Gy

- Kidney–20 Gy
- Bone marrow–250 cGy
- Ovary–200 cGy
- Testis–100 cGy

45. Alkylating agents have steep dose response (Increase dose=Increase effect)
46. Antimetabolites have linear dose response curves only over a narrow range (Increase duration=Increase effect–schedule dependent)
47. 5FU→ Myocardial ischemia

SVC SYNDROME

1. Most common cause of SVC syndrome → Lung cancer
2. Most common symptom of SVC syndrome is Dyspnea
3. Gold standard for identifying SVC obstruction is Bilateral upper extremity Venography (But doesn't identify cause of obstruction)
4. **CECT is most useful imaging to define extent of venous blockage and identify underlying cause of venous obstruction – INVESTIGATION OF CHOICE**
5. Chemotherapy is treatment of choice in SCLC, NHL, Germ cell tumor and Breast cancer associated SVC Syndrome
6. Therapy for NSCLC is endovascular stent placement and RT
7. Surgery is the treatment of choice for malignant thymoma and thymic carcinoma
8. Cyanosis that worsens when patient bends forward/supine is present in SVC syndrome
9. Most common physical finding in SVC syndrome is Thoracic/neck vein distension
10. Indications for placement of endovascular stents for SVC syndrome:
    - Previously undiagnosed NSCLC followed by RT
    - Recurrent symptomatic SVC obstruction previously treated by RT
11. Short term anticoagulation with warfarin/dual antiplatelet therapy (clopidogrel + aspirin) is recommended for 3 months after stent placement
12. Presence of dysphagia, hoarseness or stridor are adverse prognostic factors in patients with SVC Syndrome
13. Most common non malignant cause of SVC Syndrome is thrombosis in presence of central vein catheters/pacemakers
14. Most common cause of SVC Syndrome in pediatric population→ Iatrogenic
15. Ketoconazole prevents recurrent SVC Syndrome from active Histoplasmosis
16. **Relief of SVCS occurs within 7-10 days after initiation of therapy in SCLC**
17. Indications of surgery in SVC Syndrome→ Rapidly progressive disease, Retrosternal Goiter and Aortic aneurysm
18. **Preferred bypass route is between innominate/jugular vein on left side and right atrial appendage using end to end anastomosis**
19. Most common surgical approach is via sternotomy/thoracotomy with extensive resection of tumor and reconstruction of SVC
20. Venous pressures in upper extremities have commonly been recorded to be >300 mm saline in severe SVC Syndrome

SPINAL CORD COMPRESSION

- Most common cancer cause of Spinal cord compression→ Lung cancer
- Most common cause of Spinal metastasis→ Hematogenous seeding of tumor-extradural metastasis
- ***Most common site involved in Spinal cord compression→*** *Thoracic spine >Lumbosacral spine*
- 1st symptom of Spinal cord compression→ Pain which worsens with recumbency, exacerbated by flexion, Valsalva and Coughing

- MRI of entire thecal sac is preferred modality for initial evaluation of patient with suspected spinal cord compression
- Most important prognostic factor for regaining ambulation after treatment of Spinal cord compression is pretreatment neurologic status
- Corticosteroids should be started as soon as Spinal cord compression is suspected
- Rapid onset of symptoms by vertebral burst fracture should be treated immediately by removing bone fragments from spinal canal
- Most common route of tumor reaches epidural space is direct extension from metastasis to vertebral body growing into epidural space in Spinal cord compression
- Rapid progression of Spinal cord compression is seen with Lung cancer, Renal cancer and Multiple myeloma
- Thoracic disease causes bilateral radiculopathy resulting in bandlike distribution of pain
- Myelography is contraindicated in patients with coagulopathy and may worsen neurologic deficit below level of complete spinal shock
- Loss of sphincter control has poor outcome in Spinal cord compression

High yield points

- Acute emesis is the most common type of chemotherapy induced emesis
- Delayed emesis occurs due to cisplatin usually after 1-7 days
- Most common cause of death in patient with cancer is Infection
- Aprepitant is substance P/NK 1 receptor antagonist
- Most modifiable risk factor for cardiovascular and cancer is smoking
- Cancer preventing agent with high risk of stroke is alpha tocopherol
- Karnofsky performance index 70 indicates patient cares for self, unable to carry on normal activity or do active work
- Damocles syndrome–fear of relapse of malignancy
- **CONCEPT OF MICRO RNA'S and CANCER:** mir-15 and mir-16 have been shown to target Bcl-2 oncogene leading to downregulation in leukemic cells and apoptosis. P53 can transcriptionally induce mir-34 following genotoxic stress and this induction is important in mediating P53 function. Expression of miRNA is extremely specific and there is evidence that miRNA expression patterns may be useful in distinguishing lineage and differentiation state as well as cancer diagnosis and outcome prediction
- 1st tumor suppressor gene to be discovered is RB gene
- Tumor suppressor gene involved in almost all human malignancies is P53
- Most common oncogene involved in human malignancies is RAS
- Micro RNA is involved in pathogenesis of CLL
- Late adenoma to carcinoma conversion occurs due to mutation of P53
- Care taker gene–gene that preserves genome integrity
- Gate keeper gene–gene that promotes differentiation
- Increased tenascin is 10 fold increased risk of Invasive breast cancer
- Early phase–PARACRINE→ TGF beta
- PROBAND→ Index case–1st case to be diagnosed
- Macrophages of CA Pancreas are Immunosuppressive
- Alpha 4 Beta 1–Correlates Melanoma progression
- Switch NCAM Expression is associated with CRC and CA Pancreas
- Reduced NCAM Expression is associated with NSCLC, Wilms tumor and Neuroblastoma
- CXCL12→ CA breast
- Deletion BECKLIN1→ Ovarian, Breast and Prostate cancers
- Increased FAS Fraction→ CA Lung and Colon

AUTOCRINE AND PARACRINE MECHANISMS

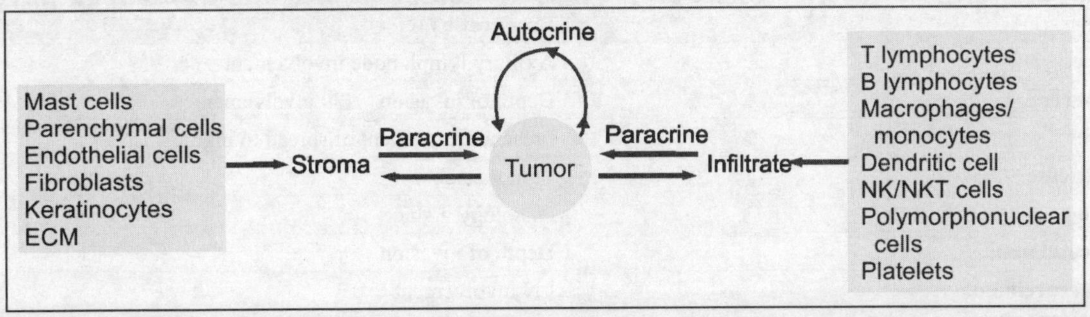

Tumor to mechanisms growth of contribution in changes

- During tumor progression, the contribution of paracrine growth mechanisms decreases, and the tumor becomes more dependent on autocrine growth mechanisms.
- At later stages, the tumor may even become independent of growth mechanisms

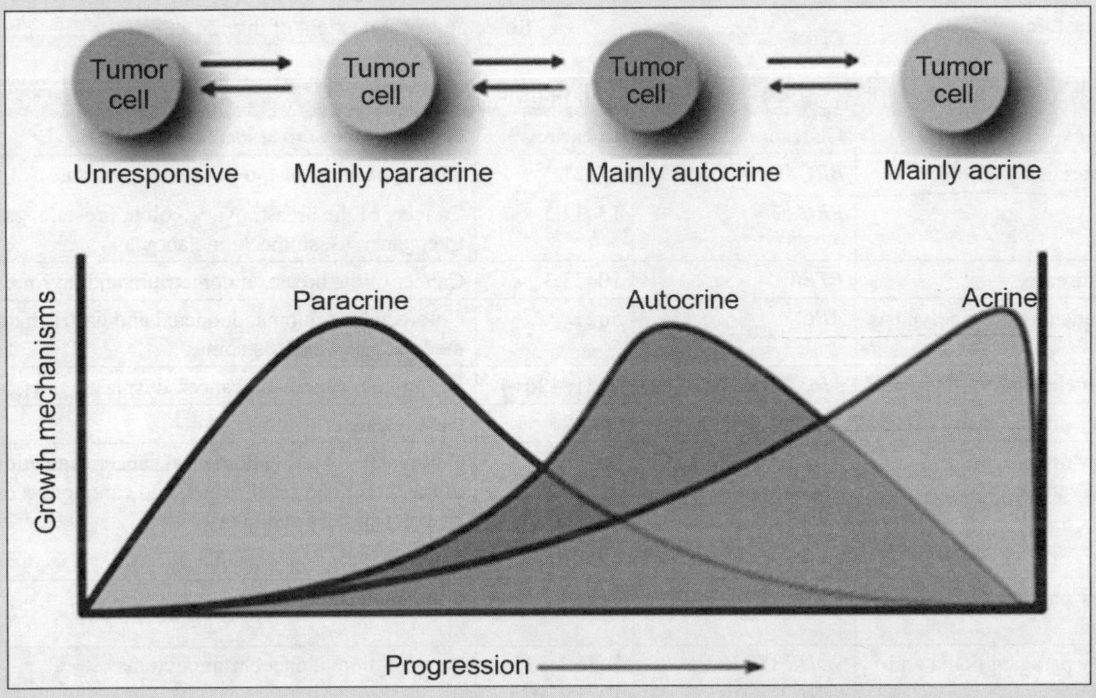

Translocation	Tumor
EWS-ATF1	Malignant melanoma of soft parts
MYC-IgH	Burkitt's lymphoma, B cell ALL
BCL1-IgH	Mantle cell lymphoma
BCL2-IgH	Follicular lymphoma
PKAR1A-RET	Thyroid carcinoma
TCRB-LCK	T cell ALL
TPM3-TRK	Colon carcinoma
FKHR/ALV-PAX3	Alveolar rhabdomyosarcoma
KHR/ALV-PAX7	Alveolar rhabdomyosarcoma
EWS-WT1	Desmoplastic small round cell tumor
BCR-ABL	Chronic myeloid leukemia
TCTA-TAL1	Acute T cell leukemia
NRG-REL	NHL
EWS-FLI1	Ewing's sarcoma

Most important prognostic markers	
Cancer	**Prognostic factor**
Breast cancer	Axillary lymph node involvement
Stomach cancer	Depth of invasion > LN involvement
Penile cancer	Presence and extent of spread to inguinal LNs
Hodgkins disease	Tumor stage
Wilms tumor	Histology > stage
Colorectal carcinoma	Depth of invasion
Endometrial carcinoma	LN involvement
Carcinoid tumor and PNET	Presence of liver metastasis
Musculoskeletal sarcomas	Tumor grade
AML	Age at diagnosis
CA bladder	Depth of tumor invasion
Renal cell carcinoma	Robson's pathologic stage
Hepatoblastoma	Resectability and extent of disease

Familial cancer syndromes			
Syndrome	**Genes**	**Locations**	**Cancer Sites and Associated Traits**
Breast/ovarian syndrome	*BRCA1*	17q21	Cancer of the breast, ovary, colon, prostate
	BRCA2	13q12.3	Cancers of the breast, ovary, colon, prostate, gallbladder and biliary tree, pancreas, stomach; melanoma
Cowden disease	*PTEN*	10q23.3	Cancer of the breast, endometrium and thyroid
Familial adenomatous polyposis	*APC*	5q21	Colorectal carcinoma, duodenal and gastric neoplasms, medulloblastomas, osteomas
Familial melanoma	*p16; CDK4*	9q21; 12q14	Melanoma, pancreatic cancer, dysplastic nevi, atypical moles
Hereditary diffuse gastric cancer	*CDH1*	16q22	Gastric cancer
Hereditary nonpolyposis colorectal cancer	*hMLH1; hMSH2; hMSH6; hPMS1; hPMS2*	3p21; 2p22-21; 2p16; 2q31.1; 7q22.2	Colorectal cancer; endometrial cancer; transitional cell carcinoma of the ureter and renal pelvis; and carcinomas of the stomach, small bowel, pancreas and ovary
Hereditary papillary renal cell carcinoma	*MET*	7q31	Renal cell cancer
Hereditary paraganglioma and pheochromocytoma	*SDHB; SDHC; SDHD*	1q36.1-p35; 1q21;11q23	Paraganglioma, pheochromocytoma
Juvenile polyposis coli	*BMPR1A SMAD4/DPC4*	10q21-q22 18q21.1	Juvenile polyps of the gastrointestinal tract, gastrointestinal malignant neoplasms
Li-Fraumeni	*p53 hCHK2*	17p13 22q12.1	Breast cancer, soft tissue sarcoma, osteosarcoma, brain tumors, adrenocortical carcinoma, Wilms tumor, phyllodes tumor (breast), pancreatic cancer, leukemia, neuroblastoma
Multiple endocrine neoplasia type 1	*MEN1*	11q13	Pancreatic islet cell tumors, parathyroid hyperplasia, pituitary adenomas
Multiple endocrine neoplasia type 2	*RET*	10q11.2	Medullary thyroid cancer, phiochromocytoma, parathyroid hyperplasia
MYH-associated adenomatous polyposis	*MYH*	1q34.3-p32.1	Cancer of the colon, rectum, breast, stomach
Neurofibromatosis type 1	*NF1*	17q11	Neurofibromas, neurofibrosarcoma, acute myelogenous leukemia, brain tumors
Neurofibromatosis type 2	*NF2*	22q12	Acoustic neuromas, meningiomas, gliomas, ependymomas
Nevoid basal cell carcinoma	*PTC*	9q22.3	Basal cell carcinoma
Peutz-Jeghers syndrome	*STK11*	19p13.3	Gastrointestinal carcinomas, breast cancer, testicular cancer, pancreatic cancer, benign pigmentation of the skin and mucosa

Contd.

Contd.

Retinoblastoma	*RB*	13q14	Retinoblastoma, sarcomas, melanoma, malignant neoplasms of the brain and meninges
Tuberous sclerosis	*TSC1; TSC2*	9q34; 16p13	Multiple hamartomas, renal cell carcinoma, astrocytona
von Hippel-Lindau syndrome	*VHL*	3q25	Renal cell carcinoma, hemangioblastomas of the retina and central nervous system, pheochromocytoma
Wilms tumor	*WT*	11p13	Wilms tumor, aniridia, genitourinary abnormalities, mental retardation

Selected IARC Group 1 pharmaceutical carcinogens

Pharmaceutical Carcinogen	Predominant Tumor Type
Azathioprine	Non-Hodgkin, lymphoma, squamous cell cancer of the skin, hepatocellular carcinoma, cholangiocarcinoma
Cyclophosphamide	Cancer of the urinary bladder, leukemia
Chlorambucil	Leukemia
Tamoxifen	Endometrial cancer
Estrogens (OCP, HRT)	Cancer of the breast and endometrium

Selected IARC Group 1 infectious carcinogens

Infectious Carcinogen	Predominant Tumor Type
Epstein-Barr virus	Bukitt lymphoma, Hodgkin disease, immunosuppression-related lymphoma, nasopharyngeal carcinoma
Hepatitis B	Hepatocellular carcinoma
Hepatitis C	Hepatocellular carcinoma
Human immunodeficiency virus type 1	Kaposi sarcoma
Human papillomavirus types 16 and 18	Cervical cancer, anal cancer
Human T cell lymphotropic virus type 1	Adult T cell leukemia
Helicobacter pylori	Gastric adenocarcinoma
Opisthorchis vivemini	Cholangiocarcinoma, hepatocelluar carcinoma
Schistosoma haematobium	Cancer of the urinary bladder

Biomarkers and biologically targeted therapies

Cancer	Biomarker	Therapy
Breast	Estrogen receptor, progesterone receptor	Tamoxifen/aromatase inhibitors
Lymphoma	CD20	Rituximab
Chronic myelogenous leukemia	*bcr-abl*	Imatinib
Gastrointestinal stromal tumor	*c-kit*	Imatinib
Non-small cell lung cancer	*EGFR* mutation	Gefitinib
Breast	*HER2/neu*	Trastuzumab
Melanoma	*BRAF*V600E mutation	Vemurafenib

Targeted treatments mapped to the hallmarks of cancer. It is noteworthy that those agents that specifically target the hallmarks of cancer are not widely used in clinical practice. This may simply reflect the novelty of these agents, but could also suggest that an approach based on hallmarks is of more relevance to cancer biologists than to oncologists

Hallmark	Drug classes	Specific drugs
Resist signals that inhibit growth	Cyclin-dependent kinase inhibitors	Dinaciclib Palbociclib Ronaciclib Seliciclib
Sustaining proliferative signaling	EGFR inhibitors	Trastuzumab Cetuximab
Avoid immune detection/destruction	Immune activators: antagonists of CTLA4, PD1, PD-L1 OX40 agonists	Ipilumumab Pembrolizumab Nivolumab MEDI6383

Contd.

Contd.

Obtain replicative immortality	Telomerase inhibitors	Imetelstat
Evoke inflammation	Anti-inflammatory drugs	Aspirin
Acquire ability to invade	Inhibition of Wnt/P-catenin	Resveratrol
Acquire ability to disseminate and implant	IGF-1 inhibitors	Linsitinib
Acquire angiogenic competence	Inhibitors of VEGF	Ramucirumab Bevacizumab Aflibercept
Genomic instability	PARP inhibitors	Olaparib Niraparib Rucaparib Veliparib
Evade apoptosis	BH3 mimetics	Navitoclax Venetoclax
Deregulate cellular energy supply and transfer	Aerobic glycolysis inhibitors	Metformin

SPECIAL TOPICS

- **EPIGENETICS:** Heritable changes in gene expression→Histone methylation, Histone acetylation, Histone phosphorylation
- Epigenetic dysregulation plays central role in malignancy

Trials

Phase	Conducted On	Purpose
I	Healthy volunteers	Safety and tolerability **Know maximum tolerable doses**
II	Patients	Establish Therapeutic efficacy
III	Several centres	Confirm Therapeutic efficacy
IV	Practicing physicians	Know rare and long term adverse effects

Lead time bias

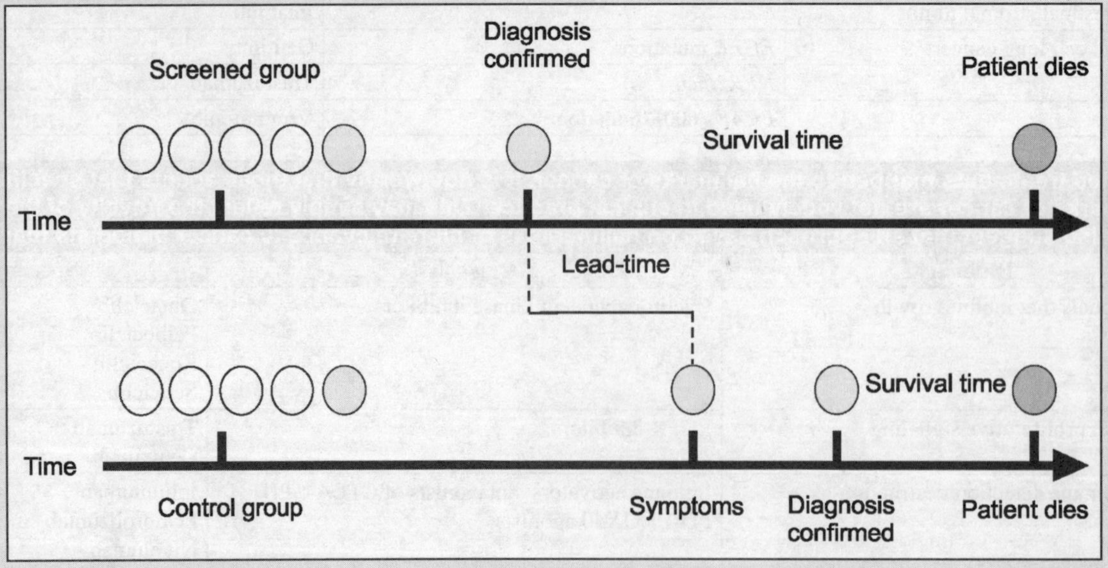

Contd.

Contd.

LAG tme bias

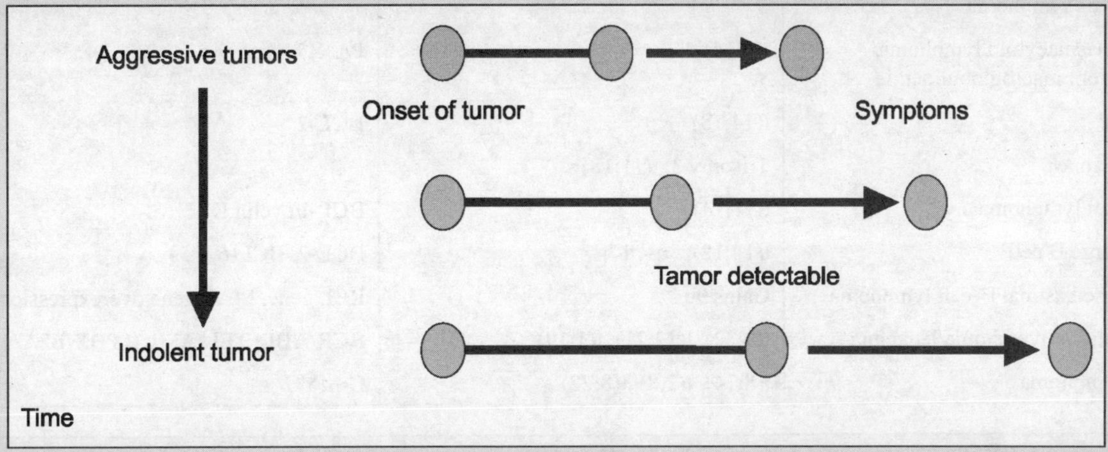

Overdiagnosis bias

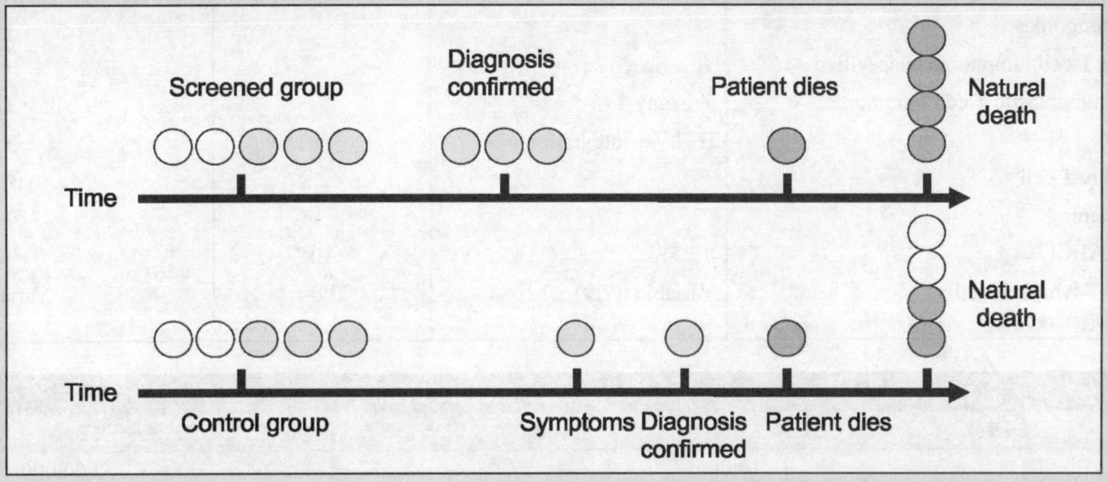

Hodgkin's lymphoma

Subtype	Morphology	Immunophenotype	Typical features
Nodular sclerosis	Lacunar cells	CD 15 and CD 30 +ve	Good prognosis, mediastinal involvement
Mixed cellularity	Mononuclear cells	CD 15 and CD 30 +ve	Poor prognosis, EBV +ve Stage III or IV
Lymphocyte rich	Mononuclear cells	CD 15 and CD 30 +ve	Good prognosis, EBV +ve
Lymphocyte depletion	Reticular variant	CD 15 and CD 30 +ve	**Poorest prognosis, Maximum** EBV +ve, **HIV infected**
Lymphocyte predominant	Pop corn cells	CD 15 and CD 30 –ve **CD 20 +ve**	**Best prognosis**

Skin involvement in Lymphoma
1. **Myocosis fungoides**–50% of all skin lymphomas, First sign of the disease is 1/more patchy, scaly red skin lesions
2. **Sezary syndrome**–Generalized erythroderma, very itchy red rash looks like Sunburn
3. **ALCL–primary cutaneous anaplastic large cell lymphoma**→good prognosis, Tumors on skin which may ulcerate
4. **Lymphomatoid papulosis**–Benign, Slow growing self limited

Histology	Cytogenetics	Oncogene/Protein
Chronic lymphocytic leukemia/small lymphocytic lymphoma	Trisomy 12[a], 13q–, 11q–, 17p–	
Lymphoplasmacytoid lymphoma/ Waldenstrom macroglobulinemia	t(9;14)	PAX-5
Follicular[b]	t(14;18)	BCL-2
Marginal zone[c]	Trisomy 3, t(11;18)	
Mantle cell lymphoma	t(11;14)	BCL-I/cyclin D1
Diffuse large B cell[d]	t(14;18), 3q–, 17p–	BCL-2, BCL-6, P53
Primary mediastinal B-cell lymphoma	Gains 9p	REL gene, MAL gene overexpression
Lymphoblastic lymphoma/leukemia	t(9;22), t(12;21), t(1;19)	BCR/ABL, TEL/AML1, PBX/E2A
Burkitt lymphoma	t(8;14), t(2;8), t(8;22)	C-MYC

Histology	Cytogenetics	Oncoprotein	TCR Gene Rearrangements
T-CLL/T-PLL	Inv14, Trisomy 8q	Bcl-3	+
Mycosis fungoides			+
Peripheral T-cell lumphoma unspecified	9p–, 5p–, 12q–		+
Angioimmunoblastic T-cell lymphoma[a]	Trisomy 3 or 5		+
ATL	HTLV-1 integration +		+
Enteropathy T cell			β+
Hepatosplenic			δγ+
Systemic ALCL[bc]	t(2;5)	Alk	+
Precursor T-lymphoblastic lymphoma/leukemia	Variable t(7;9)	Tcl-4	Variable

Prognostic factors in all

Factor	Good	Bad
WBC	<10,000	>2,00,000
Age	2-9 years	<1 year, >10 years
Gender	Female	Male
Lymph node enlarged	–	+
Hepatomegaly	–	+
Splenomegaly	–	+
Testicles enlarged	–	+
CNS involved	–	+
Ploidy	Hyperploidy	Hypoploidy
Subtype of ALL	**L1, Early pre B cell ALL**	**L2, Pre B cell ALL, Mature B cell ALL**
Markers	Trisomy 4,10,17 t(12,21) (TEL-AML1)	t(9,22) (BCR-ABL) t(4,11) (MLL-AF4)
Remission status	<14 days	>14 days

Genetic disorders associated with chromosomal instability that result in immunodeficiency and predisposition to cancer

Disorder	Gene Defect	Immune Defects	Cancers Reported
Ataxia telangiectasia	*ATM*[60]	IgA deficiency, ↓ T cells	Lymphoma, leukemia, hepatocarcinoma, genitourinary carcinoma, skin cancer
Nijmegen breakage syndrome	*NBS1*[64]	Hypogammaglobulinemia, lymphopenia	Myeloid leukemia, lymphoma
Bloom's syndrome	*BLM*[65]	Hypogammaglobulinemia, natural killer cell deficiency	Lymphoma, epithelial cancer
Werner's syndrome	*WRN*[66]	Antibody deficiency?	Lymphoma

TUMOR MARKERS

Serum, Plasma		
CA 15-3, CA 27-29	Breast	Monitoring; recurrence
HER-2	Breast	Monitoring
Circulating tumor cells (Cell Search; whole blood)	Breast	Prognosis in metastatic disease
CA 125	Ovarian	Monitoring second-look evaluation
CA 19-9	Pancreatic	Monitoring
Total PSA, complexed PSA (cPSA)	Prostate	Detection in men aged ≥50 years in conjunction with DRE; monitoring prognosis
Free PSA	Prostate	Aid in distinguishing prostate cancer from benign prostate conditions in men ≥50 years with a total PSA of 4-10 ng/mL and nonsuggestive DRE in conjunction with total PSA (% free PSA)
Prostatic acid phosphatase	Prostate	Monitoring
Carcinoembryonic antigen	Colorectal, breast, lung	Monitoring, prognosis
AFP	Nonseminomatous testicular	Monitoring
AFP-L3	Hepatocellur	Risk assessment
Des-γ-carboxy prothrombin	Hepatocellular	Risk assessment
Thyroglobulin	Thyroid	Monitoring (in patients without thyroglobulin autoantibodies)
Soluble mesothelin-related peptides	Mesothelioma	Monitoring
β-human chorionic gonadotropin	None	Detection of pregnancy (not approved as a tumor marker)
Urine		
BTA stat, BTA TRAK	Bladder	Management in conjunction with cystoscopy
NMP-22	Bladder	Diagnosis in symptomatic patients or those with risk factors; recurrence
Tumor cell markers (ImmunoCyt)	Bladder	Management in conjunction with urine cytology and cystoscopy
Tissue		
Estrogen and progesterone receptors	Breast	Assessing the likelihood of response to therapy; prognosis and management
HER-2	Breast	Identify patients eligible for trastuzumab (Herceptin) treatment
EGFR	Colorectal	Identify patients eligible for cetuximab treatment

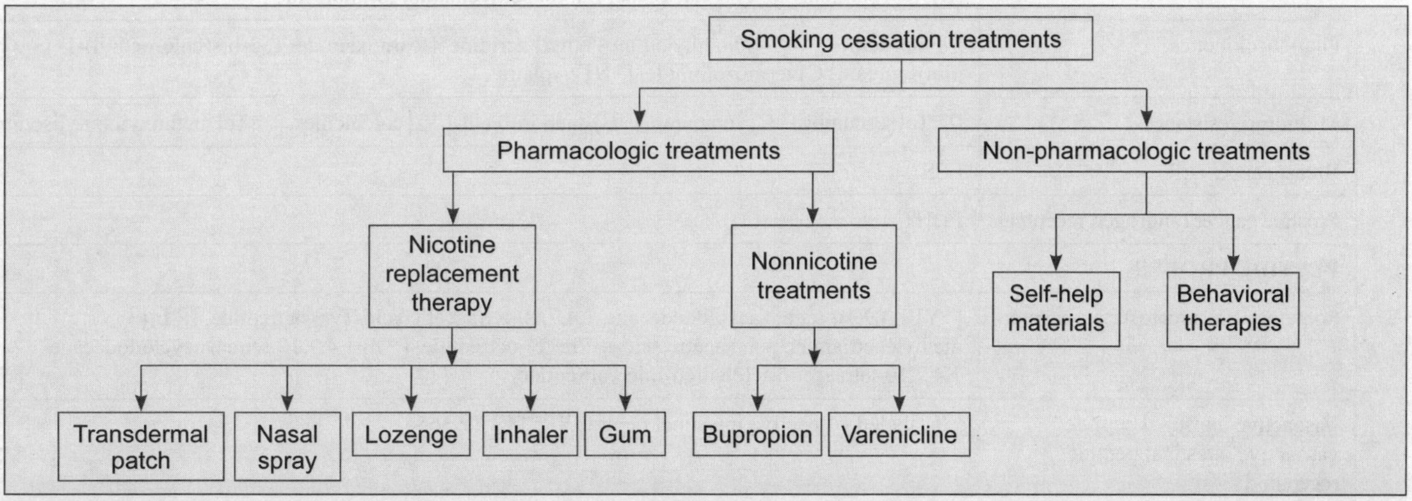

Common predisposing conditions and associated malignancies

Condition	Genes Tested	Associated Malignancy
Cryptorchid testis		Testicular
Chronic ulcerative colitis		Colon
Familial adenomatous polyposis	*APC*	Colon and rectum

Contd.

Contd.

Hereditary non-polyposis colon cancer	*MSH2* *MSH6* *MLH1* *PMS1* *PMS2*	Colon and rectum
Family history of colon cancer		Colon and rectum
Multiple endocrine neoplasia Type 1	*MEN1*	Pancreatic islet cell, anterior pituitary
Multiple endocrine neoplasia Type 2	*RET gene*	Medullary cancer of the (types II and III) thyroid
Leukoplakia		Squamous
Family history of breast cancer	*BRCA1 and BRCA2*	Breast and ovary
Family history of ovarian cancer	*BRCA1 and BRCA 2*	Ovary and breast

American Society of Anesthesiologists Physical Status Classification

Class	Description
I	Healthy patient
II	Mild systemic disease, no functional limitation
III	Severe systemic disease, definite functional limitation
IV	Severe systemic disease that is a constant threat to life
V	Moribund patient unlikely to survive 24 hours with or without operation

Imaging probes used to visualize molecular targets and processes in cancer

Molecular Target/Process	Imaging Probes
SMALL MOLECULE PROBES	
Proliferation	2-[^{11}C]JThymidine, FLT, 1-(2'-deoxy-2'-fluoro-β-D-arabinofuranosyl) thymine, 2'-deoxy-2'-fluoro-5-fluoro-1-β-D-arabinofuranosyluracil, [^{124}I] iododeoxyuridine
Apoptosis	[^{99m}Tc] Annexin V, [^{18}F] Annexin V
Hypoxia	[^{18}F] misonidazole, 2-(2-nitro-1H-imidazol-1-yl)-N-(2,2,3,3,3-pentafluoropropyl) acetamide, fluoroerythro-nitroimidazole, fluoroetanidazole, diacetyl-bis (N^4-methylthiosemicarbazone) copper (II), [^{124}I) iodo-azomycingalactoside, fluoroazomycinarabinofuranoside
Pharmacokinetics	5-Fluorouracil, *N*-[2-(dimethylamino) ethyl] acridine-4-carboxamide, 1, 3-bis(chloroethyl)-1-nitrosourea, [^{11}C] termozolomide, [^{11}N] cisplatin
Multidrug resistance	[^{99m}Tc] sestamibi, [^{11}C] verapamil, [^{11}C] daunorubicin, [^{11}C] colchicines, [^{99tm}Tc] methoxyiobutylisonitrile
Breast cancer (ER)	FES
Prostate cancer (androgen receptor)	FDHT
PEPTIDE PROBES	
Somatostatin/somatostatin receptor	[^{90}Y] 1,4,7,10-tetraazacyclododecane-1,4,7,10-tetraacetic acid-Tyr^3-octreotide, [^{111}In] diethylenetriamine pentaacetic acid-D-Phe(1)-octreotide, [^{90}Y] 1,4,7,10-tetraazacyclododecane-1,4,7,10-tetraacetic acidlanreo-tide/vapreotide
Vasoactive intestinal peptide/ vasoactive intestinal peptide receptor-1	^{123}I-labeled vasoactive intestinal peptide, [^{99m}TC] TP 3654
Bombesin, gastrin-releasing peptide/gastrin-releasing peptide receptor	^{99m}Tc-labeled bombesin
Cholecystokinin, gastrin/ cholecystokinin receptor	^{111}In-labeled diethylenetriamine pentaacetic acid-minigastrin
Angiogenesis	^{18}F-labeled Arg-Gly-Asp peptide targeted to $\alpha_\gamma\beta_3$ integrin

Contd.

Contd.

Cathepsin proteases	Prosense (VM 102)
ANTIBODY PROBES	
Angiogenesis	Paramagnetic nanoparticles using antibodies to integrin $\alpha_\gamma\beta_3$, the integrin $\alpha_\gamma\beta_3$ ligand, vascular cell adhesion molecule 1, E-selectin
CEA	Arcitumomab (CEAscan), satumomab
Prostate-specific membrane antigen	Capromab pendetide (Prosta Scint)
CD20	^{131}I-labeled tositumomab (Bexxar), ^{90}Y-labeled ibritumomab tiuxetan (Zevalin) (FDA approved)
CD22	Bectumomab

CHEMOPREVENTION

- Agents used to target high risk individuals, individuals with precancerous lesions and prevention of second primaries or recurrences

Agents
• Retinoids and Vitamin A
• Vitamin E
• COX 2 inhibitors
• Tyrosine kinase inhibitors
• ONYX 015 Inhibitors

- **Retinoids** act by modulating gene expression→ Effect on premalignant, Malignant growth, differentiation and Apoptosis
- **Beta carotene** acts as an antioxidant and prevents cancer evolution→ Less toxic
- **Selenium and Vitamin E**–Antioxidant→ Prevents cancer by reducing free radical damage

COX 2 inhibitors
• Aspirin inhibits inflammatory effects of mediators of tumors
• **Sulindac:** Pan COX inhibitor–Antineoplastic effect
• **Celecoxib:** Inhibits COX 2 but not COX 1

PALLIATIVE CARE

- Timon and Reilly estimate that approximately 20% of head and neck cancer patients would qualify for palliative care input at the time of initial diagnosis, with an average survival of 5 months

Shuman et al. suggest following situations for review regarding need for palliative care:
- Unresectable locoregional disease and/or distant metastasis at initial presentation
- Patients with recurrent unresectable locoregional disease and/or distant metastasis after treatment
- Patients unable to have anticancer treatments due to:

  Disease stage, comorbidity, functional status and/or individual preference

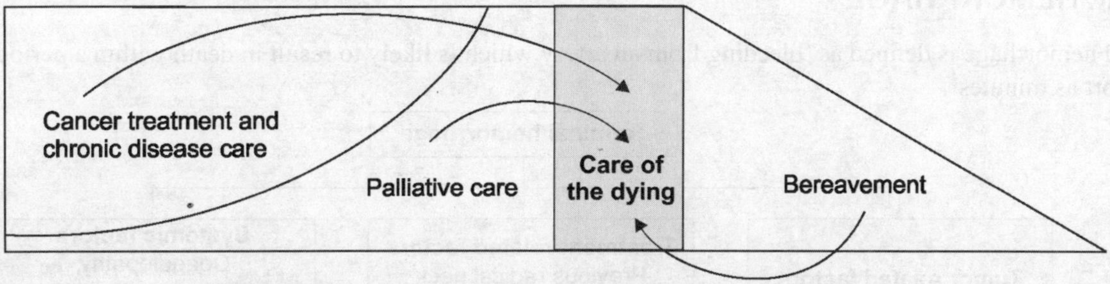

Involvement of palliative care within disease trajectory

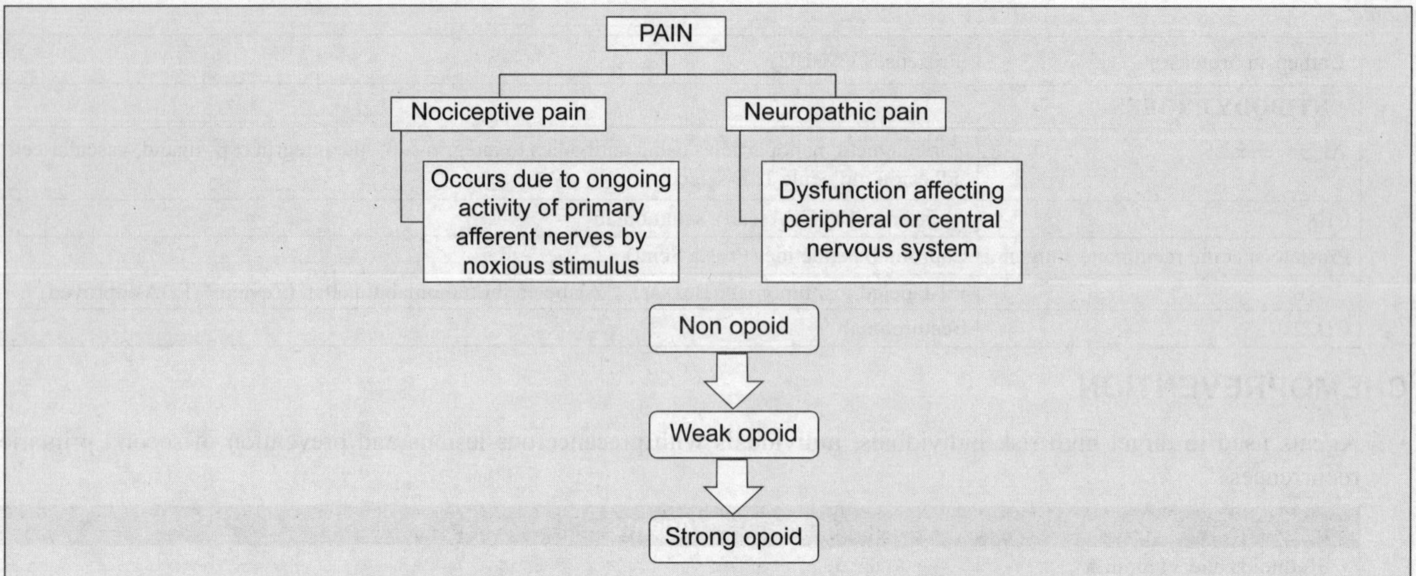

Opioid of choice for moderate to severe pain remains morphine

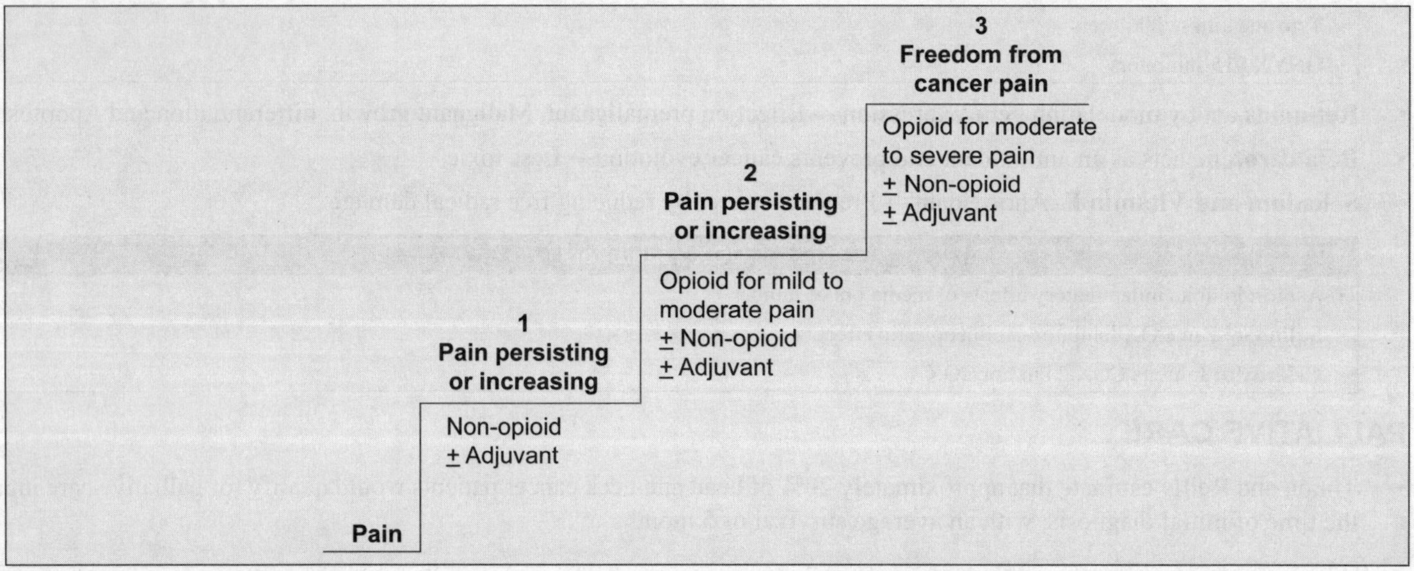

TRANSDERMAL PATCHES

- Should only be used when pain control has been established and is generally stable
- Tend to be changed every 72 hours so they don't have as much flexibility in terms of dose titration
- Buprenorphine patch have a maximum dose range (up to 20 mcg which is equivalent to just under 50 mg oral morphine

TERMINAL HEMORRHAGE

- Terminal hemorrhage is defined as 'bleeding from an artery which is likely to result in death within a period of time that may be as short as minutes

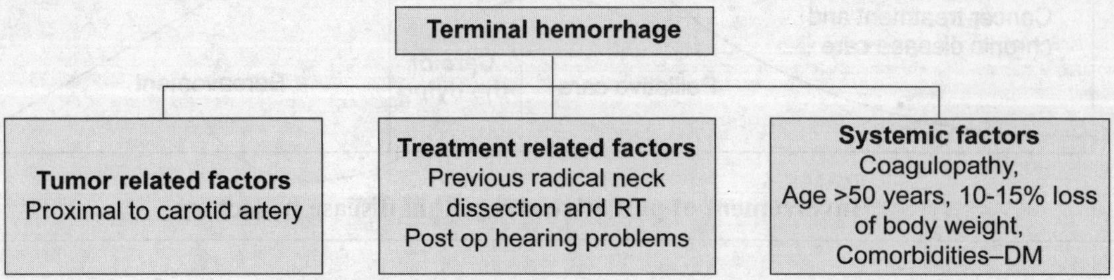

MUST READ

- ***Hamartoma***→Cell with abnormal differentiation but present at normal location
- ***Choristoma***→Cells with normal differentiation but present at abnormal location
- ***Anaplasia*** (Absence of differentiation)→Hallmark of malignant transformation
- ***Metastasis***→Most reliable feature of a malignant tumor
- Most carcinogenic UV rays to reach the earth: UVB (280-320 nm)
- Carcinogenic potential of a chemical is tested by: Ames test
- *Vimentin* is the marker of mesenchymal cells/Sarcoma
- *Desmin* is the marker of muscle cells
- Almost all cancer can metastasize except:
  - Glioma
  - Rodent ulcer/Basal cell cancer of skin
- Which phase of cell cycle is considered as point of no return: S-phase
- The phosphorylation of this gene acts as a molecular ON-OFF switch for the cell cycle: RB gene
- Rosettes pattern on histopathology is characteristically seen in: RB
- Familial Retinoblastoma is also associated with increased risk of: Osteosarcoma
- NF-1 gene encodes for: Neurofibromin protein
- NF-2 gene encodes for: Merlin protein
- In Malignant melanoma, HMB 45 is a more specific marker whereas S-100 is more sensitive marker
- *Oncogene:* RAS, ABL, MYC, SIS, INT-2, KIT
- *Tumor suppressor gene:* RB, p^{53}, NF, BRCA, APC
- RET gene mutation is associated with: Medullary CA of Thyroid
- Most radiosensitive cell in the blood: Lymphocyte
- Least radiosensitive cell: Platelet
- Spontaneous regression of tumor is seen in: Neuroblastoma
- Most radiosensitive tissue of the body: Bone marrow
- Least radiosensitive cell of the body: Neurons
- Most radiosensitive blood cell: Lymphocyte
- Least radiosensitive blood cell: Platelet
- Amifostine is: Radio protector
- National cancer control Program was launched in the year: 1975
- Gold standard in diagnosing synovial sarcoma: t (X:18)

- ***Adjuvant chemotherapy is of definitive value in:***
  - Breast CA
  - Colorectal CA
- ***CF of Neuroblastoma:***
  - Orbital metastasis lead to: Raccon eye
  - Cutaneous metastasis lead to: Blueberry muffin lesions
  - Paraneoplastic features: Opsomyoclonus (Dacing eye, Dancing feet syndrome)
- ***Trousseau sign (Migratory thrombophlebitis) is seen in:***
  - Pancreatic CA
  - Bronchogenic CA
  - Colon CA
- ***Bone Metastasis:***
  - Purely osteolytic: Kidney (expansile)
  - Purely osteoblastic: Prostrate
  - IOC: Bone scan
- ***Pulsatile secondaries are seen in:***
  - Follicular carcinoma Thyroid
  - RCC
- ***Sentinel LN Biopsy is usually done in:***
  - CA Breast
  - CA Penis
  - Malignant melanoma
  - Vulvar cancer
- ***Pure β – emitters:***
  - Strontium-90
  - Yttrium-90
  - P_{32}
  - Tritium-H_3
- ***Isotopes used as Permanent interstitial implants:***
  - Palladium 103
  - Gold (Au) 198
  - Iodine 125
- ***Isotopes used as temporary intersitial implant:***
  - Iridium 192
  - Caesium 137
- ***Intensity modulated Radiotherapy (IMRT) is most suitable for:***
  - Prostate cancer
  - CA cervix
- ***Most radiosensitive tumors:***
  - Lung tumor: Small cell CA

- Kidney tumor: Wilm's tumor
- Bone tumor: Ewing's sarcoma and Multiple myeloma
- Brain tumor: Medulloblastoma
- Ovarian tumor: Dysgerminoma
- Testicular tumor: Seminoma

Most Common

- Most common gene mutation present in human cancers: P^{53}
- Most common cancer due to excessive UV light exposure: Basal cell CA
- Most common Paraneoplastic syndrome: Hypercalcemia
- Most common tumor to produce metastasis to cervical LN: Nasopharyngeal CA
- Most common tumor responsible for secondaries in the neck with no obvious primary malignancy: Nasopharyngeal CA
- Most common primary malignancy causing bone metastasis: CA Prostate
- Most common cause of osteoblastic secondaries in male: CA Prostate
- Most common tumor metastasize to bone in females: CA Breast
- Most common cause of osteoblastic secondaries in females: CA Breast
- **Most common malignancy of childhood: Brain tumor**
- 2nd Most common malignancy of childhood: Neuroblastoma
- Most common intra abdomen (solid) tumor in childhood: Neuroblastoma
- Most common tumor associated with superior vena cava syndrome: Lung cancer
- Most common site for lymphoma in the GIT Stomach
- Most common site of gastric lymphoma: Antrum
- Most common type of gastric lymphoma: Diffuse large B-cell lymphoma
- Most common tumor of the brain: Metastatic brain tumor
- Most primary site for metastatic brain tumor: CA lung > CA Breast
- Most common type of metaplasia in Barrett's Esophagus: Intestinal metaplasia
- Most common site of CA oral cavity: Tongue
- Most common retropetitoneal tumor: Liposarcoma
- Most common site of Rhabdomyosarcoma: Orbit
- Most common site for distant metastasis: Liver
- Most common cancer caused by Ionizing radiation: Papillary CA of Thyroid and Leukemia (except CLL)
- Most cancer in India: CA oral cavity
- Most common cancer
  - Males: Prostrate > Lung
  - Females: Breast > Lung

Cell Cycle Check Points

Cell cycle check points	
G_1–S	G_2–M
• Checks for DNA damage and inhibits replication of cells with mutated DNA • Controlled by p53	• Activation by ionizing radiation • Controlled by Cyclin-B

Differences Between Metaplasia, Dysplasia and Anaplasia

Features	Metaplasia	Dysplasia	Anaplasia
Pleomorphism	Absent	Present	Present
Reversibility	Reversible	Reversible in early stage	Irreversible
Mitotic figure	Absent	Typical appearance	Atypial appearance

Autosomal Dominant and Autosomal Recessive Cancer Syndrome

AD Cancer Syndrome	AR Cancer Syndrome
• Cowden syndrome (PHH gene) • FAP • HNPCC→due to defective DNA repair gene • Li Fraumeni syndrome • Melanoma • MLN 1 and 2 • NF – 1 and 2 • Peutz-Jeghers syndrome • Retinoblastoma • VHL Syndrome	• Ataxia telangiectasia • Bloom syndrome • Fanconi anemia • Xeroderma pigmentosum

Tumor Markers

Tumor Markers	Cancer
AFP	Liver cell cancer NSGCT of Testis
Placental ALP	Seminoma
CEA	Colon, Pancreas, Lung
CA-15-3	Breast cancer
CA-19.9	Colon cancer, Pancreas
CA-125	Ovarian cancer
Gastrin	Pancreatic neuroendocrine tumor
Bcl-2	Follicular lymphoma
Chromogranin	Neuroblastoma
NSE	Neuroblastoma
HMB-45	Malignant melanoma
hCG	Gestational trophoblastic tumor Germ cell tumor
Inhibin	Granulosa cell tumor

Radiosensitivity of Tumor

Radiosensitivity of tumor		
High sensitive	**Relatively resistant**	**Highly resistant**
• Seminoma • Ewing's sarcoma • Wilm's tumor • Multiple myeloma • Lymphoma	• CA cervix	• Pancreatic carcinoma • Osteosarcoma • Melanoma

Radiosensitivity of Cell Cycle Check Point

Phase of cell cycle	Comment
$G_2M>G_2$	Most sensitive to radiation
Late 'S' phase	Most resistant to radiation

Micro-organisms Associated with Cancers

Micro-organisms Associated with Cancers		
Pathogen	**Associated malignancy**	**Comment**
H. pylori	• Gastric MALT Lymphoma	• B cell origin • Associaed with t (11:18)
HBV	• HCC	• Encodes HB_x protein
HCV	• HCC • Lymphoplasmacytic lymphoma	
HPV	• Squamous cell carcinoma of Cervix • Laryngeal Carcinoma • HPV 16>18	• Associated with E_6 and E_7 gene expression • E_6 protein causes inactivation of P_{53}
HTLV-1	• Tropical spastic paraparesis	
EBV	• Post-transplant lymphoproliferative disorder • Hodgkin lymphoma • B-cell lymphoma • Burkitt's lymphoma–African type • Nasopharyngeal Carcinoma	• CD-21 on B cell surface acts as a target molecule • Associated with LMP gene expression • Associated with t (8:14)
HHV-8	• Multicentric Castleman disease	
	• Primary effusion lymphoma	
	• Kaposi sarcoma	• Proliferation of spindle cells that express markers of both endothelial and smooth muscle cells
C. sinensis	• Cholangiocarcinoma	
Opisthorchis viverrini	• Cholangiocarcinoma	
Schistosoma haematobium	• Squamous cell carcinoma of Urinary bladder	
Schistosoma japonicum	• Colorectal carcinoma	

Genes and Their Associated Tumors

Genes	Chromosome	Associated tumor
ABL	9	CML
APC	5q	Stomach carcinoma Colan carcinoma FAP
B-catenin		HCC, Hepatoblastoma
BRCA 1 and 2	17 and 13	Breast carcinoma Ovarian carcinoma
Cyclin-D	11	Mantle cell lymphoma
E. cadherin	16	Stomach carcinoma Colon carcinoma
ERB		Squamous cell carcinoma of lung
FMS		Leukemia
INT-2		• Stomach CA
C-KIT/CD 117		• GIST

Contd.

Contd.

K RAS		12	• Colon carcinoma
RET		10	• MEN 2A/2B • Familial medullary carcinoma of thyroid
MYC	***C-myc***		• Burkitt's lymphoma
	L-myc	8	• SCLS
	N-myc		• Neuroblastoma
NF2		22	• Acoustic schwannoma
P_{16} INK 4a			• Malignant melanoma
P_{53}		17	• Li Fraumeni syndrome
RB		13	• Retinoblastoma • Osteosarcoma
WT1		11p13	• Wilm's tumor

LUNG CANCER

- Most common tumor of lung→Primary malignant tumor/CA
- Most common benign tumor of lung→Hamartoma
- Hamartoma is characterized by:
  - Popcorn calcification→Pathognomonic
  - Marble like feel of the tumor
- Most common recurrent hemoptysis→Bronchial adenoma
- Most common causes of cancer death in both M and F→Lung CA
- Most common envrionment pollutant of natural origin responsible for lung CA→Radon
- Most common nerve involved in Pancoast tumor→C8 T1, 2
- Most common site of distant Metastasis in lung CA→Liver > Bone
- Most common source of metastastic lung CA→Colon CA
- Most common site of visceral metastasis from lung CA→Liver > Lung
- CA of lung Most common associated with SVC syndrome→Small cell lung CA
- Most common endocrine organ to be involved by metastasis from CA lung→Adrenals
- CA lung which can metastasize to opposite lung→Adeno CA
- Most common tumor to metastasize to heart→Ca lung
- Ca lung most responsive to chemotherapy→Small cell Ca
- Most common type of Ca lung associated with hypokalemia→Small cell
- Most common symptom of CA Lung→Cough
- Highest risk of lung Ca→Smoking + Arsenic exposure
- Most common site of primary in a patient presenting with secondaries to adrenals→Melanoma > Lungs
- Solitary fibrous tumor→not associated with asbestosis
  - CD - 34 +ve and kertain -ve
- IOC to look for mediastinal involvement→CT scan
- Screening test→History + Physical exam + S. Alkaline Phosphatase
- TOC of CA of superior pulmonary sulcus producing Pancoast's syndrome is→RT + Surgery
- Most common anticancer drug for treatment of NSCLS→Etoposide + Cisplatin

TOC in localised NSCLC	
Sx (Pulmonary resection)	RT
Stage I and II	Stage I and II who refuse Sx Stage III disease Not fit for Sx resection

TOC in SCLC	
CT +/- RT of Sx	High dose RT to whole brain for mets

LUNG CANCERS

	Squamous cell Ca	Adeno CA	Small cell CA	Large cell CA
Most common	• Most common cancer in India • Most common lung CA in smokers	• Most common CA of lung – world wide/in non smokers/Women	• Least common type	
M-F	• M>F	• F>M	• M>F	
Location	• Central	• Peripheral	• Central	• Peripheral
Prognosis	• Best prognosis		• Worst–most rapidly growing and most aggressive lung CA	
Cavity	• Cavitation +st		• +st	
Genetics	• Over expression of EGFR and P53 mutation	• k-ras mutation	• Expression of BCI-2 gene	
Association	• Smoking–strongest • Pancoast Tumor • Highest resectability rate • Presence of keratinization on H/P	• Present as fluffly infiltrate • Trans bronchlal spread (Bronchioalveolar type) • Pleural involvement • Cells are +ve for mucin and Thyroid transcription factor-1 (TTF-1)	• Lymphocyte like oat cell also known as oat cell CA • Least resectability rate • Most early and widely metastasizing tumor • Smoking • MG, Lambert Eaton syndrome • Salt and Pepper appear on H/P	• Pleural involvement • CNS involve (Most common with this variety)
Paraneoplastic syndrome	• Most common paraneoplastic syndrome associated is hypercalcemia and hypophosphatemia due to PTHrP • Most common Lung CA associated with clubbing • Most common type of lung Ca in male • Most common cause of Pancoast tumor	• Most common paraneoplastic syndrome associated is Hematological syndrome like: – Trousseau's syndrome (Migratory venous thrombophlebitis) • Most common type in young patient • Seen in bronchoalveolar Ca especially • Most common CA spread by aerosol transmission • Most common cancer arising from pulmonary scar	• MCC of paraneoplastic syndrome, extra thoracic mets among Lung Ca • Hyponatremia with SIADH→ DI • Ectopic secretion of ACTH l/t hypokalemia (Low K') • Ectopic GHRH secretion, AVP • Cushing's syndrome • Ectopic calcitonin, ANF, GRP • Most resistant to combined modality treatment • Hilar lymphadenopathy is typical • EM shows +se of Neurosecretory granules: chromogranin, Synaptophysin, leu-7 • Azzopardi effect is frequently seen • Best serum marker: NSE	• Tender gynaecomastia • Ectopic GH secretion • Also known as Anaplastic CA

TUMORS OF GASTROINTESTINAL TRACT

<table>
<tr><th></th><th>CA-Esophagus</th><th>CA-Stomach</th><th>CA-Colon/Colorectal</th></tr>
<tr><td>General</td><td>• SqCC is the Most common type in:
– India and worldwide
– In upper 1/3rd
– Middle 1/3rd
• Adeno CA is the Most common type in
– In Western world
– In lower 1/3rd
• Most common site→Middle 1/3rd</td><td>• Most common type is Adenocarcinoma, Most common site in India→Distal stomach
• Most common site of diffuse CA →Fundus
• Overall incidence is decreasing
• CA stomach is the most common cause of:
– Krukenberg tumor
– Sister Mary Joseph nodule
• Most common Lymphatic drainage - Celiac LN</td><td>• Most common site: Rectum f/b sigmoid colon
• Mucin producing tumor are associated with bad prognosis
• HIV infected persons may be at slightly ↑ed risk</td></tr>
<tr><td>Risk factors</td><td>• RF for sq. CC
– Tabacco and alcohol
– Hot beverages and food
– Prolonged esophagitis
– Achalasia, Plummer Vinson syndrome
– Nitrates, Caustics ingestion
– Deficiency of Vitamin A, C, Zn
– Tylosis et palmaris
– Amplification of EGFR
– Esophageal diverticula
– External Beam radiation
• RF for Adenocarcinoma
– Barrett's esophagus – most important RF
– Tobacco
– Over expression of p53, amplification of C-ERB B2 and nuclear translocation of β - catenin
– Obesity, GERD
– Scleroderma</td><td>• Envionmental factors:
– H. pylori infection →Intestinal type
– Nitrites in diet, Preservative
– Nutritional deficiency–Vit, C, E
– Smoking
• Genetic factors:
– Blood gp–A
– FAP, HNPCC, Li-Fraumeni syndrome
– Familial Gastric cancer syndrome due to E. cadherin mutation →Diffuse type of CA
• Host factors:
– Chronic atrophic gastritis
– Intestinal metaplasia
– Menetrier disease
– Gastric ulcer
– Barrett's esophagus
– Achlorhydria and Pernicious anemia
– Post gastrectomy
– Adenoma</td><td>• Envrionmental factors:
– ↑Calorie intake and obesity
– Smoking, Alcohol and fatty diet
– Ureterosigmoidostomy, Low fiber diet
– IBD (UC > CD)
– Pelvic irradiation
– Acromegaly
– Strep Bovis infection
• Genetic factors:
– Mutation in p53 and K-RAS
– HNPCC (Lynch syndrome)→AD condition
○ Mutation in DNA repair gene MSH-2 and MLH-1 l/t microsatellite instability
○ Affects Rt/Ascending colon
○ Better prog. (MMR gene also involve)
– FAP: Mutation in APC gene present on long arm of chr. 5 (5q)→ CA develops in100% of patient
• Pathways:
– APC/β - catenin pathway
– Microsatellite instability pathway involve MSH 2 and MLH-1 gene</td></tr>
<tr><td>Types</td><td>• H. pylori CAG-A strain is protective in adeno CA</td><td>• Based on Histology:
– Intestinal type
– Diffuse type→Signet ring appearance
• Based on Depth of invasion:
– Early→Mucosa and submucosa ± LN Better prognosis
– Late→Invasion of muscular layer Poor prognosis</td><td>• Most common type →Adenocarcinoma
• Risk of malignancy is more in villous adenoma
• Cholecystectomy has been associated with a mod. ↑risk of proximal colon CA
• Most common prognostic indicator: Stage OR[A] LN status</td></tr>
<tr><td>Clinical features</td><td>• Progressive dysphagia - more for solids
• Most common symptom – Dysphagia
• M > F</td><td>• Most common location – antrum of the stomach
• Paraneoplastic syndrome
– Trousseau's syndrome
– Acanthosis nigricans
• Most common symptoms→Pain</td><td><table>
<tr><th>Rt.Sided/Proximal</th><th>Left Sided/Distal</th></tr>
<tr><td>• Fungating/ Ulcerative type</td><td>• Obstructive type</td></tr>
<tr><td>• Bleeds readily</td><td>• Napkin ring configuration</td></tr>
<tr><td>• Melena</td><td>• Diarrhea, constipation</td></tr>
<tr><td>• Good prognosis</td><td>• Poor prognosis</td></tr>
</table></td></tr>
</table>

Contd.

Contd.

Metastasis		• Liver (1st organ affected) • Ovary (Krukenberg tumor) • Periumbilical LN (Sister Mary nodule) • Peritoneal cull-de-sac (Blumer's shelf) • Left supraclavicular LN (Virchow's LN)	• Most common site →Liver > Lung • ***(Solitary liver mets is not a C/I to Sx)*** • Incidence of mets is related to depth of invasion[(A)]
Investigations	• IOC-Endoscopy and Biopsy • Ba swallow→'Rat-tail appearance' • EUS→IOC for staging (T-stage)	• Endoscopy with biopsy and brush cytology→IDC • CT scan→IOC for staging • IOC to know the depth of invasion = EUS • Peritoneal dissemination →Best assessed by laparoscopy	• Tumor marker→*CEA and CA - 19-9* • **Colonoscopy**–Napking ring appearance • Radiolog IOC-Double contrast Ba enema which shows ***"Apple core"*** deformity • **Colonoscopy**→*Gold stand for Δ* • Endorectal coil MRI-Radiological IOC in CA Rectum
Treatment	• SqCC is a chemoradio-sensitive • TOC for CA in situ = EMR • Cervical SqCC→Definitive chemoradiation • Chemo→Epirubicin + Cisplatin + 5FU • Approach for transhiatal esophag-ectomy→Abdomen and Neck incision • Best indicator of survival–TNM stage • Prognosis depends upon: – Depth of invasion (T) – No. of LN (involved (N) – Loation of tumor	• Surgery is the primary modality of treatment as it is curative • Relatively radioresistant tumor • Protective factors: – Antioxidants–Vit A and B – Aspirin ↓ es the risk • Alcohol is not a risk factor • Prognosis depends on: – LN status – Depth of tumor invasion	• Right sided colonic obstruction→ – Resection with ileo tranverse anastomosis • Sigmoid colon/Descending colon: – Hartmann's operation – Sigmoidectomy with primary colorectal anastomosis – Abd. colectomy with ileorectal anastomosis • Chemo: 5 FU, Leucovorin, Oxaliplatin (FOLFOX) • ***Factor ↓ ing the risk:*** – ↑intake of dietary fiber – Intake of ω-3FA (fish) – NSAIDS esp. Aspirin – Intake of folic acid and Ca^{+2} – HRT (Estrogen) • Prophylactic colectomy is standard therapy in patient with APC mutation but it does not ↓ risk for cancer due to adenoma at other sites • Patient screening is done with sigmoidoscopy • Screening guidelines as per ACS: – FOBT annually and FSS every 5 years beginning at age 50 for asymptomatic individuals OR – Colonoscopy/DCBE (total colon examination) every 10 years

TUMORS OF HEPATOBILIARY SYSTEM AND PANCREAS

	HCC	Cholangiocarcinoma	CA-GB	CA-Pancreas
General	• Most common primary malignant tumor of Liver • Most common solid organ cancer • Most common cause of death in patient with cirrhosis • Its worldwide incidence parallel with the prevalence of Hepatitis B • Most common primary malignancy in children→ Hepatoblastoma	• Most common site → Hilum • Extrahepatic – 90% • Intrahepatic – 10%	• 6th - 7th decade of life • Women > Men • Most common site of origin→ Fundus • > 90% patient of CA GB have gallstone • Risk of CA in patient with Gallstone→ 0.3-3% • Aggressive malignancy with poor progosis	• M > F • Most common site– Head

Contd.

Contd.

Risk factors	• Chronic Hepatitis with HBV (HBx protein) > HCV • Alcoholismn • Aflatoxin→toxin B_1 • Hereditary Hemochromatosis • Smoking • Cirrhosis: Most common risk factor • *High risk causes are:* – HBV, HCV – Hemochromatosis – Alcohol • *Low risk causes are:* – NAFLD – PBC • α_1 AT deficiency • Thorotrast • Wilson's disease	• PSC • Liver flukes→ – C. sinensis – Opisthorchis viverrini • Choledocholithiasis • Contrast material–thorotrast • Chronic alcoholic liver disease • Choledochal cyst • Caroli's disease • Recurrent pyogenic Cholangitis • Typhoid infection • Cigarette smoking	• **Gallstone** (Choledocholithiasis) → Most common risk factor • Choledochal cyst • Porcelain GB • GB Polyp > 10 mm • Typhoid infection • PSC (Primary sclerosing cholangitis) • Obesity • C. sinensis infection [acquired by eating fish] • GB stone > 3 cm esp. ↑↑ risk	• Smoking • Obesity • Alcohol • Chronic pancreatitis • DM • *Hereditary RF:* – PJ syndrome – Ataxia telangiectasia – CF – BRCA - 2 – Lynch syndrome HNPCC – FAP – Hereditary Pancreatitis • Genetic factors: – K-RAS and Her 2 new overexpression are earliest to occur – K-RAS (95%) Most common mutation f/b P16 (90%); and P53 (75%)
Types		• ***Klatskin tumor:*** – Most common subtype – Located at the junction of Right and left hepatic ducts – Hilar CC • Macroscopically–Most common type is sclerosing	• Adenocarcinoma – 80-90% • Histological type → Papillary has got best prognosis	• Most common → Ductal adenocarcinoma CA {PDAC}
Clinical features	• More prevalent in Asia and Sub Sahara • Most common symptom → Abdominal pain > weight loss • **Paraneoplastic syndromes** – Hypercholesterolemia = Most common – Hypercalcemia • Vascular bruit = 25%	• Painless jaundice→ Most common	• RUQ pain mimicking cholecystitis and cholelithiasis • Jaundice and abdominal mass	• Most common symptom of CA Head Jaundice • A palpable distended GB 1/3rd of patient with periampullary CA–Courvoisiter law • Left supraclavicular LN= Virchow's LN→Troisier sign • Sister Mary Joseph node • Blumer shelf • Migratory thrombophlebitis/ Trousseau syndrome seen
Metastasis	• Strong propensity for vascular invasion esp. portal vein		• Most common mode of spread → Direct invasion • Direct hepatic invasion > LN mets	
Investigations	• ↑αFp (Tumor marker) in ~ 70% • CT chest → Lung mets	• Tumor marker → Cytokeratin 7, 8, 19 + ve and -ve for cytokeratin 20	• Best tumor marker–CA 19-9	• Tumor marker → CA 19-9 [most sensitive] and CEA • IOC → MDCT

Contd.

Contd.

<table>
<tr>
<td></td>
<td><ul><li>Okuda staging → For prognosis</li><li>Other marker → PIVKA -2</li><li>If focal lesion 1-2 cm → Both CT + MRI should be done</li><li>If focal Lesion > 2 cm → Either CT or MRI done</li><li>Biopsy proof → Usually not required</li></ul></td>
<td><ul><li>↑↑ CA 19-9 → Poor prognostic factor</li></ul></td>
<td></td>
<td><ul><li>ERCP→Double duct sign</li><li>Biopsy → not necessary</li><li>Inverted 3 sign → Periampullary CA</li></ul></td>
</tr>
<tr>
<td>Mx</td>
<td><ul><li>HCC derives its blood supply from Hepatic artery</li><li>MILAN Criteria → For liver transplantation</li><li>CLIP system is applicable for Hep C related HCC</li><li>Barcelona staging→Treatment guidance</li></ul></td>
<td></td>
<td></td>
<td><ul><li>Metastatic → Gemcitabine, Folifirinox</li><li>CA Head → Pylorus preserving pancreaticoduodenectomy (Whipple's)</li><li>CA Body and tail → Distal pancreatectomy and enbloc splenectomy</li><li>Best prognosis → Periampullary/CA head of pancreas</li><li>Most common complication of Whipple procedure → Delayed Gastric emptying</li><li>Components of Whipple's → GJ, CJ, PJ</li></ul></td>
</tr>
<tr>
<td>Treatment</td>
<td><ul><li>Resection →
– Ideal in Child Pugh stage A or B
– Only 15-20% of HCC is resectable due to multicentricity, Bilobar involv
– Portal vein invasion, lymphatic mets</li><li>RFA (Radiofrequency ablation)
PCTAE (Percutaneous transarterial embolization), Sorafenib → For unresectable HCC</li><li>Fibrolamellar Variant of HCC
– Seen in young adults
– M = F
– No associated with HBV or Cirrhosis
– Better prognosis
– No ↑ of AFP (different, from HCC),</li></ul></td>
<td>Perihillar → CBD resection + LN + Hepatic resection
Intrahepatic → Hepatic resection
Distal: Whipple's procedure</td>
<td>If Δ of CA GB made after cholecystectomy
<table>
<tr><th>Stage</th><th></th><th>T/t</th></tr>
<tr><td>T_{1a}→</td><td>Tumor invading lamlna propria</td><td>Conservative and
5-FU is sufficient</td></tr>
<tr><td>T_{1b}→</td><td>Tumor invading muscularis</td><td>Margin -ve → FU
Margin + ve → Extended cholecystectomy</td></tr>
<tr><td>T_2→</td><td></td><td>Extended cholecystectomy</td></tr>
<tr><td>T_3</td><td></td><td>Radical cholecystectomy</td></tr>
</table></td>
<td></td>
</tr>
</table>

Contd.

Contd.

	– Affects left labe of liver commonly – Spread by lymphatic route – Tumor marker→ Neurotensin, – Tumor is well circumscribed easily resectable (but it is non-encapsulated) – ↑ Vit B_{12} binding globullin Recurrence → Common Screening in high risk → USG α FP > 400 ng/ml has high sensitivity			

COLORECTAL POLYPS

	HNPCC/Lynch syndrome	FAP/Gardner syndrome	Turcot's syndrome
Inheritance	• AD	• AD	• AD
Clinical features	• Small no of colorectal polyp • Muir-Torre Variant [A] – Sebaceous adenoma – Keratoacanthoma	• > 100 polyps • Congenital hypertrophy of Rentinal epithelium • Osteoma • Desmoid tumor • Epidermoid cyst	• Colorectal Polyps (may resemble classic FAP) • Brain tumors – Cerebellar medulloblastoma – Glioblastoma
Malignancy risk	• Colorectal CA → 70-80% • Endometrial CA→30-60%	• Colorectal CA ~ 100%	
Screening	• Colonscopy at age 20-25 years	• Flexible proctosigmoidoscopy at age 10-12 years	
Mx	• Prophylactic colectomy • Genes involved MMR → MLH 1 MSH-2 • Δ = Amsterdam criteria	• Prophylactic Total colectomy • APC (Chr: 5) (5q) • Usual age: 15-40 years	• Proctocolectomy gene involved=APC

TUMORS OF GENITOURINARY SYSTEM

	Wilms tumor–Nephroblastoma	RCC – Hypernephroma, Grawitz tumor	Testicular Carcinoma
General	• Most common Primary renal tumor of childhood • Peak age 2.5 years • Usually unilateral	• Most common malignant cancer of the kidney • More commonly affects upper pole • M > F • Arises from PCT/cortex commonly	• Seminoma (GCT) is – **Most common** tumor of testes – **Most common** primary bilateral testicular tumor – Most radiosensitive testicular carcinoma • **Most common** ~ in infants and children < 3 years → Yolk sac tumor • **Most common** ~ in prepubertal children→Teratoma • **Lymphoma is:** – Most common testicular carcinoma in patient > 60 years – Most common bilateral testicular carcinoma in patient > 60 years – Most common secondary testiclar CA

Contd.

Contd.

Risk factors	Associated syndromes with Wilm's tumor: • **WAGR syndrome** Deletion of two genes WT-1 and PAX-6, both located at chromosomes 11 p 13 'A' = Aniridia • **Denys Drash syndrome** Gonadal dysgenesis, male pseudohermaphroditism • **Beckwith-Wiedemann Syndrome** – Organomegaly, Macroglosia – Genetic locus is present in band p15.5 of chr. 11 called "WT-2" – Hemihypertrophy	• Hypertension • Obesity • Tobacco smoking - MI risk factor • Estrogen therapy • Asbestos exposure • Tuberus sclerosis • VHL syndrome-chr 3p • CRF (d/t Analgesic Nephropathy) • Acquired cystic diseases • Genetic basis – t (x:1), Trisomy -7, 16, 17→ Papillary type of RCC – VHL gene → Clear cell CA – Hypodiploidy → Chromophobe cancer	• **For GCT's** – Cryptorchildism - straongest association (10%) – Higher the testes greater the risk – ↑ risk is seen in both testes – **Most common** tumor seen is semilnoma – Orchidopexy does not ↓ the risk • Testicular feminization syndrome • Klinefelter syndrome • Male CA Breast • Rt side > Lt. side
Types		• Histologically, RCC is most often a mixed adenocarcinoma	• **Most common** histological type → Mixed > Seminoma • **Most common** histological type of testicular lymphoma → Diffuse histiocytic lymphoma • Best prognosis → Yolk sac tumor • Worst prognosis → *Hurricane tumor* (Type of choriocarcinoma testis)
Clinical features	• Most common is asymptomatic abdominal mass or swelling • Traid – Abdominal mass – Hematuria – Fever	• Classical triad includes→ – Hematuria → Earliest and **Most common** symptom – Palpable mass – Flank pain • Nonreducible varicocele (L > R)	• Painless swelling in one gonads • 5% GCT may present with Gynecomastia • Secondary Hydrocele • 1-2 % are Bilateral
Metastasis	• Most common lungs	• **Most common**–lungs → Pulsating secondaries • Tendency to invade Renal vein and extend into IVC upto Rt. side heart	• GCT spread by stepwise lymphatic fashion
Investigations		• IOC-CT • Inferior venocavogram	• FNAC → C/I
Treatment	Transperitioneal radical nephrectomy ↓ If unfavorable histology start RT → Within 10 days CT → After 5 days	• TOC → Partial/Total nephrectomy • Refractory to cytotoxic agents • IVC involvement does not means inoperability • Metastatic RCC → **Sunitinib** • CT with Vinblastine • Size ≤ 4 cm–Partial nephrectomy • Relatively radioresistant tumor	• Chemo → BEP regimen (Bleo + Etopo + Cisplatin) • Tumor Marker – α–FP → Yolk sac, Embryonal CA, Teratoma (YET) – β-hCG → Chorio CA, Embryonal CA, Seminoma (CE seminoma) – PLAP → Seminoma (Placental ALP) – GGT → Seminoma – ↑ AFP → Yolk sac tumor

Contd.

Contd.

	• Post chemo Rx based staging system in Wilm's→ SIOP • Presence of anaplasia leads to emergence of resistance to chemotherapy • **SIOP approach→** Preoperative / primary chemo → Rx (Nephrectomy) → Post chemo staging → Preoperative chemo/radio	• Paraneoplastic syndrome associated with RCC – Polycythemia l/t ↑ ESR (Most common) – Stauffer syndrome → non metastatic hepatic dysfunction due to ↑ IL-6 – Hypertension Anemia Fever – Hypercalcemia – due to PTHrp – Cushing's syndrome–due to corticosteroids – Amyloidosis eosinophilia or leukamoid reaction	• NSGCT are more aggressive than SGCT • Schiller dual bodies → Yolk sac Endodermal sinus tumor
	• Most common prognostic factor: Histology • Overall prognosis → Good	• Most common prognostic factor → Pathological staging • Sarcoid change in any RCC in associated with worsening of prognosis	

CARCINOMA OF URINARY BLADDER, PENIS AND PROSTATE

	CA-Urinary Bladder	CA-Penis	CA-Prostate
General	• M > F 6th and 7th decade • Most common site → Trigone and adjacent posterolateral wall	• Most common in 6th decade but 40% patients are <40 years	• Most common cancer of male • Most common cause of bone secondaries (osteoblastic) • Most common zone of developing CA prostate – Peripheral zone (BHP Most common develops in Transitional zone) • Most common lobe involved - Posterior (BHP → Median) (Most common cause of obteoblastic secondaries in female → CA Breast)
Risk factors	• *Transitional cell CA →* – Smoking → MI risk factor – Naphthylamine, Benzidine , aniline dyes, acrolein – Schistosoma haematobium – Phenacetin and chlornaphazine – Cyclophosphamide – Pelvic irradiation – Dye leather printing industry workers – Analgesic Nephropathy • *Sq. cell CA → (Biharzial CA)* – S. hematobium → Sq CC > TCC – Urinary calculi – [Irradiation]	• Most common poor hygiene • Phimosis – 50% • Smegma • HPV infection – 16, 18, 31, 33 • Premalignant lesions for CA – Buschke-Lowenstein tumor: – Verrucous CA, locally malignant – Does not metastasize – Leukoplakia – Balanitis Xerotica Obliterans • Carcinoma in situ → Precancerous lesions – Bowen's disease – Erythroplasia of Queyrat	• Advancing age • ↑ fat diet • *Factors which ↓ the risk:* – Lycopene – Vitamin A and E – Selenium • Most common genetic alteration – hyper methylation of glutathione transferase (GSTP-1) located on chr. 11

Contd.

Contd.

	– Long term indwelling catheters – Chronic UTI – Bladder diverticula • *Adeno CA* – Ectopia vesicae – Urachal remnants – Associated with intestinal metaplasia		
Types	• TCC → Most common appears as papillary or exophytic lesions • Sq. CC → Adenocarcinoma • 9 p gene deletion → SF Papillary tumor • 17 p gene deletion → Invasive CA	• Most common Type → Sq. C.C. (80%), originates Most common from glans • Buschke - Lowenstein tumor (verrucous CA) is a well differentiated variant of Sq. CC • "Neonatal" circumcision confers immunity against CA Penis, HIV, STD	• Most common type → Adenocarcinoma • Δ of CA prostate is based on absent of Basal cell layer
Clinical features	• Most common symptom → Painless hematuria – Hematuria is gross and intermittent • Vesical irritability l/t frequency urgency	• Most common and earliest symptom of metastatic CA Penis → Priapism • Most common cause of death – bleeding caused by erosion of femoral artery • Hypercalcemia • No pain	• Being peripheral it is asymptomatic initially • DRE: Median sulcus obliterated
Metastasis	• Lymphatic → Pelvic LN (obturator) • Hematogenous → Liver	• Lymphatics → Inguinal LN (Most common)	• Local→Seminal vesicle and base of UB • Hematogenous → Bones (Osteoblastic secondaries) Lymphatics → Obturator LN • Spread to vertebrae is due to internal • Vertebral plexus of veins (Baton's)
Investigations	• Urine microscopy for malignant cells → for screening and to detect recurrence • Best investigation→ Cystoscopy and Biopsy	• Sentinel LN biopsy of Penile CA → CABANA procedure [SLN biopsy was 1st done in CA Penis] • Incisional biopsy • IOC staging → MRI	• Best screening protocol → PSA + DRE • PSA velocity >0.75 ng/mL/yr indicates carcinoma • TRUS guided biopsy best investigation
Treatment	• Tis → Intravesical BCG • Ta → Complete TUR • Tb_1 → Complete TUR f/b intravesical chemotherapy/ immunotherapy • T_{2-4} → Radical cystectomy or Neoadjuvant CT f/b radical cystectomy • Invasion of the detrusor muscle (muscularis mucosa) is associated with worst prognosis	• Lesion involving glans or distal shaft → Partial penectomy with 2 cm margin • Lesion involving proximal shaft or 2 cm margins are not achieved → Total penectomy with perineal urethrostomy • Bilateral illioinguinal LN dissection for metastatic LN disease • Preputial penile CA → Wide excision	• For metastatic disorder – GnRH analogs (Goserelin) are used • T1a → Incidentally found tumors at TURP, Mx= Regular Follow up • Tumor markers – Prostatic acid phosphatase (PAP) – not prostate specific – Alkaline phosphatase – PSA → Prostate specific (not cancer specific, ↑ also in BHP) – Normal value ≤ 4 ng/ml – > 20 ng/ml is diagnostic of CA – Used for monitoring after radical prostatectomy • Grading is done by Gleason's scoring

BONE TUMORS

	Osteochondroma/Exostosis	Osteoid Osteoma	Enchondroma	Chondroblastoma
General	• Most common Benign tumor of bone • Not a true neoplasm • Characterized by growth arising from the surface of bone • Growth origin from-growth plate • Growth of tumor stops with ceassation of growth at epiphyseal plate after skeletal maturity: It is not at true neoplasm	• Most common true Benign tumor of bone • It is a Benign circumscribed lesion		• Occurs in skeletally immature persons • GCT is the adult counterpart of chondroblastoma
Presentation	• Teenage or young adult • Presents with painless swelling • Most common site - knee > humerus • Site : Metaphyseal • Rapid increase in size and appearance of pain is suggestive of malignant transformation into chondrosarcoma (Most common malignancy associated with it) • ***Occurrence of pain suggests*** – Bursitis at tip of swelling – # through stalk of osteochondroma – Tethering of neighbour structures – Malignant transformation	• 10-30 years of age gp • Most common site - Tibia > femur • Site - Diaphyseal • Presents with nagging pain, worst at night and is relieved by salicylates or other NSAIDs	• Mostly solitary lesions • Most common site: Phalanges and Metatarsals • Usually asymptomatic • Other bones affected are: Femur, Humerus, ribs • Multiple enchondroma seens in: – Ollier's disease – Maffuci's syndrome along with multiple hemangioma	• Age 10-20 years • Most common site: Proximal humerus (Codman's tumor) • Site: Epiphysis of long bones • Presents with the pain in the adjacent joints
Pathology	• **Cartilage cap** is +st surrounding pedicle of bone. Cap consist of simple hyaline cartilage	• Formation of small nidus of osteoid tissue surrounded by a reactionary zone of dense sclerosis (Sclerotic new bone formation)		• Large collection of chondroblasts set off by the surrounding matrix of immature fibrous tissue • Scattered giant cells within the stroma
X-ray	• Pathognomic • Well defined exostosis emerging from metaphysis • Medullary cavity of tumor is in continuation with that of bone • Cartilage cap is not seen on X-Ray	• Small radiolucent area surround by dense sclerosis • Local sclerotic thickening of shaft that may obscure the central nidus • CT scan → double dot sign/**"dot within dot"** sign	• Well defined radiolucent area at the junction of metaphysis and diaphysis • In mature lesions – flecks of whips of calcification present within lucent area → Pathognomonic feature	• Well defined lytic lesions (radiolucent area) in epiphysis • Stippled calcification which give rise to mottled appearance • Tumor is centric
Treatment	• Asymptomatic → Left untreated • Symptomatic → Excised	• Wide black excision along with internal fixation ± Bone graft	• Not always necessary	

	GCT/Osteoclastoma	Ewing's Sarcoma	Ostesogenic Sarcoma/Osteosarcoma
General	• It is an osteolytic tumor • Arises from epiphysis • Most common site lower end of femur > upper end of tibia > lower end of radius and upper end of humerus • Age 20-40 years • Locally very aggressive tumor	• High malignant sarcoma arising in the bone marrow (medulla) • Most common site Diaphysis of femur, tibia and humerus • Derived from primitive neuroectoderm • Age 10-15 years • Very primitive tumor with poor differentiation	• Highly malignant tumor arising within bone • Origin → Metaphysis • Most common site → lower end of femur > upper end of tibia > proximal humerus • Arises from primitive bone forming cells • Age 10-25 years • Most common Primary malignant tumor of bone in children
Presentation	• Pain at the site of tumor • Egg-cracking sensation on palpation • May be associated with secondary aneurysmal bone cyst (ABC)	• Presents with throbbing pain and swelling in the mid shaft (diaphysis) • Fever, warm swelling, tenderness → So it can mimic osteomyelitis	• 1st symptom–local pain which gradually ↑ in swelling • 10% have pulmonary metastasis at the time of presentation • Hematogenous metastasis
Pathology	• Presence of tumor giant cell is the hallmark	• Small round cell tumor with scant cytoplasm • Glycogen rich cytoplasm, so PAS+ve • Diastase sensitive • Homer Wright rosette appearance • Expresses MIC-2 which differentiate it from other round cell tumors	• Two types: 1. Primary 2. Secondary: (Predisposing factor) – Paget's disease – Bone infarction – Radiation – Chronic osteomyelitis
Radiology	• Solitary lytic lesions of the bone • Eccentric location • Expansion of overlying cortex • **Soap-bubble** appearance • No calcification within tumor • No/Minimal reactive sclerosis around tumor	• Onion skin periosteal reaction • Sunray appearance and Codman's Δ (Both are more common in osteogenic sarcoma)	• Periosteal reaction – irregular type • Codman's Δ (due to subperiosteal new bone formation) and Sunray appearance are typical for OGS • Irregular destruction in the metaphysis overshadowed by new bone formation
Diagnosis and treatment	• Enblock excision/Complete resection • Curettage and bone grafting • Excision and reconstruction by: – Turn-O-Plastry technique – Arthrodesis using fibula – Arthroplasty • Irradiation for spinal involvement • *TOC for different sites:* – Lower end of ulna upper end of fibula → Excision of tumor – Lower end of radius → Excision with reconstruction using I/L fibula – Around knee → Excision with prosthesis replacement or arthrodesis	• ES is highly radiosensitive – melts like snow by RT but can recur • TOC = RT + CT + Surgery • *Prognostic indicators*: Poor in: – Distant metastasis: Worst prognosis – Proximal location – Fever, Size, Older age, Male gender – mAb to cell surface gp Encoded by mic-2 gene is a useful screening measure – CD 99, 57, 100 +VE, NSE +VE, MIC-2 +VE – Associated with t (7:22) – t (11:22) seen in 80-95% tumor	• Δ is made by: – X-ray: (Use for staging) – Bone scan: Skip lesions – MRI and CT: Extent of tumor – CT Chest: For pulmonary metastasis – Biopsy of the lesion • Treatment it is radioresistant – Neoadjuvant chemotherapy f/b surgery (limb salvage surgery mostly) f/b postoperative CT

OGS	Parosteal OGS	Periosteal OGS
Age gp	In older individual (3-4 decade)	Same
Origin	Metaphysis	Diaphysis
Location	Cortical surface*	
Treatment	Local resection	Same as OGS

* *Sparing of medullary cavity for a long time–characteristic*

PART TWO: CHAPTER-WISE MCQs

CHAPTER 56

BASICS OF ONCOLOGY

GENETICS, RADIATION, CHEMOTHERAPY, MOLECULAR BIOLOGY AND ALLIED ASPECTS

PART 1

1. **Pectoralis major myocutaneous flap is based on the:**

   (a) Lateral thoracic artery
   (b) Perforating branch of thoracoabdominal artery
   (c) Dorsal scapular artery
   (d) Perforating branches of internal mammary artery

   Ans: (b) Perforating branch of thoracoabdominal artery

2. **Average time taken for total resorption of suture material of PDS (polydioxanone):**

   (a) 180 days
   (b) 90 days
   (c) 60 days
   (d) 600 days

   Ans: (a) 180 days

3. **Following oncogenic viruses are DNA viruses *except:***

   (a) EBV
   (b) HCV
   (c) KSHV
   (d) HPV 16

   Ans: (b) HCV

4. **Most common site for intraoral Kaposi's sarcoma in immunosuppressed patients is:**

   (a) Floor of mouth
   (b) Lips
   (c) Tongue
   (d) Hard palate

   Ans: (d) Hard palate

5. **Modified radical neck dissection includes the following *except:***

   (a) Preservation of spinal accessory nerve
   (b) Preservation of IJV
   (c) Preservation of submandibular gland
   (d) Preservation of sternomastoid muscle

   Ans: (c) Preservation of submandibular gland

6. **Thalamotomy, a neuroablative procedure is useful in relief of cancer pain from:**

   (a) Unilateral neuropathic pain in chest and lower extremity
   (b) Bone metastasis in endocrine dependent tumors
   (c) Nasopharynx and Trigeminal pain
   (d) Unilateral pain below waist

   Ans: (a) Unilateral neuropathic pain in chest and lower extremity

7.

P	HCG		W	Ovarian cancer
Q	NSE		X	Small cell ca lung
R	CD 30		Y	Gonadal germ cell tumor
S	CA 125		Z	Hodgkin's lymphoma

Choose the best match between tumor marker and cancers:

(a) PQRS = WXZY
(b) PQRS = WYZX
(c) PQRS = YZXW
(d) PQRS = YXZW

Ans: (d) PQRS = YXZW

8. **Select true statement:**

(a) Evaluation of extent of disease is Staging
(b) Karnofsky performance scale of 0 and ECOG performance scale of 0–both indicate normal functional capacity
(c) Duke's classification for colorectal cancer is an anatomical staging based on TNM
(d) TNM staging can be used for lymphoma

Ans: (a) Evaluation of extent of disease is Staging

9. **Correct pair of drug with mode of action is:**

(a) Capecitabine–Inhibits Dihydrofolate reductase
(b) Pemetrexed–Topoisomerase inhibitor
(c) Cytarabine–Inhibits DNA polymerase
(d) Doxorubicin–Depolymerise microtubules

Ans: (c) Cytarabine–Inhibits DNA polymerase

10. **Which one is FALSE regarding emesis in cancer patients?**

(a) IV dexamethasone and prochlorperazine can be given for relief
(b) Ondansetron is one of the most effective antiemetic drug
(c) Nausea and vomiting are less with drugs like dacarbazine, meclorethamine and streptozotocin
(d) Delayed emesis occurs upto a week after chemotherapy usually with cisplatin

Ans: (c) Nausea and vomiting are less with drugs like dacarbazine, meclorethamine and streptozotocin

11. **Splenectomised patients are at increased risk of the following infections:**

(a) All the below infections
(b) Neisseria meningitides
(c) Capnocytophaga canimorsus
(d) Babesia

Ans: (a) All the below infections

12. **The following are true regarding Frey's syndrome *except:***

(a) Due to inappropriate regeneration of parasympathetic fibres
(b) Complication of parotid surgery
(c) Preventable
(d) Results in tears from eyes after stimulation by taste or smell

Ans: (d) Results in tears from eyes after stimulation by taste or smell

13. **In treatment of liver and pancreatic lesion, ideal instrument is:**

(a) Radiofrequency ablation
(b) Harmonic scalpel
(c) CUSA
(d) Cryoablation

Ans: (c) CUSA

14. One of the key features in diagnosis of SIADH is:

(a) Hyponatremia corrected by fluid restriction but not by normal saline

(b) Fractional urea excretion > 55%. Hyponatremia corrected by fluid restriction but not by normal saline

(c) Urine osmolarity > 100 mOsm/kg of water

(d) Plasma uric acid < 4 mg/dL

Ans: (c) Urine osmolarity > 100 mOsm/kg of water

15. Immunohistochemical stain for CD 56 is seen in:

(a) Non Hodgkin's lymphoma
(b) Malignant melanoma
(c) Neuroendocrine tumors
(d) Vascular neoplasm

Ans: (c) Neuroendocrine tumors

16. Following are true regarding radical parotidectomy *except:*

(a) Removal of all parotid tissue
(b) No neck dissection
(c) Sectioning of facial nerve through main trunk
(d) Masseter removal

Ans: (b) No neck dissection

17. Superior vena caval syndrome is caused by the following *except:*

(a) Lymphoma
(b) Malignancy lung
(c) Central vein catheter
(d) Massive pleural effusion

Ans: (d) Massive pleural effusion

18. A patient with head and neck cancer has following features–Tumor size in its maximum dimension is 4.5 cms; no extraparenchymal extension; lymph node involved in single ipsilateral node 2 cms in greatest diameter; no distant metastasis. Which of the following statements is true?

(a) Lymph node represents N2

(b) TNM would be T1N1M0

(c) Tumor represents T2

(d) Tumor size means Stage III irrespective of lymph node status

Ans: (d) Tumor size means Stage III irrespective of lymph node status

19. Most common cancer of lower lip is:

(a) Minor salivary gland cancer
(b) Squamous cell cancer
(c) Mucosal melanoma
(d) Basal cell carcinoma

Ans: (b) Squamous cell cancer

20. According to RECIST 1.1 criteria for tumor response assessment partial response:

(a) <30% reduction in sum of longest diameter of target lesions

(b) 20% or more reduction in sum of the longest diameter of target lesions

(c) 30% or more reduction in sum of the longest diameter of target lesions

(d) <20% reduction in sum of the longest diameter of target lesions

Ans: (c) 30% or more reduction in sum of the longest diameter of target lesions

21.

P	Androgen	W	Angiosarcoma liver
Q	Phenacetin	X	Bladder cancer
R	Vinyl chloride	Y	Carcinoma renal pelvis
S	Aromatic amines	Z	Prostate cancer

Match carcinogen and cancer. Choose best combination:

(a) PQRS = WYXZ (b) PQRS = ZYWX

(c) PQRS = ZWYX (d) PQRS = XZWY

Ans: (b) PQRS = ZYWX

22. **According to American Society of Anesthesiologists classification, ASA III refers to:**

(a) Patient with mild systemic disease

(b) Patient who has incapacitating disease that is constant threat to life

(c) Patients with severe systemic disease that limits activity but is not incapacitating

(d) Moribund patient not expected to survive 24 hours with or without an operation

Ans: (c) Patients with severe systemic disease that limits activity but is not incapacitating

23. **Level II cervical lymph node basin is subdivided into IIA and IIB by:**

(a) Spinal accessory nerve (b) Sternomastoid

(c) Internal jugular vein (d) Posterior belly digastric

Ans: (a) Spinal accessory nerve

24. **First solid cancer to undergo genomic sequencing was:**

(a) Wilms' tumor (b) Gastric sarcoma

(c) Malignant melanoma (d) Gastric carcinoma

Ans: (c) Malignant melanoma

25. **Tumor lysis syndrome results in all the following *except:***

(a) Hyperphosphatemia (b) Metabolic alkalosis

(c) Hyperkalemia (d) Hyperuricemia

Ans: (b) Metabolic alkalosis

26. **Which of the following is not a very high risk category for thromboembolism in surgical patients?**

(a) Hip arthroplasty (b) Hip fracture surgery

(c) Major surgery <40 years (d) Cancer

Ans: (c) Major surgery <40 years

27. **In which of the following tumors is histological grade incorporated?**

(a) Breast cancer (b) Soft tissue sarcoma

(c) Renal cell carcinoma (d) Lung cancer

Ans: (b) Soft tissue sarcoma

28. **Range of UV light that is more damaging to DNA:**

(a) 320–400 nm (b) >400 nm

(c) 290–320 nm (d) 240–290 nm

Ans: (d) 240–290 nm

29. Which of following is not a component of SIRS:

(a) Temp > 38 degrees
(b) Systolic BP < 90 mm Hg
(c) Temp < 35 degrees
(d) WBC > 12000/mm^3

Ans: (b) Systolic BP < 90 mm Hg

30. Most significant delayed toxicity following Germ cell tumor chemotherapy:

(a) Cardiovascular toxicity
(b) Neurotoxicity
(c) Infertility
(d) Pulmonary toxicity

Ans: (a) Cardiovascular toxicity

31. The following metabolic abnormality occurs when jejunum is used in urinary intestinal diversion:

(a) Hypochloremic metabolic alkalosis
(b) Hypokalemic metabolic acidosis
(c) Hyperchloremic metabolic acidosis
(d) Hypokalemic metabolic alkalosis

Ans: (c) Hyperchloremic metabolic acidosis

32. Which interferons are indicated in hairy cell leukemia and AIDS related Kaposi sarcoma?

(a) IFN gamma 1b
(b) IFN beta 1a
(c) IFN beta 1b
(d) IFN gamma 2b

Ans: (d) IFN gamma 2b

33. A researcher intending to study possible factors causing lung cancer, visited chest hospital and collected data from patients and their records regarding lung cancer and factors like smoking, blood group, occupation and dietary pattern. Which one of the following best describes study method?

(a) Cohort study
(b) Ecologic study
(c) Cross-sectional study
(d) Case control study

Ans: (c) Cross-sectional study

34. Which one of the following is not anti-angiogenic?

(a) Fibroblast growth factor
(b) Angiostatin
(c) Thrombospondin-1
(d) Endostatin

Ans: (a) Fibroblast growth factor

35. Gross spillage from GIT during surgery is classified as:

(a) Clean-contaminated wound
(b) Dirty wound
(c) Clean wound
(d) Contaminated wound

Ans: (d) Contaminated wound

36. Following are consequences of pneumoperitoneum *except:*

(a) Tachycardia
(b) Increased urine output
(c) Acidosis
(d) Increase in respiratory rate

Ans: (b) Increased urine output

37. The following are pro-inflammatory mediators *except:*

(a) IL-6
(b) IL-10
(c) IL-2
(d) IL-1

Ans: (b) IL-10

38. Which is not a part of oral cavity?

(a) Hard palate
(b) Soft palate
(c) Ant 2/3rd tongue
(d) Retromolar trigone

Ans: (b) Soft palate

39. MALDI-Matrix assisted laser desorption is a type of:

(a) Edman reaction
(b) Atomic absorption
(c) Molecular biology
(d) Mass spectrometers

Ans: (d) Mass spectrometers

40. Harmonic scalpel vibrates at a frequency of:

(a) 1,00,000 times/sec
(b) 55,000 times/sec
(c) 1,10,000 times/sec
(d) 5000 times/sec

Ans: (b) 55,000 times/sec

41. In mammalian cell cycle, synthesis of DNA occurs during:

(a) S-phase
(b) M phase
(c) G2 phase
(d) G1 phase

Ans: (a) S-phase

42. An opoid antagonist which achieves defecation within 90 minutes of administration in a patient on opoids:

(a) Methylnaltrexone
(b) Polyethylene Glycol
(c) Liquid paraffin
(d) Magnesium and sulphate salts

Ans: (a) Methylnaltrexone

43. All of the following chemotherapeutic agents are alkylating agents *except*:

(a) Cyclophosphamide
(b) Capecitabine
(c) Carboplatin
(d) Carmustine

Ans: (b) Capecitabine

44. Semon's law is related to which of the following?

(a) Facial palsy
(b) Hypoglossal palsy
(c) Palatal palsy
(d) Vocal cord palsy

Ans: (d) Vocal cord palsy

45. Cancer outcomes measures all *except:*

(a) Response of tumor to treatment
(b) Duration of response
(c) Increase in survival
(d) Symptom free period

Ans: (c) Increase in survival

46. Following statement about metastasis is not true:

(a) In breast cancers, ER +ve tumors preferentially spread to bone; ER -ve tumors metastasize more aggressively to visceral organs
(b) Pancreatic cancer aggressively spread to liver, lungs and surrounding viscera
(c) Various types of sarcomas mainly metastasize to liver
(d) Gliomas seldom display high propensity for distance organ metastasis

Ans: (c) Various types of sarcomas mainly metastasize to liver

47. Select wrong combination:

(a) ER-Exemestane
(b) HER2-Lapatinib
(c) KRAS-Panitumumab
(d) Tyrosine kinase inhibitor-Bevacizumab

Ans: (d) Tyrosine kinase inhibitor-Bevacizumab

48. Which of the following is a biomarker for tumor angiogenesis?

(a) VEGF
(b) EGFR
(c) Bcl-2
(d) Ki 67

Ans: (a) VEGF

49. Most common direct genetic association with head and neck SCC exists with which of the following?

(a) Xeroderma pigmentosum
(b) Fanconi anemia
(c) Ataxia telangiectasia
(d) Lynch II syndrome

Ans: (b) Fanconi anemia

50. Correct order of mitosis is:

(a) Metaphase, prometaphase, prophase, anaphase, telophase
(b) Prometaphase, metaphase, prophase, telophase, anaphase
(c) Prophase, prometaphase, metaphase, anaphase, telophase
(d) Prophase, prometaphase, metaphase, telophase, anaphase

Ans: (c) Prophase, prometaphase, metaphase, anaphase, telophase

51. Protective antibody in Hepatitis B infection is:

(a) Anti HBc IgM
(b) Anti HBc IgG
(c) Anti HBs
(d) Anti HBe

Ans: (c) Anti HBs

52. Which of the following statements is true regarding meta-analysis?

(a) Meta-analysis on therapeutic studies include both randomized and non-randomized trials
(b) Meta-analysis on therapeutic studies includes only published trials
(c) Subset analysis cannot be meaningfully addressed by meta-analysis
(d) Meta-analysis assess therapeutic effectiveness based on average results pooled across trials

Ans: (d) Meta-analysis assess therapeutic effectiveness based on average results pooled across trials

53. Which among the following statements regarding apoptosis is wrong?

(a) Apoptosis is Type I programmed cell death
(b) Bcl-2 is a protein that inhibits apoptosis
(c) P53 is an apoptosis promoter
(d) Apoptosis is Type II programmed cell death

Ans: (d) Apoptosis is Type II programmed cell death

54. Obesity is defined as BMI greater than:

(a) 20 kg/m^2
(b) 25 kg/m^2
(c) 30 kg/m^2
(d) 35 kg/m^2

Ans: (c) 30 kg/m^2

55. A 60 years old man presents with abdominal pain, vomiting and altered sensorium. Chest X-ray shows right lung mass. Most likely metabolic abnormality is:

(a) Hypokalemia
(b) Hyperkalemia
(c) Hypocalcemia
(d) Hypercalcemia

Ans: (d) Hypercalcemia

56. All statements given below are true for cancer screening programmes *except:*

(a) Natural history of disease should present a window of opportunity for early detection

(b) Effective treatment should be available that favourably alters natural history

(c) Screening programmes require regular monitoring and evaluation

(d) Sensitivity of tests should be greater than specificity

Ans: (d) Sensitivity of tests should be greater than specificity

57. Wasting of intrinsic muscles of hand other than thenars can be expected to follow injury of the:

(a) Ulnar nerve (b) Radial nerve

(c) Brachial nerve (d) Axillary nerve

Ans: (a) Ulnar nerve

58. Irradiation of blood products is done to prevent which of the following complications of blood transfusion?

(a) Allergic reactions (b) Transfusion associated graft-versus-host disease

(c) Allo-immunisation (d) CMV transmission

Ans: (b) Transfusion associated graft-versus-host disease

59. Shamblin classification is for:

(a) Parapharyngeal tumors (b) Carotid body tumors

(c) Nasopharyngeal tumors (d) None of the above

Ans: (b) Carotid body tumors

60. Which one of the following monoclonal antibody is approved for use in head and neck cancers along with radiotherapy?

(a) Trastuzumab (b) Pertuzumab

(c) Cetuximab (d) Rituximab

Ans: (c) Cetuximab

61. Which of the following is not a vascular supply to sternomastoid flap?

(a) Occipital artery (b) Superior thyroid artery

(c) Facial artery (d) Transverse cervical artery

Ans: (c) Facial artery

62. According to American association of trauma organ injury severity scale more than 1 cm of renal cortical laceration with collecting system rupture is classified as:

(a) Grade 1 (b) Grade 2

(c) Grade 3 (d) Grade 4

Ans: (c) Grade 3

63. Incidence of second primary tumor in upper aerodigestive tract is:

(a) 2.7–4% per year (b) 1% per year

(c) 10% per year (d) 7.2–11% per year

Ans: (a) 2.7–4% per year

64. Causes of respiratory acidosis may be all *except*:

(a) Malignant hyperthermia
(b) Hyperalimentation solutions
(c) Salicylate overdose
(d) Status asthmaticus

Ans: (c) Salicylate overdose

65. Drug which is a synthetic anticoagulant that selectively inhibits coagulation factor Xa:

(a) Enoxaparin
(b) Dalteparin
(c) Fondaparinux
(d) Warfarin

Ans: (c) Fondaparinux

66. Bolus of morphine when used for intravenous PCA in adults is:

(a) 3–6 mg
(b) <1 mg
(c) 0.5–2.5 mg
(d) Up to 10 mg

Ans: (c) 0.5–2.5 mg

67. Ideal age for repair of isolated cleft lip is:

(a) Immediately after birth
(b) At 4–6 months of age
(c) At the time child starts to speak
(d) At 4–6 years of age before starting school

Ans: (b) At 4-6 months of age

68. Prophylactic surgery can prevent cancer in all *except:*

(a) Ulcerative colitis
(b) Familial renal cancer
(c) Familial ovarian cancer
(d) Cryptorchidism

Ans: (d) Cryptorchidism

69. Metabolic derangements in severe burns are all *except:*

(a) Increased corticosteroid secretion
(b) Hyperglycemia
(c) Increased gastric acid secretion
(d) Neutrophil dysfunction

Ans: (c) Increased gastric acid secretion

70. An adult who sustained burns of both lower limbs along with genitalia has:

(a) 18%
(b) 19%
(c) 36%
(d) 37%

Ans: (d) 37%

71. In hyponatremia with neurological symptoms 3% saline should be used until symptoms improve or sodium level is 130 meq/L; at the rate of:

(a) 0.5 meq/L
(b) 1 meq/L
(c) 1.5 meq/L
(d) 2 meq/L

Ans: (d) 2 meq/L

72. Which of the following statement is true regarding subclavian steal syndrome?

(a) Reversal of blood flow in ipsilateral vertebral artery
(b) Reversal of blood flow in contralateral vertebral artery
(c) Reversal of blood flow in contralateral carotid artery
(d) Bilateral reversal of blood flow in vertebral arteries

Ans: (a) Reversal of blood flow in ipsilateral vertebral artery

73. Allen's test is useful in evaluating:

(a) Thoracic outlet compression
(b) Presence of cervical rib
(c) Integrity of palmar arch
(d) Digital blood flow

Ans: (c) Integrity of palmar arch

74. What is true regarding Trendelenberg operation?

(a) Stripping of superficial varicose vein
(b) Saphenofemoral ligation alone
(c) Ligation of perforators
(d) Ligation of short saphenous vein

Ans: (b) Saphenofemoral ligation alone

75. Most common minor salivary gland tumor in oral cavity:

(a) Adenocarcinoma
(b) Mucoepidermoid carcinoma
(c) Adenoid cystic carcinoma
(d) Acinic cell carcinoma

Ans: (c) Adenoid cystic carcinoma

76. Most common site of intraabdominal abscess is:

(a) Subphrenic
(b) Paracolic
(c) Pelvis
(d) Retroperitoneal

Ans: (c) Pelvis

77. Regarding Hirschsprung disease all are true *except:*

(a) Absence of ganglionic cells in neural plexus of dilated segment of bowel
(b) Most common in infancy and childhood
(c) May involve small intestine rarely
(d) Rectal biopsy is diagnostic

Ans: (a) Absence of ganglionic cells in neural plexus of dilated segment of bowel

78. A man brought to casuality after a road traffic accident. He sustained multiple rib fractures with severe paradoxical chest movement. Management is:

(a) Tracheostomy and oxygen administration
(b) Wire fixation of rib fractures
(c) Strapping of chest wall
(d) Intermittent positive pressure ventilation

Ans: (d) Intermittent positive pressure ventilation

79. Best investigation for ectopic gastric mucosa of Meckel's diverticulum is:

(a) Fluoroscopy
(b) Occult blood in stool
(c) Ultrasound examination
(d) Radionuclide scan

Ans: (d) Radionuclide scan

80. Most common site of ischemic colitis is:

(a) Hepatic flexure
(b) Transverse colon
(c) Splenic flexure
(d) Sigmoid colon

Ans: (c) Splenic flexure

81. Mayos operation is done for:

(a) Spigelian hernia
(b) Richer's hernia
(c) Femoral hernia
(d) Umbilical hernia

Ans: (d) Umbilical hernia

82. Most frequent isolate of organisms that populate hands of ICU personnel:

(a) Staph. Epidermidis (b) MSSA
(c) Acinetobacter (d) Klebsiella

Ans: (a) Staph. Epidermidis

83. Staghorn renal calculus is made of:

(a) Oxalate (b) Phosphate
(c) Uric acid (d) Cystine

Ans: (b) Phosphate

84. Liver transplantation was 1st done by:

(a) Starzl (b) Huggins
(c) Carrel (d) Bernard

Ans: (a) Starzl

85. Cock's peculiar tumor is:

(a) Infected sebaceous cyst of scalp (b) A malignant tumor of scalp
(c) A metastatic tumor of scalp (d) An ulcer following osteomyelitis of scalp

Ans: (a) Infected sebaceous cyst of scalp

86. Cardiac toxicity manifests in 1–5% of patients treated with doxorubicin:

(a) Arrhythmias (b) MI
(c) Cardiomyopathy (d) Sick sinus syndrome

Ans: (c) Cardiomyopathy

87. Concept of spatial co-operation in oncology refers to:

(a) Interaction between tumor metastasis and host environment
(b) Combining different modalities of therapy to treat a particular cancer
(c) Interaction between primary tumor and host
(d) Both (a) and (c)

Ans: (b) Combining different modalities of therapy to treat a particular cancer

88. Which of the following technique of imaging gives maximum radiation exposure to patient?

(a) X-ray chest (b) CT chest
(c) Lung perfusion scan (d) Thyroid scan

Ans: (b) CT chest

89. Substrate depleted earliest in postoperative period is:

(a) Branched chain amino acids (b) Ketone
(c) Glycogen (d) Glucose

Ans: (c) Glycogen

90. Indications for laparotomy include all the following *except:*

(a) Hemodynamic instability produces source control
(b) Abdominal compartment syndrome
(c) Uncertain viability of bowel in mesenteric vascular ischemia
(d) Penetrating injury caused by knife

Ans: (d) Penetrating injury caused by knife

91. Which of the following is not a branch of internal iliac artery?

(a) Middle rectal artery
(b) Superior rectal artery
(c) Inferior vesical artery
(d) Superior vesical artery

Ans: (b) Superior rectal artery

92. Following statements regarding finasteride are true *except:*

(a) Used in medical treatment of BPH
(b) Impotence is an infrequent adverse effect
(c) It blocks conversion of dihydrotestosterone to testosterone
(d) It is 5-Alpha reductase inhibitor

Ans: (c) It blocks conversion of dihydrotestosterone to testosterone

93. Management of CSF rhinorrhoea is:

(a) Nasal packing only
(b) Nasal packing and foot end elevation
(c) Antibiotics and semi-sitting position
(d) Immediate surgery for all patients

Ans: (c) Antibiotics and semi-sitting position

94. When using sterilization by steam under pressure (autoclave):

(a) Viruses, such as HBV and HIV are not linked
(b) Biological indicators of sterilization are used for monitoring of sterilization
(c) A prevacuum cycle is not essential for prepacked instruments
(d) Temperature should be 121°C for hold time of 15 min

Ans: (d) Temperature should be 121°C for hold time of 15 min

95. Marginal mandibulectomy is absolutely contraindicated in which of the following situations?

(a) When cancellous part of bone is involved
(b) Old age patient
(c) Lesions in close proximity to mandible
(d) Edentulous patients

Ans: (a) When cancellous part of bone is involved

96. Which statement is true?

(a) FDG-PET is associated with false negative rate of 20% for detection of lymph node metastasis
(b) Bone scans are indicated in all stages of breast cancer
(c) MRI screening decreases mortality rates from breast cancer
(d) None of the above

Ans: (a) FDG-PET is associated with false negative rate of 20% for detection of lymph node metastasis

97. Behcet's disease is:

(a) Oral ulceration is the primary criterion
(b) Genital ulcers are painless
(c) Systemic steroids have no effect on outcome
(d) Testis and epididymis are never inflamed

Ans: (a) Oral ulceration is the primary criterion

98. In spina bifida:

(a) Risk of 2nd sibling having the same condition is 20%
(b) Women should commence 0.4 mg folic acid on confirmation of pregnancy
(c) Myelomeningocele accounts for 90% of open spinal dysraphic states
(d) Arnold-Chiari malformation is an occasional associated anomaly

Ans: (c) Myelomeningocele accounts for 90% of open spinal dysraphic states

99. Cancer susceptibility syndromes caused by activation of proto-oncogenes include all *except:*

(a) Costello syndrome
(b) Hereditary papillary renal cell cancer
(c) MEN 1
(d) Familial melanoma

Ans: (c) MEN 1

100. Alfred Knudson's revolutionary hypothesis: "2 hit hypothesis" modelled based on:

(a) Wilms' tumor
(b) Retinoblastoma
(c) Breast cancer
(d) CML

Ans. (b) Retinoblastoma

101. Risk factors associated with 7 days operative mortality–Relative odds of Dying is greatest in:

(a) ASA III-V vs ASA I-II
(b) Emergency vs Elective
(c) Age > 80 years vs <60 years
(d) Number of anesthetic drugs: 1-2 vs >3

Ans: (a) ASA III-V vs ASA I-II

102. First elective abdominal operation was performed in 1809 by:

(a) Ephraim McDowell
(b) Jane Todd Crawford
(c) John Collins Warren
(d) Albert Theodore Billroth

Ans: (a) Ephraim McDowell

103. Tumor markers are least useful for:

(a) Diagnosis
(b) Differential diagnosis
(c) Monitoring
(d) Prognosis, Prediction

Ans: (a) Diagnosis

104. The first description of PMMF for head and neck reconstruction was by:

(a) David Soutar
(b) Harold Gilles
(c) Stephan Ariyan
(d) McGregor

Ans: (c) Stephan Ariyan

105. Tumor suppressor genes and syndromes mismatched:

(a) Li-Fraumeni syndrome–TP53
(b) Cowden's syndrome–PTEN
(c) Hereditary papillary renal cancer–MET
(d) Xeroderma pigmentosum–P57/K1P2

Ans: (d) Xeroderma pigmentosum–P57/K1P2

106. Most common cause of death in patients with cancer of oral cavity:

(a) Distant metastasis
(b) Malignant cachexia
(c) Locoregional failure
(d) Any of the above

Ans: (c) Locoregional failure

107. Incidence of a disease is:

(a) Amount of a disease
(b) No. of cases of a disease
(c) No. of each cases of a disease each decade divided by total population
(d) No. of new cases of disease in a specified period of time divided by total population

Ans: (d) No. of new cases of disease in a specified period of time divided by total population

108. The following antibody is used in immunohistochemistry to identify epithelial cell:

(a) Vimentin (b) Desmin

(c) Cytokeratin (d) S 100

Ans: (c) Cytokeratin

109. Which is not a prognostic factor?

(a) HER 1 (b) PLAP

(c) VEGF (d) LDH

Ans: (b) PLAP

110. Which of the following chemicals in tobacco smoke is not a carcinogenic?

(a) PAH-polycyclic aromatic hydrocarbons (b) N-nitrosamine

(c) Nicotine (d) Benzopyrine

Ans: (c) Nicotine

111. Primary route of SCC invasion of edentulous mandible is:

(a) Tooth sockets (b) Cortical deficiencies

(c) Inferior alveolar nerve (d) All of the above

Ans: (b) Cortical deficiencies

112. Hallmarks of cancer that govern transformation of normal cell to malignant cell were described by:

(a) Watson and Crick (b) Vogelstein

(c) Hanahan and Weiberg (d) Sir Benjamin Gompertz

Ans: (c) Hanahan and Weiberg

113. Potential adverse effect of Tamoxifen include:

(a) Reduced bone mineral density (b) Bone marrow suppression

(c) Interstitial lung disease (d) Increased incidence of thromboembolism

Ans: (d) Increased incidence of thromboembolism

114. Bariatric surgery can resolve or improve the following comorbid conditions in most patients:

(a) DM, HTN (b) Sleep apnoea, hyperlipedemia

(c) All of the above (d) None of the above

Ans: (c) All of the above

115. Hormone responsible for release of stored milk (let down) is:

(a) Oxytocin (b) Prolactin

(c) Estrogen (d) Progesterone

Ans: (a) Oxytocin

116. Source of bleeding in duodenal ulcer is:

(a) Gastroduodenal artery (b) Right gastric artery

(c) Coeliac axis (d) Left gastric artery

Ans: (a) Gastroduodenal artery

117. Which one of the following is not considered as high grade tumor in carcinoma parotid?

(a) Malignant pleomorphic adenoma
(b) Squamous cell carcinoma
(c) Acinic cell carcinoma
(d) Adenocarcinoma

Ans: (c) Acinic cell carcinoma

118. Intention to treat analysis of a phase 3 clinical trial means:

(a) Treatment initiated should be delivered uniformly to all patients for intention treat analysis
(b) All eligible randomized patients will be included in the analysis
(c) Early deaths should be excluded from the analysis
(d) Patients with poor compliance can distort the results hence should be excluded from the analysis

Ans: (b) All eligible randomized patients will be included in the analysis

119. Warburg effect describes:

(a) Sculpturing of normal tissues as a result of cell death
(b) Inhibition of antihistone deacetylase
(c) Paracrine signalling causing increased leakiness of basement membrane
(d) Inefficient energy production in cancer cells by anerobic glycolysis

Ans: (d) Inefficient energy production in cancer cells by anerobic glycolysis

120. As per trimodal pattern of death in trauma, immediate death (prehospital) occurs in:

(a) 20%
(b) 30%
(c) 50%
(d) 70%

Ans: (c) 50%

121. Only chemotherapeutic agent has been proven to cause bladder cancer:

(a) Cyclophosphamide
(b) 5-FU
(c) Adriamycin
(d) Vincristine

Ans: (a) Cyclophosphamide

122. GHARBI classification is used in:

(a) Hydatid cyst
(b) Cholangiosarcoma
(c) Splenic cyst
(d) Liver abscess

Ans: (a) Hydatid cyst

123. Vitamin B^{12} is absorbed in:

(a) Stomach
(b) Jejunum
(c) Ileum
(d) Colon

Ans: (c) Ileum

124. All are programmed cell death *except:*

(a) Apoptosis
(b) Autophagy
(c) Necroptosis
(d) Endocytosis

Ans: (d) Endocytosis

125. Contraindications of limb salvage surgery are following *except:*

(a) Major neurovascular tumor involvement
(b) Healed pathological fracture after neoadjuvant chemotherapy
(c) Inadequate soft tissue cover
(d) Poorly planned biopsy with contamination of normal tissue components

Ans: (b) Healed pathological fracture after neoadjuvant chemotherapy

126. All syndromes associated with increased predisposition to cancer due to defect in DNA repair mechanisms *except:*

(a) Ataxia telangiectasia
(b) Fanconi's anemia
(c) Xeroderma pigmentosum
(d) VHL

Ans: (d) VHL

127. Singer's nerve:

(a) Recurrent laryngeal nerve
(b) Internal branch of superior laryngeal nerve
(c) External branch of superior laryngeal nerve
(d) Vagus nerve

Ans: (c) External branch of superior laryngeal nerve

128. All are biological activators of angiogenesis *except:*

(a) VEGF
(b) Ang 1
(c) Tie 2
(d) Angiostatin

Ans: (d) Angiostatin

129. Most important factor influencing prognosis in cancer head and neck:

(a) Lymph node metastasis
(b) Site of tumor
(c) Tumor at surgical margins
(d) Perineural spread

Ans: (b) Site of tumor

130. Feeding vessel for deltopectoral flap is:

(a) Pectoral branch of thoracoacromial artery
(b) Pectoral branch of internal mammary artery
(c) Lateral thoracic artery
(d) None of the above

Ans: (b) Pectoral branch of internal mammary artery

131. Historically 1st chemotherapeutic drugs used in clinical setting are:

(a) Alkylating agents
(b) Antimetabolites
(c) Anthracyclines
(d) Taxanes

Ans: (a) Alkylating agents

132. Kadish classification is for:

(a) Tracheostomal recurrence
(b) Olfactory neuroblastoma
(c) Nasopharyngeal carcinoma
(d) Carotid body tumor

Ans: (b) Olfactory neuroblastoma

133. Regarding confidence interval all are true *except:*

(a) Width of confidence interval depends on sample size
(b) Wide confidence interval indicates higher precision of result
(c) If confidence interval doesn't include 1, observed association is statistically significant
(d) Calculation of confidence interval assumes that variability in data can be described adequately by statistical methods

Ans: (b) Wide confidence interval indicates higher precision of result

134. Primary CNS neoplasm associated with EBV is:

(a) Oligodendroglioma
(b) Primary CNS lymphoma
(c) GBM
(d) Ependymoma

Ans: (b) Primary CNS lymphoma

135. What threshold is used to define critical weight loss in cancer patients?

(a) 10% of baseline body weight in 3 months
(b) 10 lbs in 1 month
(c) 10% of lean mass in 6 months
(d) 10% of baseline body weight in 6 months

Ans: (d) 10% of baseline body weight in 6 months

136. Metabolic abnormality in cancer cachexia:

(a) Increased gluconeogenesis
(b) Increased lipoprotein lipase activity
(c) Decreased hepatic protein synthesis
(d) Decreased body glucose consumption

Ans: (a) Increased gluconeogenesis

137. Universally unethical euthanasia:

(a) Physician assisted
(b) Involuntary active
(c) Voluntary active
(d) Passive

Ans: (b) Involuntary active

138. Trotter's triad includes all *except:*

(a) Conductive deafness
(b) Ipsilateral palatal palsy
(c) Diplopia
(d) Pain on side of face

Ans: (c) Diplopia

139. Workhorse flap for head and neck reconstruction:

(a) PMMF
(b) Deltopectoral flap
(c) Nasolabial flap
(d) Microvascular free flap

Ans: (a) PMMF

140. According to AJCC Staging System for Paranasal sinus tumors, Orbital floor involvement comes under which T staging?

(a) T1
(b) T2
(c) T3
(d) T4

Ans: (c) T3

141. Li-Fraumeni syndrome is a hereditary cancer syndrome associated with germ line mutations in:

(a) Cyclin D1
(b) ATM
(c) BRCA 1
(d) P53

Ans: (d) P53

142. WHO factfile on cancer states all of the following *except:*

(a) >30% of cancer could be prevented mainly by not using tobacco, having healthy diet being physically active and moderating use of alcohol
(b) Tobacco use is single largest preventable cause of cancer in the world causing 22% of cancer deaths

(c) 1/5th of all cancers worldwide are caused by chronic infection, e.g., HPV causes cervical cancer and HBV causes liver cancer

(d) Cancers of major public health relevance, such as breast and prostate can be cured if targeted chemotherapy was made available to all

Ans: (d) Cancers of major public health relevance, such as breast and prostate can be cured if targeted chemotherapy was made available to all

143. Retrovirus are:

(a) RNA virus that have capacity to synthesize ds DNA from viral ss RNA genome

(b) DNA virus that have capacity to synthesize ds DNA from viral ss RNA genome

(c) RNA virus that have capacity to synthesize ss DNA from viral ss RNA genome

(d) DNA virus that have capacity to synthesize ss DNA from viral ss RNA genome

Ans: (a) RNA virus that have capacity to synthesize ds DNA from viral ss RNA genome

144. Pathogenesis of increased risk of cancer in HIV is:

(a) Due to insertion of viral genome at critical locations of cellular genome leading to chimeric proteins that are procarcinogenic

(b) HIV infection causes immune deficiency in infected patients which contributes to development of cancer

(c) HIV reverse transcriptase activates many cellular oncogenes during viral replication

(d) HIV genome contains oncogenes that are transcribed in infected cells causing cancer

Ans: (b) HIV infection causes immune deficiency in infected patients which contributes to development of cancer

145. Obesity is defined as BMI greater than:

(a) 20 kg/m^2

(b) 25 kg/m^2

(c) 30 kg/m^2

(d) 35 kg/m^2

Ans: (c) 30 kg/m^2

146. HPV has been linked with:

(a) Ca cervix

(b) Penile cancer

(c) Oropharyngeal ca

(d) All of the above

Ans: (d) All of the above

147. Regarding high linear energy transfer wrong statement is:

(a) Dose response in this is nonlinear

(b) Ionisation tracks through an individual cell are few

(c) High density of this type of exposure increases probability of complex effects

(d) All of the above

Ans: (a) Dose response in this is nonlinear

148. Convincing evidence for obesity association is seen in all *except:*

(a) Kidney cancer

(b) Esophageal adenocarcinoma

(c) Endometrial cancer

(d) Ovarian cancer

Ans: (d) Ovarian cancer

149. Imatinib mesylate is indicated in:

(a) Adult patients with myelodysplastic/myeloproliferative diseases associated with PDGFR gene rearrangements

(b) Patients with kit (CD 117) +ve GIST that can't be surgically removed and/or have spread to other parts of the body

(c) Newly diagnosed adult and pediatric patients with Philadelphia chromosome +ve CML in chronic phase
(d) All of the above

Ans: (d) All of the above

150. All trans-retinoic acid is used in:
(a) Acute promyelocytic leukemia in people who don't respond to other treatments
(b) GIST
(c) Lung cancer
(d) All of the above

Ans: (d) All of the above

151. CT contrast perfusion and dynamic contrast MRI may be useful in evaluating:
(a) Response of antiangiogenic agents
(b) Response of alkylating agents
(c) Overall survival
(d) Degree of tumor necrosis

Ans: (a) Response of antiangiogenic agents

152. Immunity most responsible for host response to tumor development is:
(a) Humoral immunity
(b) B cell mediated immunity
(c) T cell mediated immunity
(d) Antibody mediated immunity

Ans: (c) T cell mediated immunity

153. Regarding HPV vaccine true is:
(a) Prevents development of cervical cancer
(b) Induces regression of cervical cancers
(c) Prevents development of cervical cancer in patients infected with HPV 16 and 18
(d) Prevents infection with HPV 16 and 18

Ans: (d) Prevents infection with HPV 16 and 18

154. About hemorrhagic cystitis is true:
(a) Mesna acts by providing free sulfhydryl group that binds to metabolize and neutralize it
(b) Bladder protection with mesna is mandatory in all receiving cyclophosphamide
(c) Mesna should be given in divided doses to total 100% of total dose of cyclophosphamide/ifosfamide
(d) Hemorrhagic cystitis is caused by direct damage to bladder wall by cyclophosphamide/ifosfamide

Ans: (a) Mesna acts by providing free sulfhydryl group that binds to metabolize and neutralize it

155. Which of the following is not an intraepithelial marker of invasive cancer?
(a) Actinic keratosis
(b) Bronchial dysplasia
(c) Colorectal adenoma
(d) Junctional nevus

Ans: (d) Junctional nevus

156. Best measurement for nicotine dependence:
(a) Age of smoking initiation
(b) No. of cigarettes smoked per day
(c) Time from waking up to 1st cigarette smoking
(d) Total years of smoking

Ans: (c) Time from waking up to 1st cigarette smoking

157. A healthy 85 years old man was found to have an elevated PSA level. He had no neurologic symptoms. Evaluation and biopsy revealed localized prostate cancer with low gleason score. This is an example of:

(a) Tertiary prevention
(b) Primary prevention
(c) Case finding
(d) Secondary prevention

Ans: (d) Secondary prevention

158. An individual who has received all 3 doses of HBV vaccine and who has never had HBV infection would be expected to have which of the following serologic markers?

(a) HBcAb
(b) HBsAb
(c) HBeAb
(d) HBeAb and HBsAb

Ans: (b) HBsAb

159. Which of the following histopathological features of surgical margin in head and neck cancers is not a high risk for recurrence?

(a) CIS at margin
(b) Pushing tumor borders
(c) Surgical margin <5 mm
(d) Invasive carcinoma at margin

Ans: (b) Pushing tumor borders

160. Cornerstone chemotherapeutic agent in modern management of head and neck cancer is:

(a) Methotrexate
(b) Cisplatin
(c) 5-FU
(d) Cetuximab

Ans: (b) Cisplatin

161. Most common genetic alteration in the progression of head and neck cancer is:

(a) Inactivation of p16 gene
(b) Inhibition of CDK
(c) Mutation of p53 gene
(d) None of the above

Ans: (a) Inactivation of p16 gene

162. Neoadjuvant chemotherapy is used in management of all of the following *except:*

(a) Breast cancer
(b) Osteosarcoma
(c) Ovarian cancer
(d) CNS lymphoma

Ans: (d) CNS lymphoma

163. As per Gompertzian growth kinetics, the growth rate of a tumor peaks when the tumor is approximately .... of maximum size.

(a) 90%
(b) 37%
(c) 50%
(d) 75%

Ans: (b) 37%

164. Which of the following is most appropriate outcome measure for case control study?

(a) Odd's ratio
(b) Relative risk
(c) Risk ratio
(d) Attributable risk

Ans: (a) Odd's ratio

165. Apparent increase in survival due to early detection of cancer screening without actual increase in survival is called as:

(a) Lead time bias
(b) Selection bias
(c) Over diagnosis
(d) Length bias

Ans: (a) Lead time bias

166. Specificity of a test is ability to detect:

(a) True +ve (b) True –ve

(c) False +ve (d) False –ve

Ans: (b) True –ve

167. Power of the study (ability to detect an effect if present) is inversely related to:

(a) Alpha error (b) Beta error

(c) P-value (d) Number of patients

Ans: (b) Beta error

168. Supplemental oxygen is indicated when:

(a) PaO_2 is <100 mm Hg and SpO_2 <98% while at rest breathing room air

(b) PaO_2 is <60 mm Hg and SpO_2 <90% while at rest breathing room air

(c) PaO_2 is <80 mm Hg and SpO_2 <96% while at rest breathing room air

(d) PaO_2 is <70 mm Hg and SpO_2 <94% while at rest breathing room air

Ans: (b) PaO_2 is <60 mm Hg and SpO_2 <90% while at rest breathing room air

169. Removal of epidural catheter in patients on LMWH prophylaxis:

(a) 10 hours prior to 1st dose of LMWH/2 hours after a dose of LMWH with no subsequent dosing for another 10 hours

(b) 4 hours prior to 1st dose of LMWH/12 hours after a dose of LMWH with no subsequent dosing for another 4 hours

(c) 6 hours prior to 1st dose of LMWH/8 hours after a dose of LMWH with no subsequent dosing for another 6 hours

(d) 2 hours prior to 1st dose of LMWH/10 hours after a dose of LMWH with no subsequent dosing for another 2 hours

Ans: (d) 2 hours prior to 1st dose of LMWH/10 hours after a dose of LMWH with no subsequent dosing for another 2 hours

170. Clinical trials demonstrating efficacy of HPV vaccine used following surrogate end points *except:*

(a) Prevention of HPV acquisition (b) Long-term persistence of HPV

(c) Development of genital warts (d) Development of cancer cervix

Ans: (a) Prevention of HPV acquisition

171. Which of the following statement regarding p-value of a test is correct?

(a) Probability of detecting true positive result

(b) Probability of getting false positive result/probability of observed effect being due to chance

(c) Probability of detecting clinically relevant effect

(d) Probability of accepting null hypothesis

Ans: (b) Probability of getting false positive result/probability of observed effect being due to chance

172. Single port access laparoscopy is being used to perform:

(a) Cholecystectomy (b) Liver biopsy

(c) Colon resection (d) All of the above

Ans: (d) All of the above

173. Which of following statement regarding abdominal trauma is false?

(a) Zone I haematoma should always be explored (b) Zone II haematoma is most commonly from kidney

(c) Zone III haematoma is difficult to control (d) Zone III haematoma should always be explored

Ans: (d) Zone III haematoma should always be explored

174. Smokeless tobacco causes:

(a) Esophageal cancer
(b) Pancreatic cancer
(c) Cancer of oral cavity
(d) All of the above

Ans: (d) All of the above

175. Knudson's hypothesis-false statement:

(a) Regarding cancer susceptibility
(b) Validated in patients with retinoblastoma
(c) Postulates that different genes are involved in familial and sporadic forms of tumor
(d) Also called two-hit hypothesis

Ans: (a) Regarding cancer susceptibility

176. Therapy specifically directed towards helping patient's ability to perform daily activities:

(a) Speech therapy
(b) Physical therapy
(c) Occupational therapy
(d) Recreational therapy

Ans: (c) Occupational therapy

177. Premenopausal woman on adjuvant tamoxifen therapy should avoid:

(a) Soy supplements
(b) Fish oil
(c) Tea tree oil
(d) Kava

Ans: (a) Soy supplements

178. Which among the following is not correctly matched?

(a) Cisplatin-Nephrotoxicity
(b) Paclitaxel-Neuropathy
(c) Carboplatin-Thrombocytopenia
(d) Cetuximab-Cardiotoxicity

Ans: (d) Cetuximab-Cardiotoxicity

179. Which of the following is not true concerning clinical trial?

(a) Sample size of clinical trial is fixed and determined before trial begins
(b) A well chosen control group provides a baseline against which to measure effects of experimental treatment
(c) Clinical trials test a clearly stated hypothesis using a predefined analysis plan
(d) Clinical trials are prospectively planned experiments involving human subjects

Ans: (a) Sample size of clinical trial is fixed and determined before trial begins

180. Which of the following is not true regarding meta-analysis?

(a) Meta-analysis based on individual patient data is more precise than meta-analysis based on summarized p-values
(b) Combines results of several studies that address a set of related research hypothesis
(c) Subset analysis can be better addressed by meta-analysis
(d) Meta-analysis on therapeutic studies usually includes both randomized and non-randomized trials

Ans: (d) Meta-analysis on therapeutic studies usually includes both randomized and non-randomized trials

181. Which among the following is not considered as high grade tumor in carcinoma parotid?

(a) Acinic cell carcinoma
(b) SCC
(c) Adenocarcinoma
(d) Malignant pleomorphic adenoma

Ans: (a) Acinic cell carcinoma

182. Radiosurgery is used in treatment and is effective in:

(a) Diffuse fibrillary astrocytoma
(b) Pineal germinoma
(c) Choroid plexus carcinoma
(d) Vestibular schwannoma

Ans: (d) Vestibular schwannoma

183. Commonly used chemotherapeutic agents for adjuvant therapy of Ca colon include all *except:*

(a) 5FU
(b) Oxaliplatin
(c) Doxorubicin
(d) Capecitabine

Ans: (c) Doxorubicin

184. All of the following structures are removed in radical neck dissection *except:*

(a) Submandibular gland
(b) External jugular vein
(c) Thyroid gland
(d) Internal jugular vein

Ans: (c) Thyroid gland

185. Gas gangrene is caused by:

(a) Pseudomonas
(b) Clostridium perfringes
(c) Clostridium welchii
(d) E. coli

Ans: (b) Clostridium perfringes

186. In axillary nerve paralysis, all the following are true *except:*

(a) Deltoid muscle is wasted
(b) Extension of shoulder with arm abducted to 90 degrees is impossible
(c) Small area of numbness is present over shoulder region
(d) Patient cannot initiate abduction

Ans: (d) Patient cannot initiate abduction

187. Which of following is the primary treatment of Pott's paraplegia?

(a) ATT
(b) Posterior instrumentation
(c) Posterior decompression
(d) Posterior spinal fusion

Ans: (a) ATT

188. Which of the following is seen in tumor lysis syndrome?

(a) Hypouricemia
(b) Hypokalemia
(c) Hypophosphatemia
(d) Hypocalcemia

Ans: (d) Hypocalcemia

189. Mechanism of action of paclitaxel is:

(a) Cell cycle non-specific agent
(b) Microtubule stabiliser
(c) Microtubule inhibitor
(d) Alkylating agent

Ans: (c) Microtubule inhibitor

190. True about Warthin's tumor are all *except:*

(a) Almost exclusively in tail of parotid
(b) Bilateral tumors are often seen
(c) More common in females
(d) Also known as adenolymphoma

Ans: (c) More common in females

191. True about cancer cachexia are all *except:*

(a) Cachexia means bad condition
(b) Interleukins and Interferons contributes
(c) Progestational agents are mainstay of therapy for anorexia
(d) Present only in advanced stage

Ans: (d) Present only in advanced stage

192. Definite factors delaying wound healing include all *except:*

(a) Hypoxia
(b) Anemia
(c) Aging
(d) Hypoalbuminemia

Ans: (b) Anemia

193. All are true about retinoblastoma gene *except:*

(a) Tumor suppressor gene
(b) Located on 13q14
(c) Autosomal recessive
(d) Transmitted as highly penetrant mutations in RB gene

Ans: (c) Autosomal recessive

194. Which of following statement is true regarding surgical site infection?

(a) Use of mechanical drain constitute clean contaminated wound
(b) Uncontrolled spillage of viscous may lead to SSI in 10–20% of cases
(c) Apparent inflammation occurs in clean contaminated wound
(d) Minimum of 48 hours antibiotic coverage is required in clean wounds

Ans: (a) Use of mechanical drain constitute clean contaminated wound

195. All are true about cystic hygroma *except:*

(a) Cystic spaces lined by endothelium
(b) 50% of them present at birth
(c) Most of them regress after waitful watching
(d) Bleomycin has been used effectively in treatment

Ans: (c) Most of them regress after waitful watching

196. A 48 years old man hit by truck was brought to Emergency room in anxious state. On examination airway patent, BP–90/50 mm Hg, PR–130 bpm, RR–32 bpm. All of the following statements are true *except:*

(a) Patient must have lost 30–40% of total blood
(b) Crystalloids suffices treatment
(c) Urine output is important parameter in management
(d) Pulse pressure will be low

Ans: (b) Crystalloids suffices treatment

197. All are true about blood transfusion *except:*

(a) James Blundell performs 1st successful documented human transfusion
(b) Landsteiner discovers ABO system
(c) Cryoprecipitate is rich in Factor VIII and Fibrinogen
(d) One point platelet precipitate increase platelets counts by 25000–30000

Ans: (d) One point platelet precipitate increase platelets counts by 25000–30000

198. SIRS definition contains all *except:*

(a) Temp <36 degrees
(b) Heart rate >90
(c) BP <90 mm Hg
(d) RR >20 bpm

Ans: (c) BP <90 mm Hg

199. All are true about trachea-esophageal fistula *except:*

(a) Type C is most common
(b) Male predominance
(c) 'A' in VACTERL stands for abdominal anomalies
(d) Maternal polyhydramnios often present

Ans: (c) 'A' in VACTERL stands for abdominal anomalies

200. True about tumor markers in general are all *except:*

(a) Correlates with amount of tumor burden
(b) Prognosticate disease
(c) Best for screening in most of cancers
(d) Predicts response to therapy

Ans: (c) Best for screening in most of cancers

201. Father of modern surgery:

(a) Alexis Carrel
(b) Ambriose Pare
(c) Kocher
(d) Halsted

Ans: (b) Ambriose Pare

202. All are features of acute adrenal insufficiency *except:*

(a) Hyponatremia
(b) Metabolic alkalosis
(c) Hypoglycemia
(d) Hyperkalemia

Ans: (b) Metabolic alkalosis

203. Surgical and Anesthetic risk scores are all *except:*

(a) ASA
(b) Hinchey score
(c) POSSUM
(d) Anerobic threshold

Ans: (b) Hinchey score

204. Spider leg deformity in excretory urogram occurs in:

(a) Hydronephrosis
(b) Polycystic kidney disease
(c) Ureterocele
(d) Renal agenesis

Ans: (b) Polycystic kidney disease

205. Most common stone in UTI:

(a) Phosphate
(b) Urate
(c) Cysteine
(d) Calcium oxalate

Ans: (a) Phosphate

206. Best approach for surgical repair of injury to abdominal aorta above level of renal artery involving SMA, Celiac trunk and suprarenal branch:

(a) Right medial visceral rotation
(b) Left medial visceral rotation
(c) Right lateral visceral rotation
(d) Left lateral visceral rotation

Ans: (b) Left medial visceral rotation

207. Most common complication of varicose vein stripping is:

(a) Infection
(b) Hemorrhage
(c) Ecchymosis
(d) Thromboembolism

Ans: (c) Ecchymosis

208. True about burn resuscitation is:

(a) Colloid is preferred in 1st 24 hours
(b) Colloid preferred if burnt area >15% of TBSA
(c) Urine output should be maintained at 50–60 ml/hr
(d) Half of calculated fluid is given in initial 16 hours

Ans: (c) Urine output should be maintained at 50–60 ml/hr

209. Clinical triad of normal pressure hydrocephalus are all *except:*

(a) Magnetic gait
(b) Dementia
(c) Urinary urgency
(d) Diplopia

Ans: (d) Diplopia

210. Contralateral neck lymph node (<6 cm) in head and neck cancers is:

(a) N1
(b) N2b
(c) N2c
(d) N3

Ans: (c) N2c

211. Radical neck dissection includes all *except:*

(a) Cervical lymph nodes
(b) Sternocleidomastoid
(c) Phrenic nerve
(d) IJV

Ans: (c) Phrenic nerve

212. LD flap is based on:

(a) Pectoral branches
(b) Thoracodorsal artery
(c) Internal mammary artery
(d) Subscapular artery

Ans: (b) Thoracodorsal artery

213. All are features of SIRS *except:*

(a) Temperature greater than/equal to 38 degrees
(b) Heart rate less than/equal to 90 beats/minute
(c) $PaCO_2$ less than/equal to 32 mm Hg or mechanical ventilation
(d) WBC greater than/equal to 12,000/L or Band forms greater than/equal to 10%

Ans: (b) Heart rate less than/equal to 90 beats/minute

214. Clinical findings of superior vena caval syndrome include all *except:*

(a) Venous distension of neck
(b) Ascites
(c) Cyanosis
(d) Facial edema

Ans: (b) Ascites

215. All are proinflammatory mediators *except:*

(a) IL-1
(b) IL-6
(c) IL-9
(d) TNF Alpha

Ans: (c) IL-9

216. All are signs of head injury *except:*

(a) Bilateral raccoon eyes
(b) Battle's sign
(c) CSF Rhinorrhea
(d) Mobius sign

Ans: (d) Mobius sign

217. All are true about Nasopharyngeal carcinoma *except:*

(a) Most common in Chinese population
(b) 3:1 preponderance in men
(c) 20% of patients younger than 30 years of age
(d) WHO type III includes SCC

Ans: (d) WHO type III includes SCC

218. Oftumumab is a:

(a) Chimeric
(b) Humanized
(c) Human
(d) Morine

Ans: (c) Human

219. PARP inhibitors all are true *except:*

(a) Based on principles of synthetic lethality
(b) Approved by BRCA related breast cancers and TNPC
(c) They were originally developed as chemoprotectors
(d) Pazopanib is a prototype

Ans: (d) Pazopanib is a prototype

220. All are non-steroidal Aromatase Inhibitors *except:*

(a) Anastrazole
(b) Letrazole
(c) Exemestane
(d) Fadrazole

Ans: (c) Exemestane

221. Bortezomib is a:

(a) Tyrosine kinase inhibitor
(b) Alkylating agent
(c) Proteosome inhibitor
(d) Histone deacetylase inhibitor

Ans: (c) Proteosome inhibitor

222. All are true about platinum agents *except:*

(a) Cisplatin is cis-diammine-dichloroplatin
(b) Cisplatin is more effective in upper digestive tract malignancy like oesophagus and stomach
(c) Oxaliplatin is more effective in colorectal cancer
(d) Sataraplatin is a new parenteral platinum analogue

Ans: (d) Sataraplatin is a new parenteral platinum analogue

223. All are true about anthracyclines *except:*

(a) Dexrazoxan is a metal chelator that reduces anthracyclin induced myocardial toxicity
(b) Idarubicin is a synthetic derivative of daunorubicin
(c) Epirubicin is an epimer of doxorubicin
(d) Cardiotoxicity is more with epirubicin than that compared to doxorubicin

Ans: (d) Cardiotoxicity is more with epirubicin than that compared to doxorubicin

224. All drugs are included in Nitrogen mustard *except:*

(a) Cyclophosphamide
(b) Ifosphamide
(c) Carmustine
(d) Melphalan

Ans: (c) Carmustine

225. Preoperative RT in head and neck cancer is indicated in all *except:*

(a) Fixed neck node
(b) Open biopsy for posterior neck node
(c) Node greater than 6 cm (N3 disease)
(d) Use of gastric pull up for reconstruction

Ans: (c) Node greater than 6 cm (N3 disease)

226. Obesity is risk factor for all cancers *except:*

(a) Breast cancer (b) Prostate cancer
(c) Ovarian cancer (d) Lung cancer

Ans: (c) Ovarian cancer

227. RECIST 1.1 includes all *except:*

(a) Measurable lesion includes unidirectional longest diameter >/= 10 mm
(b) Measurable node defined as 15 mm in long axis
(c) Measurable largest lesion up to 5 total 2 organ
(d) Base line sum includes sum of diameter of target lesion short axis nodes

Ans: (b) Measurable node defined as 15 mm in long axis

228. Splice variants of VEGF-A are all *except:*

(a) VEGF 121 (b) VEGF 166
(c) VEGF 189 (d) VEGF 206

Ans: (b) VEGF 166

229. Resistance to anti-angiogenic drugs are due to all *except:*

(a) Proangiogenic growth factor redundancy (b) Co-option of normal organ vasculature
(c) Selection of non-hypoxia resistant cells (d) Vascular remodeling

Ans: (c) Selection of non-hypoxia resistant cells

230. All are tyrosine kinase receptors *except:*

(a) PDGF (b) EGF
(c) FGF (d) TGF-B

Ans: (d) TGF-B

231. EBV is associated with all *except:*

(a) Immunoblastic lymphoma (b) Leiomyosarcoma
(c) Adult T cell lymphoma (d) Gastric cancers

Ans: (c) Adult T cell lymphoma

232. UV-A has wavelength of:

(a) 290–320 nm (b) 240–290 nm
(c) 320–400 nm (d) 400–490 nm

Ans: (c) 320–400 nm

233. Angiodysplasia is common:

(a) Rectum (b) Sigmoid colon
(c) Transverse colon (d) Ascending colon and caecum

Ans: (d) Ascending colon and caecum

234. In renal trauma meteorism refers to:

(a) Haematuria (b) Passing of clots
(c) Abdominal distension (d) Hypotension

Ans: (c) Abdominal distension

235. Sterile pyuria is a feature of:

(a) Wilms' tumor (b) TB kidney
(c) RCC (d) Renal trauma

Ans: (b) TB kidney

236. Ciclosporin is an example for following agent, use in immunosuppression in transplants:

(a) Steroid (b) Anti-proliferative agent
(c) Calcineurin inhibitor (d) Rapamycin inhibitor

Ans: (c) Calcineurin inhibitor

237. Shock produced by massive pulmonary embolism is following type:

(a) Cardiogenic (b) Obstructive
(c) Distributive (d) Endocrine

Ans: (b) Obstructive

238. Infliximab is a monoclonal antibody used in treatment of:

(a) Breast cancer (b) Lymphoma
(c) Leukemia (d) Crohn's disease

Ans: (d) Crohn's disease

239. Major cause for acute pancreatitis worldwide:

(a) Gallstones (b) Alcohol
(c) Trauma (d) ERCP

Ans: (a) Gallstones

240. External laryngeal nerve injury results in:

(a) Hoarseness (b) Stridor
(c) Loss of quality and strength (d) Aspiration

Ans: (c) Loss of quality and strength

241. Following is not true about JNAF:

(a) Benign tumor always cause significant local destruction
(b) Surgery after embolisation is primary treatment
(c) These are vascular lesion found exclusively in females
(d) Radiation is reserved for unresectable angiofibroma and recurrences

Ans: (c) These are vascular lesion found exclusively in females

242. All are true about Zevalin *except:*

(a) Radiolabelled monoclonal antibody (b) Ibritumomab covalently binds to Y90
(c) Tositumomab covalently binds to I131 (d) Used in CD20+NHL

Ans: (c) Tositumomab covalently binds to I131

243. Most common brain tumor is:

(a) Metastatic tumors (b) Glioma
(c) Meningioma (d) Acoustic neuroma

Ans: (a) Metastatic tumors

244. Ideal timing of unilateral primary cleft lip repair is:

(a) Soon after birth
(b) 5–6 months
(c) 12–15 months
(d) 2 years

Ans: (b) 5–6 months

245. Which of the following tumor is caused by EBV?

(a) JNAF
(b) NPC
(c) Inverted papilloma
(d) Ca larynx

Ans: (b) NPC

246. Bjork flap is described in:

(a) Tracheostomy
(b) Laryngectomy
(c) Pharyngeal reconstruction
(d) Maxillectomy

Ans: (a) Tracheostomy

247. All the following are premalignant conditions of oral cavity *except:*

(a) Oral submucosal fibrosis
(b) Syphilitic glossitis
(c) Chronic hyperplastic candidiasis
(d) Keratosis pharyngis

Ans: (d) Keratosis pharyngis

248. Which of the following is not a technique to prevent Frey's syndrome following parotidectomy?

(a) Sternomastoid muscle flap
(b) Digastrics muscle flap
(c) Temporalis fascial flap
(d) Insertion of artificial membrane between skin and parotid gland

Ans: (b) Digastrics muscle flap

249. External branch of superior laryngeal nerve innervates:

(a) Posterior cricoarytenoid
(b) Lateral cricoarytenoid
(c) Thyroarytenoid
(d) Cricothyroid

Ans: (d) Cricothyroid

250. In case of keloids all are true *except:*

(a They grow beyond the borders of original wound
(b) More prevalent in patients with darkly pigmented skin
(c) They frequently regress spontaneously with time
(d) They appear to have a genetic predisposition

Ans: (c) They frequently regress spontaneously with time

251. Adverse effects such as hyperkalemia, muscle pain anaphylaxis and malignant hyperthermia are common with which of the following muscle relaxant?

(a) Suxamethanium
(b) Vecuronium
(c) Atracarium
(d) Rocuronium

Ans: (a) Suxamethanium

252. Which of the following anastomosis is at high risk for anastomotic leak?

(a) Small bowel
(b) Ileocolic
(c) Ileorectal
(d) Colorectal

Ans: (d) Colorectal

253. Which of the following radiological investigation is contraindicated in patients with metallic implants like aneurismal clips and pacemakers?

(a) MRI (b) CT
(c) USG (d) PET

Ans: (a) MRI

254. One of the complications of uterine artery embolism for uterine fibroids:

(a) Dysfunctional uterine bleeding (b) Severe pain due to uterine ischemia
(c) Failure to conceive (d) Ischemic injury to ureter

Ans: (b) Severe pain due to uterine ischemia

255. Cooper's ligament repair is known as:

(a) McVay repair (b) Shouldice repair
(c) Bassing's repair (d) Stoppa-rives repair

Ans: (a) McVay repair

256. Drugs approved by US-FDA based on principles of epigenetic therapy are all *except:*

(a) 5-Azacytidine (b) Vorinostat
(c) Depsipeptide (d) 3-Azacytidine

Ans: (d) 3-Azacytidine

257. Most common lymphoma arising in small intestine:

(a) MALT lymphoma (b) Peripheral T cell/EATL
(c) Burkitt's lymphoma (d) Diffuse large B cell lymphoma

Ans: (d) Diffuse large B cell lymphoma

258. One mCi is equivalent to:

(a) 27 MBq (b) 37 MBq
(c) 47 MBq (d) 57 MBq

Ans: (b) 37 MBq

259. What is dosage of 18FDG used in PET Scan?

(a) 1 mCi (b) 10 mCi
(c) 100 mCi (d) 50 mCi

Ans: (b) 10 mCi

260. Dasatinib is:

(a Tyrosine kinase inhibitor (b) VEGF inhibitor
(c) Monoclonal antibody (d) EGFR inhibitor

Ans: (a) Tyrosine kinase inhibitor

261. Palifermin is used in prevention of:

(a) Mucositis (b) Xerostomia
(c) Halitosis (d) Vomiting

Ans: (a) Mucositis

262. Aprepitant is used in management of:

(a) Constipation
(b) Post chemotherapy alopecia
(c) Diarrhea
(d) Chemotherapy induced vomiting

Ans: (d) Chemotherapy induced vomiting

263. T1N1MO in majority of head and neck squamous cell cancer is:

(a) Stage I
(b) Stage II
(c) Stage III
(d) Stage IV

Ans: (c) Stage III

264. Wavelength of UV-C ranges between:

(a) 210–240 nm
(b) 240–290 nm
(c) 290–320 nm
(d) None of the above

Ans: (b) 240–290 nm

265. First line of management of T4 carcinoma larynx is:

(a) Radiotherapy
(b) Chemotherapy
(c) CT + RT
(d) Surgery + postop RT

Ans: (d) Surgery + postop RT

266. Arc of Riolan connects:

(a) Right and Middle colic artery
(b) Left colic and Inferior mesenteric artery
(c) Middle and Left colic artery
(d) Superior and Inferior haemorrhoidal artery

Ans: (c) Middle and Left colic artery

267. Which is false regarding Barrett's disease?

(a) Barrett's mucosa predisposes to SCC esophagus
(b) Risk of cancer is 0.5% per year
(c) Prevalence in general population is 2–7%
(d) Intestinal type of mucosa with goblet cells is most common histopathological finding

Ans: (a) Barrett's mucosa predisposes to SCC esophagus

268. Most common complication of Bevacizumab is:

(a) Hypertension
(b) Hyperglycemia
(c) Rashes
(d) GI perforations

Ans: (a) Hypertension

269. Retrosphenoidal syndrome occurs due to involvement of which cranial nerve?

(a) I
(b) II-VI
(c) VII-IX
(d) IX-XII

Ans: (b) II-VI

270. Boundaries of Gastrinoma triangle are all *except:*

(a) Cystic duct and CBD confluence
(b) Gallbladder and cystic duct junction
(c) Junction of neck and head of pancreas
(d) 2nd and 3rd part of duodenum

Ans: (b) Gallbladder and cystic duct junction

271. In transhiatal vs transthoracic esophagectomy most common complication associated with transhiatal esophagectomy is:

(a) Pulmonary complications (b) Anastomotic leak
(c) Bleeding (d) Tracheal stenosis

Ans: (b) Anastomotic leak

272. Regarding thoracic outlet syndrome all are true *except:*

(a) Vascular symptoms are more common than neurological symptoms
(b) Symptoms are often worsened by carrying heavy weights or lifting arms above head height
(c) Diagnostic tests include Roo's and Adson's manoeuvre
(d) Onset of symptom is precipitated by trauma in 1/3rd of patients

Ans: (a) Vascular symptoms are more common than neurological symptoms

273. During surgery on submandibular gland:

(a) Incision on lower border of mandible is safe
(b) Submandibular gland is seen to wrap around posterior border of mylohyoid
(c) Facial artery and vein are divided as they course through deep part of gland
(d) Hypoglossal nerve is seen to loop under submandibular duct

Ans: (b) Submandibular gland is seen to wrap around posterior border of mylohyoid

274. Tri-Incisional esophagectomy is also known as:

(a) Ivor-Lewis esophagectomy (b) Orringer esophagectomy
(c) McKeown esophagectomy (d) Thoracoabdominal esophagectomy

Ans: (c) McKeown esophagectomy

275. All are true regarding HPV related carcinomas of head and neck *except:*

(a) Mainly involves oropharynx (b) Carry poor prognosis
(c) Respond better to therapy such as radiotherapy (d) Occurs in relatively young individuals

Ans: (b) Carry poor prognosis

276. Stomach tube made during esophagectomy is primarily based on:

(a) Left gastric artery (b) Right gastric artery
(c) Left gastroepiploic artery (d) Right gastroepiploic artery

Ans: (d) Right gastroepiploic artery

277. Ideal length of Hunt-Lawrence pouch is:

(a) 10 cm (b) 15 cm
(c) 20 cm (d) 25 cm

Ans: (b) 15 cm

278. Abbe/Eslander flap is used for reconstruction of:

(a) Nose (b) Lip
(c) Ear (d) Tongue

Ans: (b) Lip

279. Level VII neck nodes are:

(a) Superior mediastinum nodes
(b) Pre occipital nodes
(c) Posterior neck nodes
(d) Central compartment nodes

Ans: (a) Superior mediastinum nodes

280. Strap muscles of thyroid is innervated by:

(a) Ansa cervicalis
(b) Hypoglossal nerve
(c) C4-C5 nerve root
(d) Cervical plexus

Ans: (a) Ansa cervicalis

281. Superior parathyroid develops from which branchial pouch?

(a) II
(b) III
(c) IV
(d) V

Ans: (c) IV

282. For patients with stage II and III rectal cancer for whom tumoral downsizing is advantageous/sphincter preservation is desired, what is preferred preoperative treatment?

(a) Short course radiotherapy (5.5 Gy) alone
(b) Long course chemoradiotherapy (1.8 Gy/day)
(c) Neoadjuvant chemotherapy
(d) Long course radiotherapy

Ans: (b) Long course chemoradiotherapy (1.8 Gy/day)

283. Which of these cancer predisposition syndromes don't have associated physical stigmata?

(a) Beckwith-Wiedemann syndrome
(b) Fanconi anaemia
(c) Li-Fraumeni syndrome
(d) VHL

Ans: (c) Li-Fraumeni syndrome

284. Most common malignancy in HIV patient:

(a) Kaposi sarcoma
(b) Adenoma of stomach
(c) Astrocytoma
(d) CNS lymphoma

Ans: (a) Kaposi sarcoma

285. TRUE about medulloblastoma is:

(a) Highly radiosensitive
(b) Surgery is only treatment
(c) Occurs in adult age group
(d) Chemotherapy is not useful

Ans: (a) Highly radiosensitive

286. Bony metastasis is a common feature with the following *except:*

(a) Carcinoma breast
(b) Carcinoma lung
(c) Oropharyngeal carcinoma
(d) Carcinoma prostate

Ans: (c) Oropharyngeal carcinoma

287. Alfa fetoprotein increases in all the following *except:*

(a) Hepatocellular carcinoma
(b) Seminoma of the testes
(c) Gastrointestinal neoplasms
(d) Embryonal carcinoma

Ans: (b) Seminoma of the testes

288. Expansible lytic osseous metastases are characteristic of primary malignancy of:

(a) Kidney (b) Bronchus

(c) Breast (d) Prostate

Ans: (a) Kidney

289. Alfa fetoprotein is increased in:

(a) Hepatoblastoma (b) Neuroblastoma

(c) Seminoma (d) Renal cell carcinoma

Ans: (a) Hepatoblastoma

290. For which malignancy, intensity modulated radiotherapy (IMRT) is the most suitable?

(a) Lung (b) Prostate

(c) Leukemias (d) Stomach

Ans: (b) Prostate

291. Tumor with perineural invasion:

(a) Adenocarcinoma (b) Adenoid cystic Carcinoma

(c) Basal cell Carcinoma (d) Squamous cell Carcinoma

Ans: (b) Adenoid cystic Carcinoma

292. Most common intra-abdominal tumor below 2 years age:

(a) Neuroblastoma (b) Wilms' tumor

(c) Hepatoblastoma (d) Lymphoma

Ans: (a) Neuroblastoma

293. Bile as it leaves liver is composed of:

(a) 50% of water (b) 10% of bile salts

(c) 20% of bile pigments and cholesterol (d) <1% fatty acids

Ans: (d) <1% fatty acids

294. In which of the following head and neck cancers, lymph node metastasis is least common?

(a) Tongue (b) Buccal mucosa

(c) Hard palate (d) Lower alveolus

Ans: (c) Hard palate

295. Phrygian cap is:

(a) Cap like adrenals over kidney (b) Gallbladder anomaly

(c) Hepatic duct anomaly (d) Diverticulum of right atrium

Ans: (b) Gallbladder anomaly

296. Which of the following carcinoma is familial?

(a) Breast (b) Prostate

(c) Cervix (d) Vagina

Ans: (a) Breast

297. Barrett's esophagus is defined by:

(a) Squamous metaplasia (b) Intestinal metaplasia

(c) Squamous dysplasia (d) Intestinal dysplasia

Ans: (b) Intestinal metaplasia

298. Transhiatal oesophagectomy was planned for adenocarcinoma of lower end of esophagus. The approach would be in the following order:

(a) Abdomen – neck
(b) Abdomen – thorax – neck
(c) Neck – thorax – abdomen
(d) Abdomen – thorax

Ans: (a) Abdomen – neck

299. Investigation of choice for dysphagia for solids is:

(a) Barium swallow
(b) Endoscopy
(c) X-ray chest
(d) CT scan

Ans: (b) Endoscopy

300. After oesophagectomy best substitute of oesophagus is:

(a) Stomach
(b) Jejunum
(c) Left colon
(d) Right colon

Ans: (a) Stomach

301. Uses of tumor marker are all *except:*

(a) Screening of a cancer
(b) Risk determination
(c) Confirmation of diagnosis of cancer
(d) Monitoring the treatment of cancer

Ans: (c) Confirmation of diagnosis of cancer

302. All are resected in Whipple's operation *except:*

(a) Duodenum
(b) Head of pancreas
(c) Portal vein
(d) Common bile duct

Ans: (c) Portal vein

303. Obesity is a risk factor for which of the following type of cancer?

(a) Renal
(b) Endometrial
(c) Esophageal adenocarcinoma
(d) All options are correct

Ans: (d) All options are correct

304. Preferred method of defunctioning for a low rectal anastomosis is:

(a) Right transverse loop colostomy
(b) Loop ileostomy
(c) Sigmoid loop colostomy
(d) Rectal tube

Ans: (b) Loop ileostomy

305. Which of the following targeted agents is not a tyrosine kinase inhibitor that influences the human epidermal growth factor receptor (HER) family signaling pathway by binding to the intracellular domain of receptors?

(a) Gefitinib
(b) Erlotinib
(c) Trastuzumab
(d) Laptinib

Ans: (c) Trastuzumab

306. Possible intervention to treat breathlessness in end stage cancer patients are all *except:*

(a) Fanning the face
(b) Opioids
(c) Bronchodilators
(d) Benzodiazepines

Ans: (d) Benzodiazepines

307. Laryngeal cancer involving both vocal cords with no neck nodes belongs to:

(a) Stage I
(b) Stage II
(c) Stage III
(d) Stage IV

Ans: (a) Stage I

308. The immunomodulating monoclonal antibody alemtuzumab is associated with which infectious complication?

(a) Cytomegalovirus (CMV) infection
(b) Pneumocystis (carinii) jiroveci pneumonia (PCP)
(c) Invasive fungal infection
(d) All options are correct

Ans: (d) All options are correct

309. All of the following are serum tumor markers *except:*

(a) NSE
(b) CEA
(c) AFP
(d) CK

Ans: (d) CK

310. Right gastric artery is a branch of:

(a) Right gastroduodenal
(b) Common hepatic
(c) Coeliac axis
(d) Right hepatic

Ans: (b) Common hepatic

311. Which of the following short-acting opioids used for breakthrough cancer related pain has the most rapid onset of action?

(a) Morphine
(b) Oxycodone
(c) Methadone
(d) Transmucosal fentanyl

Ans: (d) Transmucosal fentanyl

312. Human papilloma virus (HPV) infection is associated with which type of cancer?

(a) Cervical
(b) Anogenital
(c) Head and neck
(d) All options are correct

Ans: (d) All options are correct

313. Most sensitive to radiation therapy among the following is:

(a) Glioma
(b) Dysgerminoma
(c) Osteosarcoma
(d) Squamous carcinoma

Ans: (b) Dysgerminoma

PART 2

314. Apoptosis is characterized by all *except:* (NEET SS PATTERN 2017)

(a) Condensation of chromatin
(b) Nuclear and cytoplasmic blebbing
(c) Cellular shrinkage
(d) Autophagy

Ans: (d) Autophagy

Apoptosis	Necrosis
Membrane blebbing	Loss of membrane integrity-disruption
Cellular shrinkage	Swelling of cytoplasm and mitochondria
Apoptotic bodies–membrane bound vesicles	Complete cell lysis; no vesicles
Condensation of chromatin; DNA fragmentation	Nuclear disruption

315. First to show the signs of radiation damage among the following is:

(a) Kidney
(b) Muscle
(c) Nerves
(d) Small intestine

Ans: (d) Small intestine

316. Bladder tolerates radiation of:

(a) 45-50 Gy
(b) 85-90 Gy
(c) 100 Gy
(d) 30 Gy

Ans: (a) 45-50 Gy

RADIATION TOLERANCE DOSES (DEVITA, 10th e.d, p.155)

Organ Involved	Tolerable Dose (Gy)
Bladder	40-50
Anus, Great vessels	30
Brachial plexus	60-66
Brainstem	55-60
Kidney	50
Spinal cord	50
Lung	45
Stomach, Esophagus, Heart	60
Small intestine	50
Colon	55
Rectum	60
Liver	50

317. Log kill hypothesis implies all of following *except:*

(a) Treatment will be effective if tumors are treated at level of micrometastases
(b) Chemotherapy works by first order kinetics and kills a constant fraction of cells rather than constant number of cells
(c) It is basis for use of intermittent chemotherapy and rationale for use of combination chemotherapy
(d) It is not basis for use of adjuvant chemotherapy

Ans: (a) Treatment will be effective if tumors are treated at level of micrometastases

Log Kill Hypothesis/Skipper Exponential Tumor Growth
• Cytotoxic actions of anticancer drugs follow first-order kinetics
• Destruction of cancer cells by chemotherapeutic agents follows first-order kinetics mean that a given dose of drug destroys a **constant fraction or proportion of a cell population** rather than a constant number of cells
• They kill a **fixed percentage of tumor cells,** not a fixed number
• Log-kill hypothesis also proposes that the **magnitude of tumor cell kill by anticancer drugs is a logarithmic function**
Gompertzian Model of Tumor Growth
• A pattern of cell growth in tumors in which there is increased doubling time and decreased growth fraction as a function of time
Norton Simon Model
• Chemotherapy results in a rate of regression in tumor volume that is proportional to the rate of growth for an unperturbed tumor of that size
Goldie Coldman Model
• According to this hypothesis, even the smallest detectable cancers would contain at least one drug-resistant clone; therefore, the best chance of cure would be to use all effective chemotherapy drugs

318. Trastuzumab antibody against HER-2/neu gene active against which malignancy?

(a) Breast Ca
(b) Cervical Ca
(c) Uterine Ca
(d) Ovarian Ca

Ans: (a) Breast Ca

TRASTUZUMAB

- Trastuzumab-HERCEPTIN→anti HER 2 antibody
- **Indications:** Carcinoma breast (adjuvant/metastatic) and metastatic adenocarcinomas of stomach/GE junction that overexpress HER 2 protein
- **DOSE LIMITING SIDE EFFECT:** Cardiomyopathy

319. Dosage of carboplatin in treatment of ovarian cancer calculated by:

(a) Dose (mg) : Target AUC * (GFR + 25)
(b) Dose (mg) : Target AUC + (GFR * 25)
(c) Dose (mg) : Target AUC * (GFR + 50)
(d) Dose (mg) : Target AUC * GFR

Ans: (a) Dose (mg) : Target AUC * (GFR + 25)

CARBOPLATIN

- **Calvert formula**→Dose (mg) : Target AUC × (GFR + 25)
- Target AUC – area under curve
- 4-6 for previously treated patients and 5-7 for previously untreated patients

320. Total radiation dose to point A and B in treatment of cervical cancer:

(a) 75-90 Gy; 45-65 Gy
(b) 45-65 Gy; 75-90 Gy
(c) 20-60 Gy; 70-90 Gy
(d) 30-60 Gy; 70-90 Gy

Ans: (a) 75-90 Gy ; 45-65 Gy

Radiotherapy in CA Cervix	
Point A	**Point B**
2 cm above and 2 cm lateral to external os	2 cm above and 5 cm lateral to external os
PARACERVICAL/PARAMETRIAL Nodes	OBTURATOR Nodes

321. Each unit of packed RBC's should increase hematocrit in 70 kg adult by:

(a) 2-3%
(b) 3-4%
(c) 4-5%
(d) 5-6%

Ans: (b) 3-4%

GUIDELINES FOR BLOOD TRANSFUSION

- Accepted 3% increase in hematocrit to 1 "unit" of blood transfused is based on a calculation from total blood volume and hematocrit of blood transfused
  - Approximately 300 +/- 25 mL
  - Hematocrit: 70 +/- 5%
- ***One unit of pRBCs should increase hemoglobin by approximately 1 gm/dl***
- ***One pRBC unit will raise the hematocrit of standard adult patient by 3%***

322. Cancer cachexia can be managed using combinations of following *except:*

(a) Parenteral nutrition (b) Enteral nutrition
(c) Synthetic progestins (d) FFP

Ans: (d) FFP

TREATMENT OF CACHEXIA

- Provide small frequent feedings-6 times a day
- **Appetite stimulants:** Megestrol acetate, Dexamethasone, Metaclopramide, Antidepressants, Methylphenidate
- **Other measures:** Enteral and parenteral nutrition may be given in severe cachexia patients

323. All are alkylating agents *except:*

(a) Cyclophosphamide (b) Melphalan
(c) Ifosfamide (d) Doxorubicin

Ans: (d) Doxorubicin

DOXORUBICIN:

- Doxorubicin belongs to antitumor antibiotic group
- Side effect is cardiomyopathy
- Belong to anthracycline group

324. All are microtubule inhibitors *except:*

(a) Paclitaxel (b) Vincristine
(c) Ixabepilone (d) Topotecan

Ans: (d) Topotecan

TOPOTECAN

- Hycamtin-Ovarian cancer after failure of response to cisplatin therapy
- Dose limiting side effect: **Myelosuppression**

325. Only drug which is US-FDA approved for treatment of relapsed cervical cancer:

(a) Paclitaxel (b) Irinotecan
(c) Topotecan (d) Liposomal doxorubicin

Ans: (c) Topotecan

LIST OF FDA APPROVED DRUGS

Drug	Cancer
Alecensa (alectinib)	ALK +ve metastatic non-small cell lung cancer
Cotellic (cobimetinib)	**BRAF, V600E/V600K +ve melanoma**

Contd.

Contd.

Darzalex (daratumumab)	Multiple myeloma
Empliciti (elotuzumab)	Multiple myeloma after receiving prior therapies
Farydak (panobinostat)	Multiple myeloma
Ibrance (palbociclib)	**ER +ve, HER 2 –ve breast cancer**
Lenvima (levatinib)	Thyroid cancer
Lonsurf (trifluridine and tipiracil)	Metastatic colorectal cancer
Ninlaro (Ixazomib)	Multiple myeloma
Odomzo (sonidegib)	**Locally advanced basal cell carcinoma**
Onivyde (irinotecan liposomal)	Metastatic pancreatic cancer following gemcitabine based therapy
Opdivo (nivolumab)	Metastatic squamous non-small cell lung cancer
Portazza (necitumumab)	Metastatic squamous non-small cell lung cancer
Tagrisso (osimertinib)	EGFR T790M mutation +ve non-small cell lung cancer
Unituxin (dinutuximab)	High risk neuroblastoma
Varubi (rolapitant)	Delayed nausea and vomiting associated with chemotherapy
*Yondelis **(trabectedin)***	Liposarcoma/**Leiomyosarcoma**

326. Following are published clinical trials solid cancers. Select incorrect one:

(a) FUTURE trial-Endometrial cancer
(b) AURELIA trial-Cervical cancer
(c) OCEANS trial-Ovarian cancer
(d) LACE trial-Cervical cancer

Ans: (b) AURELIA trial-Cervical cancer

Trails of oncology		
Trial	**Cancer**	
FUTURE	Endometrial cancer	
AURELIA	Ovarian cancer (Recurrent)	Platinum resistant
OCEANS	Ovarian cancer (Recurrent)	Platinum sensitive
LACE	Cervical cancer	
AVAglio	Metastatic renal cell cancer	Bevacizumab + IFN alpha
FOLFIRI	Metastatic colorectal cancer	Aflibercept+5-FU+Irinotecan
VELOUR	Metastatic colorectal cancer	Aflibercept+5-FU+Irinotecan
DECISION	Differentiated thyroid cancer	RAI
COMPARZ	Metastatic RCC	Pazopinib and sunitinib
SUMMIT	Multiple myeloma	Bortezomib
CREST	Multiple myeloma	Bortezomib
VISTA	Multiple myeloma	Bortezomib+velcade+melphalan+prednisolone
CORRECT	Metastatic colorectal cancer	Regorafenib

327. GOG-0218 and ICON7 studies assessed combination of following drugs *except* for:

(a) Lipodoxorubicin
(b) Bevacizumab
(c) Carboplatin
(d) Paclitaxel

Ans: (a) Lipodoxorubicin

GOG-0218 and ICON 7 TRIALS

- Trials done for Advanced epithelial ovarian tumors
- Included drugs like Bevacizumab in combination with carboplatin and paclitaxel

328. HPV all are true *except:*

(a) Member of papovaviridae
(b) DNA Virus
(c) 31, 33 are high risk types
(d) Can infect skin, mucous membrane and fibroblasts

Ans: (d) Can infect skin, mucous membrane and fibroblasts

HUMAN PAPILLOMA VIRUS

- HPV is a non-enveloped DNA virus with protein capsid
- High affinity for lower ano-genital tract-cutaneous and mucosotropic

Low Risk Type	High Risk Type
HPV 6 and 11	HPV 16,18,31,33,45,58
Causes genital warts and subclinical HPV infection	Causes high grade CIN progress to invasive cancer

329. Optimal vaccine schedule for HPV vaccine:

(a) 0, 2, 6 months
(b) 0, 1, 6 months
(c) 0, 6 months
(d) 0, 1 months

Ans: (a) and (b)

HPV VACCINE

Gardasil	Cervirax
Quadrivalent	Bivalent
HPV-6,11,16,18	HPV-16,18
0,2,6 months	**0,1,6 months**
Against ca cervix and genital warts	Against ca cervix
Intramuscular	Intramuscular

330. Following are matched correctly *except:*

(a) Age specific incidence rate–It is the number of new cancers that occur over specified time among individuals of a particular age group divided by population in that same age group
(b) Age adjusted incidence rate–It is obtained by summing weighted averages of incidence rates for each age stratum
(c) Relative survival is defined as ratio of observed survival rate for patient group to survival rate for population with similar demographic characteristics
(d) Prevalence is number of new cases of disease in population within a specified time period

Ans: (d) Prevalence is number of new cases of disease in population within a specified time period

- Number of new cases of disease in population within a specified time period is defined as incidence not prevalence

331. Hereditary breast ovarian cancer associated with which genes:

(a) BRCA 1, BRCA 2
(b) HNPCC
(c) TP53
(d) VHL

Ans: (a) BRCA 1, BRCA 2

HEREDITARY BREAST OVARIAN CANCER

- Occurs due to mutation of BRCA 1 and BRCA 2
- 0.125-0.20% of general population carry this mutations
- Life time risk: 40% for BRCA 1, 20% for BRCA 2
- **Average age of onset of ovarian cancer:**
  - 49-53 years for BRCA 1
  - 55-58 years for BRCA 2
- Most of them are epithelial and non-mucinous type (serous)
- Ovarian cancers with BRCA 1 and BRCA 2 have better prognosis compared to those without mutations-respond well to platinum compounds

332. No role of radiation in management of which of the following gynecologic cancers:

(a) Primary treatment of vulvar cancer
(b) Primary treatment of cervical cancer
(c) Curative treatment of cervical cancer metastases
(d) Postsurgical adjunctive therapy of endometrial cancer

Ans: (c) Curative treatment of cervical cancer metastases

333. Which is not a particle radiation?

(a) Photons
(b) Electrons
(c) Protons
(d) Helium ions

Ans: (a) Photons

334. Radionuclides not used in brachytherapy include?

(a) Cobalt
(b) Cesium
(c) Iridium
(d) Phosphorus

Ans: (d) Phosphorus

335. Technique used to reduce risk of radiation induced ovarian failure during treatment in premenopausal women:

(a) Omental sling
(b) Ovarian transposition
(c) Ovarian transplantation
(d) All of the above

Ans: (b) Ovarian transposition

336. Not a criterion for diagnosing radiation-induced cancer:

(a) Occurs with radiation doses exceeding 60 Gy
(b) Located within previously irradiated region
(c) Pathology is different from original malignancy
(d) Diagnosed atleast few years after completion of therapy

Ans: (a) Occurs with radiation doses exceeding 60 Gy

337. Paclitaxel is:

(a) Cell cycle non specific agent
(b) Cell cycle specific agent that acts during M phase
(c) Cell cycle specific agent that acts during G2 phase
(d) Cell cycle specific agent that acts during G1 phase

Ans: (b) Cell cycle specific agent that acts during M phase

PACLITAXEL

- It is a cell cycle specific agent acts during M phase
- **INDICATIONS:** CA breast, ovary, lung, Esophagus and AIDS related Kaposi's sarcoma
- **TOXICITY:** Neutropenia, Hypersensitivity, peripheral neuropathy are dose limiting side effects. Alopecia–90% total and sudden within 3 weeks of treatment

PART 3

338. All are programmed cell death *except:*

(a) Apoptosis
(b) Autophagy
(c) Necroptosis
(d) Endocytosis

Ans: (d) Endocytosis

ENDOCYTOSIS

- Endocytosis is a process of uptake of extracellular materials by cells through general process
- Heterophagy is a process of digestion of extracellular material taken up by cells

339. Gross spillage from GIT during surgery is classified as:

(a) Clean-contaminated wound
(b) Dirty wound
(c) Clean wound
(d) Contaminated wound

Ans: (d) Contaminated wound

SURGICAL SITE INFECTION

SSI Rates Relating to Wound Contamination

Type of Surgery	Infection Rate (%)	Rate Before Prophylaxis
Clean no (viscus opened)	1–2	The same
Clean-contaminated (viscus opened, minimal spillage)	< 10	Gastric surgery up to 30% Biliary surgery up to 20%
Contaminated (open viscus with spillage or inflammatory disease)	15–20	Variable but up to 60%
Dirty (pus or perforation, or incision through an abscess)	< 40	Up to 60% or more

340. Following are consequences of pneumoperitoneum *except:*

(a) Tachycardia
(b) Increased urine output
(c) Acidosis
(d) Increase in respiratory rate

Ans: (b) Increased urine output

PNEUMOPERITONEUM

Physical + Chemical + Biological Effect = Pneumoperitoneum

Physical effects	Chemical effects	Biologic effects
Mechanical effects	Gas	Hypothermia
Abdominal compliance	Desiccation	Tissue disruption
Intra-abdominal pressure	Hypoxia	Increase peritoneal viscosity
Time	Acidosis	Acidosis
Patient position		Hypoxia

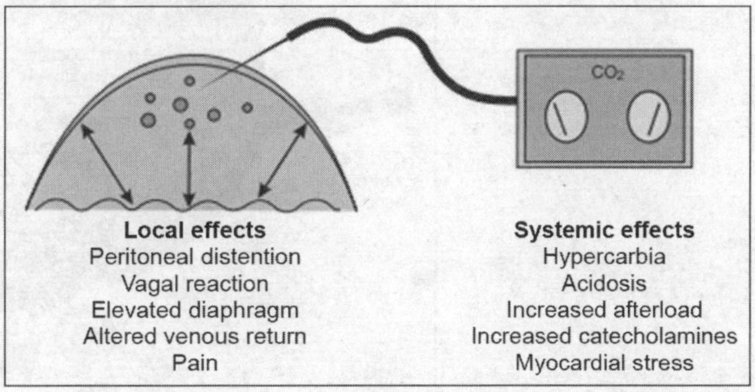

341. The following are pro-inflammatory mediators *except:*

(a) IL-6
(b) IL-10
(c) IL-2
(d) IL-1

Ans: (b) IL-10

PROINFLAMMATORY MEDIATORS

Inflammatory Mediators of Shock	
Proinflammatory	**Anti-Inflammatory**
Interleukin-1 α/β	Interleukin-4
Interleukin-2	Interleukin-10
Interleukin-6	Interleukin-13
Interleukin-8	Prostaglandin E2
Interferon	TFFb
TNF	
PAF	

342. Harmonic scalpel vibrates at a frequency of:

(a) 1,00,000 times/sec
(b) 55,000 times/sec
(c) 1,10,000 times/sec
(d) 5000 times/sec

Ans: (b) 55,000 times/sec

HARMONIC SCALPEL

- Harmonic scalpel is an instrument that uses ultrasound technology to dissect tissue in bipolar fashion with only minimal collateral tissue damage
- **The device vibrates at a high frequency, approximately 55,000 times/second, to cut tissue**
- High frequency vibration of tissue molecules generates stress and friction in the tissue, which in turn generates heat and denaturation of protein
- Because of this unique capability to dissect tissue and coagulate small blood vessels all at once, with minimal energy transfer to surrounding tissue, the device has gained recognition among surgeons
- It has been used in many different types of minimally invasive surgery and its application has also been extended to many open procedures

343. In mammalian cell cycle, synthesis of DNA occurs during:

(a) S-phase
(b) M phase
(c) G2 phase
(d) G1 phase

Ans: (a) S-phase

CELL CYCLE

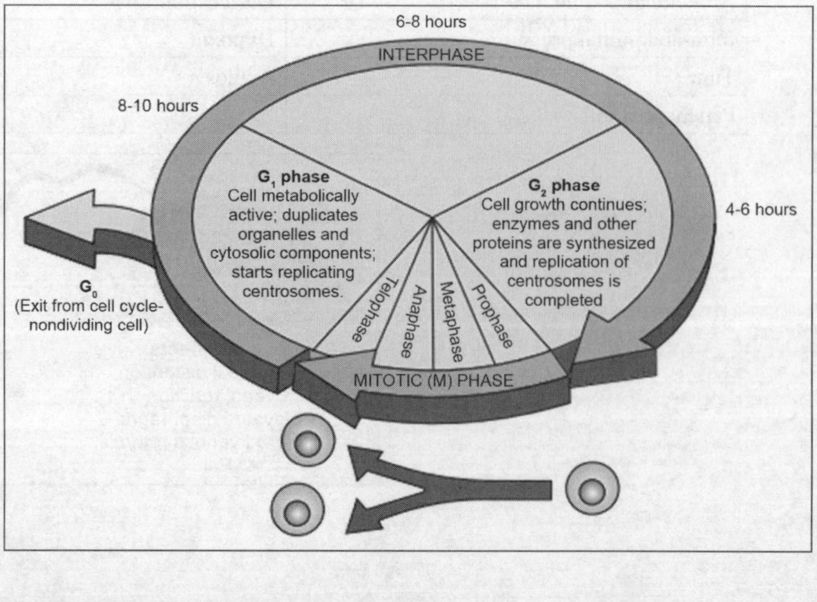

344. An opoid antagonist which achieves defecation within 90 minutes of administration in a patient on opoids:

(a) Methylnaltrexone (b) Polyethylene Glycol
(c) Liquid paraffin (d) Magnesium and sulphate salts

Ans: (a) Methylnaltrexone

- Methylnaltrexone (MNTX) is a quaternary derivative of naltrexone
- It does not cross the blood-brain barrier in humans
- Antagonizes only peripherally located opioid receptors while sparing centrally mediated analgesic effects of opioid pain medications
- **Most patients achieving defecation within 90 minutes of administration**

345. All of the following chemotherapeutic agents are alkylating agents *except:*

(a) Cyclophosphamide (b) Capecitabine
(c) Carboplatin (d) Carmustine

Ans: (b) Capecitabine

- Capecitabine is an antimetabolite that gets converted to 5 FU to become active

346. Correct pair of drug with mode of action is:

(a) Capecitabine–Inhibits Dihydrofolate reductase (b) Pemetrexed–Topoisomerase inhibitor
(c) Cytarabine–Inhibits DNA polymerase (d) Doxorubicin–Depolymerise microtubules

Ans: (c) Cytarabine–Inhibits DNA polymerase

- **Capecitabine** is an **oral fluoropyrimidine carbamate**
- **Pemetrexed** is **pyrrolopyrimidine, multitargeted antifolate analogue** that targets multiple enzymes involved in folate metabolism, including thymidylate synthase (TS), dihydrofolate reductase (DHFR), glycinamide ribonucleotide (GAR) formyltransferase, and aminoimidazole carboxamide (AICAR) formyltransferase
- **CYTARABINE-Ara-C** enters cells via nucleoside transport proteins, the most important one being the equilibrative inhibitor-sensitive (es) receptor. Once inside the cell, ara-C requires activation for its cytotoxic effects
- **Anthracyclines** are flat, planar molecules that are relatively hydrophobic. They poison Top2 by intercalating DNA with high affinity and stabilize the DNA-Top2 cleavable complexes, leading to DNA double-strand breaks

347. Which one is FALSE regarding emesis in cancer patients?

(a) IV dexamethasone and prochlorperazine can be given for relief
(b) Ondansetron is one of the most effective antiemetic drug
(c) Nausea and vomiting are less with drugs like dacarbazine, meclorethamine and streptozotocin
(d) Delayed emesis occurs upto a week after chemotherapy usually with cisplatin

Ans: (c) Nausea and vomiting are less with drugs like dacarbazine, meclorethamine and streptozotocin

- **Delayed CINV has been best characterized in relation to cisplatin**
- **Hesketh classification**

Emetic Risk (Estimated Incidence without Prophylaxis)	Antineoplastic Agent
High (> 90%)	Cisplatin Mechlorethamine Streptozotocin Cyclophosphamide ($\geq$ 1,500 mg/m^2) Carmustine Dacarbazine

348. In treatment of liver and pancreatic lesion, ideal instrument is:

(a) Radiofrequency ablation
(b) Harmonic scalpel
(c) CUSA
(d) Cryoablation

Ans: (c) CUSA

- Ultrasound (Cusa) dissector is most common method used for division of the **parenchyma**
- This allows parenchyma to be divided, leaving vessels and bile duct branches to be diathermied or ligated depending on their size
- Dissection continues on an even plane until the hepatic vein branches are approached from within the liver parenchyma, when they are ligated and divided

349. One of the key features in diagnosis of SIADH is:

(a) Hyponatremia corrected by fluid restriction but not by normal saline
(b) Fractional urea excretion > 55%. Hyponatremia corrected by fluid restriction but not by normal saline
(c) Urine osmolarity > 100 mOsm/kg of water
(d) Plasma uric acid < 4 mg/dL

Ans: (c) Urine osmolarity > 100 mOsm/kg of water

Diagnostic Criteria for SIADH
Essential diagnostic features:
• Decreased serum osmolality (< 275 mOsm/kg)
• Urine osmolality > 100 mOsm/kg in the setting of serum hypotonicity
• Euvolemic clinical examination
• In the setting of normal dietary sodium intake, urine sodium > 40 mmol/L
• Normal thyroid, adrenal, renal, cardiac function
• No recent use of diuretics

350. Which was the 1st robot approved by FDA for clinical use?

(a) DAVINCHI
(b) ROBODOC
(c) ZEUS
(d) AESOP

Ans: (d) AESOP

ROBOTICS

- **In 1990 the AESOP system produced by Computer Motion became the first system approved by Food and Drug Administration (FDA) for its endoscopic surgical procedure (Clinical use)**
- In 2000, the da Vinci Surgery System broke new ground by becoming the **first robotic surgery system approved by the FDA for general laparoscopic surgery**

351. Which among the following statements regarding apoptosis is wrong?

(a) Apoptosis is Type I programmed cell death
(b) Bcl-2 is a protein that inhibits apoptosis
(c) P53 is an apoptosis promoter
(d) Apoptosis is Type II programmed cell death

Ans: (d) Apoptosis is Type II programmed cell death

MECHANISMS OF CELL DEATH

- Apoptosis (or Type I programmed cell death) is a genetic pathway for rapid and efficient killing of unnecessary or damaged cells
- **Autophagy is sometime referred to as type II programmed cell death**
- Programmed necrotic cell death, called necroptosis, induced by interaction of death domain receptors with their respective ligands under conditions of defective or inhibited downstream apoptotic machinery
- **Necroptosis is potently inhibited by the Ripl kinase inhibitors, necrostatins**

352. Obesity is defined as BMI greater than:

(a) 20 kg/m² (b) 25 kg/m²

(c) 30 kg/m² (d) 35 kg/m²

Ans: (c) 30 kg/m²

OBESITY AND CANCER

- BMI/Quetelet's index = Weight (Kg)/Square of height (m²)
- BMI> 30 Kg/m² is defined as obesity.
- In US population it was 35.5% in adult men and 35.8% in adult women

353. Irradiation of blood products is done to prevent which of following complications of blood transfusion?

(a) Allergic reactions (b) Transfusion associated graft-versus-host disease

(c) Allo-immunisation (d) CMV transmission

Ans: (b) Transfusion associated graft-versus-host disease

TRANSFUSION ASSOCIATED GRAFT-VERSUS-HOST DISEASE

All blood products must be irradiated to prevent inadvertent engraftment of "contaminating" allogeneic lymphocytes from the transfused unit that may cause lethal transfusion-associated graft-versus-host disease

354. Drug which is a synthetic anticoagulant that selectively inhibits coagulation factor Xa:

(a) Enoxaparin (b) Dalteparin

(c) Fondaparinux (d) Warfarin

Ans: (c) Fondaparinux

FONDAPARINUX

- **Fondaparinux** is a synthetic molecule consisting of the highly active pentasaccharide sequence. **A synthetic factor Xa inhibitor**
- Fondaparinux, like the LMWHs, is almost exclusively metabolized by the kidneys, and should be avoided or used with caution in patients with severe renal impairment
- Predictable pharmacokinetics allow for weight based dosing
- A particularly long half-life (17–21 hours) allows for once-daily dosing, but the absence of necessary charge characteristics leads to a lack of binding to protamine sulfate; therefore, no effective neutralizing agent exists

355. Ideal age for repair of isolated cleft lip is:

(a) Immediately after birth (b) At 4-6 months of age

(c) At the time child starts to speak (d) At 4-6 years of age before starting school

Ans: (b) At 4-6 months of age

ISOLATED CLEFT LIP REPAIR

- Cleft lip repair at 3 months
- Cleft palate repair before 1 year, or before speech development begins
- Alveolar bone graft when permanent dentition begins and after orthodontic preparation
- Possible septorhinoplasty in the late teenage years

356. Metabolic derangements in severe burns are all *except:*

(a) Increased corticosteroid secretion (b) Hyperglycemia

(c) Increased gastric acid secretion (d) Neutrophil dysfunction

Ans: (c) Increased gastric acid secretion

METABOLIC DERANGEMENTS IN SEVERE BURNS

- **Marked and sustained increases in catecholamine, glucocorticoid, glucagon and dopamine secretion are thought to initiate the cascade of events leading to the acute hypermetabolic response, with its ensuing catabolic state**
- **Severe burn injury results in decreased gastric acid production in the acute shock period**
- A 10- to 50-fold elevation of plasma catecholamine and corticosteroid levels occurs in major burns, which persist up to 3 years post-injury
- Increases in catabolism result in loss of total body protein, decreased immune defenses and decreased wound healing
- Liver increases its size by 225% of normal by 2 weeks post burn and remains enlarged at discharge at 200% of normal
- Gastrointestinal complications including acute stress ulcerations occur after burn injury. Causes of acute gastric derangements are multiple, and tissue ischemia in the acute period of burn shock may promote breakdown of the gastric mucosal protective barrier
- Neutrophil dysfunction occurs in severe burns

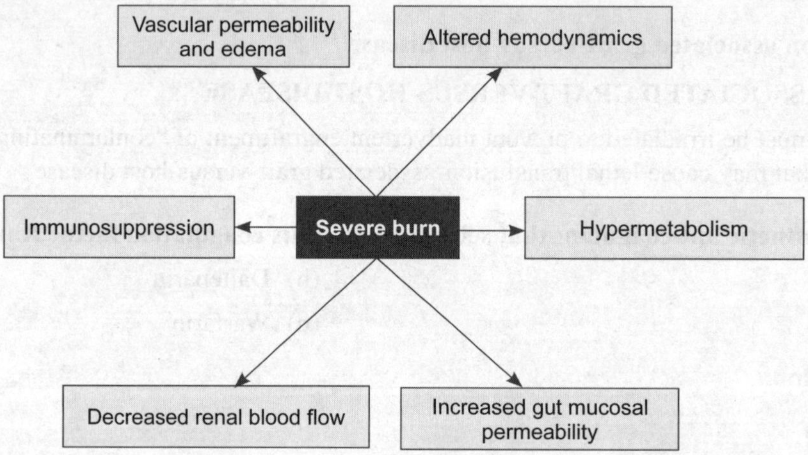

357. In hyponatremia with neurological symptoms 3% saline should be used until symptoms improve orsodium level is 130 mEq/L; at the rate of:

(a) 0.5 mEq/L (b) 1 mEq/L

(c) 1.5 mEq/L (d) 2 mEq/L

Ans: (d) 2 mEq/L

- **SEVERE HYPONATREMIA :**

  In general, 3% hypertonic saline infusion rate should not exceed 0.5 mL/kg body weight/hr; higher rates represent miscalculated sodium deficit/mathematical error
- **The goal is not to correct the serum sodium by more than 10–12 mEq/L over the first 24 hours**
- Hypertonic saline in hypervolemic patients can be hazardous, resulting in worsening volume overload, pulmonary edema and ascites
- The total increase in these patients **should not exceed 10–12 mEq/L in 24 hours or <20–25 mEq/L over 48 hours**
- Thereafter, the hypertonic saline is stopped, and the serum sodium is allowed to rise more slowly (e.g., over several days) in response to continued restriction of free water
- In all cases, serum sodium should be corrected only halfway to normal in the initial 24 hours (120–125 mEq/L) to prevent the complications listed above
- **TREATMENT:**

  Acutely to resolve neurologic symptoms especially seizures by raising serum sodium acutely by 5 mEq/L

  Sodium dose needed to increase serum sodium by 5 mEq/L is calculated and 3% saline is administered over 3 to 4 hours, raising serum sodium no more rapidly than 2 mEq/L/hour

358. Allen's test is useful in evaluating:

(a) Thoracic outlet compression
(b) Presence of cervical rib
(c) Integrity of palmar arch
(d) Digital blood flow

Ans: (c) Integrity of palmar arch

Special Hand Tests

Test	Technique	Significance
Allen's test	Elevate the hand and apply digital pressure on the radial and ulnar arteries to occlude them. Ask the patient to make a fist several times. The tips of the finger should go pale. Release each artery in turn and observe the return of colour	Tests the adequacy of the blood supply to the hand from the radial and ulnar arteries and the arcade between them
Tinel's test	Tap over the nerve of interest. Tingling may indicate nerve compression	Identifies compression of a peripheral nerve
Phalen's test	Place the wrist in maximum flexion with the elbows extended	Compression of the medial nerve causes paraesthesia
Froment's sign	Ask the patient to grip a sheet of paper between the index finger and thumb of both hands. Grip the paper yourself similarly. Ask the patient to resist as you attempt to pull the paper away	A positive test indicated by flexion of the thumb interphalangeal joint suggests weakness of the adductor pollicis muscle supplied by the ulnar nerve. Recruitment of the median nerve-innervated flexor pollicisbrev is explains the thumb posture

359. Which of the following statement is true regarding subclavian steal syndrome?

(a) Reversal of blood flow in ipsilateral vertebral artery
(b) Reversal of blood flow in contralateral vertebral artery
(c) Reversal of blood flow in contralateral carotid artery
(d) Bilateral reversal of blood flow in vertebral arteries

Ans: (a) Reversal of blood flow in ipsilateral vertebral artery

SUBCLAVIAN STEAL SYNDROME

- **Subclavian steal syndrome may occur if it is first part of the subclavian artery that is obstructed, with vertebral artery providing a collateral circulation into arm by reversing its direction of flow**
- Cause periods of cerebral ischaemia, classic syndrome of syncopal attack and visual disturbance associated with arm exercise and a diminished blood pressure in the affected limb is rare
- Asymptomatic reversal of flow in the vertebral artery is much more common

360. What is true regarding Trendelenberg operation?

(a) Stripping of superficial varicose vein
(b) Saphenofemoral ligation alone
(c) Ligation of perforators
(d) Ligation of short saphenous vein

Ans: (b) Saphenofemoral ligation alone

TRENDELENBURG'S OPERATION

- **Ligation of the long saphenous vein at the groin: performed to remove weakened portions of varicose veins**
- Perthes modified trendelenberg test that advocated a groin incision and a ligation of the GSV at the saphenofemoral junction (SFJ)

361. A man brought to casualty after a road traffic accident. He sustained multiple rib fractures with severe paradoxical chest movement. Management is:

(a) Tracheostomy and oxygen administration
(b) Wire fixation of rib fractures
(c) Strapping of chest wall
(d) Intermittent positive pressure ventilation

Ans: (d) Intermittent positive pressure ventilation

FLAIL CHEST

- **Flail chest is often associated with an underlying pulmonary contusion and should be supported with pain relief, stabilization of the chest wall, or even mechanical ventilation**

- Rib fractures are perhaps the most common traumatic injury sustained after blunt chest wall trauma
- Symptoms include pain on inspiration and localized point tenderness
- Plain films can confirm the diagnosis
- Fractures of the first or second ribs may occur after significant trauma or high-velocity injury. Because of the size and thickness of the first rib, tremendous force is needed to fracture this rib
- **Currently, treatment consists of oxygen administration, adequate analgesia (including opiates) and physiotherapy**
- If a chest tube is *in situ,* intrapleural local analgesia can be used as well
- **Ventilation is reserved for cases developing respiratory failure despite adequate analgesia and oxygen**
- Surgery to stabilise flail chest is currently in use again; it may be useful in selected group with isolated or severe chest injury and pulmonary contusion who have been shown to benefit from internal operative fixation of the flail segment

362. Mayos operation is done for:

(a) Spigelian hernia (b) Richer's hernia
(c) Femoral hernia (d) Umbilical hernia

Ans: (d) Umbilical hernia

UMBILICAL HERNIORRHAPHY

- If the defect is small, a primary herniorrhaphy can be performed. If the defect is large, the repair is best performed with prosthetic buttressing of the abdominal wall
- **Classic primary repair is that described by Mayo**
- A transverse elliptical incision is made around the umbilicus and the subcutaneous tissues are dissected off rectus sheath to expose the neck of the sac
- Neck is incised to expose the contents. Intestine is returned to the abdomen and any adherent omentum

363. Most frequent isolate of organisms that populate hands of ICU personnel:

(a) Staph. Epidermidis (b) MSSA
(c) Acinetobacter (d) Klebsiella

Ans: (a) Staph. Epidermidis

Organism	% Total cultures
Gram-positive cocci	
Staph. epidermidis	100%
Staph. aureus (MSSA)	7%
Gram-negative Bacilli	21%
Acinetobacter spp.	
Klebsiella spp.	
Enterobacter spp.	
Pseudomonas spp.	
Serratia spp.	
Yeasts and fungi	16%
Candida spp.	

364. Liver transplantation was 1st done by:

(a) Starzl (b) Huggins
(c) Carrel (d) Bernard

Ans: (a) Starzl

- Murray performed successful kidney transplant between identical twins
- Calne demonstrated the efficacy of azathioprine in preventing rejection of kidney allografts
- Starzl performed the first human liver transplant
- Starzl and colleagues used anti-lymphocyte globulin immunosuppresion
- Lillehei and Kelly performed the first human whole-organ pancreas transplant (along with a kidney transplant)
- Barnard performed the first human heart transplant
- Derom performed the first human lung transplant
- Collins developed Collins' solution, a new kidney preservation solution
- Sutherland and Najarin performed the first human pancreatic islet transplant
- Calne introduced ciclosporin into clinical practice
- Reitz and Shumway performed the first successful human heart-lung transplant
- Cosimi and colleagues reported the first use of a therapeutic monoclonal antibody (OKT3) in transplantation
- Belzer and colleagues developed University of Wisconsin (UW) solution, a new liver and pancreas preservation solution
- Starzl demonstrated the clinical efficacy of FK506 (tacrolimus)
- Ratner and colleagues first described laparoscopic living donor nephrectomy

365. Cock's peculiar tumor is:

(a) Infected sebaceous cyst of scalp
(b) A malignant tumor of scalp
(c) A metastatic tumor of scalp
(d) An ulcer following osteomyelitis of scalp

Ans: (a) Infected sebaceous cyst of scalp

COCK'S PECULIAR Tumor

- Complication found commonly in sebaceous cyst of scalp
- Infection in the cyst and ulceration on the surface of the sebaceous cyst
- Chronic irritation may lead to formation of a granuloma on the surface of the sebaceous cyst mimic an epithelioma
- **This appearance of the cyst is called a Cock's peculiar tumor of scalp**

366. Cardiac toxicity manifests in 1–5% of patients treated with doxorubicin:

(a) Arrhythmias
(b) MI
(c) Cardiomyopathy
(d) Sick sinus syndrome

Ans: (c) Cardiomyopathy

- Anthracyclines are responsible for cardiac toxicities, and special considerations are necessary to minimize this severe side effect
- **Acute doxorubicin cardiotoxicity is reversible and clinical signs include tachycardia, hypotension, electrocardiogram changes and arrhythmias**
- It develops during or within days of anthracycline infusion, and its incidence can be significantly reduced by slowing doxorubicin infusion rates
- Incidence of cardiomyopathy is related to both cumulative dose and schedule of administration, and predisposition to cardiac damage includes a previous history of heart disease, hypertension, radiation to the mediastinum, age younger than 4 years, prior use of anthracyclines or other cardiac toxins, and coadministration of other chemotherapy agents
- ***Chronic and delayed cardiotoxicity is more common and more severe because it is irreversible***
- Chronic cardiotoxicity with congestive heart failure peaks at 1 to 3 months but can occur even years after therapy

Mechanisms of Myocardial Damage:

- Classical mechanism is by the direct generation of reactive oxygen species (ROS) during the electron transfer from the semiquinone to quinone moieties of anthracycline, which leads to myocardial damage

367. Concept of spatial co-operation in oncology refers to:

(a) Interaction between tumor metastasis and host environment
(b) Combining different modalities of therapy to treat a particular cancer
(c) Interaction between primary tumor and host
(d) Both (a) and (c)

Ans: (b) Combining different modalities of therapy to treat a particular cancer

SPATIAL COOPERATION

- Spatial cooperation was the initial rationale for combining chemotherapy with radiation therapy
- Action of radiation and chemotherapeutic drugs is directed toward different anatomic sites

368. Substrate depleted earliest in postoperative period is:

(a) Branched chain amino acids
(b) Ketone
(c) Glycogen
(d) Glucose

Ans: (c) Glycogen

METABOLISM IN SURGICAL PATIENTS:

- Metabolic response to surgery (and other trauma) is a result of neuroendocrine stimulation that sharply accelerates protein breakdown, stimulates gluconeogenesis and produces glucose intolerance
- **Glycogen stores are rapidly depleted because of fall in insulin and rise in glucagon levels in plasma**

Metabolic Response to Starvation
• Low plasma insulin
• High plasma glucagon
• Hepatic glycogenolysis
• Protein catabolism
• Hepatic gluconeogenesis
• Lipolysis: Mobilization of fat stones
• Adaptive ketogenesis
• Reduction in resting energy expenditure (15-20 kcal kg^{-1} day^{-1})

369. Indications for laparotomy include all the following *except:*

(a) Hemodynamic instability produces source control
(b) Abdominal compartment syndrome
(c) Uncertain viability of bowel in mesenteric vascular ischemia
(d) Penetrating injury caused by knife

Ans: (d) Penetrating injury caused by knife

INDICATIONS FOR LAPAROTOMY

Clinical Indications for Laparotomy Following Blunt Trauma

Manifestation	Pitfall
Unstable vital signs with strongly suspected abdominal injury	Alternate sources shock
Unequivocal peritoneal irritation	Unreliable
Pneumoperitoneum	Insensitive and non-specific; may be due to cardiopulmonary source or invasive procedures (DPL, laparoscopy)
Evidence of diaphragmatic injury	Nonspecific
Significant gastrointestinal bleeding	Uncommon, unknown accuracy

370. Management of CSF rhinorrhoea is:

(a) Nasal packing only
(b) Nasal packing and foot end elevation
(c) Antibiotics and semi-sitting position
(d) Immediate surgery for all patients

Ans: (c) Antibiotics and semi-sitting position

MANAGEMENT OF CSF RHINORRHOEA

- Antibiotics for prevention of meningitis and patient kept in semi-sitting position
- Nasal pack is usually avoided in CSF leak patients
- Immediate surgery is not necessary in all patients
- Most leaks spontaneously heal without repair
- Conservative management consists of a 7–10 day trial of bed rest with the head of the bed elevated approximately 15–30°. This angle of inclination is sufficient to reduce the CSF pressure at basal cisterns
- Coughing, sneezing, nose blowing, and heavy lifting should be avoided as much as possible
- Stool softeners should be used to decrease the strain and increased ICP associated with bowel movements
- Acetazolamide can be a useful adjunct in the treatment of patients with spontaneous CSF rhinorrhea associated with elevated intracranial pressure
- It is logical to assume that the communication between a sterile environment (intracranial vault) and a nonsterile environment (sinonasal cavity) will ultimately result in infection of the sterile compartment
- This has led to the use of prophylactic antibiotics in patients with CSF rhinorrhea

371. When using sterilization by steam under pressure (autoclave):

(a) Viruses, such as HBV and HIV are not linked
(b) Biological indicators of sterilization are used for monitoring of sterilization
(c) A prevacuum cycle is not essential for prepacked instruments
(d) Temperature should be 121°C for hold time of 15 min

Ans: (d) Temperature should be 121°C for hold time of 15 min

STEAM UNDER PRESSURE (AUTOCLAVE)

- Sterilization in an autoclave is most effective when the organisms are either contacted by the steam directly or are contained in a small volume of aqueous (primarily water) liquid
- **Steam at a pressure about 15 psi; attaining temperature (121°C) will kill all organisms and endospores in about 15 minutes**
- In preparing items for autoclaving, containers should be unsealed and articles should be wrapped in materials that allow steam penetration
- **Large packages of dressings and large flasks of media require extra time for heat to penetrate them**
- Likewise, packing many articles close together in an autoclave lengthens the processing time to as much as 60 minutes to ensure sterility
- Wrapping objects in aluminum foil is not recommended because it may interfere with steam penetration

372. Behcet's disease is:

(a) Oral ulceration is the primary criterion
(b) Genital ulcers are painless
(c) Systemic steroids have no effect on outcome
(d) Testis and epididymis are never inflamed

Ans: (a) Oral ulceration is the primary criterion

BEHCET'S DISEASE

International Study Group Diagnostic Criteria for Behcet's Disease	
Recurrent oral ulceration	Minor aphithous, major aphthous, or herpetiform ulceration observed by physician or patient that recurred at least 3 times in one 12-month period
Plus 2 of the following criteria:	
Recurrent genital ulceration	Aphthous ulceration or scarring observed by physician or patient
Eye lesions	Anterior uveitis, posterior uveitis, or cells in vitreous on slit lamp examination; or retinal vasculitis observed by ophthalmologist
Cutaneous lesions	Erythema nodosum observed by physician or patient, pseudofolliculitis or papulopustular lesions; or acneiform nodules observed by physician in postadolescent patients not receiving corticosteroid treatment
Positive pathergy test	Read by physician at 24-48 hours

CHAPTER 57

GENITOURINARY ONCOLOGY

NEET SS PATTERN MCQs

1. **Which of the following drug can cause bladder cancer?**
   (a) Sirolimus (b) Cyclophosphamide
   (c) Methotrexate (d) Taxanes
   Ans: (b) Cyclophosphamide

2. **Sipuleucel T vaccine recently approved by FDA in treatment of:**
   (a) Renal cancer (b) Bladder cancer
   (c) Testicular cancer (d) Prostate cancer
   Ans: (d) Prostate cancer

3. **In prostate cancer, the mechanism of action of ketoconazole is:**
   (a) Androgen receptor antagonist (b) GNRH receptor antagonist
   (c) GNRH receptor agonist (d) Adrenal ablation
   Ans: (d) Adrenal ablation

4. **T3 in Renal cell cancer denotes:**
   (a) Invades Gerota fascia (b) Invades adrenal gland
   (c) Extends into IVC (d) Tumor size > 10 cm
   Ans: (c) Extends into IVC

5. **Regarding paraneoplastic syndromes of renal cell carcinoma true statement is:**
   (a) IL8 is the cause for Stauffer syndrome
   (b) Hyperlipidemia is the most common paraneoplastic syndrome
   (c) Hypercalcemia is due to increased PTH production
   (d) Hypertension is always aldosterone mediated
   Ans: (c) Hypercalcemia is due to increased PTH production

6. **Drug that is used for intravesical therapy perioperatively is:**
   (a) Mitomycin C (b) BCG
   (c) Epirubicin (d) Doxorubicin
   Ans: (a) Mitomycin C

7. **BCG is used in:**
   (a) Muscle invasive bladder cancer (b) In situ tumors
   (c) Nonmuscle invasive bladder cancer (d) PUNLMP
   Ans: (c) Nonmuscle invasive bladder cancer

8. Papillary urothelial neoplasms of low malignant potential (PUNLMP), true regarding this:

(a) Mitomycin C is the only drug given

(b) BCG course to be completed and follow up therapy needed

(c) Needs Deep re-excision and biopsy

(d) Random biopsies

Ans: (a) Mitomycin C is the only drug given

9. Lasers used in bladder cancer treatment are:

(a) KTP
(b) CO_2
(c) Holmium:YAG
(d) Nd:YAG laser

Ans: (d) Nd:YAG laser

10. Patient underwent anterior pelvic exenteration for muscle invasive bladder cancer and plan for orthotopic neobladder repair is contraindicated in all *except:*

(a) Age >75 years
(b) Tumor invading the wall of vagina
(c) Lymph node invasion
(d) Pre-existing HUN

Ans: (a) Age >75 years

11. Most common testicular tumor in children is:

(a) Seminoma
(b) Choriocarcinoma
(c) Yolk sac tumor
(d) Embryonal carcinoma

Ans: (c) Yolk sac tumor

12. Most common benign renal tumor which is hyperdense and appears as RCC:

(a) Oncocytoma
(b) Juxtaglomerular tumor
(c) Rhabdomyoma
(d) Metanephric adenoma

Ans: (a) Oncocytoma

13. Treatment of metastatic bladder cancer:

(a) Interferon
(b) MVAC
(c) AC
(d) Cisplatin

Ans: (b) MVAC

14. Most common site of urethral cancer:

(a) Penile
(b) Bulbomembranous
(c) Prostatic
(d) Fossa navicularis

Ans: (b) Bulbomembranous

15. Stage T2 Ca penis:

(a) Urethral involvement
(b) Corporal involvement
(c) Prostatic involvement
(d) Prepuce involvement

Ans: (b) Corporal involvement

16. Gold standard of treatment TCC involving renal pelvis:

(a) Radical nephroureterectomy
(b) Pelvi-ureterectomy
(c) Radical nephrectomy
(d) Conservative nephrectomy

Ans: (a) Radical nephroureterectomy

17. Wilms tumor not associated with:

(a) WAGR
(b) Denys-Drash
(c) Beckwith-Wiedemann
(d) Trisomy 13

Ans: (d) Trisomy 13

18. Combination chemotherapy tried by southwest oncology group in penile cancer:

(a) Cisplatin, Methotrexate and Bleomycin
(b) Ifosfamide, Paclitaxel and Cisplatin
(c) Vincristine, Bleomycin and Methotrexate
(d) Paclitaxel and Carboplatin

Ans: (a) Cisplatin, Methotrexate and Bleomycin

19. In case of non-seminomatous germ cell tumor, Retroperitoneal lymphadenectony is indicated when diameter of post chemo residual disease is more than:

(a) 1 cm
(b) 2 cm
(c) 3 cm
(d) 5 cm

Ans: (a) 1 cm

20. Indication for bone scan in carcinoma prostate:

(a) PSA >20 ng/ml and biopsy Gleason score >7
(b) T3 and T4 Stage
(c) Symptoms Suggestive of metastatic disease
(d) All of the above

Ans: (d) All of the above

21. Infection with Schistosoma hematobium predisposes to:

(a) CA Bladder
(b) CA Pancreas
(c) CA Stomach
(d) Cholangiocarcinoma

Ans: (a) CA Bladder

22. Incidence of bilaterality in Wilm's tumor:

(a) 20–25%
(b) 5–10%
(c) 2–3%
(d) 12–14%

Ans: (b) 5–10%

23. Which of the following is risk factor for CNS involvement in patients with testicular cancer?

(a) Large volume pulmonary metastases
(b) HCG >1,00,000
(c) Pure choriocarcinoma histology
(d) All of the above

Ans: (d) All of the above

24. Surgical pathology shows gleason score 6 tumor in both lobes of prostate. There is a focal surgical margin +ve. There is no evidence of seminal vesicle/lymph node invasion. His postoperative PSA is undetectable and he has good continence. Most appropriate next step is:

(a) Adjuvant radiotherapy
(b) Pelvic CT scan
(c) Prostascinti scan
(d) Repeat surgical exploration with possible re-excision of prostatic bed

Ans: (a) Adjuvant radiotherapy

25. Initial standard of care for metastatic renal cell cancer is:

(a) Sorafenib
(b) Pazopanib
(c) Sunitinib
(d) None

Ans: (c) Sunitinib

26. Selection criteria for implantation in carcinoma prostate are all *except:*

(a) PSA Level < 15 ng/ml
(b) Gleason score < 7
(c) Clinical stage T1c-T2a
(d) Gland size < 60 cm^3

Ans: (d) Gland size < 60 cm^3

27. Abiraterone acetate is used in treatment of:

(a) Lung cancer
(b) Pancreatic cancer
(c) Colonic cancer
(d) Prostate cancer

Ans: (d) Prostate cancer

28. All of the following are associated with hereditary renal cell carcinoma *except:*

(a) von Hippel-Lindau syndrome
(b) Hereditary papillary renal carcinoma
(c) Hereditary leiomyomatosis
(d) Kaizen syndrome

Ans: (d) Kaizen syndrome

29. All of the following are features of Birt-Hogg-Dube syndrome *except:*

(a) Cutaneous nodules on face and neck (hair follicle tumors, fibrofolliculoma)
(b) Pulmonary cysts
(c) Renal tumors
(d) Brain tumors

Ans: (d) Brain tumors

30. In renal cell carcinoma, tumor grossly extends into renal vein/segmental branches/vena cava below diaphragm is:

(a) T3a
(b) T3b
(c) T4a
(d) T4b

Ans: (b) T3b

31. All of the following are used in management of metastatic renal cell carcinoma *except:*

(a) Sunitinib
(b) Sorafenib
(c) Dasatinib
(d) Temsirolimus

Ans: (c) Dasatinib

32. All of the following are risk factors for carcinoma penis *except:*

(a) Leukoplakia
(b) Balanitis xerotica obliterans
(c) Buschke Lowenstein tumor
(d) Chancroid

Ans: (d) Chancroid

33. True about Spermatocytic seminoma:

(a) Seen generally in older men
(b) Express placental alkaline phosphatase
(c) Metastatic potential is high
(d) Secretes high amount of AFP

Ans: (a) Seen generally in older men

34. Extragonadal germ cell tumor comprises:

(a) 10%
(b) 20%
(c) 30%
(d) 40%

Ans: (a) 10%

35. All are exceptions for radiotherapy in patients with clinical stage I and non-bulky clinical stage II seminoma *except:*

(a) Horseshoe kidney
(b) A second metachronous testicular germ cell tumor
(c) Inflammatory bowel disease
(d) Undescended testis

Ans: (d) Undescended testis

36. Which of the following statement is true in management of prostate cancer which is confined to prostate gland?

(a) Active surveillance is a valid approach
(b) Prostatectomy has been shown to be superior to radiotherapy
(c) Radiotherapy causes impotence in 50% of patients
(d) Prostatectomy leads to long-term incontinence in 5% patients

Ans: (a) Active surveillance is a valid approach

37. Young male patient with germ cell tumor is on bleomycin, etoposide and cisplatinum. What side effect would make you to stop treatment?

(a) Peripheral neuropathy
(b) Neutropenic septicemia
(c) Interstitial lung disease
(d) High tone hearing loss

Ans: (c) Interstitial lung disease

38. Which germ cell tumor is associated with widespread hematogenous metastasis and high levels of HCG?

(a) Pure choriocarcinoma
(b) Yolk sac tumor
(c) Embryonic cell carcinoma
(d) Seminoma

Ans: (a) Pure choriocarcinoma

39. Which of the following is reasonable treatment after orchiectomy for patients with Stage IA non-seminomatous germ cell tumor?

(a) Radiotherapy
(b) Observation
(c) Bilateral RPLND with suprahilar dissection
(d) All of the above

Ans: (b) Observation

40. Gleason's scoring is done in:

(a) Carcinoma prostate
(b) Carcinoma pancreas
(c) Carcinoma kidney
(d) Carcinoma cervix

Ans: (a) Carcinoma prostate

41. True about transitional cell carcinoma of urinary bladder:

(a) Smoking predisposes
(b) Schistosoma infection predisposes
(c) Aniline dye workers are at increased risk
(d) All options are correct

Ans: (d) All options are correct

42. A patient presented with a hard swelling in his right testis. All are true statements *except:*

(a) Trans scrotal biopsy is needed
(b) High inguinal exploration should be done
(c) Scrotal ultrasound is done
(d) Serum AFP and Beta HCG are measured

Ans: (a) Trans scrotal biopsy is needed

43. Treatment options for stage I non-seminomatous germ cell tumor (NSGCT) include all of the following *except:*

(a) Surveillance or watchful waiting
(b) Retroperitoneal lymph node dissection (RPLND)
(c) Adjuvant chemotherapy
(d) High dose chemotherapy

Ans: (d) High dose chemotherapy

44. Is cytoreductive nephrectomy recommended for patients with metastatic renal cell carcinoma (RCC) before cytokine or targeted therapy?

(a) Yes
(b) No
(c) Depends on stage of the disease
(d) Depends on patient characteristics

Ans: (a) Yes

45. Which of the following statements about testicular cancer is False?

(a) Survivors are at substantial risk for second cancers
(b) Survivors with second cancers have poorer survival than patients with comparable first cancers
(c) It is incurable, except in a small percentage of men
(d) Treatment can limit treatment options for second cancers

Ans: (c) It is incurable, except in a small percentage of men

46. Which of the following chemopreventive agents has been shown to lower prostate cancer occurrence?

(a) Finasteride
(b) Lycopene
(c) Selenium
(d) All options are correct

Ans: (a) Finasteride

47. A 63 years old man with a remote history of tobacco use presents with hematuria. He undergoes a transurethral resection (TUR), which reveals T1, superficial bladder cancer. What is his risk for bladder cancer recurrence in the next 5 years without further therapy?

(a) 10%
(b) 30%
(c) 40%
(d) 70%

Ans: (d) 70%

CHAPTER 58 THORACIC ONCOLOGY

MULTIPLE CHOICE QUESTIONS

1. **A 67-year-old male with history of chronic smoking hemoptysis with cough. Bronchoscopic biopsy from centrally located mass shows undifferentiated tumor histopathologically. Most useful IHC marker to make proper diagnosis would be:**

   (a) Cytokeratin (b) Parvalbumin
   (c) HMB-45 (d) Hep-par 1

   Ans: (a) Cytokeratin

2. **Neuroendocrine lesions of lung are:**

   (a) Carcinoid (b) Alveolar carcinoma
   (c) Hamartoma (d) Asthma

   Ans: (a) Carcinoid

3. **Which of the following is true about lung cancer?**

   (a) Squamous cell variant accounts for 70% of all lung cancers
   (b) Oat cell variant typically presents with cavitation
   (c) Oat cell tumor is associated with hilar adenopathy
   (d) Adenocarcinoma variant is typically central in location

   Ans: (c) Oat cell tumor is associated with hilar adenopathy

4. **Hypersecretory granules are seen in which of the following carcinoma:**

   (a) Adenocarcinoma (b) Small cell carcinoma
   (c) Large cell carcinoma (d) Squamous cell carcinoma

   Ans: (b) Small cell carcinoma

5. **Not true about lung cancer is:**

   (a) K-ras mutations are more common in SCLC than in NSCLC
   (b) Chromosome 3p allele loss is one of the most common event on lung cancer pathogenesis
   (c) EGFR is another name for HER1
   (d) Although overexpression of c-KIT is common in SCLC, imatinib was not associated with high response rate in phase II trials in SCLC

   Ans: (a) K-ras mutations are more common in SCLC than in NSCLC

6. **Which of the following tumor is most commonly associated with SVC syndrome?**

   (a) Lymphoma (b) Small cell lung cancer
   (c) Metastasis (d) NSCLC

   Ans: (b) Small cell lung cancer

7. A 60-year-old male presented to emergency with breathlessness, facial swelling and dilated veins on chest wall. Most common cause is:

(a) Thymoma
(b) Lung cancer
(c) Hodgkin's lymphoma
(d) SVC Obstruction

Ans: (d) SVC Obstruction

8. All of the following statements about non small cell lung cancer are true *except:*

(a) Contralateral mediastinal nodes are contraindication to surgical resection
(b) Single agent chemotherapy is preferred for patients >79 years with advanced disease
(c) Squamous cell carcinoma is most common NSCLC among Asian population
(d) Geftinib is most effective for female smokers with adenocarcinoma variety

Ans: (d) Geftinib is most effective for female smokers with adenocarcinoma variety

9. Ramesh 40-year-male presents with polyuria, pain abdomen, nausea, vomiting, altered sensation was found to have bronchogenic carcinoma. Electrolyte abnormality seen in him would be:

(a) Hypokalemia
(b) Hyperkalemia
(c) Hypocalcemia
(d) Hypercalcemia

Ans: (d) Hypercalcemia

10. True statement about adenocarcinoma lung are:

(a) Common in females
(b) Not associated with smoking
(c) Central involvement is common
(d) Upper lobe involvement is common

Ans: (a) Common in females

11. Rasool is brought to emergency department following a seizure. Serum electrolytes demonstrate serum sodium of 128 mEq/L. Urine osmolarity is higher than serum osmolarity. Chest X-ray demonstrates lung mass. Which of the following forms of lung cancer is more likely to cause described electrolyte imbalance:

(a) Adenocarcinoma
(b) Bronchoalveolar carcinoma
(c) Large cell carcinoma
(d) Small cell carcinoma

Ans: (d) Small cell carcinoma

12. Scar in lung tissue develops into:

(a) Adenocarcinoma
(b) Oat cell carcinoma
(c) Squamous cell carcinoma
(d) Columnar cell carcinoma

Ans: (a) Adenocarcinoma

13. A 75-year-old man with significant smoking history of presents to emergency department with complaints of dyspnea and truncal, arm and facial swelling for 1 week. Physical examination shows facial erythema and edema with prominent thoracic and neck veins. On chest X-ray there is mass in right mediastinum with adenopathy. Which of the following is most likely diagnosis?

(a) Adenocarcinoma
(b) Hodgkin's lymphoma
(c) Large cell carcinoma
(d) Small cell carcinoma

Ans: (d) Small cell carcinoma

14. APUD cells are seen in:

(a) Bronchial carcinoid
(b) Bronchial adenoma
(c) Hepatic adenoma
(d) Villous adenoma

Ans: (a) Bronchial carcinoid

15. True about oat cell carcinoma lung:

(a) Secrete ectopic hormone
(b) Variant of small cell carcinoma
(c) Causes SIADH
(d) All

Ans: (d) All

16. Most common site of metastasis in lung carcinoma is:

(a) Brain
(b) Adrenals
(c) Kidney
(d) Testis

Ans: (b) Adrenals

17. Which of the following has no infectious etiology?

(a) NPC
(b) HCC
(c) NSCLC
(d) Gastric ca

Ans: (c) NSCLC

18. In a 56-year-old chronic smoker there was a mass in bronchus which is successfully resected. This mass is most likely to be +ve for:

(a) Cytokeratin
(b) Vimentin
(c) Epithelial membrane cadherin
(d) Leukocyte

Ans: (a) Cytokeratin

19. Which of the following statements about small cell carcinoma is true:

(a) Bone metastasis is uncommon
(b) Peripheral location
(c) Paraneoplastic syndrome with PTH raised
(d) Chemosensitive

Ans: (d) Chemosensitive

20. Lung to lung metastasis is seen in:

(a) Adenocarcinoma lung
(b) Squamous cell carcinoma
(c) Small cell carcinoma
(d) Neuroendocrine tumor

Ans: (a) Adenocarcinoma lung

21. True about carcinoma bronchus:

(a) 75% are Squamous Cell Carcinoma
(b) Cavitation is most common in oat cell carcinoma
(c) Perihilar lymphadenopathy is most common in oat cell carcinoma
(d) Peripheral nodule is more commonly seen in Squamous cell carcinoma

Ans: (c) Perihilar lymphadenopathy is most common in oat cell carcinoma

22. True about lung carcinoma is:

(a) Adenocarcinoma is most common
(b) SCC is most common
(c) Originates from type II pnemocytes
(d) SCC is peripheral

Ans: (a) Adenocarcinoma is most common

23. A 65-year-old miner has lost 7 kgs weight in 2 months, has presented with cough and blood streaked sputum. He was treated for primary tuberculosis 10 years ago. He also has dropping of his left eyelid for 1 month. On physical examination there is ptosis of left eye and papillary miosis. Chest X-ray revealed round opacification in left upper apical lobe. What is most probable diagnosis:

(a) Secondary tuberculosis
(b) Adenocarcinoma
(c) SCC
(d) Asbestosis

Ans: (c) SCC

24. A 70-year-old otherwise healthy former smoker presents with persistent cough and hemoptysis of 2-month duration. Further workup reveals a 3 cm cavitating hilar mass, multiple bilateral parenchymal lung nodules and a 2 cm hypodense lesion in the right hepatic lobe. Biopsies of lung and liver masses are consistent with squamous cell lung carcinoma. Tumor molecular analysis shows the absence of EGFR, KRAS mutations and ALK fusion. MRI brain shows no evidence of metastatic disease. Which of the following combinations would be the best choice for first-line chemotherapy?

(a) Cisplatin and gemcitabine
(b) Cisplatin and pemetrexed
(c) Carboplatin, paclitaxel and bevacizumab
(d) Carboplatin, pemetrexed and bevacizumab

Ans: (a) Cisplatin and gemcitabine

- Histology of NSCLC is important in treatment selection. Patients with squamous histology have shown showed improved survival with cisplatin/gemcitabine as initial chemotherapy treatment compared with pemetrexed/cisplatin
- Bevacizumab is ***not recommended*** in patients who are at ***increased risk of bleeding***: *Squamous histology, tumor location close to major blood vessels, tumor necrosis, cavitation or pre-existing hemoptysis*

25. Which of the following is true regarding screening for lung cancer in a 54-year-old man with 20 pack-year history of smoking who quit 3 years ago?

(a) Annual low dose CT screening is expected to result in reduction in lung cancer related mortality
(b) Annual low-dose CT screening is expected to result in a reduction in all-cause mortality
(c) Chest X-ray and sputum cytology are expected to result in a reduction in all-cause mortality
(d) None of these

Ans: (d) None of these

- National Lung Screening Trial, randomized trial ***compared annual screening by low dose chest CT scanning with chest X-ray*** for three years found a reduction in lung cancer related mortality and all cause mortality in high risk patients screened with low dose CT scan

(High-risk population-defined by NLST as individuals between 55-74 years of age with atleast 30 pack-year cigarette smoking and former smokers who had quit within previous 15 years)

26. A 70-year-old otherwise healthy woman came to medical attention with long-standing cough. CT scan showed a 4 cm left hilar mass and right hilar lymphadenopathy. The patient underwent bronchoscopy, right video-assisted thoracic surgery, wedge biopsy and cervical mediastinoscopy with biopsy. Pathology showed lung adenocarcinoma with involvement of right hilar lymph nodes. Tissue is inadequate for molecular analyses. Which of the following is the best treatment option?

(a) Surgical resection of the primary mass and lymph nodes followed by adjuvant chemoradiation
(b) Concurrent chemotherapy and radiation
(c) Neoadjuvant chemotherapy followed by surgery
(d) Sequential chemotherapy and radiation

Ans: (b) Concurrent chemotherapy and radiation

Patient has stage IIIB disease (T2N3). Stage IIIB lung cancers are not amenable to curative surgical resection unless they are highly selected

- For patients with stage IIIB disease with good performance status, combined modality therapy with chemotherapy and radiation is recommended
- Concurrent chemotherapy and radiation is superior to sequential therapy

27. A 61-year-old nonsmoking man is found to have a 4 cm right upper-lobe lesion that is biopsied and found to be adenocarcinoma. CT of the chest showed enlarged ipsilateral mediastinal and subcarinal lymphadenopathy with subsequent biopsy confirming AC. CT of the head and abdomen showed no evidence of distant metastases. You stage his cancer as stage IIIA (T2N2). He has no other comorbidities and his performance status is 0. Which is the most appropriate recommendation?

(a) Concurrent chemoradiotherapy followed by consolidation erlotinib
(b) Induction therapy with platinum doublet followed by surgery and then radiation
(c) Carboplatin with paclitaxel and bevacizumab for 4-6 cycles and then observation
(d) Concurrent chemotherapy plus radiation therapy

Ans: (d) Concurrent chemotherapy plus radiation therapy

28. A 52-year-old Asian nonsmoking woman presents with persistent cough and is found to have bilateral pulmonary nodules. Biopsy confirms adenocarcinoma of the lung with mutational analysis confirming epidermal growth factor receptor exon 19 deletions. She has no other comorbidities and her performance status is 1. Which is most appropriate first-line anticancer agent?

(a) Carboplatin with paclitaxel
(b) Erlotinib
(c) Erlotinib with carboplatin and paclitaxel
(d) Carboplatin with paclitaxel and bevacizumab

Ans: (b) Erlotinib

29. Most common mechanism of resistance in patients who progress after first-line EGFR tyrosine kinase inhibitor therapy?

(a) Secondary T790M mutations in EGFR
(b) Bypass signaling via c-MET amplification
(c) Histologic transformation, NSCLC to small-cell lung cancer
(d) Secondary L747S mutation in EGFR

Ans: (a) Secondary T790M mutations in EGFR

30. A 61-year-old nonsmoking man is found to have a 4 cm right upper-lobe lesion. He returns for followup after biopsy confirmed metastatic non-small-cell lung cancer. He has *pain in his right upper quadrant abdomen from tumor burden*, but otherwise has no significant comorbidities and his performance status is 1. Among the available choices, which is the most appropriate second-line therapy?

(a) Increase the dose of afatinib
(b) Continue afatinib and add erlotinib
(c) Stop afatinib and start carboplatin/paclitaxel/ docetaxel
(d) Stop afatinib and start carboplatin/paclitaxel

Ans: (d) Stop afatinib and start carboplatin/paclitaxel

31. A 71-year-old woman with a past medical history of insulin-dependent diabetes presents with dyspnea on exertion. CT of the chest shows bilateral nodules with mediastinal lymphadenopathy. A bronchoscopy with biopsy of the mediastinal lymph nodes and of a pulmonary nodule returns positive for adenocarcinoma. Molecular testing is completed and EML4-ALK translocations are found. Patient is initiated on crizotinib 250 mg twice daily and has a near complete response after 3 months of therapy. Nine months into therapy, she begins complaining of increasing exertional dyspnea. Repeated CT of chest shows patchy bilateral interstitial opacities with no increase in lymphadenopathy and no distant metastases. Her performance status is 1. Which is the next best step in management?

(a) Hold crizotinib and restart in 2 weeks
(b) Increase dose of crizotinib
(c) Stop crizotinib indefinitely
(d) Continue crizotinib and add carboplatin/pemetrexed

Ans: (c) Stop crizotinib indefinitely

32. Stage 3 Thymoma as per staging system of MASAOKA indicates:

(a) Microscopic invasion into capsule
(b) Macroscopic invasion into surrounding fatty tissue only
(c) Macroscopic invasion into pericardium, lung and great vessels
(d) Macroscopic invasion into surrounding fatty tissue and mediastinal pleura

Ans: (c) Macroscopic invasion into pericardium, lung and great vessels

33. **Masaoka staging system is used for one of the following neoplasms:**

(a) Neuroblastoma (b) Burkitt's lymphoma
(c) GIST (d) Thymoma

Ans: (d) Thymoma

34. **A highly effective pleurodesis with overall response rates ranging from 80-100% can be obtained from:**

(a) Tetracyclin intrapleural administration (b) Intrapleural effusion of tissue plasminogen activator
(c) Asbestosis free, gas sterilized talc insuffulations (d) Bleomycin intrapleural administration

Ans: (c) Asbestosis free, gas sterilized talc insuffulations

35. **All of the following statements are true regarding carcinoid tumors *except:***

(a) Gastrin is a growth factor for some gastric carcinoids
(b) Carcinoid syndrome is more commonly with mid gut carcinoid tumors than hind gut tumors
(c) In atypical carcinoid syndrome plasma 5-HT levels are normal
(d) Bronchial carcinoids are related to smoking

Ans: (d) Bronchial carcinoids are related to smoking

36. **A 51 years old woman had dull anterior chest pain. She is a lifelong nonsmoker. Her medical history is significant for Hashimoto's thyroiditis for which she has been taking levothyroxine for 1 year. Examination is unremarkable. Lab tests showed normal blood counts, LDH, AFP and Beta HCG. Chest X-ray shows clear lung fields with retrosternal density. CT Scan shows 4 cm smooth anterior mediastinal mass. Most likely diagnosis:**

(a) Small cell lung cancer (b) Thymoma
(c) Pericardial cyst (d) NSGCT

Ans: (b) Thymoma

37. **Patient develops a new pulmonary infiltrate and becomes febrile. Primary routine culture of expectorated sputum has been evaluated and results have not been helpful. What is next test likely to yield most diagnostic information with least patient risk:**

(a) FNAC (b) BAL
(c) Open lung biopsy (d) Thoracocentesis

Ans: (a) FNAC

38. **Regarding malignant pleural effusions, true is:**

(a) Usually asymptomatic
(b) Usually transudates from tumor obstruction
(c) Surgical pleurodesis offers higher success rate in their management than chemical pleurodesis
(d) Thoracocentesis is definitive treatment

Ans: (c) Surgical pleurodesis offers higher success rate in their management than chemical pleurodesis

39. **Which of the following statement is true of small cell lung cancer?**

(a) Surgery is most important treatment modality
(b) Limited stage disease describes disease less than T2N1M0
(c) Approximately 80% of patients respond to chemotherapy
(d) Prophylactic cranial irradiation has been shown to prolong survival

Ans: (c) Approximately 80% of patients respond to chemotherapy

40. All of the following statements about smoking and lung cancer are true *except:*

(a) Smoking increases risk of all histological types of lung cancer

(b) Risk of developing lung cancer increases with number of cigarettes smoked

(c) Risk of developing lung cancer drops to the level of never smokers within 3 years of stopping smoking

(d) Duration of smoking is strongest determinant of lung cancer in cigarette smokers

Ans: (c) Risk of developing lung cancer drops to the level of never smokers within 3 years of stopping smoking

41. Masaoka staging is used for:

(a) Melanoma
(b) Thymoma
(c) Germ cell tumor
(d) Neuroblastoma

Ans: (b) Thymoma

42. Which of the following is not true about peritoneal mesothelioma?

(a) Associated with residents of lower income countries

(b) Asbestos exposure is a notable cause

(c) Females are more affected than males

(d) Risk factor remain after exposure even if the cause is removed

Ans: (a) Associated with residents of lower income countries

43. Most common type of lung cancer is:

(a) SCC
(b) Adenocarcinoma
(c) Small cell carcinoma
(d) Large cell carcinoma

Ans: (b) Adenocarcinoma

44. On immunohistochemistry, malignant mesothelioma is +ve for:

(a) Calretinin
(b) Ber-EP4
(c) Moc-31
(d) TTF-1

Ans: (a) Calretinin

45. For patients with stage II and III rectal cancer for whom tumoral downsizing is advantageous/sphincter preservation is desired, what is preferred preoperative treatment?

(a) Short course radiotherapy (5.5 Gy) alone
(b) Long course chemoradiotherapy (1.8 Gy/day)
(c) Neoadjuvant chemotherapy
(d) Long course radiotherapy

Ans: (b) Long course chemoradiotherapy (1.8 Gy/day)

46. Which of the following malignancies has best long term survival outcome after resection of lung metastasis?

(a) Sarcoma
(b) Melanoma
(c) Breast cancer
(d) Germ cell tumor

Ans: (d) Germ cell tumor

47. Pancoast tumor is seen with cancer of:

(a) Apical lobe of lung
(b) Lingual lobe of lung
(c) Thyroid
(d) Pyriform fossa

Ans: (a) Apical lobe of lung

48. Which of the following carcinomas most frequently metastasizes to brain?

(a) Small cell carcinoma of lung (b) Prostate cancer

(c) Rectal carcinoma (d) Endometrial cancer

Ans: (a) Small cell carcinoma of lung

49. A 68 years old woman with a history of heavy tobacco use is found to have a solitary lung nodule on chest computed tomography. Pathology from a recent bronchoscopy reveals adenocarcinoma. What further staging work up is necessary for this patient before surgical resection?

(a) Brain MRI (b) PET/CT scan

(c) Mediastinoscopy (d) None

Ans: (b) PET/CT scan

50. Is the following statement True or False?

In patients with extensive small cell lung cancer (SCLC) who respond to chemotherapy, administration of prophylactic cranial irradiation has been shown to reduce the risk for brain metastases and improve overall survival:

(a) True (b) False

(c) Cannot comment (d) Depends on patient characteristics

Ans: (a) True

51. Which of the following statements about malignant pleural mesothelioma (MPM) is False?

(a) The incidence of MPM is declining in developing countries

(b) Chemotherapy is mainstay of treatment for most patients who present with inoperable MPM

(c) Randomized trials have now confirmed that combining antifolates with platinum-based therapy confers survival benefit

(d) No standard therapy has yet been defined as the second-line treatment of choice for MPM

Ans: (a) The incidence of MPM is declining in developing countries

52. What is a contraindication to the use of bevacizumab in patients with metastatic non small cell lung cancer (NSCLC)?

(a) Previous hemoptysis (b) Brain metastases

(c) Anticoagulation (d) All options are correct

Ans: (d) All options are correct

53. A 56-year-old never-smoker presents to her primary care physician with dyspnea and cough. A chest X-ray identifies multiple pulmonary masses and a new pleural effusion. Further imaging, including a CT scan of her chest/abdomen, confirm multiple lung nodules, a pleural effusion, and lesions in her bones and liver. A biopsy is positive for adenocarcinoma with the epidermal growth factor receptor (EGFR) mutation deletion 19. You recommend treatment with:

(a) Cisplatin-gemcitabine (b) Erlotinib

(c) Arboplatin-paclitaxel (d) Crizotinib

Ans: (b) Erlotinib

54. A 66-year-old woman with a 30-pack-year smoking history who quit smoking last year when her brother was diagnosed with lung cancer comes to your clinic for assessment. She is concerned about developing lung cancer and would like to be screened. You recommend:

(a) No screening because there is no cancer evidence (b) Annual chest X-ray

(c) Annual low dose CT (d) Annual PET

Ans: (c) Annual low dose CT

55. You are evaluating a 70-year-old former smoker in your clinic who has been diagnosed with squamous cell lung cancer after biopsy of a right upper lobe lung mass. His workup included a PET scan that showed a fluorodeoxyglucose (FDG) 5.4 cm right upper lobe mass and FDF-avid mediastinal adenopathy at level 4R. He is seen for surgical evaluation. You recommend:

(a) No surgery, because he has N2 disease on imaging

(b) Endobronchial ultrasound (EBUS) or mediastinoscopy for sampling of lymph nodes

(c) Concurrent chemoradiation therapy

(d) Surgery followed by adjuvant chemotherapy

Ans: (b) Endobronchial ultrasound (EBUS) or mediastinoscopy for sampling of lymph nodes

56. A 50-year-old never-smoking patient with stage IV non-small cell lung cancer adenocarcinoma histology who has progressed after multiple lines of chemotherapy presents to your clinic for a second opinion. He has a repeat biopsy and his tumor is positive for the ALK fusion. You recommend treatment with:

(a) Crizotinib
(b) Gefitinib
(b) Laptinib
(d) Cetuximab

Ans: (a) Crizotinib

CHAPTER 59

BONE AND STS

MULTIPLE CHOICE QUESTIONS

1. **Classical osteosarcoma arises from:**
   (a) Medulla of diaphysis
   (b) Medulla of metaphysis
   (c) Medulla of epiphysis
   (d) Cotex of metaphysis

   Ans: (b) Medulla of metaphysis

2. **True regarding giant cell tumor of bone:**
   (a) Pulmonary metastasis can occur in 1–2% of patients
   (b) Local recurrence is extremely uncommon after bone curettage alone
   (c) Typically arises in metaphysis of lung bone
   (d) Usually occur after 45 years age

   Ans: (a) Pulmonary metastasis can occur in 1–2% of patients

3. **Enneking staging system is used for:**
   (a) Bone sarcoma
   (b) Retroperitoneal sarcoma
   (c) GIST
   (d) Soft tissue sarcoma

   Ans: (a) Bone sarcoma

4. **Strongest predictor for patient outcome in soft tissue sarcoma is:**
   (a) Histological type
   (b) Grade
   (c) Site
   (d) Size

   Ans: (b) Grade

5. **Most common histologic type of radiation associated sarcoma:**
   (a) Pleomorphic MPH
   (b) Angiosarcoma
   (c) Leiomyosarcoma
   (d) Fibrosarcoma

   Ans: (a) Pleomorphic MPH

6. **A 50 years old lady presents with 5 cm swelling in subcutaneous plane on lateral aspect of right thigh. Appropriate step would be:**
   (a) FNAC
   (b) MRI
   (c) Incision biopsy
   (d) Excision biopsy

   Ans: (b) MRI

7. **Strongest predictor of outcome in soft tissue sarcoma is:**
   (a) Histological type
   (b) Grade
   (c) Nodal status
   (d) Size

   Ans: (b) Grade

8. Which of following sites of soft tissue sarcomas has best prognosis?

(a) Visceral (b) Head and neck

(c) Retroperitoneal (d) Extremity

Ans: (d) Extremity

9. True regarding soft tissue sarcoma is:

(a) Tumor grading can be done with FNAC

(b) Open biopsy incision should be oriented transversely to long axis of limb

(c) Adequate hemostasis should be attained after biopsy

(d) Resection of tumors should be through zone of reaction around tumor

Ans: (c) Adequate hemostasis should be attained after biopsy

10. Most important feature that distinguishes osteosarcoma from other tumors that arise from primitive mesenchymal cell is:

(a) A sunburst pattern on X-ray (b) Production of osteoid

(c) Specificity of chromosomal translocation by karyotyping (d) Metaphyseal rather than diaphyseal origin

Ans: (b) Production of osteoid

11. All are true about synovial cell sarcoma *except:*

(a) Occurs in young adults

(b) Mainly arises from synovial membrane

(c) Typically found in para-articular areas of tendon sheaths and joints

(d) Calcification with/without ossification is seen up to 10% of cases

Ans: (c) Typically found in para-articular areas of tendon sheaths and joints

12. All of the following are contraindications for limb salvage surgery in bone tumors *except:*

(a) Pathological fractures (b) Inappropriate biopsy sites

(c) Infection (d) Involved adjacent joint capsule

Ans: (d) Involved adjacent joint capsule

13. Tikhoff-Linberg resection is done for osteosarcoma of:

(a) Femur (b) Scapula

(c) Tibia (d) Radius

Ans: (b) Scapula

14. All of following are true about parosteal osteosarcoma *except:*

(a) Accounts 4% of all osteosarcoma (b) Arises from bone cortex

(c) Generally occurs in younger individuals (d) Better prognosis than classical osteosarcoma

Ans: (c) Generally occurs in younger individuals

15. All of the following statements regarding malignant bone tumors are true *except:*

(a) Most of the osteosarcoma and Ewing's sarcoma require neoadjuvant chemotherapy

(b) Chondrosarcomas are less sensitive to radiotherapy and chemotherapy

(c) Most of the malignant tumors need amputation

(d) Survival with limb sparing is similar to amputation

Ans: (c) Most of the malignant tumors need amputation

CHAPTER

60 ENDOCRINE ONCOLOGY

MULTIPLE CHOICE QUESTIONS

1. **The following abnormalities are seen in MEN 2B *except:***
   (a) Cutaneous lichen amyloidosis (b) Megacolon
   (c) Pheochromocytoma (d) Mucosal melanoma

   Ans: (a) Cutaneous lichen amyloidosis

2. **Following are true about Hurthle cell tumor *except:***
   (a) Variants of follicular neoplasm (b) Has good prognosis
   (c) Contains Ascanazy cells (d) Poor prognosis

   Ans: (b) Has good prognosis

3. **Which of the following is false regarding pancreatic endocrine tumors?**
   (a) VIPomas are associated with hyperkalemia (b) Gastrinomas are associated with ZES
   (c) Majority of insulinomas are benign (d) Migratory necrolytic erythema is seen in glucaganomas

   Ans: (a) VIPomas are associated with hyperkalemia

4. **According to AJCC TNM Classification, Anaplastic carcinoma thyroid with distant metastasis (M1) is classified as:**
   (a) Stage IV A (b) Stage IV B
   (c) Stage IV D (d) Stage IV C

   Ans: (d) Stage IV C

5. **Orphan Annie nuclei is a histological feature of:**
   (a) Papillary cancer thyroid (b) Medullary cancer thyroid
   (c) Mucoepidermoid cancer (d) Malignant melanoma

   Ans: (a) Papillary cancer thyroid

6. **Treatment options in metastatic malignant phaeochromocytoma include all *except:***
   (a) Debulking surgery
   (b) I^{131} MIBG
   (c) Cyclophosphamide, Vincristine, dacarbazine chemotherapy
   (d) Mitotane

   Ans: (d) Mitotane

7. **What should be the serum TG level after total thyroidectomy (without residual normal thyroid tissue)?**
(a) <10 ng/ml (b) <5 ng/ml
(c) <3 ng/ml (d) <2 ng/ml
Ans: (d) <2 ng/ml

8. **Which is not a lab finding of hypoparathyroidism?**
(a) Hypocalcemia (b) Hypophosphatemia
(c) Hyperphosphatemia (d) Metabolic alkalosis
Ans: (b) Hypophosphatemia

9. **An 11 years old presents to your clinic because of family history of medullary carcinoma thyroid. Physical examination is normal. Which of the following tests do you perform?**
(a) Urine VMA (b) Serum insulin
(c) Serum gastrin (d) Serum glucagon
Ans: (a) Urine VMA

10. **Which among the following is not a part of MEN 2B?**
(a) Medullary carcinoma thyroid (b) Pheochromocytoma
(c) Mucosal ganglioneuroma (d) Parathyroid hyperplasia
Ans: (d) Parathyroid hyperplasia

11. **Isotope used in radioiodine uptake studies in thyroid cancer:**
(a) I^{132} (b) I^{131}
(c) I^{125} (d) All of the above
Ans: (b) I^{131}

12. **To obtain optimal uptake of radioiodine post thyroidectomy TSH level must be:**
(a) >10 (b) >20
(c) >30 (d) >15
Ans: (c) >30

13. **MEN 2A syndrome involves all *except:***
(a) Marfanoid status (b) Medullary Ca
(c) Pheochromocytoma (d) Parathyroid hyperplasia
Ans: (a) Marfanoid status

14. **Thyroideaima artery is a branch of:**
(a) Superior thyroid artery (b) Inferior thyroid artery
(c) Innominate artery (d) Transverse cervical artery
Ans: (c) Innominate artery

15. **In 40 years old male with T4N1bM0 papillary carcinoma thyroid, stage grouping will be:**
(a) Stage I (b) Stage II
(c) Stage III (d) Stage IV
Ans: (a) Stage I

16. On FNAC solitary thyroid nodule risk of malignancy is:

(a) <1% (b) 1–10%
(c) 10–15% (d) 15–25%

Ans: (b) 1–10%

17. Most common cause of primary hyperparathyroidism is:

(a) Single adenoma (b) Double adenoma
(c) 4 gland hyperplasia (d) Parathyroid carcinoma

Ans: (a) Single adenoma

18. Sullivan modification of Mac Farlane system is used for staging of:

(a) Parathyroid carcinoma (b) Anaplastic thyroid carcinoma
(c) Adrenocortical carcinoma (d) Pituitary tumors

Ans: (c) Adrenocortical carcinoma

19. Verner Morrison syndrome is caused by:

(a) PPoma (b) VIPoma
(c) Insulinoma (d) Glucagonoma

Ans: (b) VIPoma

20. Indication of surgery in adrenal incidentaloma is:

(a) >3 cm size (b) >4 cm size
(c) Non-functional tumor (d) Associated with hypertension

Ans: (b) >4 cm size

21. Course of medullary carcinoma thyroid is more virulent in:

(a) MEN 1 (b) MEN 2A
(c) MEN 2B (d) Familial MTC

Ans: (c) MEN 2B

22. True about anaplastic thyroid carcinoma:

(a) 6% of all thyroid cancers (b) Slow growing and can be curable
(c) Treatment mainly with radioactive iodine (d) Always stage IV

Ans: (d) Always stage IV

23. A 52 years female patient presents with symptoms of pheochromocytoma. She also has thyroid carcinoma. Her thyroid carcinoma is most likely to be:

(a) Anaplastic (b) Medullary
(c) Follicular (d) Papillary

Ans: (b) Medullary

24. A patient with long standing multinodular goiter develops hoarseness of voice and also recent rapid increase in size of the swelling. Likely diagnosis is:

(a) Follicular carcinoma (b) Papillary carcinoma
(c) Medullary carcinoma (d) Anaplastic carcinoma

Ans: (d) Anaplastic carcinoma

25. Needle biopsy of a solitary thyroid nodule in a young woman with palpable cervical lymph nodes on the same side demonstrates amyloid in stroma of the lesion. Likely diagnosis is:

(a) Medullary carcinoma thyroid (b) Follicular carcinoma thyroid

(c) Thyroid adenoma (d) Multinodular goitre

Ans: (a) Medullary carcinoma thyroid

26. A patient present with a history of headache and flushing. He has a family history of his relative having died of a thyroid tumor. The investigation that would be required for this patient would be:

(a) Chest X-ray (b) Measurement of 5 HIAA

(c) Measurement of catecholamine (d) Intravenous pyelography

Ans: (c) Measurement of catecholamine

27. A 26 years woman presents with a palpable thyroid nodule and needle biopsy demonstrates amyloid in the stroma of the lesion. A cervical lymph node is palpable on the same side as the lesion, the preferred treatment should be:

(a) Removal of the involved node, the isthmus and the enlarged lymph node

(b) Removal of the opposite lobe and the enlarged lymph node

(c) Total thyroidectomy and modified neck dissection on the side of the enlarged lymph node

(d) Total thyroidectomy and irradiation of the cervical lymph nodes

Ans: (c) Total thyroidectomy and modified neck dissection on the side of the enlarged lymph node

28. RET proto-oncogene mutation is a hallmark of which of the following tumors?

(a) Medullary carcinoma thyroid (b) Astrocytoma

(c) Paraganglioma (d) Hurthle cell tumor thyroid

Ans: (a) Medullary carcinoma thyroid

29. What is the most common histological type of thyroid carcinoma?

(a) Anaplastic (b) Medullary

(c) Follicular (d) Papillary

Ans: (d) Papillary

30. All of the following are features of MEN 2A *except:*

(a) Pituitary tumor (b) Pheochromocytoma

(c) MCT (d) Neuromas

Ans: (a) Pituitary tumor

31. Type 1 MEN involves all *except:*

(a) Pancreas (b) Adrenal

(c) Pituitary (d) Parathyroid

Ans: (b) Adrenal

32. A 36-year-old female with symptoms of hyperparathyroidism, pancreas tumor adrenal cortical hyperplasia, pituitary tumors, islet cell tumors with cutaneous angiofibromas:

(a) MEN 1 (b) MEN 2A

(c) MEN 2B (d) MEN 2C

Ans: (a) MEN 1

33. All of the following are features of MEN 2A *except:*

(a) Pituitary tumor
(b) Pheochromocytoma
(c) Medullary carcinoma thyroid
(d) Parathyroid hyperplasia

Ans: (a) Pituitary tumor

34. Which of the following endocrine tumors is most commonly seen in MEN 1:

(a) Insulinoma
(b) Gastrinoma
(c) Glucagonoma
(d) Somatostatinoma

Ans: (b) Gastrinoma

35. Most common pancreatic tumor seen in MEN 1:

(a) Insulinoma
(b) Gastrinoma
(c) Glucagonoma
(d) Somatostatinoma

Ans: (b) Gastrinoma

36. Pancreatitis, Pheochromocytoma and Pituitary tumor may be associated with:

(a) Medullary carcinoma thyroid
(b) Papillary carcinoma thyroid
(c) Anaplastic carcinoma thyroid
(d) Follicular carcinoma thyroid

Ans: (a) Medullary carcinoma thyroid

37. All are associated with MEN 2 *except:*

(a) Pheochromocytoma
(b) Islet cell hyperplasia
(c) Medullary carcinoma thyroid
(d) Parathyroid adenoma

Ans: (b) Islet cell hyperplasia

38. Multiple mucosal neuromas are associated with:

(a) Medullary carcinoma thyroid
(b) CA ovary
(c) CA testis
(d) CA pancreas

Ans: (a) Medullary carcinoma thyroid

39. A patient presents with intermittent headache. On examination there is hypertension and thyroid nodule. Which of the following steps is to be taken next?

(a) Urine HIAA
(b) Urine VMA and aspiration of thyroid nodule
(c) USG Abdomen
(d) 2D Echocardiography

Ans: (b) Urine VMA and aspiration of thyroid nodule

40. A 25-year-old woman has recurrent episodes of headache and sweating. Her mother had renal calculi and died after having neck mass. Physical examination reveals thyroid nodule but no clinical sign of thyrotoxicosis. Before performing thyroid surgery surgeon should order:

(a) Measurement of thyroid hormones
(b) Serial determination of serum calcium, phosphorous and alkaline phosphatase

(c) 24-hour urine for 5 HIAA excretion

(d) Serial 24-hour urine test for catecholamines, metanephrines and VMA

Ans: (d) Serial 24-hour urine test for catecholamines, metanephrines and VMA

41. A 20-year-old male presented with chronic constipation, headache and palpitations. On examination he had marfanoid habitus, neuromas of tongue, medullated corneal nerve fibres and nodule of 2*2 cm in left lobe of thyroid. The patient is case of:

(a) Sporadic MCT
(b) Familial MCT
(c) MEN 2A
(d) MEN 2B

Ans: (d) MEN 2B

CHAPTER 61

BREAST CANCER

MULTIPLE CHOICE QUESTIONS

1. **In TNM Staging for breast cancer, involvement of which one of the following is not classified as T4a?**
   (a) Pectoralis major (b) Serratus anterior
   (c) Ribs (d) Intercostal muscles

   Ans: (a) Pectoralis major

2. **Oncotype DX assay is microassay used for prognostication in recurrence of:**
   (a) ER –ve breast cancer (b) Hormone refractory prostate cancer
   (c) ER +ve breast cancer (d) Hormone sensitive prostate cancer

   Ans: (c) ER +ve breast cancer

3. **What is level I lymph node in axillary dissection for carcinoma breast?**
   (A) Lymph node inferior to axillary vein
   (B) Lymph node lateral to pectoralis minor
   (C) Lymph node posterior to pectoralis minor
   (a) Only (A) and (B) are correct (b) Only (C) is correct
   (c) Only (A) is correct (d) Only (B) and (C) are correct

   Ans: (a) Only (A) and (B) are correct

4. **In Breast Imaging Reporting and Data System (BIRADS), Category I is:**
   (a) Negative (b) Probably benign
   (c) Incomplete assessment (d) Benign finding

   Ans: (a) Negative

5. **Mutation of which of these genes doesn't predispose to an increased risk of developing breast cancer?**
   (a) APC (b) BRCA 2
   (c) CDH 2 (d) BRCA 1

   Ans: (a) APC

6. **Relative risk of more than 4-fold increase in breast cancer includes following factors *except:***
   (a) Radiation exposure before the age of 30 (b) CHEK 2 mutation
   (c) BRCA 1 and 2 mutation (d) Atypical hyperplasia

   Ans: (b) CHEK 2 mutation

7. **Which of the following is prognostic as well as predictive factor in breast cancer?**
   (a) Grade (b) ER/PR status
   (c) No. of +ve lymph nodes (d) Lymphovascular invasion

   Ans: (b) ER/PR status

8. Following statement about Oncotype Diagnosis is not true:

(a) Assays can be done in formalin fixed paraffin embedded tissue

(b) A panel of 16 cancer related genes and 5 reference genes were used to develop an algorithm to compute a recurrence score

(c) Found that Oncotype Diagnosis assay was strong predictor of benefit from CMF in NSABP-B20 for patients with high scores

(d) Score ranging from 0 to 10 that can be used to estimate odds of recurrence over 10 years from diagnosis

Ans: (d) Score ranging from 0 to 10 that can be used to estimate odds of recurrence over 10 years from diagnosis

9. Management of lobular neoplasia breast is:

(a) Surveillance (b) Chemoprevention

(c) Prophylactic bilateral mastectomy (d) All of the above

Ans: (d) All of the above

10. Which type of carcinoma breast is characterized by "Indian file" pattern?

(a) Infiltrating duct carcinoma (b) Medullary carcinoma

(c) Tubular carcinoma (d) Invasive lobular carcinoma

Ans: (d) Invasive lobular carcinoma

11. In histologic grading of breast cancer, all of the following factors are used *except:*

(a) Tubule formation (b) Nuclear pleomorphism

(c) Mitotic activity (d) Necrosis

Ans: (d) Necrosis

12. Invasive lobular carcinoma – all are true *except:*

(a) More likely to occur in older patients (b) Tend to be ER and PR negative

(c) Associated with lower S-phase fraction (d) ERBB2, p53 and EGFR –ve

Ans: (b) Tend to be ER and PR negative

13. Which statement regarding screening for breast cancer is most true?

(a) Teaching women to perform a through BSE has been shown to have a measurable impact on breast cancer mortality rates

(b) Monthly BSE is a crucial component of breast cancer screening programs

(c) High quality CBE provides 5-20% additional benefit in mortality reduction, beyond that achieved by mammographic screening alone

(d) Physician's CBE is redundant and is unnecessary for patients who receive annual mammograms

Ans: (c) High quality CBE provides 5-20% additional benefit in mortality reduction, beyond that achieved by mammographic screening alone

14. With regard to breast imaging reporting and data system (BI-RADS) for categorizing mammography findings, which of the following is most true?

(a) BI-RADS score of zero means mammogram is normal (b) BI-RADS score of one means mammogram is normal

(c) BI-RADS score of three represents benign finding (d) BI-RADS score of four represents malignancy

Ans: (b) BI-RADS score of one means mammogram is normal

15. A woman with a T3N2 breast cancer would be best served by:

(a) Surgery (b) Neoadjuvant chemotherapy

(c) Adjuvant chemotherapy (d) Radiation therapy

Ans: (b) Neoadjuvant chemotherapy

16. In breast cancer, basal like tumors typically lack:

(a) ER (b) PR

(c) Her-2 Neu (d) All of the above

Ans: (d) All of the above

17. Stewart Treves syndrome:

(a) Epitheloid angiosarcoma (b) Radiation induced angiosarcoma

(c) Angiosarcoma in the context of lymphoedema (d) Idiopathic angiosarcoma

Ans: (c) Angiosarcoma in the context of lymphoedema

18. Oncotype DX Assay, recurrence score 18-30 denotes:

(a) Low risk (b) Intermediate risk

(c) High risk (d) None of the above

Ans: (b) Intermediate risk

19. Tamoxifen is indicated in:

(a) ER +ve premenopausal breast cancer (b) ER and PR –ve postmenopausal breast cancer

(c) Both A and B (d) None of the above

Ans: (a) ER +ve premenopausal breast cancer

20. Most appropriate adjuvant endocrine therapy in postmenopausal ER/PR +ve breast cancer:

(a) Tamoxifen for 5 years (b) Bicalutamide for 5 years

(c) Letrozole for 5 years (d) Goserelin for 5 years

Ans: (a) Tamoxifen for 5 years

21. Which statement regarding screening for breast cancer is true?

(a) BSE (Breast self examination) is crucial component of breast cancer screening programs

(b) CBE (Clinical breast examination) every 1 to 3 years from 20 years of age is recommended by American Cancer Society

(c) Latina women are at lower risk for developing aggressive breast cancer than general population

(d) Older women are more likely to develop triple –ve negative disease

Ans: (b) CBE (Clinical breast examination) every 1 to 3 years from 20 years of age is recommended by American Cancer Society

22. Following statements regarding Paget's disease of breast are true *except:*

(a) Paget cells within epidermis is pathognomonic (b) May occur with underlying invasive cancer/DCIS

(c) Never occur alone without underlying invasive cancer (d) Represents in situ cancer of epidermis of nipple

Ans: (c) Never occur alone without underlying invasive cancer

23. High risk factors for development of breast cancer include following *except:*

(a) BRCA 1 and 2 mutations (b) Atypical hyperplasia

(c) Radiation exposure before 30 years (d) History of documented fibroadenoma excision

Ans: (d) History of documented fibroadenoma excision

24. BRCA 1 mutation carriers typically develop:

(a) Low grade ER +ve, HER 2 neu –ve breast cancer (b) High grade ER –ve, HER 2 neu –ve breast cancer

(c) High grade ER –ve, HER 2 neu +ve breast cancer (d) Low grade ER +ve, HER 2 neu +ve breast cancer

Ans: (b) High grade ER –ve, HER 2 neu –ve breast cancer

25. Standard radiation doses to the conserved whole breast include all *except:*

(a) 50 Gy in 25 Fractions
(b) 40 Gy in 15 Fractions
(c) 39 Gy in 13 Fractions
(d) 42.5 Gy in 16 Fractions

Ans: (c) 39 Gy in 13 Fractions

26. All are true regarding Annual MRI recommended based on evidence per ASCO guidelines in breast cancer *except:*

(a) BRCA mutation
(b) Personal history of breast cancer including DCIS
(c) Untreated 1st degree relative of BRCA carrier
(d) Lifetime risk of breast cancer is 20–25%

Ans: (b) Personal history of breast cancer including DCIS

27. True about phyllodes tumor breast is:

(a) Malignant ranges from 10–20%
(b) Approximately 20% recur if excised with margin of few mm
(c) Role of radiotherapy and chemotherapy is clear
(d) Average age at diagnosis is 2nd decade

Ans: (b) Approximately 20% recur if excised with margin of few mm

28. HER 2/neu chromosome is located on:

(a) 17q12
(b) 13q21
(c) 17q22
(d) None

Ans: (a) 17q12

29. Which of the following is a contraindication to breast conserving surgery?

(a) Small lump to breast ratio
(b) Breast tumor size <5 cm
(c) Previous history of radiation to chest wall
(d) Young age

Ans: (c) Previous history of radiation to chest wall

30. Which is not true regarding BRCA mutation in breast cancer?

(a) BRCA 1 tumors are high grade as compared to BRCA 2
(b) BRCA 1 tumors are hormone receptor +ve
(c) BRCA 1 tumors are aneuploid
(d) BRCA 1 breast cancer has increased S phase fraction

Ans: (b) BRCA 1 tumors are hormone receptor +ve

31. In breast reconstructive surgery after mastectomy which is not true regarding TRAM flap?

(a) May be based on pedicled superior epigastric artery
(b) Can be transferred as free flap
(c) It is a type of myocutaneous flap
(d) It uses supraumbilical fat

Ans: (d) It uses supraumbilical fat

32. Mammography can detect carcinoma breast in about:

(a) 55%
(b) 65%
(c) 75%
(d) 85%

Ans: (d) 85%

33. BRCA 1 is located on chromosome:

(a) 17q
(b) 13q
(c) 14p
(d) 17p

Ans: (a) 17q

34. All are established indications for magnetic resonance imaging screening for detection of breast cancer *except:*

(a) BRCA mutation
(b) Untested first degree relative of BRCA carrier
(c) Life time risk of breast cancer 20–25%
(d) LCIS

Ans: (d) LCIS

35. Which is true regarding Paget's disease of breast?

(a) Accounts for about 1% of all breast malignancies
(b) Best treated by radiation therapy
(c) Classified as T4 disease as per TNM Staging
(d) Risk of lymph node metastasis is 30%

Ans: (a) Accounts for about 1% of all breast malignancies

36. All of the following are good risk factors for non-seminatous germ cell tumors *except:*

(a) Non-pulmonary visceral metastases absent
(b) Gonadal/retroperitoneal primary tumor
(c) AFP between 1000 and 10,000 ng/mL
(d) HCG between 500 and 5000 mIU/mL

Ans: (c) AFP between 1000 and 10,000 ng/mL

37. Which of the following statements is true regarding adjuvant treatment for early breast cancer?

(a) RT is indicated after breast conserving surgery only if >4 nodes +ve/tumor is close to resection margin
(b) Aromatase inhibitors are replacing tamoxifen in premenopausal women due to better outcomes and greater tolerability
(c) Combination chemotherapy reduces recurrence and improves survival in selected patient groups
(d) No survival benefit has been demonstrated with use of trastuzumab in adjuvant setting

Ans: (c) Combination chemotherapy reduces recurrence and improves survival in selected patient groups

38. Presence of which marker is poor prognosis variable for patients with breast cancer:

(a) CEA
(b) C-erb B-2
(c) AFP
(d) RB1

Ans: (b) C-erb B-2

39. Sentinel lymph node biopsy is an important part in the management of the following condition:

(a) Carcinoma prostate
(b) Carcinoma breast
(c) Carcinoma lung
(d) Carcinoma nasopharynx

Ans: (b) Carcinoma breast

40. BRCA 1 gene is located on:

(a) Chromosome 13
(b) Chromosome 11
(c) Chromosome 17
(d) Chromosome 22

Ans: (c) Chromosome 17

41. Breast cancer which is multifocal and bilateral:

(a) Ductal
(b) Lobular
(c) Mucoid
(d) Colloid

Ans: (b) Lobular

42. Best prognosis amongst following histological variants of breast carcinoma is seen with:

(a) Infiltrating ductal
(b) Mucinous
(c) Lobular
(d) Medullary

Ans: (b) Mucinous

43. Peau d'orange appearance of the mammary skin is due to:

(a) Intraepithelial cancer
(b) Sub-epidermal cancer
(c) Lymphatic permeation
(d) Vascular embolisation

Ans: (c) Lymphatic permeation

44. True about lymphatic spread of carcinoma breast:

(a) Axillary nodes are most commonly involves
(b) Internal mammary nodes are also involved
(c) If supraclavicular lymph node is involved then it is N3
(d) All options are correct

Ans: (d) All options are correct

45. True about breast carcinoma in men:

(a) Estrogen receptor positive
(b) Gynaecomastia is not a risk factor
(c) Seen in young males
(d) Radiotherapy contraindicated due to close proximity to the chest wall

Ans: (b) Gynaecomastia is not a risk factor

46. For carcinoma breast best chemotherapeutic regimen among the following is:

(a) Cyclophosphamide, Methotrexate, 5-fluorouracil
(b) Methotrexate, Cisplantin
(c) Cisplantin, Adriamycin, Steroid
(d) Methotrexate, Adriamycin, Steroid

Ans: (a) Cyclophosphamide, Methotrexate, 5-fluorouracil

47. A 30 years old lady presented with unilateral breast cancer associated with axillary lymph node enlargement. Modified radical mastectomy was done. Further treatment plan will be:

(a) Observation and follow up
(b) Sequential anthracylcine and taxane based chemotherapy followed by tamoxifen based on estrogen/progesterone receptor status
(c) Only anthracycline based chemotherapy followed by tamoxifen
(d) Tamoxifen only

Ans: (b) Sequential anthracylcine and taxane based chemotherapy followed by tamoxifen based on estrogen/ progesterone receptor status

48. Absolute contraindication of conservative breast cancer therapy is:

(a) Large pendulous breast
(b) History of previous radiation
(c) Axillary node involvement
(d) 3rd trimester of pregnancy

Ans: (b) History of previous radiation

49. True about treatment of early breast carcinoma:

(a) Aromatase inhibitors are replacing tamoxifen in premenopausal women
(b) Postmastectomy radiation therapy is given when 4 or more lymph nodes are positive
(c) Tamoxifen is not useful in post menopausal women
(d) In premenopausal women multidrug chemotherapy is given in selected patients

Ans: (b) Postmastectomy radiation therapy is given when 4 or more lymph nodes are positive

50. Cystosarcoma phylloides is treated by:

(a) Simple mastectomy
(b) Radical mastectomy
(c) Modified radical mastectomy
(d) Antibiotic with conservative treatment

Ans: (a) Simple mastectomy

51. On which of the following does prognosis in male breast carcinoma depends on?

(a) Duration of disease
(b) Nipple discharge
(c) Ulceration of nipple
(d) Lymph node status

Ans: (d) Lymph node status

52. The risk factor for increased incidence of relapse in stage I, carcinoma breast includes all *except:*

(a) Negative estrogen/receptor status
(b) High S phase fraction
(c) Aneuploidy
(d) Decreased Her-2 neu oncogene expression

Ans: (d) Decreased Her-2 neu oncogene expression

53. In breast carcinoma good prognostic marker among the following is:

(a) ER positive
(b) Her-2 Neu positive
(c) CD 44 positive
(d) p53 positive

Ans: (a) ER positive

54. The most important prognostic factor in breast carcinoma is:

(a) Histological grade of the tumor
(b) Stage of the tumor at the time of diagnosis
(c) Status of estrogen and progesterone receptors
(d) Over expression of p53 tumor suppressor gene

Ans: (b) Stage of the tumor at the time of diagnosis

55. Which one predisposes to breast cancer?

(a) Adenosis
(b) Fibrosis
(c) Blue domed cysts
(d) Epithelial hyperplasia

Ans: (d) Epithelial hyperplasia

56. Complication of post mastectomy lymph accumulation is:

(a) Metastases of cancer
(b) Recurrence
(c) Lymphangio sarcoma
(d) Pain

Ans: (c) Lymphangio sarcoma

57. Malti, 45 years female patient with a family history of breast carcinoma, showed diffuse micro calcification on mammography. Intraductal carcinoma in situ was seen on biopsy. Most appropriate management is:

(a) Quadrantectomy
(b) Radical mastectomy
(c) Simple mastectomy
(d) Chemotherapy

Ans: (c) Simple mastectomy

58. What percentage of all breast cancer cases is related to germ line mutations?

(a) 5%
(b) 10%
(c) 25%
(d) 40%

Ans: (b) 10%

59. All of the following statements regarding prophylactic bilateral salpingo-oophorectomy (PBSO) in BRCA mutation carriers are true *except:*

(a) It reduces the risk for ovarian cancer by about 80% in this population
(b) It reduces the risk for breast cancer by about 50% in this population
(c) It reduces overall mortality in this population
(d) Hormone replacement therapy is not recommended after PBSO-related early surgical menopause

Ans: (d) Hormone replacement therapy is not recommended after PBSO-related early surgical menopause

CHAPTER 62

HEAD AND NECK

MULTIPLE CHOICE QUESTIONS

1. **Which of the following statements is true regarding parotid gland tumors?**

(a) Majority are malignant
(b) Pleomorphic adenoma is most common
(c) Pleomorphic adenoma is managed by total parotidectomy
(d) 10 percent of pleomorphic adenoma are bilateral

Ans: (b) Pleomorphic adenoma is most common

Pleomorphic adenoma is the most common benign tumor of salivary glands and is also overall most common tumor of salivary glands

2. **All of the following regarding thyroglossal cyst are true *except:***

(a) May contain functional thyroid tissue
(b) Infection is a significant risk
(c) Malignancy may develop within cyst
(d) Management consists of simple cystectomy

Ans: (d) Management consists of simple cystectomy

- *Mangament includes Sistrunk's operation*

3. **A 12-week-old male patient presents with large posterolateral neck mass extending into axilla that transilluminates. Optimal management is:**

(a) Radiation therapy
(b) Repeat needle aspirations
(c) Radical wide excision
(d) Conservative excision

Ans: (d) Conservative excision

- *Surgery should include no damage to nerves adjacent to mass so it is conservative excision for cystic hygroma*

4. **A 54-year-old man presents with tender left neck mass with a draining sinus. Microscopic examination reveals sulfur granules. Optimal management is:**

(a) Penicillin
(b) Fluconazole
(c) Ciprofloxacin
(d) Radiation

Ans: (a) Penicillin

Actinomycosis–Treatment of choice is penicillin followed by surgical drainage

5. **Management of carotid body tumor is:**

(a) Radiographic embolization
(b) Radiation therapy
(c) Chemotherapy
(d) Surgical excision in periadventitial plane

Ans: (d) Surgical excision in periadventitial plane

Treatment is surgical excision in periadventitial plane

6. **A 35-year-old man presents with new dark mole on face anterior to tragus as well as clinically suspicious palpable neck nodes. Excisional biopsy confirms melanoma. Optimal management is:**
(a) Wide reexcision of primary tumor and MRND
(b) MRND only
(c) Wide reexcision of primary tumor, MRND and superficial parotidectomy
(d) Wide excision of primary tumor and sentinel node biopsy

Ans: (c) Wide reexcision of primary tumor, MRND and superficial parotidectomy

In case of suspicious palpable nodes, Option (c) is best answer

7. **A 65-year-old man presents with a persistent firm lateral neck mass that measures approximately 2.5 cm. Careful history and physical examination of head and neck are negative. Next step in management is:**
(a) PET
(b) CT head and neck
(c) FNAC neck mass
(d) Excision of neck mass

Ans: (c) FNAC neck mass

Though it is most likely to be malignant in that age group, Perform FNAC and confirm it

8. **Branchial cleft cysts if enlarged should be removed because of which of the following?**
(a) Prone to become secondarily infected
(b) Prone to cause acute airway obstruction
(c) Possible premalignant concerns
(d) Association with severe halitosis

Ans: (a) Prone to become secondarily infected

Prone to get infected secondarily

9. **All are true about tracheostomy *except:***
(a) Should be performed in patients anticipated to be intubated more than 2 weeks
(b) Usually spontaneously close within 2 months of removal
(c) Improves patient discomfort as compared to long term oropharyngeal intubation
(d) Doesnot obligate patient to loss of speech

Ans: (b) Usually spontaneously close within 2 months of removal

Usually spontaneously close within 2 weeks after removal

10. **A 55-year-old woman presents with complaint of a mass overlying angle of the right mandible. She says mass has been slowly enlarging over past 2-3 years and that mass is painless. On physical examination it is firm and overlies angle of the right mandible and area between angle and tragus. Neurological examination is completely normal. Which of the following mass is most likely it represents:**
(a) Mucoepidermoid cancer of parotid
(b) Acute parotitis
(c) Pleomorphic adenoma
(d) Hemangioma of parotid

Ans: (c) Pleomorphic adenoma

History is consistent with benign neoplasm of parotid

11. **An 85-year-old ventilator dependent male was endotracheally intubated 10 days ago. He remains unresponsive and is not a candidate for early extubation. ICU attending elects to perform Tracheostomy at bed side. During procedure copious dark blood is encountered:**
(a) Anterior jugular vein
(b) External jugular vein
(c) Internal jugular vein
(d) Middle thyroid vein

Ans: (a) Anterior jugular vein

Injury to anterior jugular vein while doing procedure

12. **A 43-year-old teacher underwent left parotidectomy. Upon awakening from surgery, paralysis of left lower lip was observed. This complication was most likely due to injury to which of the following?**

(a) Parotid duct
(b) Facial nerve-Temporal branch
(c) Facial nerve-Cervical branch
(d) Platysma muscle

Ans: (c) Facial nerve-Cervical branch

Injury to cervical branch (marginal mandibular branch)

13. **While shaving a 45-year-old teacher notices a marble sized mass beneath his left ear. Mass is eventually excised revealing which of the following benign parotid gland lesions?**

(a) Glandular hypertrophy secondary to Vitamin A deficiency
(b) Cystic dilatation
(c) Mikulicz's disease
(d) Warthin's tumor

Ans: (d) Warthin's tumor

Benign parotid tumor-Out of the options it is Warthin's tumor

14. **Following a vacation a 43-year-old man notices shortness of breath. He is a nonsmoker. His wife points out that his face became puffy. On examination BP is normal. His pupils are equal and respond to light. Dilated veins are noted around shoulders, upper chest and face. X-ray of chest reveals an opacity in superior mediastinum. Most likely diagnosis is:**

(a) Thymoma
(b) Neurogenic tumor
(c) Lymphoma
(d) Pheochromocytoma

Ans: (b) Neurogenic tumor

Most common cause of primary mediastinal tumor is neurogenic tumor and 10% of which are malignant

15. **A 54-year-old construction worker has smoked 2 packs of cigarettes daily for past 25 years. He notes swelling in his upper extremity and face along with dialted veins in this region CT scan and venogram performed. What is most likely cause of obstruction?**

(a) Aortic aneurysm
(b) Metastasis
(c) Bronchogenic carcinoma
(d) Chronic fibrosing mediastinitis

Ans: (c) Bronchogenic carcinoma

Bronchogenic carcinoma accounts for 70-80% of cases of SVC obstruction

16. **A 32-year-old male janitor complains of swollen face during past week. A CT scan reveals an expanding hematoma in superior mediastinum. Mediastinal tamponade is most likely to manifest as which of the following?**

(a) Hypertension
(b) Increased pulse pressure during inspiration
(c) Paresis of right arm
(d) Venous congestion in upper extremity

Ans: (d) Venous congestion in upper extremity

In mediastinal tamponade, Hypotension, dyspnea, cyanosis and decrease in pulse pressure will be evident

17. **After suffering a respiratory tract infection, a 64 years old female biochemist develops chronic lung disease requiring intubation in ICU for 8 weeks period. Tracheal stenosis is noted. What is most likely cause of tracheal stenosis?**

(a) Prolonged intubation
(b) Tuberculosis
(c) Scleroderma
(d) Riedel thyroiditis

Ans: (a) Prolonged intubation

Prolonged intubation causes pressure necrosis over tracheal tube causing tracheal stenosis

18. Identify the patient and find true statement:

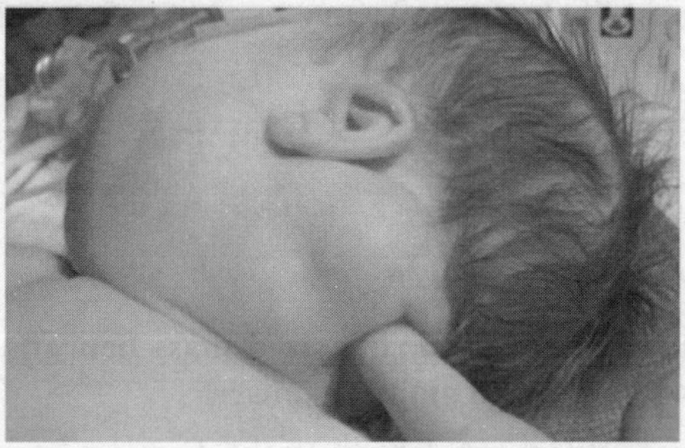

(a) It arises from sweat glands in neck
(b) Usually an anterior midline structure
(c) May occur in mediastinum
(d) Premalignant

Ans: (c) May occur in mediastinum

Occasionally cystic hygroma are seen in mediastinum

19. A 24-year-old computer technician notes a progressive increase in size of his left jaw. After X-rays are taken and a biopsy is done, diagnosis of ameloblastoma is established. What should be next step in management?

(a) Radiotherapy
(b) Laser beam therapy
(c) Currettage and bone graft
(d) Excision of lesions with 1-2 cm of normal mandible

Ans: (d) Excision of lesions with 1-2 cm of normal mandible

Treatment of choice of ameloblastoma is excision of lesions with 1-2 cm of normal mandible

20. A 62-year-old man undergoes excision of cylindroma of submandibular gland. Which of following is most likely to be injured?

(a) Maxillary branch of trigeminal nerve
(b) Lingual nerve
(c) Vagus nerve
(d) Frontozygomatic branch of facial nerve

Ans: (b) Lingual nerve

Lingual nerve is most likely to be injured accidentally while doing surgery

21. A 40-year-old woman is suspected of having carotid body tumor. Which one of the following is most characteristic of tumor?

(a) Secrete catecholamines
(b) More common at sea level
(c) Arise from structures that respond to changes in blood volume
(d) Arise from structures that respond to changes in PO_2

Ans: (d) Arise from structures that respond to changes in PO_2

Carotid body tumor responds to changes in PO_2 levels

22. Following surgical resection of large thyroid mass, a patient complains of persistent hoarseness and weak voice. What is most likely cause of these symptoms?

(a) Traumatic intubation
(b) Prolonged intubation
(c) Injury to RLN
(d) Injury to Superior laryngeal nerve

Ans: (c) Injury to RLN

Iatrogenic injury to RLN. Is cause of persistent hoarseness and weak voice

23. A 33-year-old female noted a discharge from a sinus in overlying skin below right angle of mandible. She recalls previous episodes of fullness and mild pain in this region over past several years. What is most likely cause?

(a) Thyroglossal cyst
(b) Branchial cyst
(c) Teratoma
(d) Myeloma

Ans: (b) Branchial cyst

Branchial arch remnants form cysts/fistulas in lateral neck

24. After undergoing left thyroid operation a 42-year-old opera singer notes change in speech but she has difficulty in singing high pitched notes. Which nerve is likely to be injured?

(a) Pharyngeal branch of vagus
(b) Glossopharyngeal
(c) External laryngeal nerve
(d) RLN

Ans: (c) External laryngeal nerve

Cricothyroid is supplied by External laryngeal nerve branch which controls pitch

25. A 5-year-old boy has a neck mass noticed by mother which is present since many months and is slowly getting larger. Mass is slightly to left of the midline. Ultrasound picture is shown below. What is most likely diagnosis?

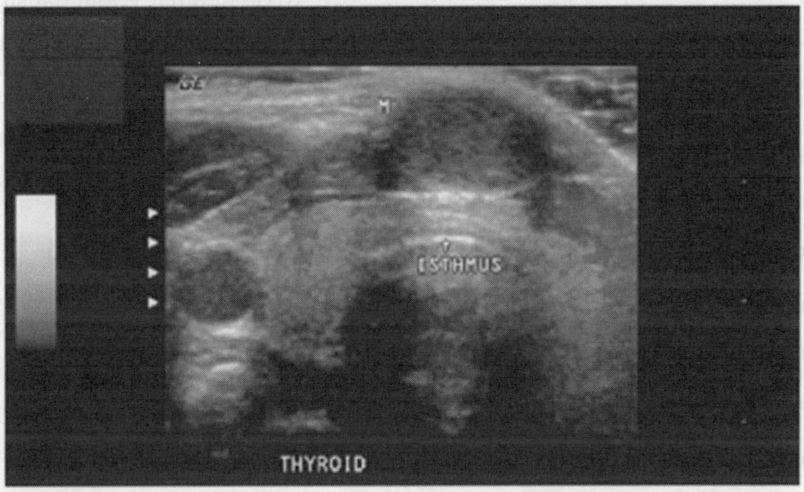

(a) Metastases from parathyroid carcinoma
(b) Chondroma
(c) Thyroglossal cyst
(d) Laryngocele

Ans: (c) Thyroglossal cyst

Ultrasound showed hypoechogenic mass anterior and superior to thyroid, it is thyroglossal cyst

26. A 5-year-old girl presents with difficulty in breathing. On examination of oral cavity a 3 cm mass is found in midline on posterior aspect of tongue. Most likely diagnosis is:

(a) Lingual tonsil
(b) Lingual thyroid
(c) Foreign body stuck to tongue
(d) Dermoid

Ans: (b) Lingual thyroid

Lingual thyroid cause difficulty in breathing

27. Plunging ranula occurs when mucocele herniates beneath–muscle into submental space:

(a) Genioglossus
(b) Geniohyoid
(c) Platysma
(d) Mylohyoid

Ans: (d) Mylohyoid

Plunging ranula herniates beneath Mylohyoid muscle

28. A 40-year-old woman presents with weight loss, palpitations and exophthalmos. On physical examination, thyroid gland is diffusely enlarged. Blood tests revealed hyperthyroidism. Which is not a treatment of hyperthyroidism?

(a) Methimazole
(b) Lugol's iodine
(c) I^{131}
(d) Steroids

Ans: (d) Steroids

Steroids are not a part of treatment of hyperthyroidism

29. Levels of neck nodes bounded anteriorly by laryngeal strap muscles, posterior border of sternocleidomastoid posteriorly, horizontal plane of cricoid cartilage inferiorly and level of hyoid bone superiorly is referred to level:

(a) Ia
(b) II
(c) III
(d) IV

Ans: (c) III

Level 3 nodes correspond to that triangle

30. Complete surgical resection (Thyroidectomy) is 1st line therapy for which of following:

(a) Reidel's thyroiditis
(b) Toxic nodular goiter causing compressive symptoms
(c) Acute suppurative thyroiditis
(d) Hashimoto's thyroiditis

Ans: (b) Toxic nodular goiter causing compressive symptoms

1st line therapy for Toxic nodular goiter causing compressive symptoms is surgery

31. Which is associated with aberrant right subclavian artery?

(a) Non recurrent right laryngeal nerve
(b) Absence of right thyroid lobe
(c) Non recurrent left laryngeal nerve
(d) Non recurrent right external branch of superior laryngeal nerve

Ans: (c) Non recurrent left laryngeal nerve

Non recurrent left laryngeal nerve is associated with aberrant right subclavian artery

32. Following parotidectomy your patient has sweating in his retroauricular region while eating. This is most likely caused by:

(a) Recurrent tumor
(b) Cross-innervation of the vagus and sympathetic nerves to the skin
(c) Cross-innervation of the auriculotemporal nerve and sympathetic nerves to the skin
(d) Cross-innervation to the glossopharyngeal nerve and sympathetic nerves to the skin

Ans: (c) Cross-innervation of the auriculotemporal nerve and sympathetic nerves to the skin

Frey's syndrome is abnormal cross-innervation of auriculotemporal nerve and sympathetic nerves to the skin

33. A 48-year-old male with massive head trauma does not have a gag reflex. Which nerve is responsible for the sensory nerve fibers that carry this reflex?

(a) Marginal mandibular nerve
(b) Recurrent laryngeal nerve
(c) Facial nerve
(d) Glossopharyngeal nerve

Ans: (d) Glossopharyngeal nerve

The afferent limb of the gag reflex comes from the glossopharyngeal nerve (cranial nerve IX)

34. Normally embedded in fat and located within 2 cm circumscribed area that is cranial to intersection of inferior thyroid artery and RLN applies to:

(a) Superior parathyroid gland
(b) Inferior parathyroid gland
(c) Thymus
(d) Pyramidal lobe of thyroid

Ans: (a) Superior parathyroid gland

Superior parathyroid is cranial to intersection of ITA and RLN

35. Otic ganglion lies under:

(a) Foramen spinosum
(b) Foramen ovale
(c) Maxillary nerve
(d) Stylomastoid foramen

Ans: (b) Foramen ovale

It lies under foramen ovale

36. Following are indications for tracheostomy *except:*

(a) Nasopharyngeal carcinoma
(b) Thyroid tumor impinging on larynx
(c) Major facial fractures involving airway
(d) Epiglottitis

Ans: (a) Nasopharyngeal carcinoma

In NPC, tracheostomy is done if necessary, before oncological resection as it doesn't compromise oral airway

37. A patient develops chylous fistula following a left neck dissection. Which of the following treatments is least likely to result in fistula closing?

(a) Endovascular embolization of thoracic duct
(b) Enteral diet with predominantly medium chain fatty acids
(c) Surgical re-exploration
(d) Enteral diet with long chain fatty acids

Ans: (d) Enteral diet with long chain fatty acids

Long chain fatty acids should not be administered during chylous leak

38. Which jaw cyst is premalignant?

(a) Nasopalatine cyst
(b) Radicular cyst
(c) Odontogenic keratocyst
(d) Dentigerous cyst

Ans: (c) Odontogenic keratocyst

Odontogenic keratocyst is a premalignant lesion

39. Painless ulcer of the tongue is due to:

(a) Dyspepsia
(b) Syphilis
(c) Tuberculosis
(d) None of the above

Ans: (b) Syphilis

Syphilitic ulcers are painless

40. All are True statements about carotid body tumor *except:*

(a) Non-chromaffin paraganglioma
(b) Good prognosis
(c) Rarely metastasizes
(d) Similar to mixed parotid tumor

Ans: (d) Similar to mixed parotid tumor

Not similar to mixed parotid tumor

41. Cystic hygroma is known to occur in all *except:*

(a) Calf
(b) Neck
(c) Axilla
(d) Mediastinum

Ans: (a) Calf

Calf is not the site for cystic hygroma

42. Blow out carotid is characteristically seen with:

(a) Thyroidectomy
(b) Radical neck dissection
(c) Flap necrosis
(d) Sistrunk operation

Ans: (b) Radical neck dissection

Radical neck dissection results in blow out carotid

43. Adson's test is positive in:

(a) Cervical rib
(b) Cervical spondylosis
(c) Cervical fracture
(d) Cervical dislocation

Ans: (a) Cervical rib

Adson's test is +ve in cervical rib

44. Which of the following does not move on deglutition?

(a) Sublingual dermoid
(b) Thyroid nodule
(c) Pretracheal lymph node
(d) Thyroglossal cyst

Ans: (a) Sublingual dermoid

Except sublingual dermoid rest all move with deglutition

45. Best view for mandible is:

(a) Antero-posterior
(b) Lateral
(c) Oblique
(d) Orthopentomogram

Ans: (d) Orthopentomogram

OPG is best view for mandible

46. Mandible is commonly fractured:

(a) At the neck of the condyle
(b) Through the angle
(c) Through the canine fossa
(d) At the middle

Ans: (a) At the neck of the condyle

Most common site of fracture mandible is condylar neck of mandible (condyle> angle>body>symphysis)

47. Millards 'Rule of Ten' includes all *except:*

(a) 10 lbs
(b) 10 weeks of age
(c) 10 gm% hemoglobin
(d) 10 months of age

Ans: (d) 10 months of age

Rule of 10 given by Wilhelmmesen and Musgrave→Age >10 weeks, Weight >10 pounds, Hb >10gm%

48. Ideal time for cleft lip repair surgery:

(a) 3-6 weeks
(b) 6-12 weeks
(c) 1-1.5 years
(d) 3-4 years

Ans: (b) 6-12 weeks

Ideal time for cleft lip surgery is 6-12 weeks

49. Posterior triangle LN is what level?

(a) Level I
(b) Level II
(c) Level V
(d) Level IV

Ans: (c) Level V

Level V contains posterior triangle nodes

50. A nerve injured in radical neck dissection leads to loss of sensation in medial side of the arm, nerve injured is:

(a) Long thoracic nerve
(b) Thoracodorsal nerve
(c) Dorsal scapular nerve
(d) Medial cutaneous nerve of arm

Ans: (d) Medial cutaneous nerve of arm

Medial cutaneous nerve of thigh injured during radical neck dissection leads to loss of sensation in medial side of arm

51. Targeted therapy has been most difficult to design for:

(a) Amplified genes
(b) Mutated genes
(c) Tumor suppressor genes
(d) Fusion genes

Ans: (c) Tumor suppressor genes

52. Most common tumor suppressor gene muatation in HNSCC is:

(a) p53
(b) FAT1
(c) PTEN
(d) NOTCH 1

Ans: (a) p53

53. RET/PTC formation is an example of:

(a) Unbalanced translocation
(b) Balanced translocation
(c) LOH
(d) Genetic amplification

Ans: (b) Balanced translocation

- RET gene is affected by point mutations in Hirschsprung disease
- Higher rates of RET/PTC3 rearrangements compared with sporadic PTC in adults in radiation induced childhood PTC

54. Prognosis of unresectable medullary carcinoma patients is best assessed with use of:

(a) Calcitonin doubling time
(b) Serial cross sectional imaging
(c) Serial PET scans
(d) Serum calcium monitoring

Ans: (a) Calcitonin doubling time

55. In patients with differentiated thyroid cancer metastatic to the lateral side of neck, which preoperative investigation should be considered?

(a) USG
(b) PET
(c) CECT neck
(d) Radioiodine scan

Ans: (a) USG

56. Rate of incidental malignancy in MNG is:

(a) <5%
(b) 5-10%
(c) 10-30%
(d) 30-50%

Ans: (c) 10-30%

57. Next step in managing a patient with normal clinical examination results and a rising thyroglobulin level after surgery for thyroid cancer is:

(a) Elective neck dissection
(b) USG
(c) Therapeutic radioiodine
(d) Tyrosine kinase inhibitor therapy

Ans: (b) USG

58. Children who are seen with papillary thyroid cancer are at high risk of:

(a) Locally advanced primary tumors
(b) Bony metastases
(c) Pulmonary metastases
(d) Local recurrence

Ans: (c) Pulmonary metastases

59. Papillary thyroid metastasis to the Delphian nodes has been shown to be associated with:

(a) Low survival rates
(b) High rates of recurrence
(c) Extrathyroidal extension
(d) Reduced rates of lateral neck metastases

Ans: (c) Extrathyroidal extension

60. True regarding pleomorphic adenoma are all *except:*

(a) Slow growing
(b) Encapsulated
(c) 75-80% of parotid tumors
(d) More common males

Ans: (d) More common males

61. True statement regarding warthins tumor:

(a) Common in male
(b) Most malignant
(c) Coldspot in tc 99 scan
(d) Most common tumor of minor salivary gland

Ans: (a) Common in male

62. Percentage of malignant tranformation in Pleomorphic Adenoma:

(a) 15
(b) 20
(c) 10
(d) 5

Ans: (d) 5

- Actually it is 1.5% for 5 years and 9.5% for 10 years
- On an average bailey mentions it as 5%

PART THREE: PREVIOUS MCQs

CHAPTER

63

MULTIPLE CHOICE QUESTIONS (PAPERS)

PAPER 1

1. A child is diagnosed to have condition "Recurrent parotitis of childhood". Treatment of choice is: (NEET SS 2018)

(a) Observation
(b) Parotidectomy
(c) Analgesics
(d) Antibiotics

Ans: (d) Antibiotics

- *Recurrent parotitis of childhood is a distinct clinical entity of unknown aetiology and variable prognosis*
- Characterized by rapid swelling of one or both parotid glands, in which the symptoms are made worse by chewing and eating
- Systemic upset with fever and malaise is variable
- Symptoms usually last from 3 to 7 days, and are then followed by quiescent period of weeks to several months
- Children usually present between 3 and 6 years
- Diagnosis is based on the characteristic history and confirmed by sialography
- **This shows a characteristic punctate sialectasis likened to a 'snowstorm'**
- Condition is difficult to manage if it becomes established and so the initial treatment is important
- *Condition responds to regular endoscopic washouts and long courses of antibiotics*
- Suspicion is that in some cases condition is caused by an incompetent punctum that leads to soiling of the parotid ducts with contaminated oral fluids

(Bailey, 27th Edition, Page 786)

2. Which of the following blade size is used for abdominal incision?

(a) 10
(b) 11
(c) 22
(d) 15

Ans: (c) 22

- The 22-blade is often used for abdominal incisions
- The 11-blade for arteriotomy
- The 15-blade for minor surgical procedures

(Bailey, 27th Edition, Page 85)

3. Which of the following statements are not true about Acute Rejection of transplant?

(a) Usually occurs during the first 6 months after transplantation
(b) Mediated predominantly by lymphocytes
(c) Acute rejection is characterised by mononuclear cell infiltration of the graft

(d) Acute antibody mediated rejection is easy to treat effectively

Ans: (d) Acute antibody mediated rejection is easy to treat effectively

- Usually occurs during the first 6 months after transplantation but may occur later. It is mediated predominantly by T lymphocytes, but alloantibodies may also play an important role
- Acute rejection is characterised by mononuclear cell infiltration of the graft
- The mononuclear cell infiltrate is heterogeneous and includes cytotoxic T cells, B cells, natural killer (NK) cells and activated macrophages
- Antibody-mediated damage may also be present, as evidenced by the deposition of the complement component C4d within the graft microvasculature
- All types of organ allograft are susceptible to acute rejection (typically occurring in around 20-30% of grafts)
- Most episodes of acute cellular rejection can be reversed by additional immunosuppressive therapy
- Acute antibody-mediated rejection is more difficult to treat effectively and may require plasmaphoresis or immunoadsorption

(Bailey, 27th Edition, Page 1536)

4. True about Freiberg disease:

(a) Ischemic necrosis of Epiphysis
(b) Settles with rest
(c) Excision of proximal phalangeal head of 2nd Metatarsal
(d) All of the above

Ans: (d) All of the above

- Freiberg's disease is an ischaemic necrosis of the epiphysis, resulting in pain and swelling of the joint
- It will often settle with rest
- Re-shaping osteotomies or excision of the proximal phalangeal head for severe adult cases with joint destruction
- Excision of the whole metatarsal head should never be performed

(Bailey, 27th Edition, Page 527)

5. All are true about Turf toe injury *except:*

(a) Seen in football players
(b) Associated with Sesamoiditis and Stress fracture at MTP joint
(c) Grade 4 fracture requires surgery
(d) Injection of steroids is not done as there is risk of AVN

Ans: (d) Injection of steroids is not done as there is risk of AVN

- Acute injuries (turf toe) can be managed non-operatively or surgically depending on the grade of the injury and occupation of the patient
- Grade 4 acute fracture may require surgery
- Chronic conditions are indistinguishable and range from stress fracture to avascular necrosis and sesamoiditis but are probably all the same phenomenon
- Management includes offloading with orthotics and injections of steroids and, rarely, shaving/excision. Excision surgery carries a high risk

(Bailey, 27th Edition, Page 527)

6. Regarding hallux valgus true is:

(a) Associated with Bunion
(b) All patients need surgery
(c) Affects men usually
(d) All of the above

Ans: (a) Associated with Bunion

- Affects women more often than men
- Patients with hallux valgus have inherited a tendency to develop the condition
- Not all patients need surgery
- Choice of operation is determined by the severity of the deformity and presence or absence of any arthritis

(Bailey, 27th Edition, Page 525)

7. Most common neurological condition associated with pes cavus is:

(a) Charcot-Marie-tooth disease
(b) Myasthenia gravis
(c) Multiple sclerosis
(d) Amyotropic lateral sclerosis

Ans: (a) Charcot-Marie-tooth disease

- Pes cavus needs neurological investigation
- About 80% of cases of pes cavus are associated with neurological disease
- Most common cause is Charcot-Marie-Tooth disease
- Unilateral pes cavus–think diastematomyelia/tumor

(Bailey, 27th Edition, Page 531)

8. Blood supply to majority of spinal cord is from:

(a) Anterior spinal artery
(b) Posterior spinal artery
(c) Lateral spinal artery
(d) None of the above

Ans: (a) Anterior spinal artery

- Blood supply of the spinal cord is derived from vertebral, deep cervical, intercostal and lumbar arteries
- Arteries of the spinal cord include the anterior spinal artery and two posterior spinal arteries, with ***anterior spinal artery supplying the majority of the vascular supply to the spinal cord***
- Radicular artery of Adamkiewicz makes a major contribution to the anterior spinal artery, supplying the lower spinal cord
- It originates on the left in 80% of people, usually accompanying the ventral root of T9, T10 or T11 but can originate anywhere from T5 to L5

(Bailey, 27th Edition, Page 471)

9. Which of the following is not a developmental neurological spine abnormality?

(a) Spina bifida
(b) Arnold chiari malformation
(c) Spinal dyraphism
(d) Scoliosis

Ans: (d) Scoliosis

- Scoliosis is a Bony disorder
- Rest all are Neurological spine abnormality

(Bailey, 27th Edition, Page 471)

10. Root value/level for Knee jerk:

(a) L2
(b) L3
(c) L4
(d) L5

Ans: (c) L4

- Biceps reflex–C5
- Triceps reflex–C7
- Knee jerk–L4

(Bailey, 27th Edition, Page 439)

11. Thenar muscle wasting is seen with injury to:

(a) Median nerve (b) Ulnar nerve

(c) Radial nerve (d) Branchial nerve

Ans: (a) Median nerve

- Thenar wasting–Median nerve palsy
- Hypothenar wasting–Ulnar nerve palsy
- Intrinsic wasting–Ulnar nerve plasy

(Bailey, 27th Edition, Page 443)

12. Boutonniere's deformity is seen in:

(a) Rheumatoid arthritis (b) Osteoarthritis

(c) Gouty arthritis (d) Psoriatic arthritis

Ans: (a) Rheumatoid arthritis

- Boutonniere's deformity, Swan neck deformity, Z deformity of thumb, Ulnar drift–Rheumatoid arthritis
- Heberden nodes, Bouchard nodes–Osteoarthritis

(Bailey, 27th Edition, Page 443)

13. False about Non recurrent RLN is:

(a) Seen in 0.5% to 1% of patients

(b) Usually on right side

(c) Associated with a retroesophageal right subclavian artery

(d) Nerve separates from vagus after descending into chest, passes directly to larynx

Ans: (d) Nerve separates from vagus after descending into chest, passes directly to larynx

- Nerve separates from vagus **BEFORE** descending into chest, passes directly to larynx
- Seen in 0.5% to 1% of patients
- Usually on right side
- Associated with a retroesophageal right subclavian artery

(Bailey, 27th Edition, Page 811)

14. Most common fungal cause of pharnygitis is:

(a) Aspergillosis

(b) Candida

(c) Rhizopus

(d) Absida

Ans: (b) Candida

- ***Candida albicans*** is most common fungal organism to cause pharyngitis
- This organism is a normal component of the oral flora, but under conditions of immunosuppression, broad-spectrum antibacterial therapy, poor oral hygiene, or vitamin deficiency, it may become pathogenic
- Whitish-cheesy or creamy mucosal patches are observed with underlying erythema
- Diagnosis is easily established by Gram's stain of this material, revealing budding yeast and pseudohyphae

- Oral (-azole) and topical (nystatin) antifungals are usually effective and immunosuppressed patients may require prophylactic therapy

(Schwartz, 10th Edition, Page 571)

15. Most common site of mandibular fracture is: (NEET SS 2017)

(a) Condyle (b) Angle

(c) Body (d) Symphysis

Ans: (a) Condyle

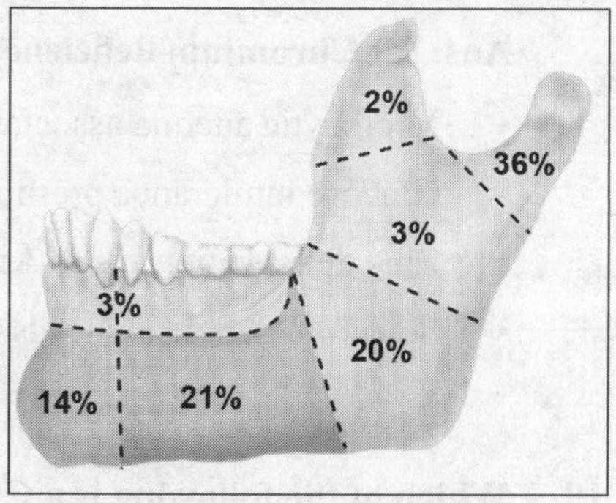

- Fractures most often involve the angle, body, or condyle, and in most cases, two or more sites are almost always involved

(Schwartz, 10th Edition, Page 576)

16. Grade 2 obesity is interpreted by which values:

(a) 30-34.9 Kg/m² (b) 35-39.9 Kg/m²

(c) 25-29.9 Kg/m² (d) >40 Kg/m²

Ans: (b) 35-39.9 Kg/m²

Interpretation of BMI
• Severely underweight: <16.5 kg/m²
• Underweight: 16.5-18.4 kg/m²
• Normal weight: 18.5-24.9 kg/m²
• Overweight: 25-29.9 kg/m²
• Obesity grade I: 30-34.9 kg/m²
• Obesity grade II: 35-39.9 kg/m²
• Obesity grade III: ≥40 kg/m²

(Sabiston, 20th Edition, Page 108)

17. Contraindications to Enteral nutrition include all *except:*

(a) Intractable vomiting refractory to medical management (b) Severe short bowel syndrome

(c) Low output intestinal fistulas (d) Enteral nutrition needed <7 days

Ans: (c) Low output intestinal fistulas

Contraindications to Enteral Nutrition
• Intractable vomiting, diarrhea refractory to medical management
• Paralytic ileus
• High-output intestinal fistulas (too distal to bypass with feeding tube)
• GI obstruction, ischemia
• Diffuse peritonitis
• Severe shock or hemodynamic instability
• Severe GI hemorrhage
• Severe short bowel syndrome (<100 cm of small bowel remaining)
• Severe GI malabsorption (e.g., EN failed, as evidenced by progressive deterioration in nutritional status)
• Inability to gain access to GI tract
• Need for EN is expected for <7 days

(Sabiston, 20th Edition, Page 112)

18. Which of the following trace elements leads to Glucose intolerance?

(a) Selenium deficiency
(b) Zinc deficiency
(c) Copper deficiency
(d) Chromium deficiency

Ans: (d) Chromium deficiency

- Microcytic anemia associated with copper deficiency
- Glucose intolerance presumably related to chromium deficiency
- Zinc deficiency leads to Acrodermatitis enteropathica
- Selenium deficiency leads to Keshan disease

(Schwartz, 10th Edition, Page 58)

19. Which of the following is a CLASS III wound?

(a) Hernia repair
(b) Cholecystectomy
(c) Penetrating abdominal trauma
(d) Perforated diverticulitis

Ans: (c) Penetrating abdominal trauma

Class	Examples	Infection Rates
I (Clean)	Hernia repair, breast biopsy specimen	1%–2%
II (Clean/Contaminated)	Cholecystectomy, Elective GI surgery Colorectal surgery	2.1%–9.5% 4%–14%
III (Contaminated)	Penetrating abdominal trauma, large tissue injury, enterotomy during bowel obstruction	3.4%–13.2%
IV (Dirty)	Perforated diverticulitis, necrotizing soft tissue infections	3.1%–12.8%

(Schwartz, 10th Edition, Page 148)

20. Contraindications to Emergency thoracotomy include:

(a) Patients sustaining witnessed penetrating trauma to torso with <15 min of prehospital CPR
(b) Cardiac tamponade with hypotension
(c) Penetrating trauma: CPR >15 min and no pupillary response
(d) Patients sustaining witnessed blunt trauma with <10 min of prehospital CPR

Ans: (c) Penetrating trauma: CPR >15 min and no pupillary response

Indications	Contraindications
Salvageable postinjury cardiac arrest: • Patients sustaining witnessed penetrating trauma to the torso with <15 min of prehospital CPR • Patients sustaining witnessed blunt trauma with <10 min of prehospital CPR • Patients sustaining witnessed penetrating trauma to the neck or extremities with <5 min of prehospital CPR **Persistent severe postinjury hypotension (SBP ≤60 mm Hg) due to:** • Cardiac tamponade • Hemorrhage—intrathoracic, intra-abdominal, extremity, cervical • Air embolism	Penetrating trauma: CPR >15 min and no signs of life (pupillary response, respiratory effort, motor activity) Blunt trauma: CPR >10 min and no signs of life or asystole without associated tamponade

(Schwartz, 10th Edition, Page 167)

21. Which laryngeal site is the most at risk of developing radionecrosis?

(a) Cricoid
(b) Thyroid lamina
(c) Arytenoid
(d) Epiglottis

Ans: (c) Arytenoid

- Chondroradionecrosis occurs in approximately 5% of patients with laryngeal cancer
- Most common cartilage affected is the arytenoid cartilage

(Bailey, Textbook of Otolaryngology, 2nd Edition, Page 1968)

22. Development of a cutaneous malignancy is associated with chronic exposure to:

(a) Ammonia
(b) Arsenic
(c) Chromium
(d) Benzene

Ans: (b) Arsenic

- Chronic exposure to arsenic (as seen in Fowlers solution) has been associated with the development of multiple squamous and basal cell carcinomas
- Predisposing factors for BCC include exposure to arsenical compounds, coal tar, aromatic hydrocarbons, ionising radiation and genetic skin cancer syndromes
- IR causes SCC, as do chemical carcinogens (arsenicals, tar) and infection with HPV 5 and 16

(Bailey, 27th Edition, Page 604)

23. Which of the following is best suitable as Muscle relaxant in Renal failure? (NEET SS 2018)

(a) Succinyl choline
(b) Vecuronium
(c) Rocuronium
(d) Atracurium

Ans: (d) Atracurium

- Atracurium is best suitable for Renal failure patients

(Bailey 27th Edition, Page 273)

24. Which of the following is placed under High risk of DVT?

(a) Maxillofacial surgery
(b) Urological surgery
(c) Total knee replacement
(d) Gynecological surgery

Ans: (c) Total knee replacement

Low Risk	Medium Risk	High Risk
Maxillofacial surgery Neurosurgery Cardiothoracic surgery	Inguinal hernia surgery Abdominal surgery Gynecological surgery Urological surgery	Pelvic elective and trauma surgery Total knee and hip replacement

(Bailey, 27th Edition, Page 296)

25. All of the following are examples of absorbable suture, *except:*

(a) Polyglactin
(b) Poliglecaprone 25
(c) Polypropylene
(d) Polydioxanone

Ans: (c) Polypropylene

- Prolene (polypropylene) suture is nonabsorbable, as are silk nylon, and polyester (Dacron, Ethibond)

- The other materials listed are absorbable

PROLENE

- Monofilament (Dyed/Undyed)–Polymer of propylene
- Infinite tensile strength
- Non absorbable, Low tissue reactions, No contraindications
- **Frequent uses:** Cardiovascular surgery, Plastic surgery, Ophthalmic surgery, General surgical subcuticular skin closure

(Bailey, 27th Edition, Page 92)

26. All are consequences of metabolic response to starvation *except:*

(a) Low plasma insulin
(b) High plasma glucagon
(c) Protein anabolism
(d) Hepatic Glycogenolysis

Ans: (c) Protein anabolism

Metabolic Response to Starvation
• Low plasma insulin • High plasma glucagon • Hepatic glycogenolysis • Protein catabolism • Hepatic gluconeogenesis, Adaptive ketogenesis • Lipolysis: Mobilisation of fat stores (Increased fat oxidation)–overall decrease in protein and carbohydrate oxidation • Reduction in resting energy expenditure (from approximately 25-30 kcal/kg per day to 15-20 kcal/kg per day

(Bailey, 27th Edition, Page 279)

27. Apfel scoring is used for:

(a) Patient Controlled Analgesia
(b) Post operative nausea and Vomiting
(c) Hypothermia
(d) Pulmonary embolus

Ans: (b) Post operative nausea and Vomiting

Characteristics	Points
Female	1
History of motion sickness or PONV	1
Non smoker	1
Post operative opoid treatment is planned	1
Total	

28. Which of the following describes Day surgery?

(a) Not admitted to a ward facility
(b) Admission of up to 72 hours
(c) Surgery not requiring full sterile theatre facilities
(d) Admitted and discharged within 12-hour day

Ans: (d) Admitted and discharged within 12-hour day

- Outpatient surgery: Not admitted to a ward facility
- Procedure room surgery: Surgery not requiring full sterile theatre facilities
- Day or same-day surgery: Admitted and discharged within 12-hour day
- Overnight stay: 23-hour admission with early morning discharge
- Short-stay surgery: Admission of up to 72 hours

(Bailey, 27th Edition, Page 301)

29. Which of the following is stain for Collagen?

(a) PAS
(b) Prussian blue
(c) Reticulin
(d) Van Gieson

Ans: (d) Van Gieson

Stains
• **PAS:** Glycogen, fungi
• **D-PAS:** Mucin
• **Peris Prussian blue:** Iron
• **Reticulin:** Reticulin fibres, fibrosis
• **Van Gieson:** Collagen
• **Congo red:** Amyloid
• **Ziehl-Neelsen:** Mycobacteria

(Bailey, 27th Edition, Page 245)

30. Dot in the circle sign is seen in:

(a) Actinomycosis
(b) Erysipelas
(c) Mycetoma
(d) Gas gangrene

Ans: (c) Mycetoma

- 'Dot-in-circle sign', which indicates the presence of grains, is highly characteristic seen in MRI
- MRI usually shows multiple 2-5 mm lesions of high signal intensity, which indicates granuloma, interspersed within a low intensity matrix denoting the fibrous tissue

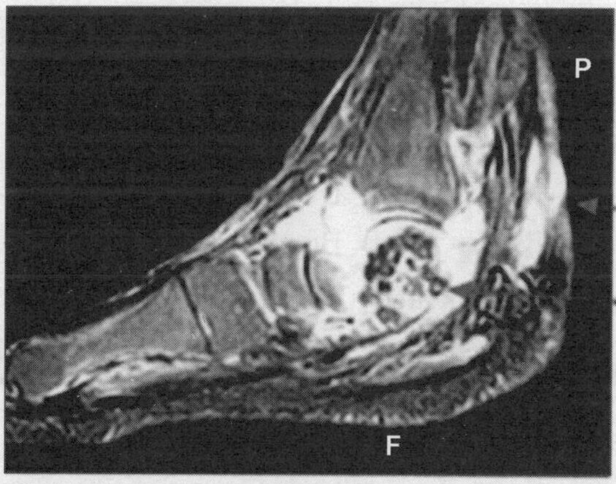

(Bailey, 27th Edition, Page 73)

31. Which of the following is not a component of ASEPSIS wound score?

(a) Erythema
(b) Serous discharge
(c) Purulent exudate
(d) Edema

Ans: (d) Edema

Criterion	Points
ADDITIONAL TREATMENT	
Antibiotics for wound infection	10
Drainage of pus under local anaesthesia	5
Debridement of wound under general anaesthesia	10

Contd.

Contd.

SEROUS DISCHARGE	Daily 0-5
ERYTHEMA	Daily 0-5
PURULENT EXUDATE	Daily 0-10
SEPARATION OF DEEP TISSUES	Daily 0-10
ISOLATION OF BACTERIA FROM WOUND	10
STAY AS INPATIENT PROLONG	5

- Scored for 5 of first 7 days only, remainder being scored if present in first 2 months

(Bailey, 27th Edition, Page 48)

32. Which of the following is not true about Vancomycin?

(a) Glycopeptide antibiotic
(b) Most active against gram-positive aerobic and anaerobic bacteria
(c) Effective against MRSA, so are often used as prophylactic antibiotics
(d) Can be safely used in renal failure patients

Ans: (d) Can be safely used in renal failure patients

VANCOMYCIN

- Glycopeptide antibiotic
- Most active against gram-positive aerobic and anaerobic bacteria and have proved to be effective against MRSA, so are often used as prophylactic antibiotics when there is a high risk of MRSA
- Ototoxic and nephrotoxic, so serum levels should be monitored
- Effective against *C. difficile* in cases of pseudomembranous colitis

(Bailey, 27th Edition, Page 56)

33. All the statements are true about Inguinal hernia in children *except:*

(a) More common in premature boys
(b) Bilateral in 15%
(c) Usually Indirect with a patent processus vaginalis
(d) Hernial sac need not be isolated, ligated and divided

Ans: (d) Hernial sac need not be isolated, ligated and divided

Inguinal Hernia in Children

- More common in premature boys (right > left)
- Bilateral 15%
- Indirect with a patent processus vaginalis
- Groin lump that appears on straining or crying
- Incarcerated inguinal hernias can usually be reduced with gentle pressure
- In infants they can transilluminate like hydrocoele, making test redundant when distinction is difficult
- If reduction is impossible emergency surgery is needed
- In infants: Repaired promptly to prevent the risk of strangulation
- Hernial sac is isolated, ligated and divided

(Bailey, 27th Edition, Page 124)

34. Who described seromuscular suture technique of bowel anastomosis?

(a) Kocher
(b) Lembert
(c) Senn
(d) Ewald

Ans: (b) Lembert

- Lembert described his seromuscular suture technique for bowel anastomosis in 1826, while Senn advocated a two layer technique for closure
- Kocher's method utilised a two-layer anastomosis, first a continuous all-layer suture using catgut, then an inverting continuous (or interrupted) seromuscular layer suture using silk, which became mainstay of bowel anastomoses

(Bailey, 27th Edition, Page 98)

35. Which of the following is not true about DRAINS?

(a) Drains for thyroidectomy may usually be removed after 24 hours

(b) Drains for mastectomy can be removed after 5 days

(c) Drains for colorectal anastomoses should be removed at about 5-7 days

(d) Common bile duct T-tubes should remain in for 5 days

Ans: (d) Common bile duct T-tubes should remain in for 5 days

- Drains put in because of infection should be left until infection is subsiding or drainage is minimal
- Drains put in to cover perioperative bleeding may usually be removed after 24 hours, e.g., thyroidectomy
- Drains put in to drain serous collections usually can be removed after 5 days, e.g., mastectomy
- Drains put in because of infection should be left until the infection is subsiding or the drainage is minimal
- Drains put in to cover colorectal anastomoses should be removed at about 5-7 days
- *Common bile duct T-tubes should remain in for 10 days.* However, once the T-tube cholangiogram has shown that there is free flow of bile into the duodenum and that there are no retained stones, some surgeons like to clamp T-tube prior to removal. **10-day period is required to minimise the risk of biliary peritonitis after removal**

(Bailey, 27th Edition, Page 101)

36. Which of the following statement is not true?

(a) For every 6 red blood cells, give 6 FFP

(b) Most common symptom of acute transfusion reaction is pain at the site of transfusion, facial flushing and chest pain

(c) Human brain thromboplastin has an International Sensitivity Index of 1

(d) Clotting factor with lowest half life is Factor V

Ans: (d) Clotting factor with lowest half life is Factor V

- For every 6 red blood cells, give 6 FFP
- Most common symptom of acute transfusion reaction is pain at the site of transfusion, facial flushing and chest pain
- Human brain thromboplastin has an International Sensitivity Index of 1
- **Clotting factor with lowest half life is Factor VII**

(Schwartz, 10th Edition, Page 99)

37. Storage temperature of FFP is:

(a) –40 to –50°C
(b) –30°C
(c) 20–24°C
(d) 2–6°C

Ans: (a) –40 to –50°C

Blood Component	Shelf Life
FFP	–40 to –50°C
Cryoprecipitate	–30°C
Platelets	20–24°C
Packed red cells	2–6°C

(Bailey, 27th Edition, Page 21)

38. Fasciotomy is done in compartment syndrome if pressures are continuously above:

(a) 40 mm Hg
(b) 30 mm Hg
(c) 20 mm Hg
(d) 35 mm Hg

Ans: (b) 30 mm Hg

- Compartment pressures can be measured using a pressure monitor and a catheter placed in the muscle compartment
- If pressures are constantly greater than 30 mm Hg or if the above clinical signs are present, then fasciotomy should be performed
- Fasciotomy involves incising the deep muscle fascia and is best carried out via longitudinal incisions of skin, fat and fascia

(Bailey, 27th Edition, Page 28)

39. Most common site of pressure sores is:

(a) Sacrum
(b) Ilium
(c) Ischium
(d) Greater trochanter

Ans: (c) Ischium

Pressure Sore Frequency in Descending Order
• Ischium
• Greater trochanter
• Sacrum
• Heel
• Malleolus (lateral then medial)
• Occiput

(Bailey, 27th Edition, Page 29)

40. Correct Match among the following is:

(a) PECAM 1–Origin is Neutrophils
(b) P selectin–Origin is Endothelium
(c) E selectin–Origin is Platelets
(d) L selectin–Origin is Leukocytes

Ans: (d) L selectin–Origin is Leukocytes

Adhesion Molecule	Origin
PECAM 1	Endothelium, platelets, leukocytes
P selectin	Platelets and Endothelium
E selectin	Endothelium
L selectin	Leukocytes

PAPER 2

41. In necrotising infection which is often absent?

(a) Pain
(b) Crepitus
(c) Fever
(d) Skin blistering

Ans: (c) Fever

Signs and Symptoms of Necrotising Infections
• Unusual pain
• Oedema beyond area of erythema
• Crepitus
• Skin blistering
• Fever (often absent)
• Greyish drainage ('dishwater pus')
• Pink/orange skin staining
• Focal skin gangrene (late sign)
• Shock, coagulopathy and multiorgan failure

(Bailey, 27th Edition, Page 30)

42. Most abscess relating to surgical wound form during:

(a) 3-5 days (b) 5-7 days

(c) 7-10 days (d) 10-14 days

Ans: (c) 7-10 days

- Suppurative wound infections take 7-10 days to develop, and even cellulitis around wounds caused by invasive organisms (such as beta haemolytic *Streptococcus*) takes 3-4 days to develop

(Bailey, 27th Edition, Page 54)

43. Best method for detecting muscle hernia:

(a) USG (b) CECT

(c) MRI (d) Both (b) and (c)

Ans: (a) USG

Radiographs are the Best First-Line Test for Bone Lesions and Fractures
• MRI is good for diagnosing bone marrow disease, occult fractures and tendon and soft-tissue disorders
• CT enables visualisation of the fine detail of bony structures
• CT gives the best three-dimensional information on fractures
• Ultrasound has better resolution inaccessible soft tissues and can be used dynamically
• Ultrasound is the best method of distinguishing solid from cystic lesions
• Ultrasound is the only method for locating non-metallic foreign bodies
• **Ultrasound is the best method for detecting muscle hernias**

(Bailey, 27th Edition, Page 200)

44. Southampton wound trading including pus in wound include in which type?

(a) 1 (b) 2

(c) 4 (d) 3

Ans: (c) 4

Southampton Wound Grading
Normal healing–0
Normal healing with mild bruising or erythema–I
Some bruising–Ia
Considerable bruising–Ib

Contd.

Contd.

Mild erythema–Ic
Erythema plus other signs of inflammation–II
At one point–IIa
Around sutures–IIb
Along wound–IIc
Around wound–IId
Clear or haemoserous discharge–III
At one point only (<2 cm)–IIIa
Along wound (>2 cm)–IIIb
Large volume–IIIc
Prolonged (>3 days)-IIId
IVa–At one point only (<2 cm)
IVb–Along wound (>2 cm)
V–Deep or severe wound infection with or without tissue breakdown, hematoma requiring aspiration

(Bailey, 27th Edition, Page 48)

45. Incidence of cleft lip alone is:

(a) 15% (b) 30%

(c) 40% (d) 45%

Ans: (a) 15%

- Incidence of cleft lip and palate is 1:600 live births and of isolated cleft palate is 1:1000 live births
- Incidence increases in Oriental groups (1:500) and decreases in the black population (1:2000)

TYPICAL DISTRIBUTION OF CLEFT TYPES

- Cleft lip alone: 15%
- Cleft lip and palate: 45%
- Isolated cleft palate: 40%

(Bailey, 27th Edition, Page 688)

46. True about Temporal bone fracture:

(a) Transverse # are most common type (b) Majority of # are of mixed variety

(c) Transverse # cause conductive hearing loss (d) Facial nerve is commonly involved in longitudinal #

Ans: (b) Majority of # are of mixed variety

- Longitudinal (80%) are more commoner than transverse (20%)
- But majority have of mixed variety
- Transverse fracture has SNHL due to injury to labyrinth
- Longitudional fractures–conductive hearing loss due to involvement of EAC and TM
- Facial nerve involvement is more common with transverse fractures

(Bailey, 27th Edition, Page 713)

47. LABEL procedure is for:

(a) Gut
(b) Bile duct
(c) Liver
(d) Pancreas

Ans: (b) Bile duct

- LABEL procedure is Laser Assisted Bile duct Exploration by Laparoendoscopy for choledocholithiasis
- It was developed when the concept of laser stone management in urology was applied to laparoscopic biliary tree surgery

(Bailey, 27th Edition, Page 118)

48. Reperfusion injury can attenuated by all *except:*

(a) Reducing the extent of tissue hypoperfusion
(b) Reducing the duration of tissue hypoperfusion
(c) Adequate resuscitation
(d) None of the above

Ans: (c) Adequate resuscitation

- Reperfusion injury can currently only be attenuated by reducing the extent and duration of tissue hypoperfusion
- During the period of systemic hypoperfusion, cellular and organ damage progresses due to the direct effects of tissue hypoxia and local activation of inflammation
- Further injury occurs once normal circulation is restored to these tissues. The acid and potassium load that has built up can lead to direct myocardial depression, vascular dilatation and further hypotension
- Cellular and humoral elements activated by hypoxia (complement, neutrophils, microvascular thrombi) are flushed back into the circulation where they cause further endothelial injury to organs such as the lungs and the kidneys
- This leads to acute lung injury, acute renal injury, multiple organ failure and death

(Bailey, 27th Edition, Page 13)

49. Most common antibiotic associated with pseudomembranous colitis:

(a) Penicillin
(b) Cephalosporine
(c) Clindamycin
(d) Quinolones

Ans: (d) Quinolones

- Clostridium difficile is the cause of pseudomembranous colitis
- **Any antibiotic may cause this phenomenon, although the quinolones such as ciprofloxacin seem to be the highest risk, especially in elderly or immunocompromised patients**
- In its most severe form, the colitis may lead to perforation and the need for emergency colectomy with an associated high mortality

(Bailey, 27th Edition, Page 45)

50. Which of the following is Non absorbable suture?

(a) Silk is a braided type of suture
(b) Nylon is monofilament or braided type of suture
(c) Prolene is monofilament suture
(d) Teflon is monofilament type of mesh

Ans: (d) Teflon is monofilament type of mesh

- Silk is a braided type of suture
- Nylon is monofilament or braided type of suture
- Prolene is monofilament suture
- Teflon is polyfilament mesh

(Sabiston, 20th Edition, Page 234)

51. Which of the following hormones will not increase in response to stress?

(a) Corticotropin
(b) Growth hormone
(c) Vasopressin
(d) Thyroxine

Ans: (d) Thyroxine

Hormones	Changes in Secretion
Corticotropin	Increased
Growth hormone	Increased
Vasopressin	Increased
Cortisol	Increased
Thyroxine, Insulin **Triiodothryroxine**	**Decreased**

(Sabiston, 20th Edition, Page 242)

52. All the following Drugs are used in treatment of Vancomycin resistant Enterococci infection *except:*

(a) Daptomycin
(b) Tigecycline
(c) Linezolid
(d) Ceftaroline

Ans: (d) Ceftaroline

VRE	VISA
VANCOMYCIN RESISTANT ENTEROCOCCI	**VANCOMYCIN INTERMEDIATE RESISTANT STAPH AUREUS**
Daptomycin	Daptomycin
Tigecycline	Tigecycline
Linezolid	Linezolid
	Ceftaroline

(Sabiston, 20th Edition, Page 259)

53. Ostrosky-Zeichner Score is used for which of the following infection?

(a) Pseudomembranous colitis of clostridium
(b) Invasive Candidiasis
(c) Vancomycin resistant staphylococcus aureus
(d) Acinetobacter baumannii infection

Ans: (b) Invasive Candidiasis

Ostrosky-Zeichner Score
• This is a prediction rule that provides a dichotomous risk assessment based on presence of at least 3 risk factors: relative risk, 5; sensitivity, 0.27, specificity; 0.93, positive predictive value; 0.13, negative predictive value; 0.97, accuracy, 0.90
• Any systemic antibiotic (days 1-3 of the ICU stay) *or*
• Central venous catheter (days 1-3) *and*
At least two of the following:
• Total parenteral nutrition (days 1-3)
• Any renal replacement therapy (days 1-3)
• Any major surgery (days −7 to 0)
• Pancreatitis (days −7 to 0)
• Any steroid use (days −7 to −3)
• Any other immunosuppression (days −7 to 0)

(Sabiston 20th Edition, Page 266)

54. All the following are characteristics of Ebb phase *except:*

(a) Lactic acidosis
(b) Increased BMR

(c) Decreased Cardiac output
(d) Hypothermia

Ans.: (b) Increased BMR

- Ebb phase is characterised by hypovolaemia, decreased basal metabolic rate, reduced cardiac output, hypothermia and lactic acidosis

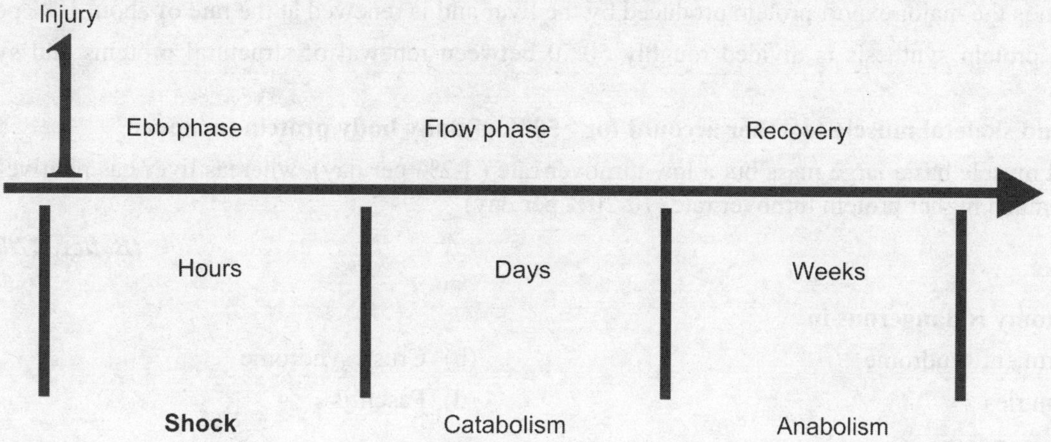

(Bailey, 27th Edition, Page 5)

55. Bright on T1 images on MRI all *except:*

(a) Fat
(b) Methaemoglobin
(c) Hemosiderin
(d) Mucinous fluid

Ans: (c) Hemosiderin

- Fat, methaemoglobin and mucinous fluid are bright on Tl-weighted images
- Water and thus most pathological processes, which tend to increase tissue water content, are bright on T2-weighted images

(Bailey, 27th Edition, Page 197)

56. All are true for simple hepatic cysts *except:*

(a) Usually solitary and more common in male
(b) Usually asymtomatic and have blue hue on laparoscopy
(c) Laparoscopic deroofing as a treatment option if symptomatic
(d) Polycystic liver more common in women

Ans: (a) Usually solitary and more common in male

SIMPLE CYSTS

- Simple cysts are generally solitary, and occur more frequently in women
- Most are incidental findings, and have a characteristic blue hue when seen at laparoscopy
- Indications for surgical intervention include symptoms, rupture, haemorrhage, infection or indeterminate diagnosis
- Surgical resection typically involves laparoscopic deroofing, with oversewing of cyst wall

POLYCYSTIC LIVER DISEASE

- Polycystic liver disease is less common and an autosomal dominant condition
- More commonly seen in women and around half of patients will also have polycystic kidneys
- Indications for surgical intervention are broadly similar to those for simple cysts, although large number of lesions means that deroofing a single cyst is unlikely to relieve symptoms

(Bailey, 27th Edition, Page 1168)

57. Renewal rate of albumin in liver is:

(a) 10%/day (b) 25% day
(c) 50% day (d) 100% a day

Ans: (a) 10%/day

- Albumin is the major export protein produced by the liver and is renewed at the rate of about 10% per day
- Hepatic protein synthesis is divided roughly 50:50 between renewal of structural proteins and synthesis of export proteins
- **Liver and skeletal muscle together account for >50% of daily body protein turnover**
- Skeletal muscle has a large mass but a low turnover rate (1-2% per day), whereas liver has relatively small mass (1.5 kg) but much higher protein turnover rate (10-20% per day)

(Bailey, 27th Edition, Page 7)

58. Late fasciotomy is dangerous in:

(a) Compartment syndrome (b) Crush syndrome
(c) Open injuries (d) Fasciitis

Ans: (b) Crush syndrome

- In crush injuries that present several days after the event, a late fasciotomy can be dangerous because dead muscle produces myoglobin which, if suddenly released into the blood stream, causes myoglobinuria with glomerular blockage and renal failure

(Bailey, 27th Edition, Page 28)

59. True about Venous drainage of Liver is:

(a) Right and middle Hepatic Vein join intrahepatic (b) Left and middle Hepatic Vein join intrahepatic
(c) Right and middle Hepatic Vein join extrahepatic (d) Left and middle Hepatic Vein join extrahepatic

Ans: (b) Left and middle Hepatic Vein join intrahepatic

- Right hepatic vein can be exposed fully outside the liver
- Middle and left veins usually join within the liver parenchyma

(Bailey, 27th Edition, Page 1154)

60. Proximal nerve degeneration occurs up to:

(a) Axon of hillock (b) Last node of ranvier
(c) Somatoplasm (d) Dendrites

Ans: (b) Last node of ranvier

- Distal to the wound, Wallerian degeneration occurs
- **Proximally, the nerve suffers traumatic degeneration as far as last node of Ranvier**
- Regenerating nerve fibres are attracted to their receptors by neurotrophism, which is mediated by growth factors, hormones and other extracellular matrix trophins
- Nerve regeneration is characterised by profuse growth of new nerve fibres which sprout from the cut proximal end
- Overgrowth of these, coupled with poor approximation, may lead to neuroma formation

(Bailey, 27th Edition, Page 25)

61. Which causes platelets aggregates to fill the wound?

(a) PDGF (b) TGF-B
(c) ADP (d) FGF

Ans: (c) ADP

- Platelets stick to the damaged endothelial lining of vessels, releasing adenosine diphosphate (ADP), which causes thrombocytic aggregates to fill the wound
- When bleeding stops, the platelets then release several cytokines from their alpha granules
- These are platelet-derived growth factor (PDGF), platelet factor IV and transforming growth factor beta (TGF beta)

(Bailey, 27th Edition, Page 24)

62. Most common cause of bleeding in hemothorax is:

(a) Intercostal vessels
(b) Internal mammary artery
(c) Superior epigastric artery
(d) Superior thoracic artery

Ans: (a) Intercostal vessels

- Most common cause of massive haemothorax in blunt injury is continuing bleeding from torn intercostal vessels
- Occasionally from the internal mammary artery secondary to fractures of the ribs
- In penetrating injury, a variety of viscera, both thoracic and abdominal (with blood leaking through hole in the diaphragm from the positive pressure abdomen into negative pressure thorax) may be involved

(Bailey, 27th Edition, Page 368)

63. Immunohistochemical Stain used for Lung Cancer is:

(a) Cytokeratin
(b) Thyroid Transcription Factor
(c) DOG-1
(d) HepPar

Ans: (b) Thyroid Transcription Factor

Immunohistochemical Stain
Cell Type/Site of Origin
• Epithelial (carcinoma): Cytokeratins
• Lymphoid (lymphoma): CD45, CD3, CD20
• Melanocytic (melanoma): S100, HMB45, Melan A
• Neuroendocrine: Synaptophysin, chromogranin
• Vascular: CD31
• Myoid: Desmin, actin
Site of Origin/Cell Type
• Prostate: Prostate-specific antigen (PSA)
• Lung: Thyroid transcription factor-1 (TTF-1)
• Thyroid: Thyroglobulin
• Colorectum: Cytokeratin 20 (CK20), CDX2
• Liver: HepPar
• Gastrointestinal stromal tumor (GIST): CD117, DOG-1
Prognosis and Treatment
• Breast and gastric carcinomas: HER2
• Neuroendocrine tumors: Ki67 labelling index
Screening for Mutations
• Colorectal carcinoma: Mismatch repair genes (MLH1,MSH2, MSH6, PMS2)

(Bailey, 27th Edition, Page 245)

64. Most common postoperative complication of tonsilectomy is:

(a) Palatal palsy
(b) Hemorrhage
(c) Injury to uvula
(d) Infection

Ans: (b) Hemorrhage

- **Main complication is hemorrhage which occurs in 3-5% patients**
- **Most common complication following tonsillectomy is hemorrhage**
- Reactionary hemorrhage is the most feared complication post tonsillectomy because of the risk of airway obstruction, shock and ultimately death

(Head and Neck Surgery, de Souza, Page 1588)

65. Vocal cord palsy is not associated with:

(a) Vertebral secondaries (b) Left atrial enlargement
(c) Bronchogenic carcinoma (d) Secondaries in mediastinum

Ans: (a) Vertebral secondaries

- Vocal cord paralysis is most commonly iatrogenic in origin following surgery to Thyroid, parathyroid, carotid or cardiothoracic structures

Right	Left	Both
• Neck trauma • Benign or malignant thyroid disease • Thyroid surgery • Carcinoma cervical oesophagus • Cervical lymphadenopathy	*i. Neck* • Accidental trauma • Thyroid disease (benign or malignant) • Thyroid surgery • Carcinoma cervical oesophagus • Cervical lymphadenopathy	Thyroid surgery Carcinoma thyroid Cancer cervical oesophagus Cervical lymphadenopathy
• Aneurysm of subclavian artery • Carcinoma apex right lung • Tuberculosis of cervical pleura • Idiopathic	*ii. Mediastum* • Bronchogenic cancer (Most common) • Carcinoma thoracic oesophagus • Aortic aneurysm • Enlarged left atrium • Intrathoracic surgery • Idiopathic	

(Dhingra, 6th Edition, Page 299)

66. Mass in ear that bleeds heavily on touch cause is:

(a) Glomus Jugulare (b) Squamous cell carcinoma mastoid
(c) Acoustic neuroma (d) Angiofibroma

Ans: (a) Glomus Jugulare

Glomus Tumor
• Glomus tumors are highly vascular tumors and bleed on Touch
• Most common site of glomus tumor in middle ear is hypotympanum
• Slow growing locally invasive, noncapsulated tumor which causes destruction of bone and facial nerve
• Highly vascular–Main Blood supply: Ascending pharyngeal artery

(Dhingra, 6th Edition, Page 109)

67. Risk of sarcoma developing in a fibroid uterus is approximately:

(a) <1% (b) 10%
(c) 30% (d) 50%

Ans: (a) <1%

- Sarcomatous change may occur in less than 0.1 percent cases
- The usual type is leiomyosarcoma
- Recurrence of fibroid polyp, sudden enlargement of fibroid or fibroid along with postmenopausal bleeding raises the suspicion

(Shaw Textbook of Gynecology, 15th Edition, Page 355;* DC Dutta, Gynecology, 6th Edition 276*)

68. Varicocele left sided in:

(a) 50% (b) 60%
(c) 70% (d) 90%

Ans (d) 90%

- Varicocoele is a common condition and 90% are left sided
- Development of a left-sided varicocoele in later life may indicate presence of a renal tumor
- They are usually asymptomatic and as such rarely need treatment
- First-line treatment is embolisation in symptomatic cases
- Varicocoeles often recur, even after surgical treatment

(Bailey, 27th Edition, Page 1502)

69. Adequate pressure for chest drain bottle to obtain gentle flow of bubbles from chest cavity:

(a) 10-20 mm Hg (b) 20-30 mm Hg
(c) 30-40 mm Hg (d) 40-50 mm Hg

Ans: (a) 10-20 mm Hg

- Indicated for a pneumothorax, pleural effusion, haemothorax or to prevent the collection of fluid or air after thoracotomy
- Once the drain has been inserted, it should be connected to an underwater sealed drain
- This system allows air to leave the pleural cavity, but it cannot be drawn back in by the negative pressure that is created in intrathoracic cavity
- During the respiratory process, it should he checked that the meniscus of the fluid is swinging, to ensure that the tube is not blocked Suction can be applied to the venting tube at the bottle whenever there is significant drainage of fluid or air expected
- **Between 10 and 20 mm of mercury is adequate to obtain a gentle flow of bubbles from the chest cavity**

(Bailey, 27th Edition, Page 100)

70. Orbital fractures–Order of frequency:

(a) Floor, medial wall, lateral wall and roof (b) Floor, lateral wall, roof, medial wall
(c) Floor, roof, medial wall, lateral wall (d) Lateral wall, medial wall, Floor, Roof

Ans: (a) Floor, medial wall, lateral wall and roof

- Bones that comprise the orbit can be fractured and in order of frequency, the floor, medial wall, lateral wall and roof may be disrupted either in combination or as isolated injuries

(Bailey, 27th Edition, Page 360)

71. Indications for damage control surgery *except:*

(a) Temperature < 34°C (b) pH < 7.2
(c) Prothrombin time >16 sec (d) Serum lactate >3 mmol/Litre

Ans: (d) Serum lactate >3 mmol/Litre

INDICATIONS OF DAMAGE CONTROL SURGERY

Anatomical	Physiological (Decline of physiological reserve)	Environmental
Inability to achieve aemostasis Complex abdominal injury Like liver, pancreas Combined vascular, solid and hollow organ injury like aortic/aval injury Inaccessible major venous injury, Like retrohepatic vena cava Demand for non-operative control of injuries like fracture pelvis Anticipated need of time-consuming procedure	Temperature <34°C pH <7.2 Serum lactate >5 mmol/L Prothrombin time (PT) >16 s PTT > 60 s >10 units blood transfused Systolic blood pressure <90 mmHg for >60 min	Operating time >60 min (core temperature loss in usually 2°C/hour) Inability to approximate abdominal incision Desire to reassess the intra-abdominal contents

(Bailey 27th Edition, Page 379)

72. Which of the following is factors of venous hypertension resulting from vascular compression including all *except?*

(a) May Thurner syndrome
(b) Pelvic tumor
(c) Pelvic radiotherapy
(d) Thrombosis

Ans: (d) Thrombosis

Dysfunction of the Venous System Causing Venous Hypertension
Venous Structural Deficit • Valvular agenesis • Valvular incompetence • Venous dilatation • Venous tortuosity • Loss of vein wall compliance • Loss of venous tone • Arteriovenous fistula
Venous Occlusion • Agenesis • Thrombosis • Iatrogenic/trauma
Venous Compression • May-Thurner syndrome • Pelvic/abdominal tumor • Pelvic/abdominal radiotherapy

(Bailey, 27th Edition, Page 971)

73. Type 2 error:

(a) True negative
(b) False negative
(c) True positive
(d) False positive

Ans: (b) False negative

- Type 1 error: Benefit is perceived when really there is none (false positive)
- Type 2 error: Benefit is missed when it was there to be found (false negative)

(Bailey, 27th Edition, Page 164)

74. Most common site for accessory breast is:

(a) Axilla (b) Groin

(c) Buttock (d) Thigh

Ans: (a) Axilla

- Accessory breasts are seen in axilla (most frequent site), groin, buttock and thigh

(Bailey, 27th Edition, Page 865)

75. Most common complication following ERCP is:

(a) Duodenal perforation (b) Sepsis

(c) Hemorrhage (d) Pancreatitis

Ans: (b) Sepsis

- **Complications specific to ERCP** include duodenal perforation (1.3%)/haemorrhage (1.4%) after scope insertion or sphincterotomy, pancreatitis (4.3%) and sepsis (3-30%); mortality rate approaches 1%

(Bailey, 27th Edition, Page 208)

76. According to tile classification most common type of pelvic ring fracture:

(a) A (b) C

(c) B (d) D

Ans: (a) A

Type A

Type A are most common fractures and are completely stable. They result from lateral compression, which causes compression fractures of pubic rami or compression fracture of sacrum posteriorly

Type B

These fractures are partially stable, and there is disruption of anterior pelvis and partial disruption of the posterior pelvis. The pelvis can open and close 'like a book', but because sacroiliac ligaments remain intact, there is no vertical displacement. Internal or external stabilisation is required. Blood loss can be significant

Type C

This fracture is completely unstable. Both anterior pelvis and entire posterior pelvic complexes are disrupted and disrupted pelvic bones are free to displace horizontally and vertically. In both type B and type C pelvic injuries, there is high risk of associated abdominal injuries (bowel perforation or mesenteric laceration) and rupture of diaphragm

(Bailey, 27th Edition, Page 377)

77. Painful arc syndrome is tested by eliciting pain during abduction from:

(a) 60 to 120 degrees (b) 60 to 90 degrees

(c) 90 to 120 degrees (d) 75 to 120 degrees

Ans: (a) 60 to 120 degrees

- Painful arc test: Ask the patient to abduct their arms from their sides. The presence of pain from 60° to 120° is positive

(Bailey, 27th Edition, Page 449)

78. "4P" Strategy for liver trauma management include all *except:*

(a) Pack (b) Push

(c) Pringle (d) Pluck

Ans: (d) Pluck

Operative Management of Liver Injuries Can Be Summarised as '4Ps'
• Push
• Pringle
• Pluck
• Pack

(Bailey and Love, 27th Edition, Page 374)

PAPER 3

79. Causes of secondary hyperparathyroidism include all *except:*

(a) Chronic renal failure
(b) Lithium induced hyperparathyroidism
(c) Persistent autonomous PTH secretion after renal transplant
(d) Hypermagnesemia induced hyperparathyroidism

Ans: (c) Persistent autonomous PTH secretion after renal transplant

Secondary Hyperparathyroidism
Chronic renal failure
25 (OH) vitamin D deficiency
Malabsorption syndromes: Celiac disease, Cystic fibrosis, Short gut syndrome, Bariatric procedures
Medications: Lithium, Diuretics (e.g., hydrochlorothiazide, furosemide)
Metabolic abnormalities: Hypermagnesemia, Hyperphosphatemia
Congenital disorders: Transient neonatal hyperparathyroidism, DiGeorge syndrome

(Sabiston, 20th Edition, Page 928)

80. A 24-year-old woman is scheduled for an elective cholecystectomy. The best method of identifying a potential bleeder is which of the following?

(a) Platelet count
(b) A complete history and physical examination
(c) Bleeding time
(d) Prothrombin time

Ans: (b) A complete history and physical examination

- A history of bleeding should alert the clinician to evaluate the underlying cause
- Bleeding time is influenced by those factors affecting platelet and capillary integrity
- Prolongation of the PT may be attributed to decreased absorption of fat-soluble vitamin K, liver impairment, or decrease in the blood components because of consumption

(Schwartz, 10th Edition, Page 88)

81. Which of the following ruptures in "penile rupture"?

(a) Tunica albuginea
(b) Tunica vaginalis
(c) Bucks fascia
(d) None of above

Ans: (a) Tunica albuginea

- Fracture of the penis is an uncommon accident, usually occurring when the erect penis is bent violently during intercourse
- The forced deformity results in a rupture of the tunica albuginea with immediate extravasation of blood from within the penis

- There is typically a loud cracking sound with immediate loss of the erection, and the rapid development of a large bruise around the penis and extending onto scrotum
- There may occasionally be an associated urethral injury
- Optimal management involves early exploration of the penis with surgical repair of the ruptured tunica albuginea

(Bailey, 27th Edition, Page 1489)

82. Success rate of intracytoplasmic sperm injection (ICSI):

(a) 10% (b) 20%

(c) 30% (d) 40 %

Ans: (c) 30%

Male Infertility
• Atrophy of the testis is associated with raised levels of follicle stimulating hormone in blood
• Testicular biopsy will show whether azoospermia is a result of obstruction or failure of sperm production
• ***If spermatozoa can be harvested they can be used in intracytoplasmic sperm injection with a fertility rate of around 30%***

(Bailey, 27th Edition, Page 1512)

83. All are included in 'Rule of 2s' radiography for trauma *except:*

(a) 2 views (b) 2 occasions

(c) 2 joints (d) 2 modalities

Ans: (d) 2 modalities

Radiographs are mainstay in initial evaluation of suspected extremity trauma
Rule of 2's should be remembered
• **2 views**–Ensure acquisition of 2 views in orthogonal planes to avoid missing a fracture out of plane on the first radiograph view. For shoulder injuries ensure at least an AP and axillary or modified axillary view
• **2 joints**–Radiographs are required of the joint above and joint below the fracture
• **2 occasions**–Sometimes the fracture may not be initially visible; a second series of radiographs should be undertaken after 10-14 days if suspicion of bony injury persists. The classic injury here is a scaphoid fracture. If initial scaphoid views are normal, consider repeating them 10-14 days later, if pain and tenderness in the anatomical snuff box persists
• **2 sides**–In paediatric injuries it can be useful to consider radiograph from opposite and uninjured side if doubt exists. With improved access to atlases of normal variants this is less important

(Bailey, 27th Edition, Page 384)

84. Ganga classification is for:

(a) Closed soft tissue injury (b) Severe open injury

(c) Paediatric fractures (d) Pelvic fractures

Ans: (b) Severe open injury

- Tscherne classification for closed injuries
- Gustilo and Anderson for open injuries
- Ganga classification of severe open injuries

(Bailey, 27th Edition, Page 385)

85. Percentage of bone metastasis in spine that are symptomatic:

(a) 5% (b) 10%

(c) 15% (d) 20%

Ans: (b) 10%

- **Carcinomas usually spread to bone by haematogenous route:**
- Spine is the third most common site for metastases, after the lung and liver
- Although most patients with metastatic cancer will have hone metastases in the spine before they die, only 10% are symptomatic

(Bailey, 27th Edition, Page 537)

86. Which has low risk of progression to malignant disease of bone and cartilage?

(a) Olliers disease (b) Chronic osteomyelitis
(c) Familial retinoblastoma syndrome (d) Maffucci syndrome

Ans: (b) Chronic osteomyelitis

Increased Risk of Malignant Disease in Bone and Cartilage		
High Risk	**Medium Risk**	**Low Risk**
Maffucci syndrome Ollier disease Familial retinoblastoma syndrome	Hereditary multiple exostosis Polyostotic Paget's disease Radiation osteitis	Chronic osteomyelitis Osteonecrosis Fibrous dysplasia, Osteogenesis imperfect, Osteoblastoma and chondroblastoma

(Bailey, 27th Edition, Page 537)

87. Minor head injury is:

(a) GCS4 or 15 with LOC (b) GCS5 with no LOC
(c) GCS-13 (d) GCS-8

Ans: (b) GCS5 with no LOC

Head Injury Classification Using Glasgow Coma Scale Score			
Minor	**Mild**	**Moderate**	**Severe**
GCS 15 with no loss of consciousness	GCS 14/15 with Loss of consciousness	GCS 9-13	GCS 3-8

(Bailey, 27th Edition, Page 329)

88. Which of the following is not useful in diagnosis of deep seated abscess?

(a) USG (b) CT
(c) Contrast radiographs (d) MRI

Ans: (c) Contrast radiographs

- Plain or contrast radiographs may not be helpful, but ultrasonography, computed tomography (CT), magnetic resonance imaging (MRI) and isotope labeled white cell scans are all useful and may allow guided aspiration without the need for surgical intervention

(Bailey, 27th Edition, Page 48)

89. At 1 year of age ____ % of boys have a non retractile foreskin.

(a) 10% (b) 30%
(c) 50% (d) 70%

Ans: (c) 50%

- At birth, the foreskin is adherent to the glans penis
- These adhesions separate spontaneously with time, allowing foreskin to become retractile
- At 1 year of age, about 50% of boys have a non-retractile foreskin. By 4 years this has declined to 10% and by 16 years to just 1 %

(Bailey, 27th Edition, Page 126)

90. Which the following is false in cellulitis?

(a) Suppurative (b) Well localised

(c) Blood culture often positive (d) All are false

Ans: (d) All are false

- **Cellulitis is a nonsuppurative, invasive infection of tissues, which is usually related to the point of injury**
- There is poor localisation in addition to the cardinal signs of spreading inflammation
- They are typically caused by organisms such as: 3-haemolytic streptococci, staphylococci and Clostridium perfringens
- Tissue destruction, gangrene and ulceration may follow, which are caused by release of proteases

(Bailey, 27th Edition, Page 46)

91. Tracheostomy reduce anatomical dead space by:

(a) 30% (b) 40%

(c) 50% (d) 70 %

Ans: (c) 50%

All forms of tracheostomy and cricothyroidotomy bypass upper airway, have following advantages

- Anatomical dead space is reduced by approximately 50%
- Work of breathing is reduced
- Alveolar ventilation is increased
- Level of sedation needed for patient comfort is decreased and, unlike endotracheal intubation, the patient may be able to talk and eat with a tube in place

(Bailey, 27th Edition, Page 747)

92. _____% of non clostridial gas producing organism causing gas gangrene post trauma.

(a) 10-20% (b) 30-40%

(c) 40-60% (d) 60-80%

Ans: (d) 60-80%

- Most common causative organism is *Clostridium perfringens*, a spore-forming, gram-positive saprophyte that flourishes in anaerobic conditions
- Other organisms implicated in gas gangrene include Clostridium bifermentansy Clostridium septicum and Clostridium sporogenes
- ***Non-clostridial gas-producing organisms such as coliforms have also been isolated in 60-85% of cases of gas gangrene***

(Bailey, 27th Edition, Page 420)

93. Power ratio is:

(a) Occipito Atlantal fracture

(b) Occipital condyle fracture

(c) Thoracic or thoracolumbar fractures

(d) Odontoid fractures

Ans: (a) Occipito Atlantal fracture

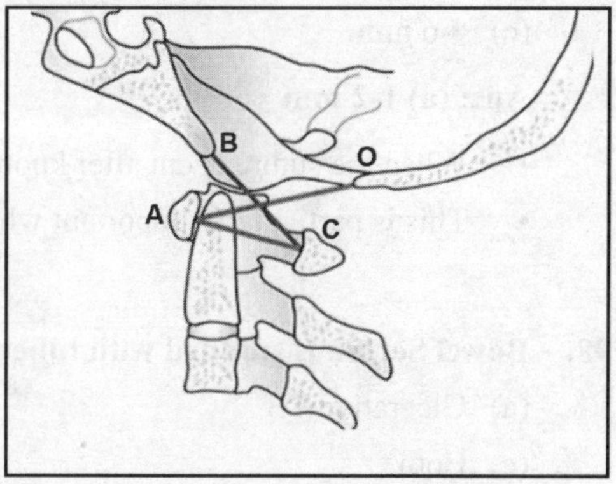

- Power's ratio is used to assess skull translation and indicates Occipito Atlantal fracture
- **Power's ratio:** BC/OA >1 indicates anterior translation, <0.75 indicates posterior translation

(Bailey, 27th Edition, Page 346)

94. Most common cause of bleeding in hemothorax is:

(a) Intercostal vessels
(b) Internal mammary artery
(c) Superior epigastric artery
(d) Superior thoracic artery

Ans: (a) Intercostal vessels

Most common cause of massive haemothorax in blunt injury is continuing bleeding from torn intercostal vessels or occasionally from internal mammary artery secondary to fractures of ribs

(Bailey, 27th Edition, Page 368)

95. During use harmonic scaple vibrate in .... range to cut tissue:

(a) 1000-2000 Hz
(b) 2000-5000 Hz
(c) 20000-50000 Hz
(d) 3000-7000 Hz

Ans: (c) 20000-50000 Hz

- Harmonic scalpel is an instrument that uses ultrasound technology to cut tissues while simultaneously sealing them
- It utilises a hand-held ultrasound transducer and scalpel which is controlled by hand switch or foot pedal
- *During use, the scalpel vibrates in the 20000-50000 Hz range and cuts through tissues, effecting haemostasis by sealing vessels and tissues by means of protein denaturation caused by vibration rather than heat*

(Bailey, 27th Edition, Page 104)

96. Thyroidectomy drain removed after:

(a) 24 hours
(b) 48 hours
(c) 72 hours
(d) 5th day

Ans: (a) 24 hour

- Drains put in to cover perioperative bleeding may usually be removed after 24 hours, e.g., thyroidectomy
- Drains put in to drain serous collections usually can be removed after 5 days, e.g., mastectomy
- Drains put in because of infection should be left until the infection is subsiding or the drainage is minimal
- Drains put in to cover colorectal anastomoses should be removed at about 5-7 days. However, it should be stressed that in no way does a drain prevent any intestinal leakage, but merely may assist any such leakage to drain externally rather than to produce life-threatening peritonitis
- Common bile duct T-tubes should remain in for 10 days

(Bailey, 27th Edition, Page 101)

97. Ends should be left how much after cutting Suture Knot of monofilament suture?

(a) 1-2 mm
(b) 2-4 mm
(c) 4-6 mm
(d) 1 cm

Ans: (a) 1-2 mm

- When the suture is cut after knotting, the ends should be left about 1-2 mm long to prevent unraveling
- This is particularly important when using monofilament material

(Bailey, 27th Edition, Page 95)

98. Bowel Serosa is studded with tubercle in:

(a) Ulcerative TB
(b) Hyperblastic TB
(c) Both
(d) None

Ans: (a) Ulcerative TB

- **Ulcerative type:** When a patient with pulmonary tuberculosis swallows infected sputum, organism colonises lymphatics of terminal ileum, causing transverse ulcers with typical undermined edges. ***Serosa is usually studded with tubercles.*** Histology shows caseating granuloma with giant cells. This pathological entity, referred to as ulcerative type, denotes severe form of the disease in which virulence of organism overwhelms host resistance
- **Hyperplastic type:** This occurs when host resistance has upper hand over Virulence of organism. It is caused by drinking infected unpasteurised milk. There is marked inflammatory reaction causing hyperplasia and thickening of terminal ileum because of its abundance of lymphoid follicles, thus resulting in narrowing of the lumen and obstruction. Macroscopically, this type may be confused with Crohn's disease. Small intestine shows areas of stricture and fibrosis, most pronounced at the terminal ileum. As a result, there is shortening of bowel with the caecum being pulled up into a subhepatic position

(Bailey, 27th Edition, Page 79)

99. Beahrs triangle border formed by all *except:*

(a) Recurrent laryngeal nerve
(b) Common carotid artery
(c) Inferior thyroid artery
(d) Superior thyroid artery

Ans: (d) Superior thyroid artery

- In terms of surgical anatomy, RLN can be located in the tracheosophageal groove where it forms one side of Beahrs' triangle (the other two sides are the carotid artery and inferior thyroid artery) or at cricothyroid joint

(Bailey, 27th Edition, Page 802)

100. Short stay surgery defined as:

(a) Admission of up to 12 hours
(b) Admission of up to 24 hours
(c) Admission of up to 48 hours
(d) Admission of up to 72 hours

Ans: (d) Admission of up to 72 hours

- **Outpatient surgery:** Not admitted to a ward facility
- **Procedure room surgery:** Surgery not requiring full sterile theatre facilities
- **Day or same-day surgery:** Admitted and discharged within the 12-hour day
- **Overnight stay:** 23-hour admission with early morning discharge
- **Short-stay surgery:** Admission of up to 72 hours

(Bailey, 27th Edition, Page 301)

101. Late post operative complication define as:

(a) Complication 6 hours within surgery
(b) Complication 6-72 hours after surgery
(c) Complication after 72 hours of surgery
(d) Complication with in 72 hours of surgery

Ans: (c) Complication after 72 hours of surgery

There are three common approaches for classification of postoperative complications of surgery:

- **Linked to time after surgery:** Immediate (within 6 hours of procedure); early (6-72 hours); late (>72 hours)
- **Generic and surgery specific**
- **Clavian-Dindo:** This system relates to surgical complications only and is used to objectively and reproducibly measure impact of surgical complication on outcome of procedure

(Bailey, 27th Edition, Page 292)

102. Rate of regrowth of nerve fibre per day:

(a) 0.5 mm
(b) 1mm
(c) 1.5 mm
(d) 2 mm

Ans: (b) 1 mm

Seddon classified nerve injuries into neurapraxia, axonotmesis and neurotmesis:

Neurapraxia–No loss of nerve sheath continuity or peripheral Wallerian degeneration. Recovery potential good may take months if the pressure is removed from the nerve

Axonotmesis–Nerve sheath remains intact, with internal nerve fibre damage with Wallerian degeneration. Neural tube (endoneurium) can guide the regenerating nerve fibres to their target. Good potential for recovery; nerve fibre regrowth is at 1 mm per day

Neurotmesis–Complete division of the nerve, nerve sheath and nerve fibre. Functionally poor outcome without surgical intervention to restore continuity of the nerve sheath

103. After major surgery maintenence fluid should be restricted to:

(a) 60% (b) 70%

(c) 80% (d) 90%

Ans: (b) 70%

- Body's response to stress is to hold on towater, which can promote hyponatraemia
- Stresses that drive the non-osmotic retention of water include trauma, head injury, chest infections and the postoperative state
- Restricting maintenance fluids to 70% can be appropriate for 24 hours after major surgery. In sick patients, raising maintenance rate is best guided by trend in daily electrolyte levels
- Urine output often decreases after major surgery without morbidity but a common response can be to increase maintenance fluids inappropriately, leading to hyponatraemia
- A postoperative bolus of fluid is appropriate if there is hypovolaemia, hypotension or poor peripheral perfusion but giving it simply because urine output is low can be inappropriate

(Bailey, 27th Edition, Page 121)

104. Down sydrome associated with which atresia?

(a) Duodenal (b) Ileal

(c) Colonic (d) Rectal

Ans: (a) Duodenal

- Duodenal atresia may take form of a membrane or proximal and distal duodenum may be completely separated
- Prenatal ultrasound finds a 'double bubble' in the fetal abdomen with polyhydramnios. There is an association with Down syndrome
- Postnatally, there is bilious vomiting if the atresia is distal to the ampulla. A plain abdominal X-ray also shows the double-bubble
- **Repair is by open duodenoduodenostomy**
- Occasionally, there is a duodenal membrane with a modest central perforation, which may delay symptoms until later childhood

(Bailey, 27th Edition, Page 133)

105. Most common cyanotic congenital heart disease:

(a) TGA (b) TAPVC

(c) TOF (d) Tricuspid atresia

Ans: (c) TOF

TETRALOGY OF FALLOT

- Most common cyanotic congenital heart disease found in children surviving to 1 year and accounts for about 4-6% of all congenital heart diseases

(Bailey, 27th Edition, Page 904)

106. Cause of non-filarial elephantiasis is:

(a) Syphilis (b) Lymphogranuloma venerum

(c) Brugia malyayi (d) All above

Ans: (b) Lymphogranuloma venerum

- Elephantiasis can occur in the absence of filariasis, most notably in sub-Saharan Africa
- Nonfilarial elephantiasis can result from fibrosis of lymphatics caused by lymphogranuloma venereum, but in many cases it is thought to arise as a consequence of persistent contact with irritant soils

(Bailey, 27th Edition, Page1510)

107. Percentage of patients with undescended testis having hernia is:

(a) 60% (b) 70%

(c) 80% (d) 90%

Ans: (d) 90%

- Around 90% of boys with an undescended testis have a patent processus vaginalis although the incidence of a clinically apparent hernia is much lower

(Bailey, 27th Edition, Page 1498)

108. Varicocele left sided in how much %?

(a) 50% (b) 60%

(c) 70% (d) 90%

Ans: (d) 90%

- Varicocele is a common condition and 90% are left-sided
- Development of left-sided varicocele in later life may indicate presence of renal tumor
- They are usually asymptomatic and as such rarely need treatment
- First-line treatment is embolisation in symptomatic cases
- Varicoceles often recur, even after surgical treatment

(Bailey, 27th Edition, Page 1502)

109. Most common cause of epididymo-orchitis in young sexually active men is:

(a) Chlamydia (b) Gonorrhoea

(c) Syphilis (d) LGV

Ans: (a) Chlamydia

- In young sexually active men, the most common cause of epididymitis is now *Chlamydia trachomatis,* but gonococcal epididymitis is still occasionally seen
- In older men with bladder outflow obstruction, epididymitis may result from a urinary infection–it is proposed that a high pressure in prostatic urethra might cause reflux of infected urine up vasa

(Bailey, 27th Edition, Page 1505)

110. Most common site of ectopic testis is:

(a) Superficial inguinal pouch (b) Deep inguinal pouch

(c) Femoral triangle (d) Root of penis

Ans: (a) Superficial inguinal pouch

- An ectopic testis has taken a non-standard path through the body and has ended up in an unusual location, most common site being the superficial inguinal pouch, which lies just inferior and medial to the superficial inguinal ring
- Other rarer ectopic sites include femoral triangle, the root of the penis and perineum

(Bailey, 27th Edition, Page 1498)

111. Adequate pressure for chest drain bottle to obtain gentle flow of bubbles from chest cavity:

(a) 10-20 mm Hg (b) 20-30 mm Hg
(c) 30-40 mm Hg (d) 40-50 mm Hg

Ans: (a) 10-20 mm Hg

Chest Drains:

- These are indicated for a pneumothorax, pleural effusion, haemothorax or to prevent the collection of fluid or air after thoracotomy. Once the drain has been inserted, it should be connected to an underwater sealed drain
- This system allows air to leave pleural cavity, but it cannot be drawn back in by the negative pressure that is created in intrathoracic cavity
- During the respiratory process, it should he checked that the meniscus of the fluid is swinging, to ensure that tube is not blocked
- Suction can be applied to venting tube at the bottle whenever there is significant drainage of fluid or air expected
- ***Between 10 and 20 mm of mercury is adequate to obtain a gentle flow of bubbles from chest cavity***

(Bailey, 27th Edition, Page 100)

112. Uncomplicated ZMC Zygomatico-orbital complex fractures are generally treated within what duration?

(a) 14 days (b) 10 days
(c) 48-72 hours (d) 24-48 hours

Ans: (b) 10 days

- Uncomplicated ZMC fractures are generally treated within 10 days of injury

(Bailey, 27th Edition, Page 359)

113. First objective in disaster management:

(a) Triage (b) Damage assessment
(c) Mobilizing resources (d) Rescue operation

Ans: (b) Damage assessment

- First objective in disaster management is an assessment of damage and number of casualties

(Bailey, 27th Edition, Page 410)

114. All of the following are Absorbable Sutures *except:*

(a) Polyglactin (b) Polyglyconate
(c) Polyglycaprone (d) Polybutester

Ans: (d) Polybutester

- Polybutester is a Monofilament may be dyed/undyed with infinite strength
- It remains encapsulated in body tissues
- Low tissue reaction
- Exhibits a degree of elasticity
- Particularly favoured for use in plastic surgery

(Bailey, 27th Edition, Page 38)

115. Inhalation agent of choice in children:

(a) Sevoflurane
(b) Desflurane
(c) Isoflurane
(d) None of the above

Ans: (a) Sevoflurane

- Inhalational induction using agents such as non-pungent sevoflurane is useful in children, needle-phobic adults and those in whom a difficult airway is anticipated)
- These patients will have a higher risk of developing airway obstruction

(Bailey, 27th Edition, Page 270)

116. Contraindication for IVRA/Bier's block is:

(a) Lignocaine
(b) Prilocaine
(c) Bupivacaine
(d) Ropivacaine

Ans: (c) Bupivacaine

- Bier's Hock produces excellent anaesthesia for short surgery, particularly for the upper limb (e.g., carpal tunnel release)
- Exsanguination using an Esmarch bandage, inflation of proximal cuff of double tourniquet is followed by intravenous injection of prilocaine into the vein on back of the hand that is being operated on
- After 5-10 minutes the distal cuff of the tourniquet is inflated and then the proximal one deflated
- Even if surgery is finished, the tourniquet should be left inflated until the local anaesthetic has hound to tissues (20 minutes), so that release of local anaesthetic into the systemic circulation does not occur
- Lignocaine can be used with caution (consider safe dose and time of tourniquet inflation) but bupivacaine should never be used for Bier's block

(Bailey, 27th Edition, Page 275)

117. Grade 3 of World Federation of Neurological Surgeons grading of SAH corresponds to GCS of:

(a) 3-9
(b) 15
(c) 7-12
(d) 13-14

Ans: (d) 13-14

Grade	GCS	Focal deficits
I	15	-
II	13-14	-
III	13-14	+
IV	7-12	+/-
V	3-9	+/-

(Bailey, 27th Edition, Page 659)

118. All are true about blooms syndrome *except:*

(a) Caused by BLM helicase gene
(b) Autosomal dominant
(c) Sensitive to UV light
(d) Causes leukemia, lymphoma

Ans: (b) Autosomal dominant

- Defect in *BLM helicase*
- *Autosomal recessive*
- Sensitivity to ultraviolet light causes Leukaemia and Lymphoma
- Active surveillance

(Bailey, 27th Edition, Page 145)

PART FOUR: PRACTICE PAPERS

CHAPTER

64

MULTIPLE CHOICE QUESTIONS (PAPERS)

PAPER 1

1. Which of the following are not included in features of malignant transformation?

(a) Acquire ability to invade
(b) Resist signals that stimulate growth
(c) Evade detection
(d) Obtain replicative immortality

Ans: (b) Resist signals that stimulate growth

Hanahan and Weinberg Features of Malignant Transformation
• Establish an autonomous lineage–Resist signals that inhibit growth, Sustain proliferative signalling
• Obtain replicative immortality
• Evade apoptosis
• Acquire angiogenic competence
• Acquire ability to invade
• Acquire ability to disseminate and implant
• Evocation of inflammation
• Evade detection/elimination
• Jettison excess baggage
• Subvert communication to and from the cellular environment
• Develop ability to change energy metabolism

(Bailey, 27th Edition, Page 140)

2. Most common malignant neoplasm in Li Fraumeni syndrome is:

(a) Soft tissue sarcoma
(b) Breast cancers
(c) Brain tumors
(d) Adrenocortical carcinoma

Ans: (b) Breast cancers

- Most common malignant neoplasm in Li Fraumeni syndrome is Breast cancer.

Defined
• A proband diagnosed with sarcoma before the age of 45 years, with
• A first-degree relative with any cancer diagnosed before the age of 45 years, plus
• An additional first or second-degree relative with either sarcoma at any age or any cancer before age of 45 years

(Sabiston, 20th Edition, Page 690)

3. Which of the following is not a component of Xeroderma pigmentosum?

(a) Early onset SCC/BCC
(b) Defective nucleotide excision repair
(c) Autosomal dominant
(d) Retinoids are used for chemoprevention

Ans: (c) Autosomal dominant

- Autosomal recessive disorder
- Caused by mutations in the genes involved in nucleotide excision repair
- Characterized by extreme photosensitivity and 2000-fold increased risk of skin cancer
- Early onset Skin cancers–SCC/BCC
- Mutations in *ras* and *p53* genes occur early in skin cancers, mainly at dipyrimidine sequences
- Retinoids are used for Chemoprevention of cancer

(Sabiston, 20th Edition, Page 695)

4. Which is correctly matched–Chemical carcinogen with predominant cancer?

(a) Aflatoxins–Pancreatic cancer
(b) Benzidine–Lung cancer
(c) Cadmium–Lung cancer
(d) Nickel–Oral cancers

Ans: (c) Cadmium–Lung cancer

Chemical Carcinogen	Predominant Cancer
Aflatoxins	HCC
Arsenic	Skin cancer
Asbestos	Lung cancer, Mesothelioma
Cadmium	Lung cancer
Chromium	Lung cancer
Benzidine	Urinary bladder
Beryllium	Lung cancer
Ethylene oxide	Leukemia, Lymphoma
Vinyl chloride	Hepatic angiosarcoma, Hepatocellular carcinoma, Brain tumors, lung cancer, Hematopoietic malignant neoplasms
Nickel	Lung cancer, Nasal cancer

(Sabiston, 20th Edition, Page 695)

5. Which of the following drugs doesn't act by forming DNA Adducts?

(a) Cisplatin
(b) Carboplatin
(c) Oxaliplatin
(d) Ifosfamide

Ans: (d) Ifosfamide

- Ifosfamide forms DNA Cross links
- Used in Small cell cancer Lung and Sarcoma

(Sabiston, 20th Edition, Page 155)

6. Which of the following is not true about CEA?

(a) Elevated CEA levels reflect the burden of tumor
(b) Elevated CEA levels occur in only 5% to 40% of patients with localized disease
(c) Most common application of CEA is in monitoring of patients for recurrent disease
(d) CEA is useful as a screening test

Ans: (d) CEA is useful as a screening test

- CEA is not useful as a screening test because of low sensitivity in early-stage disease
- Elevated CEA levels occur in only 5% to 40% of patients with localized disease
- Most common application of CEA is in monitoring of patients for recurrent disease
- CEA is most sensitive for hepatic or retroperitoneal metastasis and relatively insensitive for local, pulmonary, or peritoneal involvement

(Sabiston, 20th Edition, Page 698)

7. **Which of the following is the mechanism of action of Ronacicilb?**

(a) Resist signals that inhibit growth
(b) Sustaining proliferative signaling
(c) Obtain replicative immortality
(d) Genomic instability

Ans: (a) Resist signals that inhibit growth

TARGETED TREATMENTS MAPPED TO THE HALLMARKS OF CANCER

Hallmark	Drug Classes	Specific Drugs
Resist signals that inhibit growth	Cyclin Dependent kinase inhibitors	Dinaciclib, Palbociclib Ronaciclib, Seliciclib
Sustaining proliferative signaling	EGFR Inhibitors	Trastuzumab, Cetuximab
Avoid immune detection	CTLA 4, PD 1, PD L1	Nivolumab, Ipilumumab, Pembrolizumab
Genomic instability	PARP Inhibitors	Olaparib, Niraparib, Rucaparib,
Obtain replicative immortality	Telomerase inhibitors	Imetelstat

(Bailey, 27th Edition, Page 158)

8. **All are true regarding Ipilimumab *except:***

(a) Ipilimumab effectively prolongs T cell response
(b) Blockade can induce tumor regression
(c) Ipilimumab is the FDA approved drug that blocks CTLA 4
(d) Ipilimumab demonstrate improved disease free survival in patients with metastatic melanoma

Ans: (d) Ipilimumab demonstrate improved disease free survival in patients with metastatic melanoma

IPILIMUMAB

- Ipilimumab is a monoclonal anti-CTLA-4 antibody that was the first systemic agent to demonstrate improved overall survival in patients with metastatic melanoma
- In activated T cells, CTLA-4 receptor traffics to the extracellular membrane, where it inhibits costimulatory ligands on antigen-presenting cells and thereby prevents continued antigen-presenting cell stimulation of the T cell
- By blocking CTLA-4, ipilimumab effectively prolongs T cell response
- Ipilimumab is FDA approved for treatment of metastatic melanoma

(Sabiston, 20th Edition, Page 743)

9. **Which of the following statements are true about Ferguson-Smith syndrome?**

(a) Autosomal dominant inheritance
(b) Ch. 9q is involved
(c) Multiple self-healing squamous cell carcinomas
(d) All of the above

Ans: (d) All of the above

FERGUSON-SMITH SYNDROME: Rare, Autosomal dominant inherited abnormality on Chromosome 9q in which affected individuals develop multiple self-healing squamous cell carcinoma

KERATOACANTHOMA is involved in self healing SCC

(Bailey, 27th Edition, Page 606)

10. **Which of the following statements is not true about inverted papilloma?**

(a) Inverted papillomas can undergo malignant change
(b) Histologically the hyperplastic epithelium inverts into underlying stroma
(c) Papillomas are covered with Squamous epithelium
(d) Calcification within tumor is seen on CT with sclerosis of bone at margins of growth

Ans: (c) Papillomas are covered with Squamous epithelium

- Inverted papillomas can occur both in the nasal cavity and the nasal sinuses
- Histologically hyperplastic epithelium inverts into the underlying stroma

- Papillomas are covered with transitional epithelium and also called as Transitional cell papilloma
- Calcification within tumor may be seen on CT along with sclerosis of bone at the margins of the growth
- Inverted papillomas can undergo malignant change
- Full surgical resection is required and this can usually be performed endoscopically

(Bailey, 27th Edition, Page 723)

11. All are true about Chemodectoma *except:*

(a) Higher incidence in areas where people live at high altitudes
(b) Tumors most commonly present in the 2nd decade
(c) Approximately 10% of patients have a family history.
(d) Association with phaeochromocytoma

Ans: (b) Tumors most commonly present in the 2nd decade

- Higher incidence in areas where people live at high altitudes because of chronic hypoxia leading to carotid body hyperplasia
- Tumors most commonly present in the fifth decade
- Approximately 10% of patients have a family history.
- Asociated with phaeochromocytoma
- Tumors arise from chemoreceptor cells on the medial side of carotid bulb and at this point, tumor is adherent to carotid wall

(Bailey, 27th Edition, Page 757)

12. Who proposed the concept of *"field cancerisation"*?

(a) Slaughter
(b) Kocher
(c) Ewald
(d) Avery

Ans: (a) Slaughter

- Slaughter proposed the concept of held change or 'field cancerisation'

(Bailey, 27th Edition, Page 762)

13. Which of the following is least associated with soft tissue sarcoma?

(a) NF 1
(b) Li Fraumeni syndrome
(c) FAP
(d) MEN 1

Ans: (d) MEN 1

- NF 1, Li Fraumeni syndrome and FAP are associated with Soft tissue sarcoma

(Sabiston, 20th Edition, Page 754)

14. Which of the following statement is false about Ewing's sarcoma?

(a) Small blue cell malignant neoplasm of bone
(b) Shares common translocation, t(11;22)(q24;q12), in 10% of cases
(c) Surgical extirpation in conjunction with chemotherapy is the preferred treatment
(d) Exquisitely sensitive to chemotherapy and radiation treatment

Ans: (b) Shares common translocation, t(11;22)(q24;q12), in 10% of cases

EWING'S SARCOMA

- Small blue cell malignant neoplasm of bone with t(11;22)(q24;q12) Translocation in 85% of cases
- Tumor is exquisitely sensitive to chemotherapy and radiation treatment
- Surgical extirpation in conjunction with chemotherapy is the referred treatment

(Sabiston, 20th Edition, Page 784)

15. Which of the following is not true about Breast cancer in Men?

(a) Accounts for 0.8% of all breast cancers
(b) Gynecomastia is not a risk factor
(c) Risk factors include Klinefelter syndrome; family history; and *BRCA2* mutations
(d) 90% of breast cancers in men are invasive ductal carcinomas

Ans: (b) Gynecomastia is not a risk factor

- Accounts for 0.8% of all breast cancers, less than 1% of all newly diagnosed cancers in men, and 0.2% of cancer deaths in men
- Median age at diagnosis is 68 years
- Risk factors related to genetic predisposition include Klinefelter syndrome (47 XXY karyotype); family history; and *BRCA* gene mutations ***(BRCA2* mutations)**
- Gynecomastia is not a risk factor
- ***Contraversial point–Bailey Gynecomastia is a risk factor***
- **DEVITA**–Also mentions that it is not a risk factor

(Sabiston, 20th Edition, Page 861)

16. Transverse upper gracilis–TUG flap is based on:

(a) Superficial inferior epigastric artery
(b) Thoracodorsal artery
(c) Deep inferior epigastric artery
(d) Ascending branch of the medial circumflex femoral artery

Ans: (d) Ascending branch of the medial circumflex femoral artery

- Thoracodorsal artery–LD Flap
- Deep inferior epigastric artery–TRAM flap
- Ascending branch of the medial circumflex femoral artery–TUG flap

(Sabiston 20th Edition, Page 872)

17. Most common mutation in thyroid malignancy is:

(a) BRAF
(b) PPAR gamma
(c) p53
(d) RET

Ans: (a) BRAF

- BRAF mutation is most common mutation in thyroid malignancy
- It is seen in 40% to 50% of PTCs, including 60% of classic PTCs, 10% to 15% of follicular variant of PTC, greater than 90% of tall cell variant PTC and 25% of ATC

(Sabiston, 20th Edition, Page 901)

18. Size of Incision in MIVAP (Video assisted Parathyroidectomy) is:

(a) 1 cm
(b) 1.5 cm
(c) 0.5 cm
(d) 2 cm

Ans: (b) 1.5 cm

- In MIVAP procedure,1.5 cm transverse cervical incisionis made approximately 2 cm above the sternal notch

(Sabiston, 20th Edition, Page 933)

19. Which of the following statement is true *except?*

(a) Glucagonomas are malignant in 50% to 80% of cases
(b) 90% of somatostatinoma are malignant
(c) More than two thirds of VIPoma are malignant
(d) Neurotensinomas are usually Benign

Ans: (d) Neurotensinomas are usually Benign

- Neurotensinomas are usually malignant
- They cause hypokalemia, weight loss, hypotension, cyanosis, flushing and diabetes

(Sabiston, 20th Edition, Page 958)

20. Which of the following statement is not true regarding RET mutation?

(a) RET/PTC rearrangement is associated with Radiation induced thyroid cancers
(b) Gain of function mutation is associated with MEN 2
(c) Somatic mutations are associated with Medullary Thyroid carcinoma
(d) Gain of function mutation is associated with Hirschsprung disease

Ans: (d) Gain of function mutation is associated with Hirschsprung disease

- Loss of function mutation is associated with Hirschsprung disease
- RET/PTC rearrangement is associated with Radiation induced thyroid cancers
- Gain of function mutation is associated with MEN 2
- Somatic mutations are associated with Medullary Thyroid carcinoma

(Schwartz, 10th Edition, Page 1542)

21. A patient is found to have an adrenal tumor incidentally. Tumor is found to be functional. What is the next best step in treatment?

(a) CT every 6 monthly (b) Adrenalectomy
(c) Observation and follow up (d) Steroid administration

Ans: (b) Adrenalectomy

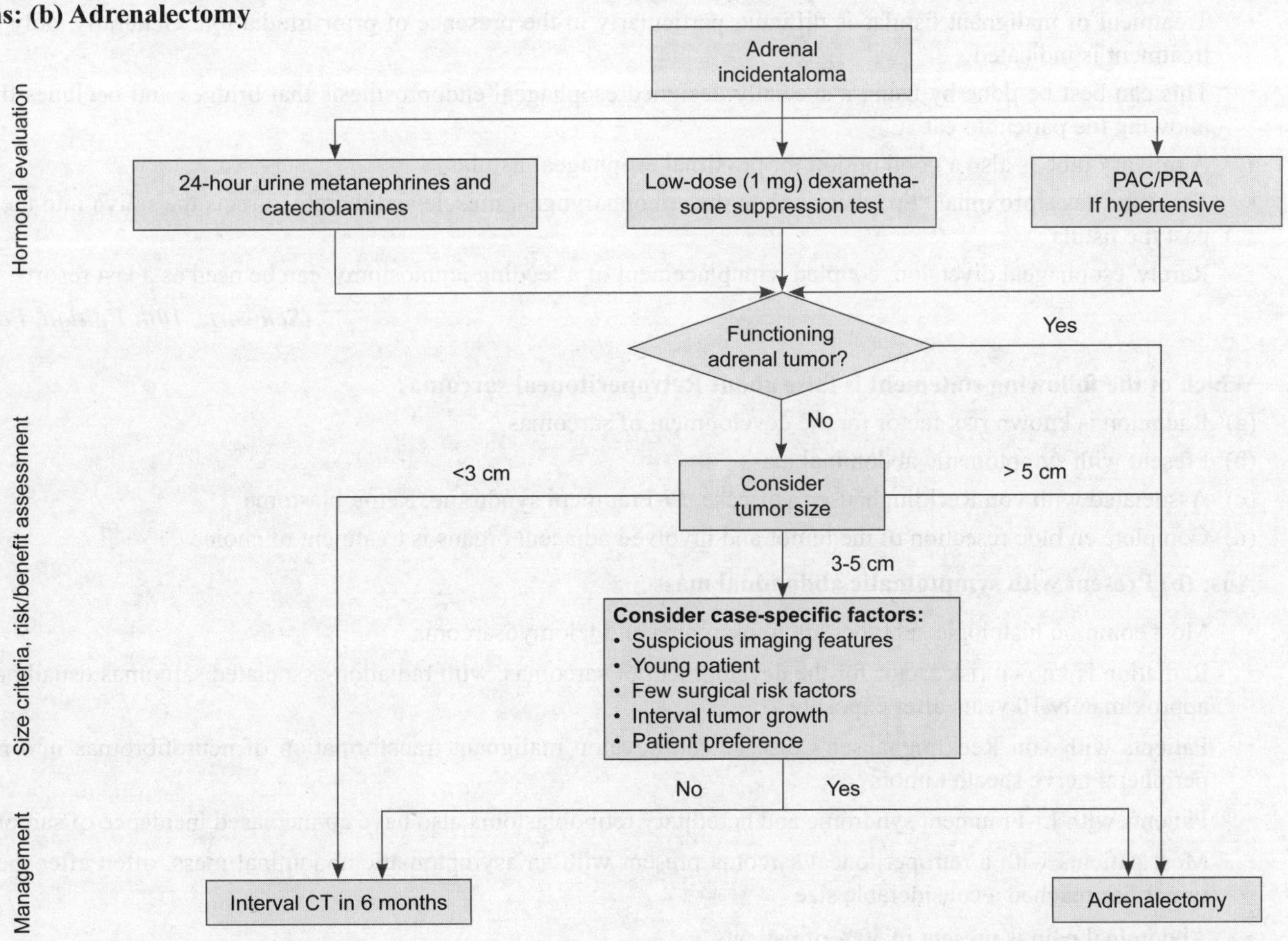

(Sabiston, 20th Edition Page 987)

22. False statement regarding Melanoma of esophagus is:

(a) Accounts for 0.1% to 0.2% of esophageal malignant neoplasms
(b) Primary melanoma is common than small cell carcinoma of the esophagus
(c) Most tumors are manifested at a late stage
(d) Prognosis is generally poor

Ans: (b) Primary melanoma is common than small cell carcinoma of the esophagus

- Primary melanoma of the esophagus is even rarer than small cell carcinoma
- Accounting for 0.1% to 0.2% of esophageal malignant neoplasms
- Similar to small cell carcinoma, most tumors are manifested at a late stage and prognosis is generally poor

(Sabiston, 20th Edition, Page 1032)

23. Which of the following statement is true about Malignant tracheosophageal fistula?

(a) Sign of curable disease
(b) An expanding metal stent is probably the best treatment
(c) Spontaneous closure gives better results in the presence of malignancy
(d) A salivary tube is not a good option for proximal esophageal fistulas

Ans: (b) An expanding metal stent is probably the best treatment

- Most acquired esophageal fistulas are to the tracheobronchial tree, and secondary to either esophageal or pulmonary malignancy
- Spontaneous closure is rare, owing to the presence of malignancy
- Treatment of malignant fistulas is difficult, particularly in the presence of prior irradiation. Generally, only palliative treatment is indicated
- This can best be done by using a specially designed esophageal endoprosthesis that bridges and occludes the fistula, allowing the patient to eat
- A salivary tube is also a good option for proximal esophageal fistulas
- This tube has a proximal "lip" that rests on the cricopharyngeal muscle and thereby directs the saliva into the tube and past the fistula
- Rarely, esophageal diversion, coupled with placement of a feeding jejunostomy, can be used as a last resort

(Schwartz, 10th Edition, Page 1024)

24. Which of the following statement is false about Retroperitoneal sarcoma?

(a) Radiation is known risk factor for the development of sarcomas
(b) Present with symptomatic abdominal mass
(c) Associated with von Recklinghausen's disease, Li-Fraumeni syndrome, Retinoblastoma
(d) Complete en bloc resection of the tumor and involved adjacent organs is treatment of choice

Ans: (b) Present with symptomatic abdominal mass

- Most common histologic subtypes are liposarcoma and leiomyosarcoma
- Radiation is known risk factor for the development of sarcomas, with radiation-associated sarcomas usually occurring approximately 10 years after exposure
- Patients with von Recklinghausen's disease can develop malignant transformation of neurofibromas into malignant peripheral nerve sheath tumors
- Patients with Li-Fraumeni syndrome and hereditary retinoblastoma also have an increased incidence of sarcoma
- Most patients with a retroperitoneal sarcoma present with an asymptomatic abdominal mass, often after the primary tumor has reached a considerable size
- Abdominal pain is present in 50% of patients

(Sabiston, 20th Edition, Page 1088)

25. Which of the following not associated risk factor with Carcinoma stomach?

(a) Low fat diet (b) High protein diet

(c) Salted meat (d) High nitrate consumption

Ans: (b) High protein diet

- High protein diet is nothing related to Carcinoma stomach
- But answer of exclusion is High potein diet

Risk Factors	
Nutritional	**Environmental**
Low fat or protein consumption	Poor food preparation (smoked, salted)
Salted meat or fish	Lack of refrigeration
High nitrate consumption	Poor drinking water–Contaminated well water
High complex carbohydrate consumption	Smoking
Medical	**Social**
Prior gastric surgery	Low social class
H. pylori infection	**Others**
Gastric atrophy and gastritis	Male sex
Adenomatous polyps	

(Sabiston, 20th Edition, Page 1214)

26. Which of the following statements is true about Small intestinal tumors?

(a) Most common site of Hemangioma is Jejunum (b) Most common site of Lipoma is Ileum

(c) Most common site of adenoma is Duodenum (d) Most common site of Adenocarcinoma is Duodenum

Ans: (c) Most common site of adenoma is Duodenum

TUMORS OF SMALL BOWEL: MOST COMMON SITE

- Lipoma–Ileum
- Hemangioma–Jejunum
- Adenoma–Ileum
- Adenocarcinoma–Duodenum
- Lymphoma–Ileum

"Twenty percent of adenomas are found in the duodenum, 30% are found in the jejunum, and 50% are found in the ileum"

(Sabiston, 20th Edition, Page 1269)

27. Large bowel can tolerate properly delivered radiation doses upto :

(a) 6000 cGy (b) 5000 cGy

(c) 4000 cGy (d) 5500 cGy

Ans: (a) 6000 cGy

- **Large bowel can tolerate radiation doses up to 6000 cGy**
- **Small bowel can tolerate below 5000 cGy only**

Radiation Enetritis (Sabiston 20th Edition, Page 1290)
• Acute radiation-induced small bowel disease usually is manifested with colicky abdominal pain, bloating, loss of appetite, nausea, diarrhea, and fecal urgency during or shortly after a course of radiotherapy
• Most patients notice symptoms during the second week of treatment, when tissue damage and inflammation are maximal, and symptoms peak by the fourth week when histologic changes are stable or improving
• Symptoms consistent with chronic radiation injury typically develop between 18 months and 6 years after a completed course of radiotherapy, but symptoms can be manifested up to 30 years after the treatment course
• **Morbidity risk increases with dosages exceeding 5000 cGy**
• *The intensity of injury is related to the dose of radiation administered, with most cases occurring in patients who have received at least 4500 cGy*
• Keeping radiation exposure to below 5000 cGy is associated with minimal long-term side effects and recommended where clinically possible **(Schwartz, Page 1163)**

(Sabiston, 20th Edition, Page 1269)

28. Not true regarding Basal cell carcinoma of anus is:

(a) Characteristic for pearly borders with central depression (b) Treated by wide local excision

(c) APR for extensive lesions or those involving the sphincter mechanism (d) Arises frequently from anal canal

Ans: (d) Arises frequently from anal canal

- Basal cell carcinoma usually arises from anal margin and not canal

Cancers	Anal Margin	Anal Canal
Squamous cell carcinoma	+	+
Verrucous carcinoma	+	–
Basal cell carcinoma	+	–
Paget's disease	+	–
Adenocarcinoma	–	+
Melanoma	–	+

(Sabiston, 20th Edition, Page 1415)

29. True statements regarding Epithelioid hemangioendothelioma of the liver:

(a) Manifests with single unilateral hepatic masses

(b) Extrahepatic metastases occur in approximately 75% of patients

(c) Most patients ultimately die of liver failure

(d) Liver transplantation is of no use

Ans: (c) Most patients ultimately die of liver failure

- Epithelioid hemangioendothelioma of the liver is a rare malignant vascular tumor that is manifested with ***multiple bilateral hepatic masses***
- ***Extrahepatic metastases occur in approximately 25% of patients*** and clinical behavior is unpredictable, with some patients having a prolonged indolent course
- Most patients ultimately die of liver failure, but *cases of successful transplantation* have been reported

(Sabiston, 20th Edition, Page 1464)

30. Which of the following statements is not true about Gallbladder cancer treatment?

(a) Polyp >10 mm has increased risk of Malignancy

(b) For T1b lesions, cholecystectomy is sufficient as long as the margins are negative

(c) For T1a lesions, cholecystectomy should suffice for therapy

(d) Goal of therapy gallbladder cancer advanced disease is Extended cholecystectomy

Ans: (d) Goal of therapy gallbladder cancer advanced disease is Extended cholecystectomy

- Many patients with gallbladder cancer will present with advanced disease and therefore the goal of therapy is palliation of symptoms in these cases
- Gallbladder polyps larger than 10 mm carry an increased risk of malignancy, cholecystectomy is treatment of choice
- For T1a lesions, cholecystectomy should suffice for therapy
- For T1b lesions, cholecystectomy is sufficient as long as the margins are negative
- With T1b lesions and perineural, lymphatic, or vascular invasion, likelihood of nodal disease increases significantly therefore an extended cholecystectomy is indicated
- For T2 Lesions, radical cholecystectomy is indicated

(Sabiston, 20th Edition, Page 1514)

31. Which of the following statements about Pancraetic cancer is not true?

(a) Loss of DPC4 is associated with metastatic disease
(b) Most common gene involved in Carcinoma Pancreas is K ras
(c) 10% of PDACs demonstrate loss of p16 function
(d) Most common Germ line mutation involved is BRCA2

Ans: (c) 10% of PDACs demonstrate loss of p16 function

- Germline mutations of the *BRCA2* gene lead to an elevated risk for pancreatic cancer, which is up to 10 times that of the general population
- *KRAS2* oncogene is activated in more than 95% of pancreatic cancers and is thought to be the initiating event in tumorigenesis
- *KRAS2* is activated by point mutation (codon 12, 13, or 61), which causes constitutive activation and loss of regulation of mitogen-activated protein kinase cell signal transduction
- Mutation of the *KRAS2* oncogene is one of the earliest genetic abnormalities identified in the progression of PanIN to PDAC and has been noted in 36% of PanIN-1 cases, 44% of PanIN-2 cases, and 87% of PanIN-3 cases
- Loss of *DPC4* function has been observed in 20% to 30% of PanIN-3 and localized cancers, whereas 78% of widely metastatic tumors show loss of *DPC4*

(Bailey, 27th Edition)

32. Which of the following statements are true about splenic tumors?

(a) Angiosarcoma of spleen is associated with thorotrast
(b) All the given statements
(c) Haemangioma is the most common benign tumor of spleen
(d) Lung cancer is the tumor that most commonly spreads to the spleen

Ans: (b) All the given statements

- Solid tumors that most frequently spread to the spleen are carcinomas of the breast and lung and melanoma
- *Lung cancer is the tumor that most commonly spreads to spleen* ***(Schwartz, 10th Edition, Page 1437)***

(Sabiston, 20th Edition, Page 1563)

33. Not true about Adenoid cystic carcinoma is:

(a) Involves trachea and mainstem bronchi
(b) More malignant than carcinoid tumors

(c) Slight male preponderance

(d) Stridor is often the presenting symptom of adenoid cystic tumors

Ans: (c) Slight male preponderance

- Adenoid cystic carcinoma is a slow-growing malignancy involving the trachea and mainstem bronchi that is similar to salivary gland tumors
- Adenoid cystic carcinoma is more malignant than carcinoid tumors
- Slight female preponderance
- Tumor typically involves lower trachea, carina, and take-off of mainstem bronchi
- **Stridor is often the presenting symptom of adenoid cystic tumors** because these tumors are most often found in the trachea and mainstem bronchi
- One third of patients have tumors that have metastasized at time of treatment
- These patients typically have involvement of the perineural lymphatics; regional nodes; or liver, bone, or kidneys
- Tumor arises from ducts in submucosa and extends proximally and distally
- Microscopic examination demonstrates cells with large nuclei and small cytoplasm and surrounding cystic spaces (pseudoacinar type); **medullary type has Swiss cheese appearance**
- Treatment is wide en bloc resection with conservation of as much lung tissue
- Radiation treatment alone may be effective in patients not amenable to surgical resection

(Sabiston, 20th Edition, Page 1600)

34. All the following statements are true about Oligodendroglioma *except:*

(a) Tumors originate from oligodendroglial cells

(b) 25% of all glial tumors

(c) Female predominance

(d) Often present clinically with seizures or hemorrhage and nonspecific mass effect

Ans: (c) Female predominance

Oligodendroglioma
• Oligodendroglioma usually originate from oligodendroglial cells
• 25% of all glial tumors
• **Male to female predominance of 3:2, observed at an average age of 40 years**
• Often present clinically with seizures or hemorrhage and nonspecific mass effect
• Overall median survival of 3 years
• **Treatment consists of surgical resection followed by chemotherapy**
• A particularly favorable response rate is associated with tumors that show allelic losses of chromosomes 1p and 19q
• Radiation therapy is considered for tumors with anaplastic transformation

(Sabiston, 20th Edition, Page 1911)

35. Which of the following mutation is associated with uveal melanoma and RCC (renal)?

(a) BAP1

(b) VHL

(c) SDH

(d) MET

Ans: (a) BAP1

BAP1 mutant disease-*Associated with chromosome* 3p21
• Breast cancer
• Uveal melanoma
• Mesothelioma
• RCC
• Other cutaneous melanocytic tumors

(Bailey, 27th Edition, Page 1418)

36. Which of the following statements is not true about Neuroblastoma?

(a) Whole chromosome 17 gain is associated with a good prognosis

(b) Deletions of chromosome 11q have associated with unfavorable patient outcome

(c) 50% of Neuroblastoma are localized to adrenal medulla

(d) N-myc is overexpressed in only 50% of localized or stage 4S neuroblastomas

Ans: (d) N-myc is overexpressed in only 50% of localized or stage 4S neuroblastomas

- *MYCN* oncogene, which is amplified at chromosome 2p24 in 25% of cases, is overexpressed in 30% to 40% of stage 3 and stage 4 neuroblastomas but only in 5% of localized or stage 4S tumors
- Deletions of chromosome 11q have been identified in 15% to 22% of neuroblastomas and are also associated with unfavorable patient outcomes and a reduced time of progression-free survival
- Whole chromosome 17 gain is associated with a good prognosis

(Sabiston, 20th Edition, Page 1887)

37. Which of the below statements are true about Vulvar cancer is:

(a) Inguinofemoral lymphadenectomy is indicated in clinical stage IA

(b) Squamous cell cancer in 90% of cases

(c) Bleeding is the most common complaint

(d) Mean age at diagnosis is 65 years

Ans: (b) Squamous cell cancer in 90% of cases

Highlights of Vulvar Cancer
• Most common type of vulvar cancer is Squamous cell carcinoma
• Most common site is labia majora (50%)
• Most common mode of spread is direct spread
• Most common site of hematogenous spread is Lung
• Most of lymphatics drain into superficial inguinal lymph nodes
• Median age of diagnosis is 65 years
• Pruritis is the most common complaint
• Inguinofemoral lymphadenectomy is indicated beyond clinical stage IA

(Schwartz, 10th Edition, Page 1696)

38. Which of the following statements are true about lymphangiosarcoma?

(a) Complication of long-standing lymphedema

(b) Usually develops more than 10 years

(c) Acute worsening of edema and appearance of subcutaneous nodules

(d) All of the above

Ans: (d) All of the above

- Lymphangiosarcoma is a rare tumor that develops as a complication of long-standing lymphedema
- Usually occurs more than 10 years
- Clinically, the patients present with acute worsening of edema and appearance of subcutaneous nodules that have propensity toward hemorrhage and ulceration
- Tumor can be treated, like other sarcomas, with preoperative chemotherapy and radiation followed by surgical excision, which usually may take form of radical amputation
- Overall, tumor has a very poor prognosis

(Sabiston, 20th Edition, Page 1855)

39. Malignant risk of Proliferative verrucous leukoplakia is:

(a) 30% (b) 40%

(c) 20% (d) 50%

Ans: (d) 50%

- Proliferative verrucous leucoplakia is a **Rare Progressive Exophytic variant** of leucoplakia, which is **frequently multifocal** and carries a **high (>50%) risk of malignant transformation**
- Diagnosis is made on the basis of combined clinical and histopathological grounds. It may be localised and typically affects gingivae or, more commonly, as a widespread varient, affects several oral mucosal sites

(Bailey and Love, 27th Edition, Page 763)

40. Most common primary malignant cutaneous tumor of hand is:

(a) Squamous cell carcinoma (b) Schwannoma

(c) Basal cell carcinoma (d) Melanoma

Ans: (a) Squamous cell carcinoma

- *Most common primary benign bone tumor of the hand and wrist–Enchondroma*
- Squamous cell carcinoma is the most common primary malignant cutaneous tumor of the hand accounting for 75% to 90% of all malignancies of the hand
- Epithelioid sarcoma is most common primary soft tissue sarcoma of the upper extremity

(Schwartz, 10th Edition, Page 1818)

41. Trastuzumab is used in: (NEET SS 2018)

(a) Metastatic HER 2 +ve breast cancer (b) Metastatic HER 2 +ve Gastric cancer

(c) Both of the above (d) None of the above

Ans: (c) Both of the above

TRASTUZUMAB: Herceptin is used against Metastatic HER2 +ve Breast and Gastric cancers

Targeted Therapies	
Avatinib, Temsirolimus, Pazopanib	RCC
Bevacizumab	Colorectal cancer, Lung cancer, Glioblastoma, NSCLC, RCC
Bosutinib, Nilotinib	CML
Cabozantinib, Vandetanib	Medullary thyroid cancer
Sunitinib	GIST, RCC, PNET
Sorafenib	HCC, RCC
Regorafenib	Colorectal cancer, GIST
Gefitinib	NSCLC

(Schwartz, 10th Edition, Page 310)

42. In Masaoka staging of Thymoma, Stage 3 is:

(a) Macroscopically completely encapsulated and microscopic no capsular invasion
(b) Macroscopic invasion into mediastinal pleura
(c) Macroscopic invasion into Pericardium, Great vessels and Lung
(d) Pleural dissemination

Ans: (c) Macroscopic invasion into Pericardium, Great vessels and Lung

Masaoka Staging	
I	Macroscopically completely encapsulated & Microscopically no capsular invasion
II	Macroscopic invasion into surrounding fatty tissue or mediastinal pleura Microscopic invasion into capsule
III	Macroscopic invasion into pericardium, Great vessels and Lung
IV	Pleural or pericardial dissemination Lymphogenous or Hematogenous metastases

(Devita, 10th Edition, Page 561)

43. Recommended screening criteria for Hereditary Gastric cancer include all *except:*

(a) Families with one or more cases of Diffuse gastric cancer
(b) Individuals with Diffuse gastric cancer before 20 years of age without family history
(c) Individuals with Diffuse gastric cancer below the age of 50 years and lobular breast cancer
(d) All of the above

Ans: (b) Individuals with Diffuse gastric cancer before 20 years of age without family history

New Recommended Screening Criteria for *CDH1* Mutations

- Families with one or more cases of DGC
- Individuals with DGC before the age of 40 years without a family history
- Families or individuals with cases of DGC (one case below the age of 50 years) and lobular breast cancer
- Cases where pathologists detect in situ signet ring cells or pagetoid spread of signet ring cells adjacent to diffuse type gastric cancer

(Devita, 10th Edition, Page 645)

44. Choriocarcinoma with Metastasis to Lungs. Stage is: (JIPMER SS 2015)

(a) I
(b) II
(c) III
(d) IV

Ans: (c) III

Stage	Component
I	Confined to uterus
II	Extends outside uterus, but limited to genital structures
III	Extends to lungs, with or without genital tract involvement
IV	All other metastatic sites

(Devita, 10th Edition, Page 1071)

45. Regarding Screening guidelines in Peutz Jeghers cancer screening incorrect is:

(a) Mammogram and breast magnetic resonance imaging (MRI) annually, Clinical breast examination every 6 monthly from 25 years
(b) Colonoscopy every 2-3 years from late teens

(c) Pelvic examination and Papanicolaou smear annually from 10 years

(d) Annual testicular examination and observation for feminizing changes from 10 years

Ans: (c) Pelvic examination and Papanicolaou smear annually from 10 years

Adopted Screening Guidelines for Peutz Jeghers Cancer Screening		
Site	**Screening Procedure**	**Initiation Age**
Breast	Mammogram and breast magnetic resonance imaging annually, Clinical breast examination every 6 monthly	**25 years**
Colon	Colonoscopy every 2–3 years	**Late teens**
Stomach	Upper endoscopy every 2–3 years	**Late teens**
Pancreas	MRCP/EUS every 1–2 years, CA-19-9 at similar intervals	**30-35 years**
Small intestine	Small-bowel visualization (CT/MRI enterography) baseline at 8–10 years with follow-up interval based on findings but at least by age 18 years, then every 2–3 years although this may be individualized, or with symptoms	**8-10 years**
Ovary	Pelvic examination and Papanicolaou smear annually	**18-20 years**
Cervix Uterus	Consider transvaginal ultrasound	
Testis	Annual testicular examination and observation for feminizing changes	**10 years**
Lung	Provide education about symptoms and smoking cessation No other specific recommendations have been made	

(Devita, 10th Edition, Page 104)

46. Anterior mediastinoscopy is useful for staging which level of lymph nodes?

(a) 5, 6
(b) 1, 2, 4, 7
(c) 4, 5, 7, 8, 9
(d) All of the above

Ans: (a) 5, 6

Mediastinal Staging Techniques	
Traditional mediastinoscopy	1, 2R, 2L, 3, 4R, 4L, Anterior 7
Videomediastinoscopy	1, 2R, 2L, 3, 4R, 4L, 5, 7, 8, 10R
Chamberlain anterior mediastinoscopy	5, 6
Video assisted thoracic surgery	R2, R4, 7, 10, 11 L2, L4, 5, 6, 7, 10, 11
Transthoracic needle aspiration/biopsy	Variable, Restricted to enlarged nodes
Transbronchial needle aspiration	2R, 2L, 3, 4R, 4L, 7, 10, 11
Endoscopic ultrasound with needle aspiration	4L, 5, 7, 8, 9
EBUS with needle aspiration	2R, 2L, 3, 4R, 4L, 7, 10, 11, 12

(Devita, 10th Edition, Page 508)

47. Absolute contraindications to Breast conservation therapy include all *except:*

(a) Radiation therapy during pregnancy

(b) Diffuse suspicious or malignant-appearing microcalcifications

(c) Positive pathologic margin

(d) Tumors >5 cm

Ans: (d) Tumors >5 cm

Absolute	Relative
Radiation therapy during pregnancy	Active connective tissue disease involving skin (scleroderma and lupus)
Diffuse suspicious or malignant-appearing microcalcifications	Tumors >5 cm
Positive pathologic margin	Focally positive margin
Widespread disease that cannot be incorporated by local excision through single incision that achieves negative margins with a satisfactory cosmetic result	*Women with a known or suspected genetic predisposition to breast cancer:* May have an increased risk of ipsilateral breast recurrence/contralateral breast cancer with BCT, prophylactic bilateral mastectomy for risk reduction may be considered

(Devita, 20th Edition, Page 1131)

48. Not true about MPNST (Malignant peripheral nerve sheath tumor) is:

(a) NF1 patients lifetime risk of developing MPNST is 8% to 13%

(b) NF1 gene is implicated in sporadic as well as NF1-associated MPNST

(c) TP53 is frequently activated in MPNST

(d) MPNST cell lines are sensitive to sorafenib at nanomolar concentrations

Ans: (c) TP53 is frequently activated in MPNST

- NF1 patients lifetime risk of developing MPNST is 8% to 13%
- NF1 gene is implicated in sporadic as well as NF1-associated MPNST
- TP53 is frequently Inactivated in MPNST
- MPNST cell lines are sensitive to sorafenib at nanomolar concentrations
- EGFR overexpression and p53 mutation cooperated to significantly increase neurofibroma and MPNST formation, effects that were enhanced by SB mutagenesis

(Devita, 20th Edition, Page 1249)

49. Incorrect Match among the following:

(a) Cowden syndrome–Follicular and Papillary thyroid carcinoma

(b) FAP–Follicular thyroid carcinoma

(c) Carney complex–Follicular and Papillary thyroid carcinoma

(d) McCune Albright syndrome–Papillary thyroid carcinoma

Ans: (b) FAP–Follicular thyroid carcinoma

Familial Cancer Syndromes Associated with Non Medullary Thyroid Cancers		
Syndrome	**Gene**	**Thyroid Tumor**
Cowden syndrome	PTEN	FTC, Rarely PTC and Hurthle cell tumors
FAP	APC	**PTC–Cribriform pattern**
Werner's syndrome	WRN	PTC, FTC, Anaplastic cancer
Carney complex 1	PRKAR 1 alpha	PTC, FTC
Mc Cune Albright syndrome	GNAS1	**PTC–Clear cell**

(Schwartz, 10th Edition, Page 1539)

50. Primary reconstructive flap of choice in Dentate mandible with Oral cancer:

(a) Iliac crest (b) Fibula

(c) Composite flap (d) PMMF

Ans: (a) Iliac crest

Site	Primary Flap
Floor of mouth	Radial forearm free flap
Lateral tongue	Radial forearm free flap/Anterolateral thigh flap
Total tongue/Glossectomy	Anterolateral thigh flap/Rectus abdominus
MANDIBLE	Dentate–Iliac crest Edentulous–Fibula
Tongue base	Radial forearm free flap
MAXILLA	Low level/Hard palate–Obturation, RFFF/ALT High–Iliac crest/Scapula
Soft palate/Tonsil	Forearm/MSAP

(Bailey, 27th Edition, Page 774)

51. Which of the following are not an indication of MRI in women at high risk breast cancer?

(a) With a known *BRCA* mutation
(b) Who have a first-degree relative with a *BRCA* mutation
(c) Who had been treated with radiation to the chest
(d) Who have an approximately 10% to 15% or greater lifetime risk of breast cancer

Ans: (d) Who have an approximately 10% to 15% or greater lifetime risk of breast cancer

Women at High Lifetime Risk (20%-25% Or Greater) of Breast Cancer
• Known *BRCA1* or *BRCA2* gene mutation • First-degree relative with *BRCA1* or *BRCA2* gene mutation, but have not had genetic testing themselves • Lifetime risk of breast cancer of ≈20%-25% or greater • Radiation therapy to the chest between the ages of 10 and 30 • Li-Fraumeni syndrome/Cowden syndrome or a first-degree relative with one of these syndromes
Women at Moderately Increased (15%-20%) Lifetime Risk
• Lifetime risk of breast cancer of 15%-20% according to risk assessment tools based mainly on family history • Personal history of breast cancer, ductal carcinoma in situ, lobular carcinoma in situ, atypical ductal hyperplasia, or atypical lobular hyperplasia • Extremely dense breasts or unevenly dense breasts when viewed by mammograms

(Devita, 10th Edition, Page 378)

52. Incorrectly matched among the following:

(a) Colorectal carcinoma–CK20+, CK7–, CDX-2+
(b) Breast–CK20–, CK7+, mammoglobin+ or ER+ or GCDFP-15+
(c) Hepatocellular- CD10+, Hepar-1+
(d) Prostate–CK20+, CK7+, PSA+

Ans: (d) Prostate–CK20+, CK7+, PSA+

Cancer	IHC
Colorectal carcinoma	CK20+, CK7–, CDX-2+
Breast carcinoma	CK20–, CK7+, mammaglobin+ or ER+ or GCDFP-15+
Hepatocellular carcinoma	CD10+, Hepar-1+
Lung/adeno/large cell carcinoma	CK20–, CK7+, TTF-1+
Lung/neuroendocrine carcinoma	CK7+, TTF1+, chromogranin+ or synaptophysin+ or CD56+
Melanoma	S100+, Melan-A+ or HMB45+
Sarcoma	Vimentin+, CK7–, S100–, desmin+, CK20–
Prostate	CK20–, CK7–, PSA+

(Devita, 10th Edition, Page 1725)

53. Callender classification is used for:

(a) Gallbladder carcinoma
(b) Lung carcinoma
(c) Intraocular melanoma
(d) Esthesioneuroblastoma

Ans: (c) Intraocular melanoma

Callender Classification
Divided uveal melanoma into three categories: • Spindle cell melanomas (spindle A, spindle B, or both) • Mixed-cell melanomas, when less than half of cells are composed of epithelioid cells • Epithelioid cell melanomas, greater than half are composed of epithelioid cells

(Devita, 10th Edition, Page 1770)

54. Treatment of choice in Symptomatic Kaposi sarcoma is:

(a) Surgery
(b) Radiotherapy
(c) Chemotherapy
(d) VEGF inhibitors

Ans: (b) Radiotherapy

- Kaposi sarcoma, a low-grade soft tissue malignant neoplasm, arises from lymphatic vascular endothelial cells in the skin
- In patients infected with HIV, HHV 8 has been identified as the causative agent of Kaposi sarcoma
- Incidence is increasing because it is most often seen in AIDS and organ transplantation
- There is also a classic variant seen on the lower extremities of older men of eastern European and Mediterranean descent
- Clinical picture is variable; asymptomatic purple to brown bruises develop and progress to spots, plaques, or nodules on both lower extremities
- Local symptoms appear late as tumors become advanced
- In AIDS patients, skin changes respond best to aggressive antiretroviral therapy
- ***Symptomatic skin lesions can be treated with radiation therapy, intralesional injection of chemotherapeutic agents, cryotherapy, or excision***

(Sabiston, 20th Edition, Page 750)

55. All are true about Thyroid lymphoma *except:*

(a) Most common thyroid lymphoma is DLBCL
(b) Diagnosis is considered in patients with goiter grown significantly in short period
(c) Thyroid lymphoma occurs four times more frequently in men
(d) Approximately half of primary thyroid lymphomas occur in setting of preexisting Hashimoto thyroiditis

Ans: (c) Thyroid lymphoma occurs four times more frequently in men

- Primary thyroid lymphoma, although rare, is being recognized more frequently
- Diagnosis is considered in patients with a goiter, especially one that has apparently grown significantly in a short period
- Other initial symptoms include hoarseness, dysphagia and fever
- Thyroid lymphoma occurs four times more frequently in women than in men
- Approximately half of primary thyroid lymphomas occur in the setting of preexisting Hashimoto thyroiditis

(Sabiston, 20th Edition, Page 911)

56. True about Cholangiocarcinoma are all *except:*

(a) Distal cholangiocarcinoma is managed by pancreaticoduodenectomy
(b) Surgical management of proximal cholangiocarcinoma involves resection of regional nodal tissue and en bloc resection of the common bile duct with hepatic parenchyma
(c) Types I and II Klatskin tumors are treated with common duct resection, cholecystectomy, and a 5- to 10-mm margin of resection
(d) Types III and IV Klatskin tumors are inoperable

Ans: (d) Types III and IV Klatskin tumors are inoperable

- Distal cholangiocarcinoma is managed by pancreaticoduodenectomy
- Surgical management of proximal cholangiocarcinoma involves resection of regional nodal tissue and en bloc resection of the common bile duct with hepatic parenchyma
- Types I and II Klatskin tumors are treated with common duct resection, cholecystectomy and a 5- to 10-mm margin of resection
- Types III and IV Klatskin tumors involve complex resection and reconstruction of portal vein, hepatic artery, or both

(Sabiston, 20th Edition, Page 1517)

57. When compared to Allopurinol, Rasburicase differs with it in all *except:*

(a) Intravenous administration (b) Rapid onset of action
(c) Interferes with metabolism of 6-mercaptopurine (d) Can lead to hemolysis in patients with G 6 PD deficiency

Ans: (c) Interferes with metabolism of 6-mercaptopurine

Allopurinol	Rasburicase
Oral	Intravenous
Slow onset	Rapid onset
Interferes with metabolism of 6 mercaptopurine	No effect on drug metabolism
No effect in patients with G 6 PD deficiency	Leads to hemolysis in patients with G6PD deficiency such as those of African or Mediterranean ancestry
1% of allergic reactions	4% to 5% incidence of immunoallergic reactions including anaphylaxis

(Devita, 10th Edition, Page 1825)

58. Which of the following malignancies cause Hypercalcemia by producing Calcitriol?

(a) Renal cell carcinoma (b) Carcinoma Breast
(c) Carcinoma Lung (d) Lymphoma

Ans: (d) Lymphoma

- Calcitriol-induced hypercalcemia typically occurs in Hodgkin lymphoma and in approximately 30% of cases of non-Hodgkin lymphoma **(Sabiston, 20th Edition, Page 926)**
- Osteolytic metastases account for 20% of cases of hypercalcemia of malignancy and breast cancer is the most frequent primary tumor

(Devita, 10th Edition, Page 1830)

59. Most common presentation of Nasopharyngeal carcinoma is:

(a) Hearing loss (b) Trotter's triad
(c) Blood stained nasal discharge (d) Cervical lymphadenopathy

Ans: (d) Cervical lymphadenopathy

- Approximately 50% of patients will present with a malignant node or nodes in the neck, indicating an advanced tumor
- Nasal complaints occur in one-third of patients and aural symptoms of unilateral deafness as a consequence of Eustachian tube obstruction and secretory otitis media occur in approximately 20%

(Bailey, 27th Edition, Page 734)

60. Most common benign cardiac tumor in children is:

(a) Atrial myxoma (b) Rhabdomyoma
(c) Adenoma (d) Leiomyoma

Ans: (b) Rhabdomyoma

- *Most common benign cardiac tumor in adult–Atrial myxoma*
- *Most common benign cardiac tumor in child–Rhabdomyoma*

(Bailey, 27th Edition, Page 912)

PAPER 2

61. Seed soil theory is given by:

(a) Ehrlich
(b) Kocher
(c) Paget
(d) Halsted

Ans: (c) Paget

- Paget pointed that there is a crucial relationship here between seed (tumor cell) and soil (distant tissue)
- Paget observed in 1889 that breast carcinoma often metastasized to the liver, lungs, bone, adrenals, or brain
- He hypothesized that tumor cells (the "seed") would grow only in selective environments (the "soil"), where conditions supported tumor growth, hence so-called seed-and-soil hypothesis

(Sabiston, 20th Edition, Page 685)

62. Which of the following statements are true about HPV virus?

(a) Epidermodysplasia verruciformis frequently develop Squamous cell carcinoma
(b) E6 protein of high-risk HPV types triggers destruction of p53
(c) Epidermodysplasia verruciformis is typically caused by HPV 5/HPV 8
(d) L1-based vaccines are used as therapeutic agents for treating cervical cancer

Ans: (a) Epidermodysplasia verruciformis frequently develop Squamous cell carcinoma

- Epidermodysplasia verruciformis is typically caused by HPV 5/HPV 8 that frequently develop Squamous cell carcinoma
- L1-based vaccines seem unlikely to serve as therapeutic agents for treating cervical cancer
- E6 protein of high-risk HPV types triggers destruction of p53

(Devita, 10th Edition, Page 72)

63. Which of the following statements are true about PARP inhibitors?

1. Inhibition of PARP would be a lethal event in cells that have inactivation of *BRCA1* or *BRCA2*
2. Based on concept of Synthetic lethality
3. BRCA-mutated cell lines showing a 100- to 1,000-fold sensitivity to PARP inhibitors

Find out correct answer:

(a) 1 and 2 are true
(b) 1, 2, 3 are true
(c) 1 and 3 are true
(d) 2 and 3 are true

Ans: (b) 1,2,3 are true

- Inhibition of PARP would be a lethal event in cells that have inactivation of *BRCA1* or *BRCA2*
- This concept, called *synthetic lethality* was tested early in development of PARP inhibitors
- Preclinical data strongly supported this concept, with *BRCA*-mutated cell lines showing a 100- to 1,000-fold sensitivity to PARP inhibitors compared with wild-type control cell lines

(Devita, 10th Edition, Page 1007)

64. **False about DFSP is:**
    (a) COL1A1-PDGFB fusion product
    (b) Associated with t(17;22) translocation
    (c) High grade
    (d) Imatinib is used for locally advanced and metastatic disease

Ans: (c) High grade

- Dermatofibrosarcoma protuberans (DFSP) is a low-grade sarcoma arising from dermal fibroblasts
- Lesions appear as smooth, flesh-colored nodules in or immediately beneath the skin and generally are manifested in patients between 20 and 50 years of age
- **Most common site–Trunk**
- Treatment consists of WLE with a 2- to 4-cm margin
- Distant metastases are uncommon and are preceded by two or more local recurrences
- Translocation t(17:22) has been found in approximately 90% of DFSP lesions
- Imatinib in patients with locally advanced or metastatic disease and as neoadjuvant therapy

(Sabiston, 20th Edition, Page 750)

65. **All are true about Melanoma *except:***
    (a) Most common histologic type is superficial spreading melanoma
    (b) Melanoma usually results more from continuous episodes of intense UV radiation
    (c) 5% to 10% of melanoma patients will have a family history of the disease
    (d) 40% may arise within preexisting lesions, including dysplastic nevi, congenital nevi and Spitz nevi

Ans: (b) Melanoma usually results more from continuous episodes of intense UV radiation

- Most common histologic type is superficial spreading melanoma
- 5% to 10% of melanoma patients will have a family history of the disease
- 40% may arise within preexisting lesions, including dysplastic nevi, congenital nevi and Spitz nevi

(Sabiston, 20th Edition, Page 724)

66. **Not true about desmoids tumors is:**
    (a) Also known as aggressive fibromatosis
    (b) Approximately 20% of FAP patients develop desmoid tumors
    (c) 15% of cases arise sporadically
    (d) Show a high likelihood of local recurrence

Ans: (c) 15% of cases arise sporadically

- Desmoids are also known as aggressive fibromatosis
- Approximately 20% of FAP patients develop desmoid tumors
- 75 to 85% of cases arise sporadic
- They usually show a high likelihood of local recurrence

(Sabiston, 20th Edition, Page 766)

67. **Majority of Primary Malignant Bone tumors belong to which Enneking staging:**
    (a) 1A (b) 1B
    (c) 2A (d) 2B

Ans: (d) 2B

- Most primary malignant bone tumors are Enneking stage 2B at diagnosis
- It means they have extended outside the bone of origin but metastases are not detectable

(Bailey, 27th Edition, Page 543)

68. Magnitude of risk of breast cancer is Highest with which of the following?

(a) CHEK 2 mutation
(b) Age >35 years for 1st birth
(c) Proliferative breast disease
(d) Radiation exposure before 30 years

Ans: (d) Radiation exposure before 30 years

Relative risk <2	Relative risk 2-4	Relative risk >4
Early menarche	One 1st degree relative with Breast cancer	Mutation BRCA 1/BRCA 2
Late menopause	CHEK 2 mutation	LCIS
Nulliparity	Age >35 years for 1st birth	Atypical hyperplasia
Estrogen plus progesterone	Proliferative breast disease	Radiation exposure before 30
HRT	Mammographic breast density	
Alcoholic use		
Post menopausal obesity		

(Devita, 10th Edition, Page 1120)

69. Which of the following is true about childhood thyroid cancer?

(a) PTC in childhood tends to be aggressive with high death rates
(b) PTC has higher incidence of metastases to nodes and lungs at presentation than adults
(c) Initial management with total thyroidectomy and cervical lymph node dissection with radioactive iodine in all cases
(d) 10% of childhood thyroid cancers are differentiated thyroid cancers

Ans: (b) PTC has higher incidence of metastases to nodes and lungs at presentation than adults

- PTC accounts for 1.5% of childhood malignancy but >90% of childhood thyroid cancers
- PTC has a higher incidence of metastases to the lymph nodes and lungs at presentation than in adults
- PTC in childhood tends to be indolent with low death rates
- Children with well-differentiated thyroid carcinoma more often than their adult counterparts have history of external irradiation to the head and neck, although majority present without such a history
- >50% of patients had exposure to ionizing radiation
- Aggressive initial management with total thyroidectomy and cervical lymph node dissection should be performed in most children with well-differentiated thyroid carcinoma
- Restrict adjuvant RAI to patients who are considered high risk with distant metastases or incomplete resection with gross residual disease

(Devita, 10th Edition, Page 1187)

70. Most common Malignant brain tumor with limited life expectancy in adults is:

(a) Meningioma
(b) Glioblastoma multiforme
(c) Pilocytic astrocytoma
(d) Optic glioma

Ans: (b) Glioblastoma multiforme

- **Most common Primary intracranial tumor–MENINGIOMA**
- Most common primary intracranial malignancy–GBM **(Sabiston, Page 1911)**
- WHO grade IV tumor, this is most commonly encountered primary brain tumor in adults
- 2 major forms: Primary and Secondary
- Primary occurs in old people with poor survival

WHO Grade	Population	Diagnosis	Pathways Affected	Hallmark Mutations or Structural Abnormalities	Notes
IV	Adult	Secondary GBM	Epigenetic dysregulation	IDH1 R132H/C/S	Progressed from lower grade gliomas
			Chromatin remodeling	ATRX mutations	
			p53 pathway	TP 53 mutations, LOH at chr 17	
			Rb pathway	Loss of RB1	
				Loss of CDKN2A	
			P13K	Loss of PTEN	
		Primary GBM	TP53 pathway	TP53 loss	
				CDKN2A loss	
				MDM1/2/4 gain	
			RB pathway	CDKN2A loss	
				RB1 loss	
				CDK 4/6 amplification	
			Receptor tyrosine kinase	EGFR amplification	
				PDGFRA amplification	
			P13K	PTEN loss	
				P13K mutation	
			RAS	NF1 loss	
			Telomere maintenance	TERT	

(Devita, 10th Edition, Page 1403)

71. All are true about Gorlin syndrome *except:*

(a) Autosomal dominant disorder

(b) Sogin hedgehog signaling pathway is involved

(c) PTCH gene defect

(d) Usually associated with Basal cell carcinoma and rhabdomyosarcoma

Ans: (d) Usually associated with Basal cell carcinoma and rhabdomyosarcoma

- Nevoid basal cell carcinoma syndrome, Gorlin syndrome, is rare **autosomal-dominant** disorder characterized by *multiple basal cell carcinomas; developmental defects, including bifid ribs and other spine and rib abnormalities; palmar and plantar pits; odontogenic keratocysts; and generalized overgrowth*
- SHH signaling pathway directs embryonic development of a spectrum of organisms
- ***Gorlin syndrome is caused by germline mutations of the tumor suppressor gene PTCH (receptor for SHH)***
- Medulloblastomas develop in approximately 5% of patients with Gorlin syndrome
- Furthermore, approximately 10% of patients diagnosed with medulloblastoma by the age of 2 years are found to have other phenotypic features consistent with Gorlin syndrome and also harbor germ-line *PTCH* mutations
- Although Gorlin syndrome develops in individuals with germ-line mutations of *PTCH*, a subset of children with medulloblastoma harbor germ-line mutations of another gene, *SUFU*, in the SHH pathway, with accompanying LOH in the tumors
- Rhabdomyosarcoma is rarely seen with Gorlin syndrome but mouse studies suggest a possible link between PTC signaling and RMS

(Devita, 10th Edition, Page 1462)

72. Gail model for risk estimation in breast cancer include all *except:*

(a) Age at menarche

(b) No. of Biopsies taken

(c) Age at 1st liver birth

(d) Age at menopause

Ans: (d) Age at menopause

Relative Risk Estimate for Gail Model
Age at menarche
No of biopsy specimen/history of benign breast disease <50 years
No of biopsy specimen/history of benign breast disease ≥50 years
Age at first live birth

(Schwartz, 10th Edition, Page 512)

73. DCIS accounts for what percentage of male breast cancer:

(a) 5% (b) 10%
(c) 15% (d) 20%

Ans: (a) 5%

Parameter	LCIS	DCIS
Age	44-47 years	54-58 years
Incidence	2-5%	5-10%
Signs	-	Mass, pain, nipple discharge
Mammographic signs	-	Microcalcifications
Premenopausal	2/3rd	1/3rd
Incidence of synchronous invasive carcinoma	5%	2-46%
Multicentricity	60-90%	40-80%
Bilaterality	50-70%	10-20%
Axillary metastasis	1%	1-2%
MALIGNANCY	25-35%	25-70%
	Bilateral 15-20 years (interval to diagnosis)	Ipsilateral 5-10 years
	DUCTAL CARCINOMA	DUCTAL CARCINOMA

- DCIS is predominantly seen in the female breast, it accounts for 5% of male breast cancers

(Schwartz, 10th Edition, Page 520)

74. Which of the following statements is not true about Levels of lymph nodes?

(a) Level IA is bounded by the anterior belly of digastric muscle, hyoid bone and midline
(b) Level IB contains the submandibular gland
(c) Level IIA is anterior to the spinal accessory nerve
(d) Level VI is bounded by hyoid bone superiorly, external carotid arteries laterally and sternum inferiorly

Ans: (d) Level VI is bounded by hyoid bone superiorly, external carotid arteries laterally and sternum inferiorly

Boundary Level	Superior	Inferior	Anterior (medial)	Posterior (lateral)
IA	Symphysis of the mandible	Body of the hyoid	Anterior belly of the contralateral digastric muscle	Anterior belly of the ipsilateral digastric muscle
IB	Body of the mandible	Posterior belly of the diagastric muscle	Anterior belly of the digastric muscle	Stylohyoid muscle
IIA	Skull base	Horizontal plane defined by the inferior border of the hyoid bone	Stylohyoid muscle	Vertical plane defined by the spinal accessory nerve
IIB	Skull base	Horizontal plane defined by the inferior body of the hyoid bone	Vertical plane defined by the spinal accessory nerve	Lateral border of the sternocleidomastoid muscle

Contd.

Contd.

III	Horizontal plane defined by the inferior body of the hyoid	Horizontal plane defined by the inferior border of the cricoids cartilage	Lateral border of the sternohyoid muscle	Lateral border of the sternocleidomastoid or sensory branches of the cervical plexus
IV	Horizontal plane defined by the inferior border of the criocoid cartilage	Clavicle	Lateral border of the sternohyoid muscle	Lateral border of the sternocleidomastoid or sensory branches of the cervical plexus
VA	Apex of the convergence of the sternocleidomastoid and trapezius muscles	Horizontal plane defined by the lower border of the cricoids cartilage	Posterior border of the sternocleidomastoid muscle or sensory branches of the cervical plexus	Anterior border of the trapezius muscle
VB	Horizontal plane defined by the lower border of the cricoid cartilage	Clavicle	Posterior border of the sternocleidomastoid muscle	Anterior border of the trapezius muscle
VI	Hyoid bone	Suprasternal notch	Common carotid artery	Common carotid artery
VII	Suprasternal notch	Innominate artery	Sternum	Trachea, esophagus, and prevertebral fascia

(AJCC, 8th Edition, Page 59)

75. Which of the following is true about salivary gland neoplasms?

(a) Risk for malignant transformation of pleomorphic adenomas is 15% within first 5 years

(b) Treatment of all salivary gland malignancies is en bloc surgical excision with RT

(c) Risk for malignant lymphoma in patients with Sjögren syndrome is 44-fold higher

(d) In adenoid cystic carcinoma extensive en bloc resection is the only treatment of choice

Ans: (c) Risk for malignant lymphoma in patients with Sjögren syndrome is 44-fold higher

- Adenoid cystic cancers are highly neurotropic; treatment consists of removal of gross tumor with radiation therapy for the microscopic disease that exists at the periphery of tumor
- Risk for malignant transformation of benign pleomorphic adenomas is 1.5% within the first 5 years, but risk increases to 9.5% when the benign tumor has been present for more than 15 years
- Risk for malignant lymphoma in patients with Sjögren syndrome is 44-fold higher than normal population
- Treatment of salivary gland malignancies is en bloc surgical excision. But not in all salivary gland tumors
- Radiation therapy is administered postoperatively for high-grade malignancies demonstrating extraglandular disease, perineural invasion, direct invasion of surrounding tissue, or regional metastases

(Sabiston, 20th Edition, Page 808)

76. Ultrasound features of thyroid malignancy include all *except:*

(a) Microcalcification (b) Hyperechogenic

(c) Intranodular vascularity (d) More taller than wide

Ans: (b) Hyperechogenic

Ultrasound Features of Malignancy
• Microcalcifications • Hypoechogenecity • Irregular margin • Loss of Halo • Solid • Intranodular vascularity • More taller than wide

(Sabiston, 20th Edition, Page 895)

77. Familial parathyroid disorder associated with cystic parathyroid tumors is:

(a) MEN 1
(b) Hyperparathyroidism-jaw tumor (HPT-JT)
(c) Familial isolated hyperparathyroidism (FIHPT)
(d) Neonatal severe hyperparathyroidism (NSHPT)

Ans: (b) Hyperparathyroidism-jaw tumor (HPT-JT)

Disorder	Inherit	Gene	Hyperparathyroidism	Associated Tumors
MEN 1	AD	MEN 1 (11q)	90% penetrance, Multiglandular	Pituitary tumor Pancreatic tumor
HPT-JT	AD	HRPT2 (1q)	Cystic parathyroid tumors (15% Risk of carcinoma)	Jaw tumor, RCC
FIHPT	AD	HRPT2/MEN 1	Adenoma/Mutiglandular	–
NSHPT	AR/AD	CASR (3q)	Markedly hyerplastic	–

78. While preparing a case with pheochromocytoma following should be taken into account *except:*

(a) Nasal congestion can actually serve as a useful indicator of adequate blockade
(b) Beta blockers are given usually after adequate alpha blockade
(c) Adverse perioperative hemodynamic changes observed most commonly with pheochromocytoma are intraoperative hypertension and postoperative hypotension
(d) Sudden withdrawal of stimulus after tumor removal leads to peripheral vasoconstriction

Ans: (d) Sudden withdrawal of stimulus after tumor removal leads to peripheral vasoconstriction

- Nasal congestion can actually serve as a useful indicator of adequate blockade
- Adverse perioperative hemodynamic changes most commonly observed with pheochromocytoma are intraoperative hypertension and postoperative hypotension
- Intraoperative hypertension may be caused by stimulation of catecholamine release by anesthetic induction agents as well as by direct manipulation of the tumor
- Postoperative hypotension may be profound. It results from a state of hypovolemia created by the presence of excess circulating catecholamines
- Sudden withdrawal of this stimulus after tumor removal leads to peripheral arteriolar vasodilation and a dramatic increase in venous capacitance, which together may precipitate cardiovascular collapse

(Sabiston, 20th Edition, Page 984)

79. Following is true about Gastrinoma *except:*

(a) ZES should be considered in all patients with intractable peptic ulcers severe esophagitis, or persistent secretory diarrhea
(b) Gastrin levels higher than 1000 pg/mL are strongly suggestive of gastrinoma
(c) 90% are located within the gastrinoma triangle
(d) 99% of patients present with diarrhea

Ans: (d) 99% of patients present with diarrhea

- Gastrin levels higher than 1000 pg/mL are strongly suggestive of gastrinoma
- ZES should be considered in all patients with intractable peptic ulcers (especially jejunal ulcers), severe esophagitis, or persistent secretory diarrhea
- 90% are located within the gastrinoma triangle
- This triangle bounded by lines connecting cystic duct, the junction between second and third portions of duodenum and junction between neck and body of pancreas
- More than 60% are located in the duodenum
- Duodenal ulcers are the most common, but jejunal ulceration may also occur; the presence of jejunal ulcers should raise suspicion for a gastrin-secreting PNET

- *Approximately 75% of patients present with abdominal pain; almost two thirds of patients with abdominal pain have diarrhea; in 10% to 20% of patients diarrhea is only symptom*

(Sabiston, 20th Edition, Page 995)

80. Which of the following statements about Staging is true for gynecological cancers?

(a) Vulvar carcinoma spreading to upper two third of vagina is Stage IIIC
(b) Vaginal carcinoma spreading to pelvic wall is Stage II
(c) Cervical carcinoma leading to hydronephrosis is Stage III
(d) Endometrial carcinoma spreading to vagina is Stage IIIA

Ans: (c) Cervical carcinoma leading to hydronephrosis is Stage III

• Vulvar carcinoma spreading to upper two third of vagina is Stage IVA
• Vaginal carcinoma spreading to pelvic wall is Stage III
• Cervical carcinoma leading to hydronephrosis is Stage III
• Endometrial carcinoma spreading to vagina is Stage IIIB

(Devita, 10th Edition, Page 1028)

81. Which of the following is not true about Fibroepithelioma of pinkus?

(a) It is a variant of BCC
(b) Typically presents on the torso and extremities
(c) Presents as a pink, smooth, dome-shaped, or pedunculated papule, plaque, or nodule
(d) Not seen on palms and soles

Ans: (d) Not seen on palms and soles

- FEP, a rare variant of BCC, typically presents on the torso and extremities, but also has been noted on the genitalia, groin, and sole of the foot
- Clinically, FEP usually presents as a pink, smooth, dome-shaped, or pedunculated papule, plaque, or nodule
- It may be difficult to distinguish clinically from amelanotic melanoma

(Devita, 10th Edition, Page 1321)

82. Cause of death in esophageal cancer is:

(a) Metastasis
(b) Cardiac complications
(c) Anastomotic leak
(d) Tracheoesophageal fistula

Ans: (a) Metastasis

- Cause of death from esophageal cancer is mainly due to metastatic disease

(Sabiston, 20th Edition, Page 1037)

83. Which of the following statements is true about desmoid tumors?

1.	Risk increases 1000 fold in patients with FAP
2.	Majority of desmoids tumors are sporadic
3.	Oral contraceptive pills are associated with these tumors
4.	Biopsy is required to establish diagnosis

(a) 1 and 2 are true
(b) 2 and 3 are true
(c) 1, 2, 3, 4 are true
(d) 1, 2, 3 are true

Ans: (c) 1, 2, 3, 4 are true

Desmoid Tumors
• Known as fibromatosis, aggressive fibromatosis or desmoid-type fibromatosis
• Risk increases 1000 fold in patients with FAP
• ***Majority of desmoids tumors are sporadic***
• Oral contraceptive pills are associated with these tumors
• Biopsy is required to establish diagnosis
• These tumors arise from fibroaponeurotic tissue and typically are manifested as a slowly growing mass
• Can be multifocal as well as locally aggressive and invasive, high propensity for recurrence
• On CT desmoid tumor appears as homogeneous mass arising from soft tissue of abdominal wall
• Resection of the tumor with a wide margin of normal tissue is considered the optimal treatment
• Abdominal wall desmoids are responsive to radiation therapy

(Sabiston, 20th Edition, Page 1073)

84. Which of the statements about gastric cancer risk is not true?

(a) Risk of development of carcinoma is 10% to 20% with adenomatous polyps
(b) Patients with pernicious anemia are at increased risk for developing gastric cancer
(c) E-cadherin mutation has 40% lifetime incidence of developing gastric cancer
(d) Lynch syndrome, which accounts for 2% to 3% of all colon and rectal cancers and is associated with an increased risk of gastric and ovarian cancers

Ans: (c) E-cadherin mutation has 40% lifetime incidence of developing gastric cancer

- Risk of development of carcinoma is 10% to 20% with adenomatous polyps
- Patients with pernicious anemia are at increased risk for developing gastric cancer
- E-cadherin mutation has 40% lifetime incidence of developing gastric cancer
- Lynch syndrome, which accounts for 2% to 3% of all colon and rectal cancers and is associated with an increased risk of gastric and ovarian cancers
- In familial adenomatous polyposis, approximately 85% of patients have fundic gland polyps, with 40% of these having some type of dysplasia and more than 50% containing a somatic adenomatous polyposis coli mutation, which places these patients at risk of developing gastric cancer
- Li-Fraumeni syndrome is an autosomal dominant disorder caused by a mutation in *p53.* These patients are at risk for gastric cancer and breast cancer

(Sabiston, 20th Edition, Page 1215)

85. Which of the following is not included in major diagnostic criteria of Gorlin syndrome?

(a) Early onset basal cell carcinoma
(b) Odontogenic keratocyst
(c) Desmoplastic medulloblastoma
(d) Cleft lip/palate

Ans: (d) Cleft lip/palate

Clinical Criteria for Diagnosis of Basal Cell Nevus Syndrome
MAJOR CRITERIA
• Early onset/multiple basal cell carcinoma
• Odontogenic keratocyst of jaw (<20 years)
• Palmoplantar pitting
• Calcification of falx cerebri
• Desmoplastic medulloblastoma
• 1st degree relative with Basal cell nevus syndrome

Contd.

Contd.

MINOR CRITERIA
• Rib anomalies
• Skeletal malformations and radiologic changes
• Macrocephaly
• Cleft lip/palate
• Ovarian/cardiac fibroma
• Lymphomesenteric cysts
• Ocular abnormalities

(Devita, 10th Edition, Page 1398)

86. Most common site of origin of chondrosarcoma of CNS is:

(a) Spheno-occiput synchondrosis
(b) Temporo-occipital synchondrosis
(c) Sphenoethmoid complex
(d) Midline

Ans: (b) Temporo-occipital synchondrosis

- Chondrosarcomas are cartilage-producing neoplasm that arise within any of the complex synchondroses in the skull base
- **Chondrosarcomas predominantly originate in more lateral skull-base structures, unlike most chordomas, which originate in the midline**

Most common site of origin is:

- Temporo-occipital synchondrosis (66%)
- Spheno-occiput synchondrosis (28%)
- Sphenoethmoid complex (6%)

(Devita, 10th Edition, Page 1447)

87. Regarding Goldie Coldman hypothesis true is:

(a) Tumor cells are genetically unstable
(b) They tend to mutate to form same cell clones
(c) Tumor cells undergo finite number of divisions
(d) Rate of regression of a tumor will depend upon its age

Ans: (a) Tumor cells are genetically unstable

- Tumors are heterogeneous, and, according to **Goldie-Coldman hypothesis,** tumor cells are genetically unstable and tend to mutate to form different cell clones
- Rate of regression of a tumor will depend upon its age–**Norton-Simon hypothesis (Bailey, 27th Edition, Page 143)**
- According to the **Hayflick hypothesis,** normal cells are permitted to undergo only a finite number of divisions **(Bailey 27th Edition Page 140)**

(Schwartz, 10th Edition, Page 312)

88. Which of the following is not true about testicular cancer?

(a) Most common solid malignancy in men age 15 to 35 years
(b) Most men are diagnosed with a symptomatic enlarging mass
(c) A major risk for the development of testicular cancer is cryptorchidism
(d) Most neoplasms arise from the germ cells

Ans: (b) Most men are diagnosed with a symptomatic enlarging mass

- Testicular cancer is the most common solid malignancy in men age 15 to 35 years
- Most men are diagnosed with an asymptomatic enlarging mass
- A major risk for the development of testicular cancer is cryptorchidism
- Most neoplasms arise from the germ cells, although non-germ cell tumors arise from Leydig's or Sertoli's cells

(Schwartz, 10th Edition, Page 1654)

89. Which of the following Bosnaik classification of renal mass is associated with malignancy?

(a) All of the below
(b) Type 4
(c) Type 1
(d) Type 2

Ans: (b) Type 4

- Bosniak classification system describes cystic renal masses according to their malignant risk and CT appearance, ranging from category I (simple cysts) to category IV (cysts associated with enhancing or solid elements)
- Category III and IV cysts are usually treated as representing cystic renal cell carcinomas

Bosnaik Renal Mass Classification

Type	Description	Malignancy Risk	Management
I	Thin-walled cyst with water density with no septations or calcifications	0%	Non surgical
II	Thin-walled cyst with few hairline septa that may contain fine or very limited thick calcifications. Also includes homogeneously hyperdense cysts <3 cm	0%	Non surgical
IIF	Multiple hairline or slightly thickened septa without measurable enhancement. May contain nodular calcification. Also includes hyperdense cysts >3 cm	5%	Followed for progression
III	Irregular or smooth thickened walls or septa with measurable enhancement	50%	Surgical
IV	Same as III, but with enhancing solid components	100%	Surgical

(Sabiston, 20th Edition, Page 2098) (Schwartz, 10th Edition, Page 1656)

90. Mollaret's meningitis occur due to which of the following brain tumors?

(a) Dermoid cyst
(b) Epidermoid cyst
(c) Teratoma
(d) Vestibular schwannoma

Ans: (b) Epidermoid cyst

- Epidermoid tumors are cystic lesions with stratified squamous epithelial walls from trapped ectodermal cell rests that grow slowly and linearly by desquamation into cyst cavity
- Cysts contain keratin, cholesterol and cellular debris
- They occur most frequently in the cerebellopontine angle and may cause symptoms due to brainstem compression
- **Recurrent bouts of aseptic meningitis may occur due to release of irritative cyst contents into the subarachnoid space (Mollaret's meningitis)**
- Treatment is surgical drainage and removal of the cyst wall
- Intraoperative spillage of cyst contents may lead to severe chemical meningitis and must be avoided by containment and aspiration

(Schwartz, 10th Edition, Page 1737)

91. Histology of which of the following bone tumor shows Staghorn Vascular spaces?

(a) Angiosarcoma
(b) Hemangioendothelioma
(c) Hemangiopericytoma
(d) Ewing's sarcoma

Ans: (c) Hemangiopericytoma

Hemangiopericytoma
• Hemangiopericytoma is usually a solitary lesion occurring in soft tissues or the axial skeleton and proximal long bones in middle-aged or elderly males
• Histology reveals branching "staghorn" vascular spaces
• The tumor cells resemble cells normally seen adjacent to capillaries
• Treatment is wide excision

(Schwartz, 10th Edition, Page 1780)

92. Which of the following statements is not true about Radiotherapy?

(a) Hyperfractionation is defined as use of >1fraction/day separated by more than 6 hours

(b) Hypofractionation refers to the administration of smaller number of larger fractions than is standard

(c) Hypofractionation might be expected to cause more late toxicity for the same antitumor effect than standard or hyperfractionation

(d) Hyperfractionation might be expected to cause more late toxicity for the same antitumor effect than standard or hyperfractionation

Ans: (d) Hyperfractionation might be expected to cause more late toxicity for the same antitumor effect than standard or hyperfractionation

Fractionation
• Hyperfractionation is defined as the use of more than one fraction per day separated by more than 6 hours with a dose per fraction that is less than standard
• Hyperfractionation is expected to produce fewer late complications for the same acute effects against both rapidly dividing normal tissues and tumors
• Overall effect is to increase the acute toxicity (which resolves) and tumor response, while not increasing the (dose-limiting) late toxicity, which can improve cure rate
• Hypofractionation refers to administration of a smaller number of larger fractions than is standard
• Hypofractionation might be expected to cause more late toxicity for the same antitumor effect than standard or hyperfractionation

(Devita, 10th Edition, Page 153)

93. Which of the following statements are true about cigarette smoking and cancer?

1.	Cigarette smoking in adenocarcinoma of the esophagus leads to a twofold increase in risk for heavy smokers
2.	Quitting smoking does not appear to decrease the risk of adenocarcinoma of esophagus
3.	Cigarette smoking is risk factor for Barrett's esophagus
4.	90% of the risk of squamous cell carcinoma of the esophagus in Western Europe and North America can be attributed to tobacco and alcohol use

(a) 1, 2 and 4 are only true

(b) 1, 2 and 3 are only true

(c) 2, 3 and 4 are only true

(d) All of the above are true

Ans: (d) All of the above are true

Esophageal Cancer-Smoking and Alcohol
• 90% of the risk of squamous cell carcinoma of the esophagus in Western Europe and North America can be attributed to tobacco and alcohol use
• Cigarette smoking in adenocarcinoma of the esophagus leads to a two-fold increase in risk for heavy smokers (more than one pack per day)
• Quitting smoking does not appear to decrease the risk of adenocarcinoma, which remains elevated for decades after smoking cessation
• This suggests that tobacco carcinogens may affect carcinogenesis early on in esophageal adenocarcinoma, and, therefore, decline in prevalence of smoking in the United States has not had an impact on the risk for the disease
• Cigarette smoking was recently identified as a risk factor for development of Barrett's esophagus
• Increasing the pack-years of smoking increased the risk of Barrett's esophagus
• Alcohol is a major contributing factor in the increased risk of esophageal squamous cell carcinoma in Western countries, likely accounting for 80% of squamous cell carcinoma of the esophagus in men in the United States

(Devita, 10th Edition, Page 575)

94. Which of the following is not true about SCC of anus?

(a) Five times more common than perianal squamous cell carcinoma

(b) Cancers of anal margin (T1) and well differentiated is treated by wide local excision

(c) Anal margin lesions that are greater than T1/node positive should be wide local excision

(d) Patients with stage IV metastatic disease may benefit from cisplatin-based chemotherapy with or without RT

Ans: (c) Anal margin lesions that are greater than T1/node positive should be wide local excision

- Squamous cell carcinoma of anal canal is five times more common than perianal squamous cell carcinoma
- Cancers of anal margin (those occurring within 5 cm of squamous mucocutaneous junction) that are small (T1) and well differentiated-treated by wide local excision
- Any anal margin lesions that are greater than T1 or node positive should be treated like primary SCC anal canal with definitive chemoradiation
- Patients with stage IV metastatic disease may benefit from cisplatin-based chemotherapy with or without radiation therapy

(Sabiston, 20th Edition, Page 1414)

95. Which of the following is not true about Hemangioma of liver?

(a) Most common benign tumor of liver
(b) Females are more commonly affected than males
(c) Mean age affected is 65 years
(d) Cavernous hemangiomas are associated with FNH

Ans: (c) Mean age affected is 65 years

Hemangioma Liver
• Hemangioma is the most common benign tumor of the liver
• It occurs in women more than in men (3 : 1 ratio)
• Mean age of approximately 45 years
• Cavernous hemangiomas have been associated with FNH and are also theorized to be congenital vascular malformations
• Enlargement of hemangiomas is by ectasia rather than by neoplasia
• They are usually solitary and less than 5 cm in diameter, and they occur with equal incidence in the right and left hemilivers
• Lesions larger than 5 cm are arbitrarily called giant hemangiomas
• Involution or thrombosis of hemangiomas can result in dense fibrotic masses that may be difficult to differentiate from malignant tumors
• Hemangiomas are usually asymptomatic and found incidentally on imaging studies
• Large compressive masses may cause vague upper abdominal symptoms. Symptoms ascribed to a liver hemangioma, however, mandate search for other disease because an alternative cause of symptoms will be found in approximately 50% cases
• Rapid expansion or acute thrombosis can occasionally cause symptoms. Spontaneous rupture of liver hemangiomas is exceedingly rare
• An associated syndrome of thrombocytopenia and consumptive coagulopathy known as Kasabach-Merritt syndrome

(Sabiston, 20th Edition, Page 1456)

96. Which of the following statements is not true about bile duct cancer?

(a) Distal bile duct tumors are treated with pylorus-preserving pancreatoduodenectomy
(b) For curative resection, location and local extension of tumor dictates extent of resection
(c) For distal bile duct tumors, endoscopic placement is often the preferred approach
(d) Adjuvant chemotherapy in the treatment of cholangiocarcinoma gives best results

Ans: (d) Adjuvant chemotherapy in the treatment of cholangiocarcinoma gives best results

- No proven role for adjuvant chemotherapy in treatment of cholangiocarcinoma
- Adjuvant radiation therapy has also not been shown to increase either quality of life or survival in resected patients
- Distal bile duct tumors are more often resectable and are treated with pylorus-preserving pancreatoduodenectomy (Whipple procedure)
- For patients with distal bile duct cancer found to be unresectable on surgical exploration, Roux-en-Y hepaticojejunostomy, cholecystectomy and gastrojejunostomy to prevent gastric outlet obstruction should be performed
- Nonoperative biliary decompression is performed for patients with unresectable disease on diagnostic evaluation
- For distal bile duct tumors, endoscopic placement is often the preferred approach
- For curative resection location and local extent of tumor dictates extent of resection

- Perihilar tumors involving the bifurcation or proximal common hepatic duct (Bismuth-Corlette type I or II) with no signs of vascular involvement are candidates for local tumor excision with portal lymphadenectomy, cholecystectomy, common bile duct excision, and bilateral Roux-en-Y hepaticojejunostomies
- If the tumor involves the right or left hepatic duct (Bismuth-Corlette type IIIa or IIIb), right or left hepatic lobectomy, respectively, should also be performed Frequently, resection of the adjacent caudate lobe is required because of direct extension into caudate biliary radicals or parenchyma

(Schwartz, 10th Edition, Page 1337)

97. All are true about Squamous cell carcinoma urinary bladder *except:*

(a) Squamous cell tumors are of solid variety
(b) Nearly always associated with no muscle invasion
(c) Most prevalent form of bladder cancer of endemic bilharzia
(d) Chronic irritation caused by stone disease in the bladder as a result of metaplasia

Ans: (b) Nearly always associated with no muscle invasion

- Squamous cell tumours tend to be solid and are nearly always associated with muscle invasion.
- This is most prevalent form of bladder cancer in areas where bilharzia is endemic
- Squamous cell tumors may be associated with chronic irritation caused by stone disease in the bladder as a result of metaplasia

(Bailey, 27th Edition, Page 1448)

98. In Finger's MOST mnemonic, all are true *except:*

(a) M=Melanoma
(b) O=Oral mucosal involvement
(c) S=Subretinal fluid
(d) T=Thickness of ≥ 2 mm

Ans: (b) O=Oral mucosal involvement

- Dr. Finger created the **mnemonic MOST** where Melanoma + Orange pigment + Subretinal fluid + Thickness of ≥2 mm
- Choroidal melanoma invades and destroys the overlying retinal pigment epithelium, accumulations of orange pigment (lipofuscin and melanolipofuscin) can be visualized on the surface of a choroidal melanoma
- Choroidal melanoma-associated incontinent tumor blood vessels leak serum beneath the retina, seen as overlying retinal pigment epithelial detachments or subretinal fluid
- Lastly, choroidal melanomas are typically ≥ 2 mm thick

(Devita, 10th Edition, Page 1772)

99. True about Stauffer's syndrome is:

(a) Non metastatic dysfunction
(b) Reversible hepatitis
(c) Associated with Renal cell carcinoma
(d) All of the above

Ans: (d) All of the above

- Stauffer's syndrome is non metastatic hepatic dysfunction which results from Renal cell carcinoma
- Reversible hepatitis is seen without metastasis

(Sabiston, 20th Edition, Page 2097)

100. Which of the following immunotherapy is not correctly matched?

(a) Cetuximab–Colorectal cancer
(b) Nivolumab–Melanoma
(c) Ipuimumab–Metastatic melanoma
(d) Alemtuzumab–NHL

Ans: (d) Alemtuzumab–NHL

- Cetuximab–Colorectal cancer
- Bevacizumab–Colorectal cancer
- Nivolumab–Melanoma
- Ipuimumab–Metastatic melanoma
- Alemtuzumab–CML
- Tositumomab–NHL
- Pembrolizumab–Melanoma

(Sabiston, 20th Edition, Page 719)

101. Fish-eye lesion is seen on ERCP in:

(a) Mucinous cystadenoma pancreas
(b) Intraductal papillary mucinous neoplasms
(c) Serous cystadenoma pancreas
(d) Pancreatic pseudocyst

Ans: (b) Intraductal papillary mucinous neoplasms

- ERCP, mucin can be seen extruding from the ampulla of Vater, a so-called *fish-eye lesion* that is virtually diagnostic of IPMN

(Schwartz 10th Edition, Page 1411)

102. Most common site of leiomyosarcoma of large intestine:

(a) Proximal colon
(b) Mid colon
(c) Distal colon
(d) Rectum

Ans: (d) Rectum

- Leiomyosarcoma is rare in the gastrointestinal tract
- When this malignancy occurs in the large intestine, rectum is most common site
- Symptoms include bleeding and obstruction
- A radical resection is indicated for these tumors
- Most common sites affected overall are retroperitoneum and peritoneal cavity namely, uterus and about 25% rise from the trunk and extremities **(Sabiston, 20th Edition, Page 770)**

(Schwartz, 10th Edition, Page 1216)

103. Which area have highest rate of second Head and neck squamous cell cancer among following?

(a) Larynx
(b) Hypopharynx
(c) Oral cavity
(d) Oropharynx

Ans: (b) Hypopharynx

- Patients with hypopharyngeal cancer have highest rate of synchronous malignancies and highest rate of development of second HNSCC primaries of any of head and neck sites

104. Which of the following is most reproducible biomarker for metastasis in Uveal melanoma?

(a) Tumor size
(b) Growth pattern
(c) Tumor infiltrating lymphocytes
(d) All of the above

Ans: (a) Tumor size

- Uveal melanoma size or largest tumor dimension has been the most reproducible biomarker for choroidal melanoma metastasis
- Choroidal melanomas are typically dome or mushroom shaped but 5% grow in a diffuse pattern
- These diffuse melanomas are low-lying tumors often with indistinct or irregular margins that are more difficult to treat

- Iris melanomas can also occur as the diffuse variant, starting as a solitary tumor then evolving to multifocal lesions after treatment

(Devita, 10th Edition, Page 1778)

105. Most common clinical symptom of Superior vena cava syndrome is:

(a) Chest pain (b) Cough

(c) Dyspnea (d) Dysphagia

Ans: (c) Dyspnea

Symptoms	Findings
Dyspnea Facial swelling Cough Arm swelling Chest pain Dysphagia	Venous distension of neck and chest wall Facial edema Cyanosis Plethora of face Arm edema

(Devita, 10th Edition, Page 1805)

106. Which of the following factors don't favour VATS?

(a) Number of nodules < 3 (b) Size of nodule <5 cm

(c) Peripheral (d) Lower lobar location

Ans: (d) Lower lobar location

Factor	Favor VATS	Favor Thoracotomy with manual palpation
No of nodules	<3	>3 or equal to 3
Size of largest nodule	<5 cm	>5 cm
Size of smallest nodule	>1.5 cm	<1.5 cm
Location	Peripheral	Central
Histology	Colorectal	Melanoma
Pulmonary function	Marginal	Normal
Previous chest RT	Never	Yes
Lobar location	Upper/middle	Lower

(Devita, 10th Edition, Page 1848)

107. Most important adverse effect of Denosumab is:

(a) Osteonecrosis (b) Vitamin D deficiency

(c) Impaired teeth development (d) Thrombocytopenia

Ans: (a) Osteonecrosis

- Most important adverse event associated with denosumab is osteonecrosis of jaw
- Denosumab is a fully human monoclonal antibody that binds and neutralizes RANKL with high affinity and specificity to inhibit osteoclast function and bone resorption

(Devita, 10th Edition, Page 1869)

108. Limbic encephalitis is a paraneoplastic syndrome most commonly associated with:

(a) Small cell lung cancer (b) Testicular germ cell tumors

(c) Thymoma (d) Teratoma

Ans: (a) Small cell lung cancer

- Limbic encephalitis is most commonly associated with Small cell lung cancer
- Others include Testicular germ cell cancer, Breast cancer, Thymoma, Teratoma and Hodgkin lymphoma

(Devita, 10th Edition, Page 1894)

109. Radiation induced delayed pericarditis typically occurs after how many years after mediastinal irradiation?

(a) 5 years (b) 10 years

(c) 1 year (d) 2 years

Ans: (c) 1 year

- ***Radiation induced pericarditis typically occurs within 1st year after mediastinal irradiation***
- Common range is from 4 months to several years after treatment
- Pericardial disease presents either as an acute pericarditis, as a pericardial effusion that may be asymptomatic, or as a combination of both
- Symptoms of delayed acute pericarditis are indistinguishable from those of other types of pericarditis and usually consist of fever, pleuritic chest pain, pericardial friction rub, ST-T segment changes, and a decrease of QRS voltage in the ECG
- Acute radiation induced pericarditis does not lead to a significant risk of late pericardial damage and is not an indication for interrupting the radiation course

(Devita, 10th Edition, Page 2018)

110. Clinical diagnosis of PJS may be made when any one of the following *except:*

(a) Any number of PJS polyps in an individual who also has characteristic mucocutaneous pigmentation

(b) Any number of PJS polyps detected in 1 individual has family history of PJS in close relatives

(c) Characteristic mucocutaneous pigmentation in an individual with family history of PJS in close relatives

(d) One histologically confirmed PJS polyps

Ans: (a) Any number of PJS polyps in an individual who also has characteristic mucocutaneous pigmentation

Clinical diagnosis of PJS may be made when any one of the following is present
• Two or more histologically confirmed PJS polyps
• Any no. of PJS polyps detected in one individual with family history of PJS in close relatives
• Characteristic mucocutaneous pigmentation in an individual with family history of PJS in close relatives
• Any no. of PJS polyps in an individual who also has characteristic mucocutaneous pigmentation

(Devita, 10th Edition, Page 1103)

111. All the following statements are true about Oncocytoma *except:*

(a) Loss of chromosome 1 and Y

(b) Mutated genes include mitochondrial genes like COX1 and COX2

(c) Gross appearance is circumscribed and mahogany colour

(d) Commonly associated with necrosis

Ans: (d) Commonly associated with necrosis

Oncocytoma
• Loss of chromosome 1 and Y chromosome and *CCND1* rearrangement
• Gross appearance of tumor is Mahogany colour, Circumscribed, Occasional central scar and
• **Rarely associated with necrosis**
• HISTOLOGY: Polygonal cells with abundant eosinophilic cytoplasm with uniform, round nuclei

(Bailey, 27th Edition, Page 1417)

112. Testing for fumarate hydratase is done for identifying which of the following RCC?

(a) Hereditary papillary renal cell carcinoma type 1
(b) Hereditary papillary renal cell carcinoma type 2
(c) Clear cell carcinoma
(d) Chromophobe carcinoma

Ans: (a) Hereditary papillary renal cell carcinoma type 1

Approach to diagnosis of familial RCC

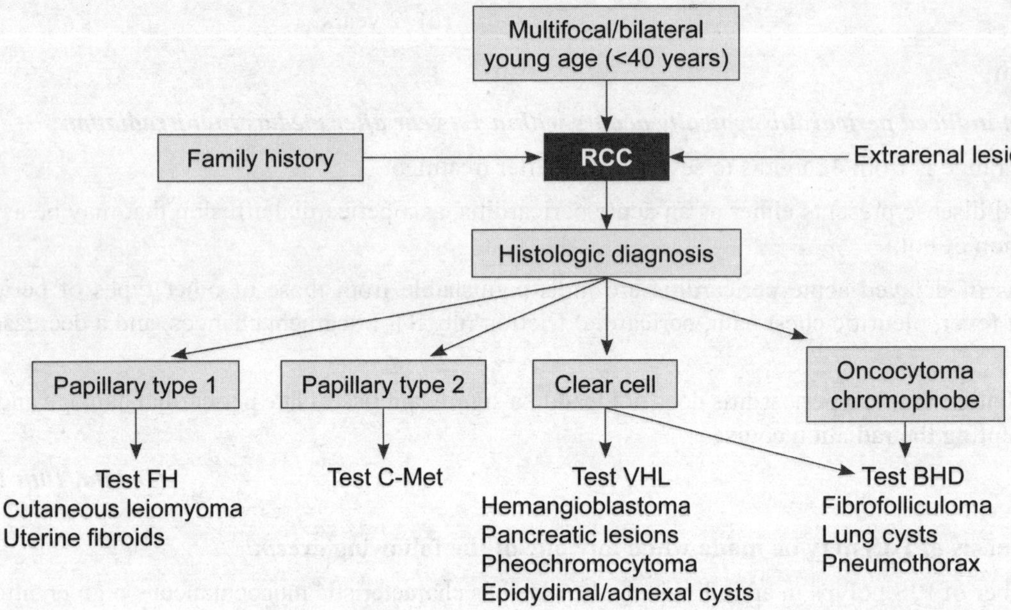

(Devita, 10th Edition, Page 921)

113. Most common type of male urethral carcinoma is:

(a) Transitional cell carcinoma
(b) Squamous cell carcinoma
(c) Adenocarcinoma
(d) Carcinoid tumor

Ans: (b) Squamous cell carcinoma

- **80% of male urethral cancers are squamous cell, 15% are urothelial (transitional cell), and approximately 5% are adenocarcinomas or undifferentiated tumors**
- Anatomic location of urethral cancer largely determines the histologic type
- **Carcinomas of prostatic urethra are urothelial in 90% and squamous in 10%; carcinomas of penile urethra are squamous in 90% and urothelial in 10%**
- Adenocarcinomas of urethra arise from metaplasia of mucosa or from periurethral glands
- Bulbomembranous urethra is most commonly involved (60%), followed by the penile urethra (30%) and the prostatic urethra (10%)

(Devita, 10th Edition, Page 981)

114. Which of the following is not true about poor risk of germ cell tumor?

(a) Non seminomatous tumor with mediastinal primary site
(b) Seminomatous tumor with mediastinal primary site
(c) Non seminomatous tumor with AFP >10,000 ng/Ml
(d) Non seminomatous tumor with Nonpulmonary visceral metastases

Ans: (b) Seminomatous tumor with mediastinal primary site

Risk Group	Seminoma	Non Seminoma
Good	Any hCG Any LDH Non pulmonary visceral metastases absent Any primary site	AFP <1,000 ng/mL hCG <5,000 mIU/mL LDH <1.5 × ULN Nonpulmonary visceral metastases absent Gonadal or retroperitoneal primary site
Intermediate	Non pulmonary visceral metastases present Any hCG Any LDH Any primary site	AFP 1,000–10,000 ng/mL hCG 5,000–50,000 mIU/mL LDH 1.5–10.0 × ULN Non pulmonary visceral metastases absent Gonadal or retroperitoneal primary site
Poor	No	Mediastinal primary site Non pulmonary visceral metastases present (e.g., bone, liver, brain) AFP >10,000 ng/mL hCG >50,000 mIU/mL LDH >10 × ULN

(Devita, 10th Edition, Page 995)

115. Which of the following statements are true about Lymphoma *except?*

(a) Can be bilateral
(b) Painful enlargement of testis
(c) Most common secondary malignancy of testis in >50 years old
(d) Occurs due to advanced systemic disease

Ans: (b) Painful enlargement of testis

Lymphoma
• Lymphoma presents as painless enlargement of the testicle
• It can be bilateral
• **Most common secondary malignancy of testis in men older than 50 years**
• It typically occurs in advanced systemic disease
• Often accompanied by central nervous system or bone marrow involvement

(Devita, 10th Edition, Page 1003)

116. Hallmark of Kaposi sarcoma is:

(a) Increased proliferation of VEGF
(b) Hyperproliferation of KSHV infected spindle cells
(c) Induces c-Kit and endothelial-to-mesenchymal transformation
(d) Increased CD57+ and decreased CD28+ T cells

Ans: (b) Hyperproliferation of KSHV infected spindle cells

- Hallmark of Kaposi sarcoma is Hyperproliferation of KSHV infected spindle cells
- KSHV encoded G-protein–coupled receptor (vGPCR, also known as ORF74) induces production of vascular endothelial growth factor (VEGF) and other angiogenic factors
- In patients with controlled HIV, KS is associated with a T-cell immunosenescense phenotype marked by increased CD57+ and decreased CD28+ T cells
- KSHV also induces c-Kit and endothelial-to-mesenchymal transformation

(Devita, 10th Edition, Page 1782)

117. All the following statements are true about cancer associated Hemolytic uremic syndrome *except:*

(a) Occurs as a manifestation of cancer

(b) Occurs as a complication of mitomycin C

(c) Occurs in setting of bone marrow transplantation

(d) Patients usually don't present with fever but present with hemolytic anemia and uremia

Ans: (d) Patients usually don't present with fever but present with hemolytic anemia and uremia

In patients with cancer, HUS occurs as:

- Manifestation of the cancer itself
- Complication of chemotherapy
- Setting of bone marrow transplantation
- More recently as a problem in patients receiving antibodies and immunotoxins
- Clinical manifestations of fulminant HUS include the classic pentad of microangiopathic hemolytic anemia, thrombocytopenia, fever, rapidly progressive renal failure, and neurological deficits

(Devita, 10th Edition, Page 1830)

118. All are true about Paget's disease of vulva *except:*

(a) Intraepithelial disease of unknown etiology

(b) Affects mostly black premenopausal women

(c) Causes chronic vulvar itching and is sometimes associated with an underlying invasive vulvar adenocarcinoma or invasive cancers of the breast, cervix, or gastrointestinal tract

(d) Treatment is surgical removal by wide local resection of the involved area with a 2 cm margin

Ans: (b) Affects mostly black premenopausal women

Paget's Disease
• Paget's disease of the vulva is an intraepithelial disease of unknown etiology that affects **mostly white postmenopausal women in their sixth decade of life**
• It causes chronic vulvar itching and is sometimes associated with an underlying invasive vulvar adenocarcinoma or invasive cancers of the breast, cervix, or gastrointestinal tract
• Grossly, the lesion is variable but usually confluent, raised, erythematous to violet, and waxy in appearance. Biopsy is required for diagnosis; disease is intraepithelial and characterized by Paget's cells with large pale cytoplasm
• Treatment is assessment for other potential concurrent adenocarcinomas, and then surgical removal by wide local resection of the involved area with a 2 cm margin
• Free margins are difficult to obtain because the disease usually extends beyond the clinically visible area
• Intraoperative frozen section of the margins can be done; however, Paget's vulvar lesions have a high likelihood of recurrence even after securing negative resection margins

(Schwartz, 10th Edition, Page 1680)

119. Which of the following statements are true about Wilms' tumor *except?*

(a) Usually presents in the first five years of life

(b) Typically presents with an abdominal mass

(c) May cause haematuria, abdominal pain or fever

(d) Metastasises to liver

Ans: (d) Metastasises to liver

Nephroblastoma (Wilms' tumor)
• Usually presents in the first five years of life
• Typically presents with an abdominal mass
• May cause haematuria, abdominal pain or fever
• Metastasises to the lung

(Bailey, 27th Edition, Page 1422)

120. Most common benign tumor of spleen is:

(a) Cysts of spleen
(b) Lipoma
(c) Nodular hyperplasia
(d) Hemangioma

Ans: (d) Hemangioma

- Haemangioma is the most common benign tumor of spleen
- May rarely develop into a haemangiosarcoma that is managed by splenectomy

(Bailey, 27th Edition, Page 1185)

121. All are true about Colonic cancer *except:*

(a) One third of patients will have liver metastases at the time of diagnosis
(b) 50% will account for the majority of deaths
(c) Lung is the most common site of metastasis
(d) Haematogenous spread is most commonly to the liver via the portal vein

Ans: (c) Lung is the most common site of metastasis

Colorectal Cancer
• Involvement of the lymph nodes by the tumor progresses from those closest to the bowel along the course of lymphatics to central nodes
• However, this orderly process does not always occur. Haematogenous spread is most commonly to the liver via the portal vein
• One third of patients will have liver metastases at the time of diagnosis and 50% will develop them at some point, accounting for the majority of deaths
• Lung is next most common site; metastasis to ovary, brain, kidney and bone is less common

(Bailey, 27th Edition, Page 1262)

PAPER 3

122. Renal cell carcinoma involving adrenal gland is T staged according to AJCC 8th edition is:

(a) I
(b) II
(c) III
(d) IV

Ans: (d) IV

T Staging of Renal Cell Carcinoma	
TX	Primary tumor cannot be assessed
T0	No evidence of primary tumor
T1a	Tumor < 4 cm in greatest dimensión, limited to kidney
T1b	Tumor > 4 cm but < 7 cm in greatest dimension limited to the kidney
T2a	Tumor > 7 cm but < 10 cm in greatest dimensión, limited to the kidney
T2b	Tumor > 10 cm limited to the kidney
T3a	Tumor extends into the renal vein or its segmental branches or invades the pelvicalyceal system or invades perirenal and/or renal sinus fat but not beyond Gerota's fascia
T3b	Tumor extends into the vena cava below the diaphragm
T3c	Tumor extends into the vena cava above the diaphragm or invades the wall of the vena cava
T4	Tumor invades beyond Gerota's fascia (including contiguous extensión into ipsilateral adrenal gland)

(Sabiston, 20th Edition, Page 2098)

123. All are components of Cancer of liver Italian Program score *except:*

(a) Unilocular <50% extension of tumor is scored as Zero
(b) Massive or extension >50% is scored as Two
(c) AFP >400 ng/dL is scored as Zero
(d) Portal vein thrombosis is scored as One

Ans: (c) AFP >400 ng/dL is scored as Zero

- Score ranges from 0 to 6; score of 4 to 6 is generally considered advanced disease
- Score of 0 to 3 has potential for long-term survival

Cancer of Liver Italian Program Score

Clinical Parameter	Cut Off Values	Points
Child pugh class	A	0
	B	1
	C	2
Tumor morphology	Uninodular <50% extension	0
	Multinodular <50% extension	1
	Massive or extension >50%	2
AFP level	<400 ng/dL	0
	>400 ng/dL	1
Portal vein thrombosis	No	0
	Yes	1

(Sabiston, 20th Edition, Page 1460)

124. Standard management of muscle invasive bladder cancer is:

(a) MVAC regimen
(b) Radical cystoprostatectomy
(c) TURBT
(d) Radiotherapy

Ans: (a) MVAC regimen

- **Standard management of MIBC is radical cystoprostatectomy**
- In male patient, radical cystectomy involves removal of the entire urinary bladder en block with the perivesical fat, prostate, seminal vesicles and pelvic lymph nodes
- In female patient, radical cystectomy typically involves en bloc removal of female pelvic viscera

(Sabiston, 20th Edition, Page 2100)

125. Median survival of metastatic prostatic carcinoma is:

(a) 1 year
(b) 2 years
(c) 3 years
(d) 4 years

Ans: (c) 3 years

- **Survival depends on stage and grade of disease**
- **T1 and T2:** Progression rate of well-differentiated T1a prostate cancer is very low: 10-14% after eight years. For moderately differentiated tumors, the rate is about 20%. For T1b and T2 tumors, the rate is in excess of 35%
- **T3 and T4 (MO):** About 50% progress to bony metastases after 3-5 years
- **M1:** Median survival of men with metastatic disease is about 3 years

(Bailey, 27th Edition, Page 1470)

126. Which of the following is not true about endometrial carcinoma?

(a) Type I tumors are estrogen-dependent endometrioid histology
(b) Type II endometrial cancers have favourable prognosis
(c) Type 2 tumors are of nonendometrioid, serous/clear cell histology
(d) Postmenopausal bleeding is the most common presentation of type I disease

Ans: (b) Type II endometrial cancers have favourable prognosis

- Endometrial adenocarcinomas are divided into type I and type II
- ***Type I tumors are estrogen-dependent endometrioid histology and have a relatively favorable prognosis***
- ***Type II endometrial cancers are estrogen-independent, aggressive, and characterized by nonendometrioid, serous, or clear cell histology***
- Postmenopausal bleeding is the most common presentation of type I disease and often permits early-stage diagnosis, resulting in a favorable prognosis
- Transvaginal ultrasonography (TVUS) often reveals a thickened endometrial stripe
- Uterine cancer is surgically staged and is graded based on the degree of histologic differentiation of the glandular components
- Grade is an important prognostic factor, independent of stage

(Schwartz, 10th Edition, Page 1700)

127. Which of the following statements are not true about HPV infection in Cervical cancers?

(a) HPV 16 and 18 cause approximately 70% of cervical cancers
(b) 90% of precancerous lesions (CIN II/III) occur as a result of HPV infection
(c) FDA approved vaccination to women between 9 and 26 years age for prevention of cervical, vulvar and vaginal cancer
(d) HPV 6 and 11 cause 90% of genital warts

Ans: (b) 90% of precancerous lesions (CIN II/III) occur as a result of HPV infection

- HPV 16 and 18 cause approximately 70% of cervical cancers
- 50% of precancerous lesions (CIN II/III) occur as a result of HPV infection
- FDA approved vaccination to women between 9 and 26 years age for prevention of cervical, vulvar and vaginal cancer
- HPV 6 and 11 cause 90% of genital warts

(Schwartz, 10th Edition, Page 1681)

128. Which of the following molecular methods are correctly matched for cancer mutation analysis?

(a) KRAS and BRAF mutations in solid tumors are analyzed by High resolution melting curve analysis
(b) KIT mutations in GIST and melanoma are analyzed by sanger sequencing
(c) EGFR exon 19 deletions in NSCLC are analyzed by fragment analysis
(d) All of the above

Ans: (d) All of the above

- KRAS and BRAF mutations in solid tumors are analyzed by **High resolution melting curve analysis**
- KRAS, BRAF and EGFR mutations in solid tumors are also analyzed by **PCR**
- KIT mutations in GIST and melanoma are analyzed by **sanger sequencing**
- EGFR exon 19 deletions in NSCLC are analyzed by fragment analysis
- ALK translocation in NSCLC, EWSR1 translocation in soft tissue tumors, HER2 amplification in breast cancer, 1p/19q deletion in oligodendroglioma are analyzed by **FISH**

(Devita, 10th Edition, Page 51)

129. All are true about GIST *except:*

(a) Succinate dehydrogenase (SDH)-deficient WT GISTs typically occur in young females

(b) Wild type GISTs harbor mutations KIT or PDGFRA mutations

(c) A negative stain for SDHB identifies the subgroup of SDH-deficient WT GISTs

(d) Gain-of-function mutations of oncogenes located on chromosome 4 coding for type III receptor tyrosine kinases KIT and PDGFRA can be found in approximately 80% of GISTs

Ans: (b) Wild type GISTs harbor mutations KIT or PDGFRA mutations

- Succinate dehydrogenase (SDH)-deficient WT GISTs typically occur in young females
- Wild type GISTs do not harbor mutations KIT or PDGFRA mutations
- A negative stain for SDHB identifies the subgroup of SDH-deficient WT GISTs
- Gain-of-function mutations of oncogenes located on chromosome 4 coding for type III receptor tyrosine kinases KIT and PDGFRA can be found in approximately 80% of GIST

(Devita, 10th Edition, Page 746)

130. Life time risk of small bowel cancer in HNPCC is:

(a) 5%
(b) <5%
(c) >5%
(d) 50%

Ans: (b) <5%

Risk Factor	Life Time Risk
FAP	2-5%
HNPCC	1-4%
Peutz Jeghers syndrome	15 fold
MUTYH associated polyposis	4%
Crohn's disease	2%

(Devita, 10th Edition, Page 738)

131. Wrong match among following about Life time Risk of colorectal cancer is:

(a) FAP-100% Colorectal cancer
(b) AFAP-70% Colorectal cancer
(c) MAP-80% Colorectal cancer
(d) Juvenile polyposis syndrome- 90% Colorectal cancer

Ans: (d) Juvenile polyposis syndrome-90% Colorectal cancer

Colorectal Cancer–Life Time Risk				
FAP	AFAP	MAP	PJS-Peutz Jeghers syndrome	JPS- Juvenile polyposis syndrome
100%	70%	80%	39%	40-50%

(Devita, 10th Edition, Page 814)

132. Which of the following is true about treatment of HCC in patients with Performance score >2 and Child pugh score?

(a) Liver resection
(b) Liver transplantation
(c) Sorafenib
(d) Best supportive care

Ans: (d) Best supportive care

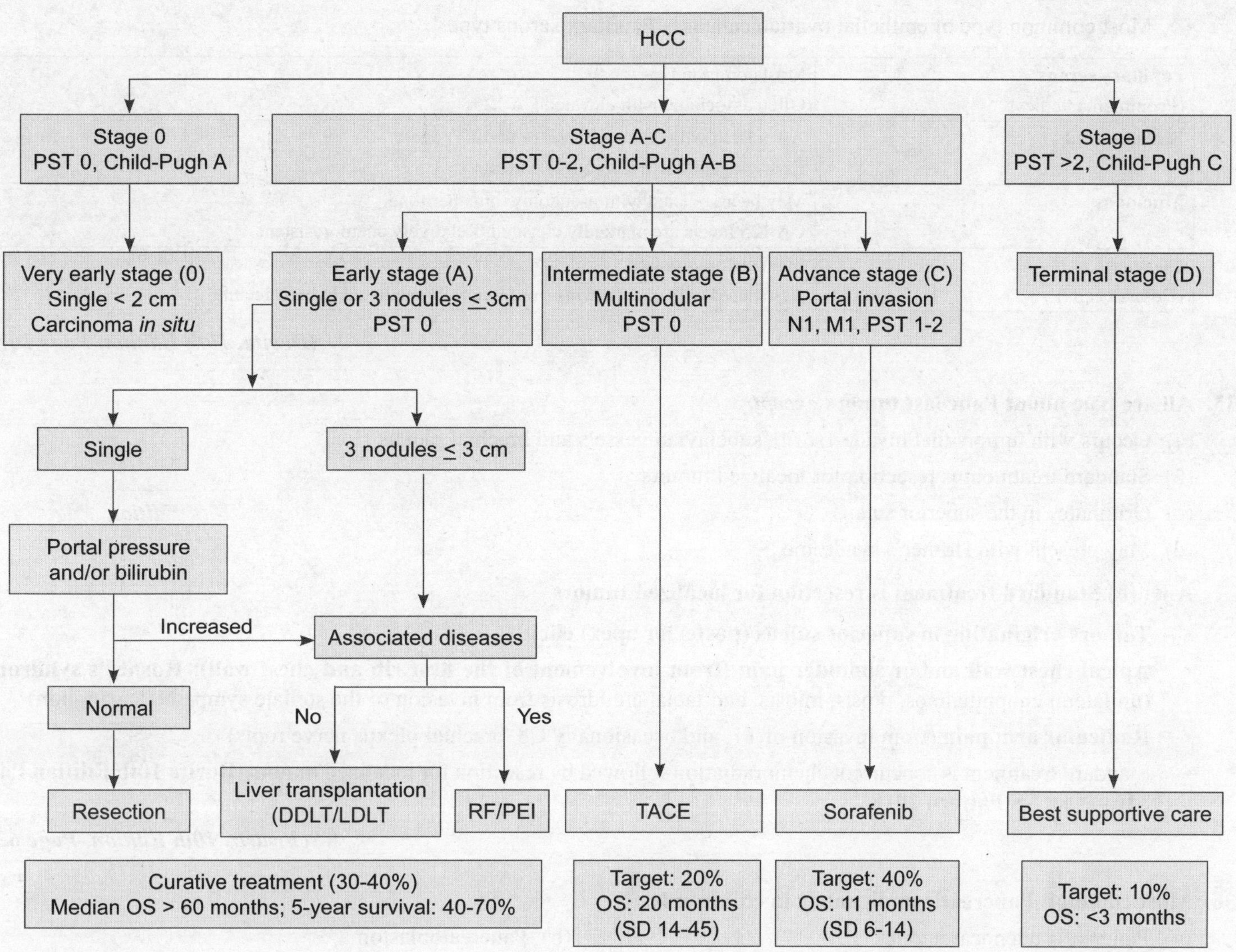

(Bailey, 27th Edition, Page 1174)

133. Which of the following risk factors are associated with Cholangiocarcinoma?

(a) Primary sclerosing cholangitis
(b) Choledochal cysts
(c) Hepatolithiasis
(d) All of the above

Ans: (d) All of the above

- Risk factors associated with cholangiocarcinoma include primary sclerosing cholangitis, choledochal cysts, ulcerative colitis, hepatolithiasis, biliary-enteric anastomosis, and biliary tract infections with Clonorchis or in chronic typhoid carriers
- Features common to most risk factors include biliary stasis, bile duct stones and infection
- Other risk factors associated with cholangiocarcinoma are liver flukes, dietary nitrosamines, Thorotrast and exposure to dioxin

(Sabiston, 20th Edition, Page 1335)

134. Most common type of epithelial ovarian cancer is:

(a) Papillary serous
(b) Endometroid
(c) Mucinous
(d) Clear cell

Ans: (a) Papillary serous

- Most common type of epithelial ovarian cancer is Papillary serous type

Papillary serous (Psommoma bodies)	Most common type Often associated with elevated CA 125
Endometroid	Associated with endometriosis or uterine cancer Early stage disease in younger patients
Mucinous	May be associated with pseudomyxoma peritonei CA 125 levels are markedly elevated, Relatively chemoresistant
Clear cell (Hobnail cells)	Most chemoresistant Associated with endometriosis or humorally mediated hypercalcemia

(Devita, 10th Edition, Page 1077)

135. All are true about Pancoast tumors *except:*

(a) Occurs with tumors that invade 1st rib, subclavian vessels and brachial plexus
(b) Standard treatment is resection for localized tumors
(c) Originates in the superior sulcus
(d) May present with Horner's syndrome

Ans: (b) Standard treatment is resection for localized tumors

- **Tumors originating in superior sulcus (posterior apex) elicit**
- **Apical chest wall and/or shoulder pain (from involvement of the first rib and chest wall); Horner's syndrome** (unilateral enophthalmos, ptosis, miosis, and facial anhidrosis from invasion of the stellate sympathetic ganglion)
- **Radicular arm pain** (from invasion of T1, and occasionally C8, brachial plexus nerve roots)
- Standard treatment is concurrent chemoradiation followed by resection for localized tumors **(Devita 10th Edition Page 516)–Neet SS Pattern 2018**

(Schwartz, 10th Edition, Page 623)

136. Most common Pancreatic malignancy in children is:

(a) Pancreatic adenocarcinoma
(b) Pancreatoblastoma
(c) Acinic cell carcinoma
(d) Solid pseudopapillary tumors

Ans: (b) Pancreatoblastoma

- Pancreatoblastoma is most common pancreatic malignancy in children
- **Usually occurs in first 8 years of life**
- These tumors have been associated with the Beckwith-Wiedemann and FAP syndromes
- Elevated levels of serum α-fetoprotein and hormones have been described
- Cures are often achievable with resection in children, although one-third of patients present with metastatic disease
- Microscopically, these tumors contain acinar cells, but other cell types like neuroendocrine, ductal origin
- Acquire relatively few mutations (~15 per tumor), SMAD4 and CTNNB1 that are typical
- ***Kras mutations have not been reported***

(Devita, 10th Edition, Page 661)

137. Which of the following is not true about Medulloblastoma?

(a) CTNNB1 mutation is associated with WNT group of medulloblastoma
(b) PTCH1 mutation is associated with SHH group of medulloblastoma
(c) Group 4 medulloblastoma is associated with poor prognosis
(d) WNT group has good prognosis

Ans: (c) Group 4 medulloblastoma is associated with poor prognosis

Subtypes of Medulloblastoma					
Group	**Progenitor Cell**	**Growth**	**Prognosis**	**Characteristic Mutations**	**Structural Events**
WNT	Lower rhombic lip	4th ventricle, with dorsal brainstem infiltration	Good	*CTNNB1 (91%), DDX3X, SMARCA4, MLL2, TP53*	Monosomy 6
SHH	Cerebellar granule neuron precursors of the external granule layer	Cerebellar hemispheres	Intermediate	*PTCH1, SUFU, SMO, TP53, MLL2, DDX3X*	Genome instability, including frequent amplification of *MYCN* and *GLI2*, deletion of *PTCH1*
Group 3	Cerebellar granule neuron precursors of the external granule layer, neural stem cells	~30% metastatic at diagnosis (47% for infants)	Poor		Genome instability, including *MYC* amplification, *MYC/PVT1* fusions, somatic copy number alteration in TGFB signaling members including amplification of *OTX2*
Group 4	Unknown	~30% metastatic at diagnosis (36% for infants)	Intermediate	*KDM6A*	Genome instability, including *SNCAIP* tandem duplication, *MYCN* amplification

(Devita, 10th Edition, Page 1048)

138. All are true about Extragonadal germ cell tumors *except:*

(a) Occurs in 1 in 35,000 live births

(b) Most common germ cell tumors in infants and newborns

(c) Approximately 80% of tumors are diagnosed within first month of life

(d) Affects usually boys

Ans: (d) Affects usually boys

- Sacrococcygeal teratoma occur in 1 in 35,000 live births
- **Most common germ cell tumors in infants and newborns, more commonly affect girls**
- Approximately 80% of these tumors are diagnosed within first month of life
- *Four types of sacrococcygeal teratomas have been defined on basis of the abdominopelvic extent and the presence or absence of external extension*
- Surgery is mainstay of therapy for sacrococcygeal tumors and should include removal of coccyx to minimize local recurrence
- Children with benign sacrococcygeal tumors have an excellent outcome with surgery alone, but recurrences that often contain a yolk sac component are seen in 11% of patients with mature teratomas and in 4% of patients with immature teratomas
- Patients with malignant yolk sac tumors located in the abdomen and pelvis are highly responsive to chemotherapy and have an excellent survival (approximately 90%) when treated with platinum-containing regimens

(Devita, 10th Edition, Page 1496)

139. Most common histological cause of carcinoma of unknown primary is:

(a) Squamous cell carcinoma

(b) Adenocarcinoma

(c) Typical Neuroendocrine carcinoma

(d) Poorly differentiated carcinoma

Ans: (b) Adenocarcinoma

- Most common histological cause of carcinoma of unknown primary is Adenocarcinoma

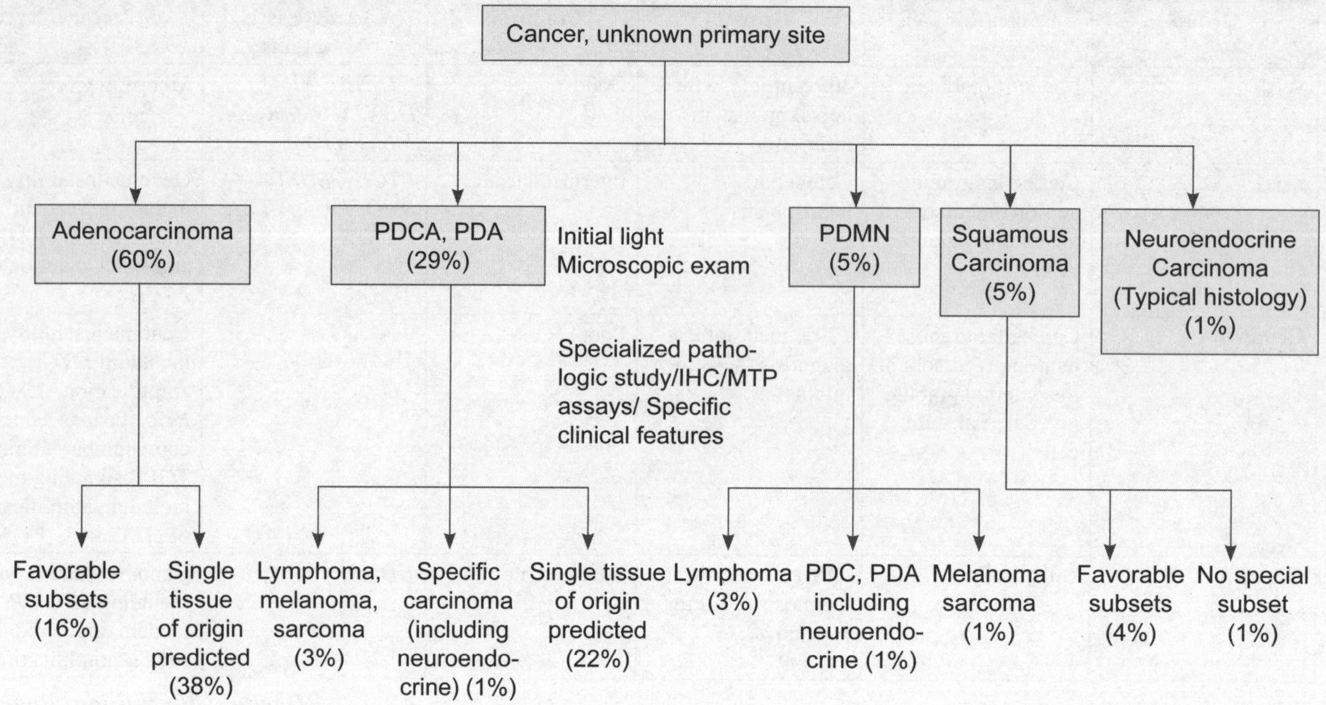

(Devita, 10th Edition, Page 1721)

140. Severe wasting in Cancer is due to:

(a) IL 6
(b) IL 1
(c) TNF alpha
(d) INF gamma

Ans: (a) IL 6

IL 1	Induces anorexia, early satiety, peripheral proteolysis, potentiates release of IL-6
IL 6	Severe wasting
TNF alpha	Lipolysis, muscle degradation, increased glucose turnover
Proteolysis-inducing factor	Skeletal muscle degradation
Lipid mobilizing factor	Lipolysis
Interferon-γ	Potentiates lipolysis, decreases protein synthesis

(Devita, 10th Edition, Page 2106)

141. All are true about chronic postsurgical pain syndromes *except:*

(a) Postmastectomy pain syndrome
(b) Postoperative frozen shoulder
(c) Phantom limb pain
(d) Plexopathy associated with intra-arterial infusion

Ans: (d) Plexopathy associated with intra-arterial infusion

Treatment-Related Chronic Pain Syndromes	
Postchemotherapy Pain Syndromes	**Chronic Post radiation Pain Syndromes**
Chronic painful peripheral neuropathy	Plexopathies
Avascular necrosis of femoral or humeral head	Radiation-induced brachial and lumbosacral plexopathies
Plexopathy associated with intra-arterial infusion	Radiation-induced peripheral nerve tumors
Raynaud's Phenomenon	Chronic radiation myelopathy

Contd.

Contd.

	Chronic radiation enteritis and proctitis Burning perineum syndrome Osteoradionecrosis
Chronic Postsurgical Pain Syndromes	**Chronic Pain Associated with Hormonal Therapy**
Postmastectomy pain syndrome Postradical neck dissection pain Postthoracotomy pain Postoperative frozen shoulder Phantom limb pain Phantom breast pain Phantom anus pain Phantom bladder pain Stump pain Postsurgical pelvic floor myalgia	Gynecomastia with hormonal therapy for prostate cancer

(Devita, 10th Edition, Page 2087)

142. Most common cause of primary hyperaldosteronism is:

(a) Aldosterone producing adenoma
(b) Adrenal cortex carcinoma
(c) Bilateral adrenal hyperplasia
(d) Familial type 1 hyperaldosteronism

Ans: (a) Aldosterone producing adenoma

Cause	Selective Screening	Non Selectible Screening
Aldosterone producing adenoma	60%	30%
Bilateral adrenal hyperplasia	35%	65%
Aldosterone producing carcinoma	<1%	<1%
Familial type 1 hyperaldosteronism	<1%	<1%
Familial type 2 hyperaldosteronism	<1%	<1%

(Sabiston, 20th Edition, Page 973)

143. Most common benign tumor of esophagus is:

(a) Adenoma
(b) Polyps
(c) Cysts
(d) Leiomyoma

Ans: (a) Adenoma

Leiomyoma	Esophageal Cysts (Congenital/Acquired)	Fibrovascular Polyps
Most common in men **Distal 2/3rd is most common site** Usually solitary **Surgical enucleation** is the treatment of choice	**Congenital**–Upper third, 1st year **Acquired-** Lower esophagus, Obstruction of excretory ducts and glands Extramucosal resection/Enucleation is the treatment of choice	Most common in men Most common site is cervical esophagus Surgical resection is the treatment of choice for > 8 cm size

(Bailey, 27th Edition, Page 1032)

144. Which amongst following statements is correct regarding prevalence of breast cancers?

(a) Hereditary breast cancer accounts for 2% of cases

(b) Presence of the BRCA gene confers a 25% risk of developing breast cancer

(c) Lobular carcinoma *in situ* (LCIS) confers a 20% risk of developing breast cancer

(d) LCIS occurs predominantly in women after menopause

Ans: (c) Lobular carcinoma in situ (LCIS) confers a 20% risk of developing breast cancer

- Hereditary breast cancer accounts for 5-10% of breast cancer cases and is mainly caused by BRCA gene mutations
- Presence of this gene confers a 60-85% risk of developing breast cancer
- Lobular carcinoma *in situ* arises from the epithelium of breast lobules and confers a twenty percent risk of developing cancer in either breast
- **LCIS occurs predominantly in premenopausal women**
- It is usually an incidental histological finding and has no typical radiologic or physical manifestations
- Invasive ductal carcinoma accounts for the majority of all breast cancer cases, followed by invasive lobular carcinoma (5-15%). Other types (medullary, mucinous, tubular) are rare and accounts for about in 2-6% of breast cancers

(Devita, 10th Edition, Page 1107)

145. Most important determinant of oncologic outcome in upper tract urothelial carcinoma is:

(a) Stage
(b) Number of tumors
(c) Location
(d) Tumor size

Ans: (a) Stage

- **Most well-established current predictors of survival in patients with upper tract urothelial tumors are stage and grade**
- The most significant decrease in survival is seen in T3 tumors and higher-grade tumors are more likely to invade the surrounding tissues, hence presenting with higher stage
- Although there have been studies showing differences in prognosis based on tumor number, location, size and architecture, these criteria are evolving and warrant further investigation

(Devita, 10th Edition 981, Campbell, 11th Edition)

146. A fair-skinned 68-year-old woman has sharply demarcated 2 cm ulcerated skin lesion in an old burn scar on her forearm. Most appropriate treatment for this patient:

(a) Topical chemotherapy
(b) Topical biologic therapy
(c) Surgical excision with frozen section
(d) Mohs micrographic surgery

Ans: (c) Surgical excision with frozen section

- **Cutaneous squamous cell carcinoma (SCC)** appears most frequently on sun-exposed areas, with two-thirds occurring on the head or neck; typical locations include exposed portion of ears, lower lip at the vermillion border, the paranasal areas, the maxillary skin and the dorsum of the hands
- Risk factors for cutaneous SCC include fair skin; light-colored eyes; prior actinic keratosis; xeroderma pigmentosum; and exposure to nitrates, arsenicals and hydrocarbons
- Other risk factors associated with the disease are chronic excessive sun exposure, immunosuppression, previous trauma and burns
- Aggressiveness of these cancers is related to underlying cause, location and size of lesion
- **It is increased in lesions arising in areas of previous burns (Marjolin ulcer) or trauma and in lesions of the lips and perineum**
- Excision of cutaneous SCC, generally with margins of 4 to 5 mm, should be accompanied by frozen section evaluation of the surgical margins
- These tumors are radiosensitive. Surgery is preferred for tumors arising in scarred, traumatized, or previously irradiated skin

- Large lesions may require adjuvant radiotherapy after surgical excision
- Mohs surgery may be used for lesions with clinically indistinct margins
- Regional LN dissection for SCC is performed for clinically evident (palpable) disease

(Schwartz, 10th Edition, Page 1817)

147. Which patient would not benefit from postmastectomy radiotherapy?

(a) A 49-year-old patient with inflammatory breast cancer
(b) A 25-year-old patient with DCIS
(c) A 57-year-old patient with a T1N2 infiltrating ductal carcinoma
(d) A 48-year-old patient with a 2.5 cm breast mass involving the underlying pectoral muscle

Ans: (b) A 25-year-old patient with DCIS

- Postmastectomy irradiation has been found to reduce the risk for local or regional recurrence by approximately two-thirds and to reduce breast cancer in all three studies
- Nodal irradiation is recommended after mastectomy for patients with four or more positive nodes, with large cancers (>5 cm) or very aggressive histology (diffuse vascular invasion) and with the extranodal extension of breast cancer
- Other indications include positive surgical margins; inflammatory breast cancer; or involvement of the skin, pectoral fascia, or skeletal muscle
- Radiation therapy is not indicated after mastectomy for DCIS, regardless of its size

(Sabiston, 20th Edition, Page 853)

148. A 75-year-old woman has a 1.2 cm mass in her right breast on physical examination that is found to be an infiltrating ductal carcinoma, and ER/PR positive, on core biopsy. Her axilla is clinically negative, as is her review of systems. She has multiple medical problems and wants to have as little done as possible. Which factor is not significantly associated with lymph node metastasis in elderly patients?

(a) Age
(b) Tumor location
(c) Tumor size
(d) Lymphovascular invasion

Ans: (b) Tumor location

- Nodal evaluation in elderly women with breast cancer remains controversial
- The risk associated with lymph node evaluation must be balanced with the benefit of staging and local control
- A recent large, prospective, multicenter trial found that on multivariate analysis, patient age, tumor size and lymphovascular invasion were significant factors predicting **lymph node metastasis**
- Patient race, palpable tumor, tumor grade, histologic subtype and tumor location were not found to be significant
- These findings suggest that some **elderly breast cancer** patients with a low likelihood of lymph node metastasis may be spared lymph node evaluation
- HER-2/neu status is not an indicator of the lymph node status

(Sabiston, 20th Edition, Page 845)

149. Most common malignancy found in childhood is:

(a) Lymphoma
(b) Leukemia
(c) Neuroblastoma
(d) Nephroblastoma

Ans: (b) Leukemia

- Approximately 40% of childhood malignancies are leukemia
- Most common solid tumor in children younger than 2 years is neuroblastoma, which accounts for 6%-10% of all childhood cancers
- In children older than 2 years, the most common solid tumor is Wilms tumor

(Devita, 10th Edition, Page 1465)

150. Which of the following is associated with a good prognosis in neuroblastoma?

(a) N-MYC amplification
(b) Age > 13 years
(c) Age < 1 year
(d) Stromal poor tumor cells on histology

Ans: (c) Age < 1 year

- Neuroblastoma is the most common solid extracranial tumor in the pediatric population
- Tumor arises from neural crest cells and is most commonly found in the adrenal medulla
- It may also be found anywhere along the sympathetic chain
- Presentation is generally insidious
- Commonly, a large abdominal mass is found
- Masses within the thoracic cavity can present with Horner syndrome (miosis, ptosis, anhidrosis and occasionally enophthalmos).
- Workup should include evaluating urinary VMA and homovanillic acid (HVA)
- **CT scans most frequently demonstrate a mass with calcifications**
- Metaiodobenzylguanidine (MIBG) scanning may be used to help identify metastatic disease
- **Tumor should be biopsied**
- Unfavorable findings associated with poor prognosis include stroma-poor tumors, MYC-N amplification and high MKI
- Patients diagnosed at less than 1 year of age have significantly improved outcomes compared with older children
- Survival is based on age at diagnosis, histologic subtype, MYC-N status and extent of disease
- Management is often multimodal and includes surgical excision, systemic chemotherapy, and occasional immunotherapy
- Stage 4S is a unique group of patients <18 months of age with a small primary tumor and metastatic disease limited to liver, skin, or bone marrow, but not the lymph nodes
- Many of these patients experience spontaneous regression of their disease
- Some require aggressive therapy, but the overall survival rates are fairly high

(Sabiston, 20th Edition, Page 1887)

151. A 75-year-old woman with recurrent breast cancer undergoes CT of the chest, abdomen and pelvis for metastatic workup. She is found to have 7 cm liver mass. Triple phase CT shows hypervascular lesion with peripheral to central enhancement. It is thought to be hemangioma. She denies abdominal pain or any episodes of jaundice. Reasonable indication for Surgery is:

(a) Disseminated intravascular coagulation
(b) Hemorrhage
(c) High-output cardiac failure
(d) All of the above

Ans: (d) All of the above

- Hepatic hemangiomas are the most common benign hepatic tumor
- **No risk of malignant degeneration and are often found incidentally**
- They typically appear as hypervascular lesions with initial peripheral enhancement followed by late central enhancement, which follows direction of blood flow into lesion
- Biopsy is not necessary and furthermore carries the risk of hemorrhage
- Asymptomatic uncomplicated hemangiomas are simply observed
- Indications for surgical resection include symptoms from mass effect, consumptive coagulopathy manifesting as DIC (seen in Kasabach-Merritt syndrome), high-output cardiac failure from arteriovenous shunting, or rupture and hemorrhage
- Enucleation can generally be performed, without formal liver resection being necessary

(Sabiston, 20th Edition, Page 1456)

152. Contraindication to resection of an adenocarcinoma of bile duct is:

(a) Tumor location in distal CBD
(b) Tumor location at bifurcation of bile duct
(c) Invasion of right and left portal vein
(d) Invasion of right portal vein and right hepatic artery

Ans: (c) Invasion of right and left portal vein

- **Cancers of the extrahepatic bile ducts** usually carry poor prognosis because these tumors are frequently beyond confines of surgical resection at time of diagnosis
- Substantial palliation can often be achieved with therapy directed at relief of biliary obstruction
- Prognosis is related to tumor location, resectability and histologic pattern
- **Proximal lesions at or near hepatic bifurcation are most common but are also least often resectable and therefore have less favorable prognosis**
- Aggressive resection of proximal lesions, usually hepatic resection can improve survival
- **Hilar cholangiocarcinoma (Klatskin tumor) is considered unresectable if there is metastatic disease, bilateral involvement of portal vein or hepatic artery, or bilateral extension of tumor to second order biliary radicles**
- Distal lesions resectable by pancreaticoduodenectomy have best prognosis with 5-year survival rate of approximately 30%-50%

(Sabiston, 20th Edition, Page 1513)

153. Which of the following is NOT considered an etiologic factor for soft tissue sarcoma?

(a) Viral infection
(b) Previous radiation exposure
(c) Scar tissue from previous injury
(d) Retroperitoneal fibrosis

Ans: (d) Retroperitoneal fibrosis

- Only retroperitoneal fibrosis is not an etiologic factor associated with development of a soft-tissue sarcoma
- When a patient presents with retroperitoneal fibrosis, a malignancy such as a soft-tissue sarcoma is in differential diagnosis, but that does not mean it constitutes an etiologic factor
- Remaining choices-viral infection, previous radiation exposure, scar tissue from a previous injury and Gardner syndrome are all etiologic factors with soft-tissue sarcomas

(Schwartz, 10th Edition, Page 1466)

154. A healthy 55-year-old man undergoes resection of a 2.0 cm bladder tumor in a posterior wall bladder diverticulum. Pathology demonstrates a pT1G3 bladder tumor with associated areas of carcinoma in situ. Muscularis mucosa is involved, but there is no definite muscularis propria in specimen. Optimal management includes:

(a) Repeat resection to stage the cancer
(b) Intravesical BCG therapy
(c) Partial cystectomy with excision of the diverticulum
(d) Radical cystectomy and neobladder urinary diversion

Ans: (d) Radical cystectomy and neobladder urinary diversion

- This patient should be strongly considered for radical cystectomy
- Partial cystectomy is not a good option because of presence of CIS, which indicates a high risk of field effect disease and subsequent recurrence
- Deeper biopsies will risk perforation and would be unlikely to influence management
- **Understaging is common with tumors in diverticuli, and high-grade invasive tumors like this are best managed with radical cystectomy to ensure local disease control and optimize outcomes on a long-term basis**

(Devita, 10th Edition, Page 900)

155. Partial cystectomy is appropriate in which of the following?

(a) 4-cm T2 lesion in the trigone
(b) 1-cm T2 lesion in the dome

(c) 3-cm T2 lesion in the dome with carcinoma in situ (CIS) in one location
(d) 1-cm T2 lesion with pelvic lymphadenopathy on imaging

Ans: (b) 1-cm T2 lesion in the dome

- In setting of muscle-invasive bladder cancer, partial cystectomy can be considered in very select patients. In those with small lesions and a lack of concurrent CIS, results of partial cystectomy approach those of radical cystectomy

(Devita, 10th Edition, Page 900, Campbell, 11th Edition)

156. According to Haggitt classification for polyps, which of the following is not true?

(a) A level 0 polyp refers to noninvasive carcinoma *in situ*
(b) All level IV polyps must be treated with segmental resection
(c) Endoscopic excision is adequate treatment for level I and level II polyps
(d) A wide-based sessile polyp with carcinoma at tip of the polyp only is considered a level III polyp

Ans: (d) A wide-based sessile polyp with carcinoma at tip of the polyp only is considered a level III polyp

- Haggitt classification for colonic polyps is used to characterize polyps for treatment
- Level 0 polyps refer to carcinoma *in situ* and are considered noninvasive. They can be treated with excision only
- Level I polyps contain carcinoma that invades the muscularis mucosa into the submucosa, but remains contained within the head of the polyp
- Level II polyps contain carcinoma that invades junction between stalk and the adenoma itself. Both level I and II polyps can generally be adequately treated with endoscopic excision
- Level III polyps invade the stalk. These can occasionally be excised endoscopically depending on margin obtained
- Carcinoma in level IV polyp invades submucosa of bowel but remains above muscularis propria. Wide-based sessile polyps with any carcinoma are also considered level IV. All level IV polyps require segmental resection

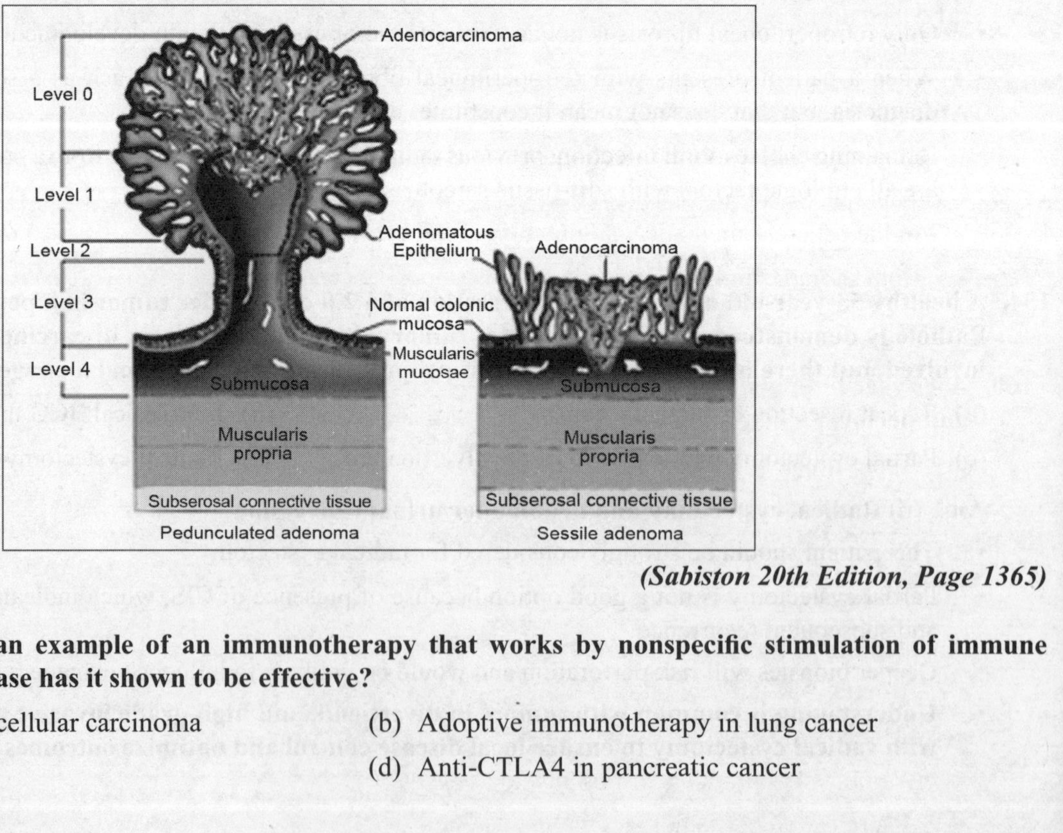

(Sabiston 20th Edition, Page 1365)

157. Which of the following is an example of an immunotherapy that works by nonspecific stimulation of immune reactions, and in which disease has it shown to be effective?

(a) Cancer vaccine in hepatocellular carcinoma
(b) Adoptive immunotherapy in lung cancer
(c) IL-2 in melanoma
(d) Anti-CTLA4 in pancreatic cancer

Ans: (c) IL-2 in melanoma

- **IL-2 is glycoprotein produced by activated peripheral blood lymphocytes and recombinant IL-2 in high doses can result in tumor cell regression**
- FDA-approved IL-2 for treatment of melanoma and renal cell carcinoma given the activity that has been shown in clinical trials

- Its activity stems from the nonspecific stimulation of the immune system
- Although anti-CTLA-4 therapies also work by nonspecific stimulation of immune reactions, they have not been shown to be effective in pancreatic cancer
- Cancer vaccines and adoptive immunotherapy have not been shown to be effective in lung cancer or hepatocellular carcinoma

(Devita, 10th Edition, Page 162)

158. Which of the following statements is CORRECT regarding pulmonary carcinoid tumors?

(a) Patients usually present with carcinoid syndrome
(b) Surgery has a curative potential for resectable localized tumors
(c) Adjuvant chemotherapy is the standard of care following complete surgical resection
(d) Most pulmonary carcinoids are atypical carcinoids

Ans: (b) Surgery has a curative potential for resectable localized tumors

- Only 2% of patients with pulmonary carcinoid present with carcinoid syndrome
- Approximately 30% of patients are asymptomatic at presentation
- Ninety percent of pulmonary carcinoids are typical, while 10% are atypical
- Surgery is the treatment of choice for carcinoid tumors
- There is no role for adjuvant chemotherapy, following complete resection for carcinoid tumors

(Devita, 10th Edition, Page 550)

159. MEN-associated gastrinomas are most frequently found in what anatomic location?

(a) Head of the pancreas
(b) Gallbladder
(c) Gastric antrum
(d) Duodenum

Ans: (d) Duodenum

- Majority of gastrinomas occur within the so-called gastrinoma triangle
- This space is bounded by confluence of the cystic and common hepatic ducts superiorly, junction of the head and neck of the pancreas medially, and junction of the second and third portions of the duodenum inferiorly
- Both sporadic and MEN-associated gastrinomas occur most frequently within duodenum

(Sabiston, 20th Edition, Page 954)

160. A 47-year-old patient presents with a slowly enlarging right parotid mass. You are suspicious for neoplastic process and perform a FNAC. Which of the following is true about parotid neoplasms?

(a) Approximately 75%–80% of parotid gland tumors are malignant
(b) Most common parotid tumor is mucoepidermoid carcinoma
(c) Pleomorphic adenoma is seen bilaterally in 50% of patients
(d) Smoking is an etiologic risk factor for Warthin's tumor

Ans: (d) Smoking is an etiologic risk factor for Warthin's tumor

- Around 75%–80% of parotid tumors are benign
- Most common parotid tumor is pleomorphic adenoma
- Warthin's tumor, not pleomorphic adenoma, is seen bilaterally in 12% of patients with a Warthin's tumor
- A surgical biopsy is not recommended due to a high risk of recurrence
- Warthin's tumor is second most common benign salivary gland tumor and is associated with smoking as a risk factor
- About 70% of salivary gland tumors occur in parotid gland, of which 75%–80% are benign

- Most common benign parotid tumor is pleomorphic adenoma followed next in incidence by **Warthin's tumor,** which is associated with smoking and an increased rate of being found bilaterally (12%)

(Sabiston, 20th Edition, Page 807)

161. Which of the following abnormalities is both paraneoplastic syndrome associated with HCC, and may also be caused by end-stage liver failure?

(a) Hypoglycemia (b) Erythrocytosis
(c) Hypercalcemia (d) Hypercholesterolemia

Ans: (a) Hypoglycemia

- Most of paraneoplastic syndromes are biochemical abnormalities without associated clinical consequences
- Most important ones include hypoglycemia (caused by end-stage liver failure), erythrocytosis, hypercalcemia, hypercholesterolemia, dysfibrinogenemia, carcinoid syndrome, increased thyroxin-binding globulin, sexual changes (gynecomastia, testicular atrophy, and precocious puberty) and porphyria cutanea tarda
- Pathogenesis of hypoglycemia is unclear but may be related to production of insulin-like growth factor I by the tumor

(Sabiston, 20th Edition, Page 1459)

162. Which tumor is associated with hydrocephalus and sudden death?

(a) Colloid cyst (b) Glioblastoma multiforme
(c) Lymphoma (d) Pilocytic astrocytoma

Ans: (a) Colloid cyst

- Colloid cysts represent 0.5 to 2% of all brain tumors and occur in the anterior part of the third ventricle near the foramen of Monro
- These lesions can be associated with the development of hydrocephalus and rapid clinical deterioration
- Sudden death has been reported but is rare, and likely involves the colloid cyst acting as a ball valve and suddenly shifting and occluding cerebrospinal fluid outflow
- **Occur in roof of third ventricle believed to represent embryonic endoderm remnants**

(Bailey 27th Edition Page 667, Schwartz, 10th Edition, Page 1751)

163. A 7-year-old boy presents with skull mass. Skeletal survey shown in this image reveals multiple other bony osteolytic lesions. Most likely diagnosis is: *(JIPMER SS 2015)*

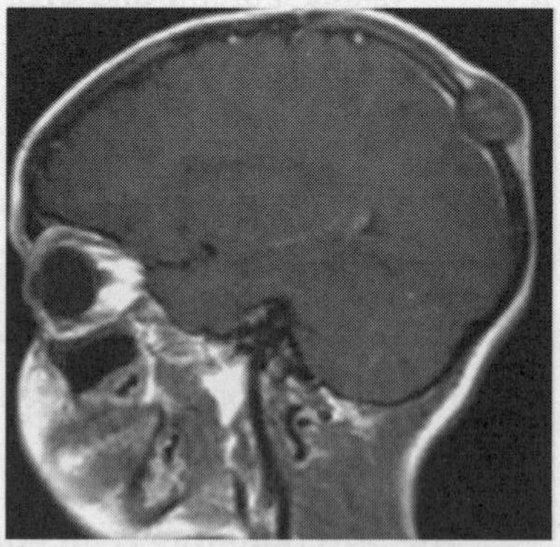

(a) Dermoid cyst (b) Epidermoid tumor
(c) Eosinophilic granuloma (d) Osteoma

Ans: (c) Eosinophilic granuloma

- Eosinophilic granuloma of skull can occur as solitary lesions or as part of a more generalized disease process of the lymphoreticular system termed Langerhans cell histiocytosis (LCH)
- In LCH, the involved tissue is infiltrated with large numbers of histiocytes (similar to Langerhans cells seen in skin and other epithelia), which are often organized as granulomas
- The cause is unknown
- Of all LCH bone lesions, 79% are solitary eosinophilic granulomas, 7% involve multiple eosinophilic granulomas, and 14% belong to other forms of more systemic LCH
- ***Isolated single eosinophilic granulomas can occur in ribs or skull, pelvis, mandible, humerus and other sites***
- They are diagnosed primarily in children between the ages of 5 and 15 years
- Because of the associated pain and tenderness, they may be confused with Ewing's sarcoma or with an inflammatory process such as osteomyelitis

- Healing may occur spontaneously, but typical treatment is limited surgical resection with a 2 cm margin
- ***Multiple osteolytic lesions are seen in a child points out to be only eosinophilic granuloma***

(Schwartz, 10th Edition, Page 666)

164. A 60-year-old woman with recent onset of diabetes mellitus undergoes an abdominal CT as part of trauma evaluation and is found to have an incidental 5 cm mass in the tail of the pancreas. Which of the following would confirm the suspicion of a glucagonoma:

(a) C-peptide assay (b) Erythematous skin rash
(c) Hypokalemia (d) Watery diarrhea

Ans: (b) Erythematous skin rash

- C-peptides assays are elevated in insulinomas
- Hypokalemia and watery diarrhea are features of VIPomas
- Necrolytic migratory erythema is typical of glucagonomas, which in turn are mostly located in tail of pancreas

(Sabiston, 20th Edition, Page 957)

165. True about Pancreatic adenocarcinoma is:

(a) Tumors of head present at an advanced unresectable stage
(b) Ampullary adenocarcinomas often present late
(c) Ampullary carcinomas account for their worse prognosis
(d) Back pain suggests possibility of retroperitoneal infiltration

Ans: (d) Back pain suggests possibility of retroperitoneal infiltration

- More than 85% of pancreatic cancers are ductal adenocarcinomas
- Tumors arising from the ampulla or from the distal common bile duct can present as a mass in the head of the pancreas, and constitute around a third of all tumors in that area
- ***More than 85% of patients with ductal adenocarcinoma are unsuitable for resection at time of presentation***
- Ampullary adenocarcinomas often present early with biliary obstruction
- Their natural history is distinctly more favourable compared with pancreatic ductal adenocarcinoma
- Ampullary carcinomas are relatively small when diagnosed, which may account for their better prognosis
- Occasionally, other malignant neoplasms can arise at the ampulla, such as carcinoid tumors and high-grade neuroendocrine carcinomas

(Bailey, 27th Edition, Page 1234)

166. All are true about lymphangioma *except:*

(a) Cavernous lymphangiomas almost invariably occur in neck or axilla
(b) Very commonly seen in the retroperitoneum
(c) Simple capillary lymphangiomas tend to occur subcutaneously in head and neck region and axilla
(d) Lymphangiosarcoma is rare tumor that develops as a complication of long-standing lymphedema

Ans: (b) Very commonly seen in the retroperitoneum

- Majority of these benign tumors are present at birth, and 90% of them can be identified by end of first year of life
- Cavernous lymphangiomas almost invariably occur in neck or the axilla and very rarely in retroperitoneum
- Simple capillary lymphangiomas tend to occur subcutaneously in head and neck region as well as in axilla
- Rarely, however, they can be found in the trunk within the internal organs or connective tissue in and about the abdominal or thoracic cavities

- Treatment of lymphangiomas should be surgical excision, with care taken to preserve all normal surrounding infiltrated structures
- Lymphangiosarcoma is a rare tumor that develops as a complication of long-standing (usually more than 10 years) lymphedema

(Sabiston, 20th Edition, Page 1855)

167. Which of the following is true about CLL?

(a) Most frequent finding is lymphadenopathy

(b) When the spleen is enlarged, it may be massive or barely palpable below costal margin

(c) Splenectomy is indicated to improve cytopenias and was shown to be 75% effective in either CLL or nonmalignant Hodgkin's disease

(d) All of the above

Ans: (d) All of the above

- Chronic lymphocytic leukemia (CCL) is currently considered a subtype of NHL
- Main characteristic of CLL is a progressive accumulation of old and nonfunctional lymphocytes
- Symptoms of CLL are nonspecific and include weakness, fatigue, fever without illness, night sweats, and frequent bacterial and viral infections
- Most frequent finding is lymphadenopathy. When the spleen is enlarged, it may be massive or barely palpable below the costal margin
- Splenectomy is indicated to improve cytopenias and was shown to be 75% effective in a combined group of patients who had either CLL or nonmalignant HD
- Splenectomy may facilitate chemotherapy in patients whose cell counts were prohibitively low before spleen removal
- Palliative splenectomy also is indicated for symptomatic splenomegaly

(Schwartz, 10th Edition, Page 1435)

168. Which is included in referral criteria for hereditary melanoma genetic counseling?

(a) Parent with multiple skin cancers

(b) Pancreatic cancer and melanoma on the same side of the family

(c) Three or more siblings with actinic keratosis

(d) Two relatives on the same side of the family with melanoma and prostate cancer

Ans: (b) Pancreatic cancer and melanoma on the same side of the family

- Approximately 5% of melanomas occur in high-risk families
- Melanoma suppressor gene that has highest frequency and penetrance is a germline mutation in CDKN2A which is present in approximately 25% of melanoma-prone families and also associated with pancreatic cancer

(Devita, 10th Edition, Page 1396)

169. Which gene is associated with hereditary nonpolyposis colorectal cancer?

(a) APC

(b) MYH

(c) STK11

(d) MSH2

Ans: (d) MSH2

- Germline mutations in the MMR genes *MSH2, MLH1* and *MSH6* account for 90% of all patients with HNPCC

- APC gene mutation is commonly associated with FAP. *MYH* associated polyposis is a rare inherited syndrome with increased for colorectal cancer

(Devita, 10th Edition, Page 821)

170. Biopsy was performed and showed small cell lung cancer. Which is best initial modality of treatment for this patient?

(a) Surgery
(b) Radiation therapy
(c) Chemotherapy
(d) SVC stent

Ans: (c) Chemotherapy

- Combination chemotherapy with an appropriate regimen is treatment of choice for small cell lung cancer and non-Hodgkin lymphoma
- Radiation therapy of the lesion and adjacent nodal areas may enhance control after initial response to chemotherapy
- Surgery is not a good option for this patient with extensive-stage small cell lung cancer, and an SVC stent may be used in case of lack of response or relapsed obstruction after initial therapy
- Although radiation therapy could be used for immediate symptomatic relief, combination chemotherapy is highly effective and preferable as initial therapy, avoiding large radiation field and also addressing the metastatic lesions
- Non-small cell lung cancer causing superior vena cava syndrome is best treated with radiation therapy

(Devita, 10th Edition, Page 1804)

171. A 26-year-old man presents with cough and a left testicular mass. Work-up reveals multiple retroperitoneal lymph nodes and several lung nodules. Serum hCG is 80 mIU/mL, AFP is normal. Pathologic diagnosis of the testicular mass is pure seminoma. What is best management decision?

(a) Two cycles of BEP
(b) Three cycles of BEP
(c) Four cycles of BEP
(d) Three cycles of EP

Ans: (b) Three cycles of BEP

- Patient has good risk metastatic seminoma (no visceral disease)
- Thus standard of care would include three cycles of BEP. In an attempt to avoid bleomycin exposure, potential equivalent therapy would include four cycles of EP, not three
- Two cycles of BEP would be insufficient and four, excessive for good risk disease

(Devita, 10th Edition, Page 996)

172. A 57-year-old previously healthy business executive presents with gradually increasing obstructive jaundice. An ultrasound of the liver shows dilated intrahepatic ducts, but the CBD is normal. An ERCP shows a filling defect at level of the common hepatic duct. Endoscopic brush biopsies are taken, and histology confirms cholangiocarcinoma. In discussing these findings, the surgeon should inform the patient that:

(a) This tumor affects men more commonly than women
(b) The tumor is a result of gallstones
(c) The tumor is best treated with a stent to relieve obstructive jaundice
(d) Weight loss is common in this condition

Ans: (a) This tumor affects men more commonly than women

- **Unlike most biliary disease conditions, cholangiocarcinoma condition affects men more commonly than women**
- Primary sclerosing cholangitis, *C. sinensis* and choledochal cysts may play an etiological role in some cases, but gallstones are not involved in the pathogenesis of this tumor
- Patients present with obstructive jaundice; pain and weight loss are less common
- Proximal tumors (Klatskin) are most common and they require excision of hepatic duct bifurcation and reconstruction with a Roux-en-Y limb of jejunum
- Tumors of the distal duct can be resected by performing a Whipple pancreatoduodenectomy

- Patients who are not operative candidates (those with advanced disease or those who cannot withstand a major operation) should undergo palliative endoscopic stent placement to relieve the obstruction

(Devita, 10th Edition, Page 726)

173. Most common presentation for appendiceal adenocarcinoma is:

(a) Palpable abdominal mass
(b) Acute appendicitis
(c) Ascites
(d) Incidental finding during unrelated abdominal surgery

Ans: (b) Acute appendicitis

- Primary adenocarcinoma of the appendix presents most commonly as acute appendicitis
- For this reason, it is always important to check final pathology of appendiceal specimen
- Patients are at increased risk of synchronous neoplasms, particularly in colon and so examination of large intestine should be done with full colonoscopy
- Definitive treatment consists of a right colectomy regardless of the size of the tumor. If the final pathology reveals appendiceal cancer, the patient should be taken back for a right colectomy
- 5-year survival rate after curative resection was 61% and 31%
- Remaining answer choices are not typically common presentation of appendiceal adenocarcinoma

(Sabiston, 20th Edition, Page 1308)

174. A 40-year-old female alcoholic is suspected of having a hepatic mass. Percutaneous ultrasound guided liver biopsy is contraindicated in which of the following:

(a) Hepatocellular carcinoma
(b) Metastatic carcinoma
(c) Cirrhosis
(d) Hepatic adenoma

Ans: (d) Hepatic adenoma

- Tru-cut needle liver biopsy allows pathologic diagnosis of liver lesions
- Needle biopsy is contraindicated if hemangioma is suspected and in adenomas, because of risk of bleeding
- Other potential complications of percutaneous needle biopsy are pain, pneumothorax, and bile peritonitis
- Needle biopsy can diagnose posthepatic and postnecrotic cirrhosis, malignant tumors, and hepatitis and can determine the need for treatment in hepatitis C

(Sabiston, 20th Edition, Page 1455)

175. Percentage of tumor cells that can give rise to metastases is:

(a) <0.01%
(b) 1%
(c) 20%
(d) >80%

Ans: (a) <0.01%

- By using radioactive nucleotides incorporated into tumor DNA, it has been shown that less than 0.01% of tumor cells can give rise to metastases

(Devita, 10th Edition, Page 30)

176. A 35-year-old female is currently being treated with pazopanib (CYP3A4 substrate). She is admitted for seizure management and the consult team recommends initiation of phenytoin. What effect may concurrent administration have on pazopanib concentrations?

(a) Decrease pazopanib concentration
(b) Increase pazopanib concentration
(c) No change in pazopanib concentration
(d) None, if the pazopanib is taken with food

Ans: (a) Decrease pazopanib concentration

- Anticonvulsant drugs such as phenytoin and carbamazepine can induce drug-metabolizing enzymes (e.g., CYP450 isoenzymes) and thereby increase anticancer agent clearance
- Suppression of CYP activity, with agents such as ketoconazole, may lead to a rise in plasma concentrations
- It is not advisable to attempt to manipulate extent of drug absorption, by way of ingesting food, to overcome drug-drug interactions

(Devita, 10th Edition, Page 295)

177. A 60-year-old woman complains of early satiety and undergoes an upper endoscopy. A small mass is seen in the antrum with sparing of the mucosa. GIST is suspected. CT scan of chest, abdomen, and pelvis is performed. What does she require next?

(a) Fulguration of the tumor
(b) Distal gastrectomy
(c) Laser therapy followed by radiation therapy
(d) Chemotherapy alone

Ans: (b) Distal gastrectomy

- If the mass is deemed resectable, the goal of surgery is resection with grossly negative margins
- Precautions should be taken to prevent rupture of the mass. Radiation and chemotherapy have traditionally been ineffective
- Clinical trials with the drug imatinib mesylate (Gleevec) are promising

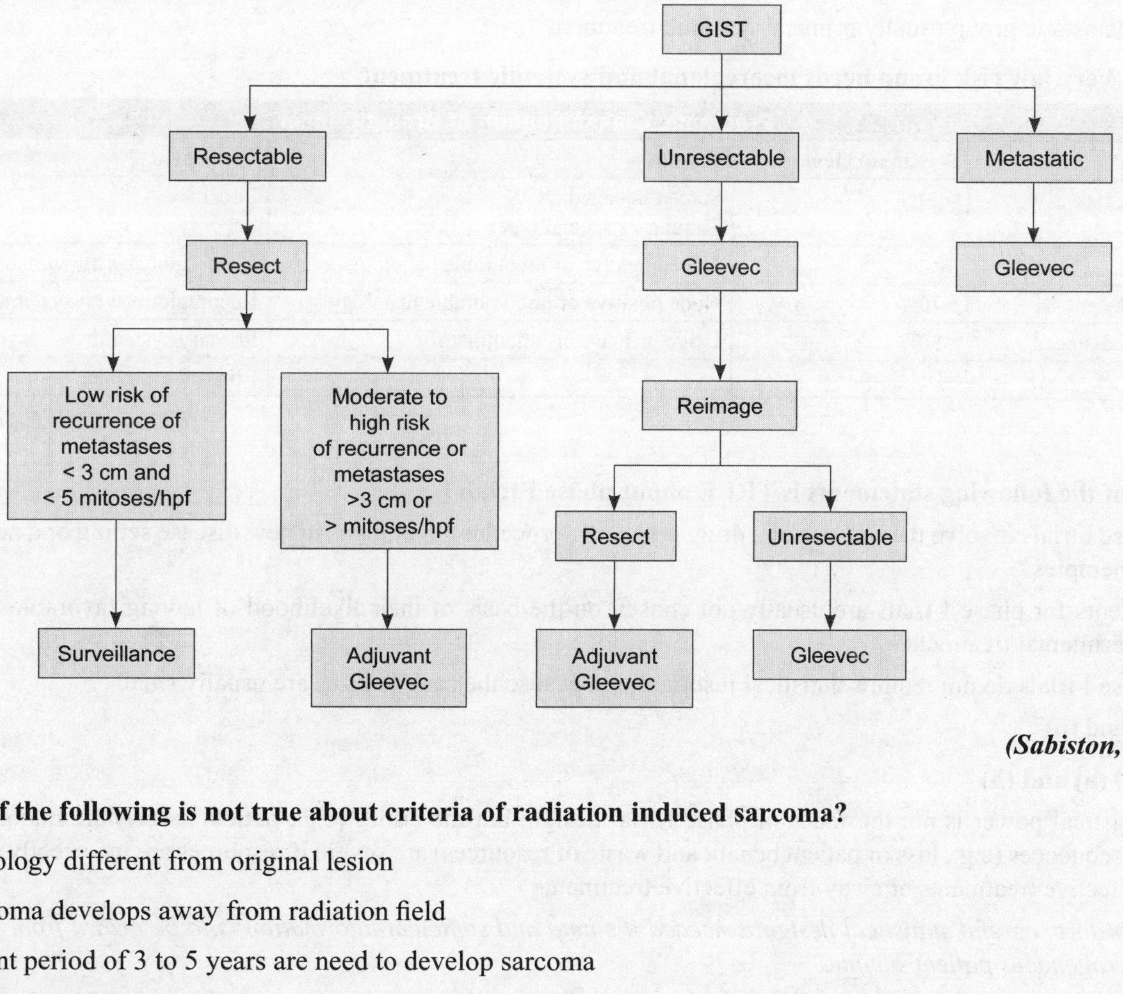

(Sabiston, 20th Edition)

178. Which of the following is not true about criteria of radiation induced sarcoma?

(a) Histology different from original lesion
(b) Sarcoma develops away from radiation field
(c) Latent period of 3 to 5 years are need to develop sarcoma
(d) All of the above

Ans: (b) Sarcoma develops away from radiation field

Three criteria for diagnosis sarcoma of radiation induced sarcoma are
• Histology different from the original lesion
• Sarcoma develops in the irradiated field
• Latent period of 3 to 5 years exists between radiation and sarcoma development

(Schwartz, 10th Edition, Page 1779)

179. Most common malignant tumor of eyelids is:

(a) Basal cell carcinoma (b) Rhabdomyosarcoma
(c) Squamous cell carcinoma (d) Malignant melanoma

Ans: (a) Basal cell carcinoma

- ***Most common malignant tumor of eyelids is Basal cell carcinoma***

(Bailey, 27th Edition, Page 674)

180. All are true about pragmatic classification of Carcinoma breast *except:*

(a) 5-year survival rate of very low risk primary breast cancer is >90%
(b) In locally advanced breast cancer primary systemic therapy is given
(c) Very low risk group needs locoregional and systemic treatment
(d) In metastatic group usually primary systemic treatment

Ans: (c) Very low risk group needs locoregional and systemic treatment

Pregmatic Classsification of Breast Cancer

Group	5-year survival rate	Example	Treatment
Very low risk	>90%	Screen detected DCIS Tubular or special types	Local
Low risk	70-90%	Node negative or favourable histology	Locoregional with/without systemic
High risk	<70%	Node positive or unfavourable histology	Locoregional with systemic
Locally advanced	<30%	Large primary or inflammatory	Primary systemic
Metastatic	–	–	Primary systemic

(Bailey, 27th Edition, Page 875)

181. Which of the following statements is TRUE about phase I trials?

(a) Phase I trials involve the first use of a drug, device, or procedure in humans in new disease setting or a new combination of therapies
(b) Patients for phase I trials are usually not chosen on the basis of their likelihood of having favorable response to the experimental treatment
(c) Phase I trials do not require statistical justification because the sample sizes are usually small
(d) (a) and (b)

Ans: (d) (a) and (b)

- Statistical power is not the focus of phase I trial design, but the issues (e.g., patient safety) are major and long-term consequences (e.g., loss of patient benefit and waste of resources) are severe if resources are incorrectly directed toward ineffective treatments or away from effective treatments
- *Therefore, careful statistical design is needed if sound and sufficient information is to be drawn from small and often heterogeneous patient samples*

(Devita, 10th Edition, Page 399)

PAPER 4

182. Most common histology of Carcinoma of Unknown primary is:

(a) Adenocarcinoma
(b) Squamous cell carcinoma
(c) Unclassified neoplasm
(d) Carcinosarcoma

Ans: (a) Adenocarcinoma

Histopathology	Percentage of CUP patients
Adenocarcinoma	60%
SCC	5%
Others Poorly differentiated carcinoma Poorly differentiated neoplasm Unclassified neoplasm	35%

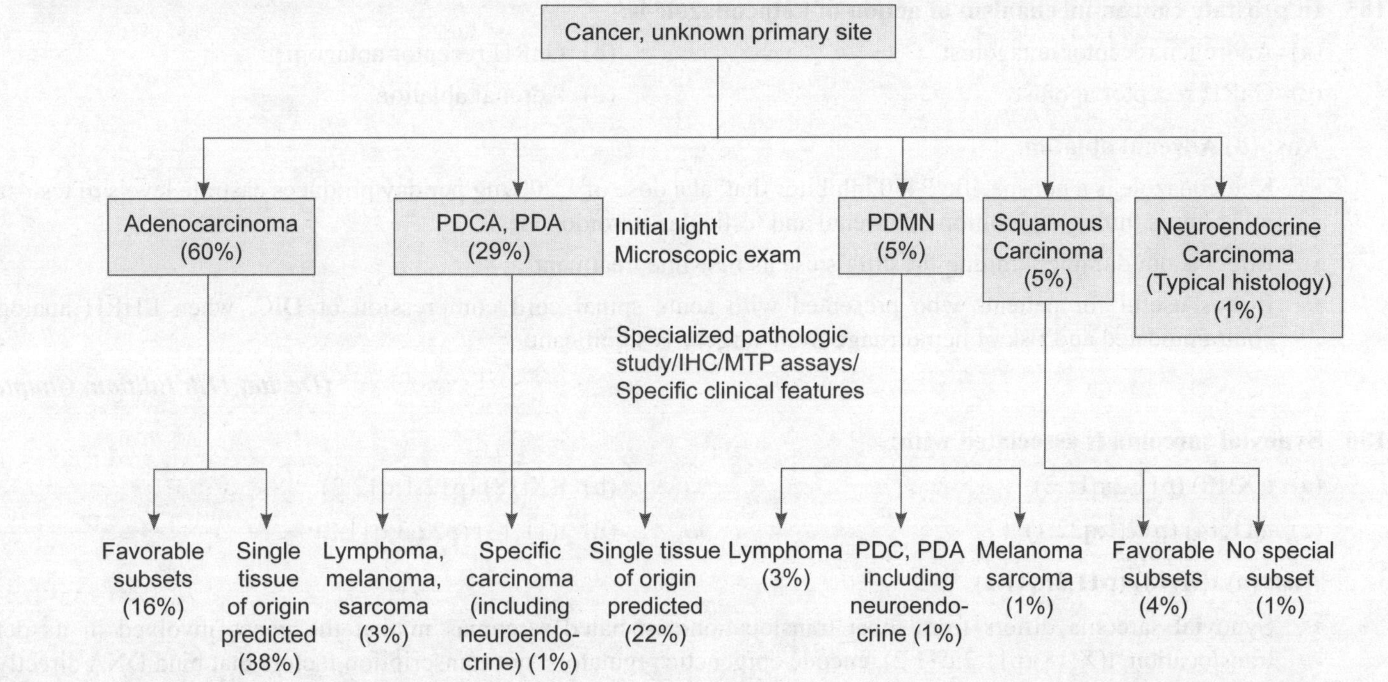

(Devita, 11th Edition, Chapter 108)

183. Which of the following immunohistochemical markers is not correctly matched?

(a) CK_7+, CK_{20}+ is seen in Urothelial tumors
(b) CK_7+, CK_{20}– is seen in Lung adenocarcinoma
(c) CK_7–, CK_{20}+ is seen with Colorectal carcinoma
(d) CK_7+, CK_{20}– is seen with Squamous cell lung carcinoma

Ans: (d) CK_7+, CK_{20}- is seen with Squamous cell lung carcinoma

Approach to Immunohistochemical Markers Used in Cancer of Unknown Primary Site		
Ck_7	**Ck_{20}**	**Primary Tumor**
+	+	Urothelial tumors, ovarian mucinous adenocarcinoma, pancreatic adenocarcinoma and cholangiocarcinoma
+	–	Lung adenocarcinoma, breast carcinoma, thyroid carcinoma, endometrial carcinoma, cervical carcinoma, salivary gland carcinoma, cholangiocarcinoma, pancreatic carcinoma
–	+	Colorectal carcinoma, Markel cell carcinoma

Contd.

Contd.

–	–	Hepatocellular carcinoma, renal cell carcinoma, prostate carcinoma, squamous cell and small-cell lung carcinoma, head and neck carcinoma

(Devita, 11th Edition, Chapter 108)

184. Sipuleucel T vaccine recently approved by FDA in treatment of:

(a) Renal cancer
(b) Bladder cancer
(c) Testicular cancer
(d) Prostate cancer

Ans: (d) Prostate cancer

- Sipuleucel-T is an autologous active cellular immunotherapy that includes an acid phosphatase specific, replication-competent adenovirus that is co-transfected with granulocyte-macrophage colony-stimulating factor
- Mononuclear cells are harvested by leukopheresis, transfected with the viral construct, and maintained in culture under an adequate number of defined mononuclear cell fraction has developed to enable reinfusion to patient

(Devita, 11th Edition, Chapter 70)

185. In prostate cancer, mechanism of action of ketoconazole is:

(a) Androgen receptor antagonist
(b) GnRH receptor antagonist
(c) GnRH receptor agonist
(d) Adrenal ablation

Ans: (d) Adrenal ablation

- Ketoconazole is a nonspecific P450 inhibitor that, at a dose of 1,200 mg per day produces castrate levels of testosterone in 24 hours through inhibition of adrenal and testicular steroidogenesis
- Effect is not durable, limiting the drug's use as first-line treatment
- It was useful for patients who presented with acute spinal cord compression or DIC, when LHRH analogs are contraindicated and risk of hemorrhage from surgery is significant

(Devita, 11th Edition, Chapter 70)

186. Synovial sarcoma is associated with:

(a) t(X:18) (p11.2;q11.2)
(b) t(X:18) (p12.1;q12.2)
(c) t(11;14) (p17.1;q22.1)
(d) t(11;13) (p22.3;q11.2)

Ans: (a) t(X:18) (p11.2;q11.2)

- Synovial sarcoma differs from most translocation-associated sarcomas in that the genes involved in its defining translocation, t(X;18)(p11.2;q11.2), encode epigenetic regulators, not transcription factors that bind DNA directly
- The translocation fuses the widely expressed SS18 (also known as *SYT*) gene with an *SSX* gene normally expressed only in testis
- In the fusion oncoprotein, SS18, which forms part of the BAF chromatin remodeling complex, retains all but the last eight amino acids from its C-terminal transcriptional activation domain

(Casciato Manual of Oncology, 7th Edition, Page 458)

187. Risk factors associated with Adenocarcinoma Esophagus is:

(a) Achalasia
(b) Caustic injury
(c) Barrett's esophagus
(d) Tylosis

Ans: (c) Barrett's esophagus

Predisposing Factors	
Squamous cell carcinoma	**Adenocarcinoma**
• Alcohol	• Barret's esophagus
• Cigarette	• Obesity

Contd.

Contd.

• Carcinogens–nitrates, opiates smoked, fungal toxins • Physical agents–hot tea, lye ingestion, radiation strictures, **Chronic achalasia** • Plummer vinson syndrome • Tylosis palmaris et plantaris • Dietary deficiency of molybdenum, zinc, vitamin A • Coeliac sprue • Achalasia Cardia	• Scleroderma • High Protein and Fat diet • Smoking

In Achalasia the most common cancer is SCC, but adenocarcinoma can develop below the air fluid level in mediastinum in middle third Esophagus**

(Bailey and Love, 27th Edition, Page 1087)

188. Mechanism of action of Cytarabine is:

(a) Inhibits Dihydrofolate reductase
(b) Topoisomerase inhibitor
(c) Inhibits DNA polymerase
(d) Depolymerise microtubules

Ans: (c) Inhibits DNA polymerase

CYTARABINE

- **Ara-C** enters cells via nucleoside transport proteins, the most important one being the equilibrative inhibitor-sensitive (es) receptor
- Once inside the cell, ara-C requires activation for its cytotoxic effects
- First metabolic step is the conversion of ara-C to ara-C monophosphate (ara-CMP) by the enzyme deoxycytidine kinase (dCK) with subsequent phosphorylation to the di- and tri-phosphate metabolites, respectively
- Ara-CTP is **potent inhibitor of DNA polymerases** which, in turn, interferes with DNA chain elongation, DNA synthesis and DNA repair

(Devita, 11th Edition, Page 543)

189. Fibro-epithelioma of Pinkus, a rare variant of BCC presents typically on:

(a) Head and neck region
(b) Torso and extremities
(c) Sun exposed areas of face
(d) Trunk

Ans: (b) Torso and extremities

- Fibroepithelioma of Pinkus (FEP), a rare variant of BCC, typically presents on torso and extremities but also has been noted on the genitalia, groin and sole of the foot
- Clinically, FEP usually presents as pink, smooth, dome-shaped, or pedunculated papule, plaque, or nodule
- Characterized histologically by a polypoid lesion in which basaloid cells grow downward from the surface in a network of anastomoses of cords of cells in loose connective tissue
- FEP tends to have an indolent prognosis similar to superficial BCC

(Devita, 11th Edition, Page 2624)

190. False statement regarding Barrett's esophagus is:

(a) 10% of GERD cases develop Barrett's esophagus
(b) It has 40 fold increased risk of Adenocarcinoma
(c) Incidence of Adenocarcinoma is 5% per year in Barrett's esophagus
(d) Intestinal metaplasia occurs

Ans: (c) Incidence of Adenocarcinoma is 5% per year in Barrett's esophagus

- Incidence of malignancy is 1% per year
- 70% are men

Treatment	
Type	**Opinion**
No dysplasia	Follow up 2-3 yearly once
Low grade dysplasia	6 monthly interval for 1 year and then annually
High grade dysplasia	Unfit–Ablative therapy FIT- Esophagectomy
Early adenocarcinoma	Esophagectomy

(Sabiston, 20th Edition, Page 1050)

191. Which of the following is not true about Small intestinal lymphoma?

(a) Most common neoplasia in children <10 years
(b) Most common site of small intestinal lymphoma is duodenum
(c) If asymptomatic then undergo chemotherapy
(d) Symptomatic cases should undergo surgical resection

Ans: (b) Most common site of small intestinal lymphoma is duodenum

Small Intestinal Lymphoma
• Most common neoplasia in children <10 years • ***Most common site–Ileum***
Treatment
• Asymptomatic–Chemotherapy • Symptomatic–Surgical resection • B cell lymphoma–More chemosensitive • T cell lymphoma–Surgical resection

(Devita, 11th Edition, Page 1607)

192. Not true regarding Gastric MALToma is:

(a) Early stage tumor with no high risk features require H. pylori eradication
(b) Cases with transmural invasion suggest poor prognosis
(c) Patients with nodal disease may have failure of H. pylori eradication
(d) Chemoradiation alone is treatment of choice for high risk MALToma

Ans: (d) Chemoradiation alone is treatment of choice for high risk MALToma

Management of Gastric Maltoma	
Early stage with no t(11,18) or Bcl 10 expression	***H. pylori eradication with careful follow up*** Repeat endoscopy every 2 months to ensure infection clearance Biannual surveillance for 3 years to look for tumor regression
Transmural invasion *Nodal disease* *Large cell phenotypic transformation t(11,18)* *Bcl–10 expression* *H. pylori –ve*	Predicts failure after H.pylori eradication Suggests poor prognosis ***Chemoradiation +/- Surgery***
If persistent MALT lymphoma after H. pylori therapy If without evidence of H. pylori infection	*External beam Radiotherapy–Best response* *If RT contraindicated Rituximab is advised*
Median time for remission–15 Months	

(Sabiston, 20th Edition, Page 1229)

193. Which of the following is not true regarding Pancreatic cancer?

(a) Investigation of choice in Pancreatic cancer is MDCT
(b) Percutaneous fine needle aspiration cytology is done only for Unresectable tumors
(c) All
(d) EUS differentiates between chronic lymphadenitis from metastatic lymph node involvement

Ans: (d) EUS differentiates between chronic lymphadenitis from metastatic lymph node involvement

- Investigation of choice–MDCT
- Percutaneous fine needle aspiration cytology is done only for unresectable/metastatic lesions
- EUS can't differentiate between chronic pancreatitis and CA Pancreas
- EUS can't differentiate chronic lymphadenitis from metastatic lymph node involvement

(Devita 11th Edition, Page 1469)

194. Most common pancreatic malignancy in children is:

(a) Pancreatic adenocarcinoma
(b) Pancreatoblastoma
(c) Frantz tumor
(d) Lymphoma pancreas

Ans: (b) Pancreatoblastoma

Pancreatoblastoma is Most Common Pancreatic Malignancy in Children

- Usually occurs in 1st 8 years of life
- Associated with the Beckwith-Wiedemann and familial adenomatous polyposis syndromes
- Elevated levels of serum α-fetoprotein and hormones
- Cures are often achievable with resection in children
- One-third of patients present with metastatic disease
- Cases have been reported in adults as well, with survival after resection that is comparable to conventional PDA
- Microscopically, these tumors contain acinar cells, but other cell types (neuroendocrine, ductal) are often present
- Pancreatoblastomas have been whole-exome sequenced in only two adult cases
- They acquire relatively few mutations (approximately 15 per tumor) and *SMAD4* and *CTNNB1* mutations are typical

(Devita, 11th Edition, Page 1466)

195. Anti Hu Antibodies are associated with which of the following Cancer induced Paraneoplastic Syndrome?

(a) Small cell lung cancer
(b) Carcinoma Ovary
(c) Thymoma
(d) Hodgkin's lymphoma

Ans: (a) Small cell lung cancer

Onconeural Antibodies and Associated Syndromes and Malignancies

Onconeural antibody	Paraneoplastic syndrome	Most common malignancy
Anti Hu	Limbic encephalitis Paraneoplastic cerebellar degeneration Subacute sensory neuronopathy Autonomic neuropathy Chronic gastrointestinal pseudo obstruction	*Small cell lung cancer*
Anti Yo	Paraneoplastic cerebellar degenration	*Ovary and Breast*
Anti CV2	Limbic Encephalitis Paraneoplastic cerebellar degeneration Subacute sensory neuropathy Autonomic neuropathy Chronic gastrointestinal pseudo obstruction	*Small cell lung cancer,* *Thymoma*

Contd.

Contd.

Anti Ri	Paraneoplastic cerebellar degeneration Brainstem encephalitis Opsoclonus myoclonus	***Breast, Small cell lung cancer***
Anti Ma2	Limbic Encephalitis	***Testicular***
Anti amphiphysin	Sensory neuropathy Stiff person syndrome	***Small cell lung cancer, Breast cancer***
Anti Tr	Paraneoplastic cerebellar degeneration	***Hodgkin's Lymphoma***

(Devita, 11th Edition, Page 3506)

196. All of the following are Contraindications to surgery in Gallbladder cancer *except?*

(a) Regional metastasis (b) Extension to porta hepatis

(c) Significant Ascites (d) Occlusion of major vessels

Ans: (a) Regional metastasis

CONTRAINDICATIONS TO SURGERY

- Distant metastases, Extensive involvement of porta hepatis causing jaundice, Significant Ascites and Encasement/Occlusion of major vessels

(Devita, 11th Edition, Page 1586)

197. Which of the following breast pathological subtype is associated with Familial diffuse type of gastric cancer?

(a) Medullary (b) Ductal adenocarcinoma – No special type

(c) Ductal adenocarcinoma–special types (d) Lobular adenocarcinoma

Ans: (b) Ductal adenocarcinoma–No special type

- BRCA 2 mutation at chromosome 13q–results in Breast cancer and Ovarian cancer
- BRCA 2 results in Triple positive Ductal Adenocarcinomas of NST commonly
- BRCA 2 also results in Male breast cancers
- BRCA 2 can also cause other cancers like Prostate, Colon and Gastric Cancers

(Devita, 11th Edition, Page 2244)

198. Which of the following is not true about Birt Hogg Dubé syndrome?

(a) Bilateral multifocal tumors (b) Associated with chromophobe RCC and oncocytoma

(c) Chromosome 17p11 (d) Associated with hepatic cysts

Ans: (d) Associated with hepatic cysts

- Birt-Hogg-Dubé syndrome–Bilateral multifocal tumors with both *chromophobe RCC and oncocytoma* histology along with cutaneous fibrofolliculomas, pulmonary cysts and spontaneous pneumothorax–Chromosome 17p11 encodes folliculin protein

(Devita, 11th Edition, Page 1828)

199. Fong score and outcome of colorectal liver metastasis include all *except:*

(a) Number of lesions more than 1

(b) Size of largest colorectal liver metastasis not more than 3

(c) Time to develop CRLM >1year

(d) CEA > 200 ng/Ml

Ans: (b) Size of largest colorectal liver metastasis not more than 3

- Each factor is scored 0 or 1, with a median survival of 74 months reported for patients scoring 0, and 14 months for those with five risk factors

Fong score and outcome of CRLM
• Extension of 1° colorectal carcinoma into the serosa • Time to develop CRLM >1 y • Number of lesions >1 • Size of largest CRLM > 5 cm • CEA >200 ng/mL

- *Each factor is scored 0 or 1, with a median survival of 74 months reported for patients scoring 0 and 14 months for those with five risk factors*

(Bathedsa Book of Clinical Oncology, Page 119)

200. Which of the following is not true about Hepatoblastoma?

(a) AFP is usually elevated in 85-90%

(b) Associated with FAP

(c) Most of them are Symptomatic

(d) Patients Without metastasis should undergo Complete resection

Ans: (c) Most of them are Symptomatic

HEPATOBLASTOMA

- **Most common primary hepatic tumor in children**
- Median age is 18 months
- Associated with FAP
- Generally Asymptomatic
- **AFP is usually elevated in 85-90%**

TREATMENT

- **Without metastasis-Complete resection**
- **Chemotherapy followed by surgery**
- Pulmonary metastasis–Resect hepatic tumor and chemotherapy/Resect pulmonary mets

(Devita, 11th Edition, Page 1555)

201. Spoke wheel appearance is seen with:

(a) Gastric carcinoids (b) Small bowel carcinoids

(c) Appendiceal carcinoids (d) Rectal carcinoids

Ans: (b) Small bowel carcinoids

SPOKE WHEEL APPEARANCE

- *In small bowel carcinoids on CT Scan due to extensive mesenteric fibrosis and calcification*

(Devita, 11th Edition, Page 1247)

202. Which of the following is not true about Mucinous tumors of Appendix?

(a) If ruptures it results in development of pseudomyxoma peritonei

(b) Cytoreductive surgery combined with IPHC is Treatment of choice for PMP

(c) Frankly malignant

(d) Direct peritoneal seeding from appendiceal contents

Ans: (c) Frankly malignant

- Not frankly malignant

- If ruptured, can result in intraperitoneal spread and the development of pseudomyxoma peritonei (PMP)
- Pseudomyxoma peritonei is a consequence of perforation and direct peritoneal seeding from appendiceal contents
- Avoid rupture if mucocele or mucinous neoplasm is suspected on preoperative imaging or diagnosed intraoperatively
- **Treatment of PMP – cytoreductive surgery combined with IPHC**

(Sabiston, 20th Edition, Page 1308)

203. Renal cell carcinoma involving adrenal gland is staged according to AJCC 8th edition is:

(a) I (b) II
(c) III (d) IV

Ans: (d) IV

T Staging of Renal Cell Carcinoma	
TX	Primary tumor cannot be assessed
T0	No evidence of primary tumor
T1a	Tumor < 4 cm in greatest dimensión, limited to kidney
T1b	Tumor > 4 cm but < 7 cm in greatest dimension limited to the kidney
T2a	Tumor > 7 cm but < 10 cm in greatest dimensión, limited to the kidney
T2b	Tumor > 10 cm limited to the kidney
T3a	Tumor extends into the renal vein or its segmental branches or invades the pelvicalyceal system or invades perirenal and/or renal sinus fat but not beyond Gerota's fascia
T3b	Tumor extends into the vena cava below the diaphragm
T3c	Tumor extends into the vena cava above the diaphragm or invades the wall of the vena cava
T4	Tumor invades beyond Gerota's fascia (including contiguous extensión into ipsilateral adrenal gland)

(Sabiston, 20th Edition, Page 2098)

204. All are true about Pancoast tumors *except:*

(a) Occurs with tumors that invade 1st rib, subclavian vessels and brachial plexus
(b) Standard treatment is resection for localized tumors
(c) Originates in the superior sulcus
(d) May present with Horner's syndrome

Ans: (b) Standard treatment is resection for localized tumors

- **Tumors originating in superior sulcus (posterior apex) elicit:**
  Apical chest wall and/or shoulder pain (from involvement of the first rib and chest wall); Horner's syndrome (unilateral enophthalmos, ptosis, miosis and facial anhidrosis from invasion of the stellate sympathetic ganglion)
  Radicular arm pain (from invasion of T1 and occasionally C8, brachial plexus nerve roots)
- Standard treatment–Concurrent chemoradiation followed by resection (localized tumors)

(Schwartz, 10th Edition, Page 623; Devita, 10th Edition, Page 516)

205. Not an etiologic factor for soft tissue sarcoma:

(a) Viral infection (b) Previous radiation exposure
(c) Scar tissue from previous injury (d) Retroperitoneal fibrosis

Ans: (d) Retroperitoneal fibrosis

- Only retroperitoneal fibrosis is not an etiologic factor associated with development of a soft-tissue sarcoma
- When patient presents with retroperitoneal fibrosis, malignancy such as soft-tissue sarcoma is in differential diagnosis that doesn't mean it constitutes an etiologic factor
- Remaining choices–Viral infection, previous radiation exposure, scar tissue from a previous injury and Gardner syndrome are all etiologic factors with soft–tissue sarcomas

(Schwartz, 10th Edition, Page 1466)

206. Which of the following is not true about pancreatic endocrine tumors?

(a) VIPomas are associated with hyperkalemia
(b) Gastrinomas are associated with ZES
(c) Majority of insulinomas are benign
(d) Migratory necrolytic erythema is seen in glucaganomas

Ans: (a) VIPomas are associated with hyperkalemia

PANCREATIC ENDOCRINE TUMORS

- **Gastrinoma, or Zollinger-Ellison syndrome (ZES),** is a rare disease caused by a NET (gastrinoma) in **pancreas or duodenum**
- **Insulinomas** are seldom malignant and represent most common functioning NET of pancreas
- **VIPomas** are the cause of the classic Verner-Morrison syndrome. These endocrine tumors secrete vasoactive intestinal peptide, which can cause watery diarrhea, **hypokalemia,** and achlorhydria (WDHA)
- In **glucaganoma,** patients typically present with a syndrome that includes diabetes and a characteristic rash known as necrolytic migratory erythema
- **Somatostatinomas** may be associated with von Recklinghausen's disease; those tumors so associated are mostly duodenal or ampullary in origin and less likely to be associated with a hormonal syndrome or metastatic at the time of diagnosis

(Devita, 10th Edition, Page 1178)

207. Most frequently involved anatomic location in MEN associated gastrinomas?

(a) Head of the pancreas
(b) Gallbladder
(c) Gastric antrum
(d) Duodenum

Ans: (d) Duodenum

- Majority of gastrinomas occur within the so-called gastrinoma triangle
- This space is bounded by confluence of the cystic and common hepatic ducts superiorly, junction of the head and neck of the pancreas medially, and junction of the second and third portions of the duodenum inferiorly
- Both sporadic and MEN-associated gastrinomas occur most frequently within duodenum

(Sabiston, 20th Edition, Page 954)

208. Warburg effect describes:

(a) Sculpturing of normal tissues as a result of cell death
(b) Inhibition of antihistone deacetylase
(c) Paracrine signalling causing increased leakiness of basement membrane
(d) Inefficient energy production in cancer cells by anerobic glycolysis

Ans: (d) Inefficient energy production in cancer cells by anerobic glycolysis

WARBURG EFFECT

- Necrosis is derived from the Greek word nekros for corpse and it involves rapid swelling of the cell, loss of plasma membrane integrity and release of the cellular contents into the extracellular environment, resulting in an acute inflammatory response
- Necrosis is largely viewed as an accidental and unregulated cellular event triggered by cellular trauma (direct physical injury), acute energy depletion, or extreme stress
- Recently, a type of programmed necrotic cell death, called necroptosis, has been identified as induced by interaction of death domain receptors with their respective ligands under conditions of defective or inhibited downstream apoptotic machinery
- Necroptosis depends on the serine/threonine kinase activity of the death domain receptor-associated adaptor Ripl and its relative Rip3
- **Necroptosis is potently inhibited by Ripl kinase inhibitors, necrostatins**

- Harnessing necroptosis to induce cell death in cancer is an exciting new prospect, the exploitation of which will require a deeper mechanistic insight into the process and its regulation
- Regarding necrosis as a therapeutic end point, tumor cell fate in response to treatment with DNA-damaging agents depends on the effect of the DNA repair protein poly(ADPribose) polymerase (PARP) on cellular metabolism. PARP activation by DNA-damaging alkylating agents causes PARPmediated f3-nicotinamide adenine dinucleotide (NAD) consumption, ATP depletion, and metabolic stress
- Glycolytic state (Warburg effect) and inefficient mode of energy production in most cancer cells renders them sensitive to this ATP depletion in response to PARP activation, resulting in induction of necrotic cell death of apoptosis-defective tumor cells
- **Tumor cells with defects in both apoptosis and autophagy may be particularly susceptible to death by necrosis as loss of autophagy potential deprives cells of an alternate energy source for maintenance of metabolism and viability in metabolic stress that is compounded by the Warburg effect**

(Devita, 10th Edition, Page 32)

209. A 40-year-old patient came with cough with hemoptysis and occasional chest pain. On further radiological investigation it is diagnosed to be malignant lesion. Biopsy was performed and showed small cell lung cancer. Best initial modality of treatment for this patient?

(a) Surgery
(b) Radiation therapy
(c) Chemotherapy
(d) SVC stent

Ans: (c) Chemotherapy

- Combination chemotherapy with an appropriate regimen is treatment of choice for Small cell lung cancer and non-Hodgkin lymphoma
- Radiation therapy of the lesion and adjacent nodal areas may enhance control after initial response to chemotherapy
- Surgery is not a good option for this patient with extensive-stage small cell lung cancer, and an SVC stent may be used in case of lack of response or relapsed obstruction after initial therapy
- Although radiation therapy could be used for immediate symptomatic relief, combination chemotherapy is highly effective and preferable as initial therapy, avoiding large radiation field and also addressing the metastatic lesions
- Non-small cell lung cancer causing superior vena cava syndrome is best treated with radiation therapy

(Devita, 10th Edition, Page 1804)

210. Not true about Criteria of Radiation induced sarcoma:

(a) Histology different from original lesion
(b) Sarcoma develops away from radiation field
(c) Latent period of 3 to 5 years are needed to develop sarcoma
(d) Histology same from original lesion

Ans: (b) Sarcoma develops away from radiation field

Three criteria for diagnosis sarcoma of radiation induced sarcoma are:
• Histology different from the original lesion
• Sarcoma develops in the irradiated field
• Latent period of 3 to 5 years exists between radiation and sarcoma development

(Schwartz, 10th Edition, Page 1779)

211. Oncotype DX Assay, recurrence score >31 denotes:

(a) Low risk
(b) Intermediate risk
(c) High risk
(d) No risk

Ans: (c) High risk

ONCOTYPE DX ASSAY

- Oncotype DX Assay predicts the benefit of hormonal therapy in patients
- Oncotype DX test is used to estimate a woman's risk of recurrence of early-stage, hormone-receptor-positive breast cancer, as well as how likely she is to benefit from chemotherapy after breast cancer surgery

Recurrence score	Risk	Benefit of chemotherapy
<18	Low	Small and will not outweigh the risks
18-30	Intermediate	Unclear
>31	High	Greater than the risks

(Devita, 10th Edition, Page 1112)

212. Not true about Paget's disease of the anal canal is:

(a) It is a rare intraepithelial adenocarcinoma in an area of squammous epithelium

(b) It has been proposed to be derived from pluripotent epidermal stem cells

(c) More common in younger individuals and associated with an underlying carcinoma in 50-86% of patients

(d) Presence of PAS positive Paget cells confirms the diagnosis

Ans: (c) More common in younger individuals and associated with an underlying carcinoma in 50-86% of patients

- Paget's disease is more common in older individuals
- Associated with an underlying carcinoma in 50-86% of patients
- Portends a poor prognosis

(Sabiston, 20th Edition, Page 1414)

213. Which of the following patients would most likely benefit from robotic-assisted versus laparoscopic surgery or colorectal cancer?

(a) A 75-year-old admitted with a lower gastrointestinal bleed, bound to have a bleeding cecal tumor on colonoscopy

(b) A 60-year-old man with a low rectal cancer Abutting prostate on EUS

(c) A 64-year-old man with no significant medical history with a descending colon mass

(d) A 55-year-old man admitted with obstipation with obstructing sigmoid tumor

Ans: (b) A 60-year-old man with a low rectal cancer Abutting prostate on EUS

- Robotic-assisted laparoscopic surgery is rarely applied to emergent operations
- Laparoscopic approach is rarely preferred in an urgent colorectal operation including obstipation due to an obstructing colon cancer
- Studies suggest that robotic assistance may be of no added benefit in routine colon resections, but selective application in complex rectal cancer procedures may prove to have long-term benefits

(Recent Advances in Surgery-Pubmed.com)

214. In Carcinoma head of pancreas, Nausea and vomiting is due to:

(a) External Compression of duodenum
(b) Portal vein infiltration
(c) Proliferation infiltration of tumor into duodenum
(d) Chemotherapy related

Ans: (a) External Compression of duodenum

- Pancreatic adenocarcinoma develops in the ductal cells and are called Ductal Adenocarcinoma
- ***Most commonly occur on the Right side, i.e., Head and Uncinate Process (60-70%)*** than left side, Body and Tail of pancreas (20-25%)

Features of Carcinoma Head of Pancreas
• Jaundice 75%
• Weight loss 51%
• Abdominal pain 39%
• Nausea/vomiting 13%
• Pruritus 11%
• Fever 3%
• Gastrointestinal bleeding 1%
• For tumors at the body and tail of pancreas, Pain (most common) and weight loss are the presenting features as they present at a late advanced stage
• Regarding Nausea and vomiting, they occur due to tumor extrinsic compression of duodenum C loop presenting a state of Gastric outlet obstruction
• In unresectable cases, these patients should be offered Endoluminal duodenal metal stent as palliation

(Sabiston, 20th Edition, Page 1544)

215. Which of the following is most common presenting feature of appendiceal adenocarcinoma is:

(a) Palpable abdominal mass
(b) Acute appendicitis
(c) Ascites
(d) Incidental finding during unrelated abdominal surgery

Ans: (b) Acute appendicitis

- Primary adenocarcinoma of the appendix presents most commonly as acute appendicitis
- For this reason, it is always important to check final pathology of appendiceal specimen
- Patients are at increased risk of synchronous neoplasms, particularly in colon and so examination of large intestine should be done with full colonoscopy
- Definitive treatment consists of a right colectomy regardless of the size of the tumor. If the final pathology reveals appendiceal cancer, the patient should be taken back for a right colectomy
- 5-year survival rate after curative resection was 61% and 31%
- Remaining answer choices are not typically common presentation of appendiceal adenocarcinoma

(Sabiston, 20th Edition, Page 1308)

216. According to AJCC, 8th edition, Staging of 2 cm size Pancreatic cancer if it involves portal vein is:

(a) T1
(b) T2
(c) T3
(d) T4

Ans: (a) T1

AJCC 8th edition has brought the following changes with regard to carcinoma pancreas
• 1 is subdivided into T1a, T1b and T1c based on size
• T2 and T3 are categorized based on size and not on extrapancreatic involvement anymore
• T4 is a radiological staging done by the relationship to vessels
• Nodal staging has N1 and N2 subdivisions unlike before N1 alone
• Portal vein or SMV involvement will not change the staging as per AJCC 7 and AJCC 8th edition. Staging Decided based on the Tumor size only
• Borderline resectable lesion is lesion involvement > 180 degrees of PV/SMV or <180 degree involvement of Coeliac axis/SMA

(AJCC, 8th Edition, Manual Page 342)

217. Not true about Primary peritoneal serous carcinoma include:

(a) Type of adenocarcinoma
(b) Constitutes 50% of all Epithelial ovarian carcinoma
(c) Associated with older age at diagnosis
(d) Obesity is also associated factor

Ans: (b) Constitutes 50% of all Epithelial ovarian carcinoma

PRIMARY PERITONEAL SEROUS CARCINOMA

- Rare type of primary peritoneal adenocarcinoma
- **Constitutes 7-20% of all epithelial ovarian carcinoma**
- Risk factors for primary peritoneal carcinoma are similar to those for ovarian and fallopian tube cancer, including *BRCA* mutation and low parity
- ***Also been associated with older age at diagnosis and increased rates of obesity when compared with ovarian cancer***
- *Simulates ovarian cancer in its clinical features and is seen especially in women who have previously undergone hysterectomy and bilateral salpingooophorectomy*
- At laparotomy, extensive disease is seen in upper abdomen, particularly in omentum
- Microscopic/small macroscopic cancer deposits are seen on surface of ovaries, but more extensive involvement of uterosacral ligaments, pelvic peritoneum or omentum is seen
- *Histologically resemble moderately to poorly differentiated serous ovarian carcinoma*
- Primary peritoneal endometrioid carcinoma is less common
- **Treatment:** Chemotherapy and/or radiotherapy with intraperitoneal radioisotopes and external beam therapy

(Handbook of Gynecological Oncology)

218. Which of the following is not true about Placental site trophoblastic tumor?

(a) Arises from trophoblasts of placental bed
(b) Associated with modestly elevated serum Beta hCG levels
(c) Presents with vaginal bleeding
(d) No lymphatic invasion occurs

Ans: (d) No lymphatic invasion occurs

PLACENTAL SITE TROPHOBLASTIC TUMOR (PSTT)

- Arises from the intermediate trophoblasts of placental bed
- Composed mainly of cytotrophoblastic cells
- Associated with modestly elevated serum b-hCG levels
- Identification of a high proportion of free b-hCG (>30%) is considered diagnostic
- Patient presents with vaginal bleeding
- Local invasion into myometrium and lymphatics occurs
- **Hysterectomy is the preferred treatment**

(Devita, 11th Edition, Page 2193)

219. Indication for bone scan in carcinoma prostate:

(a) PSA >20 ng/ml and biopsy Gleason score >7
(b) T3 and T4 Stage
(c) Symptoms suggestive of metastatic disease
(d) All of the above

Ans: (d) All of the above

PROBABILITY OF BONE SCAN WITH PSA IN CA PROSTATE

- PSA < 10 ng/ml→ <1%
- PSA < 10-50 ng/ml→10%
- PSA >50 ng/ml→ 50%
- Bone scan is used to assess hormonal and chemotherapy in men with metastatic disease
- All the above options signify metastatic disease

(Devita, 10th Edition, Page 941)

220. All are true about pragmatic classification of Carcinoma breast *except:*

(a) 5-year survival rate of very low risk primary breast cancer is >90%

(b) In locally advanced breast cancer primary systemic therapy is given

(c) Very low risk group needs locoregional and systemic treatment

(d) In metastatic group usually primary systemic treatment

Ans: (c) Very low risk group needs locoregional and systemic treatment

Pregmatic Classification of Breast Cancer

Group	5-year survival rate	Example	Treatment
Very low risk	>90%	Screen detected DCIS, Tubular/special types	Local
Low risk	70-90%	Node negative or favourable histology	Locoregional with/without systemic
High risk	<70%	Node positive or unfavourable histology	Locoregional with systemic
Locally advanced	<30%	Large primary or inflammatory	Primary systemic
Metastatic	–	–	Primary systemic

(Bailey, 27th Edition, Page 875)

221. What is the risk of malignancy when RMI (Risk of malignancy index) is >250?

(a) 25%

(b) 50%

(c) 75%

(d) 100%

Ans: (c) 75%

Risk of Malignancy Index

RMI = U × M × CA 125

U = USG score (1 point each for: multi-locular cyst; solid areas; metastasis; ascites; bilateral lesions)

M = 3 (postmenopausal women)

CA-125 level in U/mL

Risk of cancer is 75% when the RMI value is > 250

(Handbook of Gynecological Oncology)

222. A 70 years old male came with complaints of pain in the right hypochondrium. On examination the patient had a mass abdomen in the right upper quadrant. Ultrasound of the abdomen done which showed a 10 × 10 cm mass in the right lobe of liver. Which of the following tumor marker would be helpful?

(a) CA 19-9

(b) ALP

(c) AFP

(d) Calcitonin

Ans: (c) AFP

***Huge Liver mass** in an **elderly male** is more likely to be **Hepatocellular Carcinoma,** for which measurement of **Serum Alpha FetoProtein** will be helpful*

ALPHA FETOPROTEIN

- It is an **Oncofetal antigen** that is elevated during **fetal period** and **falls after birth.** However it is synthesised by **hepatocytes** in small numbers
- **Elevated in:**
  - Hepatocellular carcinomas
  - Nonseminomatous Germ cell tumors
  - Gastric, Pancreatic, Colorectal and Lung cancers
  - Benign conditions like Hepatitis, Inflammatory bowel disease and Cirrhosis
- AFP is neither highly sensitive or specific for HCC, but it is elevated in >80% of patients

- AFP has prognostic values and are used in monitoring response to therapy
- Normal level is <25 ng/mL
- It reflects tumor size, with serum levels >400 ng/mL are associated with larger tumors
- It also has a prognostic value; AFP correlates with tumor stage and prognosis
- It is rate of increase, i.e., AFP doubling time increases are associated with poor prognosis
- It also predicts the recurrence potential of the tumors
- Normally, after resection the AFP should drop below 10 ng/mL
- When the preoperative AFP level is more than 100 ng/mL and the postoperative level did not fall below 20 ng/mL have high recurrence rates
- Also helps in monitoring response to chemotherapy; fall in AFP noted with use of chemotherapy
- AFP levels doesn't correlate with tumor regrowth after chemoembolization treatment
- AFP is less sensitive and specific for tumors less than 2 cm and the sensitivity and specificity increases for tumors more than 2 cm and with increasing levels
- To differentiate between benign and malignant lesions less than 2 cm, Des-carboxyprothrombin (DCP) levels are raised in 40% of HCC lesions less than 2 cm

(Sabiston, 20th Edition, Page 699)

223. Gallbladder carcinoma is M1 stage which of the following lymph nodes are involved?

(a) Superior mesenteric lymph nodes
(b) Aortic lymph nodes
(c) Celiac lymph nodes
(d) Pancreato-duodenal lymph nodes

Ans: (b) Aortic lymph nodes

Presence of tumor in the periaortic lymph nodes of the celiac axis indicates that the tumor is beyond the limits of normal resection

- Regional lymph nodes are the hepatic hilus nodes (including nodes along common bile duct, hepatic artery, portal vein and cystic duct), celiac and superior mesenteric artery nodes
- Lymphatic drainage normally occurs into peripancreatic nodes located along veins

Staging of Gallbladder Cancer	
T1	T1a–Invades Lamina propria T1b–Invades Muscular layer *(Water shed area for Gallbladder cancer management)*
T2	T2a–Invades Perimuscular connective tissue on peritoneal side without serosal involvement T2b–Invades Perimuscular connective tissue on hepatic side with no extension into liver
T3	Perforates serosa (visceral peritoneum) and/or directly invades liver or adjacent organ like stomach, duodenum, colon, pancreas, omentum or extrahepatic bile ducts
T4	Invades main portal vein/hepatic artery or invades two/more extrahepatic organs/structures
N1	1-3 Regional lymph nodes
N2	4/more Regional lymph nodes

<table>
<tr><th></th><th>N0</th><th>N1</th><th>N2</th><th>M1</th></tr>
<tr><td>T1</td><td>I</td><td rowspan="4">IIIB</td><td rowspan="5">IVB</td><td rowspan="5">IVB</td></tr>
<tr><td>T2a</td><td>IIa</td></tr>
<tr><td>T2b</td><td>IIb</td></tr>
<tr><td>T3</td><td>IIIA</td></tr>
<tr><td>T4</td><td colspan="2">IVA</td></tr>
</table>

(CSDT, 13th Edition, Page 600)

224. All of the following are indications of diagnostic laparoscopy in a patient with carcinoma pancreas *except:*

(a) Tumor located in the head of the pancreas
(b) Tumor size 4 cm
(c) CA 19-9 level 200 U/mL
(d) Inconclusive findings on CECT abdomen

Ans: (a) Tumor located in the head of the pancreas

Indications of diagnostic laparoscopy in Carcinoma pancreas
• Tumor located in body or tail of pancreas
• CA-19-9 level >100 U/mL
• Tumor size >3 cm
• Diagnostic uncertainty on CECT

(Sabiston, 20th Edition, Page 1544)

225. Ideal preferred treatment for carcinoma of the gallbladder in majority is:

(a) Radical resection that includes gallbladder in continuity with the right hepatic lobe and regional lymph node dissection

(b) Radiation therapy

(c) Chemotherapy

(d) Palliative

Ans: (d) Palliative

Many patients with gallbladder cancer will present with advanced disease and therefore the goal of therapy is palliation of symptoms

- Radical resection, radiation therapy, and chemotherapy have been effective only anecdotally
- ***Most believe that the dismal prognosis of carcinoma of the gallbladder does not justify anything more than palliative treatment***
- About 88% of patients are dead within a year of diagnosis and only about 4% are alive after 5 years, regardless of the type of treatment
- Those whose surgeon was unaware of the presence of the tumor at the time of cholecystectomy (approximately 12% of cases) are most likely to survive long term
- There are insufficient data to support conclusively the proposition that the patient with unexpected carcinoma found on histologic examination should undergo reoperation with intent for radical excision
- There also are indirect suggestions that the prognosis of gallbladder carcinoma may be improving, but it is not clear if this is spontaneous or due to either earlier diagnosis or surgical management

(Sabiston, 20th Edition, Page 1514)

226. Following are risk factors for developing Gastric Adenocarcinoma *except:*

(a) Multifocal mucosal atrophy

(b) Intestinal metaplasia

(c) Partial gastrectomy

(d) PGDFRA mutation

Ans: (d) PGDFRA mutation

Factors Associated With Increased Risk for Developing Stomach Cancer
Nutritional
Low fat or protein consumption
Salted meat or fish
High nitrate consumption
High complex carbohydrate consumption
Environmental
Poor food preparation (smoked, salted)
Lack of refrigeration
Poor drinking water (e.g., contaminated well water)
Smoking
Social
Low social class

Contd.

Contd.

Medical
Prior gastric surgery
H. pylori infection
Gastric atrophy and gastritis
Adenomatous polyps
Other
Male sex

- Germline mutations in CDH 1 which encodes for E–cadherin
- BRCA 2 mutation–Familial gastric cancer
- Familial gastric cancer–usually diffuse

(Sabiston, 20th Edition, Page 1214)

227. With regard to adenocarcinoma of the small bowel, all of the following statements are correct *except:*

(a) Small bowel adenocarcinoma is found in decreasing order of frequency in ileum, jejunum and duodenum
(b) Villous adenomas of the small bowel are commonly found in the duodenum around the Ampulla of Vater
(c) Adenocarcinoma of the duodenum usually occurs earlier than small bowel adenocarcinoma elsewhere in the jejunum and ileum
(d) Villous adenomas of the duodenum are frequently associated with familial adenomatous polyposis

- Germline mutations in CDH 1 which encodes for E–cadherin.
- *BRCA 2* mutation–Familial gastric cancer.
- Familial gastric cancer–usually diffuse.

Ans: (a) Small bowel adenocarcinoma is found in decreasing order of frequency in ileum, jejunum and duodenum

- Adenocarcinomas constitute approximately 50% of malignant tumors of the small bowel
- Peak incidence is in 7th decade of life and most series show slight male predominance
- Most of these tumors are located in the duodenum and proximal jejunum
- Those arising in association with Crohn's disease tend to occur at a somewhat younger age and more than 70% arise in the ileum
- Tumors of duodenum tend to be manifested somewhat earlier than those in the most distal intestine because of the earlier presentation of symptoms, which are usually jaundice and chronic bleeding
- Adenocarcinomas of the jejunum and ileum usually produce symptoms that may be more nonspecific and include ***vague abdominal pain and weight loss***
- Intestinal obstruction and chronic bleeding can also occur
- Perforation is uncommon
- As with adenocarcinomas in other organs, survival of patients with small bowel adenocarcinomas is related to the stage of disease at the time of diagnosis
- Unfortunately, diagnosis is often delayed and the disease is advanced at the time of surgery secondary to various factors (e.g., vagueness of symptoms, absence of physical findings, lack of clinical suspicion because of the rarity of these lesions)

(Sabiston, 20th Edition, Page 1277)

228. All the following are protective factors against ovarian cancer *except:*

(a) Use of OCP's
(b) Tubal ligation
(c) Preganancy
(d) BRCA1/2 mutations

Ans: (d) BRCA1/2 mutations

- **Use of oral contraceptives and tubal ligation are protective**

Protective Factors for Ovarian Malignancy
• Combined oral contraceptives
• Pregnancy
• Tubal ligation, hysterectomy
• Breastfeeding

- Carriers of a BRCA1 or 2 mutation have a 20% to 40% lifetime risk

(Devita, 11th Edition, Page 2197)

229. Length of colon resection for colon cancer is based on:

(a) Size of primary tumor
(b) Need to remove regional lymph nodes
(c) Performance status
(d) Grade of primary tumor

Ans: (b) Need to remove regional lymph nodes

COLON RESECTION

- *For invasive carcinomas of the colon, stages I through III, the surgical approach will be dictated by the* ***size and location of lesions in the colon***
- Location will determine what region of bowel is removed and the extent of its resection is dictated by its vascular and lymphatic supply
- Objective in treatment of carcinoma of the colon is to remove the primary tumor along with its lymphovascular supply
- Because the lymphatics of the colon accompany main arterial supply, length of bowel resected depends on which vessels are supplying the segment involved with cancer
- Number of lymph nodes recovered in the surgical specimen has long served as a proxy for the oncologic adequacy of resection
- **Minimum of 12 lymph nodes in the resected specimen are necessary for adequate staging**
- If unexpected metastatic disease is encountered at the time of a laparotomy, the decision about whether to proceed with resection of the primary tumor depends on the volume of distant disease, location and size of the primary tumor, the operation required to remove the primary tumor and the operative approach

(Schwartz, 10th Edition, Page 1212)

230. Which of following skin tumors have least tendency for metastases?

(a) Squamous cell carcinoma
(b) Melanoma
(c) Basal cell carcinoma
(d) Sebaceous carcinoma

Ans: (c) Basal cell carcinoma

BASAL CELL CARCINOMA

- Although overall prognosis of the vast majority of BCC is excellent, some tumors exhibit infiltrative growth patterns and extensive subclinical spread
- Most significant predictors were anatomic location on the nose of any type of BCC; morpheaform BCC on the cheek; recurrent BCC in men; any tumor located on neck in men; any tumor located on ear helix, eyelid, or temple and increasing preoperative size
- Invasive BCC can migrate along the perichondrium, periosteum, fascia, or tarsal plate
- This type of spread accounts for higher recurrence rates in tumors involving eyelid, nose and scalp
- Embryonic fusion planes likely offer little resistance and can lead to deep invasion and tumor spread, with very high rates of recurrence
- Most susceptible areas include the inner canthus, philtrum, middle to lower chin, nasolabial groove, preauricular area, and retroauricular sulcus
- **PNI** is infrequent in BCC and occurs most often in recurrent, clinically aggressive lesions

- In all cases, PNI was associated with recurrent tumors that were most often located in the periauricular and malar areas
- Clinically, PNI may present with paresthesia, pain, and weakness or, in some cases, paralysis
- Metastatic BCC is rare, with incidence rates varying from 0.0028% to 0.1%
- This concept of stromal dependence may explain the low incidence of metastatic BCC. Metastases, when reported, have involved the lung, lymph nodes, esophagus, oral cavity and skin.
- Although long-term survival has been reported, the prognosis for metastatic BCC is generally poor, with an average survival of 8 to 10 months following diagnosis
- Platinum-based chemotherapy or molecularly targeted *Smoothened* inhibitors may provide benefit as salvage therapy for metastatic BCC

(Devita, 10th Edition, Page 1320)

231. Which of the following statements is not true?

(a) Type 1 epithelial ovarian cancers include low grade serous, endometroid, mucinous varieties

(b) Type 2 epithelial ovarian cancers include high grade serous and endometroid varieties

(c) Type 2 epithelial ovarian cancers are associated with P53 mutations

(d) Type 1 epithelial ovarian cancers are more aggressive than Type 2

Ans: (d) Type 1 epithelial ovarian cancers are more aggressive than Type 2

- **Type 1 epithelial ovarian cancers:** Low grade serous, endometroid, mucinous, clear cell, transitional cell carcinomas. Associated with serous and mucinous cystadenomas. Serous has BRAF and K-RAS mutations. **Mucinous has K-RAS mutations–80%**
- **Type 2 epithelial ovarian cancers:** High grade serous, endometroid and undifferentiated carcinomas. More aggressive. TP53 muatations

(Handbook of Gynecological Oncology)

232. Which of the following differentiates between Borderline tumors from benign cystadenomas of Ovary by all *except?*

(a) Epithelial budding

(b) Single layered epithelium

(c) Increased mitotic activity

(d) Nuclear atypia

Ans: (b) Single layered epithelium

Borderline tumors are differentiated with benign cystadenomas by
• Epithelial budding
• Multilayering of epithelium
• Increased mitotic activity
• Nuclear atypia

(Handbook of Gynecological Oncology)

233. Which of the following is not True about Fallopian tube cancer?

(a) Infertility and Nulliparity are predisposing factors

(b) OC pills and Breastfeeding are protective factors

(c) Most frequent change detected is Gains at 3q

(d) Life time risk of Fallopian tube cancers in BRCA carriers is 30%

Ans: (d) Life time risk of Fallopian tube cancers in BRCA carriers is 30%

Predisposing Factors
• Infertility, nulliparity and family history of ovarian cancer, early menarche and late menopause
• **Women with BRCA1 or BRCA2 mutations are at high risk**

- Protective factors include oral contraceptive use, multiparity, breastfeeding and tubal ligation
- Most frequent changes detected in FTCA are gains at 3q (70%) and 8q (75%), with high-level amplifications (Genetic change)

Lifetime risk of fallopian tubal cancer in BRCA mutation carriers is 0.6% to 3%

(Handbook of Gynecological Oncology)

234. Treatment of choice of Squamous cell carcinoma Anal canal with more than T1 and N+ Stage is:

(a) Wide local excision
(b) APR
(c) Chemoradiotherapy
(d) Radiotherapy

Ans: (c) Chemoradiotherapy

SCC Anal Margin	SCC Anal canal
Small T1→WLE	T1 within 5cm→WLE
>T1, N+, Advanced→CRT+APR	>T1, N+→ CRT
	(Nigro regimen)

(Sabiston, 20th Edition, Page 1412)

235. Which of the following is not True about Carcinoid tumors?

(a) Appendiceal carcinoids are more common in females
(b) Type 3 gastric carcinoids are more common in females
(c) Maximum malignant potential is associated with pancreatic carcinoids
(d) Somatostatin receptor scintigraphy with in^{111} labelled pantreotide has shown lesser sensitivity than CT scan

Ans: (d) Somatostatin receptor scintigraphy with in^{111} labelled pantreotide has shown lesser sensitivity than CT scan

- Appendiceal carcinoids are more common in females
- Type 3 gastric carcinoids are more common in men
- Maximum malignant potential is associated with pancreatic carcinoids
- Somatostatin receptor scintigraphy with in^{111} labelled pantreotide has shown higher sensitivity than CT scan

(Sabiston, 20th Edition, Page 1272)

236. Not True about Phase trials is:

(a) Phase I trial is conducted on Healthy volunteers
(b) Phase I trials gives information about maximum tolerable doses
(c) Phase II trials gives information about Establishing therapeutic efficacy
(d) Phase IV trials confirms therapeutic efficacy

Ans: (d) Phase IV trials confirms therapeutic efficacy

Phase	Conducted on	Purpose
I	Healthy volunteers	Safety and tolerability **Know maximum tolerable doses**
II	Patients	Establish Therapeutic efficacy
III	Several centres	Confirm Therapeutic efficacy
IV	Practising physicians	Know rare and long term adverse effects

(Devita, 11th Edition, Page 903)

237. Not true about Mesothelioma is:

(a) Most commonly seen with Pleura
(b) Associated with asbestosis exposure
(c) Good prognosis
(d) 20% occur in peritoneum

Ans: (c) Good prognosis

MESOTHELIOMA

- Most common occurs in pleura
- Occurs with asbestosis exposure
- Poor prognosis
- 20% occur in peritoneum

(Sabiston, 20th Edition, Page 1607)

238. Not true about Malignant mucosal melanoma is:

(a) Most common site of head and neck mucosal melanoma is sinonasal region
(b) Most common site of laryngeal mucosal melanoma is Supraglottic region
(c) Majority of mucosal melanomas may be associated with BRAF mutations
(d) More advanced and Poor prognosis

Ans: (c) Majority of mucosal melanomas may be associated with BRAF mutations

- Most common site of mucosal melanoma is head and neck
- Most common site of head and neck mucosal melanoma is sinonasal region
- Most common site in sinonasal region is nasal cavity (80%)
- Anterior portion of nasal septum accounts for most cases of nasal cavity mucosal melanoma
- Maxillary sinus is the most common site involved among paranasal sinus
- ***Most common site of laryngeal mucosal melanoma is Supraglottic region***
- Majority of mucosal melanomas may be associated with *KIT* amplifications
- Occult location–Patients tend to present with more advanced disease and have a poor prognosis

(Sabiston, 20th Edition, Page 747)

239. Which of the following is not true about Cyclophosphamide?

(a) Causes Carcinoma bladder
(b) Alkylating agent
(c) Myelosuppression that involves platelets
(d) Causes cardiac toxicity

Ans: (c) Myelosuppression that involves platelets

CYCLOPHOSPHAMIDE

- Alkylating agent
- FDA→Lymphoma, Leukemia, Multiple myeloma, Advanced Mycosis fungoides, Neuroblastoma, Ovarian adenocarcinoma, Retinoblastoma and CA Breast
- Hemorrhagic cystitis and Renal tubular necrosis and secondary malignancies (Acute leukemia and CA Bladder), Cardiac toxicity and SIADH
- Consider vigorous hydration and MESNA therapy with high dose cyclophosphamide
- Myelosuppression: PLATELET SPARING IS CHARACTERISTIC of cyclophosphamide
- Women-High incidence of amenorrhea and ovarian atrophy
- Immunosuppresssion→suppressed B cell function, Depleted B lymphocytes, Suppressed lymphocytic function

(Devita, 11th Edition, Page 506)

240. Most common cancer to cause Opsoclonus in children is:

(a) Neuroblastoma (b) ALL

(c) AML (d) Carcinoma lung

Ans: (a) Neuroblastoma

- Most common cancer to cause opsoclonus in children–Neuroblastoma
- Most common cancer to cause opsoclonus in Adults–Carcinoma lung

(Devita, 11th Edition, Page 3505)

241. Translocation seen with Ewing's sarcoma is:

(a) t(x,18) (b) t(11,22)

(c) 3p- (d) 12p-

Ans: (b) t(11,22)

Chromosomal Markers
• t(x,18)→Synovial sarcoma
• t(11,22)→Ewing's sarcoma
• 3p– →Small cell carcinoma lung, RCC
• 1p– →Neuroblastoma
• 12p– →GCT

(Devita, 11th Edition, Page 2463)

242. Next line management in patients with <4 cm incidentaloma with benign imaging features is:

(a) Repeat imaging in 3-6 months (b) Biochemical evaluation annually

(c) Adrenalectomy (d) Both A and B

Ans: (d) Both A and B

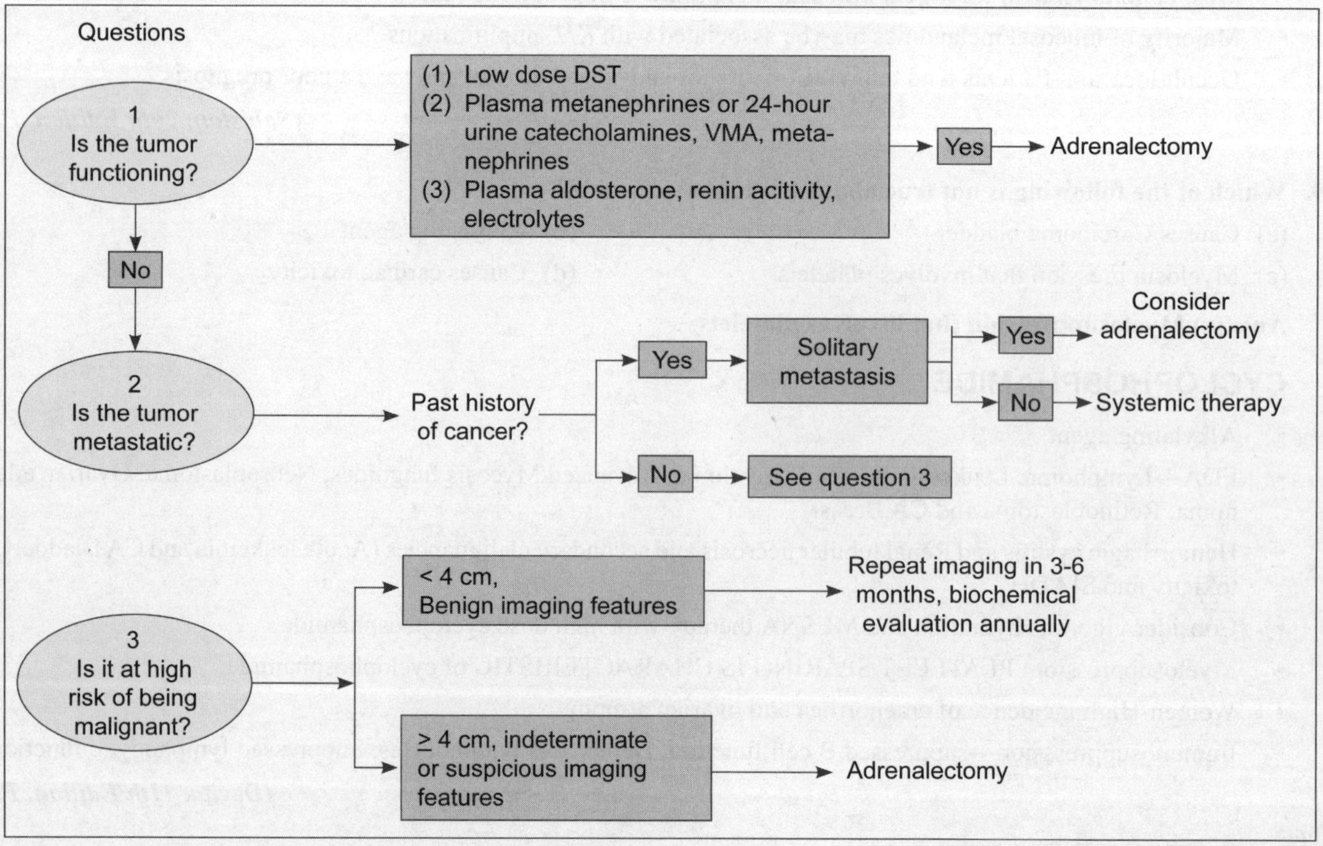

(Schwartz, 10th Edition, Page 1589)

PAPER 5

243. All of the following are worrisome features of IPMN *except:*

(a) Enhancing cyst wall (b) Jaundice

(c) Pancreatitis (d) Main duct 5-9 mm

Ans: (b) Jaundice

A Summary of Worrisome and High-Risk Features of Intraductal Papillary Mucinous Neoplasm

Worrisome Features	High-Risk Features
Main duct 5-9 mm	Main duct >1 cm
Nonenhancing mural nodule	Enhancing solid component
Thickened, enhancing cyst wall	Jaundice
BD-IPMN size >3 cm	
Abrupt caliber change in main duct with upstream atrophy	
Lymphadenopathy	
Pancreatitis	

(Sabiston, 20th Edition, Page 1539)

244. Negative CEA, High amylase and Negative mucin is suggestive of:

(a) Pseudocyst pancreas (b) Serous cystadenoma pancreas

(c) Mucinous cystadenoma pancreas (d) IPMN

Ans: (d) IPMN

Defining Characteristics of Pseudocysts and Pancreatic Cystic Neoplasms

Characteristics	Pseudocyst	SCN	MCN	IPMN
Epidemiology				
Gender	F=M	F≫M (4:1)	F⋙M (10:1)	F=M
Age (years)	40-60	60-70	50-60	60-70
Imaging Findings				
Location	Evenly distributed	Evenly distributed	Head ≪ body/tail	Head > diffuse > body/tail
Appearance	Round, thick-walled large cyst; gland atrophy ± calcification	Multiple small cysts separated by internal septations with central starburst calcification	Thick-walled, septated macrocyst with smooth contour; ± solid component, eggshell calcifications	Poorly demarcated, lobulated, polycystic mass with dilation of main or branch ducts
Communication with ducts	Yes	No	Very rare	Yes
Cyst Fluid Analysis				
Cytology	Inflammatory cells	Scant glycogen-rich cells, with positive periodic acid-Schiff stain	Sheets and clusters of columnar, mucin-containing cells	Tall, columnar, mucin-containing cells
Mucin stain	Negative	Negative	Postive	Positive
Amylase	Very high	Low	Low	High
CEA	Low	Low	High	High

(Sabiston, 20th Edition, Page 1538)

245. Lymph node along splenic artery in carcinoma stomach staging belongs to:

(a) 10
(b) 11
(c) 13
(d) 15

Ans: (b) 11

LN number	
1	Right cardia
2	Left cardia
3	Lesser curve
4sa	Short gastric
4sb	Left gastroepiploic
4d	Right gastroepiploic
5	Suprapyloric
6	Infrapyloric
7	Left gastric artery
8a	Anterior hepatic artery
9	Coeliac artery
10	Splenic hilum
11	Splenic artery
19	Infradiaphragmatic
20	Oesophageal hiatus
110	Loweroesophagus
111	Supradiaphragmatic

(Bailey and Love, 27th Edition, Page 1138)

246. A 43-year-old male patient comes with 5 cm thyroid lump involving level 6 lymph nodes. FNAC suggestive of Papillary thyroid carcinoma TNM staging of patient will be:

(a) Stage I
(b) Stage II
(c) Stage III
(d) Stage IV

Ans: (a) Stage I

- A patient who presents at younger than 45 years old is stage 1 regardless of T stage and N stage as long as there are no distant metastases

(Sabiston, 20th Edition, Page 904)

247. Most common site for Metastases from Malignant Phyllodes is:

(a) Bone
(b) Stomach
(c) Lungs
(d) Brain

Ans: (c) Lungs

- Malignant phyllodes tumors are characterized by features such as stromal overgrowth, cellular atypia and high number of mitoses
- These tumors are treated similarly to soft tissue sarcomas that occur on trunk or extremities
- Complete surgical excision of entire tumor with a margin of normal tissue is advised
- When tumor is large with respect to the size of breast, total mastectomy may be required
- If mastectomy is performed and margins are –ve, radiation therapy is not recommended
- If margins are concerning or close, if the tumor involves fascia or chest wall, or if tumor is very large (>5 cm), irradiation of the chest wall is considered

- If only wide local excision is performed, adjuvant radiation therapy is recommended As with other soft tissue sarcomas, regional lymph node dissection is not required for staging or locoregional control.
- ***Metastases from malignant phyllodes tumors occur via hematogenous spread; common sites of metastasis include lung, bone, abdominal viscera and mediastinum***

(Sabiston, 20th Edition, Page 842)

248. Development of a cutaneous malignancy is associated with chronic exposure to:

(a) Ammonia (b) Arsenic
(c) Chromium (d) Benzene

Ans: (b) Arsenic

- Chronic exposure to arsenic (as seen in Fowler's solution) has been associated with the development of multiple squamous and basal cell carcinomas
- Predisposing factors for BCC include exposure to arsenical compounds, coal tar, aromatic hydrocarbons, ionising radiation and genetic skin cancer syndromes
- IR causes SCC, as do chemical carcinogens (arsenicals, tar) and infection with HPV 5 and 16

(Bailey, 27th Edition, Page 604)

249. Most common malignant neoplasm in Li-Fraumeni syndrome is:

(a) Soft tissue sarcoma (b) Breast cancers
(c) Brain tumors (d) Adrenocortical carcinoma

Ans: (b) Breast cancers

- Most common malignant neoplasm in Li-Fraumeni syndrome is Breast cancer

Defined
• A proband diagnosed with sarcoma before the age of 45 years, with
• A first-degree relative with any cancer diagnosed before the age of 45 years, plus
• An additional first or second-degree relative with either sarcoma at any age or any cancer before age of 45 years

(Sabiston, 20th Edition, Page 690)

250. In Masaoka staging of Thymoma, Stage 1 is:

(a) Macroscopically completely encapsulated and microscopic no capsular invasion
(b) Macroscopic invasion into mediastinal pleura
(c) Macroscopic invasion into Pericardium, Great vessels and Lung
(d) Pleural dissemination

Ans: (a) Macroscopically completely encapsulated and microscopic no capsular invasion

Masaoka Staging	
I	Macroscopically completely encapsulated and Microscopically no capsular invasion
II	Macroscopic invasion into surrounding fatty tissue or mediastinal pleura Microscopic invasion into capsule
III	Macroscopic invasion into pericardium, Great vessels and Lung
IV	Pleural or pericardial dissemination Lymphogenous or Hematogenous metastases

(Devita, 10th Edition, Page 561)

251. Choriocarcinoma confined to Uterus. Stage is:

(a) I (b) II
(c) III (d) IV

Ans: (c) III

Stage	Component
I	Confined to uterus
II	Extends outside uterus, but limited to genital structures
III	Extends to lungs, with or without genital tract involvement
IV	All other metastatic sites

(Devita, 10th Edition, Page 1071)

252. Diarrhea in Medullary thyroid carcinoma is due to:

(a) 5 hydroxytryptamine (b) Prostaglandins

(c) Calcitonin (d) Both A and B

Ans: (d) Both A and B

- Diarrhea is a feature in 30% of cases and this may be due to 5-hydroxytryptamine or prostaglandins produced by tumor cells
- MTC are tumors of the parafollicular (C cells) derived from neural crest, rather than the cells of the thyroid follicle as are other primary thyroid carcinomas
- Cells are not unlike those of a carcinoid tumor and on histological analysis a characteristic amyloid stroma is seen
- High levels of serum calcitonin and carcinoembryonic antigen are produced by many medullary tumors, which should be tested for in suspected cases
- Calcitonin levels fall after resection and rise again with recurrence, making it a valuable tumor marker in the follow-up of patients with this disease

(Bailey and Love, 27th Edition, Page 820)

253. Guidelines for EMR in Early gastric cancer include all *except:*

(a) Tumor limited to mucosa (b) No ulceration

(c) Tumor smaller than 3 cm (d) No lymphovascular invasion

Ans: (c) Tumor smaller than 3 cm

General guidelines for endoscopic resection of Early gastric cancer are as follows:
• Tumor limited to the mucosa • No lymphovascular invasion • Tumor smaller than 2 cm • No ulceration • Well or moderately well differentiated histopathology
Any of these listed findings on initial biopsy or during endoscopic resection is an indication for gastrectomy with lymph node dissection

(Sabiston, 20th Edition, Page 1222)

254. Primary reconstructive flap of choice in Dentate mandible with Oral cancer:

(a) Iliac crest (b) Fibula

(c) Composite flap (d) PMMF

Ans: (a) Iliac crest

Site	Primary Flap
Floor of mouth	Radial forearm free flap
Lateral tongue	Radial forearm free flap/Anterolateral thigh flap

Contd.

Contd.

Total tongue/Glossectomy	Anterolateral thigh flap/Rectus abdominus
MANDIBLE	Dentate–Iliac crest Edentulous–Fibula
Tongue base	Radial forearm free flap
MAXILLA	Low level/Hard palate–Obturation, RFFF/ALT High–Iliac crest/Scapula
Soft palate/Tonsil	Forearm/MSAP

(Bailey, 27th Edition, Page 774)

255. Risk of Malignancy in type 3 Bosnaik renal cysts is:

(a) 0% (b) 5%
(c) 50% (d) 100%

Ans: (c) 50%

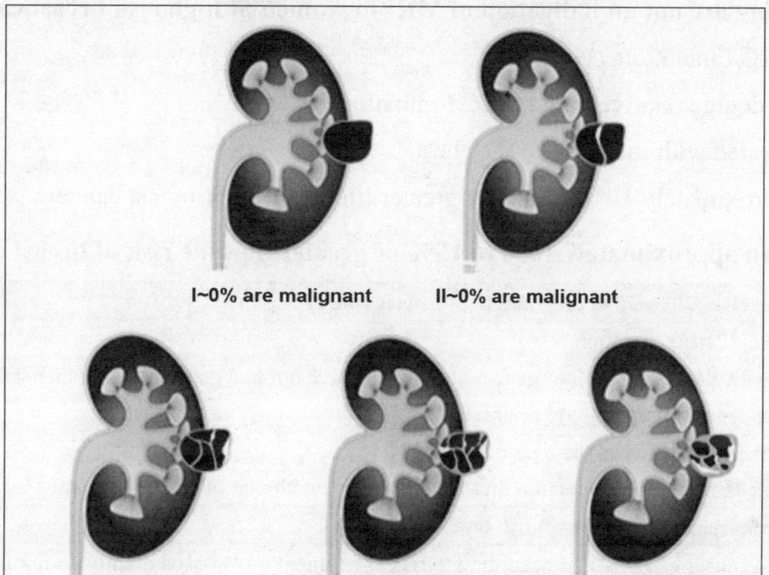

(Bailey and Love, 27th Edition, Page 1390)

256. All are true about HNPCC *except:*

(a) Most common genes affected are MLH1 and MSH2
(b) Life time risk of developing Colorectal cancer is 80%
(c) Most cancers develop in distal colon
(d) Females have 30-50% chances of developing Endometrial cancer

Ans: (c) Most cancers develop in distal colon

- HNPCC is characterised by an increased risk of colorectal cancer and also cancers of endometrium, ovary, stomach and small intestine
- Autosomal dominant condition
- Caused by a mutation in one of the DNA mismatch repair genes
- Most commonly affected genes are *MLHI* and *MSH 2*
- Lifetime risk of developing colorectal cancer is 80%
- Mean age of diagnosis is 45 years
- Most cancers develop in the proximal colon
- Females have a 30-50% lifetime risk of developing endometrial cancer

(Bailey and Love, 27th Edition, Page 1260)

257. Tumor deposits in mesentery in Carcinoma colon as per AJCC staging is:

(a) N1a (b) N1c

(c) N2c (d) M1

Ans: (b) N1c

N1a	Metastasis in one regional lymph node
N1b	Metastasis in two or three regional lymph nodes
N1c	Tumor deposit(s) in the subserosa, mesentery, or nonperitonealized pericolic or perirectal tissues without regional nodal metastasis
N2	Metastasis in four or more regional lymph nodes
N2a	Metastasis in four to six regional lymph nodes
N2b	Metastasis in seven or more regional lymph nodes

(Sabiston, 20th Edition, Page 1374)

258. Which of the following are not an indication of MRI in women at high risk breast cancer?

(a) With a known *BRCA* mutation

(b) Who have a first-degree relative with a *BRCA* mutation

(c) Who had been treated with radiation to the chest

(d) Who have an approximately 10% to 15% or greater lifetime risk of breast cancer

Ans: (d) Who have an approximately 10% to 15% or greater lifetime risk of breast cancer

Women at high lifetime risk (20%-25% or greater) of breast cancer
• Known *BRCA1* or *BRCA2* gene mutation
• First-degree relative with *BRCA1* or *BRCA2* gene mutation, but have not had genetic testing themselves
• Lifetime risk of breast cancer of ≈20%-25% or greater
• Radiation therapy to the chest between the ages of 10 and 30
• Li-Fraumeni syndrome/Cowden syndrome or a first-degree relative with one of these syndromes
Women at moderately increased (15%-20%) lifetime risk
• Lifetime risk of breast cancer of 15%-20% according to risk assessment tools based mainly on family history
• Personal history of breast cancer, ductal carcinoma *in situ,* lobular carcinoma *in situ,* atypical ductal hyperplasia, or atypical lobular hyperplasia
• Extremely dense breasts or unevenly dense breasts when viewed by mammograms

(Devita, 10th Edition, Page 378)

259. Characteristics of Ideal tumor markers include all *except:*

(a) Should be expressed exclusively by particular tumor

(b) Collection of specimen for tumor marker assay should be easy

(c) Assay itself should be reproducible

(d) It should be Rapid and Expensive

Ans: (d) It should be Rapid and Expensive

Ideal Tumor Marker Has Three Defining Characteristics
• First marker should be expressed exclusively by the particular tumor
• Second, collection of the specimen for the tumor marker assay should be easy
• Third, the assay itself should be reproducible, rapid and inexpensive
• Currently, there is no one marker that fulfils all these criteria for any cancer, nor is there any specific cancer for which there are biomarkers that completely describe its behavior

(Sabiston, 20th Edition, Page 697)

260. Not a nuclear microscopic feature of malignancy is:

(a) Enlargement
(b) Pleomorphism
(c) Hypochromaticity
(d) Chromatin clumping

Ans: (c) Hypochromaticity

Microscopic Features of Malignancy

• Metastasis
• Invasion
  • Of surrounding tissue
  • Vascular
  • Perineural
• Architectural abnormalities
• Necrosis
• Numerous mitotic figures
• Atypical mitotic figures
• Nuclear abnormalities
  • Pleomorphism
  • Enlargement
  • Hyperchromaticity
  • Chromatin clumping
• Nucleolar enlargement and multiplicity

(Bailey and Love, 27th Edition, Page 239)

261. Most common presentation of Nasopharyngeal carcinoma is:

(a) Hearing loss
(b) Trotter's triad
(c) Blood stained nasal discharge
(d) Cervical lymphadenopathy

Ans: (d) Cervical lymphadenopathy

- Approximately 50% of patients will present with a rnalignant node or nodes in the neck, indicating an advanced tumor.
- Nasal complaints occur in one-third of patients and aural symptoms of unilateral deafness as a consequence of Eustachian tube obstruction and secretory otitis media occur in approximately 20%

(Bailey, 27th Edition, Page 734)

262. Siewert classification is for classifying:

(a) Lung cancers
(b) Adrenal carcinoma
(c) Gastroesophageal Junctional tumors
(d) Neuroendocrine tumors

Ans: (c) Gastroesophageal Junctional tumors

SIEWERT CLASSIFICATION

- GEJ cancers (i.e., tumors with a definitive component involving the EGJ) are no longer classified by the AJCC as gastric cancers per se
- Siewert and Stein classified adenocarcinomas of the EGJ (Siewert classification) into three distinct clinical entities

Junctional cancer	Description
Type I	Adenocarcinoma of the distal oesophagus arising in an area of specialized intestinal metaplasia and which may infiltrate the oesophago-gastric junction
Type II	True carcinoma of the cardia arising from the cardiac epithelium or short segments with intestinal metaplasia at the oesophagogastric junction; this entitiy is also often referred to as 'junctional carcinoma'
Type III	Sub-cardial gastric carcinoma which infiltrates the oesophagogastric junction and distal oesophagus from below

(Devita, 10th Edition, Page 620)

263. True about Spermatocytic seminoma is:

(a) Seen generally in older men
(b) Express placental alkaline phosphatase
(c) Metastatic potential is high
(d) Secretes high amount of AFP

Ans: (a) Seen generally in older men

SPERMATOCYTIC SEMINOMA

- Spermatocytic seminoma, however, is the one variant of seminoma that has a different natural history and is even of uncertain relation to other germ cell tumors
- Spermatocytic seminoma usually occurs in **older individuals** and has **low metastatic potential.**
- Orchiectomy is the only treatment required
- Unlike all other germ cell tumors, spermatocytic seminoma is not associated with ITGCN
- Its relation to other GCTs is not clear
- It is not associated with IGCNU or bilaterality, does not express placental alkaline phosphatase or OCT3/4 and has not shown the same genetic abnormalities as other GCTs. Metastatic potential is minimal

(Devita, 10th Edition, Page 1285)

264. Which is true regarding Paget's disease of breast?

(a) Accounts for about 1% of all breast malignancies
(b) Best treated by radiation therapy
(c) Classified as T4 disease as per TNM Staging
(d) Risk of lymph node metastasis is 30%

Ans: (a) Accounts for about 1% of all breast malignancies

PAGET'S DISEASE OF BREAST

- It frequently presents as a chronic, eczematous eruption of the nipple, which may be subtle but may progress to an ulcerated, weeping lesion
- Paget's disease usually is associated with **extensive DCIS** and may be associated with an **invasive cancer**
- A **palpable mass may or may not be present**
- A nipple biopsy specimen will show a population of cells that are identical to the underlying DCIS cells (pagetoid features or pagetoid change)
- Pathognomonic of this cancer is the presence of large, pale, vacuolated cells **(Paget cells)** in the rete pegs of the epithelium
- Paget's disease may be confused with superficial spreading melanoma
- Differentiation from pagetoid intraepithelial melanoma is based on the presence of S-100 antigen immunostaining in melanoma and carcinoembryonic antigen immunostaining in Paget's disease
- Surgical therapy for Paget's disease may involve lumpectomy or mastectomy, depending on the extent of involvement of the nipple-areolar complex and the presence of DCIS or invasive cancer in the underlying breast parenchyma

(Schwartz, 10th Edition, Page 1658)

265. More than ....% of cancers of uterine cervix are associated with HPV.

(a) 50%
(b) 90%
(c) 75%
(d) 40%

Ans: (b) 90%

HPV ASSOCIATED CERVICAL CANCERS

- HPV can be identified in more than 99% of cervical cancers and infection with HPV is now accepted as a necessary cause of most cervical cancers
- It appears that most of the covariables historically associated with an increased risk of cervical cancer are surrogates for sexually transmitted HPV infection

- Women who have coitus at a young age, who have multiple sexual partners, or who bear children at a young age are at increased risk
- Promiscuous sexual behavior in male partners is also a risk factor

(Devita, 10th Edition, Page 1025)

266. Pectoralis major myocutaneous flap is based on the:

(a) Lateral thoracic artery (b) Perforating branch of thoracoabdominal artery
(c) Dorsal scapular artery (d) Perforating branches of internal mammary artery

Ans: (b) Perforating branch of thoracoabdominal artery

- Deltopectoral flap–Internal mammary artery
- PMMF–Acromiothoracic artery
- Lattismus dorsi flap–Lateral thoracic vessels/thoracodorsal artery
- Sternomastoid flap–Occipital and superior thyroid artery
- Trapezius flap–Occipital artery
- Platysmal flap–Submental and transverse cervical artery

(Stell and Maren Head and Neck Surgery, 5th Edition, Page 945)

267. Li-Fraumeni syndrome is associated with germline mutations in:

(a) Cyclin D1 (b) ATM
(c) BRCA 1 (d) p53

Ans: (d) p53

LI-FRAUMENI SYNDROME

- LFS1: Mutations in TP53
- LFS2: Mutations in CHEK2
- Classical LFS malignancies–sarcoma, cancers of the breast, brain and adrenal glands–comprise about 80% of all cancers that occur in this syndrome
- Most common malignancies are early onset breast cancer and sarcomas followed by brain tumor, leukemia, lung tumor and then gastric cancers
- High risk for multiple primary malignancies and 60% of carriers develop second tumor and 4% develop third malignancy
- 70% of them carry p53 gene mutations

(Devita, 10th Edition, Page 1160)

268. Germline mutation of which tumor suppressor gene is most frequently associated with hereditary pancreatic cancer?

(a) BRCA 2 (b) PALB 2
(c) K ras (d) P 53

Ans: (a) BRCA 2

HEREDITARY PANCREATIC CANCER

- K-ras is present in approximately 95% of all pancreatic cancer with frequent inactivation of several tumor suppressor genes (p53, DPC4, p16 and BRCA2)
- Nearly 90% of all cases have p16 mutations, 55 to 75% have p53 mutations and 50% have DPC4 mutations
- Frequency of DNA repair gene inactivations, which include BRCA2, MLHl, FANC-C and FANC-G, is relatively low

(Devita, 10th Edition, Page 687)

269. On immunohistochemistry, malignant mesothelioma is +ve for:

(a) Calretinin (b) Ber–EP4

(c) Moc–31 (d) TTF–1

Ans: (a) Calretinin

MALIGNANT MESOTHELIOMA

- Most malignant mesotheliomas (50–60%) are of the epithelial type, approximately 10% are sarcomatoid and remainder are biphasic malignant mesotheliomas
- For epithelial mesotheliomas, positive stainings for pankeratin and calretinin and negative stainings for three epithelial markers are considered sufficient for diagnosis

(Devita, 10th Edition, Page 1743)

270. Most common genetic mutation in Nevoid basal cell carcinoma syndrome is:

(a) PTCH (b) STK11

(c) TSC (d) RECQL4

Ans: (a) PTCH

NEVOID BASAL CELL CARCINOMA SYNDROME

- NBCCS is a rare autosomal dominant genetic disorder characterized by a mutation in the human patched *(PTCH1)* gene and predisposition to multiple BCC and other tumors, as well as a wide range of developmental defects
- Patients with this syndrome may exhibit a broad nasal root, borderline intelligence, odontogenic keratocysts of the jaw, palmar and plantar pits, calcification of the falx cerebri, medulloblastomas, and multiple skeletal abnormalities in addition to a few to thousands of BCCs
- Tumor development in patients with NBCCS is related to sun exposure, as BCCs develop most frequently in sun-exposed areas
- Clinical course is commonly benign prior to puberty; nonetheless, after puberty individual lesions may progressively enlarge and ulcerate
- Individuals with NBCCS are exceedingly sensitive to ionizing radiation. Hundreds of BCCs were reported in children treated with RT for medulloblastoma
- NBCCS confirms a classic two-hit model of carcinogenesis–tumors develop in cells sustaining two genetic alterations
- First alteration or hit is inheritance of a mutation in a TSG and the second is inactivation of normal homologue by environmental mutagenesis or random genetic rearrangement

Sporadic BCCs would arise in cells that underwent two somatic events, resulting in the inactivation of NBCCS TSG PTCH1

(Devita, 10th Edition, Page 1320)

271. AMICO CRITERIA for risk categorization in prostatic cancer includes all *except:*

(a) Blood PSA level (b) Gleason grade

(c) T stage (d) PSA velocity

Ans: (d) PSA velocity

D'Amico, *et al.* Risk Stratification for Clinically Localized Prostate Cancer	
Low risk	Diagnostic PSA < 10.0 ng/mL and Highest biopsy Gleason score ≤ 6 and Clinical stage T1c or T2a

Contd.

Contd.

Intermediate risk	Diagnostic PSA ≥ 10 but < 20 ng/mL or Highest biopsy Gleason score = 7 or Clinical stage
High risk	Diagnostic PSA ≥ 20 ng/mL or Highest biopsy Gleason score ≥ 8 or Clinical stage T2c/T3

(Campbell Urology 11th Edition)

272. Most common 1st metastatic site for ocular melanoma:

(a) Liver
(b) Skin
(c) Brain
(d) Lung

Ans: (a) Liver

INTRAOCULAR MELANOMA

- Melanomas are the most common primary intraocular malignancy in adults
- Represent 5% of all melanomas
- Choroidal and ciliary body melanomas constitute about 95% of all uveal melanomas
- Uveal melanoma has a unique metastatic predilection for the liver
- Liver is involved in 71 to 94% of uveal melanoma patients with metastases and is the sole or initial site of metastases in more than 50% of these patients
- Hepatic metastases are recognized as a poor prognostic marker for response to treatment and survival
- Overall 1 year survival after the development of metastasis is only 13%, and median survival estimates range from 2 to 9 months

(Devita, 10th Edition, Page 1770)

273. Which of the following factors is not considered when considering patient for Genetic counseling for risk assessment of Familial Breast or Ovarian cancer?

(a) Breast cancer younger than 40 years age
(b) Family member with male breast cancer
(c) Bilateral breast cancer
(d) Low grade papillary serous carcinoma of Ovary

Ans: (d) Low grade papillary serous carcinoma of Ovary

Factors That Should be Considered When Considering Referring a Patient for Genetic Counseling for Risk Assessment of Familial Breast or Ovarian Cancer
• Breast Cancer at younger than 40
• Family member with a male breast cancer
• Premenopausal breast cancer and a first- or second-degree relative with breast or ovarian cancer or two relatives of any degree or age
• Breast cancer or ovarian cancer in a family of Ashkenazi Jewish heritage
• High-grade papillary serous carcinoma of the ovary, fallopian tube or primary peritoneal cancer at any age
• Two primary cancers of the breast or breast and ovary at any age
• A known mutation within the family
• Bilateral breast cancer

(Handbook of Gynecological Oncology)

274. Which of the following statements is not true?

(a) In hyperfractionation, dose per fraction is reduced
(b) In accelerated fractionation, Total dose is reduced
(c) In hypofractionation, dose per fraction is Increased
(d) In hyperfractionation, Total dose is reduced

Ans: (d) In hyperfractionation, Total dose is reduced

Types of fractionation	Characteristics	Rationale	Results
Hyperfractionation	Total dose: Same Dose per fraction: Reduced Number of fractions: Increased Overall time: same	Reduce dose per fraction reduces late effects Higher total dose increase tumor kill	Local control: Better Acute toxicity: Higher Late toxicity: Less
Accelerated fractionation	Total dose: Reduce Dose per fraction: Reduced/same Number of fractions: Same Overall time: Reduced	Reduced time reduces tumor repopulation Reduce dose per fraction reduces late effects	Local control: Better Acute toxicity: Higher Late toxicity: Less
Hypofractionation	Total dose: Reduced Dose per fraction: Increased Number of fractions: Reduced Overall time: Reduced	Reduced time Repopulation reduced	Local control: Less Acute toxicity: Less Late toxicity: Higher

(Perez and Brady, Principles of Radiotherapy, 4th Edition)

275. Which of the following is not a radiosensitizer?

(a) Metronidazole
(b) Cisplatin
(c) GM CSF
(d) Hydroxyurea

Ans: (c) GM CSF

Radiosensitizers	Radioprotectors
Metronidazole, misonidazole	Amifostine
Hyperbaric oxygen	Pentoxyphyline
Cisplatin	II-1
5 FU	GM-CSF
Gemcitabine hydroxyurea	

(Devita, 11th Edition, Page 427)

276. Which of the following is not a Contraindication to Radiotherapy in Gynecological cancers?

(a) Uterovaginal prolapse
(b) Severe Anemia
(c) Sepsis
(d) Diabetes

Ans: (d) Diabetes

Contraindications to Radiotherapy
• Severe anaemia • Poor general health • Sepsis • Pregnancy • Presence of fibroids in the uterus • Tubo-ovarian mass • Uterovaginal prolapsed • Presence of genital fistulae

(Perez and Brady, Principles of Radiotherapy, 4th Edition)

277. Which of the following is not included in High risk factors for Endometrial cancers?

(a) Late menopause
(b) Nulliparity
(c) Multiparity
(d) Obesity

Ans: (c) Multiparity

'High Risk' Factors for Endometrial Cancer
• Late menopause
• Nulliparity
• Unopposed estrogen therapy
• History of persistent anovulation (PCOS)
• History of irregular and excessive premenopausal bleeding
• Obesity, diabetes, hypertension
• Personal or family history of breast, ovary, colon or endometrial cancer
• Atypical endometrial hyperplasia (p. 331)
• Tamoxifen therapy
• Radiation menopause

(Handbook of Gynecological Oncology)

278. Which of the following is not a Tumor Associated Antigens?

(a) MUC1
(b) CEA
(c) BRCA 2
(d) HER 2/NEU

Ans: (c) BRCA 2

- **HER-2/NEU:** Transmembrane protein of HER family amplified in 20–30% ovarian cancers and breast cancer
- **Folate-Binding Protein:** FBP functions as a transmembrane transporter of folate expressed more than 80 times normal in ovarian malignancies
- **MUC-1:** High molecular weight glycoprotein expressed on membranes of glandular epithelial cancer cells including ovary, breast and gastrointestinal malignancies
- **CEA:** Over-expressed in more than 50% of ovarian mucinous carcinomas and about 15% in other ovarian malignancies
- **p53:** Tumor suppressor gene mutated in 30–50% of ovarian cancers
- **Sialyl–Tn:** Common in mucinous tumors and is extremely immunogenic

(Devita, 11th Edition, Page 461)

279. Which of the following is not true about Leiomyosaroma?

(a) More common in African Americans
(b) Median age at diagnosis is early 50s
(c) Usually present as stage IV disease
(d) Vascular invasion and extrauterine tumor spread are associated with worse prognosis

Ans: (c) Usually present as stage IV disease

LEIOMYOSARCOMA

- ***More common in African Americans***
- Usually present as stage I disease with abnormal bleeding or a pelvic mass
- Median age at diagnosis is Early 50s–**(Younger than other uterine sarcomas)**
- Vascular invasion and extrauterine tumor spread are associated with worse prognosis
- **Approximately 85% of women diagnosed with a leiomyosarcoma have clinical stage I or II disease**

(Handbook of Gynecological Oncology)

280. Short latency aggressive papillary carcinoma thyroid is associated with which of the 'following Oncogene?

(a) RET/PTC 1 (b) RET/PTC 2

(c) RET/PTC 3 (d) RET/PTC 4

Ans: (c) RET/PTC 3

- Short latency aggressive papillary cancer is associated with ret/PTC 3 oncogene and later developing, possibly less aggressive, cancers with RET/PTC 1

(Bailey and Love, 27th Edition, Page 816)

281. Syndromes associated with hereditary breast cancer are all *except:*

(a) Li-Fraumeni syndrome (b) Peutz-Jeghers syndrome

(c) Cowden disease (d) Cronkhite Canada syndrome

Ans: (d) Cronkhite Canada syndrome

Incidence of sporadic, familial and hereditary breast cancer	
Sporadic breast cancer	65%-75%
Familial breast cancer	20%-30%
Hereditary breast cancer	5%-10%
• ***BRCA1***	45%
• ***BRCA2***	35%
• **p53** (Li-Fraumeni syndrome)	1%
• **STK11/LKB1** (Peutz-Jeghers syndrome)	<1%
• **PTEN** (Cowden disease)	<1%
• **MSH2/MLH1** (Muir-Torre syndrome)	<1%
• **ATM** (Ataxia-telangiectasia)	<1%
• **Unknown**	20%

(Schwartz, 10th Edition, Page 514)

282. Which of the following is not an Ectodermal manifestations of FAP?

(a) Desmoid tumor (b) Pilomatrixoma

(c) CHRPE (d) Epidermoid cyst

Ans: (a) Desmoid tumor

Extracolonic manifestations of FAP
Endodermal derivatives
• Adenomas and carcinomas of duodenum, stomach, small intestine, thyroid and biliary tree
• Fundic gland polyps
• Hepatoblastoma
Ectodermal derivatives
• Epidermoid cysts
• Pilomatrixoma
• Congenital hypertrophy of the retinal pigment epithelium (CHRPE)
• Brain tumors
Mesodermal derivatives
• Desmoid tumors
• Osteomas
• Dental problems

(Bailey and Love, 27th Edition, Page 1260)

283. According to Hayflick hypothesis maximum no. of divisions for normal human cells is:

(a) 10-20 (b) 20-40

(c) 40-60 (d) 60-80

Ans: (c) 40-60

- According to the Hayflick hypothesis, normal cells are permitted to undergo only a finite number of divisions.
- For humans this number is between 40 and 60

(Bailey and Love, 27th Edition, Page 140)

284. A tumor of 1cm diameter will contain ....cells.

(a) 10^3 (b) 10^6

(c) 10^9 (d) 10^{12}

Ans: (c) 10^9

- A tumor 10 mm in diameter will contain about 10^9 cells
- Since $2^{30} = 10^9$ this implies that it would take 30 generations to reach the threshold of clinical detectability and as $2^{45} = 3 \times 10^{13}$, it will take fewer than 15 subsequent generations to produce a tumor that, through sheer bulk alone, would be fatal

(Bailey and Love, 27th Edition, Page 142)

285. Indications for Post op Radiotherapy in Head and Neck cancer include all *except:*

(a) Close or +ve margins (b) Extracapsular extension

(c) N2a or greater cervical node (d) T1 or T2 tumor

Ans: (d) T1 or T2 tumor

INDICATIONS FOR POSTOPERATIVE RT

- Close (<5 mm) or positive margins
- ECE
- N2a or greater cervical node classification
- Invasion of the soft tissues of the neck
- Lymph-vascular invasion
- PNI
- T3 or T4 tumor classification
- >5 mm of subglottic invasion

(Devita, 10th Edition, Page 430)

286. Renal cell carcinoma with poor prognosis is:

(a) Clear cell carcinoma (b) Papillary carcinoma

(c) Chromophobe carcinoma (d) Collecting duct carcinoma

Ans: (a) Clear cell carcinoma

- Clear cell carcinoma has worse prognosis than papillary or chromophobe RCC

(Bailey and Love, 27th Edition, Page 1417)

287. Strongest predisposing factor for Basal cell carcinoma is:

(a) Ionizing radiation (b) UV radiation

(c) Genetic skin cancer syndromes (d) Arsenical compounds

Ans: (b) UV radiation

BASAL CELL CARCINOMA

- Longest predisposing factor to BCC is UVR
- Occurs in the elderly or the middle-aged after excessive sun exposure, with 95% occurring between the ages of 40 and 80 years
- Incidence of BCC rises with proximity to the equator, although 33% arise in parts of the body not usually sunexposed
- Other predisposing factors include exposure to arsenical compounds, coal tar, aromatic hydrocarbons, ionising radiation and genetic skin cancer syndromes
- White skinned people are almost exclusively affected
- BCC is more common in men than women

(Bailey and Love, 27th Edition, Page 604)

288. What percentage of cases have metastasis in Cutaneous Squamous cell carcinoma?

(a) 2% (b) 10%

(c) 50% (d) 80%

Ans: (a) 2%

SQUAMOUS CELL CARCINOMA

- Associated with ultraviolet radiation, chronic inflammation and chemical carcinogens
- High- and low-risk squamous cell carcinoma
- Metastasis in 2% cases

(Bailey and Love, 27th Edition, Page 606)

289. All are true about Carcinoma Breast in pregnancy *except:*

(a) Radiotherapy is avoided (b) Chemotherapy is avoided in 1st trimester

(c) Most tumors are Hormone receptor +ve (d) All the above are true

Ans: (c) Most tumors are Hormone receptor +ve

TREATMENT IS SIMILAR WITH SOME PROVISOS

- Radiotherapy should be avoided during pregnancy, making mastectomy a more frequent option than breast conservation surgery
- Chemotherapy should be avoided during the first trimester but appears safe subsequently

Most tumours are hormone receptor negative and so hormone treatment, which is potentially teratogenic, is not required

- Becoming pregnant subsequent to a diagnosis of breast cancer appears not to alter the likely outcome, but women are usually advised to wait at least 2 years as it is within this time that recurrence most often occurs
- Risk of developing breast cancer with oral contraceptive use is only slight, and disappears 10 years after stopping the oral contraceptive pill

(Bailey and Love, 27th Edition, Page 881)

290. Tumor size over which size should be considered to have metastatic potential in GIST?

(a) 3 cm (b) 5 cm

(c) 7 cm (d) 10 cm

Ans: (b) 5 cm

- Tumors over 5 cm in diameter should be considered to have metastatic potential
- If easily resectable, surgery is the primary mode of treatment

(Bailey and Love, 27th Edition, Page 1140)

291. Which of the following is incorrect about APBI (Accelerated partial breast irradiation)?

(a) APBI is delivered in an abbreviated fashion and lower total dose than standard course of whole breast radiation
(b) Suitable patients include women of 60 or more
(c) Suitable patients include those with tumor margins 2 mm or greater
(d) Suitable patients include those with multifocal disease

Ans: (d) Suitable patients include those with multifocal disease

- APBI is delivered in an abbreviated fashion (twice daily for 5 days) and at a lower total dose compared with the standard course of 5 to 6 weeks of radiation (50 Gray with or without a boost) in the case of whole breast irradiation
- ASTRO guidelines describe patients "suitable" for APBI to include women 60 years of age or older with a unifocal, T1, ER-positive tumor with no lymphovascular invasion, and margins of at least 2 mm

(Schwartz, 10th Edition, Page 539)

292. A 25-year-old male presented with painless testicular swelling and with history of fever and weight loss. All the following investigations are indicated in this patient *except:*

(a) USG scrotum
(b) CT abdomen and pelvis
(c) Chest X-ray
(d) Transscrotal biopsy

Ans: (d) Transscrotal biopsy

- Painless testicular swelling in a 25-year-male with history of fever and weight loss amounts to a diagnosis of Malignant Testicular swelling, i.e., Testicular cancer
- Diagnosis of testicular cancer includes history and physical examination of the both testes, abdomen examination to rule out para aortic nodes
- Radiological imaging in the form of ultrasonogram will have a better accuracy in identifying the tumor in both the testes
- To confirm the histopathological evidence of testicular cancer, Orchidectomy in form of High inguinal Orchidectomy to be done after a Maneuver known as CHEVASU Maneuver
- ***Transscrotal biopsy is contraindicated*, as Tunica albuginea will be breached during biopsy***
- Since Tunica albuginea is a natural barrier to testicular cancer, following biopsy, this will be breached and extend into the scrotum
- Before orchidectomy, Serum tumor markers specific for testicular cancers like AFP, LDH and Beta HCG to be quantified
- If tumor markers are elevated, metastatic work up to be done, to rule out lung metastases and liver metastases and nodal metastases
- Chest X-ray PA view can pick up cannon ball metastases, if in doubt CT scan of the abdomen and pelvis and Thorax to be done

(Bailey and Love, 27th Edition, Page 1507)

293. Carcinoma breast is diagnosed in 2nd trimester of pregnancy. Which should not be done?

(a) Breast conservation surgery/BCS
(b) Chemotherapy
(c) Modified radical mastectomy
(d) 30 focal radiotherapy to local area

Ans: (d) 30 focal radiotherapy to local area

- Pregnant women with breast cancer often present at later stage of disease because breast tissue changes that occur in hormone-rich environment of pregnancy obscure early cancers
- However, they have a prognosis, stage by stage, that is similar to that of nonpregnant women with breast cancer
- Ultrasonography and needle biopsy specimens are used in the diagnosis of these nodules
- Mammography is rarely indicated because of its decreased sensitivity during pregnancy and lactation; however, the fetus can be shielded if mammography is needed

- Breast surgery can be safely performed in all trimesters of pregnancy; however, patients and surgeons may choose to wait until after the 12th week of gestation when the risk of spontaneous abortion may be lower
- A modified radical mastectomy can be performed during the first and second trimesters of pregnancy
- During the third trimester, lumpectomy with axillary node dissection can be considered if adjuvant radiation therapy is deferred until after delivery
- Lactation is suppressed
- Chemotherapy administered during the first trimester carries a risk of spontaneous abortion and a 12% risk of birth defects
- There is no evidence of teratogenicity resulting from administration of chemotherapeutic agents in the second and third trimesters
- For this reason, many clinicians now consider the optimal strategy to be delivery of chemotherapy in second and third trimesters as a neoadjuvant approach, which allows local therapy decisions to be made after the delivery of the baby
- If the patient meets criteria for post mastectomy radiation therapy or they have had breast-conserving surgery, radiation therapy should be administered and this is recommended only after delivery of fetus
- Radiation exposure during pregnancy may result in fetal death, malformations, growth and/or mental impairment, and induction of cancers or hereditary defects

(Schwartz, 10th Edition, Page 554)

294. A patient is diagnosed with Liposarcoma of 8 × 6 × 4 cm involving the posterior part of thigh. Treatment of choice in this patient is:

(a) Above thigh amputation
(b) Extra compartmental excision
(c) Chemotherapy
(d) Wide local excision

Ans: (d) Wide local excision

- Among soft tissue sarcoma, the most common site is Extremity sarcoma*, among extremities, the most common site being Thigh
- Most common histological variant of STS is Liposarcoma* (previously MFH, i.e., Malignant fibrous Histiocytoma which has been reclassified as High grade undifferentiated pleomorphic sarcoma)
- Nowadays, the treatment goal is to do function sparing resection of the tumors and not amputation

PRINCIPLES OF SURGERY

- Wide Local Excision is to remove the tumor with approximately 1 to 2 cm of surrounding normal soft tissue outside the Pseudocapsule (Zone of compressed reactive tissue that surrounds the soft tissue sarcoma)
- Tumor adjacent to or displacing major neurovascular structures, these need not be resected, but adventitia or perineurium should be removed
- In cases of Bony invasion, Bone resection is required to obtain an adequate surgical margin and to achieve adequate local control
- For locally advanced tumors, repair of bone defects, vascular reconstruction, tendon transfers and soft tissue reconstruction using regional or free flaps have resulted in good functional outcomes
- All patients undergoing resection for extremity sarcomas should undergo physical therapy beginning immediately after surgery and continuing until maximum function is achieved
- **Amputation (In 5% of tumors):**

  Tumors that cannot be completely resected by any other means

  Without evidence of metastatic disease

  Have propensity for good long term functional rehabilitation

(Sabiston, 20th Edition, Page 763)

295. A 45 years old male having multiple sexual partners presents with lesion in the anus. Biopsy reveals early stage of squamous cell carcinoma of anus. Correct management for this patient is:

(a) Wide local excision
(b) APR
(c) Chemoradiation nigro regimen
(d) Antiviral therapy

Ans: (c) Chemoradiation nigro regimen

- Historically, treatment consisted of surgery alone or radiation therapy alone
- Epithelial or subepithelial tumors were locally excised, and more advanced lesions underwent APR
- Introduction of multimodality therapy combining chemotherapy and radiation therapy promised to preserve continence, to avoid colostomy, and to offer similar or improved survival
- Nigro was the first to promote radiation therapy with chemotherapy as definitive treatment for squamous cell cancers of the anal canal
- Current protocol includes infusional 5-FU with mitomycin C and external beam radiation to pelvis with a minimum dose of 45 Gy. The inguinal nodes, pelvis, anus and perineum should be included in the radiation fields
- Patients with advanced and residual disease after 45 Gy, or node-positive disease are usually treated with an additional 9 to 14 Gy for a total dose of 54 to 59 Gy

(Sabiston 20th Edition, Page 1414)

296. A 47-year-old patient presents with a slowly enlarging right parotid mass. You are suspicious for neoplastic process and perform an FNAC. Which of the following is true about parotid neoplasms?

(a) Approximately 75%–80% of parotid gland tumors are malignant
(b) Most common parotid tumor is mucoepidermoid carcinoma
(c) Pleomorphic adenoma is seen bilaterally in 50% of patients
(d) Smoking is an etiologic risk factor for Warthin's tumor

Ans: (d) Smoking is an etiologic risk factor for Warthin's tumor

- Around 75%–80% of parotid tumors are benign
- Most common parotid tumor is pleomorphic adenoma
- Warthin's tumor, not pleomorphic adenoma, is seen bilaterally in 12% of patients with a Warthin's tumor
- A surgical biopsy is not recommended due to a high risk of recurrence
- Warthin's tumor is second most common benign salivary gland tumor and is associated with smoking as a risk factor
- About 70% of salivary gland tumors occur in parotid gland, of which 75%–80% are benign
- Most common benign parotid tumor is pleomorphic adenoma followed next in incidence by **Warthin's tumor,** which is associated with smoking and an increased rate of being found bilaterally (12%)

(Sabiston, 20th Edition, Page 807)

297. Which of the following abnormalities is both paraneoplastic syndrome associated with HCC and may also be caused by end-stage liver failure?

(a) Hypoglycemia
(b) Erythrocytosis
(c) Hypercalcemia
(d) Hypercholesterolemia

Ans: (a) Hypoglycemia

- Most of paraneoplastic syndromes are biochemical abnormalities without associated clinical consequences
- Most important ones include hypoglycemia (caused by end-stage liver failure), erythrocytosis, hypercalcemia, hypercholesterolemia, dysfibrinogenemia, carcinoid syndrome, increased thyroxin-binding globulin, sexual changes (gynecomastia, testicular atrophy, and precocious puberty), and porphyria cutanea tarda
- Pathogenesis of hypoglycemia is unclear but may be related to production of insulin-like growth factor I by the tumor

(Sabiston, 20th Edition, Page 1459)

298. Seed soil theory is given by:

(a) Ehrlich (b) Kocher

(c) Paget (d) Halsted

Ans: (c) Paget

- Paget pointed that there is a crucial relationship here between seed (tumor cell) and soil (distant tissue)
- Paget observed in 1889 that breast carcinoma often metastasized to the liver, lungs, bone, adrenals, or brain
- He hypothesized that tumor cells (the "seed") would grow only in selective environments (the "soil"), where conditions supported tumor growth, hence so-called seed-and-soil hypothesis

(Sabiston, 20th Edition, Page 685)

299. Which of the following Anticancer drug causes Hemolytic uremic syndrome?

(a) Cyclophosphamide (b) Mitomycin C

(c) Cisplatin (d) Hydroxyurea

Ans: (b) Mitomycin C

In Patients with Cancer, HUS Occurs as:

- Manifestation of the cancer itself
- Complication of chemotherapy–Mitomycin C
- Setting of bone marrow transplantation
- More recently as a problem in patients receiving antibodies and immunotoxins

(Devita, 10th Edition, Page 1830)

300. Death in esophageal cancer usually occurs due to:

(a) Metastasis (b) Cardiac complications

(c) Anastomotic leak (d) Tracheoesophageal fistula

Ans: (a) Metastasis

- Cause of death from esophageal cancer is mainly due to metastatic disease

(Sabiston, 20th Edition, Page 1037)

301. WDHA syndrome seen in:

(a) Insulinoma (b) VIPoma

(c) Gastrinoma (d) GLucagonoma

Ans: (b) VIPoma

- VIP is a small peptide normally found in the brain, G cells of the antrum, adrenal medulla, gut mucosa, pancreatic neurons, and D2 cells of the pancreas
- First described by Verner and Morrison in 1958, VIP omas usually arise from pancreatic islet D2 cells and release high levels of VIP
- This syndrome is also known as WDHA (watery diarrhea, hypokalemia, achlorhydria) syndrome or pancreatic cholera
- **VIPomas** are the cause of the classic Verner-Morrison syndrome. These endocrine tumors secrete vasoactive intestinal peptide, which can cause watery diarrhea, hypokalemia and achlorhydria

(Sabiston, 20th Edition, Page 956; Devita, 10th Edition, Page 1178)

302. Which of the following is not considered a high risk condition for Oral cavity Cancer?

(a) Erythroplakia
(b) Speckled Erythroplakia
(c) Discoid lupus erythematosus
(d) Chronic hyperplastic candidiasis

Ans: (c) Discoid lupus erythematosus

Conditions Associated with Malignant Transformation		
High risk lesions	**Intermediate risk**	**Low/equivocal**
Erythroplakia	Oral submucous fibrosis	Oral lichen planus
Speckled leukoplakia	Syphillitic glossitis	DLE
Chronic hyperplastic candidiasis	Sideropenic dysphagia	Discoid keratosis congenita

(Bailey and Love, 27th Edition, Page 707)

PART FIVE: RECENT MODEL PAPERS

CHAPTER

65 MULTIPLE CHOICE QUESTIONS

PAPER 1 (SET 1)

1. **Abscopal effect of radiation is:**

(a) Cytokine mediated systemic immune response
(b) Adaptive immunity
(c) Tumor killing within radiation field
(d) More seen in hyperfractionated therapy

Ans: (a) Cytokine mediated systemic immune response

Explanation

The abscopal effects of radiation (i.e., tumor cell killing outside of the radiation field) have been attributed to the activation of antigen and cytokine release by radiation, which subsequently activates a systemic immune response against tumor cells. This response begins with the transfer of tumor cell antigens to dendritic cells and, subsequently, the activation of tumor-specific T cells and immunogenic tumor cell death. It is likely that radiation dose and fractionation influence the optimal immune response with higher doses and fewer fractions of radiation than those used in conventional fractionation schemes appearing superior in experimental models. Unfortunately, abscopal effects are uncommon because immune system evasion is an inherent characteristic of cancer cells that often dominates, even in the presence of a radiation-induced immune response

(Devita, 11th Edition, Page 427)

2. **Death of non-irradiated cells outside radiation field is:**

(a) Stuart Treves syndrome
(b) Abscopal effect
(c) Delayed hypersensitivity
(d) None of the above

Ans: (b) Abscopal effect

Explanation

As described earlier radiation induced abscopal effect–cytokine mediated immune response leads to death of tumor cells outside the radiation field

Like cisplatin, temozolomide-mediated radiosensitization does not seem to require cell cycle redistribution

Cisplatin is likely the most commonly used chemotherapeutic agent in combination with radiation. Although cisplatin was the prototype for several other platinum analogs, carboplatin is also frequently used in combination with radiation. Cisplatin, in combination with radiation and sometimes in conjunction with a second chemotherapeutic agent, is indicated for cancers of the head and neck, esophagus (with 5-fluorouracil), lung, cervix and anus

Radiosensitization by cisplatin is related to its ability to cause inter- and intrastrand DNA crosslinks. Removal of these cross-links during the repair process results in DNA strand breaks. Although there are multiple theories to explain the mechanism(s) of radiosensitization by cisplatin, two plausible explanations are that cisplatin inhibits the repair (both HRR and NHEJ) of radiation-induced DNA double-strand breaks and/or increases the number of lethal radiation induced double-strand breaks

Temozolomide in combination with radiation is standard therapy for glioblastoma. Temozolomide is an alkylating agent that forms methyl adducts at the O6 position of guanine (as well as at N7-and N3-guanine) that are subsequently improperly repaired by the mismatch repair pathway. Radiosensitization by temozolomide involves the inhibition of DNA repair and/or an increase in radiation-induced DNA double-strand breaks due to radiation-induced single-strand breaks in proximity to O6 methyl adducts

Antimetabolities–Being an analog of uracil, 5-fluorouracil is misincorporated into RNA and DNA. However, the ability of 5-fluorouracil to radiosensitize is related to its ability to inhibit thymidylate synthase, which leads to the depletion of thymidine triphosphate (dTTP) and the inhibition of DNA synthesis. This slowed, inappropriate progression through S phase in response to 5-fluorouracil is thought to be the mechanism underlying radiosensitization. Similar to 5-fluorouracil, the oral thymidylate synthase inhibitor capecitabine is also being increasingly used in combination with radiation

In addition, poly (ADP-ribose) polymerase (PARP) inhibitors have been demonstrated to preclinically induce radiosensitization, and several clinical trials combining PARP inhibitors with radiation therapy are underway

In contrast to the taxanes, the vinca alkaloids depolymerize microtubules and destroy mitotic spindles–it acts in M phase

The taxanes, paclitaxel and docetaxel, act to stabilize microtubules resulting in the accumulation of cells in G2/M, the most radiation-sensitive phase of the cell cycle. The radiosensitizing properties of the taxanes are thought to be attributable to the redistribution of cells into G2/M. Platinums and temozolamide need are not cell cycle specific they can act in any phase of cell cycle

(Devita, 11th Edition, Page 427)

3. **Incorrect match regarding site of action is:**

(a) Antimetabolites–early S phase

(b) Platinum and temozolamide–S phase

(c) Vinca alkaloids–M phase

(d) Taxanes–G2M phase

Ans: (b) Platinum and temozolamide–S phase

4. **Incorrect match is:**

(a) Photoelectric effect–diagnostic X-rays

(b) Compton effect–therapeutic X-rays

(c) Treatment isocentre–centre of radiation field

(d) Therapeutic–Bremstraullung X-rays

Ans: (c) Treatment isocentre–centre of radiation field

Explanation

As previously mentioned, effective external-beam photon treatments require higher energy beams capable of reaching deep-seated tumors with suficient fluence to make it likely that the dose deposition will kill tumor cells. To spare normal tissues and maximize targeting, beams are arranged to enter the patient from several directions and to intersect at the center of the tumor (treatment isocenter). Although machines containing collimated beams from high-intensity radioactive sources (primarily cobalt 60 [60Co]) are still in use, today's modern treatment machine accelerates electrons to high (megaelectron volt) energy and impinges them onto an X-ray production target, leading to the generation of intense beams of Bremsstrahlung X-rays. A typical photon beam treatment machine consists of a high-energy (6 to 20 MeV) linear electron accelerator, electromagnetic beam steering and monitoring systems, X-ray generation targets, high-density treatment field-shaping devices (collimators) and up to a ton of radiation shielding on a mechanical C-arm gantry that can rotate precisely around a treatment couch. These treatment delivery machines routinely maintain mechanical isocenters for patient treatments to within a sphere of 1 mm radius

As mentioned earlier, ionizing radiation kills cells via both direct and indirect mechanisms

Radiation therapy aims to instigate those ionizations and events in the tumor cells. Photons are massless, uncharged packets of energy that primarily interact with matter via electromagnetic processes. As a consequence of those interactions, an incident photon can become either entirely absorbed (giving up its energy to the ejection of an atomic electron [photoelectric effect]), create an energetic electron-positron pair (pair production), or scatter off an electron with reduction in energy and change in direction and subsequent transfer of parts of its energy *to the free electron (Compton scattering).* The secondary electrons generated as a Consequence of these interactions have residual energy, mass and most important, electric charge

Treatment beams intersect at the centre of tumor called as isocenter and not exactly means, the centre of radiation field

(Devita, 11th Edition, Page 427)

5. **False regarding IMRT:**

(a) Multiple small beams (beamlets)
(b) Intensity controlled
(c) Very less degree of freedom
(d) Useful for ca prostate treatment

Ans: (c) Very less degree of freedom

Explanation

Automation allows precise reshaping of the treatment beam for each angle of incidence, allowing not only conformation of irradiation to target volumes but also modulation of the beam intensity patterns via reconfiguration of the MLC across the fixed field (intensity modulated radiation therapy [IMRT]) or continuously as the gantry rotates about the patient (volumetric modulated arc therapy [VMAT]

The same control allows the selection and use of many differing beam angles to build up dose at the tumor location

In IMRT, as most often applied, each treatment beam portal is broken down into simple basic components called beamlets, typically 0.5 × 1 cm to 1 × 1 cm in size, evenly distributed on a grid over the cross-section of each beam. Optimization begins with precomputation of the relative dose contribution that each of these beamlets gives to every subportion of tumor and normal tissue that the beamlet traverses as it goes through the patient model. Sophisticated optimization engines and search routines then iteratively alter the relative intensities of each beamlet in all the beams to minimize a cost function associated with target and normal tissue treatment goals. These often hundreds of beamlets (each with its own intensity) provide the necessary flexibility and degrees of freedom to create dose distributions that can preferentially irradiate subportions of targets and also produce sharp dose gradients to avoid nearby organs at risk

(Devita, 11th Edition, Page 440)

6. **In radiotherapy:**

(a) Patient immobilized by meshes and foam moulds
(b) Patient immobilized by sedation
(c) Tumor localization done by laser and tattooing
(d) All of the above

Ans: (a) Patient immobilized by meshes and foam moulds

Explanation

To take advantage of the precision of modern beam delivery, it is crucial to localize the patient's tumor and normal tissue. This process can be divided into patient immobilization (i.e., limiting the motion of the patient) and localization (i.e., knowing the tumor and normal tissue location precisely in space). Although these concepts of immobilization and localization are related, they are not identical. Patients can be held reasonably comfortably in their treatment pose with the aid of foam molds and meshes (immobilization devices). Traditionally, localization has been achieved by indexing the immobilization device to the computer-controlled treatment couch and/or by positioning the patient using low-power laser alignment beams that intersect at the treatment machine isocenter

(Devita, 11th Edition, Page 434)

7. **Regarding 'kerma' and 'dose', which of the options of the following are correct?**

(a) Energy released at a point is kerma
(b) Energy absorbed at a point is dose
(c) Energy absorbed per unit mass is Gray
(d) Energy released per unit mass is kerma

Ans: (a) Energy released at a point is kerma

Explanation

Dose "deposition" is a two-step process of photon interaction (proportional to the local fluence of photons) and energy transfer to the medium via the slowing down of secondary electrons. Thus, the point where a photon interacts is not the place where the dose is actually deposited, which happens over the track of the secondary electron. Dose has a very strict definition of energy "absorbed" per unit mass (i.e., due to the slowing down charged particles) and should be distinguished from the energy released at a point, defined as kerma (e.g., energy transfer from the scattering incident photon)

(Devita, 11th Edition, Page 436)

8. **Mammosite is:**

(a) Balloon brachytherapy (b) Breast implant

(c) Radioactive element used in RT (d) All of the above

Ans: (a) Balloon brachytherapy

Explanation

APBI is an approach that treats only the lumpectomy bed plus a 1-2 cm margin, rather than the whole breast. By increasing the radiation fraction size and decreasing the target volume, this technique allows the treatment to be accomplished in a shorter period. APBI is generally defined as radiation therapy that uses daily fraction. Doses greater than 2 Gy delivered in less than 5 weeks. There are a number of approaches now available for the implementation of APBI, these include: multi-catheter interstitial brachytherapy, balloon catheter brachytherapy, 3D-CRT (conformal radiation therapy) and intra-operative radiation therapy (IORT) research and development

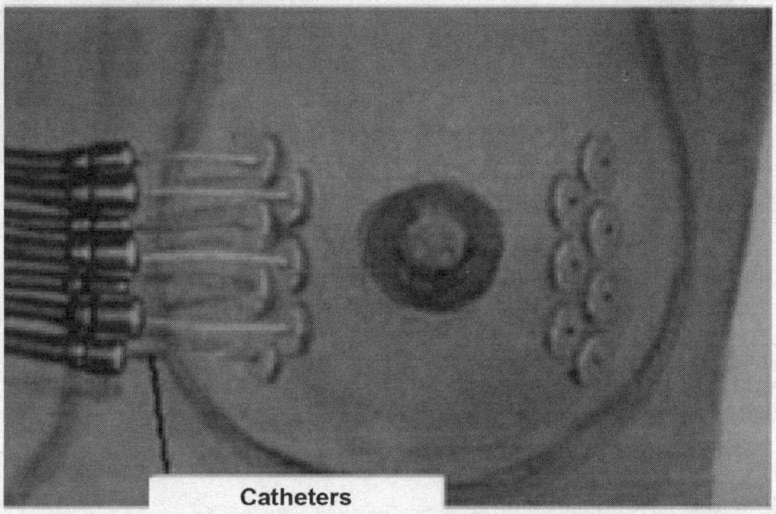

Figure 1: Diagrammatic illustration of multi-catheter interstitial brachytherapy

MAMMO SITE

Although MIB has had very encouraging results, the technical challenges limit its widespred application. The MammoSite* brachytherapy (MSB) system (Hologic, Marlborough, MA) applicator was developed to be more reproducible, easily applied and better tolerated. The mammosite catheter consists of a silicone ballon connected to a 15 cm double-lumen catherter (Figure 2) that is 6 mm in diameter. The catheter has both a small inflation channel and a channel for the passage of an Ir-192 high dose rate (HDR) brachytherapy source. The source channel runs centrally through the length of the balloon. The ballon is inflated with saline solution mixed with a small amount of contrast material to aid visualization. The ballon is inflated to a size that would completely fill the lumpectomy cavity and ensures conformance of the tissue to the balloon. An Ir-192 radioactive source, connected to a computer-cotrolled HDR remote after-loader, is inserted through the catheter into the balloon to deliver the prescription radiation dose

The MammoSite applicator can be placed into the lumpectomy cavity at the time of surgery or in separate procedure after surgery. In the latter case, the applicator can be inserted under ultrasound guidance either through the lumpectomy scar or via small separate incision. Following placement, a computed tomography (CT) scan is performed to assess the quality of the implant and for use in radiation planning. Implant quality is determined by examination of three parameters: balloon conformance to the lumpectomy cavity, distance from the surface of the balloon to the skin surface, and the symmetry of the balloon in relationship to the central catheter. Treatment planning parameters are: the diameter of the inflated balloon, the planning target volume, and the dose distribution. While a minimum balloon-to-skin distance of 5 mm is required, a threshold of at least 7 mm is strongly recommended. A longer skin distance is associated with greater improvement in cosmesis. Conformance of the balloon to the lumpectomy cavity is assessed by quantifying the volume of the planning target volume (PTV) that is filled by air or seroma fluid. Adequate conformance is considered to have been achieved when less than 10% of the PTV is composed of fluid or air. A symmetric implant in relation to the source channel is also essential for adequate dosimetry. A non-symmetrical implant can result in dose inhomogeneity in the surrounding tissues since the MSB device contains a single, central source channel that does not allow for shaping of the radiation isodose curves in the direction perpendicular to the central channel. The MSB may not be suitable in patients with small breast or for tumors located in the upper-inner quadrant because of the requirement for skin-to-cavity distances. Recently, Hologic has introduced a MammoSite Multi-lumen (4 lumen) device with the potential to eliminate some of the drawbacks of the single lumen device

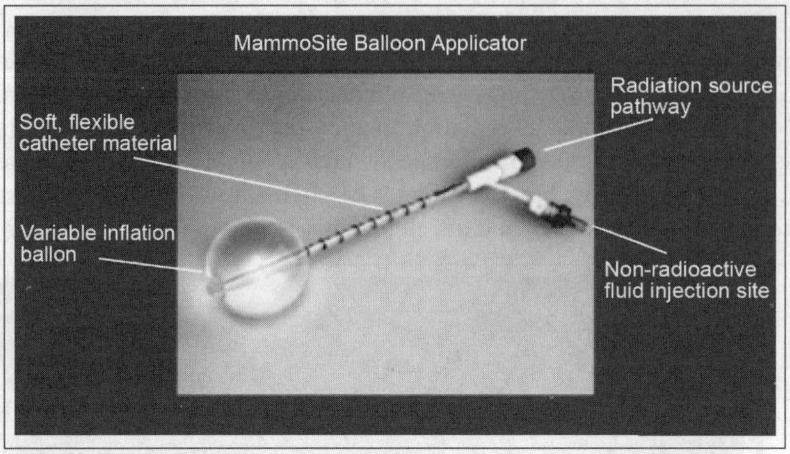

Figure 2: The MammoSite Balloon applicator (courtesy of Hologic, Marlborough)

9. **Incorrect match regarding clinical application:**

(a) Photons–IMRT
(b) Protons–head and neck tumors
(c) Protons–pediatric cancer
(d) Carbon ions–head and neck

Ans: (d) Carbon ions–head and neck

Explanation

Also true is Neutrons–refractory parotid carcinoma

Brachytherapy–prostate

Charged particles, including protons and carbon ions, are being investigated for treatment of HCC. Another high linear energy transfer method used to treat unresectable soft tissue sarcoma is carbon ion radiotherapy. Although currently available only in Europe and Asia, carbon ion radiotherapy brings together neutrons' advantage of high linear energy transfer with the capability of modulating the range of radiation in tissue available with protons

Carbon ions are used as a salvage after photon radiotherapy for recurrence of head and neck cancers and not primarily. Carbon ions are mainly used in unresectable sarcomas and hepatocellular carcinoma

(Devita, 11th Edition, Page 2525)

10. **Elotuzumab is a monoclonal antibody used in multiple myeloma which targets:**

(a) CD38
(b) SLAMF7
(c) Complement C5
(d) IL–6

Ans: (b) SLAMF7

11. **Shrinking field technique involves:**

(a) 50 Gy + 20 Gy additional boost to tumor
(b) 50 Gy + 20 Gy boost to surrounding field
(c) 20 Gy + 50 Gy boost to tumor
(d) 20 Gy + 50 Gy boost to surrounding field

Ans: (a) 50 Gy + 20 Gy additional boost to tumor

Explanation

It is common during the course of radiation to give higher doses of radiation to regions that have a higher tumor burden. For example, regions that are suspected of harboring occult disease may be targeted to receive (in once-daily 2-Gy fractions) 54

Gy, whereas, to control the gross tumor, the goal may be to administer a total dose of 70 Gy. Because the gross tumor will invariably reside within the region at risk for occult disease, it has become standard practice to deliver 50 Gy to the entire region and then an additional boost dose of 20 Gy to the tumor. This sequence is called the shrinking field technique

(Devita, 11th Edition, Page 445)

12. False regarding Stereotactic radiotherapy:

(a) 8 crossfiring beams
(b) >90% tumor control of 4-5 cm tumor
(c) Can be used for oligomets in lung and liver
(d) None of the above

Ans: (d) None of the above

Explanation

SBRT (sometimes called stereotactic ablative radiation [SABR]) is a particular form of external beam radiation that is in widespread use and is continuing to increase. SBRT uses many (typically more than eight) cross-firing beams and provides an improved method of curing early-stage lung cancer and hepatocellular cancer. This approach uses precise localization and image guidance to deliver a small number (less than five) of high doses of radiation, with the concept of ablating the tumor, rather than using fractionation to achieve a therapeutic index (see the section "Fractionation"). SBRT can provide long-term, local control rates of >90% for tumors less than 4 to 5 cm with minimal side effects

(Devita, 11th Edition, Page 444)

13. RT can be used in all *except:*

(a) Palliative
(b) Adjuvant
(c) Organ preservation
(d) Cure of multiple metastasis

Ans: (d) Cure of multiple metastasis

Explanation

Radiation can be used in all the above options which are clearly documented and also useful for cure for oligomets

(Devita, 11th Edition, Page 445)

14. Single fraction RT for bone pain in metastasis is:

(a) 4 Gy
(b) 8 Gy
(c) 2 Gy
(d) 1 Gy

Ans: (b) 8 Gy

Explanation

A single 8 Gy fraction is highly effective for many patients with bone pain from a metastatic lesion

15. Conventional RT dose per fraction is:

(a) 1.5–5.5 Gy
(b) 3.5–6.5 Gy
(c) 1.8–2.2 Gy
(d) 2.8–3.2 Gy

Ans: (c) 1.8- 2.2 Gy

Explanation

Two crucial features that influence the effectiveness of a physical dose of radiation are the dose given in each radiation treatment (i.e., the fraction) and the total amount of time required to complete the course of radiation. Standard fractionation for radiation therapy is defined as the delivery of one treatment of 1.8 to 2.25 Gy per day. This approach produces a fairly well-understood chance of tumor control and risk of normal tissue damage (as a function of volume). By altering the fractionation schemes, one may be able to improve the outcome for patients undergoing curative treatment or to simplify the treatment for patients receiving palliative therapy

(Devita, 11th Edition, Page 447)

16. **Incorrect match is:**

(a) Accelerated fractionation–duration of therapy reduced

(b) Hyperfractionation–increased acute toxicity and same late toxicity

(c) Hypofractionation–palliative

(d) Hyperfractionation–more late toxicity and same acute toxicity

Ans: (d) Hyperfractionation–more late toxicity and same acute toxicity

Explanation

Two forms of altered fractionation have been tested for patients undergoing curative treatment: accelerated fractionation and hyperfractionation. Accelerated fractionation emerged from analyses of the control of head and neck cancer as a function of dose administered and total treatment time. It was found not only that with an increasing dose, there was increasing local control but also that protraction of treatment was associated with a loss of local control that was equivalent to about 0.75 Gy per day. The data were best modeled by assuming that, approximately 2 weeks into treatment, tumor cells began to proliferate more rapidly than they were proliferating early in treatment (called accelerated repopulation). In accelerated fractionation, the goal is to complete radiation before the accelerated tumor cell proliferation occurs. The second approach to altering fractionation is called hyperfractionation. Hyperfractionation is defined as the use of more than one fraction per day separated by more than 6 hours (see the section titled "Biologic Aspects of Radiation Oncology"), with a dose per fraction that is less than standard. Hyperfractionation is expected to increase the acute toxicity (which resolves) and tumor response, while not increasing the (dose-limiting) late toxicity, which can improve cure rate. Both accelerated fractionation and hyperfractionation were superior, in a meta-analysis, to standard fractionation in the treatment of head and neck cancer with radiation alone. However, recent trials suggest that hyperfractionation combined with chemotherapy does not increase tumor control or survival compared to standard chemoradiation but does increase toxicity; therefore, the use of altered fractionation schemes has decreased dramatically over the past few years. Hypofractionation refers to the administration of a smaller number of larger fractions than is standard. Hypofractionation might be expected to cause more late toxicity for the same anti-tumor effect than standard fractionation or hyperfractionation

(Devita, 11th Edition, Page 447)

17. **False regarding acute radiotoxicity is:**

(a) Nausea and fatigue may be due to abscopal effect

(b) Acute effects stop after 1–2 weeks of RT

(c) Affects non-dividing cells

(d) None of the above

Ans: (c) Affects non-dividing cells

Explanation

Adverse effects from radiation can be divided into acute, subacute, and chronic (or late) effects. Acute effects are common, rarely serious, and usually self-limiting. Acute effects tend to occur in organs that depend on rapid self renewal, most commonly, the skin or mucosal surfaces (oropharynx, esophagus, small intestine, rectum and bladder). This is due to radiation-induced cell death that occurs during mitosis so that cells that divide rapidly show the most rapid cell loss. In the treatment of head and neck cancer, mucositis becomes worse during the first 3 to 4 weeks of therapy but then will often stabilize as the normal mucosa cell proliferation increases in response to mucosal cell loss. It seems likely that normal tissue stem cells are relatively resistant to radiation compared with the more differentiated cells because these stem cells survive to permit the normal mucosa to reepithelialize. Acute side effects typically resolve within 2 weeks of treatment completion

(Devita, 11th Edition, Page 447)

18. **True regarding subacute radiotoxicity:**

(a) Within 6 months of RT

(b) Non-reversible

(c) Not proportional to dose delivered

(d) All of the above

Ans: (a) Within 6 months of RT

Explanation

Radiation can also produce subacute toxicities in the form of radiation pneumonitis and radiation-induced liver disease. These typically occur 2 weeks to 3 months after radiation is completed. The risk of radiation pneumonitis and radiation-induced liver disease is proportional to the mean dose delivered. Thus, the 3D tools that permit the calculation of dose-volume histograms are currently used to determine the maximum safe treatment that can be delivered in terms of dose and volume. These toxicities appear to be initiated subclinically during the course of radiation as a cascade of cytokines in which TGF-β, tumor necrosis factor α, interleukin-6, and other cytokines play a role. Thus, in the future, we might look toward a combination of physical dose delivery, measured by the dose-volume histogram, the functional imaging of normal tissue damage and the detection of biomarkers of toxicity, such as TGF-β, to improve the ability to individualize therapy. Attempts to determine the genomic basis of radiation sensitivity, beyond the known rare genetic defects such as ataxia telangiectasia, have not yet been successful

(Devita, 11th Edition, Page 448)

19. Regarding late radiotoxicity, false is:

(a) Irreversible effects occurring after 6 months
(b) Includes fibrosis, fistula and parenchymal damage
(c) Consequential type involves no symptom-free period
(d) Brain necrosis is consequential toxicity

Ans: (d) Brain necrosis is consequential toxicity

Explanation

Late effects, which are typically seen 6 or more months after a course of radiation, include fibrosis, fistula formation, or long-term organ damage. Two theories for the origin of late effects have been put forth: late damage to the microvasculature and direct damage to the parenchyma

Late complications can also be divided into two categories: consequential and true late effects. The best example of a consequential late effect is fibrosis and dysphagia after high-dose chemoradiation for head and neck cancer. Here, late fibrosis or ulceration appears to be the result of the mucosa becoming denuded for a prolonged time period. Late consequential effects are distinct from true late effects, which can follow a normal treatment course of self-limited toxicity and a 6-month or more symptom-free period. Examples of true late effects are radiation myelitis, radiation brain necrosis, and radiation-induced bowel obstruction. In the past, radiation fibrosis was thought to be an irreversible condition. Therefore, an exciting recent development is that severe radiation-induced breast fibrosis is an active process that can be reversed by drug therapy (pentoxifylline and Vitamin E). Radiation therapy also causes second cancers

(Devita, 11th Edition, Page 448)

20. Combination RT utilizes all *except:*

(a) Radiosensitization
(b) Spatial additivity
(c) Symbiosis
(d) Synergism

Ans: (c) Symbiosis

Explanation

Combining chemotherapy with radiation therapy has produced important improvements in treatment outcome. Randomized clinical trials show improved local control and survival through the use of concurrent chemotherapy and radiation therapy for patients with high-grade gliomas and locally advanced cancers of the head and neck, lung, esophagus, stomach, rectum, prostate and anus. There are least two proposed reasons why chemoradiotherapy might be successful. The first is radiosensitization, meaning that the observed effect of using chemotherapy and radiation concurrently is greater than simply adding the two together. A second proposed reason to combine radiation and chemotherapy is to realize the benefit of improved local control radiation along with the systemic effect of chemotherapy, a concept called spatial additivity

By targeting the aberrant growth factor pathways that are specific to cancer cells rather than all rapidly proliferating cells, molecularly targeted therapies offer the potential to improve outcome without increasing toxicity. Even a selective cytostatic effect against the tumor would be predicted to act synergistically with radiation. The best validation of this combination has been in head and neck cancer. A phase III clinical trial demonstrated that in a cohort of 424 patients with locoregionally advanced squamous cell carcinoma of the head and neck, the addition of cetuximab nearly doubled the median survival of patients (compared to radiotherapy alone), from 28 to 54 months. This study represents the first major success achieved by the addition of an EGFR antagonist to radiotherapy. This improvement was achieved without enhanced toxicity. Notably, the rates of pharyngitis and weight loss were identical in the two arms. Local control was improved rather than the development of metastases, suggesting synergy rather than spatial additivity. Thus, the principle that can be derived from this study is that in tumors expressing high EGFR levels and that are likely to depend on aberrant EGF signaling, combining a true cytotoxic agent such as radiation with a cytostatic agent such as cetuximab has considerable promise

(Devita, 11th Edition, Page 449)

PAPER 1 (SET 2)

21. Additional testing using risk prediction tools warranted for:

(a) Mutation negative but strong family history
(b) Mutation positive but strong family history
(c) Mutation negative and no family history
(d) None of the above

Ans: (a) Mutation negative but strong family history

Explanation

Generally, testing should be focused on those in a family affected by cancer. Sometimes, this is not possible, and testing is performed on unaffected individuals. However, negative test results in an unaffected individual are uninformative for the rest of the family because these autosomal dominant mutations are only transmitted on average to half of offspring. If a disease-causing mutation is identified, "cascade testing" for that single mutation can be performed at less expense in other family members

(Devita, 11th Edition, Page 762)

22. Risk reduction with bilateral prophylactic mastectomy is:

(a) 50%
(b) 60%
(c) 90%
(d) 20%

Ans: (c) 90%

Explanation

Invasive options, including risk-reducing mastectomy (RRM) and risk-reducing salpingo-oophorectomy (RRSO), provide the largest breast cancer risk reduction. The Prevention and Observation Surgical End Points (PROSE) study group showed that RRM reduced the risk of breast cancer by 99% in BRCA1/2 patients with prior oophorectomy and 90% in women with intact ovaries

(Devita, 11th Edition, Page 757)

23. Criteria for CDH1 testing in diffuse gastric cancer includes all *except:*

(a) 2 or more gastric cancer in family with atleast one with DGC <50 years
(b) 3 or more DGC in first or second degree relative irrespective of age
(c) Any no. of DGC <40 years irrespective of family history
(d) None of the above

Ans: (d) None of the above

Explanation

New recommended screening criteria for CDH1 mutations are as follows:

1. Families with one or more cases of DGC
2. Individuals with DGC before the age of 40 years without a family history
3. Families or individuals with cases of DGC (one case below the age of 50 years) and lobular breast cancer
4. Cases where pathologists detect in situ signet ring cells or pagetoid spread of signet ring cells adjacent to DGC

(Devita, 11th Edition, Page 759)

24. Risk of lobular cancer in HDGC is:

(a) 20%
(b) 30%
(c) 40%
(d) 80%

Ans: (c) 40%

Explanation

Some individuals with CDH1 mutations choose not to pursue prophylactic gastrectomy. These individuals should undergo careful surveillance, including biannual endoscopy with multiple biopsies according to the method developed at Cambridge, beginning when they are at least 10 years younger than the youngest family member with DGC at time of diagnosis. It is recommended that any endoscopically visible lesion is targeted and that six each random biopsies are taken from the following regions: antrum, transitional zone, body, fundus and cardia

Careful white-light examination with targeted and random biopsies combined with detailed histopathology can identify early lesions and help to inform decision making with regard to gastrectomy. Additionally, because women with CDH1 mutations have a nearly 40% lifetime risk of developing lobular breast carcinoma, they should be carefully screened with annual mammography and biannual breast MRI starting at age 35 years. They should also do monthly self-examinations and have a breast examination by a physician every 6 months. The same surveillance recommendations are probably appropriate for HDGC families without identifiable CDH1 mutations, although no current guidelines for this exist

(Devita, 11th Edition, Page 761)

25. A 35-year male presented to emergency with history of high grade fever with chills of 10 days duration with multiple petechiae over the body with 3 episodes of epistaxis. On physical examination found to have multiple petechiae over the chest and limbs with active bleeding from nose with pallor. His peripheral smear shows more than 50% cells with bilobed nucleus with large azurophilic granules, with multiple auer rods, briskly staining in Sudan black. His fibrinogen level was 75 mg/dl. What is the next best step in the management of this patient?

(a) Start 3+7 chemotherapy
(b) Steroids
(c) Fresh frozen plasma or cryoprecipitate
(d) All of the above

Ans: (c) Fresh frozen plasma or cryoprecipitate

26. Common side effect of Sunitinib is:

(a) Hypertension
(b) Capillary leak
(c) Hematotoxicity
(d) Diarrhea

Ans: (a) Hypertension

27. High fat meal affects the bioavailability of all the drugs *except:*

(a) Sorafenib
(b) Vismodegib
(c) Imatinib
(d) Everolimus

Ans: (c) Imatinib

(Devita, Page 179)

28. Use of Sipleucel is:

(a) Minimally symptomatic, no visceral mets
(b) CRPC
(c) Vaccine for prevention of Ca Prostate
(d) Symptomatic bony mets with no visceral mets

Ans: (a) Minimally symptomatic, no visceral mets

Explanation

First line treatment of metastatic cancer prostate is:

- Docetaxel with 75 mg/m^2 every three weeks
- Abiraterone/ Enzalutamide with prednisone

Sipleucel T → Minimally symptomatic, no visceral mets

Radium 223 → Symptomatic bony mets with no visceral mets

29. Ruxolitinib is used to target which mutation?

(a) RET mutation
(b) JAK kinase mutation
(c) Ckit mutation
(d) HER2 Neu mutation

Ans: (b) JAK kinase mutation

(Devita, Page 238)

30. Patients with DPD deficiency will have increased side effects when exposed to which chemotherapy?

(a) Mitoxantrone
(b) 5-fluorouracil
(c) Irinotecan
(d) Oxaliplatin

Ans: (b) 5-fluorouracil

(Devita, Page 187)

31. Top 2 inhibitor therapies leads to secondary AML in what percentage of patients?

(a) 1%
(b) 3%
(c) 5%
(d) 7%

Ans: (c) 5%

(Devita, Page 226)

32. Reversing resistance to taxane chemo is:

(a) Custirsen
(b) Galenterone
(c) Cabozantinib
(d) Mitoxantrone

Ans: (a) Custirsen

33. One of the following drugs is a VEGF receptor inhibitor?

(a) Everolimus
(b) Pazopanib
(c) Ceritinib
(d) Vandetanib

Ans: (d) Vandetanib

(Devita, Page 238)

34. Due to absence of which enzyme leads to severe hematological toxicity when 6 MP is given in leukemias?

(a) MGMT mutation
(b) G-6PD deficiency
(c) TPMT deficiency
(d) DPD deficiency

Ans: (c) TPMT deficiency

(Devita, Page 186)

35. During cryotheraphy, gas used for warming is:

(a) Argon
(b) Helium
(c) CO_2
(d) N_2O

Ans: (b) Helium

36. Platinum agents act by binding preferentially to:

(a) N 7 position of Guanine
(b) C 7 position of Guanine
(c) N 7 position of Cytidine
(d) C 7 position of Thiamine

Ans: (a) N 7 position of Guanine

(Devita, Page 201)

37. PD-1 is a check point modulator expressed on:

(a) Activated B cells
(b) Activated T cells
(c) Tumor cells
(d) Macrophages

Ans: (b) Activated T cells

(Devita, Page 164)

38. The dose limiting toxicity of oxaliplatin is:

(a) Nephropathy
(b) Ototoxicity
(c) Neuropathy
(d) Myelosuppression

Ans: (c) Neuropathy

(Devita, Page 206)

39. Vismodegib–small molecule inhibitor of Hedgehog pathway is used in metastatic:

(a) Small cell carcinoma
(b) Squamous cell carcinoma
(c) Basal cell carcinoma
(d) Merkel cell carcinoma

Ans: (c) Basal cell carcinoma

(Devita, Page 269)

40. The pulmonary toxicity of which drug increases when GCSF is given along with it?

(a) Bleomycin
(b) Actinomycin–D
(c) Streptozocin
(d) Vinorelbine

Ans: (a) Bleomycin

(Devita, Page 286)

PAPER 1 (SET 3)

41. The dose of exemestane used in hormonal therapy of breast cancer is:

(a) 1 mg (b) 2.5 mg
(c) 25 mg (d) 20 mg

Ans: (c) 25 mg

(Devita, Page 284)

42. The drug which is used to increase the appetite in cachectic cancer patient is:

(a) Letrozole (b) Estradiol
(c) Megestrol (d) Octreotide

Ans: (c) Megestrol

(Devita, Page 287)

43. The monoclonal antibody which targets RANKL ligands is used to reduce the skeletal related events is:

(a) Cetuximab (b) Denosumab
(c) Cetuximab (d) Panitumumab

Ans: (b) Denosumab

(Devita, Page 305)

44. 5-Azacytidine is a demethyllating agent which is used to treat?

(a) ALL (b) AML
(c) CML (d) CLL

Ans: (b) AML

(Devita, Page 254)

45. Which is the most common adverse effect of bortezomib used in multiple myeloma?

(a) Diarrhoea (b) Neutropenia
(c) Peripheral neuropathy (d) Anemia

Ans: (c) Peripheral neuropathy

(Devita, Page 260)

46. Synthetic lethality is the mechanism used by which group of drugs?

(a) Proteasome inhibitors (b) PARP inhibitors
(c) Kinase inhibitors (d) HDAC inhibitors

Ans: (b) PARP inhibitors

(Devita, Page 264)

47. All the drugs are antibody drug conjugates *except:*

(a) Blinatumomab (b) Gemtuzumab ozogamicin
(c) Ado trastuzumab emtansine (d) Brentuximab

Ans: (a) Blinatumomab

(Devita, Page 234)

48. An BiTE-biallelic T cell engager which is approved to be used in refractory ALL is:

(a) Brentuximab
(b) Blinatumomab
(c) Bevacizumab
(d) Ramucirumab

Ans: (b) Blinatumomab

(Devita, Page 302)

49. Brentuximab vedotin is an antibody drug conjugate used to treat anaplastic large cell lymphoma and:

(a) Relapsed diffuse large b cell lymphoma
(b) Relapsed hodgkin's lymphoma
(c) Relapsed mantle cell lymphoma
(d) Relapsed CLL

Ans: (b) Relapsed Hodgkin's lymphoma

(Devita, Page 304)

50. Ramucirumab is a fully human IgG1 monoclonal antibody against:

(a) Vascular Endothelial growth factor
(b) C-kit receptor
(c) Insulin like growth factor
(d) Vascular endothelial growth factor receptor

Ans: (d) Vascular endothelial growth factor receptor

(Devita, Page 297)

51. Regorafenib is a multikinase inhibitor approved in use for all the advanced cancers *except:*

(a) Renal cell carcinoma
(b) Colorectal carcinoma
(c) Gastrointestinal stromal tumor
(d) Hepatocellular carcinoma

Ans: (a) Renal cell carcinoma

(Devita, Page 296)

52. Ramucirumab is approved in all cancers *except:*

(a) Metastatic adenocarcinoma lung
(b) Metastatic squamous cell carcinoma lung
(c) Metastatic gastric carcinoma
(d) Metastatic gastroesophageal carcinoma

Ans: (b) Metastatic squamous cell carcinoma lung

(Devita, Page 297)

53. A 60-year-old diabetic lady with stage IIIC ovarian cancer got neoadjuvant chemotherapy with paclitaxel and carboplatin for 3 cycles and underwent interval cytoreductive surgery and then now has come for adjuvant chemotherapy. She has grade 3 peripheral neuropathy which combination of drugs will be appropriate to avoid worsening of neuropathy?

(a) Paclitaxel and carboplatin
(b) Paclitaxel and cisplatin
(c) Docetaxel and cisplatin
(d) Docetaxel and carboplatin

Ans: (d) Docetaxel and carboplatin

54. A metastatic renal cell carcinoma patient was started on sunitinib–which one of the parameters to be checked regularly for him?

(a) ECG
(b) Blood pressure
(c) SPO2
(d) Lipid profile

Ans: (b) Blood pressure

(Devita, Page 295)

55. A 40-year-old lady underwent TAH + BSO for uterine fibroid in June 2017, HPE reported as leiomyosarcoma of uterus. Patient underwent radiotherapy and was kept on follow up. One year later she presented with recurrence in the abdomen with a mass of size 6×7 cms? What regimen will give her prolonged survival?

(a) Anthracycline single agent
(b) Gemcitabine and docetaxel
(c) Pazopanib
(d) Anthracycline and olaratumab

Ans: (d) Anthracycline and olaratumab

56. The most common adverse effect of infusional 5-Fluorouracil is:

(a) Mucositis
(b) Diarrhoea
(c) Neutropenia
(d) Thrombocytopenia

Ans: (a) Mucositis

(Devita, Page 213)

57. Trabectedin acts by which mechanism?

(a) By destabilizing microtubules
(b) Binding to minor groove of DNA
(c) By depolymerising the microtubules
(d) Topoisomerase 2 inhibition

Ans: (b) Binding to minor groove of DNA

58. Microsatellite Instable colorectal tumors does not respond better to which drug?

(a) 5-Fluorouracil
(b) Oxaliplatin
(c) Irinotecan
(d) Mitomycin

Ans: (a) 5-Fluorouracil

(Devita, Page 212)

59. Pemetrexed toxicity can be reduced by giving supplementation with:

(a) Vitamin B_6
(b) Vitamin B_{12}
(c) Vitamin B_3
(d) Thiamine

Ans: (b) Vitamin B_{12}

(Devita, Page 210)

60. Methotrexate acts by inhibiting all the following enzymes *except:*

(a) AICAR (aminoimidazole carboxamide)
(b) GAR (Glycinamide ribonucleotide)
(c) Dihydrofolate reductase
(d) Deoxycytidine kinase

Ans: (d) Deoxycytidine kinase

(Devita, Page 208)

PAPER 2 (SET 1)

61. PICOT framework used in:

(a) Case control study
(b) Cohort study
(c) Summary of research study
(d) None of above

Ans: (c) Summary of research study

62. Regarding Characteristic morphology of classical Hodgkin's lymphoma, all are true *except:*

(a) cHL is a lymphoid neoplasm composed of mononuclear Hodgkin's cells and multinucleated RS cells residing in an abundant cellular microenvironment
(b) Microenvironment cells are in excess than the Reed-Sternberg cells
(c) Lymphocytes are predominantly T regulatory cells
(d) Hodgkin's lymphoma is not associated EBV infection

Ans: (d) Hodgkin's lymphoma is not associated EBV infection

63. RECIST 1.1 criteria includes all *except:*

(a) Complete response if lymph node size less than 1cm
(b) Partial response if >=30% decrease longest diameters
(c) Single non-target lesion is significant
(d) 5 lesions measured with 2 per organ

Ans: (c) Single non-target lesion is significant

64. RECIST immunotherapy criteria includes all *except:*

(a) Upto 5 new lesions can be incorporated into tumor burden
(b) To be significant, new lesions should contribute to >25% of tumor burden
(c) Any non measurable lesion itself defines disease progression
(d) None of the above

Ans: (c) Any non measurable lesion itself defines disease progression

65. Bidimensional measurements used in all *except:*

(a) WHO criteria
(b) CNS RANO
(c) PRIAS study
(d) RECIST 1.1

Ans: (d) RECIST 1.1

66. Progression and partial response in WHO criteria is:

(a) 50% decrease and 25% increase
(b) 25% increase and 50% decrease
(c) 50% increase and 25% decrease
(d) 50% increase and 25% increase

Ans: (b) 25% increase and 50% decrease

67. In IWG for lymphoma, complete response involves all *except:*

(a) PET negative after treatment of a lesion which was PET avid
(b) Complete disappearance of lesion
(c) FDG PET non avid lymph node size <1.5 cm which was previously >1.5 cm
(d) Lymph node <=1 cm if previously >1.5 cm

Ans: (d) Lymph node <=1 cm if previously >1.5 cm

68. Choi criteria is based on:

(a) Density on CT scan
(b) Intensity on MRI scan
(c) Clinical benefit response
(d) FDG PET uptake

Ans: (a) Density on CT scan

69. FDG PET based response assessment includes all *except:*

(a) EORTC
(b) PERCIST
(c) SWAT
(d) None of the above

Ans: (c) SWAT

70. True clinical benefit include as:

(a) Overall survival
(b) Symptom benefit
(c) Both
(d) None

Ans: (c) Both

71. Overall response rate is:

(a) Complete response + partial response
(b) Complete response + partial response + stable disease
(c) Stable disease + partial response
(d) Complete response + stable disease

Ans: (a) Complete response + partial response

72. Forest plot utilized in:

(a) Subset analysis
(b) Interim analysis
(c) Meta analysis
(d) Publication bias

Ans: (c) Meta analysis

73. All are poor risk factors in Acute myeloid leukemia *except?*

(a) Presence of FLT-3 ITD mutation
(b) Presence of complex cytogenetics
(c) Deletion 5q abnormality
(d) Core binding factor mutations

Ans: (d) Core binding factor mutations

74. Grade A recommendation based on:

(a) RCT
(b) Analytical studies
(c) Case series
(d) Expert opinion

Ans: (a) RCT

75. Level 2 evidence based on:

(a) Meta analysis of RCT
(b) Case series
(c) Case control and cohort studies
(d) Expert opinion

Ans: (c) Case control and cohort studies

76. Strong recommendation for screening includes all *except:*

(a) Cancer cervix
(b) Colon cancer
(c) Ovarian cancer
(d) High risk for breast cancer

Ans: (c) Ovarian cancer

77. **Goal of screening is:**

(a) Reduce morbidity
(b) Prevent disease
(c) Prevent risk factors
(d) Reduce mortality

Ans: (d) Reduce mortality

78. **Screening types include all *except:***

(a) Opportunistic
(b) Programmatic
(c) Prospective
(d) Retrospective

Ans: (d) Retrospective

79. **False statement is:**

(a) PPV correlates with prevalence
(b) PPV inversely correlates with prevalence
(c) PPV changes more with specificity
(d) NPV correlates with sensitivity

Ans: (b) PPV inversely correlates with prevalence

PAPER 2 (SET 2)

80. False statement is:

(a) Lead time bias occurs in screening
(b) Length bias leads to overdiagnosis
(c) Selection bias due to healthy volunteer effect
(d) Selection bias cannot be eliminated by randomization

Ans: (d) Selection bias cannot be eliminated by randomization

81. Regarding mammographic breast screening, false is:

(a) Reduces mortality by 20-30%
(b) Increases incidence of early breast cancer
(c) Dose is 4 mSv or 0.1 cGy
(d) Started at age of 20 years

Ans: (d) Started at age of 20 years

82. False about colorectal screening:

(a) Colonoscopy done at 10 years interval
(b) 5 years interval in familial cancer syndrome
(c) 21% adenomas missed
(d) Perforation is never a complication

Ans: (d) Perforation is never a complication

83. HPV testing includes following modes *except:*

(a) Cotesting
(b) Repetitive testing
(c) Reflexive testing
(d) Stand alone

Ans: (b) Repetitive testing

84. Risk reducing BSO for HBOC syndrome is:

(a) Preferably done at 35 years
(b) Done before 35 years
(c) Reduces risk of triple negative breast cancer
(d) None of above

Ans: (a) Preferably done at 35 years

85. Tobacco is a:

(a) Group 1 carcinogen
(b) Not a carcinogen
(c) Group 3 carcinogen
(d) Group 2 carcinogen

Ans: (a) Group 1 carcinogen

86. Tobacco has a causal relationship in all cancer *except:*

(a) Prostate
(b) AML
(c) Head and neck
(d) Breast

Ans: (a) Prostate

87. Cancer index defined by:

(a) No of cigarettes
(b) Type of tobacco
(c) Pack years
(d) All of the above

Ans: (c) Pack years

88. False about nicotine is:

(a) Carcinogen
(b) Causes addiction
(c) Acts as a reinforcer
(d) Not a carcinogen

Ans: (a) Carcinogen

89. Animal fat increase risk of Cancer in all *except:*

(a) Breast (b) Prostate

(c) Colon (d) Lung

Ans: (d) Lung

90. False about carotenoids is:

(a) Increased risk of lung cancer (b) Decreased risk of skin cancer

(c) Decreased ER negative breast cancer (d) None of above

Ans: (d) None of above

91. True about physical activity is:

(a) Occupational and recreational

(b) Household activities is a type of occupational activity

(c) Sedentary behaviors is a risk factor for cancer

(d) All of above

Ans: (d) All of above

92. Physical activity in breast, false is:

(a) Decreases risk significantly more in post menopausal women than pre menopausal

(b) Independent of HRT

(c) Both of above

(d) None of above

Ans: (d) None of above

93. Obesity in breast cancer, false is:

(a) Increases risk in post menopausal women

(b) Weight gain after age 18 years increase in postmenopausal breast cancer, in the absence of HRT

(c) Higher incidence in prememopausal women

(d) Increased breast cancer mortality

Ans: (c) Higher incidence in prememopausal women

94. True about aristolochic acid is all *except:*

(a) Class 1 carcinogen (b) Causes interstitial fibrosis

(c) Upper tract urothelial cancer (d) Non specific molecular action

Ans: (d) Non specific molecular action

95. All are established carcinogen *except:*

(a) Tobacco (b) Air pollution

(c) Aristolochic acid (d) Farm weeds

Ans: (d) Farm weeds

96. Most common type of UV rays causing carcinogenesis:

(a) UV A (b) UV B

(c) UV C (d) Cyclobutane

Ans: (b) UV B

97. Most important role in tumor promoting inflammation is by:

(a) TNF alpha (b) HIF 1

(c) STAT-3 (d) All of the above

Ans: (a) TNF alpha

98. Oncogenic viruses cause:

(a) Low penetrance cancer (b) High penetrance cancer

(c) Both (d) None

Ans: (a) Low penetrance cancer

99. Which viruses are non-enveloped?

(a) HPV (b) Merkel cell polyoma virus

(c) Both (d) None

Ans: (c) Both

PAPER 2 (SET 3)

100. Cofactor for cirrhosis all *except:*

(a) Advancing age
(b) Female
(c) Alcohol
(d) Diabetes

Ans: (b) Female

101. Lifetime risk of HPV infection:

(a) 70%
(b) 15%
(c) 50%
(d) 10%

Ans: (a) 70%

102. True about HPV vaccine:

(a) Can't eradicate tumor or infection
(b) No life long immunity
(c) Can be given at birth
(d) None of the above

Ans: (a) Can't eradicate tumor or infection

103. Merkel cell polyoma virus, true is:

(a) Group 2A carcinogen
(b) Group 1 carcinogen
(c) Not associated with CLL
(d) None of the above

Ans: (a) Group 2A carcinogen

104. False statement about EBV is:

(a) Endemic Burkitt's lymphoma associated with EBV in 100% cases
(b) IgA antibodies is a risk indicator
(c) Nasopharyngeal carcinoma 100% associated with EBV in all geographic areas
(d) Exists in lytic phase

Ans: (d) Exists in lytic phase

105. False about Kaposi sarcoma:

(a) Caused by HHV–8
(b) Exists as lytic phase
(c) Expresses viral IL–6
(d) Tocilizumab can be used as anti IL–8

Ans: (d) Tocilizumab can be used as anti IL-8

106. True regarding HTLV-1 is all *except:*

(a) Only 20-50% infected will develop disease
(b) ATLL seen only in individuals who acquire infection by breastfeeding
(c) Circulating flower cells seen
(d) Lytic lesions in bone

Ans: (a) Only 20-50% infected will develop disease

107. Incorrect match is:

(a) HBV-ccc DNA
(b) HCV-non-structural proteins
(c) HBV-95% chronicity in adults
(d) HBV-integration of genome

Ans: (c) HBV-95% chronicity in adults

108. False about retroviruses:

(a) Reverse transcriptase present in most
(b) RNA virus without RT is HCV
(c) Only oncogenic retrovirus in human is HIV-1
(d) Lentivirus has a long latent period

Ans: (c) Only oncogenic retrovirus in human is HIV-1

109. Incorrect match is:

(a) DNA direct damage–high LET-particulate ions
(b) DNA indirect damage–low LET-ionizing radiation
(c) Heavy carbon ions have no impact upon by free radical scavenger or oxygen effect
(d) None of the above

Ans: (d) None of the above

110. NHEJ pathway of repair predominant in:

(a) G1
(b) G1S
(c) Early S
(d) G2

Ans: (a) G1

111. HRR pathway predominant in:

(a) Late S and G2
(b) G2
(c) Interphase
(d) G1 and G2

Ans: (a) Late S and G2

112. NHEJ pathway present in:

(a) G1
(b) G2
(c) All phases of cell cycle
(d) S phase

Ans: (c) All phases of cell cycle

113. Shoulder in survival curve denotes:

(a) Resistance by tumor cells to killing
(b) Inversely proportional to killing power of RT
(c) None of above
(d) Both of above

Ans: (d) Both of above

114. Acutely radiosensitive organs are all *except:*

(a) Skin
(b) GIT
(c) Bone marrow
(d) Bone

Ans: (d) Bone

115. Most radiosensitive is:

(a) Breast
(b) Bone marrow
(c) Spinal cord
(d) Testes

Ans: (b) Bone marrow

116. TCD50 is:

(a) Dose to kill all of tumor cells
(b) Time taken to grow to 50% of initial size
(c) Dose which controls 50% of tumor growth
(d) All of the above

Ans: (c) Dose which controls 50% of tumor growth

117. Most sensitive phase of cell cycle:

(a) G2M
(b) Late S
(c) G1
(d) Mid S

Ans: (a) G2M

118. Most resistant phase of cell cycle is:

(a) Late S and G1
(b) Mid S
(c) Early S
(d) G2

Ans: (a) Late S and G1

119. True regarding hypoxia and tumor cells:

(a) Chronic hypoxia is diffusion mediated due to large intervessel distance
(b) Acute transient hypoxia due to tumor vessel abnormality
(c) Anti VEGF therapy targets acute type of hypoxia
(d) All of the above

Ans: (d) All of the above

PAPER 3 (SET 1)

120. Drug used in chronic lymphocytic leukemia is:

(a) Ofatumumab (b) Nivolumab

(c) Alemtuzumab (d) Ramicirumab

Ans: (a) Ofatumumab

Explanation

The anti-CD20 ofatumumab is a fully human antibody that binds an epitope on CD20 distinct from that bound by rituximab and is engineered for better complement activation, although it induces less ADCC. Ofatumumab has received regulatory approval for the treatment of patients with fludarabine-refractory chronic lymphocytic leukemia (CLL). In a recently reported, planned interim analysis that included 138 CLL patients with treatment refractory disease or bulky (> 5 cm) lymphadenopathy, treatment with ofatumumab led to an overall response rate (primary end point) of 47% in patients with bulky disease and 5% in patients refractory to both alemtuzumab and fludarabine

Antibodies Approved by the U.S. Food and Drug Administration for the Treatment of Cancer

Generic Name (Trade Name)	Origin	Isotype (Conjugate)	Indication	Target
Unconjugated MAbs				
Rituximab (Rituxan)	Chimeric	IgG1	NHL	CD20
Trastuzumab (Herceptin)	Humanized	IgG1	BrCa	HER2
Alemtuzumab (Campath-1H)	Humanized	IgG1	CLL	CD52
Cetuximab (Erbitux)	Chimeric	IgG1	CRC, SCCHN	EGFR
Bevacizumab (Avastin)	Humanized	IgG1	CRC, NSCLC, RCC, GBM	VEGF
Panitumumab (Vectibix)	Human (XenoMouse)	IgG2	CRC	EGFR
Ofatumumab (Arzerra)	Human (XenoMouse)	IgG1	CLL	CD20
Denosumab (Prolia/Xgeva)	Human	IgG2	Metastasis-related SREs, ADT/AI-associated osteoporosis, GCT	RANKL
Pertuzumab (Perjeta)	Humanized	IgG1	BrCA	HER2
Obinutuzumab (Gazyva)	Humanized	IgG1	CLL, FL	CD20
Blinatumomab (Blincyto)	Murine	BiTE	ALL	CD3/CD19
Ramucirumab (Cyramza)	Human	IgG1	Gastric, colorectal, lung	VEGFR2
Daratumumab (Darzalex)	Human	IgG1	MM	CD 38
Elotuzumab (Empliciti)	Humanized	IgG1	MM	SLAMF7
Necitumumab (Portrazza)	Human	IgG1	NSCLC	EGFR
Dinutuximab (Unituxin)	Chimeric	IgG1	Neuroblastoma	GD2
Olaratumab (Latruvo)	Human	IgG1	PDGFRα	Sarcoma
Immunoconjugates				
Gemtuzumab ozogamicin (Mylotarg)	Humanized	IgG4 (Calicheamicin)	AML	CD33
Ibritumomab tiuxetan (Zevalin)	Murine	IgG1(^{90}Y)	NHL	CD20
Tositumomab (Bexxar)	Murine	IgG2A (^{131}I)	NHL	CD20
Brentuximab vedotin (Adcetris)	Chimeric	IgG1 (MMAE)	HL, sALCL	CD 30
Ado-trastuzumab emtansine (Kadcyla)	Humanized	IgG1 (DM1)	BrCa	HER2
Inotuzumab ozogamicin (Besponsa)	Humanized	IgG4 (Calicheamicin)	ALL	CD22

Alemtuzumab (Campath-1H) targets the CD52 glycopeptide, which is highly expressed on T and B lymphocytes. It has been tested as a therapeutic agent for CLL and promyelocytic leukemias, as well as other non-Hodgkin lymphomas

Alemtuzumab is an anti CD52 monoclonal antibody useful in CLL Ofatumumab will be more appropriate since it is more commonly used. Another antibody useful is obinutuzumab

(Devita, 11th Edition, Page 688)

121. False about Cetuximab is:

(a) Approved for use in metastatic colorectal cancer

(b) Superior activity when combined with irinotecan

(c) Synergistic when combined with Chemotherapy

(d) Severity of rash associated with toxicity of cetuximab

Ans: (d) Severity of rash associated with toxicity of cetuximab

Explanation

Reduced locoregional recurrence when given with chemoRT in head and neck cancer Cetuximab (Erbitux) targets the EGFR. This chimeric IgG1 binds to domain III of the EGFR, with roughly a 10-fold higher affinity than either EGF or transforming growth factor α (TGF-α) ligands and thereby inhibits ligand induced activation of this tyrosine kinase receptor. Cetuximab may also function to downregulate EGFR dependent signaling by stimulating EGFR internalization. Cetuximab is approved for the treatment of colorectal cancer and, more recently, for the treatment of squamous cell cancer of the head and neck (SCCHN). An international, multicenter, phase III trial comparing definitive radiotherapy to radiotherapy plus cetuximab in SCCHN demonstrated that EGFR blockade with radiotherapy significantly reduced the risk of locoregional failure by 32% and the risk of death by 26%

The efficacy and safety of cetuximab against colorectal cancer was demonstrated alone and in combination with irinotecan in a phase II, multicenter, randomized, and controlled trial of 329 patients. The combination of irinotecan plus cetuximab increased both the overall response and the median duration of response as compared to cetuximab alone. Additionally, patients with irinotecan-refractory disease responded to treatment with the combination regimen. Recent studies in patients with colorectal cancers have indicated that patients with KRAS mutations in codon 12 or 13 should not receive anti-EGFR therapy

Grade 2-4 cetuximab rash was associated with better survival possibly due to reduction of distant metastasis. This observation was noted mainly in p16 negative patients

Cetuximab rash associated with better survival and not toxicity of the cetuximab

(Devita, 11th Edition, Page 694)

122. Correct match with toxicity is:

(a) Cetuximab–acneiform rash

(b) Bevazicumab–hemorrhage and delayed wound healing

(c) Trastuzumab–cardiomyopathy

(d) All of the above

Ans: (d) All of the above

Explanation

In adjuvant trastuzumab trials the incidence of grade iii/iv congestive cardiac failure and cardiac related death occurred in the percentage of 0% (finHER) Trial to 4.1% (NSABP B-31) Trial

From the above discussion done in previous questions, cetuximab causes acneiform rash and bevacizumab causes bleeding and wound healing complications

123. Tumor needs independent blood supply if size more than:

(a) 2 mm (b) 3 mm

(c) 4 mm (d) 5 mm

Ans: (a) 2 mm

Explanation

Tumors can grow to a size of approximately 1-2 mm^3 before their metabolic demands are restricted due to the diffusion limit of oxygen and nutrients. In order to grow beyond this size, the tumor switches to an angiogenic phenotype and attracts blood vessels from the surrounding stroma

(Cancer Metastasis Rev. 2007 Dec, 26(3-4), 489-502)

124. Intervessel distance in tumor is:

(a) 10-40 microns (b) 40-100 microns

(c) 500 microns (d) 400 microns

Ans: (b) 40-100 microns

Explanation

Inter-vessel distance

Although the IVD does not directly contribute to the haemodynamical properties of the tumor vascular system, it is nevertheless an important attribute in determining tissue hypoxia and it is also an indicator of local metabolic burden of the tumor tissue *(Hlatky et al., 2002)*. Increased variability in this parameter was observed in the tumor tissues when compared to the normal mucosa samples, which had a very narrow range for this parameter. IVD shows a lower vessel density in the core relative to the peripheral carcinoma samples

THE ARCHITECTURE OF TUMOR VASCULATURE

Cell type	Location and host	Structure	Characteristic measurement	Method	Tumor size
Primary human colorectal adenocarcinoma	Human colon	Intervessel distance tumor center tumor surface tumor periphery Vessel diameter tumor center tumor surface tumor periphery	 134.9 µm 89.1 µm 45.7 µm 22.9 µm 16.6 µm 18.2 µm	Corrosion casts, microCT and SEM	>0.8-1.0 cm
Human colorectal carcinomas (LS 1741)	Flanks of node (nu/nu, MF1) mice	Intervessel distance Vessel diameter	45.7 µm 18.2 µm	Corrosion casts, microCT and SEM	0.88 ± 0.27 g
Primary human colorectal cancer	Human colon	Intervessel distance tumor center tumor surface tumor periphery Vessel diameter tumor center tumor surface tumor periphery	 177.7 µm 118.6 µm 54.3 µm 30.9 µm 18.3 µm 19.4 µm	Corrosion casts and SEM	>0.8-1.0 cm
Murine carcinoma (CaX)	Dorsal xenograft CBA/GyfTO	Intervessel distance Vessel diameter	112.4 µm 24.4 µm	Corrosion casts and SEM	0.15-0.9 mL

The intervessel distance is 40-100 microns

125. False statement is:

(a) No HAMA response in radioimmunoconjugate therapy

(b) Half life of IgG is 3 weeks

(c) Primary toxicity of radioimmunotherapy is dose-limiting myelosuppression

(d) Targeted radioimmunotherapy cannot be administered IV

Ans: (d) Targeted radioimmunotherapy cannot be administered IV

Explanation

Yttrium-90 ibritumomab tiuxetan (IDEC-Y2B8) is a murine immunoglobulin G1 kappa monoclonal antibody that covalently binds MX-DTPA (tiuxetan), which chelates the radioisotope yttrium-90. The antibody targets CD20, a B-lymphocyte antigen

In summary, the current labeling states that Y90 ibritumomab tiuxetan may be given at a dose of 0.4 mCi/kg to subjects with a normal platelet count, and this dose is adjusted to 0.3 mCi/kg if the baseline platelet count is 100,000–150,000/μL, with a maximum allowable dose of 32 mCi. No dosimetry-based adjustments are needed, and rituximab 250 mg/m^2 is administered on days 1 and 8 of a treatment scheme with Y90 ibritumomab tiuxetan infusion given immediately after the second dose of rituximab. Similar dosing schemas have been studied in hundreds of clinical protocols and retrospective series, largely in indolent subtypes of NHL

Adverse events were primarily hematologic and correlated with baseline extent of marrow involvement with NHL and baseline platelet count. One patient (2%) developed an anti-antibody response (human antichimeric antibody/human antimouse antibody) (HAMA). Since ibritumomab is a monoclonal antibdoy derived from mouse

Under normal circumstances, most serum proteins that are too large for renal filtration (> around 60 kDa) are removed by pinocytosis, a process that occurs in all nucleated cells as they obtain their essential nutrients from plasma. This accounts for the half-life of IgA and IgM, which is constant at around 5-6 days. By contrast, IgG has a concentration-dependent half-life of approximately 21 days due to recycling by FcRn receptors

From above discussion we can understand the false statement is Targeted radioimmunotherapy cannot be administered IV

126. IL-2 toxicity includes all *except:*

(a) Hypotension

(b) Capillary leak

(c) Hepatorenal failure

(d) Headache

Ans: (d) Headache

Explanation

High-dose (HD) IL-2 administration results in severe hypotension and a capillary leak syndrome, limiting its administration to patients with excellent organ function and performance status, age younger than 70 years, and treatment in specialized centers with specific expertise. HD IL-2 has demonstrated complete cancer regressions in about 5% to 10% of patients treated for metastatic melanoma and renal cancer; most of these have been "cured" as defined by maintaining complete regressions for >10 years. At high doses, IL-2 binds to heterodimeric IL2Rβγ receptor leading to desired expansion of tumor-killing CD8 memory effector T (CD8 T) cells. However, IL-2 also binds to its heterotrimeric receptor IL2Rαβγ with even greater affinity, which expands immunosuppressive CD4+ CD25 (IL2Rα) + Tregs. After IL-2 administration, induced cytokines are released, leading to increased capillary permeability and decreased vascular resistance, which results in a shift of fluid from the bloodstream into the extravascular space. This fluid shift ultimately leads to a hypovolemic state and excessive fluid in the extravascular space. Capillary leak syndrome-associated fluid accumulation in the extravascular spaces may manifest as generalized edema, weight gain, pulmonary congestion, pleural effusions, and ascites. Capillary leak syndrome-associated hypovolemia may cause decreased blood flow to the kidneys, gut, heart and brain, resulting in oliguria, ischemia and confusion. Usually, capillary leak syndrome affects more than one organ system simultaneously, contributing to the toxicity often observed in patients receiving high-dose IL-2. The release of cytokines after IL-2 administration has also been implicated as the cause of flu-like symptoms, such as fever, chills, myalgias and arthralgias. So IL2 causes capillary leak syndrome, hypovolemia and renal failure

Headache will be the best answer here

(Devita, 11th Edition, Page 719)

127. Germline specific tumor marker is:

(a) CEA
(b) PSA
(c) CAGE
(d) hTERT

Ans: (c) CAGE

Explanation

A cancer/testis antigen, CAGE, is widely expressed in various cancer tissues and cancer cell lines but not in normal tissues except the testis. Cancer/testis (CT) antigens, of which more than 40 have now been identified, are encoded by genes that are normally expressed only in the human germline, but are also expressed in various tumor types, including melanoma, and carcinomas of the bladder, lung and liver. These immunogenic proteins are being vigorously pursued as targets for therapeutic cancer vaccines

Andrew J. G. Simpson *Nature Reviews Cancer,* volume 5, pages 615–625 (2005, Cancer-testis antigens (CTAs) represent a novel family of immunogenic proteins. The genes MAGE, BAGE, GAGE, LAGE and NY-ESO-1 code for antigens that are recognised on various neoplastically transformed cells by autologous, cytolytic CD8 (+) T lymphocytes

Obviously CEA, PSA are not germline markers. hTERT is human Telomerase reverse transcriptase enzyme. So answer is CAGE

128. Lineage specific tumor antigen is:

(a) E6 protein
(b) EBV
(c) PSA
(d) CDK4

Ans: (c) PSA

Explanation

PSA is prostate specific, hence that is the best answer among the options

129. Cancer specific tumor antigens are:

(a) Melan
(b) gp-100
(c) PSA
(d) Beta catenin

Ans: (d) Beta catenin

Explanation

Tumor-specific unique antigens		
Antigens	**HLA Presentation**	**Peptides**
MUM-1	HLA-B44	EEKLIVVLF
CDK4	HLA-A2	ACDPHSGHFV
β-catenin	HLA-A24	SYLDSGIHF
HLA-A2	HLA-A2	Altered HLA-A2

Beta catenin is one of the tumor specific antigen

Tissue-specific differentiation antigens			
Antigens	**HLA restrictions**	**Peptides**	**Comments**
Tyrosinase	HLA-A2 HLA-A2 HLA-B44 HLA-A24 HLA-DR4 HLA-DR4	MLLAVLYCL YMNGTMSQV SEIWRDIDF AFLPWHRLF QNILLSNAPLGPQFP SYLQDSDPDSFQD	
MART-1/Melan-A gP100	HLA-A2 HLA-A2 HLA-A2 HLA-A2 HLA-A2 HLA-A2 HLA-A3 HLA-A2	AAGIGILTV KTWGQYWQV ITDQVPFSV YLEPGPVTA LLDGTATLRF VLYRYGSFSV ALLAVGATL VYFFLPDHL	Epitope generated from an intron of an incomplete splicing RNA
gP75/TRP-1 TRP-2	HLA-A31 HLA-A31	MSLQRQFLR LLGPGRPYR	Epitope was derived from an alternative ORF Mouse TRP-2 was identified as a tumor antigen for B^{16} melanoma

Melan, gp-100, PSA are tissue specific tumor antigen

(R.-F. Wang: Tumor Antigens Discovery and Cancer Therapy, Molecular Medicine, Volume 3, Number 11, November 1997)

130. Antibodies action mediated by all *except:*

(a) Antibody dependent cellular cytotoxicity (b) Phagocytosis

(c) Classical complement (d) Necrosis

Ans: (d) Necrosis

Explanation

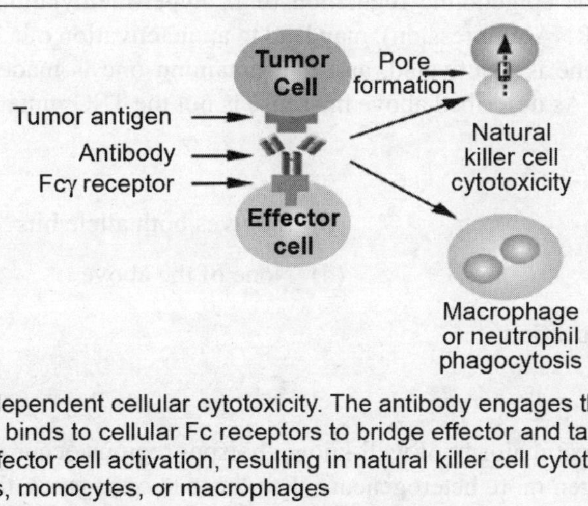

Antibody-dependent cellular cytotoxicity. The antibody engages the tumor antigen and the Fc domain binds to cellular Fc receptors to bridge effector and target cells. This bridging induces effector cell activation, resulting in natural killer cell cytotoxicity or phagocytosis by neutrophils, monocytes, or macrophages

Necrosis is not the pathway mediated through antibody mechanism

(Devita, 11th Edition, Page 691)

131. True about dendritic cells:

(a) Myeloid derived and plasmactoid derived

(b) Cross presentation to CD 8 cells

(c) Activated by CD 4 cells

(d) All of the above

Ans: (d) All of the above

Explanation

Numerous *subpopulations* of DCs have been identified to date, including interstitial DCs, dermal DCs, *Langerhans cells* (LCs), plasmacytoid DCs (pDCs), and inflammatory DCs. Dendritic cells (DCs) are the most potent professional *antigen-presenting cells* (APCs) *in vivo,* capable of both tolerance induction and the initiation of primary *T-cell* responses. A number of DC subsets have been described in both men and mice with unique functional attributes ascribed to a few. However, in general, constitutive expression of *Major Histocompatibility Complex* (MHC) class II and the high migratory capacity exhibited by a number of DC subsets contribute to the high stimulatory capacity of this cell type. Under resting conditions, DCs are considered "immature" and have been shown to induce *peripheral tolerance* by causing T-cell anergy, directing T-cell deletion or by inducing the generation of regulatory *T cells*

Dendritic cells are of many types as described and they are the classical antigen presenting cells. They can lead to anergy or t cell activation. All of the above is the best answer

132. Tumor suppressor gene mutation includes all *except:*

(a) Truncation

(b) Non-sense point mutation

(c) Missense point mutation

(d) Deletion

Ans: (c) Missense point mutation

Explanation

The two-hit model has been commonly applied to study the roles of TSGs in cancer (Knudson, 1971). Unlike oncogenes, most loss-of-function (LoF) mutations that occur in TSGs act in a recessive way in nature. In principle, both copies of a TSG need to be mutated for a TSG to completely lose its function, whereas haploinsufficient TSGs work in a dosage-sensitive manner. Mutations that may lead to LoF of their residing genes include, but are not limited to, nonsense single nucleotide variants (SNVs), SNVs disrupting canonical splicing sites, small insertions and deletions (indels) that cause frameshift and copy-number variations (CNVs) (Johnston *et al.,* 2015). In cells, mRNA carrying a nonsense mutation undergoes nonsense mediated decay (NMD) (Schweingruber *et al.,* 2013), resulting in a decrease of its expression; however, some genes may escape NMD. Other mechanisms, such as epigenomic regulation (e.g., hyper-methylation of its promoter region) and posttranscriptional regulation (e.g., microRNA suppression), may lead to an inactivation of a TSG. For the haploinsufficient mechanism in TSGs, one copy of the gene is inactivated, and the remaining one is inadequate to maintain the normal function of the gene (Davoli *et al.,* 2013). As described above missense is not the TSG mutation)

133. Oncogene mutation true is:

(a) Commonly involves hotspot mutation

(b) Involves both allele hits

(c) Most common mutated gene is RET

(d) None of the above

Ans: (a) Commonly involves hotspot mutation

Explanation

For the first time, we quantify why the great majority of well-known hotspot regions occur in oncogenes. Because hotspot regions in tumor suppressor genes are larger, more heterogeneous than those in oncogenes, they are more difficult to detect using protein sequence alone and are likely to be underreported. Our results indicate that protein structure-based 3D mutation clustering increases power to find hotspot regions, particularly in tumor suppressor genes. According to Knudson two hit hypothesis, hits involving both alleles is a feature of tumor suppressor gene, most common mutated gene is ras

(Cancer Res. 2016 Jul 1; 76(13): 3719–3731)

134. Most commonly mutated protooncogene:

(a) p53
(b) kras
(c) pi3k
(d) RET

Ans: (b) kras

Explanation

The Ki-ras gene is the most commonly mutated oncogene in sporadic colonic neoplasia. Point mutations in the K-ras gene have been observed in approximately 40% of sporadic colorectal adenomas and carcinomas

In general I could not find the direct answer for ras protooncogene. It is the most commonly mutated protooncogene in colon cancer

135. False about next gen sequencing is:

(a) Also known as massive parallel sequencing
(b) Multiple genes or the entire exome or genome can be interrogated simultaneously
(c) Most common NGS approach for cancer testing is sequencing of specific genes and mutation hotspot regions
(d) It's a type single-gene basis as in Sanger sequencing or pyrosequencing

Ans: (d) It's a type single-gene basis as in Sanger sequencing or pyrosequencing

Explanation

NGS, also known as massive parallel sequencing or deep sequencing, has revolutionized the speed, throughput, and cost of sequencing and has facilitated the discovery of clinically relevant genetic biomarkers for diagnosis, prognosis, and personalized therapeutics. By way of this technology, multiple genes or the entire exome or genome can be interrogated simultaneously in multiple parallel reactions, instead of a single-gene basis as in Sanger sequencing or pyrosequencing. Currently, the most common NGS approach for cancer testing in the clinical setting employs targeted sequencing of specific genes and mutation hotspotregions. Available panels commonly range in size from 10 to 150 genes. Copy number variations (CNVs) are genomic alterations that result in an abnormal number of copies of one or more genes. Structural genomic rearrangements such as duplications, deletions, translocations, and inversions can cause CNVs

Like single-nucleotide polymorphisms (SNPs), certain CNVs have been associated with disease susceptibility. Illumina offers a variety of array and next-generation sequencing (NGS) solutions for high-resolution copy number analysis

Indeed, the NGS machine generally makes mistakes only 0.1% of the time, but there are rare sites where the sequencer is systematically more error prone (e.g., ~1% error rate)

So all options are correct

136. Localized hypermutation is known as:

(a) Catharsis
(b) Kataegis
(c) Plexothesis
(d) None of the above

Ans: (b) Kataegis

Explanation

In *molecular biology* kataegis describes a pattern of localized *hypermutation* identified in some *cancer genomes*. The term *kataegis* is derived from the ancient Greek word for "thunder", καταιγίς *(kataegis)*. Regions of kataegis have been shown to be colocalised with regions of somatic genome rearrangements. The base *mutations* in these regions were found to be almost exclusively *cytosine* to *thymine* in the context of a TpC *dinucleotide*. It has been hypothesised that an enzyme of the APOBEC family is responsible for the process of kataegis. The direct link between the *APOBEC* deaminases and kataegistic clusters of mutations was recently obtained by expressing hyperactive deaminase in yeast cells. More recent evidence has linked the overexpression of the family member APOBEC3B with multiple human cancers, highlighting its possible contribution to genomic instability and kataegis

(Source: Internet)

137. False statement is:

(a) Chromothripsy is disorganized widespread rearrangement

(b) Chromoplexy is coordinated stepwise disruption

(c) Chromoplexy seen in prostate cancer

(d) Chromothripsy constitutes more than 50% of all tumors

Ans: (d) Chromothripsy constitutes more than 50% of all tumors

Explanation

Cancer genome sequencing has identified chromothripsis, a complex class of structural genomic rearrangements involving the apparent shattering of an individual chromosome into tens to hundreds of fragments.

An initial error during mitosis, producing either chromosome missegregation into a micronucleus or chromatin bridge interconnecting two daughter cells, can trigger the catastrophic pulverization of the spatially isolated chromosome

The resultant chromosomal fragments are re-ligated in random order by DNA double-strand break repair during the subsequent interphase. Chromothripsis scars the cancer genome with localized DNA rearrangements that frequently generate extensive copy number alterations, oncogenic gene fusion products, and/or tumor suppressor gene inactivation. Chromothripsis is the phenomenon by which up to thousands of clustered *chromosomal rearrangements* occur in a single event in localised and confined genomic regions in one or a few *chromosomes,* and is known to be involved in both cancer and congenital diseases. It occurs through one massive genomic rearrangement during a single catastrophic event in the cell's history. It is believed that for the cell to be able to withstand such a destructive event, the occurrence of such an event must be the upper limit of what a cell can tolerate and survive. The chromothripsis phenomenon opposes the conventional theory that cancer is the gradual acquisition of genomic rearrangements and somatic mutations over time

Chromothripsis was first observed in sequencing the genome of a *chronic lymphocytic leukaemia.* Subsequent investigations using genome-wide paired-end sequencing and *SNP array analysis* have found similar patterns of chromothripsis in various human cancers, e.g., *Melanomas, sarcomas* and *colorectal, lung* and *thyroid cancers.* In subsequent investigations, about 25% of studied *bone cancers* displayed evidence of chromothripsis. Chromothripsis has been linked to the generation of oncogenic fusions in supratentorial *ependymoma, chondromyxoid fibroma* and *Ewing sarcoma,* the latter two being bone tumors. Chromothripsis has been seen in 2–3% of cancers across all subtypes

Chromoplexy refers to a class of complex DNA rearrangement observed in the genomes of cancer cells. This phenomenon was first identified in *prostate cancer* by *whole genome sequencing* of prostate tumors. Chromoplexy causes genetic material from one or more chromosomes to become scrambled as multiple strands of DNA are broken and ligated to each other in a new configuration. In prostate cancer, chromoplexy may cause multiple oncogenic events within a single cell cycle, providing a proliferative advantage to a (pre-) cancerous cell. Several oncogenic mutations in prostate cancer occur through chromoplexy, such as disruption of the tumor suppressor gene *PTEN* or creation of the *TMPRSS2-ERG fusion gene*

Chromothripsis is found only in 2-3% of all cancers hence the last option saying it constituites 50% of all tumors is a false statement

(Source: Internet)

138. Most frequent somatic alteration is:

(a) Nucleotide substitution (b) Indels

(c) Copy number variation (d) All of the above

Ans: (a) Nucleotide substitution

Explanation

CANCER GENES AND THEIR MUTATIONS

Cancer genes are broadly grouped into oncogenes and tumor suppressor genes. Using a classical analogy, oncogenes can be compared to a car accelerator so that a mutation in an oncogene would be the equivalent of having the accelerator continuously pressed. Tumor suppressor genes, in contrast, act as brakes so that when they are not mutated, they function to inhibit tumorigenesis. Oncogene and tumor suppressor genes may be classified by the nature of their somatic mutations in tumors. Mutations in oncogenes typically occur at specific hotspots, often affecting the same codon or clustered at neighboring codons in different tumors. Furthermore, mutations in oncogenes are almost always missense, and the mutations usually affect only one allele, making them heterozygous. In contrast, tumor suppressor genes are usually mutated throughout the gene; a large number of the mutations may truncate the encoded protein and generally affect both alleles, causing loss of heterozygosity (LOH). Major types of somatic mutations present in malignant tumors include nucleotide substitutions, small insertions and deletions (indels), chromosomal rearrangements, and copy number alterations

(Devita, 11th Edition, Page 91)

Human cancers (n=210) including breast, lung, colorectal, gastric, testis, ovarian, renal, melanoma, glioma and acute lymphoblastic leukaemia (Supplementary Table 3) were screened for somatic mutations in the coding exons and splice junctions of the 518 protein kinase genes; a total of 274 Mb of cancer genome. Of the 210 cancers analysed 169 were primary tumors, 2 were early cultures and 39 were immortal cancer cell lines

One-thousand-and-seven somatic mutations were detected (Supplementary Table 2 and *http://www.sanger.ac.uk/genetics/CGP/Studies/)*. Of these, 921 were single base substitutions, 78 were small insertions or deletions and 8 were complex changes, usually double nucleotide substitutions. Of the single base substitutions, 620 encoded mis-sense changes, 54 caused nonsense changes, 28 were at highly conserved positions of splice junctions and 219 were synonymous (silent) mutations

So the most common form of somatic mutations are nucleotide (single base) substitutions

PAPER 3 (SET 2)

139. Regarding end point of phase 2 trial, true is:

(a) Response to drug in case of cytotoxic drugs

(b) Progression free survival is the end point used in cystostatic drugs

(c) None of the above

(d) Both

Ans: (d) Both

Explanation

Traditional RR-based endpoints have done reasonably well historically, but simpler and more robust and efficient phase II endpoints are needed, particularly when evaluating novel therapeutics. PFS, although a validated surrogate of OS in many tumors, generally results in larger phase II trials. Some investigators have attempted to improve the efficiency of RR by including coprimary endpoints (multinomial endpoints) or by exploring novel uses of tumor measurement data

Response

In cytotoxics response assessed with response to drugs and with cytostatic drugs PFS is used as an endpoint

140. Phase 3 clinical trial, false is:

(a) Patient centred

(b) Endpoint is overall survival

(c) Endpoint for adjuvant therapy in advanced stage may be disease free survival

(d) Non-randomized

Ans: (d) Non-randomized

Explanation

There is generally a role for both randomized and non-randomized trials in drug development. The non-randomized format can in some cases be used for determining which regimens are sufficiently promising for randomized phase III evaluation and in clinical settings in which outcome is uniformly poor. For major questions of public health importance, unless the expected treatment effect on outcome is very large, the need for reliable answers dictates the use of randomized phase III trials. Most of the phase III trials are randomised to find the difference between two drugs

Regarding the potential for pragmatic, Bayesian and adaptive trial designs to enhance patient centeredness within a clinical trial setting. There are characteristics specific to pragmatic, Bayesian, and adaptive clinical trials that offer potential improvements to the clinical trial process, which frequently is neither patient centered (in terms of the evidence generated, population studied) nor patient friendly (in terms of meeting information needs)

Initially, overall survial was considered as a gold standard end point of phase III trial. In recent trials with immunotherapy or Tyrosine kinase inhibitors PFS is considered the bench mark endpoint rather than OS

Appropriate endpoints for phase II include measures of anti-tumour activity such as Overall Response Rate (ORR) or reduction of a tumor marker (e.g., PSA response rate). Progression-free survival (PFS) or percent without progression at a given time are also appropriate endpoints in phase II trials, especially if they are randomised. Identification of biomarkers is important in early phase trials. New endpoints such as reduction in circulating tumor cells (CTCs) are under investigation

While OS is a preferred endpoint and not subject to bias, the survival time for patients with many types of cancer is (fortunately) quite long. This is especially true for trials of adjuvant therapy. Disease-Free Survival (DFS), also known as Relapse-Free Survival (RFS), is often used as a primary endpoint in phase III trials of adjuvant therapy. Progression-Free Survival (PFS) is used commonly as a primary endpoint in phase III trials evaluating treatment of metastatic cancer. Since the size of a trial is determined by the number of "events" and recurrence or progression of cancer usually occurs before death, trials with DFS or PFS as the primary endpoint can be evaluated earlier and require a smaller sample. Some investigators also prefer these endpoints because they are not influenced by subsequent therapies

141. All are GnRH agonists *except:*

(a) Goserelin (b) Degarelix

(c) Leuprolide (d) Triptorelin

Ans: (b) Degarelix

(Devita, Page 279)

142. False regarding clinical trial is:

(a) Power is directly proportional to sample size, follow up and size of true difference

(b) 2 sided significance level better than single sided

(c) Overall survival includes death only

(d) Disease free survival includes prevalence, disease recurrence and death

Ans: (d) Disease free survival includes prevalence, disease recurrence and death

Explanation

A one-sided significance level represents the probability, by chance alone, of obtaining a difference as large as and in the same direction as that actually observed. A two-sided significance level represents the probability of obtaining by chance a difference in either direction as large in absolute magnitude as that actually observed. The two-sided significance level is usually twice the one-sided significance level. A two-sided significance level of .05 has become widely accepted as a standard level of evidence for phase III clinical trials

The probability of obtaining a statistically significant result when the treatments differ in effectiveness is called the power of the trial. As the sample size and extent of follow-up increases, the power increases. The power depends critically, however, on the size of the true difference in effectiveness of the two treatments. When the primary endpoint is overall survival, the events are deaths; for disease-free survival curves, events are deaths or recurrences

Control groups cannot be assigned if the disease is rapidly fatal and can use only historical controls

143. True regarding clinical trial:

(a) Factorial designs used for comparison of therapy (b) Bayesian model involves larger sample size

(c) Confidence interval less useful than significance levels (d) Bayesian methods use bayes theorem

Ans: (c) Confidence interval less useful than significance levels

Explanation

In *probability theory* and statistics, Bayes' theorem (alternatively Bayes' law or Bayes' rule) describes the *probability* of an *event,* based on prior knowledge of conditions that might be related to the event. For example, if cancer is related to age, then, using Bayes' theorem, a person's age can be used to more accurately assess the probability that they have cancer, compared to the assessment of the probability of cancer made without knowledge of the person's age

The factorial design is one approach to improving the efficiency of phase III clinical trials by using the same patients to answer more than one therapeutic question. For example, consider a two-by-two factorial design involving factor A, whether drug A1 or A2 is used for induction, and factor B, whether drug B1 or B2 is used for consolidation. There are four treatment groups: A1B1, A1B2, A2B1 and A2B2. Although there are four treatment groups, the average effect of each treatment factor can be evaluated using all of the patients. To compare A1 to A2, you ignore factor B or average the factor A treatment effect over the two factor B strata

For the analysis of such trials, confidence intervals rather than statistical significance tests should be emphasized. The confidence interval for the true difference of effectiveness gives a much clearer picture of which differences are consistent with the data. Makuch and Simon and Durrleman and Simon discuss this approach for planning and monitoring therapeutic equivalence trials

144. Regarding intention to treat analysis, false is:

(a) All randomized patients included
(b) Dropouts are excluded
(c) All go through phase 3
(d) None of the above

Ans: (b) Dropouts are excluded

Explanation

INTENTION-TO-TREAT ANALYSIS

The intention-to-treat principle indicates that all randomized patients should be included in the primary analysis of the trial. For cancer trials, this has often been interpreted to mean all "eligible" randomized patients. Excluding patients from analysis because of treatment deviations, early death, or patient withdrawal can severely distort the results. Often, excluded patients have poorer outcomes than do those who are not excluded. Investigators frequently rationalize that the poor outcome experienced by a patient was due to lack of compliance to treatment, but the direction of causality may be the reverse. For example, in the Coronary Drug Project, the 5-year mortality for poor adherents to the placebo regimen was 28.3%, significantly greater than the 15.1% experienced by good adherents to the placebo regimen. In randomized trials, there may be poorer compliance in one treatment group than the other, or the reasons for poor compliance may differ. Excluding patients, or analyzing them separately (which is equivalent to excluding them), for reasons other than eligibility is generally considered unacceptable. The intention-to-treat analysis with all eligible randomized patients should be the primary analysis. If the conclusions of a study depend on exclusions, these conclusions are suspect. The treatment plan should be viewed as a policy to be evaluated. The treatment intended cannot be delivered uniformly to all patients, but all eligible patients should generally be evaluable in phase III trials

Droup outs should not be excluded they should be included in the intent to treat analysis, which is the most important factor to analyse the results

145. Publication bias is:

(a) Only favorable data published
(b) Non favorable data not published
(c) Non favorable data published in less known journal
(d) All of the above

Ans: (d) All of the above

Explanation

An additional factor to consider is that of publication bias, which denotes the preference of journals to publish positive rather than negative results. A negative result may not be published at all, particularly from a small trial. If it is published, it is likely to appear in a less widely read journal than it would if the result were positive

146. Criteria for discontinuation of TKI in chronic myeloid leukemia?

(a) Age more than or equal to 18 years of age
(b) Chronic phase CML with no previous blastic phase. They can have previous accelerated phase
(c) Prior evidence of quantifiable BCR-ABL transcript
(d) Stable molecular response MR 4 BCR-ABL less than or equal to 0.01% in 4 or more than 2 years

Ans: (b) Chronic phase CML with no previous blastic phase. They can have previous accelerated phase

147. Regarding cohort study, false is:

(a) Cumulative incidence ratio or risk ratio used
(b) Incidence density ratio or rate ratio used
(c) Exposure odds ratio used
(d) Probability odds ratio calculated

Ans: (c) Exposure odds ratio used

Explanation

In a cohort study, the incidence of disease in the exposed group and the unexposed group is compared. The incidence measure can be cumulative incidence or incidence density, depending on the availability of data. When comparing the incidence in the two groups, both relative differences and absolute differences can be assessed. In cohort studies, the relative risk of developing the disease is expressed as the ratio of the cumulative incidence in the exposed group to that in the unexposed group, which is also called cumulative incidence ratio or risk ratio

If we have data on the exact person-time of follow-up for every subject, we can also calculate an incidence density ratio (also called rate ratio) in a similar way. In addition to risk ratio and rate ratio, another relative measure called probability odds ratio can be calculated in cohort studies

The probability odds of disease is the number of subjects who developed a disease divided by the number of subjects who did not develop the disease, and the probability odds ratio is the probability odds in the exposed group divided by the probability odds in the unexposed group

Cohort design is the best way to study the natural history of a disease. There is usually a clear temporal relationship between an exposure and a disease as all the subjects are free of the disease at the beginning of the follow-up (it can be a problem if a subject has a subclinical disease such as undetected prostate cancer). Furthermore, multiple diseases can be studied with respect to the same exposure

Exposure odds ratio is used in cross-sectional studies whereas cumulative incidence ratio, incidence density ratio and probability odds ratio all calculated using cohort study

(Devita, 11th Edition, Page 346)

148. False about case-control study is:

(a) Population based control is most common
(b) Hospital based control is most commonly used
(c) Selection bias and recall bias can be observed
(d) Case is her own control in cross over study

Ans: (b) Hospital based control is most commonly used

Explanation

Case-control design is an alternative to cohort design for the evaluation of the relationship between an exposure and a disease (or any other health condition)

A case-control approach compares the odds of past exposure between cases and noncases (controls) and uses the exposure odds ratio as an estimate for relative risk

There are two main types of Case-control studies: Case-based case-control studies and case-control studies within defined cohorts. Some variations of the case-control design also exist. For instance, if the effect of an exposure is transient, sometimes a case can be used as his or her own control (case-crossover design). In case based case-control studies, cases and controls are selected at a given point in time from a hypothetical cohort (i.e., at the end of follow-up)

In general, a case-control design tends to be more susceptible to biases than a cohort design. Such biases include but are not limited to selection bias when choosing and enrolling subjects (especially controls) and recall bias when obtaining data from the subjects. The status of the subjects (i.e., case or control) may affect how they recall and report previous exposures, some of which occurred years or even decades ago

The most common types of controls include population-based controls (often selected through random digit dialing in case-control studies of cancer etiology), hospital controls and friend controls. The advantages and disadvantages of different types of controls have been nicely summarized by Wacholder *et al.*

Case-control studies are often population based, an important factor in avoiding many kinds of ascertainment bias

149. Errors in epidemiological study include:

(a) Chance
(b) Bias
(c) Confounding
(d) All of the above

Answer: (d) All of the above

Explanation

Errors can be differential (systematic) or non-differential (random)

Random error–use of invalid outcome measure that equally misclassifies cases and controls

Differential or systematic error–use of invalid measures that misclassifies cases in one direction and controls in another direction

The term bias is used for systematic error

Confounding factor is a one which is associated with both the exposure and disease but not occurring as a consequence of the exposure. Be associated with outcome but not an intermediary

Errors of measurement in epidemiological studies

Different types of bias are reporting bias, recall bias, selection bias

While the results of an epidemiological study may reflect the true effect of an exposure(s) on the development of the outcome under investigation, it should always be considered that the findings may in fact be due to an alternative explanation

Such alternative explanations may be due to the effects of chance (random error), bias or confounding, which may produce spurious results, leading us to conclude the existence of a valid statistical association when one does not exist, or alternatively the absence of an association when one is truly present

Observational studies are particularly susceptible to the effects of chance, bias and confounding, and these need to be considered at both the design and analysis stage of an epidemiological study so that their effects can be minimized

(Internet)

150. Confounding error is:

(a) Associated with exposure
(b) Associated with disease independantly
(c) Not an intermediate step
(d) All of the above

Answer: (d) All of the above

Explanation

As explained in the above question, the definition of the confounding factor is–it is associated with the exposure and disease but not an intermediary to disease

151. False statement is:

(a) Epigenetics in non-inheritable
(b) Epigenetics is modified by environment and lifestyle
(c) Metagenomics involve microbe genomes
(d) Metabolomics involve metabolites

Ans: (a) Epigenetics in non-inheritable

Explanation

Epigenetic gene silencing is a complex series of events that includes DNA hypermethylation of CpG islands within gene-promoter regions, histone deacetylation, methylation or phosphorylation, or histone demethylation. The overall level of genomic methylation is reduced in cancer (global hypomethylation), but hypermethylation of promoter regions of specific genes is a common event that is often associated with transcriptional inactivation of specific genes

Epigenetics are heritable processes that affect gene function independent of changes in DNA sequence and can play a central role in tumor development, maintenance, and response to therapy.The most studied modes of epigenetic regulation in cancer include DNA methylation and histone modification

(Devita, 11th Edition, Page 1242)

Metagenomics focuses on environmental genomics of microbiome that resides in our body, influencing the biologic functions and health status of human beings. Three examples of research have provided new insights into the etiology of cancer. One is the interaction of microbiome with colon mucosa in the development of colon cancer, in which microbiome-garnered carcinogens, immunity, and inflammation are considered to play an important role. The second one is the bacteria-involved bile acid metabolism and liver cancer. Based on animal experiments, it is hypothesized that a high-fat diet changes gut microbiota, which produce cytotoxic bile acid metabolites that are reabsorbed through the enterohepatic circulation, causing liver damage and inflammation, which have tumorigenetic effects in the long run.The third one is the metabolism of estrogen in relation to breast cancer risk. Estrogens are metabolized in the liver and excreted in bile fluid and urine. A significant amount of estrogens in the gut are reabsorbed through the enterohepatic circulation after gut bacteria with β-glucuronidase activity deconjugate the estrogen metabolites. The bacterial β-glucuronidase activity is influenced by diet and bacterial context, which in turn affect the circulating level of estrogens and subsequently the risk of breast cancer

Metabolomics is a systematic analysis of metabolome composed of small molecule metabolites, such as amino acids, free fatty acids, and sugars, in a biologic system, including cell, tissue, blood, urine, body fluid and feces

The analysis catches not only endogenous but exogenous metabolites and the exogenous ones are from environmental exposure, diet, food supplement, microbiome metabolism, substance use and iatrogenic sources

Two types of technologies are often used for analysis of metabolomes: nuclear magnetic resonance and mass spectrometry coupled with liquid or gas chromatograph. These analyses can add tremendous value to epidemiologic studies, but currently, many findings on cancer in humans are from small studies that analyzed tumor specimens or blood samples collected at or after diagnosis. Thus, most of the studies could only address diagnosis or prognosis, but not etiology. Interestingly, one study analyzed metabolomics in the blood samples of patients with pancreatic cancer collected before diagnosis, and it found that branched-chain amino acids were elevated in the samples before diagnosis, with animal experiments confirming the change as an early event

Epigenetics is a heritable process as mentioned above so false answer is the options saying epigenetis is not heritable

152. True about biomarkers:

(a) Genotypic markers change with time

(b) Genotypic markers influenced by disease and treatment

(c) Phenotypic markers change with time

(d) Phenotypic markers not influenced by disease process

Ans: (c) Phenotypic markers change with time

Explanation

Two types of molecular markers, genotypic and phenotypic markers, can be considered

Genotypic markers refer to nucleotide sequences of genomic DNA and all other molecules are considered phenotypic markers, including the chemical modifications on DNA, such as cytosine methylation. The distinction between the two is whether a marker changes its status or quantity over time. Genotypic markers generally do not change over time and are not affected by the development of a disease, whereas phenotypic markers are likely to change over time or to be influenced by the presence of a disease, either itself or treatment associated with it

If measurements of a phenotypic marker are made from the specimens that are collected after or at the time of cancer diagnosis, investigators will have difficulties determining the status of the phenotypic marker before the cancer was diagnosed

A disease condition, however, does not affect genotypic markers such as SNPs and therefore, a temporal relationship can be easily established even if the samples are collected after the disease is diagnosed

Based on this distinction, one can evaluate genotypic markers either in case-control or cohort studies, but a case-control study would be the design of choice because of efficiency and cost-effectiveness

A prospective cohort study design is ideal for phenotypic markers. Investigators, however, may use other study designs if they can demonstrate that the disease status does not influence the phenotypic markers of interest. To reduce study cost, investigators usually use nested case-control or case-cohort designs to avoid analysis of specimens from the entire cohort. The main purpose to choose a cohort study design for molecular epidemiology investigation is to ensure that biospecimens are collected before the development of a disease so that a temporal relationship between a marker and disease development can be established

So from above explanation we understand phenotypic markers change with time and not genotypic markers

(Devita, 11th Edition, Page 352; Epidemiology–Sabiston)

153. Hypothesis testing includes all *except:*

(a) Superiority trials

(b) Equivalence trial

(c) Non-inferiority trial

(d) None of the above

Ans: (d) None of the above

Explanation

When the aim of the randomized controlled trial (RCT) is to show that one treatment is superior to another, a statistical test is employed and the trial (test) is called a superiority trial (test). Often a non-significant superiority test is wrongly interpreted as proof of no difference between the two treatments. Proving that two treatments are equal in performance is impossible with statistical tools; at most, one can show that they are equivalent. In an equivalence trial, the statistical test aims at showing that two treatments are not too different in characteristics, where "not too different" is defined in a clinical manner. Finally, in a non-inferiority trial, the aim is to show that an experimental treatment is not (much) worse than a standard treatment

(Bull NYU Hosp Jt Dis. 2008;66(2):150-4)

154. Will Rogers Phenomenon is:

(a) Subject bias
(b) Stage migration
(c) Length bias
(d) Aerobic glycolysis

Ans: (b) Stage migration

Explanation

The 'Will Rogers Phenomenon' is an apparent epidemiological paradox named after a remark made by the humorist Will Rogers about migration during the American economic depression of the 1930's: "When the Okies left Oklahoma and moved to California, they raised the average intelligence level in both states." In 1985, Alvan Feinstein proposed the name 'Will Rogers Phenomenon' to describe the 'stage migration', he observed in patients with cancer. Changes in the criteria for assigning patients to the various stages of a disease can produce spurious improvements in stage-specific prognosis, even though the outcome of individual patients has not changed. In oncology, new imaging tools allowed detection of cancer metastases before they became evident clinically. In consequence, more patients are classified into the more severe metastatic disease stage from the less severe single tumor stage. Such a 'stage migration' resulted in an improved survival of patients in both the less and the more severe disease stages

155. Incorrect match is:

(a) Charges–amount spent for therapy
(b) Charges–amount requested for health services
(c) Costs–amount which is already spent to deliver health care
(d) Cost benefit–assessed in dollars

Ans: (a) Charges–amount spent for therapy

Explanation

Also correct match is:
Cost utility–assessed by quality adjusted life year
Cost effectiveness–difference in outcomes
Appropriateness–meeting standard criteria
Efficacy–testing in controlled environment
Effectiveness–outcomes in usual practice

Charges are the amount of money requested for health services and supplies. By comparison, costs are the actual amount of money spent to deliver care. The perspective of the study defines which costs are necessary to ascertain and include in the analysis. For example, although a societal perspective would include the costs of care and the direct and indirect monetary costs associated with care (e.g., travel and boarding expenses, lost productivity at work, caretaker expenses), a hospital's perspective would be more selective, not considering the patient's out-of-pocket expenses but including payer reimbursement

There are three common approaches to comparing cost outcomes. A cost-benefit analysis quantifies health benefit in terms of dollars. The great challenge with this approach is assigning a dollar value to a life or a specific health outcome. A cost-utility analysis quantifies health benefits in terms of quality-adjusted life-years (QALYs). Utilities are a measure of overall quality of life, usually scaled between 0 and 1, with 1 being perfect health, and are multiplied by survival time to determine QALYs

(Sabiston, 20th Edition, Page 196)

156. False regarding variant RCT is:

(a) Pragmatic trials involve control replaced by usual practice
(b) Step wedge design is parallel and non-sequential
(c) Factorial design tests combination therapy and synergistic effect
(d) Adaptive trial uses and adapts prior response information

Ans: (b) Step wedge design is parallel and non-sequential

Explanation

Also true is:

- Cluster RCT employed in testing safety checklist policy
- Step wedge design involves all participants to have received intervention
- Step wedge design is sequential and non parallel

VARIATIONS ON RANDOMIZED TRIALS

Although RCTs can offer the strongest evidence pointing toward causality, they are not ideal for all research questions. Numerous variations in the RCT design exist to allow assessment of effectiveness of an intervention across broad populations of patients and practice environments. The pragmatic RCT, in which the traditional "control" arm is replaced with "usual practice" is a contemporary methodology that capitalizes on the benefits of randomization but also accounts for variable practice environments and settings. In cluster-randomized trials, groups of subjects, rather than individuals, are randomly assigned. Cluster randomized trials permit researchers to study interventions that cannot be directed toward selected individuals (e.g., implementing a surgical safety checklist as a hospital policy) and can control for "contamination" across individuals in the same cluster (e.g.,one surgeon's use of preoperative antibiotics may influence another surgeon to do the same). In step-wedge randomized trials, the study intervention is sequentially rolled out to individuals or clusters of participants. The order in which participants receive the intervention is random, but all participants have received it by the end of the study. Step-wedge designs are used in situations in which a true RCT parallel design may be impractical for logistical or financial reasons or the intervention is thought to cause more good than harm (so withholding it in a true RCT would be unethical). In factorial RCTs, participants are assigned to a group that receives a combination of interventions (or non-interventions), allowing researchers to compare multiple effects with a smaller sample size than a traditional RCT. Finally, adaptive trials allow for key trial characteristics (e.g., treatment arms, eligibility and sample size) to evolve in response to information accrued in the trial itself. This trial methodology (sometimes termed personalized medicine trials) is increasingly being applied to patient-centered outcomes research where focus on certain subpopulations may evolve with the trial

Step wedge design is sequential and not parallel so false is the option saying it is paralled and non-sequential

(Sabiston, 20th Edition, Page 198)

157. Bonferroni correction employed in:

(a) Multiple comparisons in a study
(b) Eliminate crossover
(c) Eliminate confounding
(d) All of the above

Ans (a) Multiple comparisons in a study

Explanation

Two types of errors can occur with hypothesis testing. An α (or type I) error occurs when one observes a difference in outcomes when such a difference does not actually exist. If the research question and analysis have not been specified a priori or numerous statistical tests are performed on many subgroups, a type I error can occur. For example, if a threshold of 5% were considered statistically significant, 5 of 100 statistical tests could potentially demonstrate a statistically significant finding that is attributable to chance alone (a false-positive finding). If one repeats a comparative analysis in different subgroups (i.e., multiple comparisons), there are more opportunities to observe a false-positive result

When multiple comparisons are necessary, corrections (e.g., Bonferroni correction) to the P value can be made in an attempt to safeguard against type I errors. A β (or type II) error occurs when no difference in outcomes is observed when a difference truly exists (a false-negative finding). This type of error occurs when a study has insufficient power to detect true differences in outcomes between groups. Power is directly related to sample size and the size of the observed difference

(Sabiston, 20th Edition, Page 201)

158. False regarding confidence interval:

(a) Not significant if includes 1 in relative risk

(b) Not significant if includes 0 in absolute risk

(c) Significance level more useful measure than confidence level

(d) Measure of uncertainty

Ans: (c) Significance level more useful measure than confidence level

Explanation

Also true is:

Wide interval lacks precision

Tight interval means minimum uncertainty

Hypothesis testing is also possible by examining confidence interval (CI). Summary measures of the difference between groups are provided as an estimated ratio (outcomes in the study group divided by outcomes in the standard or control group) or as an absolute difference, with a 95% CI. The CI provides an estimate of the uncertainty around a given value; a wide CI indicates a lack of precision, whereas a tight (small) interval would be indicative of minimal uncertainty. When the summary measure is an odds or relative risk ratio, a CI inclusive of 1.0 indicates no statistical difference in outcomes. If the summary measure is the absolute difference or relative risk, a CI inclusive of 0 indicates no statistically significant difference

As described in earlier questions, confidence level is more useful than significance so false is the third option

(Sabiston, 20th Edition, Page 201)

PAPER 4

159. Most frequent load of mutation occurs in:

(a) Melanoma and lung
(b) Colon and breast
(c) Prostate
(d) Childhood and haematological

Ans: (a) Melanoma and lung

Explanation

Recently, the number of somatic mutations per megabase of sequencing, also known as tumor mutation burden (TMB), is being evaluated as a potential biomarker of response to immunotherapy in patients with various cancer types. The hypothesis is that antitumor immune responses can be stimulated by the numerous mutation associated neoantigens in hypermutated tumors. Some evidence suggests that TMB can predict better outcomes after anti-PD-1/PD-L1 immunotherapy in melanoma, NSCLC, as well as in other tumor types

(Devita, 11 Edition, Page 148)

160. True statement is:

(a) Mountains are in high frequency involves most of driver mutations
(b) Hills are low frequency involves few drivers
(c) Hills provide selective advantage to tumors
(d) All of the above

Ans: (c) Hills provide selective advantage to tumors

Explanation

For most cancer types, this landscape consists of a small number of "mountains" (genes altered in a high percentage of tumors) and a much larger number of "hills" (genes altered infrequently)

Data suggest that the vast majority of identified somatic DNA alterations are passenger mutations, representing harmless, biologically neutral changes that do not contribute to oncogenesis. Conversely, driver mutations confer a growth advantage on the cell in which they occur and appear to be implicated in cancer development

When specific driver mutations are catalogued, a bimodal cancer genomic landscape appears, comprising a small number of commonly mutated gene mountains among hundreds of infrequently mutated gene hills. Gene mountains correspond to the most frequently mutated genes found within breast tumors, such as TP53, CDH1, phosphatidylinositol 3-kinase (PI3K), cyclin D, PTEN and AKT. Each individual gene hill, on the other hand, is typically found in less than 5% of breast tumors. This substantial heterogeneity of DNA mutations among breast tumors may explain the wide variations in phenotypes, in terms of both tumor behavior and responsiveness to therapy. Historically, the focus of genetic research has been on the gene mountains; however, emerging data suggest that it is actually the gene hills that play a more pivotal role in breast cancer, consistent with the idea that having a large number of mutations, each associated with a small survival advantage, drives tumor progression

(Devita, 11 Edition, Page 2247)

161. False about driver mutations:

(a) Impact the phenotype
(b) Mendelian pattern
(c) Most are hills
(d) Recurring mutations

Ans: (c) Most are hills

Explanation

Driver mutations impact the phenotype and have Mendelian pattern of inheritance and most are mountains, and to differentiate between passenger and driver mutation SIFT (Sorting Intolerant From Tolerant) technology is used. The most reliable indicator that a gene was selected for and therefore is highly likely to be pathogenic is the identification of recurrent mutations, whether at the same exact amino acid position or in neighbouring amino acid positions in different patients. More than that, if somatic alterations in the same gene occur very frequently (mountains in the tumor genome landscape), these can be confidently classified as drivers. For example, cancer alleles that are identified in multiple patients and different tumor types, such as those found in KRAS, TP53, PTEN and PIK3CA, are clearly selected for during tumorigenesis. However, most genes discovered thus far are mutated in a relatively small fraction of tumors (hills), and it has been clearly shown that genes that are mutated in less than 1% of patients can still act as drivers

162. Drug used for geftinib resistant exon 20 mutation lung cancer is:

(a) Osmeritinib
(b) Ofatinib
(c) Afatinib
(d) None of the above

Ans: (a) Osmeritinib

Explanation

Identification of this resistance mechanism in tumors collected at the time of disease progression on the EGFR inhibitors erlotinib and gefitinib led to the development of osimertinib, a third-generation EGFR kinase inhibitor with clinical activity in erlotinib-resistant T790M-mutant lung cancers

(Devita, 11th Edition, Page 587)

163. False regarding liquid biopsies is:

(a) Used for screening
(b) Involves ctDNA
(c) Evaluates tumor burden
(d) Useful for monitoring response

Ans: (c) Evaluates tumor burden

Explanation

Diagnostic analysis of circulating DNA in plasma is also emerging as a novel and potentially less invasive method to detect and analyze tumor-derived DNA for mutations and translocations that are predictive biomarkers of kinase inhibitor response. This "liquid biopsy" approach circumvents the need for invasive biopsies in order to collect tumor tissue for molecular analysis. It can also facilitate the identification of emerging resistance mutations through serial sampling of plasma in patients receiving kinase inhibitors, which may allow for the early use of combinatorial therapies that prevent or delay the emergence of drug-resistant cancer cells

(Devita, 11th Edition, Page 588)

Biomarker detection can occur in either a targeted manner for specific mutations (e.g., by quantitative or digital PCR) or in an untargeted fashion by next-generation sequencing (NGS), which is particularly advantageous for revealing *tumor heterogeneity.* Therefore, liquid biopsies have generated a lot of enthusiasm because biofluid collection, especially blood, is minimally invasive and could bypass the need for an invasive, needle or surgical tissue biopsy. Additionally, the ease of collection means that repeated longitudinal analysis is possible, for instance to monitor treatment response, *development of resistance,* and to detect *minimal residual disease* (MRD) in patients. Liquid biopsies have also been suggested as a possible screening method for *early cancer detection* if the method could be made *sufficiently specific and sensitive* to detect low level biomarkers at the start of tumorigenesis

Liquid biopsy has not become diagnostic as of now and we need a tissue biopsy for diagnosis of cancer

164. False statement is:

(a) Clinical validity relates to disease or response to therapy
(b) Clinical utility relates to patient benefit
(c) Analytical validity relates to test accuracy
(d) None of the above

Ans: (d) None of above

Explanation

The ideal cancer biomarker is only associated with the disease and not the normal state. The utility of the biomarker largely depends on what the clinical effect the biomarker predicts for, how large the effect is and how strong the evidence is for the effect. Biomarkers for clinical applications require a high level of analytic validity, clinical validity and clinical utility. Analytic validity refers to the ability of the overall testing process to accurately detect and, in many cases, measure the biomarker. Clinical validity is the ability of a biomarker to predict a particular disease behavior or response to therapy. Clinical utility, arguably the most difficult to assess, addresses whether the information available from the biomarker is actually beneficial for patient care

(Devita, 11th Edition, Page 129)

165. Polymorphism is:

(a) Deleterious
(b) Present in less than 1% population
(c) Also known as nonsense mutation
(d) Present in 1% or more of population

Ans: (d) Present in 1% or more of population

Explanation

Biomarker Genetics–It is important to recognize that many genetic variations occur within the healthy population. Formally, the term polymorphism is used to describe genetic differences present in ≥1% of the human population, whereas mutation describes less frequent differences. However, in practice, polymorphism is often used to describe a nonpathogenic genetic change and mutation a deleterious change, regardless of their frequencies

(Devita, 11th Edition, Page 129)

166. Trials in prostate cancer for Enzalutamide is all *except:*

(a) Prosper
(b) Affirm
(c) Terrain
(d) Stampede

Ans: (d) Stampede

Explanation

Docetaxel trials includes:

- Stampede
- Chaarted
- Getug

167. Most common mutation in cancers is:

(a) Loss of function
(b) Gain of function
(c) Both
(d) None of above

Ans: (a) Loss of function

Explanation

Loss of function mutations, either through point mutations or deletions in tumor suppression genes such as CDKN2A and TP53 are very common in human cancers

(Devita, 11th Edition, Page 130)

168. Most common form of structural chromosomal alteration is:

(a) Point mutation
(b) Copy number variation
(c) Chromothripsy
(d) None of the above

Ans: (b) Copy number variation

Explanation

Copy number variation (CNV) is a phenomenon in which sections of the genome are repeated and the number of repeats in the genome varies between individuals in the human population. Copy number variation is a type of *structural variation:* specifically, it is a type of *duplication* or *deletion* event that affects a considerable number of base pairs. However, note that although modern genomics research is mostly focused on human genomes, copy number variations also occur in a variety of other organisms including *E. coli*. Recent research indicates that approximately two thirds of the entire human genome is composed of repeats and 4.8–9.5% of the human genome can be classified as copy number variations. In mammals, copy number variations play an important role in generating necessary variation in the population as well as disease phenotype

169. True statement is:

(a) Rb responds to external stimuli
(b) p53 responds to intrinsic stressors
(c) Beclin-1 in autophagy
(d) All of the above

Ans: (d) All of the above

Explanation

Beclin-1 is a member of the Bcl-2 family of apoptotic regulatory proteins, and its BH3 domain allows it to bind the Bcl-2/Bcl-XL proteins. Stress sensor–coupled BH3-containing proteins (e.g., Bim, Noxa) can displace Beclin-1 from its association with Bcl-2/Bcl-XL, enabling the liberated Beclin-1 to trigger autophagy, much as they can release proapoptotic Bax and Bak to trigger apoptosis. Hence, stress-transducing Bcl-2–related proteins can induce apoptosis and/or autophagy depending on the physiologic state of the cell. Through p53 and RB proteins apoptosis is effected through both intrinsic and extrinsic pathways

170. False about TGF beta is:

(a) Fibroblast proliferation
(b) Involved in angiogenesis
(c) Potent immunostimulant
(d) Implicated in EMT

Ans: (c) Potent immunostimulant

Explanation

Transforming growth factor beta (TGF-beta) plays an important role in tumor initiation and progression, functioning as both a suppressor and a promoter. The mechanisms underlying this dual role of TGF-beta remain unclear. TGF-beta exerts systemic immune suppression and inhibits host immunosurveillance. Neutralizing TGF-beta enhances CD8+ T-cell- and NK-cell-mediated anti-tumor immune responses. It also increases neutrophil-attracting chemokines resulting in recruitment and activation of neutrophils with an antitumor phenotype. In addition to its systemic effects, TGF-beta regulates infiltration of inflammatory/immune cells and cancer-associated fibroblasts in the tumor microenvironment causing direct changes in tumor cells. Understanding TGF-beta regulation at the interface of tumor and host immunity should provide insights into developing effective TGF-beta antagonists and biomarkers for patient selection and efficacy of TGF-beta antagonist treatment

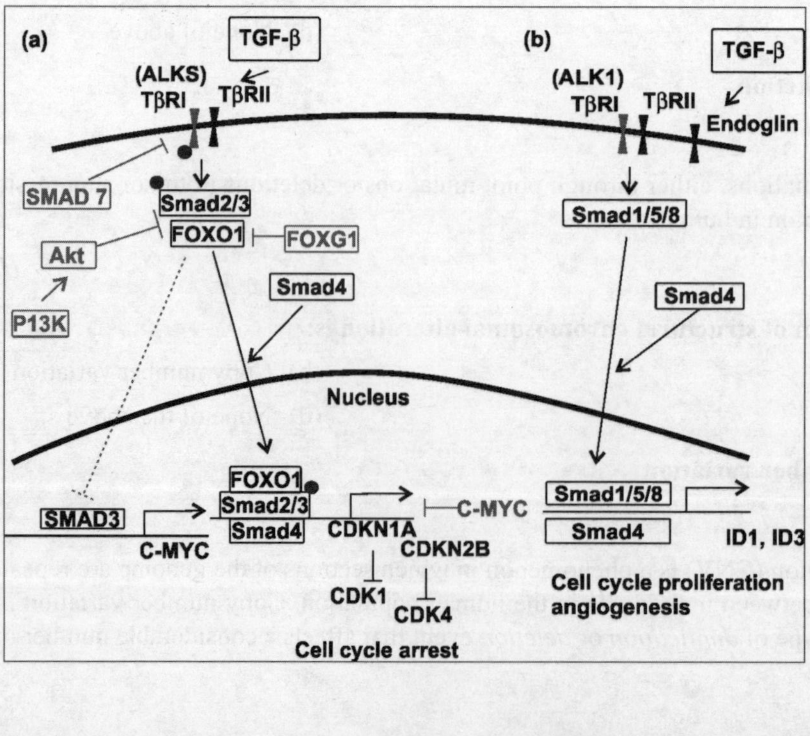

TGF-beta signaling has been shown to play an important role in EMT. In fact, adding TGF-beta to epithelial cells in culture is a convenient way to induce EMT in various epithelial cells. Although much less characterized, epithelial plasticity can also be regulated by TGF-beta-related bone morphogenetic proteins (BMPs), and BMPs have been shown to induce EMT or MET depending on the developmental context. In this review, we will discuss the induction of EMT in response to TGF-beta, and focus on the underlying signaling and transcription mechanisms

171. False about tumor vessels is:

(a) Non leaky and streamlined flow
(b) Leaky and convoluted
(c) Precocious sprouting
(d) Erratic flow with microhemorrhages

Ans: (a) Non leaky and streamlined flow

Explanation

The blood vessels produced within tumors by unbalanced mixtures of proangiogenic signals are typically aberrant: Tumor neovasculature is marked by precocious capillary sprouting, convoluted and excessive vessel branching, distorted and enlarged vessels, erratic blood flow, microhemorrhaging leading to leakage of plasma into the tissue parenchyma and abnormal levels of endothelial cell proliferation and apoptosis

(Devita, 11th Edition, Page 167)

172. Regarding epithelial-mesenchymal transition, false is:

(a) Polygonal to spindly shape
(b) Decreased motility
(c) Resistant to apoptosis
(d) Expression of matrix degrading enzymes

Ans: (b) Decreased motility

Explanation

Included among the cell-biologic traits evoked by these EMT-TFs are loss of adherens junctions concomitant with conversion from a polygonal/epithelial to a spindly/fibroblastic morphology, activation of secreted matrix-degrading enzymes, as well as increased motility and heightened resistance to apoptosis, all of which are implicated in the processes of invasion and metastasis. Several of these transcription factors can directly repress E-cadherin gene expression, thereby releasing neoplastic epithelial cells from this key suppressor of motility and invasiveness

EMT classically confers increased motility and invasion and not decreased motility

(Devita, 11 Edition, Page 169)

173. Warburg effect is:

(a) Dynamic phenomenon
(b) Tumor specific
(c) Anaerobic glycolysis
(d) Increased GLUT-4

Ans: (a) Dynamic phenomenon

Explanation

Otto Warburg first observed an anomalous characteristic of cancer cell energy metabolism. Even in the presence of oxygen, cancer cells can reprogram their glucose metabolism, and thus their energy production, leading to a state that has been termed aerobic glycolysis

Interestingly, some tumors have been found to contain two subpopulations of cancer cells that differ in their energy-generating pathways. One subpopulation consists of glucose-dependent (Warburg-effect) cells that secrete lactate, whereas cells of the second subpopulation preferentially import and utilize the lactate produced by their neighbours as their main energy source, employing part of the citric acid cycle to do so. These two populations evidently function symbiotically: The hypoxic cancer cells depend on glucose for fuel and secrete lactate as waste, which is imported and preferentially used as fuel by their more oxygenated brethren

A key signature of aerobic glycolysis is upregulation of glucose transporters, notably GLUT1, which substantially increases glucose import into the cytoplasm. Indeed, markedly increased uptake and utilization of glucose has been documented in many human tumor types, most readily by visualizing glucose uptake noninvasively using positron-emission tomography with a radiolabeled analog of glucose (18 Ffluorodeoxyglucose) as a reporter

(Devita, 11th Edition, Page 172)

174. Tumor-promoting inflammation involves:

(a) T and B lymphocytes
(b) Mast cells
(c) Both macrophages and neutrophils
(d) All of the above

Ans: (d) All of the above

Explanation

Inflammatory cells can contribute to multiple hallmark capabilities by supplying signaling molecules to the tumor microenvironment, including growth factors that sustain proliferative signaling; survival factors that limit cell death; proangiogenic factors; ECM-modifying enzymes that facilitate angiogenesis, invasion and metastasis and inductive signals that lead to activation of EMT and other hallmark-promoting programs

175. Phase 0 includes all *except:*

(a) Proof of concept
(b) Very low dose tested
(c) Measure pharmokinetic end point
(d) Measure pharmacodynamic end point

Ans: (c) Measure pharmokinetic end point

Explanation

The PD-driven phase 0 trial is a new form, designed to be a first-in-man study, often of a new agent, conducted to assess drug effect on a molecular target, by means of a pharmacodynamic (PD) assay, in a very small number of patients. Such a study is meant to be a proof of principle trial to determine whether the agent yields the PD effect predicted by pre-clinical studies. The dosage is meant to be pharmacologically active, but neither toxic nor likely to yield clinical benefit. Such a trial may be used to serve as a very early test of an agent's biologic effect, allowing for early weeding out of ineffective agents, or as an early means of determining the most promising of competing analogue agents

Rubinstein LV, Steinberg SM, Kummar S, *et al.* The statistics of phase 0 trials. Stat Med 2010;29(10):1072–1076

176. Phase 1 trial, false is:

(a) For finding out appropriate dose of drug and Subjects should have normal organ function
(b) Pharmacokinetic end point and Highest dose producing 33% toxicity is selected
(c) Subjects should have advanced disease resistant to standard therapy
(d) Diseased organ with early stage disease

Ans: (d) Diseased organ with early stage disease

Explanation

The main objectives of phase I trials have traditionally been to determine a dose that is appropriate for use in phase II and III trials and to determine information about the pharmacokinetics of distribution of the drug. Patients with advanced disease that is resistant to standard therapy but who have normal organ function are usually included in such trials. For molecularly targeted drugs, eligibility is often limited to patients whose tumors have a mutated target protein or otherwise appear driven by alteration of the target

(Devita, 11th Edition, Page 903)

177. True regarding phase 1 conventional model trial:

(a) Takes longer time and many patients

(b) Limited information on interpatient variablity and cumulative toxicity

(c) Accelerated titration model gives more parameter

(d) All of the above

Ans: (d) All of the above

Explanation

Drawbacks of conventional phase 1 trial model are:

1. They sometimes expose too many patients to subtherapeutic doses of the new drug
2. The trials may take a long time to complete
3. They provide very limited information about interpatient variability and cumulative toxicity

   More recent trial designs have been developed to address these problems
4. The accelerated titration designs permit within-patient dose escalation and use only one patient per dose level until grade 2 or greater toxicity is seen. Doses are titrated within patients to achieve grade 2 toxicity. The model includes parameters that represent the steepness of the dose-toxicity curve, the degree of interpatient variability in the location of the dose-toxicity curve, and the degree (if any) of cumulative toxicity. All these parameters are estimated from the data

The model includes parameters that represent the steepness of the dose-toxicity curve, the degree of interpatient variability in the location of the dose–toxicity curve, and the degree (if any) of cumulative toxicity. All these parameters are estimated from the data. A more limited objective is to identify a dose that is biologically active

(Devita, 11th Edition, Page 904)

178. Phase 2 trial, false statement is:

(a) Efficacy of drug tested

(b) Safety assessed

(c) Predictive biomarkers assessed and assays developed

(d) Can never be randomized

Ans: (d) Can never be randomized

Explanation

Phase 2 trials have traditionally been performed separately by tumor type in patients with the least amount of prior therapy for whom no effective therapy is available

Phase 2 trial assess the safety and efficacy

Examples of Phase 2 trials that have utilized or are utilizing an adaptive design strategy are I-SPY 2 and The BATTLE trial. I-SPY 2 is an ongoing neoadjuvant trial in breast cancer that is designed to compare the efficacy of standard therapy to the efficacy of novel drugs in combination with chemotherapy. All drugs will be evaluated within the biomarker-defined signature groups. Regimens that have a high predicted probability of being successful in a Phase 3 trial are moved forward to Phase 3 testing within sub-populations corresponding to the most promising biomarker signature(s). Regimens that have a low probability of efficacy for all biomarker signature subgroups will be dropped from further development

Phase 2 trials can be with single agent or comparing it with another drug using randomised Phase 2 trials. So in Phase 2 randomisation is done. So false statement is can never be randomised

(Devita, 11th Edition, Page 905)

PAPER 5 (SET 1)

179. Obesity plays a key epidemiological role in:

(a) Breast
(b) Colon
(c) Kidney
(d) All of the above

Ans: (d) All of the above

Explanation

In 2016, the International Agency for Research on Cancer (IARC) systematically reviewed more than 1,000 studies that investigated the relationship between obesity and cancer risk and determined there was sufficient evidence to conclude that obesity is associated with an increased risk of developing 13 different types of cancer. The increased risk of malignancy associated with obesity is strongest in endometrial cancer (relative risk, 7.1). Other cancers in which the link between obesity and risk is particularly strong include esophageal adenocarcinoma, gastric cardia, liver, renal cell and multiple myeloma (relative risks, ≥ 1.5). Cancers that are not associated with obesity are often cancers for which smoking is a strong risk factor, as smoking and obesity are inversely correlated

Strength of the Evidence for a Cancer-Preventive Effective of the Absence of Excess Adiposity, According to Cancer Site or Type

Cancer Site or Type	Strength of the Evidence in Humans	Relative Risk of the Highest BMI Category Evaluated versus Normal BMI (95% CI)
Esophagus: adenocarcinoma	Sufficient	4.8 (3.0-7.7)
Gastric cardia	Sufficient	1.8 (1.3-2.5)
Colon and rectum	Sufficient	1.3 (1.3-1.4)
Liver	Sufficient	1.8 (1.6-2.1)
Gallbladder	Sufficient	1.3 (1.2-1.4)
Pancreas	Sufficient	1.5 (1.2.-1.8)
Breast: postmenopausal	Sufficient	1.1 (1.1-1.2)
Corpus uteri	Sufficient	7.1 (6.3-8.1)
Ovary	Sufficient	1.1 (1.1-1.2)
Kidney: renal cell	Sufficient	1.8 (1.7-1.9)
Meningioma	Sufficient	1.5 (1.3-1.8)
Thyroid	Sufficient	1.1 (1.0-1.1)
Multiple myeloma	Sufficient	1.5 (1.2-2.0)
Male breast cancer	Limited	NA

(Devita, 11th Edition, Page 332)

180. Regarding obesity in breast cancer, false is:

(a) Poor survival
(b) Increased recurrence
(c) Not an independent risk factor
(d) Acts through hormonal mechanism

Ans: (c) Not an independent risk factor

Explanation

Since as per the previous explanation it is independent risk factor. It is estimated that 20% of new cancer cases and 17% of cancer-related deaths are attributable to obesity

(Devita, 11th Edition, Page 332)

181. Not a hallmark of cancer is:

(a) Self sufficiency
(b) Inducing angiogenesis
(c) Deregulating cellular energetics
(d) Mitosis

Answer: (d) Mitosis

Explanation

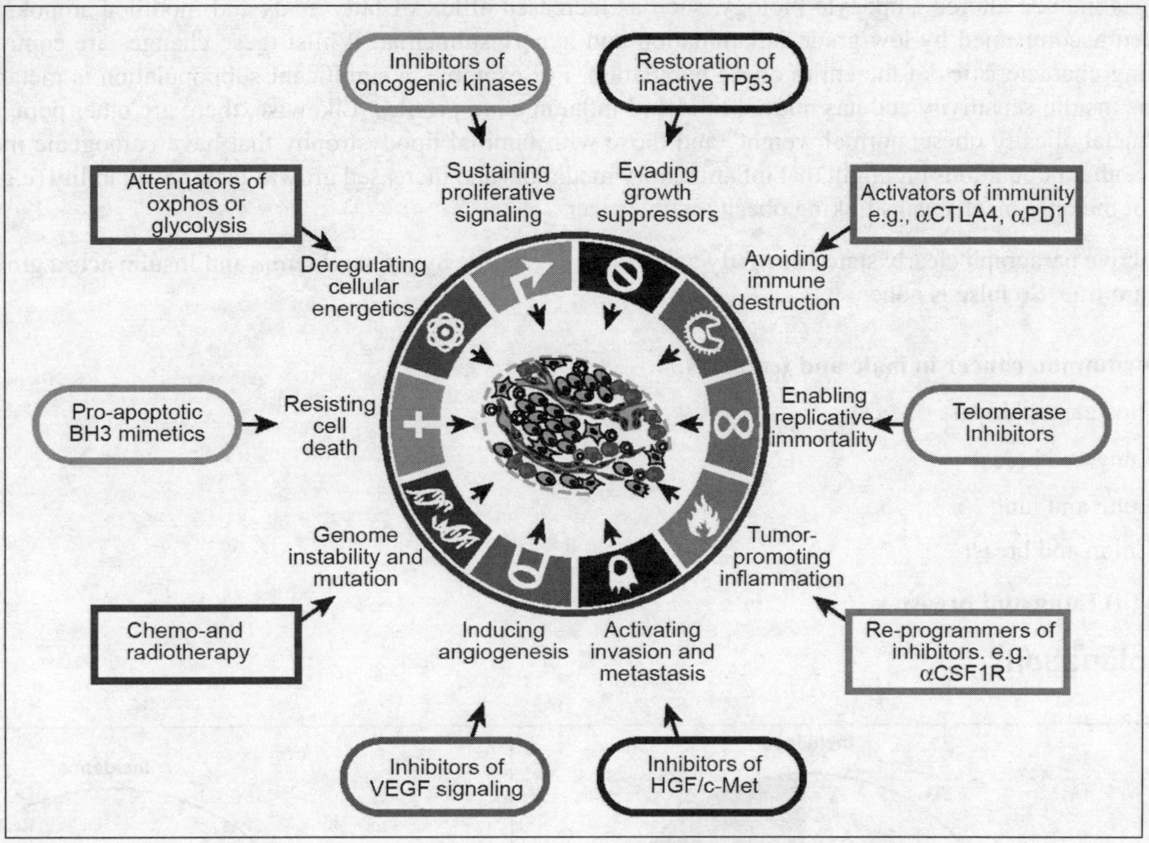

There are 8 hallmarks of cancer and 2 enabling characteristics. Mitosis is not the characteristic of cancer. It occurs any normal cell also

(Devita, 11th Edition, Page 189)

182. Emerging key enabling characteristic of cancer include all *except:*

(a) Genomic instability
(b) Tumor promoting inflammation
(c) Guardian genome mutation
(d) None of the above

Answer: (d) None of the above

Explanation

Guardian genome mutation is nothing but p53 mutation which is an important final step in carcinogenesis hence it a part of genomic instability and mutation

(Devita, 11th Edition, Page 189)

183. Regarding obesity in colon cancer, false is:

(a) FFA induced chronic hyperinsulinemia
(b) Insulin acting as a growth factor
(c) Both
(d) None

Ans: (d) None

Explanation

Obesity is defined by increased adipose mass arising from energy imbalance. The predominant cell type in adipose tissue is the adipocyte, which is the professional lipid storage cell. Alongside the adipocyte there are a number of other cell types in adipose including preadipocytes, endothelial cells and immune cells such as resident macrophages. This collective results in a highly complex organ that is central to energy homeostasis and its biology is dramatically altered in obesity. These changes include altered adipocyte biology, such as increased efflux of fatty acids and modified adipokine profile, which is often accompanied by low-grade inflammation and hyperinsulinemia. Whilst these changes are common, they are not defining characteristics of the entire obese population. For example, a significant subpopulation is metabolically healthy, retains insulin sensitivity and has normal lipid and inflammation profiles. Likewise, there are other populations, including the "metabolically obese, normal weight" and those with familial lipodystrophy that have pathogenic metabolic profiles. These other populations highlight that inflammatory mediators and increased growth factor availability (e.g., IGF-1, insulin) are not the only mechanisms linking obesity with cancer

The above paragraph clearly states free fatty acids induces chronic hyperinsulinemia and Insulin acts a growth factor, hence both are true. So false is none

184. Most common cancer in male and female is:

(a) Prostate and breast

(b) Lung and breast

(c) Lung and lung

(d) Colon and breast

Ans: (b) Lung and breast

Explanation

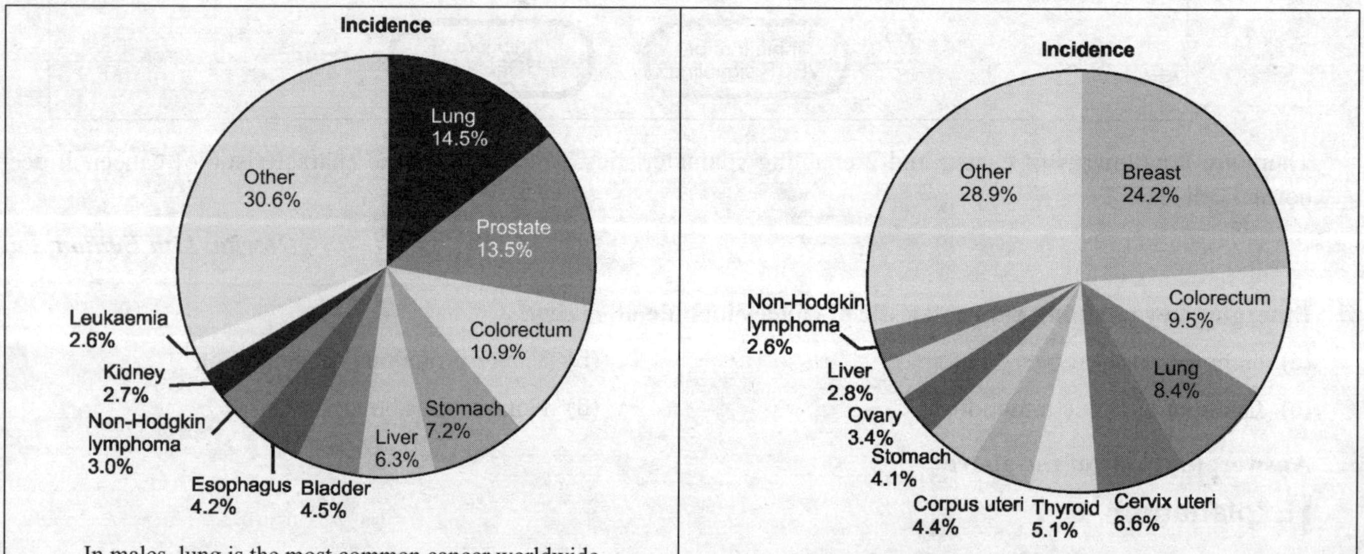

In males–lung is the most common cancer worldwide

In females–breast is the most common cancer worldwide

Globocan data 2018 says it is lung and breast

185. Regarding self-sufficiency in cancer cells true is:

(a) Paracrine factors from stroma and infiltrates

(b) Autocrine factor from stroma

(c) Acrine state never seen in cancer

(d) None of the above

Ans: (a) Paracrine factors from stroma and infiltrates

Explanation

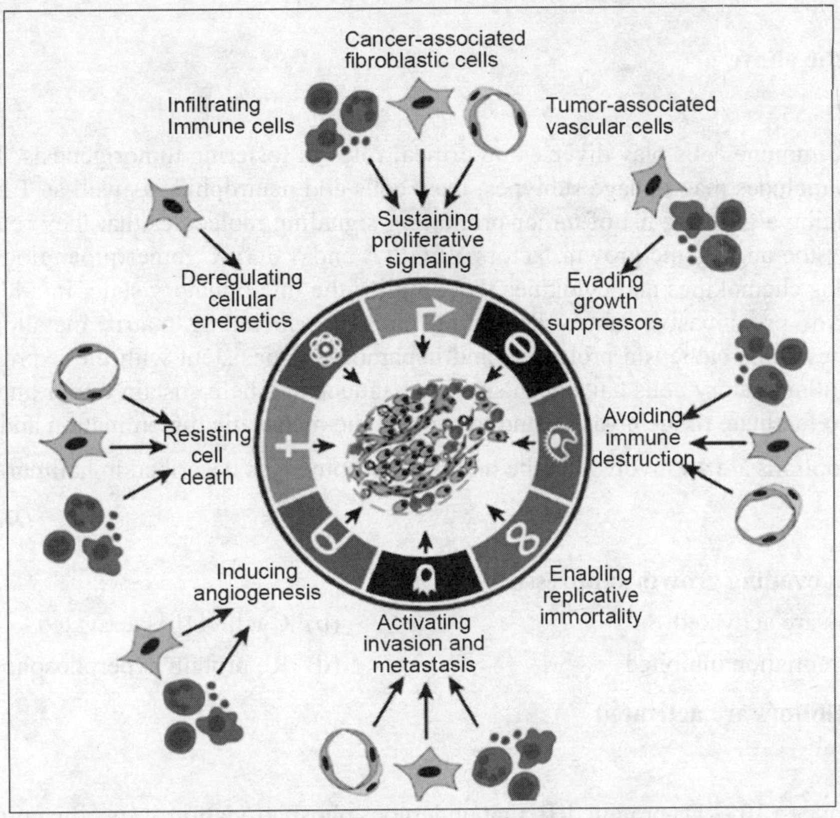

Diverse contributions of stromal cells to the hallmarks of cancer. Of the eight hallmark capabilities acquired by cancer cells, seven depend on contributions by stromal cells forming the tumor microenvironment. The stromal cells can be divided into three general classes: infiltrating immune cells, cancer-associated fibroblastic cells, and tumor-associated vascular cells. The association of these corrupted cell types with the acquisition of individual hallmark capabilities has been documented through a variety of experimental approaches that are often supported by descriptive studies in human cancers. The relative importance of each of these stromal cell classes to a particular hallmark is certain to vary according to tumor type and stage of primary tumorigenesis and malignant progression

(Devita, 11th Edition, Page 182)

186. Self sufficiency promoted by all *except:*

(a) Receptor overexpression
(b) Independent downstream signalling
(c) Negative and positive feedback mechanisms
(d) Act at transcellular level only

Ans: (d) Act at transcellular level only

Explanation

The concept that high-grade malignancy does not arise in a strictly cell-autonomous manner and that its manifestation cannot be understood through analyses of signaling occurring entirely within cancer cells. The heterotypic EMT model holds an important implication for the late stages of malignant progression: the ability of carcinoma cells in primary tumors to negotiate most of the steps of the invasion–metastasis cascade may be acquired without the requirement that these cells sustain additional function-enabling mutations beyond those that were involved previously in primary tumor formation. Thus, malignant progression may be largely orchestrated by nongenetic (i.e., epigenetic), cell-biologic processes. That indicate it does not act only at transcellular level

(Devita, 11th Edition, Page 170)

187. Tumor development by stroma includes all *except:*

(a) ECM molecules like fibronectin, laminin
(b) Receptors like integrins and heparan sulfate proteoglycans

(c) Soluble factors like VEGF Engage in intracellular signalling and cross talk
(d) None of the above

Ans: (d) None of the above

Explanation

We now know that immune cells play diverse and critical roles in fostering tumorigenesis. The roster of tumor promoting inflammatory cells includes macrophage subtypes, mast cells and neutrophils, as well as T and B lymphocytes. Studies of these cells are yielding a growing list of tumor-promoting signaling molecules that they release, which include the tumor growth factor EGF, the angiogenic growth factors VEGF-A and VEGF-C, other proangiogenic factors such as fibroblast growth factor 2, plus chemokines and cytokines that amplify the inflammatory state. In addition, these cells may produce proangiogenic and/or pro invasive matrix degrading enzymes, including matrix metallopeptidase-9 and other matrix metallopeptidases, cysteine cathepsin proteases, and heparanase. Consistent with the expression of these diverse signals, tumor-infiltrating inflammatory cells have been shown to induce and help sustain tumor angiogenesis, to stimulate cancer cell proliferation, to facilitate tissue invasion and to support the metastatic dissemination and seeding of cancer cells

Above mentioned options are all involved in the tumor development as described in hallmarks of cancer chapter

(Devita, 11th Edition, Page 180)

188. All are involved in evading growth suppressors *except:*
(a) CDK-inhibitors are activated
(b) Cyclin D1 is activated
(c) Terminal differentiation inhibited
(d) Rb protein hyperphosphorylated

Ans: (a) CDK-inhibitors are activated

Explanation

The RB1 gene encodes a 105 kDa protein, RB, that undergoes phosphorylation at specific points in the cell cycle. During G0 and G1, hypophosphorylated RB can bind to E2F transcription factors and prevent activation of S phase-promoting proteins such as cyclin E. On entry into the cell cycle, the cyclin D–cyclin dependent kinase (CDK) 4/6 complex phosphorylates RB, releasing it from the E2F proteins, allowing unbound E2F factors to recruit transcriptional activators and induce transcription of cyclin E and other cell-cycle genes

If CDK inhibitors are activated then the cell cycle is arrested, which the mechanism of action of ribociclib, palociclib and amebaciclib

The picture better demonstrate it

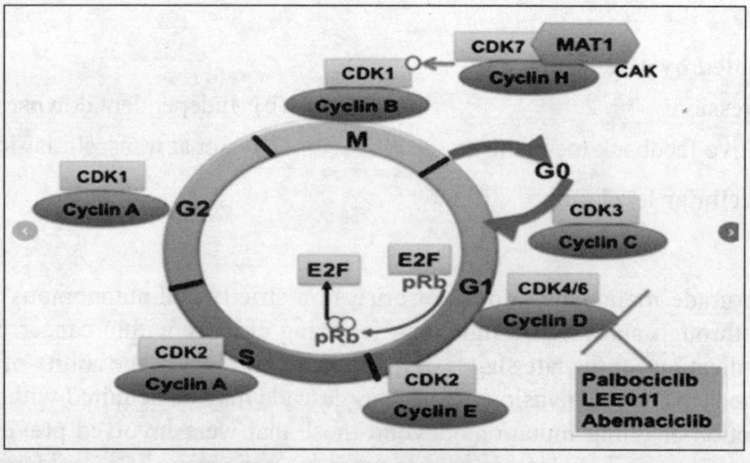

Cyclin-dependent kinases (CDKs) and their cyclin regulatory subunits. CDK-cyclin complexes with direct functions in regulating the cell cycle. CDK3/cyclin C drives cell cycle entry from G0. CDK 4/6/cyclin D complexes initiate phosphorylation of the retinoblastoma protein (pRb) and they sequester p21 Cip1 and p27kip 1 (not shown), which are both inhibitors of CDK2, thus promoting the activation of CDK2/cyclin E complex. In late G1, CDK2/cyclin E complex completes phosphorylation and inactivation of pRb, which releases the E2F transcription factors and G1/S transition takes place. DNA replication takes place in S phase. CDK2/cyclin A complex regulates progression through S phase and CDK1/cyclin A complex through G2 phase in preparation for mitosis (M). Mitosis is initiated by CDK1/cyclin B complex. The activity of CDK1/cyclin B is tightly regulated by activating phosphorylation by the CDK-activating kinase CAK (a heterodimer of cyclin H-CDK7-MAT1) and inhibitory phosphorylations by Wee1 and Myt1 on Tyr15 and Thr14 (not shown). The specific CDK4/CDK6 pharmacological inhibitors described in this study are shown

(Devita, 11th Edition, Page 223)

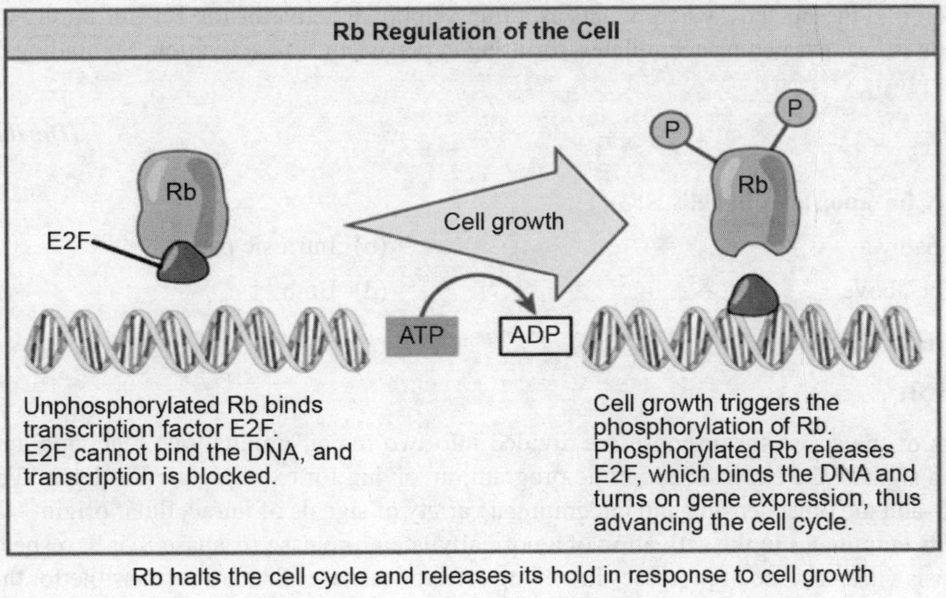

189. Cell proliferation will result in all *except:*

(a) APC mutation causing beta catenin translocation to nucleus

(b) Loss of E cadherin

(c) Wnt signalling activation

(d) Binding of beta catenin to APC

Ans: (d) Binding of beta catenin to APC

Explanation

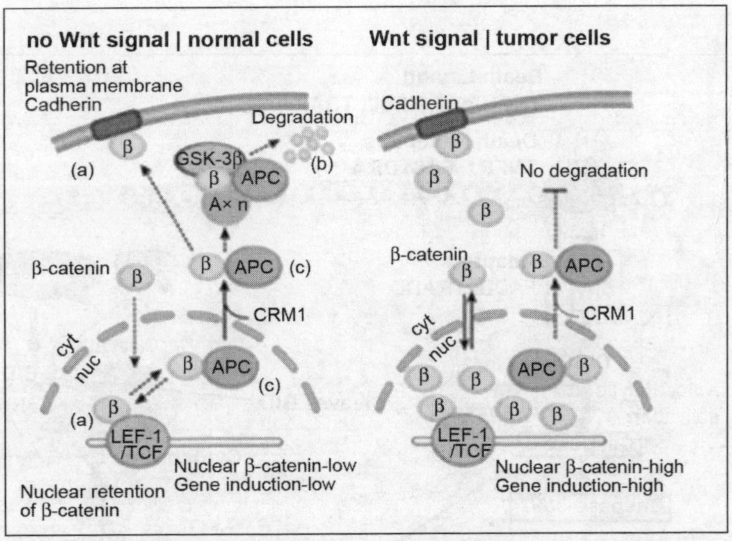

Nuclear-cytoplasmic shuttling of β-catenin. In normal, non-stimulated cells, β-catenin (indicated here as 'β') is bound to various interacting partners. Its distribution is therefore dictated by (a) retention in the nucleus, the cytoplasm and at the plasma membrane; (b) degradation in the cytoplasm; and (c) the movements of APC. In tumor cells (or Wnt-stimulated cells), β-catenin accrues to very high levels and is likely to shuttle independently of APC (wild-type or mutant). Some tumor-associated forms of β-catenin may show reduced anchorage by E-cadherin

APC regulates Wnt signaling by promoting degradation of β-catenin. APC functions in a cytoplasmic complex containing β-catenin, GSK3-β, and the scaffolding proteins axin and conductin. When APC is present, the complex forms and GSK3-β phosphorylates β-catenin on several N-terminal residues. Phosphorylated β-catenin is targeted for degradation, preventing its translocation into the nucleus, where it acts as a transcriptional activator for Tcf/Lef family transcription factors. When APC expression is lost, β-catenin accumulates, resulting in persistent Wnt activation. So binding of APC to beta catenin will not occur

(Devita, 11th Edition, Page 226)

190. Main pathway for apoptosis in cells is:

(a) Extrinsic pathway (b) Intrinsic pathway

(c) None of the above (d) Both

Ans: (b) Intrinsic pathway

Explanation

The regulators of the apoptotic response are divided into two major circuits, one receiving and processing extracellular death-inducing signals–the extrinsic apoptotic program, involving for example the Fas ligand/Fas receptor, also known as CD95L/CD95–and the other sensing and integrating a variety of signals of intracellular origin—the intrinsic program. Each of these circuits culminates in the activation of a normally latent protease (caspase 8 or 9, respectively), which proceeds to initiate apoptosis via a cascade of proteases involving effector caspases that are responsible for the execution phase of these cell death mechanisms. During this final phase, an apoptotic cell is progressively disassembled and then consumed, both by its neighbours and by professional phagocytic cells. Currently, the intrinsic apoptotic program is more widely implicated as a barrier that serves to block cancer pathogenesis

(Devita, 11th Edition, Page 163)

191. Extrinsic pathway mediated by all *except:*

(a) Fas-L and TRAIL (b) Death receptor 5

(c) Caspase 8 (d) Bax

Ans: (d) Bax

Explanation

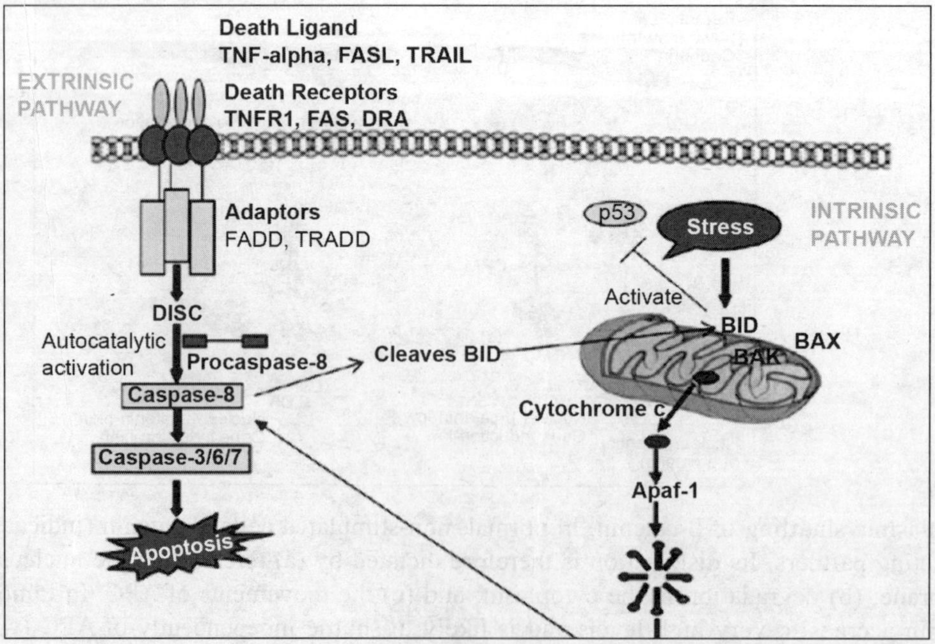

Extrinsic and Intrinsic pathway of apoptosis: In extrinsic pathway, the death ligands bind to transmembrane death receptors present on the cell destined to die. The binding of ligand to the receptors on the target cell triggers receptor clustering on the cell surface. This aggregation recruits the adaptor proteins on the cytoplasmic site of the receptors, forming death inducing signalling complex (DISC). Formation of DISC brings procaspase molecules close to one another, which facilitates their autocatalytic activation and release into the cytoplasm where they activate caspase cascade. Active caspase-8 also mediates the cleavage of proapoptotic protein, BID which subsequently releases mitochondrial proapoptotic factors linking the two pathways. In case of intrinsic pathway, stress signal causes the binding of cytoplasmic proteins, BAX and BID to the outer membrane of mitochondria. Another mitochondrial protein BAK interacts with BAX and BID causing release of cytochrome c into the cytosol. This binds to Apaf-1 which then forms apotosome that triggers the activation of procaspase-9. Activated caspase-9 further initiates the caspase cascade leading to apoptosis. Tumor suppressor p53 protein is a sensor of cellular stress and play a vital role in initiating apoptosis by transcriptionally activating proapoptotic proteins BID and BAX

Bax is involved in intrinsic pathway whereas Fas-L and TRAIL, Death receptor 5, Caspase 8 are involved in extrinsic pathway of apoptosis

192. Proapoptotic molecules include all *except:*

(a) Bax
(b) Bim
(c) Bak
(d) Bcl-XL

Ans: (d) Bcl-XL

Explanation

The molecular machinery that conveys signals between the apoptotic regulators and effectors is controlled by counterbalancing pro- and antiapoptotic members of the Bcl-2 family of regulatory proteins.The archetype, Bcl-2, along with its closest relatives (Bcl-XL, Bcl-W, Mcl-1, A1), are inhibitors of apoptosis, acting in large part by binding to and thereby suppressing two proapoptotic triggering proteins (Bax and Bak); the latter are embedded in the mitochondrial outer membrane. When relieved of inhibition by their antiapoptotic relatives, Bax and Bak disrupt the integrity of the outer mitochondrial membrane, causing the release into the cytosol of proapoptotic signaling molecules, the most important of which is cytochrome C. When the normally sequestered cytochrome C is released, it activates a cascade of cytosolic caspase proteases that proceed to fragment multiple cellular structures, thereby executing the apoptotic death program

Several abnormality sensors have been identified to play key roles in triggering apoptosis. Most notable is a DNA damage sensor that acts through the TP53 tumor suppressor; TP53 induces apoptosis by upregulating expression of the proapoptotic, Bcl-2-related Noxa and Puma proteins, doing so in response to substantial levels of DNA breaks and other chromosomal abnormalities. Alternatively, insufficient survival factor signaling (e.g.,inadequate levels of interleukin [IL]-3 in lymphocytes or of insulin-like growth factors 1 and 2 in epithelial cells) can elicit apoptosis through another proapoptotic Bcl-2–related protein called Bim. Yet another condition triggering apoptosis involves hyperactive signaling by certain oncoproteins, such as Myc, which acts in part via Bim and other Bcl-2-related proteins. Bcl-XL is inhibitor of apoptosis. Bax Bim Bak are proapoptotic

(Devita, 11th Edition, Page 164)

193. Bcl 2 family includes:

(a) Proapoptotic molecules
(b) Antiapoptotic molecules
(c) Both
(d) None

Ans: (c) Both

Explanation

As explained in the previous answer Bcl 2 family includes both antiapoptotic molecules like Bcl-XL

Bcl-W, Mcl1, A1, Proapoptotic molecules include Noxa, bim and puma, bid and bax

194. Non-apoptotic cell death includes all *except:*

(a) Necrosis causing release of inflammatory factors
(b) Autophagy regulated by becklin-1 gene
(c) Mitotic catastrophe Activating MDM2 which inhibits p53
(d) Decoy receptors for FAS-L

Ans: (d) Decoy receptors for FAS-L

Explanation

As described in the previous apoptosis answers FAS and FAS-L are the principal mechanisms by which apoptosis is initiated. Others are not related to apoptosis

195. Key cytochrome in apoptosis is:

(a) A (b) B

(c) Cytochrome-C (d) D

Ans: (c) Cytochrome-C

Explanation

When relieved of inhibition by their antiapoptotic relatives, Bax and Bak disrupt the integrity of the outer mitochondrial membrane, causing the release into the cytosol of proapoptotic signaling molecules, the most important of which is cytochrome C. When the normally sequestered cytochrome C is released, it activates a cascade of cytosolic caspase proteases that proceed to fragment multiple cellular structures, thereby executing the apoptotic death program

Cytochrome C inititates the caspases and leads to cell disintegration and cell death

196. Key regulator of apoptosis is:

(a) Rb (b) p53

(c) Caspase–3 (d) Caspase–9

Ans: (b) p53

Explanation

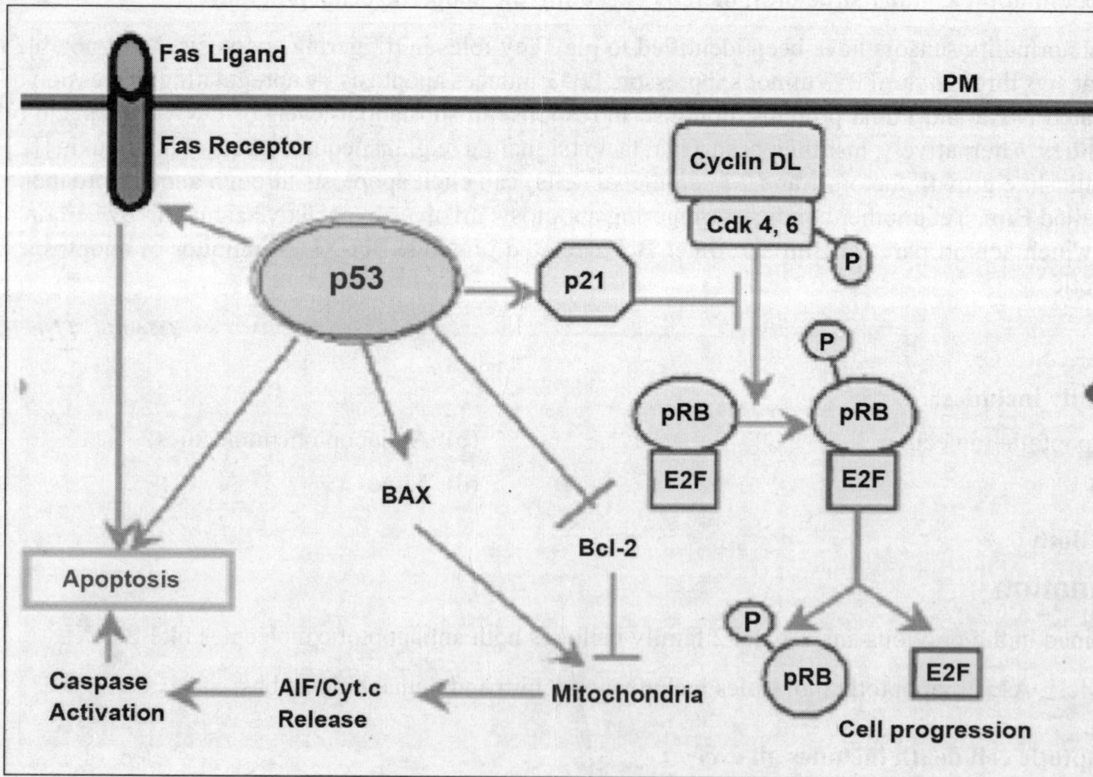

As seen in the picture p53 initiates the apoptosis and regulates it. p53 acts through RB and caspases

197. Correct pathway includes all *except:*

(a) Ras-raf-mek-erk (b) Pi3k-akt

(c) GAP inhibits ras and PTEN inhibits pi3k (d) None

Ans: (d) None

Explanation

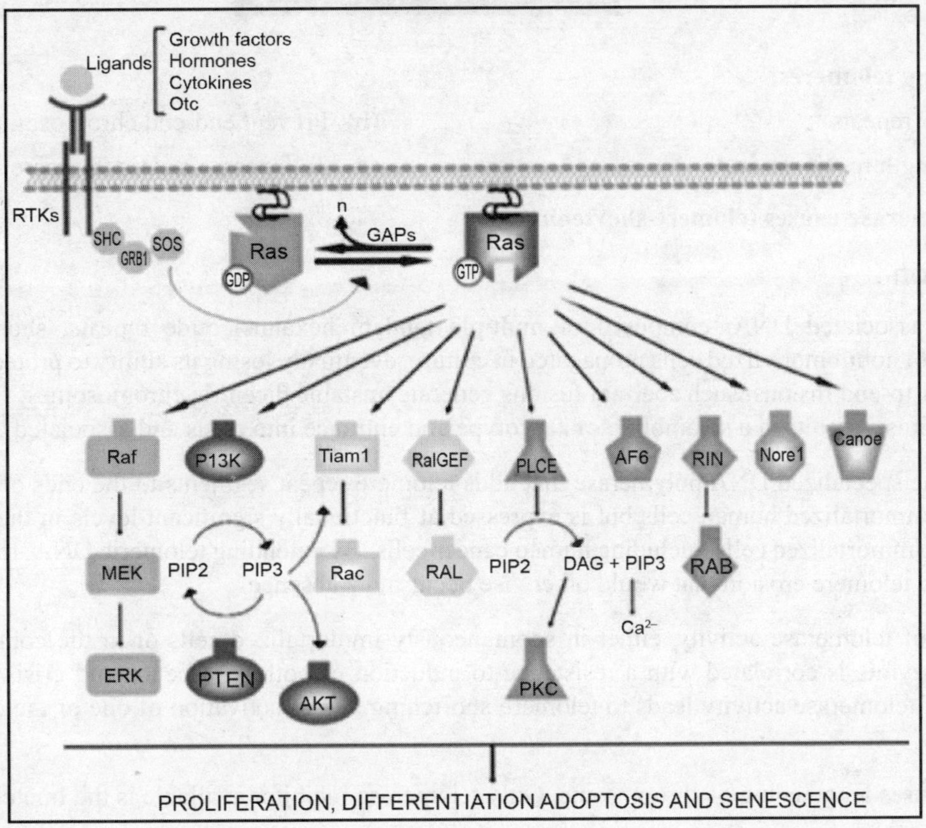

All are correctly matched pathways

198. Replicative immortality enabled by:

(a) Telomerase

(b) Recombinant based interchromosomal exchange

(c) Both of the above

(d) DNA Ligase

Ans: (a) Telomerase

Explanation

Telomerase, the specialized DNA polymerase that adds telomere repeat segments to the ends of telomeric DNA, is almost absent in nonimmortalized human cells but is expressed at functionally significant levels in the great majority (<90%) of spontaneously immortalized cells, including human cancer cells. By extending telomeric DNA, telomerase is able to counter the progressive telomere erosion that would otherwise occur in its absence

The presence of telomerase activity, either in spontaneously immortalized cells or in the context of cells engineered to express the enzyme, is correlated with a resistance to induction of both senescence and crisis/apoptosis; conversely, the suppression of telomerase activity leads to telomere shortening and to activation of one or the other of these proliferative barriers

PAPER 5 (SET 2)

199. False regarding telomeres:

(a) 6 base pair repeats
(b) Prevent end-end chromosomal fusion
(c) Critical length results in death
(d) Telomerase causes telomere shortening

Ans: (d) Telomerase causes telomere shortening

Explanation

The telomere-associated DNA, composed of multiple tandem hexanucleotide repeats, shortens progressively in the chromosomes of nonimmortalized cells propagated in culture, eventually losing its ability to protect the ends of chromosomal DNA from end-to-end fusions; such aberrant fusions generate unstable dicentric chromosomes, whose resolution during the anaphase of mitosis results in a scrambling of karyotype and entrance into crisis and associated apoptosis

Telomerase, the specialized DNA polymerase that adds telomere repeat segments to the ends of telomeric DNA, is almost absent in nonimmortalized human cells but is expressed at functionally significant levels in the great majority (<90%) of spontaneously immortalized cells, including human cancer cells. By extending telomeric DNA, telomerase is able to counter the progressive telomere erosion that would otherwise occur in its absence

The presence of telomerase activity, either in spontaneously immortalized cells or in the context of cells engineered to express the enzyme, is correlated with a resistance to induction of both senescence and crisis/apoptosis; conversely, the suppression of telomerase activity leads to telomere shortening and to activation of one or the other of these proliferative barriers

Telomerase causes lengthening of chromosome. Only telomerase inhibitor available is the Imetelstat

200. False regarding Cancer Stem Cells or cancer initiating cells:

(a) Confer chemoradioresistance
(b) CD 44, CD 133, CXCR4
(c) Constitute 50 percent of tumor cells
(d) Make up less than 10 percent of neoplastic cells

Ans: (c) Constitute 50 percent of tumor cells

Explanation

Biomarkers used to date for the detection of circulating cancer stem cells in different cancer types

Tumor type	Cell surface markers on circulating cancer stem cells
Pancreatic	CD133, CD44, CD24, CXCR4, c-Met, ALDH1, ABCG2
Breast	CD44, ANTXR1, ALDH1, CXCR4, ALDH1
Colorectal	CD133, CD44, CD44v6, CXCR4, CD26
Gastric cancer	CD44
Glioblastoma	CD133, MMP-13
Lung	CXCR4, ABCG2, CD133, ALDH1
Osteosarcoma	CD133
Retinoblastoma	ABCG2
Head and neck cancer	c-Met
Ovarian	CD133

Cancer stem cells (CSCs) are tumorigenic, able to reproduce the heterogeneous tumorigenic and nontumorigenic cell subpopulations of the original tumor population and self-renewing. CSCs were originally isolated from lymphomas, but subsequent investigation has revealed the presence of subsets of highly tumorigenic cancer cells in essentially every solid cancer type. Generally, CSCs represent a very small subpopulation in cancers, typically less than 10% of the cancer cell population. A variety of surface markers and biologic markers have been used to isolate the CSC population in HNSCC including CD44, CD133, epithelial-specific antigen (ESA) and aldehyde dehydrogenase (ALDH) activity. CSCs are critical in the growth and development of primary tumors, exhibit resistance to radiation and chemotherapy and play a role in R/M disease after treatment. CSC represent only 5-10% of the tumor cells and could self-renew as well as differentiate into all other adenoma cell types, indicating they are the CSCs. CD133, CXCR4, CD44 are markers of cancer stem cells. CSCs will not form the 50% of tumor cells

201. Antiangiogenetic factors include all *except:*

(a) Angiostatin (b) Endostatin

(c) Canstatin (d) MMP-9

Ans: (d) MMP-9

Explanation

MMP-9 is a proangiogenic protein. A variety of secreted proteins have been reported to have the capability to help shut off normally transient angiogenesis, including TSP-1, fragments of plasmin (angiostatin) and type 18 collagen (endostatin), along with another dozen candidate antiangiogenic proteins. Almost all are proteins and many are derived by proteolytic cleavage of structural proteins that are not themselves regulators of angiogenesis

Endogenous Inhibitors of Angiogenesis

Matrix Derived
- Arresten
- Canstatin
- Collagen fragments
- EFC-XV
- Endorepellin
- Endostatin
- Fibronectin fragments
- Fibulin
- Thrombospondin-1 and -2
- Tumstatin

Non-Matrix Derived

Growth factors and cytokines
- Interferons
- Interlukins
- PEDF
- Platelet factor-4

Other
- Angiostatin
- Antithrombin III (cleaved)
- Chondromodulin
- 2-Methoxyestradiol
- PEX
- Plasminogen Kringle 5
- Prolactin fragments
- Prothrombin Kringle 2
- sFit-1
- TIMPs
- Troponin I
- Vasostatin

(Devita, 11th Edition, Page 168)

202. Proangiogenetic factors include all *except:*

(a) VEGF (b) IL-6

(c) MMP-9 collagenase (d) Thrombospondin

Ans: (d) Thrombospondin

Explanation

The VEGF-A gene encodes ligands that are involved in orchestrating new blood vessel growth during embryonic and postnatal development, in the survival of endothelial cells in already-formed vessels, and in certain physiologic and pathologic situations in the adult. VEGF signaling via three alternative cognate receptor tyrosine kinases (VEGFR1 to VEGFR3) is regulated at multiple levels, reflecting this complexity of purpose. VEGF gene expression can be upregulated both by hypoxia and by oncogene signaling.Additionally, VEGF ligands can be sequestered in the ECM in latent forms that are subject to subsequent release and activation by ECM-degrading proteases (e.g., matrix metallopeptidase 9). In addition, other proangiogenic proteins, such as members of the fibroblast growth factor family, have been implicated in sustaining tumor angiogenesis.TSP-1, a key counterbalance in the angiogenic switch, also binds transmembrane receptors displayed by endothelial cells and thereby triggers suppressive signals that can counteract proangiogenic stimuli

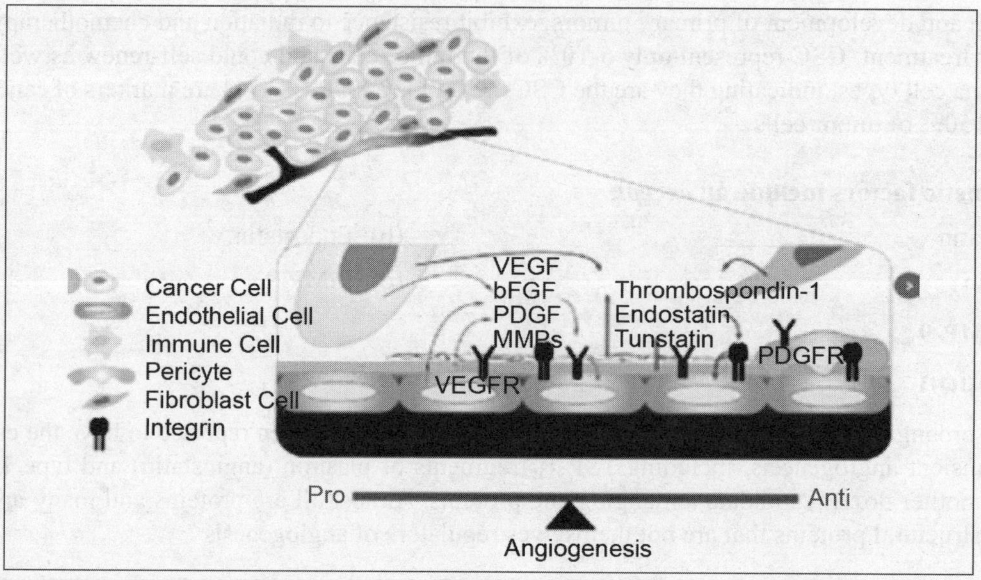

Thrombospondin is an antiangiogenic molecule

(Devita, 11th Edition, Page 168)

203. Theories of invasion and metastasis include:

(a) Seed for soil
(b) Adhesion and chemokine mediated
(c) Growth factor theory
(d) All of the above

Ans: (d) All of the above

Paget
(1899)

1700-1899: Paget proposed that metastases from specifically in organs that are "soil" to a metastatic cell's "seed"

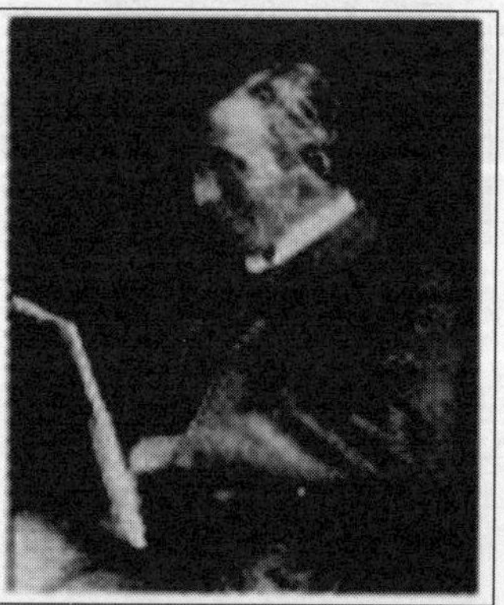

Explanation

One of the first lines of evidence associating cancer with soluble growth factors (GFs) emerged from studies performed in the 1950s, in the laboratory of Victor Hamburger, by two fellows, Rita Levi-Montalcini and Stanley Cohen. Chemokines regulate leucocyte recirculation and trafficking to sites of inflammation and infection

All the above are known theories for metastasis

(Source: Internet)

204. Growth factor implicated in metastasis.

(a) Transferrin
(b) Ferritin
(c) Both
(d) None

Ans: (a) Transferrin

Explanation

Transferrin Is an Insulin-Like Growth Factor-Binding Protein-3

The growth-enhancing effects of Tf at the cellular level are well-recognized. Tf is required for cell viability or proliferation in many cell culture systems, including cortical neuron, lymphocyte, renal cortex, liver and bladder. Tf also seems to be required for differentiation of fetal metanephric mesenchyme during embryogenesis. Tf deprivation from cells is associated with elevated indices of apoptosis. Growth and aggressiveness of malignancies are also Tf-dependent; Tf-R number is positively correlated with tumor growth rate and metastasis. In prostate cancer cells, Tf stimulates both proliferation and invasiveness; and suramin, a compound employed in metastatic prostate cancer therapy, has recently been demonstrated to exert its effects by antagonizing the binding of Tf to the Tf-R

205. Regarding invasion and metastasis, false is:

(a) Altered selectins expression results in increases invasiveness

(b) Altered integrins correlate with tumor progression

(c) Epithelial-mesenchymal transition

(d) E cadherin loss prevents invasion

Ans: (d) E cadherin loss prevents invasion

Explanation

The best-characterized alteration involves the loss by carcinoma cells of E-cadherin, a key epithelial cell-to-cell adhesion molecule. By forming adherens junctions between adjacent epithelial cells, E-cadherin helps to assemble epithelial cell sheets and to maintain the quiescence of the cells within these sheets. Moreover, increased expression of E-cadherin has been well established as an antagonist of invasion and metastasis, whereas a reduction of its expression is known to potentiate these behaviors. The frequently observed downregulation and occasional mutational inactivation of the E-cadherin–encoding gene, CDH1, in human carcinomas provides strong support for its role as a key suppressor of the invasion-metastasis hallmark capability

(Devita, Page 169)

206. Regarding invasion and metastasis, false is:

(a) Regulated by genetic and epigenetic mechanisms

(b) Basement membrane breach is the first step

(c) Occurs by intravasation-extravasation-survival-reinitiation

(d) Only mediated by epigenetic alterations

Ans: (d) Only mediated by epigenetic alterations

Explanation

Invasion and metastasis is regulated by multiple genetic and epigenetic mechanisms

207. Regarding immune evasion by cancer cells, false is:

(a) CD4 and CD8 relate to good prognosis

(b) Macrophage infiltrate relate to worse prognosis

(c) Adaptive immunity first line of defence

(d) All of the above

Answer: (d) All of the above

Explanation

In particular, deficiencies in the development or function of either CD8+ cytotoxic T lymphocytes (CTL), CD4+ TH1 helper T cells, or natural killer (NK) cells each led to demonstrable increases in tumor incidence. Moreover, mice with combined immunodeficiencies in both T cells and NK cells were even more susceptible to cancer development. The results indicated that, at least in certain experimental models, both the innate and adaptive cellular arms of the immune system are able to contribute significantly to immune surveillance and thus to tumor eradication. CXCL8 is predominantly secreted by macrophages and contributes to the immunosuppressive microenvironment by inducing PD-L1+ macrophages in gastric cancer. CXCL8 inhibitors may drive antitumor response, providing potential therapeutic effects for patients with gastric cancer. Adaptive immunity is the second line of defense

208. Correct order of immunoediting:

(a) Elimination-equilibrium-escape
(b) Escape-equilibrium-elimination
(c) Elimination-escape-equilibrium
(d) Equilibrium-escape-elimination

Ans: (a) Elimination-equilibrium-escape

Explanation

Elimination is a phase of cancer immunoediting where both the innate and adaptive immune system together detect and destroy early tumors before they become clinically visible. Normal cells (blue) are transformed into tumor cells by carcinogens and other genotoxic insults along with the failure of intrinsic tumor suppressor mechanisms (e.g. p53, ATM)

Equilibrium

The molecular mechanisms that trigger immune-mediated tumor dormancy (Equilibrium phase) are poorly understood because this phase has been difficult to model in mice and have been described only anecdotally in humans. Importantly, the balance of IL-12 promoting elimination, and IL-23 (sharing the common subunit IL-12 (p40) promoting persistence, maintains tumors in equilibrium. Although a minor tumor-promoting role for IL-10 was also uncovered, many other pathways (e.g. IL-4, IL-17A, TNF, IFN-αβ) were shown to be dispensable for this phase

Escape

Tumor cell escape can occur through many different mechanisms including: reduced immune recognition (such as the absence of strong tumor antigens, or loss of MHC class I, class I-like, or co-stimulatory molecules), increased resistance or survival (such as increased expression of STAT-3 or anti-apoptotic molecule Bcl2), or development of an immunosuppressive tumor microenvironment (cytokines such as VEGF, TGF-β; immunoregulatory molecules such as IDO, PD-1/PD-L1, Tim-3/ galectin-9, LAG-3)

So the correct order is if tumor could not be eliminated it makes an equilibrium. Finally the tumor escapes out of the immune control

209. Escape from immune system occurs by:

(a) Host related immunosuppression
(b) Activating negative immune regulators like T-regs, CTLA-4 and PD-1
(c) Activating immunosuppressants like IL-10 and TGF-beta
(d) All of the above

Ans: (d) All of the above

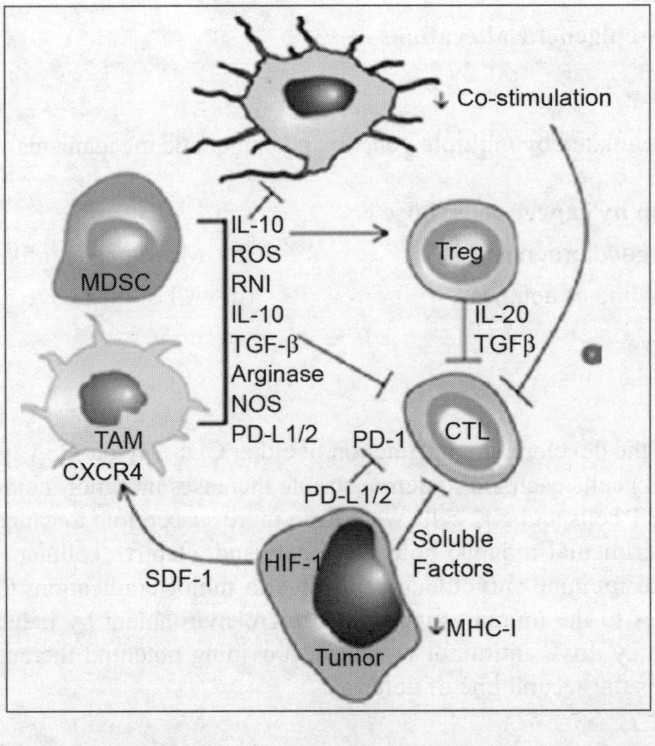

Explanation

Mechanisms of immune suppression in the tumor microenvironment. Tumors utilize multiple mechanisms for evading the immune system. Tumor cells can down-regulate expression of MHC-I, making them poor targets for CTL mediated killing. Along with myeloid-derived suppressor cells (MDSCs) and tumor-associated macrophages (TAMs), they can express PD-L1 and PD-L2, which inhibit CTL function through the PD-1 receptor. Tumors make other soluble factors that also inhibit CTLs. Hypoxia in tumors induces HIF-1, driving the production of SDF-1, which acts as a chemokine to attract MDSCs and TAMs to the tumor microenvironment through the receptor CXCR4. These MDSCs and TAMs secrete cytokines such as IL-10 that promote a regulatory phenotype among intratumoral DCs, induce Tregs and directly inhibit CTLs. Other myeloidderived factors that inhibit CTL activity include TGF-β, reactive oxygen species (ROS) and reactive nitrogen intermediates (RNI), and arginase and nitric oxide synthase (NOS), which are enzymes that deplete l-arginine, an important metabolite for CTL function

The answers given are all the mechanisms of immune evasion

210. Regarding Warburg effect, false is:

(a) Specific to tumor cells (b) Increased expression of GLUT-1

(c) Dynamic state (d) Utilized to diagnose or stage cancer

Ans: (a) Specific to tumor cells

Explanation

Otto Warburg first observed an anomalous characteristic of cancer cell energy metabolism: Even in the presence of oxygen, cancer cells can reprogram their glucose metabolism, and thus their energy production, leading to a state that has been termed aerobic glycolysis.

The existence of this metabolic specialization operating in cancer cells has been substantiated in the ensuing decades. A key signature of aerobic glycolysis is upregulation of glucose transporters, notably GLUT1, which substantially increases glucose import into the cytoplasm. Indeed, markedly increased uptake and utilization of glucose has been documented in many human tumor types, most readily by noninvasively visualizing glucose uptake using positron-emission tomography (PET) with a radiolabeled analog of glucose (18F-fluorodeoxyglucose [FDG]) as a reporter. The reprogramming of energy metabolism is seemingly counterintuitive, in that cancer cells must compensate for the ~18-fold lower efficiency of ATP production afforded by glycolysis relative to mitochondrial oxidative phosphorylation. According to one long-forgotten and a recently revived and refined hypothesis, increased glycolysis allows the diversion of glycolytic intermediates into various biosynthetic pathways, including those generating nucleosides and amino acids. In turn, this facilitates the biosynthesis of the macromolecules and organelles required for assembling new cells. Moreover, Warburg-like metabolism seems to be present in many rapidly dividing embryonic tissues, once again suggesting a role in supporting the large-scale biosynthetic programs that are required for active cell proliferation

So warburg effect is not specific to tumor cells and can happen in embroyonic tissues also

(Devita, 11th Edition, Page 172)

211. Regarding genomic instability, true is:

(a) p53 is the guardian of genome and most commonly mutated TSG

(b) ras is most commonly mutated oncogene

(c) Caretaker genes are genes involved in repair mechanism

(d) All of the above

Ans: (d) All of the above

Explanation

The role of TP53 is central in protecting the genome, leading to its being called the guardian of the genome

A diverse array of defects affecting various components of the DNA-maintenance machinery, referred to as the caretakers of the genome, have been documented. The catalog of defects in these caretaker genes includes those whose products are involved in (1) detecting DNA damage and activating the repair machinery, (2) directly repairing damaged DNA, and (3) inactivating or intercepting mutagenic molecules before they have damaged the DNA. From a genetic perspective, these caretaker genes behave much like tumor suppressor genes in that their functions are often lost during the course of tumor progression, with such losses being achieved either through inactivating mutations or via epigenetic repression. Mutant versions of many of these caretaker genes encoding functionally defective repair proteins have been introduced into the mouse germline, resulting, not unexpectedly, in increased cancer incidence, thus supporting their involvement in human cancer development

RAS proteins (KRAS4A, KRAS4B, NRAS and HRAS) function as GDP-GTP-regulated binary on off switches, which regulate cytoplasmic signaling networks that control diverse normal cellular processes. Gain-of-function missense mutations in RAS genes are found in ~25% of human cancers, prompting interest in identifying anti-RAS therapeutic strategies for cancer treatment. The three human RAS genes [i.e., Kirsten rat sarcoma viral oncogene homolog (KRAS), neuroblastoma RAS viral (v-ras) oncogene homolog (NRAS) and Harvey rat sarcoma viral oncogene homolog (HRAS)] encode four RAS proteins, with two KRAS isoforms that arise from alternative RNA splicing (KRAS4A and KRAS4B)

(Devita, 11th Edition, Page 176)

212. Cancer caused by viruses in ___ of tumors worldwide.

(a) 25
(b) 15
(c) 45
(d) 95

Ans: (b) 15

Explanation

An estimated 15 percent of all human cancers worldwide may be attributed to viruses, representing a significant portion of the global cancer burden

213. Regarding viral carcinogenesis, false is:

(a) HPV–E6 mediated p53 inhibition
(b) HBV–insertional mutagenesis and endoplasmic reticulum stress
(c) HCV–direct integration of genome
(d) HBx trascription factor

Ans: (c) HCV- direct integration of genome

Explanation

The most extensively studied early region proteins are the E6 and E7 oncogenes of HPV16 and HPV18. The E6 protein of high-risk HPV types triggers the destruction of p53 by recruiting a host cell ubiquitin-protein ligase, E6AP. Another important oncogenic function of E6 is the activation of cellular telomerase

The HBV viral genome is a relaxed circular partially double-stranded DNA of 3.2 kb. The genome exists as an episomal covalently closed circular double stranded DNA molecule in the nucleus of infected cells, although chromosomal integration of viral genomic sequences can occur during cycles of hepatocyte regeneration and proliferation. In addition to 40 to 42 nm virions, HBV-infected cells also produce non-infectious 20 nm spherical and filamentous subviral particles. The viral genome encodes four open reading frames. The presurface–surface (preS-S) region encodes three proteins from different translational initiation sites; these include the S (HBsAg), M (or pre-S2) and L (or pre-S1) proteins. The L protein is responsible for receptor binding and virion assembly. The precore–core (preC-C) region encodes the HBcAg and HBeAg. The P region encodes the viral polymerase, and the X (HBx) protein modulates host-cell signal transduction

HCV is a positive-sense, enveloped single-stranded RNA virus of the Flaviviridae family. There are seven genotypes of HCV; in the United States, about 70% of infections are caused by genotype 1. HCV replicates in the cytoplasm and does not integrate into the host cell genome. The viral RNA is 9.6 kb and encodes a single polyprotein of 3,010 amino acids that is proteolytically processed into structural and non-structural proteins. In addition to the structural roles of the core (C) protein, it has also been reported to affect various host cell functions. The envelope glycoproteins E1 and E2 mediate infectious entry through tetraspanin CD81 and other receptors on hepatocytes and B lymphocytes

HCV does not integrate in viral genome directly whereas HBV integrates directly

(Devita, 11th Edition, Page 268)

214. Cancer epigenetics include all *except:*

(a) DNA methylation
(b) Histone acetylation
(c) Genomic imprinting
(d) Insertions and deletions

Ans: (d) Insertions and deletions

Explanation

Cancer is the manifestation of both genetic and epigenetic modifications. Although cancer initiation and progression are predominantly driven by acquired genetic alterations, it is becoming clear that microenvironment-mediated epigenetic perturbations play important roles in neoplastic development. Epigenetics is defined as heritable changes in gene expression activity and expression that occur without alteration in DNA sequences but which are sufficiently powerful to regulate the dynamics of gene expression. The key processes that are responsible for epigenetic regulation are DNA methylation, modifications in chromatin (covalent modification of core histones), nucleosome positioning (physical alteration) and posttranscriptional gene regulation by noncoding RNA (micro-RNAs). A number of well characterized epigenetic modifications are linked to aberrant gene functions and altered patterns of gene expression that play critical roles in the pathobiology of cancer

Insertions and deletions are genetic alterations and others are epigenetic alterations

215. Regarding carcinogen groups, true is:

(a) Group 1 is proven human carcinogen
(b) Group 2A is possible limited evidence in humans
(c) Group 3 is inadequate evidence in humans
(d) All of the above

Ans: (d) All of the above

Explanation

International Agency for Research on Cancer

The International Agency for Research on Cancer (IARC) is part of the World Health Organization (WHO). One of its major goals is to identify causes of cancer. The most widely used system for classifying carcinogens comes from the IARC. In the past 30 years, the IARC has evaluated the cancer-causing potential of more than 900 likely candidates, placing them into one of the following groups:

Group 1: Carcinogenic to humans

Group 2A: Probably carcinogenic to humans

Group 2B: Possibly carcinogenic to humans

Group 3: Unclassifiable as to carcinogenicity in humans

Group 4: Probably not carcinogenic to humans

216. False statement is:

(a) CYP1A1 polymorphism puts light smokers at a greater risk than heavy smokers
(b) Aflatoxin is a group 1 chemical carcinogen
(c) Nucleotide excision repair dysfunction causes XER
(d) None of the above

Ans: (d) None of the above

Explanation

International Agency for Research on Cancer

Group 1: Carcinogenic to humans

Acetaldehyde (from consuming alcoholic beverages)

Acheson process, occupational exposure associated with:

Acid mists, strong inorganic

Aflatoxins

Alcoholic beverages

Aluminum production

4-Aminobiphenyl

Areca nut

Aristolochic acid (and plants containing it)

Arsenic and inorganic arsenic compounds

Asbestos (all forms) and mineral substances (such as talc or vermiculite) that contain asbestos

Auramine production

Azathioprine

Benzene

Benzidine and dyes metabolized to benzidine

Benzo[a]pyrene

Beryllium and beryllium compounds

Betel quid, with or without tobacco

Bis(chloromethyl)ether and chloromethyl methyl ether (technical-grade)

Busulfan

1,3-Butadiene

Cadmium and cadmium compounds

Chlorambucil

Chlornaphazine

Chromium (VI) compounds

Clonorchis sinensis (infection with), also known as the Chinese liver fluke

Coal, indoor emissions from household combustion

Coal gasification

Coal-tar distillation

Coal-tar pitch

Coke production

Cyclophosphamide

Cyclosporine

1,2-Dichloropropane

Diethylstilbestrol

Engine exhaust, diesel

Epstein-Barr virus (infection with)

Erionite

Estrogen postmenopausal therapy

Estrogen-progestogen postmenopausal therapy (combined)

Estrogen-progestogen oral contraceptives (combined) (**Note:** There is also convincing evidence in humans that these agents confer a protective effect against cancer in the endometrium and ovary)

Ethanol in alcoholic beverages

Ethylene oxide

Etoposide

Etoposide in combination with cisplatin and bleomycin

Fission products, including strontium-90

Fluoro-edenite fibrous amphibole

Formaldehyde

Haematite mining (underground)

Helicobacter pylori (infection with)

Hepatitis B virus (chronic infection with)

Hepatitis C virus (chronic infection with)

Human immunodeficiency virus type 1 (HIV-1) (infection with)

Human papilloma virus (HPV) types 16, 18, 31, 33, 35, 39, 45, 51, 52, 56, 58, 59 (infection with) (**Note:** The HPV types that have been classified as carcinogenic to humans can differ by an order of magnitude in risk for cervical cancer)

Human T-cell lymphotropic virus type I (HTLV-1) (infection with)

Ionizing radiation (all types)

Iron and steel founding (workplace exposure)

Isopropyl alcohol manufacture using strong acids

Kaposi sarcoma herpesvirus (KSHV), also known as human herpesvirus 8 (HHV-8) (infection with)

Leather dust

Lindane

Magenta production

Melphalan

Methoxsalen (8-methoxypsoralen) plus ultraviolet A radiation, also known as PUVA

4,4'-Methylenebis (chloroaniline) (MOCA)

Mineral oils, untreated or mildly treated

MOPP and other combined chemotherapy including alkylating agents

2-Naphthylamine

Neutron radiation

Nickel compounds

N'-Nitrosonornicotine (NNN) and 4-(N-Nitrosomethylamino)-1-(3-pyridyl)-1-butanone (NNK)

Opisthorchis viverrini (infection with), also known as the Southeast Asian liver fluke

Outdoor air pollution (and the particulate matter in it)

Painter (workplace exposure as a)

3,4,5,3',4'-Pentachlorobiphenyl (PCB-126)

2,3,4,7,8-Pentachlorodibenzofuran

Phenacetin (and mixtures containing it)

Phosphorus-32, as phosphate

Plutonium

Polychlorinated biphenyls (PCBs), dioxin-like, with a Toxicity Equivalency Factor according to

WHO (PCBs 77, 81, 105, 114, 118, 123, 126, 156, 157, 167, 169, 189)

Processed meat (consumption of)

Radioiodines, including iodine-131

Radionuclides, alpha-particle-emitting, internally deposited (**Note:** Specific radionuclides for which there is sufficient evidence for carcinogenicity to humans are also listed individually as Group 1 agents)

Radionuclides, beta-particle-emitting, internally deposited (**Note:** Specific radionuclides for which there is sufficient evidence for carcinogenicity to humans are also listed individually as Group 1 agents)

Radium-224 and its decay products

Radium-226 and its decay products

Radium-228 and its decay products

Radon-222 and its decay products

Rubber manufacturing industry

Salted fish (Chinese-style)

Schistosoma haematobium (infection with)

Semustine (methyl-CCNU)

Shale oils

Silica dust, crystalline, in the form of quartz or cristobalite

Solar radiation

Soot (as found in workplace exposure of chimney sweeps)

Sulfur mustard

Tamoxifen (**Note:** There is also conclusive evidence that tamoxifen reduces the risk of contralateral breast cancer in breast cancer patients)

2,3,7,8-Tetrachlorodibenzo-para-dioxin

Thiotepa

Thorium-232 and its decay products

Tobacco, smokeless

Tobacco smoke, second hand

Tobacco smoking

Ortho-Toluidine

Treosulfan

Trichloroethylene

Ultraviolet (UV) radiation, including UVA, UVB and UVC rays

Ultraviolet-emitting tanning devices

Vinyl chloride

Wood dust

X- and Gamma-radiation

Ionizing radiation is both a carcinogen and therapuetic agent–it is a well-known fact and answer is none of the above. Nucleotide excision repair causes xeroderma pigmentosum

217. Regarding H. pylori, true is:

(a) IL-1beta potent inhibitor of acid secretion
(b) Cag-A implicated in gastric cancer
(c) Ramicirumab is a IL-1beta receptor antagonist
(d) All of the above

Ans: (d) All of the above

Explanation

H. pylori is epidemiologically associated with non cardia gastric carcinoma and lymphoma. H. pylori infection is prevalent worldwide, and it only causes well-tolerated gastritis in most individuals. In a few patients, it causes serious pathologic lesions including atrophy, metaplasia and cancer. Two toxin-encoding genes cytotoxin associated gene A (cag A) and vacuolating gene (vac A) are present in virulent and carcinogenic strains of H. pylori (reviewed in Plottel and Blaser). IL-1 beta and TNF-alpha inhibited basal and stimulated acid secretion in a dose dependent manner; near maximal effects were seen with both at 10 ng/ml

218. All involve nearly 100 percent penetrance in germline mutation *except:*

(a) FAP/APC and Li-Fraumeni (by 60 years age)
(b) MTC/RET
(c) NF/NF-1
(d) Pheochromocytoma

Ans: (d) Pheochromocytoma

Explanation

A condition, most commonly inherited in an autosomal dominant manner, is said to show complete penetrance if clinical symptoms are present in all individuals who have the disease-causing mutation. A condition which shows complete penetrance is *neurofibromatosis type 1* – every person who has a mutation in the gene will show symptoms of the condition. The penetrance is 100%.

NF1 affects approximately 1 in 2,000 live births. The trait is inherited in an autosomal dominant fashion, with a penetrance of 100% for neurofibromas. The spectrum of other phenotypes is variable and strongly influenced by the patient's genetic background.

This study aimed to investigate the penetrance, full phenotypic spectrum and effectiveness of clinical/genetic screening in TMEM127-related PHEO.Pheochromocytoma was diagnosed in 11 carriers (32%) at a median age of 43 years. In nine patients, symptoms started at 29 years (range, 10-55 years) and two cases were asymptomatic. Tumors were multicentric in five (45%) and bilateral in five (45%) patients. Six patients (54%) had at least one adrenomedullary nodule less than 10 mm. No paragangliomas, distant metastases, or other manifestations were detected. Cumulative penetrance of pheochromocytoma was 0% at 0-20 years, 3% at 21-30 years, 15% at 31-40 years, 24% at 41-50 years and 32% at 51-65 years

Pheochromocytoma Penetrance is less whereas in other autosomal dominant familial genetic syndromes penetrance is high

PAPER 5 (SET 3)

219. Hereditary retinoblastoma constitutes:

(a) 50% (b) 40%

(c) 10% (d) 90%

Ans: (b) 40%

Explanation

Retinoblastoma is a tumor of the retinal photoreceptor precursor cells. Occurring in approximately 1 in 20,000 children, the tumors develop in affected individuals between birth and 8 years old. Retinoblastoma occurs in both an inherited and sporadic fashion, which account for approximately 40% and 60% of total retinoblastoma cases, respectively

(Devita, 11th Edition, 222)

220. Hereditary pheochromocytoma constitutes:

(a) 10% (b) 25%

(c) 50% (d) 100%

Ans: (b) 25%

Explanation

Pheochromocytoma (PCC) is a rare (approximately 0.8 cases per 100,000 population), catecholamine-secreting neuroendocrine tumor that presents with sustained or paroxysmal hypertension, headache, profuse sweating, anxiety and palpitations. Among the general population, PCCs are responsible for 0.1% to 0.6% of patients with hypertension. Approximately 25% of patients present as part of a familial disorder including MEN2, VHL type 2 (OMIM #193300), NF1 (OMIM #162200), or hereditary paraganglioma (PGL) or PCC. Because of this, genetic testing is always indicated in patients with PCC or PGL

(Devita, 11th Edition, 2347)

221. False about CEA is:

(a) Normal limit is 2.5-5 ng/ml (b) Useful for screening

(c) Predicts response to chemotherapy (d) Category 1 prognostic factor in Colorectal cancer

Ans: (b) Useful for screening

Explanation

Carcinoembryonic Antigen

An elevated preoperative CEA is a poor prognostic factor for cancer recurrence. Although there is variability in the available data regarding the level that denotes a prognostic cutoff, a preoperative CEA level >5 ng/mL is considered a category I poor prognostic indicator by the CAP consensus panel. Patients in whom the elevated CEA fails to normalize after a potentially curative operation are at particularly high risk. Several authors have presented evidence that indicates that CEA is an independent prognostic factor. In a report of 572 patients who underwent curative resection for node-negative colon cancer, the preoperative CEA level and the stage of disease predicted survival by both univariate and multivariate analyses. Given the prognostic significance of the preoperative CEA, it is reasonable to recommend that all patients who undergo operation for CRC have a serum CEA drawn prior to operation. No other serum markers have been demonstrated to be reliably prognostic or predictive in CRC. Although of little use in detecting early colorectal cancer, high preoperative concentrations of CEA correlate with adverse prognosis. Serial CEA measurements can detect recurrent colorectal cancer with a sensitivity of approximately 80%, a specificity of approximately 70% and can provide a lead time of approximately 5 months. CEA is the most frequent indicator of recurrence in asymptomatic patients and currently is the most cost-effective test for the preclinical detection of resectable disease. CEA is most useful for the early detection of liver metastasis in patients with diagnosed colorectal cancer. Overall, however, little evidence is available that monitoring of all patients with diagnosed colorectal cancer leads to enhanced patient outcome or quality of life

CEA may be elevated in other malignant and benign conditions and cannot be used as marker for screening. CEA specificity is low

(Devita, 11th Edition, 1674)

222. False about alpha feto-protein:

(a) Normal limit less than 25 ng/ml
(b) Useful for screening
(c) Proportional to tumor burden
(d) Correlates to response to chemoembolization

Ans: (d) Correlates to response to chemoembolization

Explanation

Serum α-fetoprotein (AFP), a fetal-specific glycoprotein antigen, is an HCC tumor marker. It is not specific to HCC as it may be elevated in hepatitis, pregnancy, and some germ cell tumors. AFP has variable sensitivity and has not been tested in any randomized clinical trial with a mortality endpoint. The American Association for the Study of Liver Diseases (AASLD) and the European Association for the Study of the Liver (EASL) have outlined non-invasive criteria for the diagnosis of HCC. EASL recommends that lesions that are >2 cm with characteristic radiologic features of arterial hyperenhancement on two different imaging modalities, or on one imaging modality alongside with a serum α-fetoprotein (AFP) of 400 ng/dL or more, are diagnostic of HCC and no biopsy is needed

Alpha-fetoprotein response following transarterial chemoembolization indicates improved survival for intermediate-stage hepatocellular carcinoma

Alpha-fetoprotein levels in men and non-pregnant women vary for age and race but mostly range from 0 ng/ml to 40 ng/ml

223. Regarding CA 19-9, false is:

(a) Elevated in biliary cancer
(b) Elevated in benign biliary diseases
(c) May not be elevated in biliary cancer
(d) Normal limit is 100 U/ml

Ans: (d) Normal limit is 100 U/ml

Explanation

Cancer antigen 19-9 (CA 19-9) is used to help differentiate between cancer of the *pancreas* and other conditions, as well as to monitor treatment response and recurrence. CA 19-9 may not be elevated in biliary tumors. They may present with normal values also. The reference range of serum CA 19-9 is less than 37 U/mL

224. Regarding PSA, false is:

(a) First sign in recurrence and metastatic prostate cancer
(b) Raised in relapse after Radiotherapy
(c) Raised in recurrence after radical surgery
(d) PSA values more than 4 ng is diagnostic of prostate cancer

Ans: (d) PSA values more than 4 ng is diagnostic of prostate cancer

Explanation

PSA levels are best considered as a continuum: The higher the level, the greater the likelihood that any cancer, or high-grade cancer, will be found on biopsy. The most commonly used threshold for recommending a biopsy is 3 ng/mL. A level this high is found in only 5% to 10% of men aged 45 to 69 years. As PSA levels vary, a rise in PSA to a newly "elevated" level should be verified 2 to 3 months later, after the patient has been evaluated by a medical history, DRE, and appropriate laboratory tests to exclude causes other than cancer for the "rise." The likelihood of finding cancer is about 15% to 20% in men with a normal DRE and a PSA level between 2.5 to 4 ng/mL. Among men with a PSA level of 4 to 10 ng/mL, 20% to 30% will have cancer. If the PSA level is >10 ng/mL, 60% of men will have cancer on biopsy. Many of these cancers will be low risk and can be managed conservatively without radical therapy. Higher circulating PSA levels prior to treatment are associated with larger, more extensive cancers, although there may be a wide range of levels within any clinical T, N, or M category. Although poorly differentiated cancers produce less PSA per gram than well-differentiated cancers, higher PSA levels indicate a more extensive cancer and a poorer prognosis across all Gleason grade groups. Rare, highly aggressive, poorly differentiated cancers are found in men with low PSA levels (<2 ng/mL), but patients with these cancers usually present with rapidly progressive voiding symptoms and an abnormal DRE. PSA levels rise with age because of age-related increases in prostate volume due to BPH. Adjusting the upper limit of normal for age, PSA should be <2.5 ng/mL for men aged 40 to 49 years, <3.5 for men aged 50 to 59 years, <4.5 for men aged 60 to 69 years, and <6.5 for men aged 70 to 79 years. The utility of age-specific PSA levels has been challenged in screening trials because sensitivity is lost for a small increase in specificity in older men

PSA is not a specific diagnostic marker mainly used for monitoring of treatment

225. True regarding CA-125:

(a) Expressed in normal ovarian epithelium
(b) Used as an adjunct to diagnosis
(c) Correlates with stage of ovarian cancer
(d) Increased values not an indication for second look laparotomy

Ans: (b) Used as an adjunct to diagnosis

Explanation

Cancer Antigen 125

CA 125 was discovered in 1981 by Bast *et al.* Although it is the only U.S. Food and Drug Administration (FDA)–approved biomarker for ovarian cancer detection, it is only expressed in approximately 75% of cases and principally in the serous subtype. It is not expressed by mucinous and other ovarian carcinomas, although when these diseases are metastatic to the abdominal cavity, levels of CA 125 may be aberrantly elevated but not reliably enough to accurately reflect intra-abdominal tumor burden. Additional shortcomings of CA 125 include a lack of sensitivity for detecting early-stage ovarian cancer and the potential presence of this protein at abnormally high levels in many benign gynecologic and non-gynecologic conditions. For these reasons, CA 125 is not a suitable screening test for ovarian cancer in the general population of women, and the search for more sensitive and informative biomarkers continues. Accepted uses of CA 125 include (1) helping to determine whether a pelvic mass is malignant; (2) assisting in determining whether a cancer of unknown primary origin has arisen from the ovary; (3) monitoring response of ovarian cancer to systemic chemotherapy; (4) carrying out surveillance of patients treated for ovarian cancer who are in remission; and (5) screening for ovarian cancer in high-risk populations (i.e., patients with a strong family history or BRCA1/2 mutation carriers)

Ca 125 as described earlier will not correlate with the stage in all histologies of ovarian cancer, in follow up after treatment, increasing CA 125 values is an indication for further evaluaton and second look laparotomy

(Devita, 11th Edition, 2201)

226. False statement is:

(a) Kras mutation codon 12/13 precludes EGFR targeted therapy in colorectal cancer
(b) Exon 20 mutation T 790M confers resistance to geftinib in lung cancer
(c) Deletion of exon 19 confers sensitivity to geftinib therapy in lung cancer
(d) BRAF/V600E mutation confers resistance to vemurafenib in malignant melanoma

Ans: (b) Exon 20 mutation T 790M confers resistance to geftinib in lung cancer

Explanation

KRAS AND NRAS if it is wild type–EGFR blockers–cetuximab and panitumumab should be used in colon cancers

If kras and nras is mutated-bevacizumab should be used

Exon 19 deletion is the most common mutation in adenocarcinomas of the lung. Exon 19 deletion in 45% of patients and a point mutaion in Exon 21 L858R in 40% of patients. Both mutation activate the tyrosine kinase domain and are make them sensistive to geftinib, erlotinib, afatinib, dacomatinib, osimeritinib

T790 mutation is associated with acquired resistance to EGFR TKI THERAPY and is seen in 60% of patients on treatment with geftinib, erlotinb or afatinib

BRAF V 600 Mutation is the indication for treatment with dabrafenib and vemurafenib

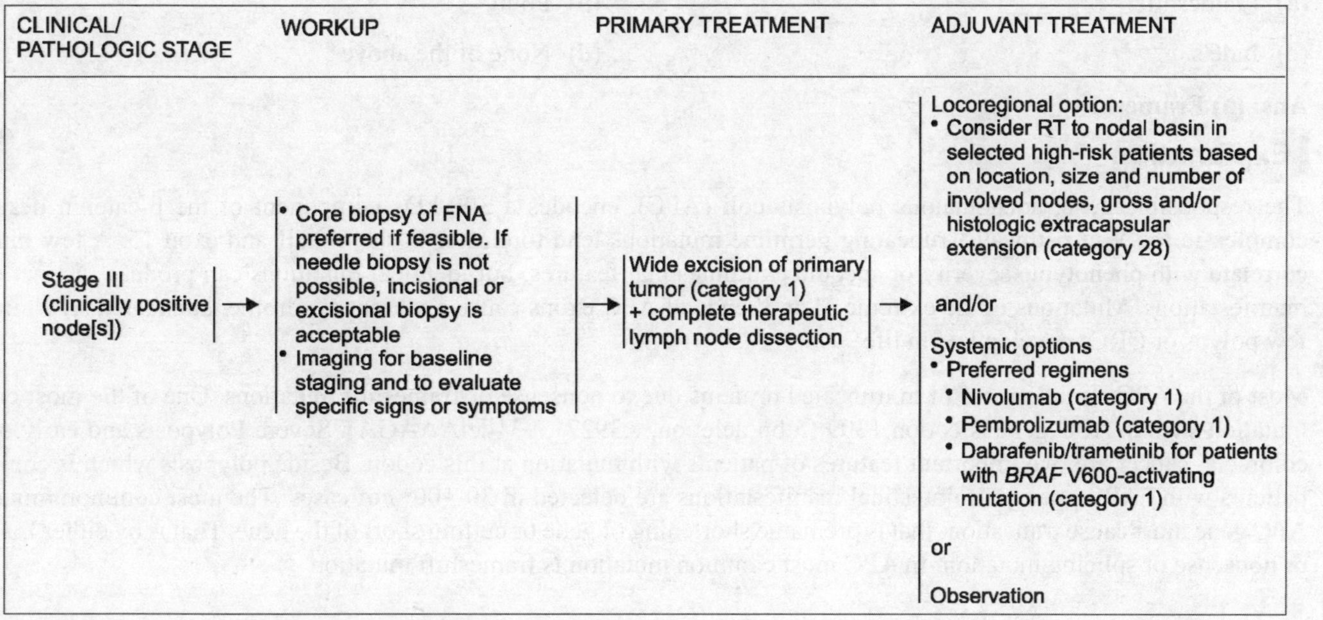

227. Truncated proteins in cancer involve all *except:*

(a) BRCA (b) APC

(c) EGFR (d) Ras

Ans (d) Ras

Explanation

Elimination of the N– or *C–terminal* portion of a protein by proteolysis or manipulation of the structural *gene,* or premature termination of protein elongation due to the presence of a termination *codon* in its structural *gene* as a result of a nonsense mutation

In APC, BRCA and EGFR genes we have truncation–that is shortening of the protein by splice site mutations or nonsense mutations or frameshift mutations. Truncation does not happen in Ras

228. Gene mutated in Li-Fraumeni:

(a) APC (b) Rb

(c) CHK-1 (d) CHK-2

Ans: (d) CHK-2

Explanation

The CHEK2 and TP53 genes are associated with Li-Fraumeni syndrome

More than half of all families with Li-Fraumeni syndrome have inherited mutations in the TP53 gene. TP53 is a tumor suppressor gene, which means that it normally helps control the growth and division of cells. Mutations in this gene can allow cells to divide in an uncontrolled way and form tumors. Other genetic and environmental factors are also likely to affect the risk of cancer in people with TP53 mutations

A few families with cancers characteristic of Li-Fraumeni syndrome and Li-Fraumeni-like syndrome do not have TP53 mutations, but have mutations in the CHEK2 gene. Like the TP53 gene, CHEK2 is a tumor suppressor gene. Researchers are uncertain whether CHEK2 mutations actually cause these conditions or are merely associated with an increased risk of certain cancers (including breast cancer)

229. Most common mutation in APC:

(a) Frameshift
(b) Point
(c) Indels
(d) None of the above

Ans: (a) Frameshift

Explanation

The responsible gene, adenomatous polyposis coli (APC), encodes a 300-kDa component of the β-catenin destruction complex in the Wnt pathway. Truncating germline mutations tend to cluster in the 5′ half and exon 15. A few mutations correlate with phenotypic severity or specific extraintestinal features, but identical mutations can produce distinct clinical manifestations. Mutations in the extreme 5′ or 3′ ends of APC exons cause a variant syndrome, attenuated APC, in which few polyps or CRCs develop late in life

Most of the APC mutations result in truncated proteins due to nonsense or frameshift mutations. One of the most common mutation sites in APC gene is codon 1309 (5 bp deletion, c.3927_3931delAAAGA). Severe Polyposis and early onset of colorectal cancer are two important features of patients with mutation at this codon. Beside polyposis which is common in patients with FAP, upper gastrointestinal manifestations are detected in 30-100% of cases. The most common mutation of APC gene must cause truncation–that is prematue shortening of gene or cutting short of the gene. That is by either frameshift or nonsense or splicing mutation. In APC most common mutation is frameshift mutation

230. False regarding attenuated FAP:

(a) Less than 100 polyps
(b) More distal colon cancer
(c) Onset delayed by 15 years
(d) None of the above

Ans: (b) More distal colon cancer

Explanation

Familial adenomatous polyposis (FAP) constitutes 1% of all CRC incidence. Hallmark features include hundreds to thousands of colonic polyps that develop in patients in their teens to 30s, and if the colon is not surgically removed, 100% of patients progress to CRC. Extracolonic manifestations include benign conditions–congenital hypertrophy of the retinal pigment epithelium, mandibular osteomas, supernumerary teeth, epidermal cysts, adrenal cortical adenomas, desmoid tumors (although these tumors may lead to obstruction)–and malignant conditions–thyroid tumors, gastric small intestinal polyps with a 5% to 10% risk of duodenal or ampullary adenocarcinoma, and brain tumors. The brain tumors may be of two types–glioblastoma multiforme or medulloblastoma–and the particular association of brain tumors and colonic polyposis is called Turcot syndrome. The colonic polyps in Turcot syndrome are fewer and larger than in classic FAP. An attenuated form of FAP harbors up to 100 colonic polyps and has a predisposition to CRC in patients when they are in their 50s or 60s. FAP is an autosomal dominant syndrome that accounts for <1% of the annual CRC burden and is caused by mutations in the tumor-suppressor APC gene. It is characterized by the presence of ≥100 adenomatous polyps in the colorectum, nearly 100% penetrance, and an inevitable risk of CRC if prophylactic colectomy is not performed. Patients with a less severe form known as AFAP usually present with <100 colorectal adenomas that tend to be proximally located. Approximately 10% to 30% of patients with clinically evident FAP/AFAP will not have an identifiable APC mutation on genetic testing, and new genetic screening methods are finding mutations associated with APC among these patients. These findings include deep intronic mutations, mosaicism, genomic rearrangements, missense mutations, as well as mutations in other genes that have yet to be identified or further characterized such as POLE, POLD1 and GREM1

(Devita, 11th Edition, Page 771)

231. False about MAP:

(a) Autosomal recessive
(b) Base pair excision repair defect
(c) APC mutation
(d) 50% penetrance

Ans: (c) APC mutation

Explanation

MAP is an autosomal recessive syndrome secondary to biallelic mutations in the MUTYH gene leading to an increase in G:C to T:A transversions within the APC and KRAS genes, and subsequently microsatellite-stable adenomas. The number of polyps in MAP is highly variable, and patients often present phenotypically as attenuated polyposis, making it difficult to differentiate MAP between AFAP and FAP MAP is an autosomal recessive disorder caused by biallelic mutation in the MUTYH gene with the number of polyps being highly variable, ranging from a few adenomas to hundreds of adenomas, making it sometimes difficult to distinguish between AFAP and classic FAP. MAP has been diagnosed in over 7% of patients with polyposis (>100 adenomas) and lack of an APC mutation, and therefore, patients with polyposis and negative APC should be tested for an MUTYH mutation. Polyps may be found throughout the colon, but, as in AFAP, there is a slight propensity to CRC proximal to the splenic flexure. It has been suggested that approximately 30% of MAP patients with CRC do not develop polyposis. The mean age at CRC diagnosis is between the late 40s and early 50s, which is later than classic FAP but similar to AFAP. The estimated cumulative risk of CRC in biallelic MUTYH mutation carriers is 80% by age 80 years (19% by age 50 years, 43% by age 60 years). Additionally, there is a 2.5 increased risk of CRC for heterozygous carriers of MUTYH mutations compared with the general population, and an even higher risk if they have a first-degree relative diagnosed with CRC. Synchronous cancers occur in up to 24% of MAP patients. In MAP APC is not mutated, there is a mutation in MUTYH gene

Al-Tassan and colleagues (2002) reported for the first time that predisposition to multiple colorectal adenomas and carcinomas can be inherited in an autosomal recessive manner. By analyzing tumor DNAs from three affected individuals of the same family, they found that APC tumor suppressor gene was somatically inactivated due to the frequent occurrence of G:C to T:A transversions. Such a pattern was suggestive of a defect in the repair system that prevents mutations caused by spontaneous oxidation of guanine to 8-oxoguanine, the most prevalent product of the oxidative stress. Accordingly, the human genes encoding for the enzymes of the BER pathway were entirely sequenced and germline biallelic mutations in MUTYH were detected in the affected members of the family. Subsequent studies have unequivocally established the association between MUTYH germline mutations and predisposition to adenomas and CRCs, confirming the preponderance of G:C to T:A transversions as a molecular feature of MAP-associated tumors. Base excision repair pathway gene is MUTYH gene. The estimated cumulative risk of CRC in biallelic MUTYH mutation carriers is 80% by age 80 years–which indicates it is not having 100% penetrance

232. True statement is:

(a) Menin gene implicated in MEN 2

(b) 90% penetrance in MEN 2

(c) MTC in MEN 2B is better prognostic than sporadic cancer

(d) Chromosome 11 in MEN 2A

Ans: (c) MTC in MEN 2B is better prognostic than sporadic cancer

Explanation

Classical MEN1 syndrome is inherited in accordance with Knudson's two-hit hypothesis, exhibiting a 90% penetrance by age 50 years in MEN1 patients with an inherited MEN1 mutant copy. Multiple endocrine neoplasia type 2 (MEN2) is a hereditary disease, further categorized as being type 2A or type 2B. Both multiple endocrine neoplasia type 2A (MEN2A) and multiple endocrine neoplasia type 2B (MEN2B) are autosomal dominant diseases, with MEN2A comprising 90% of MEN2 cases (including familial medullary thyroid cancer [MTC]) and MEN2B comprising approximately 10% of MEN2 cases.

Percent of Clinical Features by MEN 2 Subtype			
Subtype	**Medullary Thyroid Carcinoma**	**Pheochromocytoma**	**Parathyroid Disease**
MEN 2A	95%	50%	20%-30%
FMTC	100%	0%	0%
MEN 2B	100%	50%	Uncommon

MEN2A has variable penetrance as seen in the table whereas MEN1 has 90% penetrance

Multiple Endocrine Neoplasia Syndromes				
	MEN1	**MEN2A**	**MEN2B**	**MEN4**
Gene	*MEN1*	*RET*	*RET*	*CDKN1B*
OMIM#	131100	171400	162300	610755
Function	Tumor suppressor	Protooncogene	Protooncogene	Tumor suppressor
Gene location	11q13	10q11.21	10q11.21	12q13
Gene structure	10 exons	21 exons	21 exons	3 exons
Protein product	Menin (610 aa)	Ret (1,114 aa)	Ret (1,114 aa)	p27 (198 aa)
Inheritance	AD	AD	AD	AD
Prevalence	2:100,000	MEN2: 1:35,000		12 index cases reported
		70%-80% of MEN2 cases	5% of MEN2 cases	
Tumors				
Pituitary	Pituitary adenoma (30%-40%)			Pituitary adenoma (40%)
Parathyroid	Parathyroid adenoma (90%)	Parathyroid tumors (20%-30%)		Parathyroid adenoma (80%)

Menin is a protein product involved in MEN1 syndrome. Whereas in MEN 2 Syndromes it is RET protein. Chromosome 11 is involved in MEN1 whereas chr. 10 is involved in MEN2

Medullary thyroid cancer–MTC is a neuroendocrine tumor of the parafollicular or C cells of the thyroid gland. Most cases of MTC (75 percent) are sporadic, but as many as 25 percent of all MTCs are familial. Among patients with MEN2, virtually all patients develop clinically apparent MTC, often early in life. In MEN2A-associated MTC, the peak incidence of index cases is in the third decade of life, and it is usually earlier in MEN2B. Specific RET mutations are associated with characteristic age-specific penetrance of MTC, as well as characteristic prevalence of the extrathyroidal manifestations. MTCs in patients with MEN2 are multicentric and concentrated in the upper third of the thyroid gland, reflecting the normal distribution of parafollicular cells

If diagnosed as an index case, the clinical presentation and manifestations of MEN2-associated MTC are similar to those of sporadic MTC, except that sporadic MTC typically presents later in life. The most common presentation is that of a solitary thyroid nodule or cervical lymphadenopathy. Fine-needle aspiration (FNA) biopsy shows eccentrically placed nuclei that are larger and more pleomorphic than those of normal follicular cells. The cytoplasm may be slightly granular and is usually configured as a tear drop or cytoplasmic tail. If the diagnosis is suspected, immunocytologic staining for calcitonin should be performed

MTC in MEN2B has a better prognosis should be taken as the answer by exclusion

233. Action of trastuzumab is:

(a) Extracellular

(b) Intracellular

(c) Both

(d) None

Ans: (b) Intracellular

Explanation

Trastuzumab (Herceptin) is a humanized IgG1 that targets domain IV of the HER2/ErbB2 member of the EGFR/ErbB family of receptor tyrosine kinases. Gene amplification as judged by fluorescence in situ hybridization (FISH) with concomitant overexpression of HER2 protein measured by immunohistochemistry (IHC) is seen in approximately 25% of breast cancers. HER2 amplification and overexpression is now recognized to be a critical driver in a subset (7% to 34%) of gastric cancers. Trastuzumab inhibits tumor cell growth by binding to HER2 and blocking the unregulated HER2 signaling that is associated with high-level overexpression

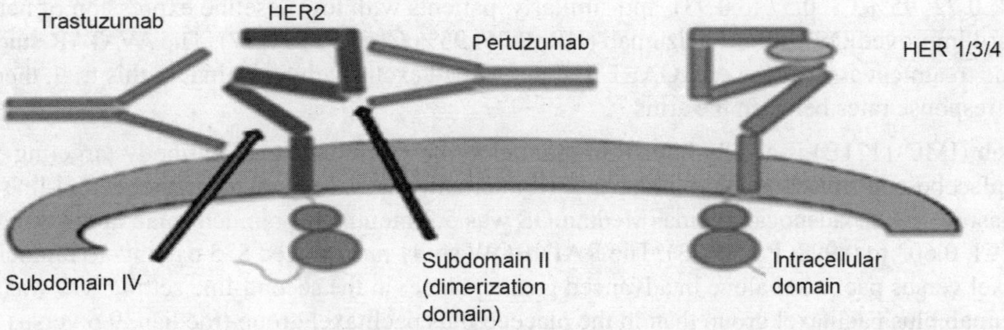

Mechanisms of Action of Trastuzumab and Pertuzumab–Trastuzumab and pertuzumab are similar in that they are both IgG 1 monoclonal antibodies that activated ADCC. Their mechanisms of action differ. Trastuzumab binds HER2 subdomain IV and inhibits activation of HER2. Pertuzumab binds HEF2 subdomain III and inhibits activation of HER2 by interaction with HER1/3/4 molecules. HER–human epidermal growth factor receptor; IgG–immunoglobulin G; ADCC–antibody-dependent cell-mediated cytotoxicity

Obviously action of trastuzumab is intracellular

234. All are immunoconjugates *except:*

(a) Brentuximab vedotin
(b) Ibrituzumab tiuxetan
(c) Trastuzumab emtansin
(d) Nivolumab

Ans: (d) Nivolumab

Explanation

Three ADCs are now approved for use in clinical practice. Ado-trastuzumab emtansine an ADC composed of the anti-HER2 MAb trastuzumab linked to DM1, is now approved for the treatment of patients with refractory HER2/neu-expressing breast cancers. The other, brentuximab vedotin, is an ADC consisting of the anti-CD30 chimeric MAb cAC10 that is linked to three to five molecules of the microtubule-disrupting agent monomethyl auristatin E (MMAE). At this point, this drug is approved for use in patients with recurrent systemic anaplastic large cell lymphoma. Inotuzumab ozogamicin is another ADC that was recently approved for treatment of patients with acute lymphoblastic leukemia (ALL). This drug is directed against CD22+ B cell found in patients with B-cell ALL. This drug is based on a similar platform as used with another ADC, gemtuzumab ozogamicin

Two anti-CD20 radioimmunoconjugates have been FDA approved for radioimmunotherapy (RIT) of non-Hodgkin lymphoma. Ibritumomab tiuxetan (Zevalin) and tositumomab (Bexxar) are murine MAbs labeled with yttrium-90(90Y) and iodine-131 (131I), respectively

Nivolumab is anti PD1 monoclonal antibody which is an immunotherapy molecule. Ibritumomab tiuxetan is a radioimmunoconjugate and brentuximab vedotin AntiCD30 and Ado trastuzumab emtasine both are antibody drug conjugates

(Devita, 11th Edition, Page 693)

235. All are useful in gastric cancer *except:*

(a) Ramicirumab
(b) Bevacizumab
(c) 5 FU
(d) All of the above

Ans: (b) Bevacizumab

Explanation

Bevacizumab

Bevacizumab is a humanized monoclonal antibody that binds the vascular endothelial growth factor ligand (VEGFA). In the AVAGAST multinational phase III trial comparing bevacizumab plus XP versus XP alone, patients were randomly assigned to XP (n = 387) or XP/bevacizumab (n = 387). The study did not meet the primary endpoint of improving OS (12.1 months with XP/bevacizumab versus 10.1 months with XP, P = .1), but bevacizumab did demonstrate improvement in PFS (6.7 versus 5.3 months, P = .004) and ORRs (46.0% versus 37.4%, P = .03). In this study, non-Asian patients appeared to benefit more than Asian patients. Furthermore, patients with high baseline plasma VEGF-A appeared to benefit from bevacizumab therapy (HR, 0.72; 95% CI, 0.57 to 0.93), and similarly, patients with low baseline expression of neuropilin 1 also showed a trend toward improved OS with bevacizumab (HR, 0.75; 95% CI, 0.59 to 0.97). The AVATAR study was a phase III trial with the same treatment arms as the AVAGAST trial performed exclusively in China. In this trial, there was no difference in OS, PFS, or response rates between the arms

Ramucirumab (IMC-1121B) is a fully human immunoglobulin G1 monoclonal antibody targeting VEGFR2. The Regard study was a placebo-controlled, double-blind, phase III international trial conducted in the second-line setting in patients with metastatic gastric or EGJ adenocarcinoma. Median OS was 5.2 months for ramucirumab and 3.8 months for placebo (HR, 0.776; 95% CI, 0.603 to 0.998; P = .0473). The RAINBOW study randomized 885 patients to ramucirumab in combination with paclitaxel versus paclitaxel alone in advanced gastric cancer in the second-line setting. OS was significantly longer in the ramucirumab plus paclitaxel group than in the placebo plus paclitaxel group (median, 9.6 versus 7.4 months; HR, 0.81; P = .017)

Bevacizumab is VEGF inhibitor but not found to be useful in gastric cancer. But VEGF receptor inhibitor ramucirumab is found to be useful in gastric cancer. Obviously 5FU is the backbone of adjuvant or metastatic chemotherapy like FOLFOX chemotherapy

(Devita, 11th Edition, Page 1425)

236. Drugs used in melanoma is:

(a) Ipilimumab
(b) Tremelimumab
(c) Pembrolizumab
(d) All of the above

Ans: (d) All of the above

Explanation

Melanoma	
Improved overall survival	Ipilimumab (vs. gp 100 peptide vaccine)
	Vemurafenib (vs. dacarbazine)
	Trametinib (vs, dacarbazine)
	Pembrolizumab (vs, ipilimumab)
	Nivolumab (vs. ipilimumab)
	Dabrafenib + trametinib (vs. dabrafenib)
	Dabrafenib + trametinib (vs. vemurafenib)
	Vermurafenib + cobimetinib (vs. vemurafenib)
	Nivolumab + ipilimumab (vs. ipilimumab)
Improved progression-free survival	Dabrafenib (vs. dacarbazine)
	Trametinib (vs. dacarbazine)
	Nab-paclitaxel (vs. dacarbazine)
	Encorafenib + binimetinib (vs. encorafenib)
	Encorafenib + binimetinib (vs. vemurafenib)
Improved response duration	T-VEC (vs. granulocyte-macrophage colony-stimulating factor)
Validated antitumor activity	High-dose interleukin-2
	TIL ACT
	Carboplatin-paclitaxel
	Dacarbazine
	Fotemustine

Another anti–CTLA-4 antibody, tremelimumab (Pfizer and MedImmune-Astra Zeneca, New York, NY), has been developed clinically in patients with metastatic melanoma. This fully human immunoglobulin G2 monoclonal antibody went through phase I, II and III testing in melanoma but failed to demonstrate improvement in OS compared to dacarbazine. Potential contributing factors were the study design, the treated population, the dosing regimen and the postrandomization use of ipilimumab in the control arm

All the three drugs are used in melanoma, hence answer is all of the above

(Devita, 11th Edition, Page 2728)

237. Drug used in Hodgkin's lymphoma (anti-CD 30):

(a) Brentuximab vedotin
(b) Pembrolizumab
(c) Bevacizumab
(d) All of the above

Ans: (a) Brentuximab vedotin

Explanation

Brentuximab vedotin (SGN-35, Adcetris), is an ADC consisting of the anti-CD30 chimeric MAb cAC10 that is linked to three to five molecules of the microtubule-disrupting agent monomethyl auristatin E (MMAE)

(Devita, 11th Edition, Page 693)

238. Drug targeting CD 33 in AML:

(a) Alemtuzumab
(b) Brentuximab
(c) Gemtuzumab ozogamicin
(d) Nivolumab

Ans: (c) Gemtuzumab ozogamicin

Explanation

More recently, the anti-CD33-directed antibody drug conjugate gemtuzumab ozogamicin that delivers the toxin calcheamicin to AML blasts has been investigated in a number of large randomized trials in addition to standard AML induction and consolidation.Overall, these trials have suggested a survival benefit for patients with favorable- and intermediate-risk AML, in particular patients with favorable risk, and this has led to the recent approval of gemtuzumab ozogamicin in AML by the U.S. Food and Drug Administration (FDA)

(Devita, 11th Edition, Page 3074)

PAPER 6 (SET 1)

239. False statement about lung cancer:

(a) Clubbing will not resolve with excision of the primary lesion

(b) Pleural fluid is an ominous feature

(c) Dyspnoea may come from lymphatic invasion

(d) Severe localised pain suggests chest wall invasion

Ans: (b) Pleural fluid is an ominous feature

Explanation

Severe localised pain suggests chest wall invasion with the infiltration of an intercostal nerve. Invasion of the apical area may involve the brachial plexus, leading to Pancoast's syndrome

Dyspnoea may come from loss of functioning lung tissue, lymphatic invasion or the development of a large pleural effusion Pleural fluid is an ominous feature and the presence of blood in a pleural effusion suggests that the pleura has been directly invaded

Clubbing and hypertrophic pulmonary osteoarthropathy accompany some lung cancer and may resolve with excision of the primary lesion

(Sabiston, Page 925)

240. Most common cardiac lesion in carcinoid syndrome:

(a) Pulmonary regurgitation
(b) Pulmonary stenosis
(c) Tricuspid regurgitation
(d) Triscuspid stenosis

Ans: (b) Pulmonary stenosis

Explanation

In carcinoid cardiac lesions usually involve right side of the heart, but left sided lesions present in 15%, lead to CCF

(Sabiston, Page 1273)

241. The best predictor of survival for patients with gastrinoma is:

(a) Lymph node metastasis
(b) Location of tumor
(c) Hepatic mets
(d) Gastrin level

Ans: (c) Hepatic mets

Explanation

The 10-year survival rate is 30% in patients with the aggressive form compared with greater than 90% in patients with the non-aggressive form

The best predictor of survival for patients with gastrinoma is the presence of liver metastases; lymph node metastases are not predictive

(Sabiston, Page 956)

242. Most common second primary site in small bowel carcinoid is:

(a) Colon
(b) Ileum
(c) Ovary
(d) Lung

Ans: (a) Colon

Explanation

Unusual observation in carcinoid tumor is second primary lesion of different histologic type. Usually synchronus adenocarcinoma in large intestine (10-20%)

(Sabiston, Page 1272)

243. Which benign lesion of duodenum mimics peptic ulcer?

(a) Hemangioma
(b) Lipoma
(c) Hyperplastic polyp
(d) Brunner gland adenoma

Ans: (d) Brunner gland adenoma

Explanation

Brunner gland adenoma usually from proximal duodenum benign hyperplastic lesion; produces symptoms mimics PUD

(Sabiston, Page 1271)

244. Most common symptomatic benign neoplasm of small bowel:

(a) Hemangioma
(b) Lipoma
(c) Stromal tumor
(d) Adenoma

Ans: (c) Stromal tumor

Explanation

Adenoma reported most commonly in aytopsy series. But stromal tumors are most common benign SI neoplasm that produce symptoms

(Sabiston, Page 1270)

245. Most common tumor of small intestine:

(a) Adenocarcinoma
(b) Lymphoma
(c) Adenoma
(d) Metastasis

Ans: (d) Metastasis

Explanation

Metastatic tumors of SI is much more common than primary neoplasm. Mets arising from ovary, cervix, kidney, stomach extra abdominal–cutaneous melanoma (Most common), breast, lung

(Sabiston, Page 1280)

246. Nodal involvement in SI GIST is …….. stage.

(a) IIIC
(b) III B
(c) III A
(d) IV

Ans (d) IV

Explanation

If N1 or M1 irrespective of mitotic rate, staged as IV

(Sabiston, Page 1280)

247. Which of the following is false regarding testicular seminoma?

(a) Active lymphocyte infiltration indicate good prognosis
(b) Two histological subtypes

(c) Main metastasis via blood

(d) Inguinal node enlarged only when scrotal skin involved

Ans: (c) Main metastasis via blood

Explanation

Seminoma most common testicular germ cell tumor. Remain localised for long term. Spread via lymphatics mainly. Inguinal node enlarged only when scrotal skin involved

Subtypes: Spermatocytic, anaplastic

(Bailey, Page 1506)

248. Which of the following is false regarding non seminomatous GCT?

(a) Yolk sac tumor secrete AFP

(b) Immature teratoma will not metastasise

(c) Different histological type coexist within a single tumor

(d) Teratoma contains cystic spaces with gelatinous fluid

Ans: (b) Immature teratoma will not metastasise

Explanation

Both immature and mature teratoma will metastasise

(Bailey, Page 1506)

249. Which of the following metastasise early via both blood and lymph?

(a) Choriocarcinoma

(b) Embryonal carcinoma

(c) Teratoma

(d) Yolk sac tumor

Ans: (a) Choriocarcinoma

Explanation

Choriocarcinoma is highly malignant that metastasise early via both lymphatics and blood

(Bailey, Page 1507)

250. Which of the following is feminizing tumor?

(a) Yolk sac tumor

(b) Tertaoma

(c) Leydig cell tumor

(d) Sertoli cell tumor

Ans: (d) Sertoli cell tumor

Explanation

Leydig cell tumor–masculanises. Sertoli cell tumor feminises

(Bailey, Page 1507)

251. Which of the following is false regarding interstitial tumor?

(a) Only 10% malignant

(b) Most prepubertal tumors secrete feminizing hormones

(c) Regression of symptoms after orchidectomy may be incomplete

(d) Well circumscribed tumor with yellow cut surface

Ans: (b) Most prepubertal tumors secrete feminizing hormones

Explanation

Most prepubertal tumors secrete androgens. Postpubertal–feminizing hormones.10% of tumors only malignant

(Bailey, Page 1507)

252. Nodes below diaphragm staged in testicular tumor staged as in older staging system, Stage ....

(a) I
(b) II
(c) III
(d) IV

Ans: (b) II

Explanation

Stage I: Tumor is confined to the testis and epididymis

Stage II: Nodal disease is present but is confined to nodes below the diaphragm

Stage III: Nodes are present above the diaphragm

Stage IV: Non-lymphatic metastatic disease (most typically within the lungs)

(Bailey, Page 1508)

253. Which of the following is false regarding testicular tumor investigation?

(a) Usg is mandatory
(b) Tumor marker raised in 50% cases
(c) CT chest, abdomen usually undertaken after orchidectomy
(d) Serum half life of AFP 3 days

Ans: (d) Serum half life of AFP 3 days

Explanation

Serum half life of AFP –5 to 7 days, Hcg half life 2-3 days

(Bailey, Page 1508)

254. Which of the following is false regarding testicular tumor examination?

(a) Lax secondary hydrocele usually obscures the underlying tumor, if present
(b) Vas is never thickened
(c) Around 5% of cases have gynaecomastia
(d) In 1–2% of cases the tumor is bilateral at the time of diagnosis

Ans: (a) Lax secondary hydrocele usually obscures the underlying tumor, if present

Explanation

On examination there is an intratesticular solid mass. If present, a lax secondary hydrocele does not usually obscure the underlying tumor

(Bailey, Page 1507)

255. Which of the following is second most common tumor of testes?

(a) Interstitial cell tumors
(b) Metastasis
(c) Lymphoma
(d) Germ cell tumor

Ans: (c) Lymphoma

Explanation

Germ cell tumors (90–95%) (these include seminoma, embryonal cell carcinoma, yolk sac tumor, teratoma and choriocarcinoma

- interstitial tumors (1–2%) (these include Leydig cell tumors)
- lymphoma (3–7%)
- other tumors (1–2%)

(Bailey, Page 1506)

256. Which of the following is false regarding stage I testicular tumor treatment after orchidectomy?

(a) NSGCT having less chance of sub clinical mets compared to seminoma

(b) In seminoma stage I, chemotherapy indicated only if relapse occurs

(c) NSGCT is radiosensitive and chemosensitive

(d) NSGCT with good prognosis can be managed with surveillance alone in stage I

Ans: (c) NSGCT is radiosensitive and chemosensitive

Explanation

NSGCTs are not radiosensitive, but they are highly sensitive to combination chemotherapy. Up to 30% of NSGCT patients with stage I disease have subclinical metastases and will relapse if surveillance alone is applied. Only around 15–20% of men with stage I seminoma have subclinical metastatic disease

(Bailey, Page 1509)

257. Following is not a chemotherapy drug for GCT:

(a) Taxanes (b) Cisplatin

(c) Bleomycin (d) Etoposide

Ans: (a) Taxanes

Explanation

Bleomycin, etoposide and cis-platinum (so called BEP chemotherapy)

(Bailey, Page 1509)

258. Recommended margin for wide local excision of 3 mm thickness melanoma:

(a) 0.5 CM (b) 1

(c) 1.5 CM (d) 2 CM

Ans: (d) 2 CM

Explanation

Thickness	Margin*
In situ	0.5 cm
<1 mm	1 cm
1-2 mm	1-2 cm†
>2-4 mm	2 cm
>4 mm	2 cm‡

(Sbaiston, Page 734)

PAPER 6 (SET 2)

259. Intransit mets with single node involvement in malignant melanoma is …….. stage acc to AJCC 8th edition.

(a) II C
(b) II B
(c) III B
(d) III C

Ans: (d) III C

(AJCC, 8th Edition, NCCN website)

260. Single most important prognostic index in melanoma:

(a) Breslow thickness
(b) Lymph node mets
(c) Ulceration
(d) Mitotic index

Ans: (b) Lymph node mets

Explanation

The presence of lymph node metastases is the single most important prognostic index in melanoma, outweighing both tumor and host factors

(Bailey, Page 612)

261. All are true about merkel cell tumor *except:*

(a) Wide local excision enough
(b) Radiotherapy needed
(c) Aggressive one
(d) Common in women

Ans: (a) Wide local excision enough

Explanation

Treatment is with wide local excision aiming for a 25–30 mm margin, followed by radiotherapy

(Bailey, Page 612)

262. Which of the following drug not used in malignant melanoma stage 4?

(a) Dabrafenib
(b) Regorafenib
(c) Trametinib
(d) Iplimumab

Ans: (b) Regorafenib

Explanation

Stage 4 malignant melanoma–targeted therapies

Dabrafenib or vemurafenib

Trametinib alone or combined with dabrafenib

Immune checkpoint inhibitors: Iplimumab, nivolimumab

(Bailey, Page 612)

263. False about subungual melanoma:

(a) Usually superficial spreading type
(b) Classical feature Hutchinson sign
(c) DD is benign racial melanonychia
(d) Malignancy is unlikely if nail fold is involved

Ans: (d) Malignancy is unlikely if nail fold is involved

Explanation

MM under the finger usually SSM rather than ALM. Malignancy is unlikely if the nail fold is uninvolved

264. Which of the following will not a chemical carcinogen causing lung cancer?

(a) Ethylene oxide (b) Beryllium

(c) Radon (d) Vinyl chloride

Ans: (a) Ethylene oxide

Explanation

Ethylene oxide causes leukemia, lymphoma

Lung cancer–beryllium, cadmium, chromium, radon, vinyl chloride

(Sabiston, Page 695)

265. All are predominant tumor caused by azathioprine *except:*

(a) Hepatocellular carcinoma (b) Leukemia

(c) Squamous cell carcinoma skin (d) NHL

Ans: (b) Leukemia

Explanation

Azathioprine causes–HCC, NHL, SCC skin, cholangio ca

Chlorambucil–leukemia

(Sabiston, Page 695)

266. ....% of all human tumors caused by virus.

(a) 15 (b) 10

(c) 20 (d) 25

Ans: (a) 15

Explanation

15% tumors caused by virus. Most of them are HPV causes cervical ca, HBV, HCV cause HCC

(Sabiston, Page 696)

267. Which of the following is false regarding virus induced tumor?

(a) Long latent period (b) Viral markers usually present in neoplastic cells

(c) Tumor virus causes persistent infection (d) Viral factors are important determinant of tumorigenesis

Ans: (d) Viral factors are important determinant of tumorigenesis

Explanation

Host factors are important determinant of tumorigenesis, not viral factors

(Sabiston, Page 696)

268. Which of the following is not a DNA based tumor marker?

(a) Single nucleotide polymorphism (b) Chromosomal translocation

(c) Over expressed transcript (d) Epigenetic changes

Ans: (c) Over expressed transcript

Explanation

RNA based tumor markers – over/under expressed transcript, regulatory RNA (micro RNA). Others are DNA based tumor markers

(Sabiston, Page 697)

269. Most common symptom of small bowel malignancy:

(a) Abdominal pain
(b) Hemorrhage
(c) Weight loss
(d) Vomiting

Ans: (a) Abdominal pain

Explanation

Malignant lesion unlike benign lesion, almost always produce symptoms. Most common is abdominal pain

Second common is weight loss. Obstruction occurs secondary to adhesion, infiltration

(Sabiston, Page 1271)

270. Which of the following type of SI lymphoma usually chemo resistant?

(a) DLBCL
(b) Both
(c) B cell
(d) T cell

Ans: (d) T cell

Explanation

B cell lymphomas are more chemosensitive than T cell lymphomas and have high remission rates with or without surgery

T cell lymphomas are traditionally more resistant to therapy and will progress to symptoms of obstruction or perforation if not resected

(Sabiston, Page 1278)

271. False regarding peritoneal mesothelioma:

(a) Complete surgical excision is usually not possible
(b) Encasement of bowel create obstruction
(c) Local invasion of abdominal wall will not occur
(d) Common in males

Ans: (c) Local invasion of abdominal wall will not occur

Explanation

Slight male predominance and a median age at presentation of approximately 50 years

In contrast to pseudomyxoma peritonei, local invasion of intra-abdominal organs, such as the liver, intestine, bladder, and abdominal wall, can occur.

Encasement of bowel can create a malignant bowel obstruction

Complete surgical resection is difficult because of the extent of disease

(Sabiston, Page 1081)

272. False regarding pseudomyxoma peritonei:

(a) APPENDIX most common primary site
(b) Females affected more
(c) Patients often asymptomatic
(d) 4th 5th decade usually affected

Ans: (b) Females affected more

Explanation

Pseudomyxoma peritonei occurs most commonly in patients who are 40 to 50 years of age and occurs with equal frequency in men and women. Patients are often asymptomatic until late in the course of their disease

Appendix Most common primary site

Others causing – ovarian adeno ca

diagnosis usually made during laparatomy

(Sabiston, Page 1080)

273. Metastasis in a single node size 4 cm with extra nodal extension in carcinoma oral cavity N stage?

(a) N2a
(b) N2b
(c) N2c
(d) N3

Ans: (d) N3

Explanation

N1- Single ipsilateral <= 3 cm
N2 a- Single ipsilateral > 3 cm <= 6 cm
b- Multiple ipsilateral none > 6 cm
c- Bilateral or contralateral none > 6 cm
N3 a- Mets in LN > 6 cm without extra nodal extension
b- Mets in a single or multiple LN with extra nodal extension

(AJCC, 8th Edition, NCCN website)

274. Which of the following gene mutation increase susceptibility to radiation induced cancer?

(a) p53
(b) BRCA
(c) MAPK
(d) Cerb B2

Ans: (a) p53

Explanation

p53 mutation increase susceptibility to malignancy induced by radiation

So, p53 mutation is a relative contraindication to radiation

(Sabiston, Page 846)

275. First investigation in suspected pheochromocytoma:

(a) Spot serum metanephrin
(b) 24 hours urinary VMA
(c) Clonidine suppression test
(d) 24 hours urinary metanephrins

Ans: (a) Spot serum metanephrin

Explanation

Initial plasma free metanephrin testing effectively exclude the diagnosis if negative

(Ref: Sabiston Page 981)

276. Prognosis for Dukes stage C 5 years survival:

(a) 50%
(b) 40%
(c) 30%
(d) 25%

Ans: (b) 40%

Explanation

Prognosis worsen as the stage advances. For Dukes stage A, 5 years survival is 90%. For stage C, 5 years survival is 40%

(Bailey, Page 1331)

277. Which of the following is most common histological type of stromal tumor of SI?

(a) Fusiform (b) Epithelioid

(c) Papillary (d) Mixed

Ans: (a) Fusiform

Explanation

Three histological sub types of stromal tumors : fusiform (77%), epithelioid (8%), mixed (15%)

(Sabiston, Page 1270)

278. Which of the following is not a high risk feature of differentiated thyroid malignancy?

(a) 45 years age (b) Male sex

(c) Extra thyroid extension (d) 3 cm size

Ans: (d) 3 cm size

Explanation

HIGH RISK

>40 years

Male

Capsular invasion, extrathyroidal extension

Regional or distant mets

>4 cm

Poorly differentiated

(Sabiston, Page 903)

PAPER 6 (SET 3)

279. Which of the following is not a component in cancer of the Liver Italian Program (CLIP)?

(a) Portal vein thrombosis
(b) Child Pugh class
(c) AST level
(d) Tumor extension

Ans: (c) AST level

Explanation

CLIP–AFP level not AST level. Others are correct

Cancer of the Liver Italian Program Score		
Clinical Parameters	**Cutoff Values**	**Points**
Child-Pugh class	A	0
	B	1
	C	2
Tumor morphology	Uninodular, <50% extension	0
	Multinodular, <50% extension	1
	Massive or extension >50%	2
AFP level	<400 ng/dL	0
	>400 ng/dL	1
Portal vein thrombosis	No	0
	Yes	1

(Sabiston, Page 1460)

280. Which of the following is not a component in Okuda staging system?

(a) Serum bilirubin
(b) Serum albumin
(c) Tumor stage
(d) Ascites

Ans: (c) Tumor stage

Explanation

The Okuda staging system is an older but simple and effective system that takes liver function and tumor-related factors into account

It adds up a single point for the presence of tumor involving more than 50% of the liver, presence of ascites, albumin level less than 3 g/dL and bilirubin level higher than 3 mg/dL

The Okuda staging system reliably distinguishes patients with a prohibitively poor prognosis from those with potential for long-term survival

(Sabiston, Page 1460)

281. False regarding fibrolamellar HCC:

(a) Recurrence common
(b) Older circumscribed and Non encapsulated
(c) Elevated neurotensin
(d) Lymph node mets predicts worse outcome

Ans: (b) Older circumscribed and Non encapsulated

Explanation

Fibrolamellar HCC is a variant of HCC with remarkably different clinical features

This tumor generally occurs in younger patients without a history of cirrhosis

The tumor is usually well demarcated and encapsulated and may have a central fibrotic area

The presence of lymph node metastases predicts a worse outcome

Resection of lymph node metastases and recurrent disease has been advocated because of a lack of alternative therapy and the possibility of long-term survival

Fibrolamellar HCC does not produce AFP but is associated with elevated neurotensin levels

(Sabiston, Page 1462)

282. Factors most useful to predict outcome in colorectal liver mets all *except:*

(a) Size of the primary tumor >5 cm
(b) LN positive primary lesion
(c) Increased CEA >200 ng/ml
(d) More than one tumor

Ans: (a) Size of the primary tumor >5 cm

Explanation

Most influential on outcome:

Size larger than 5 cm
Disease-free interval less than 1 year
More than one tumor
Lymph node positive primary, and
CEA level higher than 200 ng/mL
Size of the metastasis > 5 cm, not primary tumor

(Sabiston, Page 1467)

283. False regarding hepatoblastoma:

(a) Low birth weight may be a risk factor
(b) More common in males
(c) Associated with von Recklinghausen disease
(d) Not associated with inborn errors of metabolism

Ans: (c) Associated with von Recklinghausen disease

Explanation

Associated with Beckwith Wiedemann syndrome and FAP, not with von Recklinghausen disease. Most common primary hepatic tumor of childhood. Common in males

Not associated with hepatitis, cirrhosis, inborn errors of metabolism

(Sabiston, Page 1464)

284. False regarding cystadenoma:

(a) Fluid content is mucinous
(b) CECT–enhancement cyst wall
(c) Grows rapidly
(d) USG–nodularity, fluid filled locule

Ans: (c) Grows rapidly

Explanation

Ultrasound usually demonstrates a cystic structure with varying wall thickness, nodularity, septations, and fluid-filled locules

Importantly, contrast-enhanced CT demonstrates enhancement of the cyst wall and septa

Cystadenomas tend to grow slowly but can eventually progress to their malignant counterpart, cystadenocarcinomas

(Sabiston, Page 1469)

285. Typical peripheral nodular enhancement seen in:

(a) Hepatic adenoma
(b) Hepatoblastoma
(c) Hemangioma
(d) Focal nodular hyperplasia (FNH)

Ans: (c) hemangioma

Explanation

FNH – homogenous mass with central scar, enhances in arterial phase

Hepatic adenoma–heterogenous and hypervascular on arterial phase

Hepatoblastoma–vascular mass with speckled calcification

(Sabiston, Page 1457)

286. Risk of rupture is more with:

(a) Hepatic adenoma
(b) Hepatoblastoma
(c) Hemangioma
(d) Focal nodular hyperplasia (FNH)

Ans: (a) Hepatic adenoma

Explanation

30-50% risk of rupture with hepatic adenoma. Malignant transformation is less

(Sabiston, Page 1456)

287. Most common NET of pancreas:

(a) Insulinoma
(b) Gastrinoma
(c) Non-functional NET
(d) Functional NET

Ans: (c) Non-functional NET

Explanation

Non-functional NET S more common type and mostly malignant. Among functional NET, insulinoma is most common type

(Sabiston, Page 944)

288. Most common location of GIST:

(a) Omentum
(b) Colon
(c) Small bowel
(d) Stomach

Ans: (d) Stomach

Explanation

Stomach is the most common site for GIST
Second most common is small bowel
Arises from interstitial cells of kajal
Equal sex distribution, slight male predominance
Diagnosed by EUS

(Sabiston)

289. False regarding gastrinoma:

(a) Most common symptom abdominal pain
(b) Ryles tube aspiration stops diarrhea
(c) Only 50% occurs inside passaro triangle
(d) Most common site 1st part of duodenum

Ans: (c) Only 50% occurs inside passaro triangle

Explanation

70-90% occurs inside passaro triangle bounded by junction of cystic duct and CBD, junction of 2nd and 3rd part of duodenum, junction of neck and body of pancreas

Approximately 75% of patients present with abdominal pain

Almost two thirds of patients with abdominal pain have diarrhea

In 10% to 20% of patients, diarrhea is the only symptom

This acid-induced diarrhea is stopped by nasogastric aspiration of gastric secretions, differentiating it from other secretory diarrheas

(Sabiston, Page 954)

290. False regarding ZES:

(a) Elevated serum gastrin is enough to diagnose
(b) Most patients have peptic ulcer.
(c) Gastrin level >1000 pg/ml is diagnostic
(d) Duodenal primary tends to spread to local lymph nodes

Ans: (a) Elevated serum gastrin is enough to diagnose

Explanation

Hypergastrinemia results in peptic acid hypersecretion and refractory peptic ulcer disease. Duodenal ulcers are the most common. Elevated serum gastrin and with increased gastric acid secretion is must. BAO >15 meq/hr

(Sabiston, Page 954)

291. Best intraoperative localization of insulinoma:

(a) Portal vein sampling with arterial stimulation with calcium stimulation
(b) EUS
(c) CECT
(d) SRS scintigraphy

Ans: (a) Portal vein sampling with arterial stimulation with calcium stimulation

Explanation

SRS sensitivity is > 80% for all Pancreatic NET except insulinoma

Best intraoperative method is EUS and palpation

(Sabiston, Page 954)

292. Most common cause of death in ZES:

(a) Hepatic metastasis
(b) MODS
(c) Hypovolemic shock
(d) Sepsis

Ans: (a) Hepatic metastasis

Explanation

The 10-year survival rate is 30% in patients with the aggressive form compared with greater than 90% in patients with the non-aggressive form

The best predictor of survival for patients with gastrinoma is the presence of liver metastases; lymph node metastases are not predictive

(Sabiston, Page 956)

293. Median survival after resection in metastatic insulinoma:

(a) 6 months
(b) 1 year
(c) 3 years
(d) 5 years

Ans: (d) 5 years

Explanation

Life expectancy should be normal after complete excision of a benign insulinoma

More extensive resections are required for complete excision of malignant insulinomas

Even with metastatic disease, the median survival after resection is approximately 5 years

(Sabiston, Page 954)

294. VIPoma lesion present in the following site *except:*

(a) Pancreas
(b) Adrenal gland
(c) Kidney
(d) Bronchus

Ans: (c) Kidney

Explanation

Of lesions, 90% are found in the pancreas 10% have been described in the colon, bronchus, liver, adrenal gland, and sympathetic ganglia

Most VIPomas are diagnosed middle-age patients, but the diagnosis is made before age 10 years in approximately 10% of patients

(Sabiston, Page 956)

295. Glucagonoma presents with following features *except:*

(a) Diabetes
(b) Dementia
(c) Depression
(d) Deep vein thrombosis

Ans: (b) Dementia

Explanation

Glucagonoma syndrome is a rare syndrome, with a classic presentation of the "4 D's": diabetes, dermatitis, deep vein thrombosis and depression

(Sabiston, Page 957)

296. Which of the following is false regarding necrolytic migrating erythema:

(a) Associated with glucagonoma
(b) Approximately two third of patients
(c) Often appears as the last symptom of the syndrome
(d) Trace element deficiency probably contribute

Ans: (c) Often appears as the last symptom of the syndrome

Explanation

The characteristic skin lesion of glucagonoma, a necrolytic migrating erythema, is noted in approximately two thirds of patients often appears before other symptoms of the syndrome

The cause is believed to be severe amino acid deficiency, although trace element deficiency and general malnutrition probably contribute

Parenteral administration of amino acids was found to result in the disappearance of the skin lesions

(Sabiston, Page 957)

297. Diabetes, gall stone, steatorrhea are classical features of which pancreatic NET:

(a) Glucagonoma
(b) Gastrinoma
(c) VIPoma
(d) Somatostatinoma

Ans: (d) Somatostatinoma

Explanation

Inhibition of pancreatic enzyme and hormone secretion by unregulated hypersecretion of somatostatin causes steatorrhea, diabetes, malabsorption and cholelithiasis resulting from reduced gallbladder emptying

(Sabiston, Page 957)

298. Entities That May Mimic Soft Tissue Sarcoma all *except:*

(a) Hypertrophic scar
(b) Keloid
(c) Cyst
(d) Melanoma

Ans: (b) Keloid

Explanation

Entities That May Mimic Soft Tissue Sarcoma
Hypertrophic scar
Retroperitoneal lymphadenopathy: lymphoma, germ cell tumor, or metastasis from gastrointestinal primary
Hematoma
Myositis ossificans
Benign lipoma
Cyst
Abscess
Cutaneous malignant neoplasms, including melanoma

(Sabiston, Page 760)

PAPER 7

299. Risk of rupture is more with:

(a) Hepatic adenoma
(b) Hepatoblastoma
(c) Hemangioma
(d) Focal nodular hyperplasia (FNH)

Ans: (a) Hepatic adenoma

Explanation

30-50% risk of rupture with hepatic adenoma. Malignant transformation is less

(Sabiston, Page 1456)

300. Most common NET of pancreas:

(a) Insulinoma
(b) Gastrinoma
(c) Non-functional NET
(d) Functional NET

Ans: (c) Non-functional NET

Explanation

Non-functional NET S more common type and mostly malignant. Among functional NET, insulinoma is most common type

(Sabiston, Page 944)

301. Most common location of GIST:

(a) Omentum
(b) Colon
(c) Small bowel
(d) Stomach

Ans: (d) Stomach

Explanation

Stomach is the most common site for GIST. Second most common is small bowel. Arises from interstitial cells of kajal. Equal sex distribution, slight male predominance. Diagnosed by EUS

(Sabiston)

302. False regarding gastrinoma:

(a) Most common symptom abdominal pain
(b) Ryles tube aspiration stops diarrhea
(c) Only 50% occurs inside passaro triangle
(d) Most common site 1st part of duodenum

Ans: (c) Only 50% occurs inside passaro triangle

Explanation

70-90% occurs inside passaro triangle bounded by junction of cystic duct and CBD, junction of 2nd and 3rd part of duodenum, junction of neck and body of pancreas

Approximately 75% of patients present with abdominal pain

Almost two thirds of patients with abdominal pain have diarrhea

In 10% to 20% of patients, diarrhea is the only symptom

This acid-induced diarrhea is stopped by nasogastric aspiration of gastric secretions, differentiating it from other secretory diarrheas

(Sabiston, Page 954)

303. False regarding ZES:

(a) Elevated serum gastrin is enough to diagnose
(b) Most patients have peptic ulcer
(c) Gastrin level >1000 pg/ml is diagnostic
(d) Duodenal primary tends to spread to local lymph nodes

Ans: (a) Elevated serum gastrin is enough to diagnose

Explanation

Hypergastrinemia results in peptic acid hypersecretion and refractory peptic ulcer disease. Duodenal ulcers are the most common Elevated serum gastrin and with increased gastric acid secretion is must. BAO >15 meq/hr

(Sabiston, Page 954)

304. Best intraoperative localization of insulinoma:

(a) Portal vein sampling with arterial stimulation with calcium stimulation
(b) EUS
(c) CECT
(d) SRS scintigraphy

Ans: (a) Portal vein sampling with arterial stimulation with calcium stimulation

Explanation

SRS sensitivity is > 80% for all Pancreatic NET except insulinoma

Best intraoperative method is EUS and palpation

(Sabiston, Page 954)

305. Most common cause of death in ZES:

(a) Hepatic metastasis
(b) MODS
(c) Hypovolemic shock
(d) Sepsis

Ans: (a) Hepatic metastasis

Explanation

The 10-year survival rate is 30% in patients with the aggressive form compared with greater than 90% in patients with the non-aggressive form

The best predictor of survival for patients with gastrinoma is the presence of liver metastases; lymph node metastases are not predictive

(Sabiston, Page 956)

306. Median survival after resection in metastatic insulinoma:

(a) 6 months
(b) 1 year
(c) 3 years
(d) 5 years

Ans: (d) 5 years

Explanation

Life expectancy should be normal after complete excision of a benign insulinoma

More extensive resections are required for complete excision of malignant insulinomas

Even with metastatic disease, the median survival after resection is approximately 5 years

(Sabiston, Page 954)

307. VIPoma lesion present in the following site *except:*

(a) Pancreas (b) Adrenal gland
(c) Kidney (d) Bronchus

Ans: (c) Kidney

Explanation

Of lesions, 90% are found in the pancreas. 10% have been described in the colon, bronchus, liver, adrenal gland, and sympathetic ganglia

Most VIPomas are diagnosed middle-age patients, but the diagnosis is made before age 10 years in approximately 10% of patients

(Sabiston, Page 956)

308. Glucagonoma presents with following features *except:*

(a) Diabetes (b) Dementia
(c) Depression d) Deep vein thrombosis

Ans: (b) Dementia

Explanation

Glucagonoma syndrome is a rare syndrome, with a classic presentation of the "4 D's": diabetes, dermatitis, deep vein thrombosis and depression

(Sabiston, Page 957)

309. Which of the following is false regarding necrolytic migrating erythema:

(a) Associated with glucagonoma (b) Approximately two third of patients
(c) Often appears as the last symptom of the syndrome (d) Trace element deficiency probably contribute

Ans: (c) Often appears as the last symptom of the syndrome

Explanation

The characteristic skin lesion of glucagonoma, a necrolytic migrating erythema, is noted in approximately two thirds of patients often appears before other symptoms of the syndrome

The cause is believed to be severe amino acid deficiency, although trace element deficiency and general malnutrition probably contribute

Parenteral administration of amino acids was found to result in the disappearance of the skin lesions

(Sabiston, Page 957)

310. Diabetes, gall stone, steatorrhea are classical features of which pancreatic NET?

(a) Glucagonoma (b) Gastrinoma
(c) VIPoma (d) Somatostatinoma

Ans: (d) Somatostatinoma

Explanation

Inhibition of pancreatic enzyme and hormone secretion by unregulated hypersecretion of somatostatin causes steatorrhea, diabetes, malabsorption and cholelithiasis resulting from reduced gallbladder emptying

(Sabiston, Page 957)

311. Entities that may Mimic Soft Tissue Sarcoma all *except:*

(a) Hypertrophic scar (b) Keloid
(c) Cyst (d) Melanoma

Ans: (b) Keloid

Explanation

Entities That May Mimic Soft Tissue Sarcoma

Hypertrophic scar

Retroperitoneal lymphadenopathy: lymphoma, germ cell tumor, or metastasis from gastrointestinal primary

Hematoma

Myositis ossificans

Benign lipoma

Cyst

Abscess

Cutaneous malignant neoplasms, including melanoma

(Sabiston, Page 760)

312. False statement about Desmoid tumor:

(a) Aggressive fibromatosis
(b) Distant metastasis is common
(c) High local recurrence
(d) Second leading causes of death in FAP patients

Ans: (b) Distant metastasis is common

Explanation

Desmoid tumors, also known as aggressive fibromatosis, are an uncommon group of fibroblastic tumors that have a curious natural history in that distant metastases are extremely rare

Desmoid tumors are usually preceded by colonic polyposis in FAP patients and represent the second leading cause of death in FAP patients

Even when the tumors are adequately resected, especially in the FAP population, desmoid tumors show a high likelihood of local recurrence

(Sabiston, Page 765)

313. Which of the following is the most important primary site of angiosarcoma?

(a) Extremity
(b) Scalp
(c) Trunk
(d) Head and neck

Ans: (b) Scalp

Explanation

In decreasing order of frequency, the most important primary sites are the trunk, head and neck (particularly the scalp) and the viscera

Within the head and neck, the scalp is often the site of angiosarcoma origin

Angiosarcoma typically is diagnosed in the seventh and eighth decades

(Sabiston, Page 766)

314. Patient with GIST with SDH mutation characterized by the following feature:

(a) Older patients
(b) Good response to imatinib therapy
(c) Multiple gastric GIST
(d) None

Ans: (c) Multiple gastric GIST

Explanation

The third major molecular GIST group is characterized by SDH mutations

Patients with these mutations are generally younger, have multiple gastric GISTs and have a poor response to imatinib

(Sabiston, Page 769)

315. ...... mutations are related to GIST in patients affected by the Carney-Stratakis syndrome.

(a) c kit (b) PDGFRA

(c) BRAF (d) SDH

Ans: (d) SDH

Explanation

Overall, about 70% of GIST tumors have KIT gene mutations

Approximately 7% have PDGFRA mutations and

15% have wild-type KIT and PDGFRA genotypes. These GIST tumors are characterized by a number of other mutations affecting succinate dehydrogenase (SDH), BRAF, KRAS and NF1

SDH mutations are related to GIST in patients affected by the Carney-Stratakis syndrome, and

NF1 mutations drive GIST formation in patients with type 1 neurofibromatosis

(Sabiston, Page 768)

316. DOG1 is:

(a) Calcium-activated chloride channel (b) Chloride activated calcium channel

(c) Sodium activated chloride channel (d) Chloride activated sodium channel

Ans: (a) Calcium-activated chloride channel

Explanation

Cajal cells and GIST share common markers for CD117 and a calcium-activated chloride channel called DOG1

CD117 is another name for the KIT gene, which codes for a tyrosine kinase transmembrane receptor called c-kit

(Sabiston, Page 768)

317. American Society for Radiation Oncology Guidelines for Accelerated Partial Breast Irradiation, which of the following is not a feature for suitable group?

(a) Size < 2 cm (b) Age >60 years

(c) ER positive (d) Invasive lobular carcinoma

Ans: (d) Invasive lobular carcinoma

Explanation

American Society for Radiation and Breast Irradiation

Factor	"Suitable" Group
Patients factors	
• Age (year)	≥ 60
Tumor factors	
• Tumor size (cm)	≤ 2
• T stage	T1
• Margins	Negative by at least 2 mm
• Histology	Invasive ductal carcinoma or other favorable subtypes

Contd.

Contd.

• Pure DCIS • Grade • LVI • ER status • Multicentricity • Multifocality **Nodal factors** • N stage **Treatment factors** • Neoadjuvant chemotherapy	Not allowed Any None Positive Unicentric Clinically unifocal with total size ≤ 2 pN0 Not allowed

(Sabiston, Page 854)

318. Eggshell calcifications seen in which cystic lesion of pancreas:

(a) MCN
(b) SCN
(c) IPMN
(d) Pesudocyst

Ans: (a) MCN

Explanation

Mucinous cystic neoplasm of pancreas: Thick-walled, septated macrocyst with smooth contour; ± solid component, eggshell calcifications

(Sabiston, Page 1538)

319. Which of the following is not a high risk feature of IPMN?

(a) Jaundice
(b) Main duct > 1 cm
(c) Enhancing solid component
(d) BD-IPMN size >3 cm

Ans : (d) BD-IPMN size >3 cm

Explanation

A Summary of Worrisome and High-Risk Features of Intraductal Papillary Mucinous Neoplasm

Worrisome Features
Main duct 5-9 mm
Nonenhancing mural nodule
Thickened, enhancing cyst wall
BD-IPMN size >3 cm
Abrupt caliber change in main duct with upstream atrophy
Lymphadenopathy
Pancreatitis
High-risk imaging features of BD-IPMN include the presence of an enhancing solid component within the cyst and main pancreatic duct dilation of more than 1 cm. Patients who present with clinical signs of jaundice should also be considered at high risk

(Sabiston, Page 1539)

320. Which of the following is not a worrisome feature of IPMN?

(a) Thickened, enhancing cyst wall
(b) Lymphadenopathy
(c) Jaundice
(d) Pancreatitis

Ans: (c) Jaundice

Explanation

Worrisome Features of IPMN

Main duct 5-9 mm

Nonenhancing mural nodule

Thickened, enhancing cyst wall

BD-IPMN size >3 cm

Abrupt caliber change in main duct with upstream atrophy

Lymphadenopathy

Pancreatitis

(Sabiston, Page 1539)

321. BD IPMN 2.5 cm in size with worrisome features, in a 20 years old male, next appropriate line of management:

(a) Surgical resection
(b) EUS 6 monthly interval
(c) EUS yearly interval
(d) MRI at 3 monthly interval

Ans: (a) Surgical resection

Explanation

For those with asymptomatic cysts between 1 and 2 cm, imaging at 1 year is appropriate, followed by less frequent evaluation if no change in size has occurred during the first 2 years of surveillance

Cysts that are 2 to 3 cm should be surveyed more frequently, at 3 to 6-month intervals, to ensure stability for the first year before lengthening of the interval is considered

Given the need for long-term surveillance, resection of cysts 2 to 3 cm may be considered in young, otherwise healthy individuals

Cysts larger than 3 cm warrant closer surveillance because of the increased risk of malignancy

EUS alternating with MRI every 3 to 6 months should be performed in cases in which surgical intervention may be of high risk

Surgery should be strongly considered in young patients with long life expectancy and individuals considered to be at low surgical risk

(Sabiston, Page 1540)

322. Symptomatic BD IPMN in an old patient of size 1 cm, next line of management:

(a) CT/MRI in 2-3 years
(b) CT/MRI yearly
(c) EUS yearly
(d) Surgical resection

Ans: (d) Surgical resection

Explanation

Any patient with symptoms or high-risk features related to BD-IPMNs (e.g., jaundice, mural nodule, dilated main pancreatic duct) should undergo surgical resection because the risk of malignant disease in symptomatic patients is heightened

Overall, the risk of invasive malignant disease in the setting of BD-IPMN is approximately 10% to 15%

(Sabiston, Page 1540)

323. False statement about IPMN:

(a) Elevation of the CEA level is predictive of invasive malignant disease
(b) 50% of patients with IPMNs of the pancreas present with abdominal pain
(c) Main duct dilation of more than 5 mm is consistent with a diagnosis of MD-IPMN
(d) EUS is important secondary diagnostic study

Ans: (a) Elevation of the CEA level is predictive of invasive malignant disease

Explanation

As in MCNs and BD-IPMNs, fluid aspirates characteristically reveal an elevated CEA level (>192 ng/mL; log scale)

This elevation of the CEA level is not predictive of invasive malignant disease, only the presence of mucinous metaplasia

MRCP and EUS is important secondary diagnostic study

Unlike patients with pancreatic ductal adenocarcinomas (PDACs), 50% of patients with IPMNs of the pancreas present with abdominal pain and up to 25% present with AP, which, not surprisingly, has led to the diagnosis of chronic pancreatitis in many series

Main duct dilation >5 mm–diagnostic

>10 mm–high risk

5-9 mm–worrisome

(Sabiston, Page 1541)

324. ....Mutation results in >100-fold increase in risk of PDAC.

(a) PRSS1 (b) CDKN2A

(c) STK 11 (d) BRCA2

Ans: (c) STK 11

Explanation

PRSS1–Familial pancreatitis–Mutation results in chronic pancreatitis and 40% lifetime risk of PDAC

CDKN2A–Familial atypical mole and multiple melanoma syndrome–Mutation leads to increased risk of melanoma and >40-fold increase in risk of PDAC

STK 11–Peutz-Jeghers syndrome–Mutation results in >100-fold increase in risk of PDAC

BRCA2–Hereditary breast and ovarian cancer–Mutation results in elevated risk of breast and ovarian cancer and 10-fold increase in risk of PDAC

(Sabiston, Page 1542)

325. Late mutation occurs in pancreatic cancer:

(a) Kras (b) CDKN2.A

(c) P16 (d) DPC 4

Ans: (d) DPC 4

Explanation

DPC4 mutations occur late in the pathway from PanIN to PDAC

Loss of DPC4, which normally functions as a downstream mediator related to TGF-β, leads to decreased inhibition of cell growth and proliferation

Loss of DPC4 function has been observed in 20% to 30% of PanIN-3 and localized cancers, whereas 78% of widely metastatic tumors show loss of DPC4

(Sabiston, Page 1543)

326. Second most common symptom of periampullary carcinoma:

(a) Jaundice (b) Weight loss

(c) Abdominal pain (d) Nausea/vomiting

Ans: (b) Weight loss

Explanation

Presenting Symptoms for Periampullary Tumors of the Pancreas	
Presenting Symptoms	**Frequency (%)**
Jaundice	75
Weight loss	51
Abdominal pain	39
Nausea/vomiting	13
Pruritus	11
Fever	3
Gastrointestinal bleeding	1

(Sabiston, Page 1544)

327. High risk conditions associated with malignant transformation of oral cavity all *except:*

(a) Erythroplakia (homogenous or speckled)
(b) Proliferative verrucous leucoplakia
(c) Chronic hyperplastic candidiasis
(d) Oral submucous fibrosis

Ans: (d) Oral submucous fibrosis

Explanation

High-risk lesions

Erythroplakia (homogenous or speckled) Proliferative verrucous leucoplakia

Chronic hyperplastic candidiasis

Medium-risk lesions

- Oral submucous fibrosis
- Syphilitic glossitis

Low-risk/equivocal-risk lesions

- Oral lichen planus
- Discoid lupus erythematosus
- Discoid keratosis congenita

(Bailey, Page 761)

328. Clinical features of oral cancer that warrant investigation all *except:*

(a) Persistent oral swelling for >3 weeks
(b) Mouth ulceration for 2 weeks
(c) Sore tongue
(d) Painless neck lump

Ans: (b) Mouth ulceration for 2 weeks

Explanation

Clinical features of oral cancer that warrant investigation

- Persistent oral swelling for >3 weeks
- Mouth ulceration for >3 weeks
- Sore tongue
- Difficulty swallowing
- Jaw or facial swelling
- Painless neck lump
- Unexplained tooth mobility
- Trismus

(Bailey, Page 765)

329. Most common of the NSCLC types (Non small cell lung cancer):

(a) Adenocarcinoma (b) Squamous carcinoma

(c) Large cell undifferentiated (d) Bronchioalveloar carcinoma

Ans: (a) Adenocarcinoma

Explanation

Adenocarcinoma is now the most common of the NSCLC types, having overtaken squamous cancer

The increasing incidence is partly due to an increasing incidence in women and may be the result, in part, of a move towards lower-tar cigarettes that are inhaled more deeply to get the same effect

(Bailey, Page 925)

330. Most common small bowel neoplasm in children:

(a) Adeno carcinoma (b) Lymphoma

(c) Leiomyoma (d) GIST

Ans: (b) Lymphoma

Explanation

One third GI lymphoma occurs in small bowel. This is most common malignancy of small bowel in children. Increased risk with HIV, celiac disease

(Sabiston, Page 1278)

331. Which of the following has least five-year survival?

(a) Squamous cell carcinoma (b) Adenosquamous carcinoma

(c) Undifferentiated carcinoma (d) Small cell carcinoma

Ans: (d) Small cell carcinoma

Explanation

Five-year survival according to cell type (%)

Squamous cell carcinoma–35–50%

Adenocarcinoma–25–45%

Adenosquamous carcinoma–20–35%

Undifferentiated carcinoma–15–25%

Small cell carcinoma–0–5%

(Bailey, Page 928)

332. False statement about pneumonectomy:

(a) Reserved for peripherally placed tumors

(b) Removal of a whole lung

(c) Fixation of the tumor to the oesophagus implies irresectability

(d) Stump is usually stapled

Ans: (a) Reserved for peripherally placed tumors

Explanation

Pneumonectomy is removal of a whole lung and has a higher mortality rate (5–8%)

This procedure is reserved for either centrally placed tumors involving the main bronchus or those that straddle the fissure

The technique of stump closure is important if a bronchopleural fistula is to be avoided

The tissues are carefully handled and the stump is usually stapled and sometimes covered using pleura, pericardium or a vascular pedicle such as an intercostal muscle

Fixation of the tumor to the aorta, heart or oesophagus implies irresectability

(Bailey, Page 932)

333. Prostate cancer found incidentally following PSA measurement:

(a) T1a (b) T1b

(c) T1c (d) T2

Ans: (c) T1c

Explanation

T1a, T1b and T1c. These are incidentally found tumors in a clinically benign gland after histological examination of a prostatectomy specimen

T1a is a tumor involving less than 5% of the resected specimen; these tumors are usually well or moderately well differentiated

T1b is tumor involving >5% of the resected specimen

T1c tumors are impalpable tumors found following investigation of a raised PSA

(Bailey, Page 1470)

334. Prostate cancer with seminal vesicle extension:

(a) T2a (b) T2b

(c) T3b (d) T4

Ans: (c) T3b

Explanation

T2a disease presents as a suspicious nodule on rectal examination confined within the prostate capsule and involving one lobe

T2b disease involves both lobes

T3 tumor extends through the capsule (T3a, uni- or bilateral extension; T3b, seminal vesical extension)

T4 is a tumor that is fixed or invading adjacent structures other than seminal vesicles–rectum or pelvic side wall

(Bailey, Page 1470)

335. .... is the most accurate method of staging local disease of prostate cancer.

(a) MRI with a high tesla magnet (1.5–3 T) (b) TRUS

(c) TRUS + PSA measurement (d) TRUS + DRE + PSA measurement

Ans: (a) MRI with a high tesla magnet (1.5–3 T)

Explanation

MRI with a high tesla magnet (1.5–3 T) is the most accurate method of staging local disease

Transrectal ultrasound scanning can also be used to stage prostate cancer

Locally extensive disease (T2) can be diagnosed with increased sensitivity by TRUS compared with rectal examination, but many tumors will still be missed

This problem remains a real one in screening for early prostate cancer; in comparison with breast cancer, with mammography detecting 70–80% of tumors

TRUS plus rectal examination and measurement of PSA will detect only 30–50% of cancers that are known to be present on autopsy studies

(Bailey, Page 1472)

336. False statement about bone scan for prostate cancer:

(a) More sensitive in the diagnosis of metastases than a skeletal survey

(b) False positive in healing fracture

(c) If the PSA is <10 ng/mL, then a bone scan should not be performed

(d) Injection of technetium-99m used

Ans: (c) If the PSA is <10 ng/mL, then a bone scan should not be performed

Explanation

Once the diagnosis has been established, if metastatic spread is suspected (on the basis of a high PSA [>10 ng/mL], locally advanced disease or presence of Gleason 7 or higher) a bone scan should be carried out

If however the PSA is <10 ng/mL, then a bone scan would be performed only on clinical indications

The bone scan is performed by the injection of technetium-99m, which is then monitored using a gamma camera

It is more sensitive in the diagnosis of metastases than a skeletal survey, but false positives occur in areas of arthritis, osteomyelitis or a healing fracture

(Bailey, Page 1472)

337. Walsh modification of radical prostatectomy:

(a) Preserve urinary continence

(b) Preserve erectile function

(c) Increases impotence

(d) Avoid urethral damage

Ans: (b) Preserve erectile function

Explanation

Radical prostatectomy is suitable for localised disease and should be carried out only in men with a life expectancy of >10 years

It results in a high incidence of impotence, but a low incidence of severe stress incontinence (<2%), which may require the fitting of an artificial urinary sphincter or urethral sling

Modifications to this operation by Walsh can lead to preservation of the neurovascular bundles that lie behind the prostate

This modification has led to the preservation of erectile function in about 60–70% of cases

(Bailey, Page 1473)

338. Mahogany colour in gross appearance:

(a) Papillary

(b) Oncocytoma

(c) Collecting duct

(d) Chromophobe

Ans: (b) Oncocytoma

Explanation

Oncocytoma: Mahogany colour

- Circumscribed

- Occasional central scar
- Rarely with necrosis

(Bailey, Page 1473)

339. Nephroblastoma (Wilms' tumor) false statement:

(a) Usually presents in the first five years of life
(b) Typically presents with an abdominal mass
(c) May cause haematuria, abdominal pain or fever
(d) Metastasises to the liver common

Ans: (b) Typically presents with an abdominal mass

Explanation

Nephroblastoma (Wilms' tumor)

Usually presents in the first five years of life

Typically presents with an abdominal mass

May cause haematuria, abdominal pain or fever

Metastasises to the lung

Is best treated in a specialist pediatric oncology unit

(Bailey, Page 1422)

340. Location of insulinoma in pancreas:

(a) Head
(b) Body
(c) Tail
(d) Equally distributed

Ans: (d) Equally distributed

Explanation

Virtually all insulinomas are located in the pancreas and tumors are equally distributed within the gland

Approximately 90% are solitary and about 10% are multiple and associated with MEN 1 syndrome

(Bailey, Page 849)

341. Which of the following is not a feature of non-functioning pancreatic cancer?

(a) >5 cm
(b) Hyperdense on CT
(c) Chromogranin A negative
(d) Calcification in CT

Ans: (c) Chromogranin A negative

Differences between pancreatic cancer and non-functioning endocrine pancreatic tumors (NF-PETs)

	Pancreatic cancer	NF-PETs
Tumor size	< 5 cm	> 5 cm
CT scan	Hypodensity No calcifications	Hyperdensity Calicifications possible
Chromogranin A in blood	Negative	Positive
Somatostatin receptor scintigraphy	Negative	Positive

(Bailey, Page 852)

342. Which type of gastric neuroendocrine tumor Associated with MEN 1?

(a) Type I
(b) Type II
(c) Type III
(d) Type IV

Ans: (b) Type II

Explanation

Type I–ECLomas in chronic atrophic gastritis, hypergastrinaemia

Type II–ECLomas with hypergastrinaemia as a result of gastrinoma in MEN 1

Type III–Sporadic ECLomas not related to hypergastrinaemia

Type IV–Causative factor unknown; prognosis poor

(Bailey, Page 853)

343. Which of the following is gastric NET is large ulcerating malignancies similar to adenocarcinomas?

(a) Type I
(b) Type II
(c) Type III
(d) Type IV

Ans: (b) Type II

Explanation

Type 4 tumors present as large ulcerating malignancies similar to adenocarcinomas and should be treated accordingly. The prognosis of types 3 and 4 is poor

(Bailey, Page 854)

344. Type 3 gastric NET usually present as:

(a) Abdomen pain
(b) Diarrhea
(c) Flushing
(d) UGI bleed

Ans: (b) Diarrhea

Explanation

Type 3 tumors are rare, sporadic and solitary tumors of unknown origin

Serum gastrin is normal; upper gastrointestinal bleeding is the usual symptom that leads to endoscopy

Type 3 tumors are usually larger than 2 cm and often have lymph node and liver metastases at the time of diagnosis

Gastrectomy and lymph node dissection and resection of liver metastases is the treatment of choice

Liver metastases can also be treated by chemoembolisation

(Bailey, Page 854)

345. The most common syndrome-associated cause of death in MEN 1:

(a) Pancreatic NET
(b) Pituitary tumor
(c) Parathyroid malignancy
(d) Gastric carcinoid

Ans: (a) Pancreatic NET

Explanation

PETs occur in around 50–60% of MEN 1 patients

In such patients taking part in screening programmes, 70–90% are found to have non-functioning and functioning PETs

This high rate of detection of PETs is the result of the improvement in diagnostic procedures in the last decade, including EUS

MEN 1 PETs are the most common syndrome–associated cause of death

They are mostly multiple and often recur after surgery

(Bailey, Page 857)

346. Most common functional pancreatic NET in MEN 1:

(a) Gastrinoma
(b) Insulinoma
(c) Glucagonoma
(d) Somatostatinoma

Ans: (a) Gastrinoma

Explanation

The most common functional tumor is gastrinoma followed by insulinoma. VIPomas, glucagonomas and somatostatinomas are extremely rare

Non-functioning tumors can be asymptomatic for many years

(Bailey, Page 857)

347. MEN 2 patients with normal Calcitonin level, having low risk for medullary thyroid cancer, prophylactic thyroidectomy should be done within…. ..years of age.

(a) 1 year
(b) 5 years
(c) 10 years
(d) 20 years

Ans: (d) 20 years

Explanation

Different RET mutations are associated with early or late onset of the disease

Risk groups have been defined to determine the appropriate age for thyroidectomy high risk codons–prophylactic thyroidectomy within 1 year of age

Medium risk codons–prophylactic thyroidectomy within 6 years of age

Low risk of age–prophylactic thyroidectomy within 20 years of age

(Bailey, Page 858)

348. Which of the following breast lesion has slightly increased risk of cancer?

(a) Adenosis, sclerosing or florid
(b) Apocrine metaplasia
(c) Squamous metaplasia
(d) Papilloma with a fibrovascular core

Ans: (d) Papilloma with a fibrovascular core

Explanation

Slightly increased risk (1.5–2 times)

Hyperplasia, moderate or florid, solid or papillary

Papilloma with a fibrovascular core

Moderately increased risk (5 times)

Atypical hyperplasia (ductal or lobular)

(Bailey, Page 871)

349. Most common benign tumor of lung:

(a) Hemangioma
(b) Adenoma
(c) Hamartoma
(d) Granuloma

Ans: (c) Hamartoma

Explanation

Most benign nodules are granulomas (tuberculosis or histoplasmosis)

The most common benign tumor is a hamartoma, a developmental abnormality containing mesothelial and endothelial elements

Diagnosis (and definitive treatment) is achieved by excision of the lesion

Any of the mesodermal elements of the lung may form a mesodermal tumor (chondroma, lipoma, leiomyoma)

Deposits of amyloid may have a similar radiographic appearance to a nodule (pseudotumour)

(Bailey, Page 934)

350. A lung tumour is likely to be benign if it has not increased in size on chest radiographs for more than …… .

(a) 6 months
(b) 1 year
(c) 18 months
(d) 2 years

Ans: (c) 18 months

Explanation

Benign tumors of the lung are uncommon and account for fewer than 15% of solitary lesions seen on chest radiographs

A peripheral tumor usually causes no symptoms until it is large; a central tumor may present with haemoptysis and signs of bronchial obstruction while still small. A tumor is likely to be benign if it has not increased in size on chest radiographs for more than 2 years or it has some degree of calcification; however, a tissue diagnosis is usually pursued

(Bailey, Page 934)

351. In masaoka thymoma staging system, Macroscopic invasion into surrounding mediastinal pleura staged as:

(a) II
(b) III
(c) IV A
(d) IV B

Ans: (a) II

Explanation

Masaoka thymoma staging system

Stage I

Macroscopically completely encapsulated

Microscopically no capsular invasion

Stage II

Macroscopic invasion into surrounding fatty tissue or mediastinal pleura

Microscopic invasion into the capsule

Stage III

Macroscopic invasion into neighbouring organs (pericardium, great vessels, lungs)

Stage IV A

Pleural or pericardial dissemination

Stage IV B

Lymphogenous or haematogenous metastasis

(Bailey, Page 935)

352. The vaccines cervarix and gardasil for cervical cancer is based on immunity to:

(a) L1 Capsid protein
(b) L2 capsid protein
(c) E6 and E7 proteins
(d) All of the above

Ans: (a) L1 Capsid protein

(Devita, Page 256)

353. Which virus plays a causal role in pruritic skin rashes with a distinctive "peacock tail" histology in patients with various forms of immunosuppression?

(a) BK virus
(b) Merkel cell Virus
(c) HPyV6
(d) HPyV1

Ans: (c) HPyV6

(Devita, Page 259)

354. One of the following statements regarding EBV is not correct:

(a) Elevated antibody responsiveness to EBV antigens may offer a method for identifying individuals at greater risk of gastric cancer
(b) Elevated antibody responsiveness to EBV antigens give a clue to identify Nasopharyngeal carcinoma
(c) EBV is also associated with rare lymphoproliferative diseases of non-B-cell origin, including NK cell leukemia and nasal-type NK/T cell (angiocentric) lymphoma
(d) In sporadic Burkitt lymphoma about 80% of cases are associated with EBV

Ans: (d) In sporadic Burkitt lymphoma about 80% of cases are associated with EBV

355. The radiosensitization of the paclitaxel is due to rearrangement of the cells in:

(a) G1 phase
(b) G0 phase
(c) G2/M phase
(d) S phase

Ans: (c) G2/M phase

(Devita, Page 428)

356 If a tumor has predominant hypoxic cells, which beam of radiation therapy will be highly effective?

(a) Photons
(b) Protons
(c) Electrons
(d) Carbon ion

Ans: (d) Carbon ion

(Devita, Page 444)

357. Metagenomics involves study of:

(a) Environmental genomics of microbiome that resides in our body
(b) Systemic analysis of small molecule metabolites like amino acids, fatty acids
(c) Regarding the methylation pattern of the DNA
(d) Meta analysis of the genome wide studies

Ans: (a) Environmental genomics of microbiome that resides in our body

(Devita, Page 353)

358. Examples of precision oncology clinical trials include all *except:*

(a) Basket trial
(b) Umbrella trial
(c) Shiva trial
(d) Extreme trial

Ans: (d) Extreme trial

(Devita, Page 400)

PAPER 8

359. Axicabtagene ciloleucel is a CAR T cell therapy used against which antigen:

(a) CD20
(b) CD19
(c) CD21
(d) CD23

Ans: (b) CD19

360. All are PDL1 blockers *except:*

(a) Atezolizumab
(b) Durvalumab
(c) Pembrolizumab
(d) Avelumab

Ans: (c) Pembrolizumab

361. Mobile DNA gene delivery system used in CAR T cell therapy against B cell malignancies are:

(a) Gamma lenti virus
(b) Lenti virus
(c) Retro virus
(d) Transposon

Ans: (d) Transposon

(Devita, Page 167)

362. In stage III NSCLC after chemoradiotherapy which drug has shown increased survival benefit?

(a) Atezolizumab
(b) Pembrolizumab
(c) Durvalumab
(d) Nivolumab

Ans: (c) Durvalumab

363. A lady of metastatic carcinoma breast started on Capecitabine presented in 10 days with painful erythema, crackling, desquamation and activity is impaired–What Grade of HFS she has?

(a) Grade 1
(b) Grade 2
(c) Grade 3
(d) Grade 4

Ans: (b) Grade 2

364. All are cell cycle specific agents *except:*

(a) Docetaxel
(b) Vinca alkaloids
(c) Cyclophosphamide
(d) Methotrexate

Ans: (c) Cyclophosphamide

(Devita, Page 189)

365. The drug which has properties of both alkylating agent and antimetabolite is:

(a) Estramustine
(b) Bendamustine
(c) Carmustine
(d) Lomustine

Ans: (b) Bendamustine

(Devita, Page 197)

366. The formula which is used to calculate the carboplatin dose based on AUC is:

(a) Dubois formula
(b) Mosteller formula
(c) Calverts formula
(d) All of the above

Ans: (c) Calverts formula

(Devita, Page 204)

367. The drug which on exposure to cold leads to oropharyngeal dysesthesia is:

(a) Oxaliplatin
(b) Nedaplatin
(c) Carboplatin
(d) Cisplatin

Ans: (a) Oxaliplatin

(Devita, Page 204)

368. Which drug is relatively contraindicated in ischemic heart disease?

(a) Cytarabine
(b) Gemcitabine
(c) 5-Fluorouracil
(d) Fludarabine

Ans: (c) 5-Fluorouracil

(Devita, Page 212)

369. Renal angiopathic syndromes–HUS and TTP are one of the rare complication of the which drug?

(a) Gemcitabine
(b) Cytarabine
(c) Decitabine
(d) Cytosine Arabinoside

Ans: (a) Gemcitabine

(Devita Page 214)

370. 30-year-old male with Diffuse large B cell lymphoma and testis and paranasal sinus involvement planned for treatment. What will be next best investigation for him in management?

(a) Lumbar puncture
(b) Radiation of testis and paranasal sinuses
(c) Orchiectomy
(d) Upper and lower GI endoscopy

Ans: (a) Lumbar puncture

371. 70-year-old male presented with abdominal pain and easy fatigability and bleeding from nose and gums. On examination has large splenomegaly with HB 12.5, albumin 3.6, LDH 500, platelets 15000. Peripheral smear shows villous lymphocytes. Flow cytometry is positive for CD10, CD19, CD22, Negative for CD 102, CD 25, cyclin D1. What is the probable diagnosis?

(a) Hairy cell leukemia
(b) Splenic Marginal zone lymphoma
(c) Extranodal marginal zone lymphoma
(d) Mantle cell lymphoma

Ans: (b) Splenic Marginal zone lymphoma

(Devita, Page 1565)

372. What will be best option for the management of the above patient?

(a) Close surveillance
(b) Single agent rituximab
(c) RCHOP
(d) Rituximab and bendamustine

Ans: (b) Single agent rituximab

373. 45-year-old female got evaluated for generalised tiredness and neck nodes. Physical examination reveals generalised lymphadenopathy and splenomegaly. Flow cytometry shows CD10, CD19, CD 20, CD22 positivity and negative mum-1 and bcl-6. What is the probable diagnosis?

(a) Diffuse large B cell lymphoma–Germinal Centre B cell type
(b) Diffuse large B cell lymphoma–Activated B Cell type
(c) Mantle cell lymphoma
(d) Follicular lymphoma

Ans: (a) Diffuse large B cell lymphoma–Germinal Centre B cell type

(Devita, Page 1569)

374 A 60-year-old male from Hong Kong presented with chronic sinus pain for 5 months with fever chills and weight loss of 10 kgs. On examination has paranasal area tenderness and neck nodes, also has a skin rash. CT PNS revealed a mass in the nasal sinus. IHC of the biopsy showed CD2, CD56 and cytoplasmic CD3. What is the most probable diagnosis?

(a) Burkitt's lymphoma (b) Extranodal marginal zone lymphoma
(c) ALCL (d) Nasal NK/T cell lymphoma

Ans: (d) Nasal NK/T cell lymphoma

(Devita, Page 1576)

375. In DLBCL, if c-myc is rearranged along with BCL2, it is called as:

(a) Activated B cell lymphoma–DLBCL (b) Germinal Centre B cell type–DLBCL
(c) Double hit lymphoma (d) Triple hit lymphoma

Ans: (c) Double hit lymphoma

376. HTLV-1 is associated with which lymphoma?

(a) NK T cell lymphoma (b) Burkitt's lymphoma
(c) Adult T cell lymphoma/leukemia (d) Post Transplant Hodgkin's lymphoma

Ans: (c) Adult T cell lymphoma/leukemia

(Devita, Page 1577)

377. Bortezomib acts by which mechansism?

(a) Inhibition of MAPK pathway (b) Inhibition of PI3K/AKT pathway
(c) Inhibition of NFKB pathway (d) Inhibition of Hedgehog pathway

Ans: (c) Inhibition of NFKB pathway

(Devita, Page 259)

378. 62-year-old man came with history of worsening back pain for 2 months, with reduced urine output for few days. On physical examination has generalised edema, with altered sensorium. His creatinine is 4.3 mg/dl and serum calcium is 11.2 mg/dl. X-ray of spine shows multiple lytic lesions what is the next investigation to confirm the diagnosis?

(a) MRI spine (b) Bone scan
(c) Renal biopsy (d) Serum Protein Electrophoresis

Ans: (d) Serum Protein Electrophoresis

379. Myeloma defining events are all *except:*

(a) Presence of bone marrow clonal plasma cells of greater than or equal to 60%
(b) Serum free light chain (FLC) ratio greater than or equal to 100
(c) Presence of renal failure with creatinine more than 2 mg/dl
(d) More than one focal lesion on whole body MRI

Ans: (c) Presence of renal failure with creatinine more than 2 mg/dl

380. The most significant toxicity of anthracyclines is:

(a) Cardiac toxicity (b) Pulmonary toxicity
(c) Nephrotoxicity (d) Neurotoxicity

Ans: (a) Cardiac toxicity

(Devita, Page 225)

381. Peak incidence of pediatric ALL is:

(a) 2–5 years
(b) 4–8 years
(c) 5–10 years
(d) 10–15 years

Ans: (a) 2–5 years

(Devita, Page 1501)

382. The most common type of AML in Down syndrome patient is:

(a) AML–M2
(b) AML–M4
(c) AML–M5
(d) AML–M7

Ans: (d) AML-M7

(Devita, Page 1502)

383. The genetic alteration which occurs in the transition from intermediate adenoma to late adenoma occurs in which gene/chromosome?

(a) APC/Beta Catenin
(b) b–kras
(c) 18q
(d) p53

Ans: (c) 18q

(Devita, 10th Edition, Page 3)

384. One of the following is true regarding pediatric ALL?

(a) Most common translocation in pediatric ALL is t(12,21)
(b) Ph-positive ALL is more prevalent in children than adults
(c) In T cell ALL children with NOTCH-1 mutation have worse prognosis
(d) Early T precursor ALL has a very good prognosis

Ans: (a) Most common translocation in pediatric ALL is t(12,21)

(Devita, Page 1504)

385. A female child of 10 years old presents with extreme monocytosis, hepatosplenomegaly and increased fetal hemoglobin. Bone marrow study shows myelodysplasia and myeloproliferation. BM cytogenetics reveal monosomy 7. The most probable diagnosis is:

(a) AML–M4
(b) MDS
(c) CML
(d) Juvenile Myelomonocytic Leukemia

Ans: (d) Juvenile Myelomonocytic Leukemia

(Devita, Page 1506)

386. Based on St. Jude classification of Pediatric Non-Hodgkin's Lymphoma isolated Primary Mediastinal tumor involvement is classified as:

(a) Stage I
(b) Stage II
(c) Stage III
(d) Stage IV

Ans: (c) Stage III

(Devita, Page 1507)

387. Regarding Pediatric Non-Hodgkin's lymphoma one of the statement is false:

(a) Precursor T cell lymphoblastic lymphoma is more common than precursor B cell Lymphoblastic lymphoma
(b) Excluding children with Heriditary and Acquired Immunodeficiency Syndromes most children with NHL have no risk factors and have normal health

(c) EBV is strongly associated with lymphoma in HIV-negative children

(d) Nelarabine is used in relapsed T cell ALL

Ans: (c) EBV is strongly associated with lymphoma in HIV-negative children

(Devita, Page 1507)

388. An 8-year-old boy is brought to clinic by his parents due to jaw swelling for past 1 month. Physical examination reveals left jaw mass which displaces teeth and is impinging on trachea. Biopsy reveals sheets of atypical lymphocytes with large vacuolated areas of fat. Ki 67% is 99%. Which translocation is most common in this malignancy this boy has?

(a) t (1,14)
(b) t (8,14)
(c) t (8,22)
(d) t (2,8)

Ans: (b) t (8,14)

(Devita, Page 1508)

389. Sporadic Burkitt's lymphoma presents with:

(a) Localised head and neck masses frequently in jaw

(b) 95% of cases are associated with EBV

(c) Commonly present with right lower quadrant mass or acute abdomen secondary to ileocecal intusseception

(d) All of the above

Ans: (c) Commonly present with right lower quadrant mass or acute abdomen secondary to ileocecal intusseception

(Devita, Page 1508)

390. A 35-year-old male came to emergency with history of fever with chills, drenching night sweats for past 2 months associated with weight loss. He also complains of itchy rash over the abdomen. On examination has painless generalised lymphadenopathy. Biopsy shows large cells with prominent nucleoli. Immunophenotyping show ALK and CD30 positive, negative for B cell markers. Which is true regarding this condition?

(a) ALK positive cases are more common in older adults

(b) ALK protein is detected in minority of patients around 10% in young adults

(c) Cells are derived from mature activated T cells

(d) Prognosis of ALK positive case is worse than ALK negative case

Ans: (c) Cells are derived from mature activated T cells

(Devita, Page 1575)

391. A 10-year-girl presents with her parents to clinic with painless neck nodes of two months duration with fever chills and rigor with weight loss of 5 kgs. She has dyspnea on fast walking. On imaging she is found to have mediastinal and cervical adenopathy. Biopsy of the Lymph Nodes reveal thickened capsule and bands of fibrosis. IHC shows CD15 and CD30 positivity. The most probable malignancy in this patient could be:

(a) Hodgkin's lymphoma Mixed cellularity
(b) Hodgkin's lymphoma Nodular sclerosis
(c) Hodgkin's lymphoma Lymphocyte Rich
(d) Nodular lymphocyte Predominant Hodgkin's lymphoma

Ans: (b) Hodgkin's lymphoma Nodular sclerosis

(Devita, Page 1509)

392. What drug is given prophylactically with the use of thalidomide and lenalidomide while used in multiple myeloma?

(a) Warfarin
(b) Heparin
(c) Aspirin
(d) Apixaban

Ans: (c) Aspirin

393. A 65-year-business man with history of diabetes and hypertension since 10 years with hyperlipidemia got evaluated for abdominal distension. On physical examination was found to have massive splenomegaly. His peripheral smear shows myelocytes 15% metamyelocytes 25% neutrophils 25% basophils 10% eoisinophils 12% with lymphocytes 8%, Monocytes 5%. What best option of Tyrosine kinase inhibitor can be used in this patient?

(a) Imatinib (b) Dasatinib

(c) Nilotinib (d) Bosutinib

Ans: (a) Imatinib

(Devita, Page 1649)

394. The vaccines cervarix and gardasil for cervical cancer is based on immunity to:

(a) L1 capsid protein (b) L2 capsid protein

(c) E6 and E7 proteins (d) All of the above

Ans: (a) L1 capsid protein

(Devita, Page 256)

395. Which virus plays a causal role in pruritic skin rashes with a distinctive "peacock tail" histology in patients with various forms of immunosuppression?

(a) BK virus (b) Merkel cell Virus

(c) HPyV6 (d) HPyV1

Ans: (c) HPyV6

(Devita, Page 259)

396. One of the following statements regarding EBV is not correct?

(a) Elevated antibody responsiveness to EBV antigens may offer a method for identifying individuals at greater risk of gastric cancer

(b) Elevated antibody responsiveness to EBV antigens give a clue to identify Nasopharyngeal carcinoma

(c) EBV is also associated with rare lymphoproliferative diseases of non-B-cell origin, including NK cell leukemia, and nasal-type NK/T cell (angiocentric) lymphoma

(d) In sporadic Burkitt lymphoma about 80% of cases are associated with EBV

Ans: (d) In sporadic Burkitt lymphoma about 80% of cases are associated with EBV

397. The radiosensitization of the paclitaxel is due to rearrangement of the cells in:

(a) G1 phase (b) G0 phase

(c) G2/M phase (d) S phase

Ans: (c) G2/M phase

(Devita, Page 428)

398. If a tumor has predominant hypoxic cells, which beam of radiation therapy will be highly effective?

(a) Photons (b) Protons

(c) Electrons (d) Carbon ion

Ans: (d) Carbon ion

(Devita, Page 444)

399. Metagenomics involves study of:

(a) Environmental genomics of microbiome that resides in our body

(b) Systemic analysis of small molecule metabolites like amino acids, fatty acids

(c) Regarding the methylation pattern of the DNA
(d) Meta analysis of the genome wide studies

Ans: (a) Environmental genomics of microbiome that resides in our body

(Devita, Page 353)

400. Examples of precision oncology clinical trials include all *except:*

(a) Basket trial (b) Umbrella trial
(c) Shiva trial (d) Extreme trial

Ans: (d) Extreme trial

(Devita, Page 400)

401. In merkel cell carcinoma which immunotherapy molecule is approved?

(a) Durvalumab (b) Avelumab
(c) Pembrolizumab (d) Atezolizumab

Ans: (b) Avelumab

(Devita, Page 469)

402. The best possible treatment of malignant peritoneal mesothelioma is:

(a) Palliative chemotherapy with cisplatin and pemetrexed
(b) Cytoreductive surgery
(c) CRS with HIPEC
(d) CRS with HIPEC with long-term IV cisplatin and IP pemetrexed

Ans: (d) CRS with HIPEC with long-term IV cisplatin and IP pemetrexed

(Devita, Page 3325)

403. Among the appendiceal neoplasms which histology has the worst prognosis?

(a) Multicystic (b) Deciduoid
(c) Papillary (d) Epithelial

Ans: (b) Deciduoid

(Devita, 11th Edition, Page 3319)

404. Bone metastasis in adults are more frequent in all types *except:*

(a) Liver (b) Lung
(c) Breast (d) Prostate

Ans: (a) Liver

(Devita, Page 3456)

405. Regarding metastatic to bone all are true *except:*

(a) Bone metastastis produce pain due to release of inflammatory mediators
(b) Functional bone pain is caused by mechanical weakness of the bone
(c) Pathological fracture occurs in around 35% of breast cancer patients
(d) Pathological fracture occurs only in osteolytic bone metastasis

Ans: (d) Pathological fracture occurs only in osteolytic bone metastasis

(Devita, Page 3456)

406. What does this X-ray demonstrate?

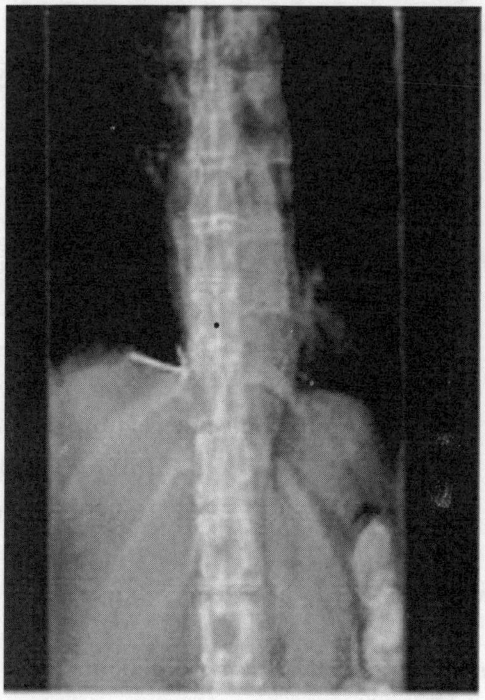

(a) Codman triangle
(b) Winking owl sign
(c) Westermark sign
(d) Volcano sign

Ans: (b) Winking owl sign

(Devita, Page 3458)

407. High grade serous carcinoma of the ovary are derived from the cell that originate in:

(a) Isthmus of the fallopian tube
(b) Peritoneum
(c) Fimbria of the fallopian tube
(d) Ovary

Ans: (c) Fimbria of the fallopian tube

408. Diffuse gastric adenocarcinoma has overlap with which cancer?

(a) Breast infiltrating ductal carcinoma
(b) Colon signet ring cell carcinoma
(c) Breast lobular carcinoma
(d) Appendiceal Mucinous Carcinoma

Ans: (c) Breast lobular carcinoma

(Devita, Page 572)

409. Which chemotherapy regimen has superior outcomes in Gastric Carcinoma given both pre and post operatively?

(a) EOX regimen
(b) FLOT regimen
(c) DOF regimen
(d) ECX regimen

Ans: (b) FLOT regimen

410. Choi criteria is used to assess response in all of the following *except:*

(a) Hepatocellular carcionoma
(b) Renal cell carcinoma
(c) Adrenocortical carcionoma
(d) Gastrointestinal Stromal Tumor

Ans: (c) Adrenocortical carcionoma

(Devita, 10th Edition, Page 311)

411. Diffuse gastric adenocarcinoma has overlap with which cancer?

(a) Breast infiltrating ductal carcinoma
(b) Colon signet ring cell carcinoma
(c) Breast lobular carcinoma
(d) Appendiceal mucinous carcinoma

Ans: (c) Breast lobular carcinoma

(Devita, 10th Edition, Page 572)

412. Which of the following herbal products to be avoided when prescribing erlotinib?

(a) Ginseng
(b) Ginko
(c) Green tea
(d) Ephedra

Ans: (c) Green tea

(Devita, Page 180)

413. Which cytogenetic abnormality is characteristic of testicular germ cell tumor?

(a) 9,22 translocation
(b) Isochromosome 12p
(c) 13q deletion
(d) 17p deletion

Ans: (b) Isochromosome 12p

414. The risk category, the mediastinal–Non-seminomatous germ cell tumor falls:

(a) Intermediate risk
(b) Good risk
(c) Poor risk
(d) None of the above

Ans: (c) Poor risk

415. For highly emetogenic chemotherapy schdeule when antiemetics are used with aprepitant, the dose of dexamethasone on day 1 prechemotherapy will be:

(a) 20 mg
(b) 12 mg
(c) 8 mg
(d) 16 mg

Ans: (b) 12 mg

416. Patient with mediastinal germ cell tumor is associated with which chromosomal abnormality?

(a) Klinefelter syndrome
(b) Down's syndrome
(c) Patau syndrome
(d) Costello syndrome

Ans: (a) Klinefelter syndrome

417. UV and ionising radiation related single stranded breaks are repaired by which mechanism:

(a) Nucleotide excision repair
(b) Non-homologous end joining
(c) Homologous recombination
(d) Mismatch repair

Ans: (a) Nucleotide excision repair

(Devita, Page 96)

PAPER 9

418. Type of leukemia associated with mediastinal GCT is:

(a) AML–M2 (b) AML–M5

(c) AML–M7 (d) AML–M4

Ans: (c) AML–M7

(Devita, 11th Edition, Page 2064)

419. The incidence of Second primary germcell tumor of the contralateral testes occurs in which percentage of survivors?

(a) 2% (b) 3%

(c) 4% (d) 5%

Ans: (a) 2%

(Devita, 11th Edition, Page 2064)

420. Etoposide associated acute leukemia has which chromosomal abnormality?

(a) 5q gene rearrangement (b) 11q gene rearrangement

(c) 17p gene rearrangement (d) 13q gene rearrangement

Ans: (b) 11q gene rearrangement

(Devita, 11th Edition, Page 2064)

421. The adverse event associated with use of vismodegib is development of:

(a) Basal cell carcinoma of skin (b) Squamous cell carcinoma of skin

(c) Renal cell carcinoma (d) Merkel cell carcinoma

Ans: (b) Squamous cell carcinoma of skin

(Devita, 11th Edition, Page 3775)

422. Risk of radiation-related cancer has been shown to increase with increasing dose for cancers of the all *except:*

(a) Breast cancer (b) Lung cancer

(c) Thyroid cancer (d) Stomach cancer

Ans: (c) Thyroid cancer

(Devita, 11th Edition, Page 3773)

423. Which germline mutation should you test for in a patient with medullary thyroid cancer and a mother with phaeochromocytoma?

(a) BRCA1 mutation (b) CHEK2 mutation

(c) Mutation of CDH1 (d) Mutation of RET proto-oncogene

Ans: (d) Mutation of RET proto-oncogene

424. Which of the following drugs blocks the heterodimerization HER-2-HER-3?

(a) Lapatinib (b) Olaparib

(c) Pertuzumab (d) Trastuzumab

Ans: (c) Pertuzumab

425. Regarding follow-up of breast cancer patients after adjuvant therapy, according to ESMO guidelines, what is recommended?

(a) Annual breast MRI for 5 years

(b) Mammography every year

(c) Chest X-ray, liver ultrasound and bone scan annually for five years

(d) Patients on tamoxifen should have an annual endovaginal ultrasonography

Ans: (b) Mammography every year

(Devita, Page 2308)

426. What is the most important endpoint to be specified in a phase I clinical trial exploring a novel agent for cancer treatment?

(a) Clinical benefit
(b) Dose-limiting toxicity
(c) Objective response rate
(d) Pharmacokinetics

Ans: (b) Dose-limiting toxicity

427. A 75-year-old man receives monochemotherapy with oral capecitabine for colon cancer metastatic to the liver. Twelve days after treatment initiation he develops grade 4 febrile neutropenia and grade 3 diarrhoea and mucositis.Which of the following drug-metabolizing enzymes is most likely to be deficient in this patient?

(a) Dihydropyrimidine dehydrogenase (DPD)

(b) O6-methylguanine methyltransferase (MGMT)

(c) Thiopurine S-methyltransferase (TPMT)

(d) Uridine diphosphate glucuronosyl-transferase 1A1 (UGT1A1)

Ans: (a) Dihydropyrimidine dehydrogenase (DPD)

428. In patients with glioblastoma multiforme which group of patients have the maximum survival?

(a) Unmethylated MGMT with radiotherapy
(b) Unmethylated MGMT with radiotherapy and temozolomide
(c) Methylated MGMT with radiotherapy
(d) Methylated MGMT with radiotherapy and temozolomide

Ans: (d) Methylated MGMT with radiotherapy and temozolomide

(Devita, Page 2797)

429. In meduloblastoma M2 represents:

(a) Presence of gross tumor nodules in the intracranially, subarachnoid or ventricular space

(b) Gross tumor nodules in spinal subarachnoid space

(c) Systemic metastasis

(d) Tumor cells in the CSF

Ans: (a) Presence of gross tumor nodules in the intracranially, subarachnoid or ventricular space

(Devita, Page 2815)

430. Mesenchymal chondrosarcomas are treated in terms of:

(a) Osteosarcoma protocols
(b) Ewing's sarcoma protocols
(c) Pleomorphic sarcoma protocol
(d) Leiomyosarcoma protocol

Ans: (b) Ewing's sarcoma protocols

431. False statement about lung cancer:

(a) Clubbing will not resolve with excision of the primary lesion

(b) Pleural fluid is an ominous feature

(c) Dyspnoea may come from lymphatic invasion

(d) Severe localised pain suggests chest wall invasion

Ans: (b) Pleural fluid is an ominous feature

Explanation

Severe localised pain suggests chest wall invasion with the infiltration of an intercostal nerve. Invasion of the apical area may involve the brachial plexus, leading to Pancoast's syndrome

Dyspnoea may come from loss of functioning lung tissue, lymphatic invasion or the development of a large pleural effusion

Pleural fluid is an ominous feature and the presence of blood in a pleural effusion suggests that the pleura has been directly invaded

Clubbing and hypertrophic pulmonary osteoarthropathy accompany some lung cancer and may resolve with excision of the primary lesion

(Sabiston, Page 925)

432. Most common cardiac lesion in carcinoid syndrome:

(a) Pulmonary regurgitation

(b) Pulmonary stenosis

(c) Tricuspid regurgitation

(d) Triscuspid stenosis

Ans: (b) Pulmonary stenosis

Explanation

In carcinoid cardiac lesions usually involve right side of the heart, but left sided lesions present in 15%, lead to CCF

(Sabiston, Page 1273)

433. The best predictor of survival for patients with gastrinoma is:

(a) Lymph node metastasis

(b) Location of tumor

(c) Hepatic mets

(d) Gastrin level

Ans: (c) Hepatic mets

Explanation

The 10-year survival rate is 30% in patients with the aggressive form compared with greater than 90% in patients with the non-aggressive form

The best predictor of survival for patients with gastrinoma is the presence of liver metastases; lymph node metastases are not predictive

(Sabiston, Page 956)

434. Most common second primary site in small bowel carcinoid is:

(a) Colon

(b) Ileum

(c) Ovary

(d) Lung

Ans : (a) Colon

Explanation

Unusual observation in carcinoid tumor is second primary lesion of different histologic type. Usually synchronus adeno carcinoma in large intestine (10-20%)

(Sabiston, Page 1272)

435. Which benign lesion of duodenum mimics peptic ulcer?

(a) Hemangioma
(b) Lipopma
(c) Hyperplastic polyp
(d) Brunner gland adenoma

Ans: (d) Brunner gland adenoma

Explanation

Brunner gland adenoma usually from proximal duodenum benign hyperplastic lesion; produces symptoms mimics PUD

(Sabiston, Page 1271)

436. Most common symptomatic benign neoplasm of small bowel…. .

(a) Hemangioma
(b) Lipoma
(c) Stromal tumor
(d) Adenoma

Ans: (c) Stromal tumor

Explanation

Adenoma reported most commonly in autopsy series. But stromal tumors are most common benign SI neoplasm that produce symptoms

(Sabiston, Page 1270)

437. Most common tumor of small intestine:

(a) Adenocarcinoma
(b) Lymphoma
(c) Adenoma
(d) Metastasis

Ans: (d) Metastasis

Explanation

Metastatic tumors of SI is much more common than primary neoplasm. Mets arising from ovary, cervix, kidney, stomach. extra abdominal–cutaneous melanoma (most common), breast, lung

(Sabiston, Page 1280)

438. Nodal involvement in SI GIST is …….. stage.

(a) III C
(b) III B
(c) III A
(d) IV

Ans: (d) IV

Explanation

If N1 or M1 irrespective of mitotic rate, staged as IV

(Sabiston, Page 1280)

439. Which of the following is false regarding testicular seminoma?

(a) Active lymphocyte infiltration indicate good prognosis
(b) Two histological subtypes
(c) Main metastasis via blood
(d) Inguinal node enlarged only when scrotal skin involved

Ans: (c) Main metastasis via blood

Explanation

Seminoma most common testicular germ cell tumor. Remain localised for long term. Spread via lymphatics mainly. Inguinal node enlarged only when scrotal skin involved. Subtypes: spermatocytic, anaplastic

(Bailey, Page 1506)

440. Which of the following is false regarding non-seminomatous GCT?

(a) Yolk sac tumor secrete AFP

(b) Immature teratoma will not metastasise

(c) Different histological type coexist within a single tumor

(d) Teratoma contains cystic spaces with gelatinous fluid

Ans: (b) Immature teratoma will not metastasise

Explanation

Both immature and mature teratoma will metastasise

(Bailey, Page 1506)

441. Which of the following metastasise early via both blood and lymph?

(a) Choriocarcinoma (b) Embryonal carcinoma

(c) Teratoma (d) Yolk sac tumor

Ans: (a) Choriocarcinoma

Explanation

Choriocarcinoma is highly malignant that metastasise early via both lymphatics and blood

(Bailey, Page 1507)

442. Which of the following is feminizing tumor?

(a) Yolk-sac tumor (b) Tertaoma

(c) Leydig cell tumor (d) Sertoli cell tumor

Ans: (d) Sertoli cell tumor

Explanation

Leydig cell tumor–masculanises. Sertoli cell tumor feminises

(Bailey, Page 1507)

443. Which of the following is false regarding interstitial tumor?

(a) Only 10% malignant

(b) Most prepubertal tumors secrete feminizing hormones

(c) Regression of symptoms after orchidectomy may be incomplete

(d) Well circumscribed tumor with yellow cut surface

Ans: (b) Most prepubertal tumors secrete feminizing hormones

Explanation

Most prepubertal tumors secrete androgens. Postpubertal–feminizing hormones. 10% of tumors only malignant

(Bailey, Page 1507)

444. Nodes below diaphragm staged in testicular tumor staged as in older staging system, STAGE:

(a) I (b) II

(c) III (d) IV

Ans: (b) II

Explanation

Stage I: Tumor is confined to the testis and epididymis

Stage II: Nodal disease is present but is confined to nodes below the diaphragm

Stage III: Nodes are present above the diaphragm

Stage IV: Non-lymphatic metastatic disease (most typically within the lungs)

(Bailey, Page 1508)

445. Which of the following is false regarding testicular tumor investigation?

(a) Usg is mandatory

(b) Tumor marker raised in 50% cases

(c) CT chest, abdomen usually undertaken after orchidectomy

(d) Serum half life of AFP 3 days

Ans: (d) Serum half life of AFP 3 days

Explanation

Serum half life of AFP–5 to 7 days, Hcg half life 2-3 days

(Bailey, Page 1508)

446. Which of the following is false regarding testicular tumor examination?

(a) Lax secondary hydrocele usually obscures the underlying tumor, if present

(b) Vas is never thickened

(c) Around 5% of cases have gynaecomastia

(d) In 1–2% of cases the tumor is bilateral at the time of diagnosis

Ans: (a) Lax secondary hydrocoele usually obscures the underlying tumor, if present

Explanation

On examination there is an intratesticular solid mass. If present, a lax secondary hydrocoele does not usually obscure the underlying tumor

(Bailey, Page 1507)

447. Which of the following is second most common tumor of testes?

(a) Interstitial cell tumors (b) Metastasis

(c) Lymphoma (d) Germ cell tumor

Ans: (c) Lymphoma

Explanation

Germ cell tumors (90–95%) (these include seminoma, embryonal cell carcinoma, yolk sac tumor, teratoma, and choriocarcinoma)

- Interstitial tumors (1–2%) (these include Leydig cell tumors)
- Lymphoma (3–7%)
- Other tumors (1–2%)

(Bailey, Page 1506)

448. Which of the following is false regarding stage I testicular tumor treatment after orchidectomy?

(a) NSGCT having less chance of sub clinical mets compared to seminoma

(b) In seminoma stageI, Chemotherapy indicated only if relapse occurs

(c) NSGCT is radiosensitive and chemosensitive

(d) NSGCT with good prognosios can be managed with surveillance alone in Stage I

Ans: (c) NSGCT is radiosensitive and chemosensitive

Explanation

NSGCTs are not radiosensitive, but they are highly sensitive to combination chemotherapy. Up to 30% of NSGCT patients with stage I disease have subclinical metastases and will relapse if surveillance alone is applied. Only around 15–20% of men with stage I seminoma have subclinical metastatic disease

(Bailey, Page 1509)

449. Following is not a chemotherapy drug for GCT:

(a) Taxanes (b) Cisplatin

(c) Bleomycin (d) Etoposide

Ans: (a) Taxanes

Explanation

Bleomycin, etoposide and cis-platinum (so called BEP chemotherapy)

(Bailey, Page 1509)

450. Recommended margin for wide local excision of 3 mm thickness melanoma:

(a) 0.5 cm (b) 1

(c) 1.5 cm (d) 2 cm

Ans: (d) 2 cm

Explanation

Thickness	Margin*
In situ	0.5 cm
<1 mm	1 cm
1–2 mm	1–2 cm†
>2–4 mm	2 cm
>4 mm	2 cm‡

(Sbaiston, Page 734)

451. Intransit mets with single node involvement in malignant melanoma is .... stage according to AJCC, 8th edition.

(a) II C (b) II B

(c) IIIB (d) IIIC

Ans: (d) IIIC

(AJCC, 8th Edition, NCCN website)

452. Single most important prognostic index in melanoma:

(a) Breslow thickness (b) Lymph node mets

(c) Ulceration (d) Mitotic index

Ans: (b) Lymph node mets

Explanation

The presence of lymph node metastases is the single most important prognostic index in melanoma, outweighing both tumor and host factors

(Bailey, Page 612)

453. All are true about merkel cell tumor *except:*

(a) Wide local excision enough
(b) Radiotherapy needed
(c) Aggressive one
(d) Common in women

Ans : (a) Wide local excision enough

Explanation

Treatment is with wide local excision aiming for a 25–30 mm margin, followed by radiotherapy

(Bailey, Page 612)

454. Which of the following drug not used in malignant melanoma stage 4?

(a) Dabrafenib
(b) Regorafenib
(c) Trametinib
(d) Iplimumab

Ans: (b) Regorafenib

Explanation

Stage 4 malignant melanoma–targeted therapies

Dabrafenib or vemurafenib

Trametinib alone or combined with dabrafenib

Immune checkpoint inhibitors: iplimumab, nivolimumab

(Bailey, Page 612)

455. False about subungual melanoma?

(a) Usually superficial spreading type
(b) Classical feature Hutchinson sign
(c) DD is benign racial melanonychia
(d) Malignancy is unlikely if nail fold is involved

Ans: (d) Malignancy is unlikely if nail fold is involved

Explanation

MM under the finger nail are usually SSM rather than ALM. Malignancy is unlikely if the nail fold is uninvolved

456. Which of the following will not a chemical carcinogen causing lung cancer?

(a) Ethylene oxide
(b) Beryllium
(c) Radon
(d) Vinyl chloride

Ans: (a) Ethylene oxide

Explanation

Ethylene oxide causes leukemia, lymphoma

Lung cancer – beryllium, cadmium, chromium, radon, vinyl chloride

(Sabiston, Page 695)

457. All are predominant tumor caused by azathioprine *except:*

(a) Hepatocellular carcinoma
(b) Leukemia
(c) Squamous cell carcinoma skin
(d) NHL

Ans: (b) Leukemia

Explanation

Azathioprine causes–HCC, NHL, SCC skin, cholangio ca

Chlorambucil–leukemia

(Sabiston, Page 695)

458. ....% of all human tumors caused by virus.

(a) 15
(b) 10
(c) 20
(d) 25

Ans: (a) 15

Explanation

15% tumors caused by virus. Most of them are HPV causes cervical ca, HBV, HCV cause HCC

(Sabiston, Page 696)

459. Which of the following is false regarding virus induced tumor?

(a) Long latent period
(b) Viral markers usually present in neoplastic cells
(c) Tumor virus causes persistent infection
(d) Viral factors are important determinant of tumorigenesis

Ans: (d) Viral factors are important determinant of tumorigenesis

Explanation

Host factors are important determinant of tumorigenesis, not viral factors

(Sabiston, Page 696)

460. Which of the following is not a DNA based tumor marker?

(a) Single nucleotide polymorphism
(b) Chromosomal translocation
(c) Overexpressed transcript
(d) Epigenetic changes

Ans: (c) Over expressed transcript

Explanation

RNA based tumor markers–over/under expressed transcript, regulatory RNA (micro RNA). Others are DNA based tumor markers

(Sabiston, Page 697)

461. Most common symptom of small bowel malignancy?

(a) Abdominal pain
(b) Hemorrhage
(c) Weight loss
(d) Vomiting

Ans: (a) Abdominal pain

Explanation

Malignant lesion unlike benign lesion, almost always produce symptoms. Most common is abdominal pain. Second common is weight loss. Obstruction occurs secondary to adhesion, infiltration

(Sabiston, Page 1271)

462. Which of the following type of SI lymphoma usually chemoresistant?

(a) DLBCL (b) Both

(c) B cell (d) T cell

Ans: (d) T cell

Explanation

B cell lymphomas are more chemosensitive than T cell lymphomas and have high remission rates with or without surgery

T cell lymphomas are traditionally more resistant to therapy and will progress to symptoms of obstruction or perforation if not resected

(Sabiston, Page 1278)

463. False regarding peritoneal mesothelioma?

(a) Complete surgical excision is usually not possible (b) Encasement of bowel create obstruction

(c) Local invasion of abdominal wall will not occur (d) Common in males

Ans: (c) Local invasion of abdominal wall will not occur

Explanation

Slight male predominance and a median age at presentation of approximately 50 years

In contrast to pseudomyxoma peritonei, local invasion of intra-abdominal organs, such as the liver, intestine, bladder and abdominal wall, can occur.

Encasement of bowel can create a malignant bowel obstruction

Complete surgical resection is difficult because of the extent of disease

(Sabiston, Page 1081)

464. False regarding pseudomyxoma peritonei:

(a) Appendix most common primary site (b) Females affected more

(c) Patients often asymptomatic (d) 4th, 5th decade usually affected

Ans: (b) Females affected more

Explanation

Pseudomyxoma peritonei occurs most commonly in patients who are 40 to 50 years of age and occurs with equal frequency in men and women. Patients are often asymptomatic until late in the course of their disease.

Appendix most common primary site.

Others causing–ovarian adeno ca

Diagnosis usually made during laparatomy

(Sabiston, Page 1080)

465. Metastasis in a single node size 4 cm with extra nodal extension in carcinoma oral cavity N stage:

(a) N2a (b) N2b

(c) N2c (d) N3

Ans: (d) N3

Explanation

N1–single ipsilateral <= 3 cm

N2 a–single ipsilateral > 3 cm <= 6 cm

b–multiple ipsilateral none > 6 cm

c–bilateral or contralateral none > 6 cm

N3 a–mets in LN > 6 cm without extra nodal extension

b–mets in a single or multiple LN with extra nodal extension

(AJCC, 8th Edition, NCCN website)

466. Which of the following gene mutation increase susceptibility to radiation induced cancer?

(a) P53 (b) BRCA

(c) MAPK (d) Cerb B2

Ans: (a) P53

Explanation

P53 mutation increase susceptibility to malignancy induced by radiation

So, p53 mutation is a relative contraindication to radiation

(Sabiston, Page 846)

467. First investigation in suspected pheochromocytoma:

(a) Spot serum metanephrin (b) 24 hours urinary VMA

(c) Clonidine suppression test (d) 24 hours urinary metanephrins

Ans: (a) Spot serum metanephrin

Explanation

Initial plasma free metanephrin testing effectively exclude the diagnosis if negative

(Sabiston, Page 981)

468. Prognosis for Dukes stage C 5 years survival:

(a) 50% (b) 40%

(c) 30% (d) 25%

Ans: (b) 40%

Explanation

Prognosis worsen as the stage advances. For Dukes stage A, 5 years survival is 90%. For stage C, 5 years survival is 40%

(Bailey, Page 1331)

469. Which of the following is most common histological type of stromal tumor of SI?

(a) Fusiform (b) Epithelioid

(c) Papillary (d) Mixed

Ans: (a) Fusiform

Explanation

Three histological sub types of stromal tumors: fusiform (77%), epithelioid (8%), mixed (15%)

(Sabiston, Page 1270)

470. Which of the following is not a high risk feature of differentiated thyroid malignancy?

(a) 45 years age (b) Male sex

(c) Extra thyroid extension (d) 3 cm size

Ans: (d) 3 cm size

Explanation

High Risk

>40 years

Male

Capsular invasion, extrathyroidal extension

Regional or distant mets

>4 cm

Poorly differentiated

(Sabiston, Page 903)

471. Which of the following is not a component in cancer of the liver Italian program (CLIP)?

(a) Portal vein thrombosis (b) Child Pugh class

(c) AST level (d) Tumor extension

Ans: (c) AST level

Explanation

CLIP–AFP level not AST level. Others are correct

Cancer of the Liver Italian Program Score		
Clinical Parameters	**Cutoff Value**	**Points**
Child-Pugh class	A	0
	B	1
	C	2
Tumor morphology	Uninodular, <50% extension	0
	Multinodular, <50% extension	1
	Massive or extension > 50%	2
AFP level	<400 ng/dL	0
	>400 ng/dL	1
Portal vein thrombosis	No	0
	Yes	1

(Sabiston, Page 1460)

472. Which of the following is not a component in Okuda staging system?

(a) Serum bilirubin (b) Serum albumin

(c) Tumor stage (d) Ascites

Ans: (c) Tumor stage

Explanation

The Okuda staging system is an older but simple and effective system that takes liver function and tumor-related factors into account

It adds up a single point for the presence of tumor involving more than 50% of the liver, presence of ascites, albumin level less than 3 g/dL and bilirubin level higher than 3 mg/dL

The Okuda staging system reliably distinguishes patients with a prohibitively poor prognosis from those with potential for long-term survival

(Sabiston, Page 1460)

473. Factors most useful to predict outcome in colorectal liver mets all *except:*

(a) Size of the primary tumor >5 cm
(b) LN positive primary lesion
(c) Increased CEA >200 ng/ml
(d) More than one tumor

Ans: (a) Size of the primary tumor >5 cm

Explanation

Disease-free interval less than 1 year

More than one tumor

Lymph node positive primary, and

CEA level higher than 200 ng/mL

Size of the metastasis > 5 cm, not primary tumor

(Sabiston, Page 1467)

474. False regarding hepatoblastoma?

(a) Low birth weight may be a risk factor
(b) More common in males
(c) Associated with von Recklinghausen disease
(d) Not associated with inborn errors of metabolism

Ans: (c) Associated with von Recklinghausen disease

Explanation

Associated with Beckwith Wiedemann syndrome and FAP, not with von Recklinghausen disease. Most common primary hepatic tumor of childhood

Common in males

Not associated with hepatitis, cirrhosis, inborn errors of metabolism

(Sabiston, Page 1464)

475. False regarding cystadenoma:

(a) Fluid content is mucinous
(b) CECT–enhancement cyst wall
(c) Grows rapidly
(d) USG–nodularity, fluid-filled locule

Ans: (c) Grows rapidly

Explanation

Ultrasound usually demonstrates a cystic structure with varying wall thickness, nodularity, septations and fluid-filled locules

Importantly, contrast-enhanced CT demonstrates enhancement of the cyst wall and septa. Cystadenomas tend to grow slowly but can eventually progress to their malignant counterpart, cystadenocarcinomas

(Sabiston, Page 1469)

476. Typical peripheral nodular enhancement seen in:

(a) Hepatic adenoma
(b) Hepatoblastoma
(c) Hemangioma
(d) Focal nodular hyperplasia (FNH)

Ans: (c) Hemangioma

Explanation

FNH–homogenous mass with central scar, enhances in arterial phase.

Hepatic adenoma–heterogenous and hypervascular on arterial phase

Hepatoblastoma–vascular mass with speckled calcification

(Sabiston, Page 1457)

PAPER 10

477. Glioblastomas with mutation in which gene has better prognosis?

(a) IDH1 mutation
(b) MGMT mutation
(c) KRAS mutation
(d) PI3CK mutation

Ans: (a) IDH1 mutation

478. NSCLC patients treated with geftinib or erlotinib after few months, mutation develops in which gene?

(a) EGFR exon 20
(b) EGFR exon 19
(c) EGFR exon 18
(d) EGFR exon 12–

Ans: (a) EGFR exon 20

479. One of the Enabling characteristics of hallmark of cancer is:

(a) Genomic instability and mutation
(b) Enabling replicative mortality
(c) Inducing angiogenesis
(d) D-evading immune destruction

Ans: (a) Genomic instability and mutation

480. The drugs which work targeting genomic instability are:

(a) Telomerase inhibitors
(b) Proapoptotic inhibitors
(c) BH3 mimetics
(d) PARP inhibitors

Ans: (d) PARP inhibitors

481. SMO and PITCH genes work through which pathway?

(a) Motor pathway
(b) PI3K pathway
(c) JAK-STAT pathway
(d) Hedgehog pathway

Ans: (d) Hedgehog pathway

482. Fragment analysis–molecular methodology is used to identify which mutation?

(a) Kras, braf mutation in solid tumors
(b) kit mutation in GIST and melanoma
(c) NPM1 mutation in AML
(d) IGH/BCL2 translocation in follicular lymphoma

Ans: (c) NPM1 mutation in AML

483. ALK rearrangement with EML-4, TFG can be detected by which technique?

(a) Dual fusion probe FISH
(b) Break apart probe FISH
(c) Fragment analysis
(d) Real time PCR

Ans: (b) Break apart probe FISH

484. Tobacco leads to cancer through which pathways?

(a) NFKB pathway
(b) DNA adduct pathway
(c) Hypermethylation pathway
(d) All of the above

Ans: (d) All of the above

485. EBV leads to which cancer?

(a) Kaposi carcinoma
(b) Castleman disease
(c) Burkitts lymphoma
(d) Adult T cell lymphoma

Ans: (c) Burkitts lymphoma

486. As per NCI CTCAE Version 5, if nausea leads to inadequate oral caloric intake or fluid intake requiring tube feeding or TPN, then the grade of nausea is:

(a) Grade 2 (b) Grade 3
(c) Grade 4 (d) Grade 5

Ans: (b) Grade 3

487. In a 45-year-old lady got evaluated for profuse PV bleeding and found to have endometrial endometriod carcinoma. She underwent TAH and BSO with pelvic and paraaortic lymphadenectomy. HPE revealed endometrial endometroid carcinoma grade 1 with 25% myometrial invasion with no lower uterine or cervical stromal involvement, nodes were negative. What will be adjuvant management for this patient?

(a) Observation (b) Vaginal brachytherapy
(c) Pelvic RT (d) Chemotherapy

Ans: (a) Observation

488. In case of extravasation, cold compress should be given to all the following drugs *except:*

(a) Anthracyclines (b) Alkylating agents
(c) Platins (d) Antibiotics

Ans: (c) Platins

489. All are prerequesites of liver transplatation in liver limited metastatic pancreatic neuroendocrine tumor *except:*

(a) Well differentiated NET with ki67% less than or equal to 10
(b) Disease should be stable for 6 months
(c) Age less than 65 years
(d) Primary tumor removed prior to transplantation atleast 6 months

Ans: (c) Age less than 65 years

490. Pre-requisites for diagnosing hepatocellular carcinoma are all *except:*

(a) AFP more than 400 ng/dl
(b) Size of the lesions more than 2 cms
(c) With classical arterial hyperenhancement and venous washout
(d) Liver biopsy is mandatory

Ans: (d) Liver biopsy is mandatory

491. For HCC, UCLS Criteria for liver transplantation all the following are correct *except:*

(a) Single lesion of less than 6.5 cms (b) Single lesion of less than 5 cms
(c) No more than 3 lesions less than or equal to 4.5 cms (d) Total diameter of lesions 8 cms

Ans: (b) Single lesion of less than 5 cms

492. FUS-DDIT3 Translocation is characteristic of which malignancy?

(a) GIST (b) Extraskeletal myxoid chondrosarcoma
(c) Myxoid round cell liposarcoma (d) Extraskeletal Ewing's sarcoma

Ans: (c) Myxoid round cell liposarcoma

493. The best first line option for a patient of 70 years old with Ivier limited, multifocal metastasis in a pancreatic tail Neuroendocrine tumor:

(a) Peptide Receptor Radionuclide Therapy (b) Long acting octreotide
(c) TACE (d) TARE

Ans: (b) Long acting octreotide

494. For appendiceal neuroendocrine tumors all are indications for right hemicolectomy *except:*

(a) Tumors more than 2 cms
(b) Invasion of the appendiceal wall
(c) Presence of tumor at the apex
(d) Lymph node metastases

Ans: (c) Presence of tumor at the apex

495. The translocation associated with synovial sarcoma is:

(a) t(2,19)
(b) t(12,22)
(c) t(X,18)
(d) t(X,17)

Ans: (c) t(X,18)

496. A patient of solitary fibrous tumor is found to have recurrent episodes of hypoglycemia. This syndrome is called as:

(a) Glucagonoma syndrome
(b) Doege Potter syndrome
(c) Li Fraumeni syndrome
(d) Von Recklinghausen syndrome

Ans: (b) Doege Potter syndrome

497. The chance of breast and ovarian cancer in women with BRCA2 syndrome are:

(a) 80% and 50%
(b) 50% and 20%
(c) 70% and 30%
(d) 82% and 25%

Ans: (b) 50% and 20%

498. Homologous recombination deficiency leads to the following changes *except:*

(a) Medium-scale state transitions
(b) Loss of Heterozygosity
(c) Telomeric Allelic Imbalance
(d) Large-scale state transitions

Ans: (a) Medium-scale state transitions

499. A 60-year-old male got evaluated for unexplained anemia and found to have right side colon carcinoma. He underwent right hemicolectomy. Histopathology showing the tumor penetrates through the muscularis propria and serosa is involved. 23 lymph nodes were negative. What adjuvant therapy is the best option for him?

(a) If MSI HIGH only observtion
(b) Capecitabine
(c) XELOX for 8 cycles
(d) Radiation

Ans: (c) XELOX for 8 cycles

500. The above mentioned patient should undergo colonoscopy once in:

(a) 2 years
(b) 3 years
(c) 4 years
(d) No need of colonoscopy

Ans: (b) 3 years

501. In a case of suspected lung cancer if the patient has voice change, what is the tumor status the patient has?

(a) T1
(b) T2
(c) T3
(d) T4

Ans: (d) T4

502. The best adjuvant management in a female of 45 years old who had underwent cytoreductive surgery for adnexal mass and HPE found to have for low grade serous ovarian carcinoma and nodes are negative, no peritoneal surface inolvement. Adjvuant management include:

(a) Only follow up and observation
(b) Adjuvant chemotherapy
(c) Hormonal therapy
(d) All of the above are correct

Ans: (b) Adjuvant chemotherapy

503. All are true about low grade serous carcinoma of the ovary *except:*

(a) KRAS and BRAF mutations are frequent
(b) No adjuvant treatment is indicated for stage IA, IB low grade serous ca ovary
(c) Adjuvant chemotherapy is indicated in stage II-IV patients
(d) TP53 mutations are very commonly found in these patients

Ans: (d) TP53 mutations are very commonly found in these patients

504. Treatment of choice for M1b low grade mucinous appendiceal malignant neoplasm:

(a) Simple appendicectomy (b) Radical right hemicolectomy
(c) Cytoreductive surgery with HIPEC (d) None of the above

Ans: (c) Cytoreductive surgery with HIPEC

505. Treatment of Stage IA Endometroid endmetrial carcinoma post TAH plus BSO and node dissection is:

(a) Vaginal brachytherapy (b) Observation
(c) EBRT (d) Chemotherapy

Ans: (b) Observation

506. The amount of pleural fluid secreted physiologically every day is:

(a) 0.05 ml/kg/hour (b) 0.001 ml/kg/hour
(c) 10 ml/kg/hour (d) 5 mgl/kg/hour

Ans: (b) 0.001 ml/kg/hour

507. The IHC marker NKX3.1 is specific for:

(a) Pancreatic adenocarcinoma (b) Prostatic adenocarcinoma
(c) Colonic adenocarcinoma (d) Ovarian adenocarcinoma

Ans: (b) Prostatic adenocarcinoma

508. In a patient of CUP, according to Culine S *et al*, patient with ECOG PS2, with liver metastases will have a median survival of:

(a) 4.2 months (b) 2.4 months
(c) 3.6 months (d) 1.2 months

Ans: (b) 2.4 months

509. Following are the agents associated with the causation of mesothelioma except:

(a) Eronite exposure (b) Thorotrast exposure
(c) SV-40 (simian virus) (d) Human papilloma virus

Ans: (d) Human papilloma virus

510. High grade serous carcinoma of the ovary are derived from the cell that originate in:

(a) Isthmus of the fallopian tube (b) Peritoneum
(c) Fimbria of the fallopian tube (d) Ovary

Ans: (c) Fimbria of the fallopian tube

511. Diffuse gastric adenocarcinoma has overlap with which cancer?

(a) Breast infiltrating ductal carcinoma (b) Colon signet ring cell carcinoma
(c) Breast lobular carcinoma (d) Appendiceal Mucinous Carcinoma

Ans: (c) Breast lobular carcinoma

512. Which chemotherapy regimen has superior outcomes in Gastric Carcinoma given both pre and post operatively?

(a) EOX regimen
(b) FLOT regimen
(c) DOF regimen
(d) ECX regimen

Ans: (b) FLOT regimen

513. Choi criteria is used to assess response in all of the following *except:*

(a) Hepatocellular carcinoma
(b) Renal cell carcinoma
(c) Adrenocortical carcinoma
(d) Gastrointestinal Stromal Tumor

Ans: (c) Adrenocortical carcinoma

514. Diffuse gastric adenocarcinoma has overlap with which cancer?

(a) Breast infiltrating ductal carcinoma
(b) Colon signet ring cell carcinoma
(c) Breast lobular carcinoma
(d) Appendiceal Mucinous Carcinoma

Ans: (c) Breast lobular carcinoma

515. Paclitaxel acts by:

(a) Destabilizing microtubules
(b) Stabilizing microtubules
(c) DNA adduct formation
(d) Depolymerise microtubules

Ans: (b) Stabilizing microtubules

516. Which cytogenetic abnormality is characteristic of testicular germ cell tumor?

(a) 9,22 translocation
(b) Isochromosome 12p
(c) 13q deletion
(d) 17p deletion

Ans: (b) Isochromosome 12p

517. The risk category, the mediastinal–Non-seminomatous germ cell tumor falls:

(a) Intermediate risk
(b) Good risk
(c) Poor risk
(d) None of the above

Ans: (c) Poor risk

518. For highly emetogenic chemotherapy schedule when antiemetics are used with aprepitant, the dose of dexamethasone on day 1 prechemotherapy will be:

(a) 20 mg
(b) 12 mg
(c) 8 mg
(d) 16 mg

Ans: (b) 12 mg

519. Patient with mediastinal germ cell tumor is associated with which chromosomal abnormality?

(a) Klinefelter syndrome
(b) Down's syndrome
(c) Patau syndrome
(d) Costello syndrome

Ans: (a) Klinefelter syndrome

520. UV and ionising radiation related single stranded breaks are repaired by which mechanism?

(a) Nucleotide excision repair
(b) Non homologous End Joining
(c) Homologous recombination
(d) Mismatch repair

Ans: (a) Nucleotide excision repair

521. The genetic alteration which occurs in the transition from intermediate adenoma to late adenoma occurs in which gene/chromosome?

(a) APC/Beta Catenin
(b) kras
(c) 18q
(d) p53

Ans: (c) 18q

522. Glioblastomas with mutation in which gene has better prognosis?

(a) IDH1 mutation
(b) MGMT mutation
(c) KRAS mutation
(d) PI3CK mutation

Ans: (a) IDH1 mutation

523. Which alkylating agent has platelet sparing effect?

(a) Ifosfamide
(b) Cyclophosphamide
(c) Melphalan
(d) Chlorambucil

Ans: (b) Cyclophosphamide

524. One of the Enabling characteristics of hallmark of cancer is:

(a) Genomic instability and mutation
(b) Enabling replicative mortality
(c) Inducing angiogenesis
(d) Evading immune destruction

Ans: (a) Genomic instability and mutation

525. The drugs which work targeting genomic instability are:

(a) Telomerase inhibitors
(b) Proapoptoptic inhibitors
(c) BH3 mimetics
(d) PARP inhibitors

Ans: (d) PARP inhibitors

526. SMO and PITCH genes work through which pathway?

(a) Motor pathway
(b) PI3K pathway
(c) JAK-STAT pathway
(d) Hedgehog pathway

Ans: (d) Hedgehog pathway

527. Fragment analysis–molecular methodology is used to identify which mutation?

(a) Kras, braf mutation in solid tumors
(b) Kit mutation in GIST and melanoma
(c) NPM1 mutation in AML
(d) IGH/BCL2 translocation in follicular lymphoma

Ans: (c) NPM1 mutation in AML

528. ALK rearrangement with EML-4, TFG can be detected by which technique?

(a) Dual fusion probe FISH
(b) Break apart probe FISH
(c) Fragment analysis
(d) Real time PCR

Ans: (b) Break apart probe FISH

529. Tobacco leads to cancer through which pathways?

(a) NFKB pathway
(b) DNA adduct pathway
(c) Hypermethylation pathway
(d) All of the above

Ans: (d) All of the above

530. EBV leads to which cancer?

(a) Kaposi carcinoma
(b) Castleman disease
(c) Burkitts lymphoma
(d) Adult T cell lymphoma

Ans: (c) Burkitts lymphoma

531. As per NCI CTCAE Version 5. If nausea leads to inadequate oral caloric intake or fluid intake requiring tube feeding or TPN, then the grade of nausea is:

(a) Grade 2
(b) Grade 3
(c) Grade 4
(d) Grade 5

Ans: (b) Grade 3

532. In which cancer Vitamin-D administration along with treatment is proved to be beneficial?

(a) Non-Hodgkin's lymphoma
(b) Hodgkin's lymphoma
(c) Breast cancer
(d) Lung cancer

Ans: (b) Hodgkin's lymphoma

533. Which germline mutation should you test for in a patient with medullary thyroid cancer and a mother with pheochromocytoma?

(a) BRCA1 mutation
(b) Mutation of CDH1
(c) Mutation of RET proto-oncogene
(d) PTEN mutation

Ans: (c) Mutation of RET proto-oncogene

534. A 54-year-old female patient was treated for high-grade serous ovarian cancer, FIGO stage IIIC, with optimal debulking. Then she received 6 cycles of adjuvant carboplatin and dose dense paclitaxel. She was in a complete remission with normal levels of CA-125 and a normal CT scan. 15 months later her general physician finds an elevated CA-125 of 300 U/ml. The patient is asymptomatic. How do you proceed?

(a) Evaluate diagnostic laparoscopy
(b) Keep patient under surveillance
(c) Restart carboplatin/paclitaxel
(d) Start second line chemotherapy and bevacizumab

Ans: (c) Restart carboplatin/paclitaxel

535. A fit 66-year-old man with moderate smoking and alcoholic beverage consumption habits is diagnosed with cT3 cN0 M0 cervical (upper third) esophageal squamous cell carcinoma. The best treatment approach is:

(a) Definitive chemoradiotherapy
(b) Definitive radiotherapy
(c) Definitive radiotherapy followed by adjuvant chemotherapy
(d) Esophagectomy followed by adjuvant chemoradiotherapy

Ans: (a) Definitive chemoradiotherapy

PART SIX: GENERAL SURGERY REVIEW

CHAPTER

66

GENERAL SURGERY

NEET SS Pattern

PART 1

1 **Risk factors associated with adenocarcinoma esophagus is:**

(a) Achalasia (b) Caustic injury

(c) Barrett's esophagus (d) Tylosis

Ans: (c) Barrett's esophagus

2. **Which of following breast pathological subtype is associated with familial diffuse gastric cancer?**

(a) Medullary (b) Ductal adenocarcinoma – No special type

(c) Ductal adenocarcinoma – special types (d) Lobular adenocarcinoma

Ans: (d) Lobular adenocarcinoma

3. **Familial adenomatous polyps include:**

(a) Cowden disease (b) Juvenile polyposis

(c) Peutz-Jeghers polyp (d) Gardner syndrome

Ans: (d) Gardner syndrome

4. **Imatinib is used in:**

(a) Colorectal cancer (b) Stomach cancer

(c) Pancreatic cancer (d) GIST

Ans: (d) GIST

5. **Patient underwent surgery for GIST and HPE revealed a 10 cm tumor with high mitotic index. Imatinib is advised for:**

(a) 1 year (b) 3 years

(c) 5 years (d) 6 months

Ans: (b) 3 years

6. **Most common malignant tumor of small intestine:**

(a) Adenocarcinoma (b) GIST

(c) Lymphoma (d) Carcinoid

Ans: (a) Adenocarcinoma

7. **A 40 years male underwent radical right hemicolectomy for ascending colon growth with serosal extension and HPE revealed moderately differentiated adenocarcinoma with free margins and no nodes positive in the 15 nodes in resected specimen. Patient insists on chemotherapy. Which of the following is recommended?**

(a) 5FU and leucovirin (b) FOLFOX 3 months

(c) FOLFOX 6 months (d) FOLFIRI

Ans: (a) 5FU and leucovirin

- Serosal involvement: T3
  Nodal involvement: Minimal nodes to be removed is 15- and all negative-N0
  Mets negative – M0
  T3N0M0–is stage II**
- No improvement in overall survival was seen with the addition of oxaliplatin in patients with stage II disease
- Hence Stage II cases if chemotherapy is given better give only 5FU+ Leucovorin
- Outcome of this MOSAIC trial established FOLFOX as the (current) routine standard treatment for patients with stage III colon cancer
- **FOLFOX (Oxaliplatin added to 5FU+ Leucovorin) is used for Stage 3 cases****
- **Irinotecan is used only for metastatic cases (FOLFIRI) for Stage 4 cases****

8. Which of following statement is false regarding desmoid tumor:

(a) It is called aggressive fibromatosis
(b) RT is the treatment option
(c) It occurs in women during the period of pregnancy or just after child birth
(d) It is associated with FAP

Ans: (b) RT is the treatment option

9. True statement regarding peritoneal mesothelioma is:

(a) Slight female preponderance at late ages
(b) Most common primary malignant neoplasm of peritoneum
(c) Preoperative diagnosis is always possible
(d) Treatment is complete surgical excision of the tumor

Ans: (b) Most common primary malignant neoplasm of peritoneum

10. Dysphagia in esophagus cancer indicates tumor has invaded:

(a) Mucosa (b) Submucosa
(c) Transmural (d) Nodal metastases

Ans: (c) Transmural

11. N2 in esophageal cancer is:

(a) Involvement of nodes in 2 stations (b) 3–6 nodes
(c) 7 or more nodes (d) 1–2 nodes

Ans: (b) 3–6 nodes

12. Tumor spread to umbilicus from intraabdominal malignancy is called:

(a) Umbilical granuloma (b) Cullen sign
(c) Caput medusa (d) Sister Mary Joseph nodule

Ans: (d) Sister Mary Joseph nodule

13. Tumors in the gastroesophageal junction belongs to which type of Siewert classification?

(a) Siewert type I (b) Siewert type II
(c) Siewert type III (d) Siewert type IV

Ans: (b) Siewert type II

14. In Lauren classification regarding diffuse gastric cancer, which is false statement?

(a) Males > females (b) Familial

(c) Poorly differentiated (d) Young age onset

Ans: (a) Males > females

15. According to Borrmann classification of gastric cancer, Type I is:

(a) Protruding (b) Excavated

(c) Flat (d) Linitis plastic

Ans: (a) Protruding

16. Lag phase required to develop gastric cancer following Vagotomy and drainage procedure:

(a) 5 years (b) 10 years

(c) 20 years (d) 8 years

Ans: (b) 10 years

17. False statement regarding the gastrointestinal stromal tumor is:

(a) It is mesenchymal origin (b) Size > 5 cm is considered malignant

(c) More common in females (d) Associated with mutation in c-kit oncogene

Ans: (c) More common in females

18. False statement regarding familial adenomatous polyposis:

(a) APC gene is tumor suppressor gene located in 5q21

(b) It is an autosomal dominant condition

(c) The penetrance is very high that more than 90% of the individuals affected

(d) Untreated patients will develop cancer by 15–20 years of age

Ans: (d) Untreated patients will develop cancer by 15–20 years of age

19. PDGFRA mutation found in:

(a) Aplastic anemia (b) ITP

(c) GIST (d) GI Lymphoma

Ans: (c) GIST

20. Mutation found in GIST is:

(a) CD117 (b) CD110

(c) CD 52 (d) CD 10

Ans: (a) CD117

21. Imatinib used in treatment of:

(a) GIST (b) Ca Esophagus

(c) Ca Colon (d) GI Lymphoma

Ans: (a) GIST

22. MAGIC trial is about:

(a) Adjuvant treatment (b) Perioperative chemotherapy

(c) Postoperative radiotherapy (d) D2 Lymphadenectomy

Ans: (b) Perioperative chemotherapy

23. **Station 8 in cancer stomach lymph node:**
(a) Left gastric (b) Common hepatic artery
(c) Proper hepatic artery (d) Celiac trunk
Ans: (b) Common hepatic artery

24. **First LN to drain colonic wall:**
(a) Epicolic mode (b) Paracolic mode
(c) Intermediate mode (d) None
Ans: (a) Epicolic mode

25. **Cancer rectum stage II (T3-T4) treatment:**
(a) Neoadjuvant CT+ RT followed by surgery (b) Surgery followed by CTRT
(c) Chemoradiation alone (d) Surgery alone
Ans: (a) Neoadjuvant CT+ RT followed by surgery

26. **Best result of rectal cancer surgery is from:**
(a) TME (b) Distal margin more than 5 cm
(c) Pelvic LN dissection (d) Maintaining of plane of dissection
Ans: (a) TME

27. **Tumor marker of colorectal cancer:**
(a) CEA (b) CA 19-9
(c) AFP (d) CA 125
Ans: (a) CEA

28. **Which of the following is not true about FAP?**
(a) Autosomal recessive (b) Screening done by colonoscopy
(c) Polyps develop in late adulthood (d) Epidermal cysts and Osteoma may occur
Ans: (a) Autosomal recessive

29. **PET-CT in carcinoma esophagus helps in the following *except:***
(a) Defining radiotherapy fields (b) Identifying lesion and location
(c) Identifying nature of carcinoma (d) Identifying distant metastasis
Ans: (c) Identifying nature of carcinoma

30. **Preferred investigation for staging carcinoma esophagus is:**
(a) Endoscopic ultrasound (b) Endoscopy
(c) MRI (d) CT scan
Ans: (a) Endoscopic ultrasound

31. **Most common small bowel tumor is:**
(a) Lymphoma (b) Metastatic tumor
(c) Carcinoid (d) GIST
Ans: (b) Metastatic tumor

32. Which of the following gastric lymphoma regresses with H. pylori eradication therapy?

(a) Burkitt's lymphoma (b) Follicular lymphoma
(c) Mantle cell lymphoma (d) MALT lymphoma

Ans: (d) MALT lymphoma

33. Carney triad is associated with:

(a) Sex chord stromal tumor of ovary (b) Merkel cell carcinoma
(c) Gastrointestinal stromal tumor (d) Small cell lung cancer

Ans: (c) Gastrointestinal stromal tumor

34. Statements regarding metal stents in biliary tract drainage are correct *except:*

(a) Don't require changing every 2 months (b) Maintain biliary drainage longer than silastic stents
(c) Can pass a new stent through an obstructed metal stent (d) Lower complication rates than plastic

Ans: (c) Can pass a new stent through an obstructed metal stent

35. In Borrmann's–classification, gastric cancer type 2 indicates:

(a) Unclassifiable tumor (b) Polypoidal/fungating tumor
(c) Ulcerating lesion infiltrating gastric wall (d) Ulcerating lesions surrounded by elevated borders

Ans: (d) Ulcerating lesions surrounded by elevated borders

36. Ivor Lewis approach for oesophageal resection in carcinoma oesophagus is:

(a) Laparotomy with cervical approach (b) Left thoracotomy and laparotomy
(c) Transhiatal cervical anastomosis (d) Right thoracotomy and laparotomy

Ans: (d) Right thoracotomy and laparotomy

37. In Japanese classification of early gastric cancer, superficial elevated type is classified as:

(a) Type IIa (b) Type IIb
(c) Type I (d) Type IIc

Ans: (a) Type IIa

38. Treatment of radiation proctitis includes all *except:*

(a) Local steroids (b) Formalin instillation
(c) Argan plasma coagulator (d) Hyperbaric oxygen

Ans: (a) Local steroids

39. D2 lymph node resection in carcinoma stomach includes:

(a) Periaortic lymph nodes (b) Lymph node along celiac axis
(c) All of the above (d) Perigastric lymph nodes

Ans: (b) Lymph node along celiac axis

40. Regarding GIST tumor, following are true except:

(a) Arise from mucosa and submucosa (b) Common in jejunum and ileum
(c) Treatment is segmental resection (d) >5 cms are considered malignant

Ans: (b) Common in jejunum and ileum

41. Which was the 1st robot approved by FDA for clinical use?

(a) DAVINCHI (b) ROBODOC

(c) ZEUS (d) AESOP

Ans: (d) AESOP

42. Which is the most common germline mutation seen in hereditary pancreatic cancer?

(a) PRSS1 mutation (b) BRCA2 mutation

(c) p16 mutation (d) ATM mutation

Ans: (b) BRCA2 mutation

43. Which among the statements regarding Amsterdam criteria II is correct?

(a) Atleast 2 relatives with HNPCC associated cancer

(b) Atleast 3 successive generations should be affected

(c) Atleast one case before age of 35

(d) Tumors should be verified histopathologically

Ans: (d) Tumors should be verified histopathologically

44. Which of the following disease carries greatest risk of tumor lysis syndrome initiating chemotherapy?

(a) ALL (b) AML

(c) CML (d) Multiple myeloma

Ans: (d) Multiple myeloma

45. A 60-year-old man with 10 years history of GERD to have MALT lymphoma, localised to gastric antrum on endoscopic biopsy. H. pylori was detected on mucosal biopsy and on urea breath test. What is the most appropriate treatment for this patient?

(a) Radiotherapy to stomach

(b) Chemotherapy with R-CVP (Rituximab, Cyclophosphamide, Vincristine)

(c) Triple therapy for H. pylori eradication

(d) Observation alone with repeat endoscopy after 6 months

Ans: (c) Triple therapy for H. pylori eradication

46. In colon cancer T1N1M0 is stage:

(a) 2A (b) 2B

(c) 3A (d) 3B

Ans: (c) 3A

47. Ideal upper limit of central venous pressure during parenchymal transaction of liver is:

(a) 5 mm Hg (b) 10 mm Hg

(c) 14 mm Hg (d) None of the above

Ans: (a) 5 mm Hg

48. Average time for an adenomatous colonic polyp to turn malignant is:

(a) 4–5 years (b) 6 months–1 year

(c) 1–2 years (d) 8–10 years

Ans: (d) 8–10 years

49. Ideal anterior plane of dissection in males with low rectal cancer is:

(a) Posterior to Denonviller's fascia (b) Anterior to Denonviller's fascia

(c) Anterior to prostatic capsule (d) None of the above

Ans: (b) Anterior to Denonviller's fascia

50. Maruyama index is used in:

(a) DCIS (b) HCC

(c) RCC (d) CA Stomach

Ans: (d) CA Stomach

51. Plummer-Vinson syndrome is associated with:

(a) Epidermoid carcinoma (b) Adenocarcinoma

(c) Signet ring cell carcinoma (d) None of the above

Ans: (a) Epidermoid carcinoma

52. HER-2 overexpression is seen in ____ % of gastric cancers.

(a) 30 (b) 20

(c) 10 (d) 40

Ans: (b) 20

53. All are risk factors for development of SCC Esophagus *except:*

(a) GERD (b) Tylosis

(c) PV syndrome (d) Achalasia

Ans: (a) GERD

54. Not an absolute contraindication for transarterial chemoembolization in HCC is:

(a) ECOG performance status (b) Mild encephalopathy

(c) Total bilirubin 5 mg/dL (d) Child-Pugh C cirrhosis

Ans: (b) Mild encephalopathy

55. Principal fuel for bowel mucosa is:

(a) Leucine (b) Isoleucine

(c) Glutamate (d) Valine

Ans: (c) Glutamate

56. HCV Infection and HCC–true is:

(a) Incidence of HCC has decreased during past few years due to better screening of blood products for HCV

(b) Incidence of HCC has decreased during past decade due to effective vaccine against HCV

(c) 1–5% of patients with chronic HCV infection will develop HCC

(d) All of the above

Ans: (c) 1–5% of patients with chronic HCV infection will develop HCC

57. HCC secondary to HCV/HBV can be due to:

(a) Cirrhosis due to infection leading to cancer

(b) Oncogene proteins produced by virus

(c) Increased amount of somatic mutations in normal hepatocytes

(d) Inhibition of normal immune response

Ans: (c) Increased amount of somatic mutations in normal hepatocyte–*Best answer among above*

58. Revised Bethesda guidelines** (Criteria to prompt microsatellite instability testing of tumors) include all *except:***

(a) Diagnosis of CRC before age 50
(b) Synchronous/Metachronous presence of CRC/other HNPCC associated cancer
(c) CRC with histopathologic features associated with MSI-H at any age
(d) CRC in two/more 1st degree relatives with HNPCC related tumors regardless of age

Ans: (c) CRC with histopathologic features associated with MSI-H at any age

59. Magic trial is related to:

(a) Rectum
(b) Stomach
(c) Sarcoma
(d) Pancreas

Ans: (b) Stomach

60. Which of the following statements regarding use of tumor markers in colorectal cancer is true?

(a) CEA is recommended as a screening for colorectal cancer
(b) Patients with K-RAS mutation in codons 12/13 have low probability of achieving benefit from anti-EGFR antibody therapy
(c) MSI predicts efficacy of adjuvant chemotherapy in CRC
(d) CEA has limited utility in post-surgical surveillance and monitoring metastatic disease

Ans: (b) Patients with K-RAS mutation in codons 12/13 have low probability of achieving benefit from anti-EGFR antibody therapy

61. Most common 1st metastatic site for ocular melanoma:

(a) Liver
(b) Skin
(c) Brain
(d) Lung

Ans: (a) Liver

62. Barrett's esophagus:

(a) 2 to 8 fold higher risk of esophageal carcinoma than normal population
(b) Patients with low grade dysplasia should undergo surveillance annual endoscopy
(c) Prevalence of Barrett's esophagus in general population undergoing endoscopy is around 5%
(d) Medical and antireflux therapies reduce risk of developing esophageal cancer

Ans: (b) Patients with low grade dysplasia should undergo surveillance annual endoscopy

63. All of the following may be protective against development of adenocarcinoma esophagus *except:*

(a) Cessation of smoking
(b) H. pylori infection
(c) Aspirin use
(d) Consumption of raw vegetables and fruits

Ans: (a) Cessation of smoking

64. Following statements are true for Lynch syndrome *except:*

(a) Responsible for at least 13–20% of total colon cancer cases
(b) Inherited as autosomal dominant disease
(c) Males are affected at higher penetrance
(d) Associated with younger age at presentation of colon cancer

Ans: (a) Responsible for at least 13–20% of total colon cancer cases

65. Surgery for gastric cancer is classified as D1 or D2 dissection based on:

(a) Extent of stomach resected
(b) Reconstruction after gastric resection
(c) Extent of lymphadenectomy
(d) Status of histopathologic margin

Ans: (c) Extent of lymphadenectomy

66. Adenocarcinoma is most common in which part of pancreas?

(a) Head
(b) Neck
(c) Body
(d) Tail

Ans: (a) Head

67. Which of following is not part of standard reconstructive anastomosis following a pancreaticoduodenectomy?

(a) Pancreatico jejunal
(b) Choledocho jejunal
(c) Gastric jejunal
(d) Choledocho pancreatic

Ans: (d) Choledocho pancreatic

68. BCLC Staging classification includes all *except:*

(a) Size of tumor
(b) Number of tumors
(c) HBV infection
(d) Child-Pugh status

Ans: (c) HBV infection

69. Gastrointestinal carcinoids are most commonly seen in:

(a) Stomach
(b) Small intestine
(c) Colon
(d) Rectum

Ans: (b) Small intestine

70. Which of the following is major prognostic factor for GIST?

(a) Tumor site
(b) Tumor ulceration
(c) Mucosal invasion
(d) Bleeding

Ans: (a) Tumor site

71. Length of colon resection for colon cancer is based on:

(a) Size of primary tumor
(b) Need to remove regional lymph nodes
(c) Performance status
(d) Grade of primary tumor

Ans: (b) Need to remove regional lymph nodes

72. KIT mutations leading to aberrant intracellular signaling pathways are typically seen in:

(a) Gastrointestinal carcinoid tumors
(b) Gastrointestinal stromal tumors
(c) Gastrointestinal melanoma
(d) Gastrointestinal lymphomas

Ans: (b) Gastrointestinal stromal tumors

73. Which of the following drugs are ineffective for colon cancer in presence of KRAS?

(a) Irinotecan
(b) Oxaliplatin
(c) Cetuximab
(d) Bevacizumab

Ans: (c) Cetuximab

74. True about anal cancer:

(a) Most common variety is adenocarcinoma treated by chemoradiation
(b) HPV 16 is detected in 90% of SCC cases
(c) Not associated with solid organ transplant recipients
(d) Benign lesions are thought to contribute to disease

Ans: (b) HPV 16 is detected in 90% of SCC cases

75. SHARP trial was study conducted on:

(a) HCC (b) RCC
(c) Colorectal cancer (d) Neuroendocrine tumor

Ans: (a) HCC

76. Localised GIST with no evidence of distant metastases are treated with good performance score:

(a) Imatinib 400 mg for 1 year (b) Surgery
(c) Sunitinib 50 mg for 1 year (d) Radiotherapy

Ans: (b) Surgery

77. Which of the following carry high risk for HCC?

(a) Wilson's disease (b) Hereditary hemochromatosis
(c) Cigarette smoking (d) Primary biliary cirrhosis

Ans: (b) Hereditary hemochromatosis

78. Magic trial true is:

(a) Indian trial
(b) Trial conducted to study different surgical techniques in CA stomach
(c) ECP was proposed and used chemotherapy regimen
(d) Trial used for GE junction and CA stomach

Ans: (d) Trial used for GE junction and CA stomach

79. Common molecular genetic alterations observed in esophageal and gastric cancers are all *except:*

(a) E-Cadherin (b) Mismatch repair instability
(c) Cyclin D1 (d) RB

Ans: (d) RB

80. Yttrium 90 microsphere treatment is useful for:

(a) Liver metastases (b) Bone metastases
(c) Brain metastases (d) LN metastases

Ans: (a) Liver metastases

81. Esophageal adenocarcinoma arises predominantly in which part of esophagus?

(a) Cervical (b) Proximal thoracic
(c) Mid thoracic (d) Distal

Ans: (d) Distal

82. Which of the following is not a risk factor for developing carcinoma stomach?

(a) Li-Fraumeni syndrome (b) HPV infection
(c) Prior gastric surgery for benign gastric ulcer disease (d) Previous radiation exposure

Ans: (b) HPV infection

83. All are true about carcinoid syndrome *except:*

(a) 80% occur in small bowel carcinoids
(b) Mainstay of treatment is Somatostatin
(c) Symptoms are not precipitated by stress and alcohol intake
(d) Liver is common site for metastasis

Ans: (c) Symptoms are not precipitated by stress and alcohol intake

84. Prognostic factors in carcinoma colon category III includes all *except:*

(a) Perineural invasion
(b) Lymphatic vessel invasion
(c) Genetic polymorphism
(d) Primary tumour location

Ans: (b) Lymphatic vessel invasion

85. Imatinib as adjuvant therapy for resected primary GIST:

(a) 800 mg daily for 3 years
(b) 400 mg daily for 1 year
(c) 400 mg daily for 3 years
(d) 800 mg daily for 1 year

Ans: (b) 400 mg daily for 1 year

86. Mutation in PTEN gene causes:

(a) Cowden syndrome
(b) Peutz-Jeghers syndrome
(c) Bloom's syndrome
(d) Nevoid basal cell syndrome

Ans: (a) Cowden syndrome

87. Best modality for T stage assessment in carcinoma esophagus is:

(a) CT
(b) EUS
(c) MRI
(d) PET scan

Ans: (b) EUS

88. T2N0M0 Carcinoma esophagus is best treated by:

(a) Surgery
(b) RT
(c) Chemoradiation
(d) Surgery + postop

Ans: (a) Surgery

89. Siewert classification is for classifying:

(a) Lung cancers
(b) Adrenal carcinoma
(c) GE junctional tumors
(d) Neuroendocrine tumors

Ans: (c) GE junctional tumors

90. Okuda staging for HCC includes all *except:*

(a) Ascites
(b) Albumin
(c) Bilirubin
(d) Prothrombin time

Ans: (d) Prothrombin time

91. Consideration for liver transplantation for HCC is:

(a) BCLC criteria
(b) CLIP staging
(c) MELD scoring
(d) Milan criteria

Ans: (d) Milan criteria

92. Fibrolamellar HCC differs from usual HCC in following *except:*

(a) Occurs in much younger age group
(b) Commonly associated with cirrhosis/viral hepatitis
(c) Affects males and females equally
(d) Higher percentage present with +ve lymph nodes

Ans: (b) Commonly associated with cirrhosis/viral hepatitis

93. All are true of preop biliary stenting *except:*

(a) Indicated when patient is being referred to high volume center and expected delay of surgery more than 1 week
(b) Increased incidence of wound infection

(c) Indicated in resectable pancreatic cancer with cholangitis
(d) Intraabdominal abscess and death rate increased with preop stent

Ans: (c) Indicated in resectable pancreatic cancer with cholangitis

94. Most common lymphoma arising in small intestine:

(a) MALT lymphoma
(b) Peripheral T cell/EATL
(c) Burkitt's lymphoma
(d) Diffuse large B cell lymphoma

Ans: (d) Diffuse large B cell lymphoma

95. All of the following syndromes are associated with adenomatous polyps *except:*

(a) Turcot syndrome
(b) Muir Torre syndrome
(c) Attenuated APC
(d) Bannayan-Ruvalcaba-Riley syndrome

Ans: (d) Bannayan-Ruvalcaba-Riley syndrome

96. All of the following are included in Amsterdam II criteria *except:*

(a) At least 3 relatives with HNPCC associated cancer
(b) Signet ring cell type colorectal cancer before 45 age
(c) FAP should be excluded
(d) Tumors should be verified histopathologically

Ans: (b) Signet ring cell type colorectal cancer before 45 age

97. Not true about CEA in carcinoma colon:

(a) It is useful as screening test
(b) Slight elevation can occur in certain benign diseases
(c) Useful as a prognostic marker in cancer colon
(d) Preoperative value is predictor of survival

Ans: (a) It is useful as screening test

98. In classification of klatskin tumor type II is:

(a) Confined to common hepatic duct
(b) Involve bifurcation without involvement of secondary intrahepatic ducts
(c) Tumours extend into either right/left secondary intrahepatic ducts
(d) Involve secondary hepatic ducts on both sides

Ans: (b) Involve bifurcation without involvement of secondary intrahepatic ducts

99. Regarding pancreatic carcinoma all are true *except:*

(a) 90% are ductal adenocarcinomas
(b) <20% occur in head of gland
(c) Usual presentation is pain, weight loss and obstructive jaundice
(d) Ultrasound has sensitivity of 60–80% in detection of tumors

Ans: (b) <20% occur in head of gland

100. All of the following are paraneoplastic syndromes associated with carcinoma stomach *except:*

(a) Acanthosis nigricans
(b) Cerebellar ataxia
(c) Hypercalcemia
(d) Cushing's syndrome

Ans: (c) Hypercalcemia

101. All of the following are features of foregut carcinoids *except:*

(a) Argentaffin –ve
(b) High 5-HT content
(c) Secrete multiple hormones
(d) Bony metastasis

Ans: (b) High 5-HT content

102. In carcinoid syndrome cardiac manifestation is characterised by:

(a) Left sided lesions are more common
(b) Mainly involve myocardium
(c) Associated with pericardial effusion
(d) Fibrous deposits cause constriction of both tricuspid and pulmonary valves

Ans: (d) Fibrous deposits cause constriction of both tricuspid and pulmonary valves

103. All are true regarding desmoids tumor *except:*

(a) Associated with FAP
(b) High metastatic potential
(c) Can arise at any site in body
(d) Most of them are extra-abdominal

Ans: (b) High metastatic potential

104. True regarding serous cystic neoplasm of pancreas:

(a) High chance of metastatic conversion
(b) More common on pancreatic head
(c) Well demarcated multicystic mass on imaging
(d) High cyst fluid CEA levels

Ans: (b) More common on pancreatic head

105. What is the best treatment of patient with FAP present with approximately 300 colorectal polyps and 15 rectal adenomas?

(a) Observation
(b) Total proctocolectomy with permanent ileostomy
(c) Proctocolectomy with ileal pouch anal anastomosis
(d) Total colectomy with ileorectal anastomosis

Ans: (c) Proctocolectomy with ileal pouch anal anastomosis

106. Germline mutation of which tumor suppressor gene is most frequently associated with hereditary pancreatic cancer?

(a) BRCA 2
(b) PALB 2
(c) K ras
(d) P 53

Ans: (a) BRCA 2

107. Which of the following biochemical abnormality is both a paraneoplastic syndrome associated with HCC and may also be caused by end stage liver failure?

(a) Hypoglycemia
(b) Erythrocytosis
(c) Hyperbilirubinemia
(d) Hypercholesterolemia

Ans: (a) Hypoglycemia

108. Most common site for lymphoma in gastrointestinal tract is:

(a) Stomach
(b) Duodenum
(c) Ileum
(d) Rectum

Ans: (a) Stomach

109. In which of the following location, carcinoid tumor is most common?

(a) Esophagus
(b) Stomach
(c) Small bowel
(d) Appendix

Ans: (c) Small bowel

110. In right radical hemicolectomy for cancer, all of the following vessels are ligated *except:*

(a) Middle colic
(b) Right colic
(c) Ileo colic
(d) Right branch of middle colic

Ans: (a) Middle colic

111. Precancerous condition of carcinoma stomach is:

(a) Peptic ulcer
(b) Gastric atrophy
(c) Achalasia cardia
(d) Curling's ulcer

Ans: (b) Gastric atrophy

112. Most common site for carcinoma stomach is:

(a) Antrum
(b) Fundus
(c) Lesser curvature
(d) Greater curvature

Ans: (a) Antrum

113. True of early gastric carcinoma:

(a) Invasion of mucosa and submucosa with neighbouring lymph node
(b) Invasion of mucosa and submucosa irrespective to lymph node spread
(c) Radical gastrectomy preferred
(d) Endoscopic removal of lesion

Ans: (b) Invasion of mucosa and submucosa irrespective to lymph node spread

114. True about gastric carcinoma are all *except:*

(a) Haematemesis present in majority of patients
(b) H. pylori association present in majority of patients
(c) D2 gastrectomy includes total gastrectomy
(d) Patients after total gastrectomy should be given vitamin B_{12}

Ans: (a) Haematemesis present in majority of patients

115. In squamous cell carcinoma of oesophagus predisposing factors include all *except:*

(a) Tylosis
(b) Smoking
(c) Lye stricture
(d) Reflux oesophagitis

Ans: (d) Reflux oesophagitis

116. True about carcinoma esophagus all *except:*

(a) Most common in middle 1/3rd
(b) Adenocarcinoma is a common variety
(c) Carcinoma develops at achalasia segment
(d) Smoking is a risk factor

Ans: (c) Carcinoma develops at achalasia segment

117. Lynch II syndrome is associated with which of the following carcinoma?

(a) Bone
(b) Colon
(c) Breast
(d) Thyroid

Ans: (b) Colon

118. True about pancreatic carcinoma:

(a) Head is the most common site
(b) Pain is the most common symptom
(c) Obstruction of bile and pancreatic secretion is not common
(d) 80% cases respond well to resection

Ans: (a) Head is the most common site

119. Inverted 3 sign is seen in:

(a) Ampullary carcinoma
(b) Insulinoma
(c) Ca head pancreas
(d) Ca stomach

Ans: (c) Ca head pancreas

120. In which case is anterior resection is the method of treatment?

(a) Ca sigmoid colon
(b) Ca rectum
(c) Ca colon
(d) Ca anal canal

Ans: (b) Ca rectum

121. A 57 years old, obese, white man has symptoms of chronic gastroesophageal reflux disease (GERD). Endoscopic evaluation reveals evidence of Barrett's esophagus with high grade dysplasia. What is the recommended management of this disease?

(a) Repeated endoscopy in 3–5 years
(b) Annual endoscopy
(c) Mucosal resection or endoscopic ablation therapies
(d) Every 3 months screening

Ans: (c) Mucosal resection or endoscopic ablation therapies

122. A 53 years old white man with no family history of colorectal cancer had his first screening colonoscopy. He was found to have a < 1 cm tubular adenoma with low-grade dysplasia. When should he schedule his next colonoscopy?

(a) 1 year
(b) 3 years
(c) 5 years
(d) 10 years

Ans: (c) 5 years

123. What is the 5-year survival rates for patients who undergo curative hepatic resection of colorectal liver metastases?

(a) <5%
(b) 10 to 20%
(c) 30 to 50%
(d) >70%

Ans: (c) 30 to 50%

124. All of the following are known to be strong risk factors for gastric cancer *except:*

(a) Helicobacter pylori infection
(b) Smoking
(c) Alcohol abuse
(d) Previous gastric surgery

Ans: (c) Alcohol abuse

125. Crow's feet refers to:

(a) Subserosal vascular anastomosis in stomach
(b) Lymphatic plexus of stomach
(c) Seen in fundus of stomach
(d) Branches of vagus nerve

Ans: (d) Branches of vagus nerve

126. All are prognostic factors in patients undergoing resection of colorectal liver metastasis *except:*

(a) Stage of primary
(b) Time from primary resection
(c) Location of metastasis
(d) Number of metastasis

Ans: (c) Location of metastasis

127. False Regarding FAP cases causing Duodenal adenoma:

(a) Spigelman stage 4 needs 2 yearly follow up
(b) 5% life time risk of cancer
(c) Spigelman classification helps in surveillance
(d) 4 Stages are there as per classification

Ans: (a) Spigelman stage 4 needs 2 yearly follow up

- Spigelman stage 4 needs to be **considered for surgery**

128. Which benign tumor is DESMIN +ve and Smooth muscle Actin +ve?

(a) Leiomyoma
(b) GIST
(c) Schwannoma
(d) All of the above

Ans: (a) Leiomyoma

Specific Features	Schwannoma	Leiomyoma	GIST
Histology	Moderately cellular Peripheral lymphoid cuff Spindle cells	Eosinophilic cytoplasm	Highly cellular
Markers	S100+, GFAP+	Desmin+, SMA+	CD117+, CD34+

129. False statement regarding Barrett's esophagus is:

(a) 10% of GERD cases develop Barrett's esophagus
(b) It has 40 fold increased risk of Adenocarcinoma
(c) Incidence of Adenocarcinoma is 5% per year in Barrett's esophagus
(d) Intestinal metaplasia occurs

Ans: (c) Incidence of Adenocarcinoma is 5% per year in Barrett's esophagus

- Incidence of malignancy is 1% per year
- 70% are men

TREATMENT

Type	Opinion
No Dysplasia	Follow up 2-3 yearly once
Low Grade Dysplasia	6 monthly interval for 1 year and then annually
High Grade Dysplasia	Unfit–Ablative therapy FIT- Esophagectomy
Early Adenocarcinoma	Esophagectomy

130. False about True wild type of GIST is:

(a) -ve for KIT Mutation
(b) -ve for PDGFRA
(c) Very rare condition
(d) DOG 1 +ve

Ans: (d) DOG 1 +ve

- DOG 1 is more sensitive in diagnosis of GIST. It has no relation to wild type GIST

131. Risk of malignancy in Meckels diverticulum is:

(a) 70 times
(b) 50 times
(c) 30 times
(d) 10 times

Ans: (a) 70 times

- Risk of malignancy in Meckels diverticulum is 70 times
- So it should be resected even though incidentally found

132. Most common tumor in appendix is:

(a) Melanoma
(b) Carcinoid
(c) Mucinous adenocarcinoma
(d) Adenocarcinoma

Ans: (b) Carcinoid

- Most common is Carcinoids

133. Which of the following polyps is not premalignant to Colorectal cancer?

(a) FAP
(b) Hamartomatous polyps of peutz jeghers syndrome
(c) Villous adenoma
(d) Tubular adenoma

Ans: (b) Hamartomatous polyps of Peutz Jeghers syndrome

- Hamartomatous polyps of PJS rarely are premalignant
- Remember that among options it is rare
- PJS can increase risk of cancers like pancreatic, ovary etc

134. Which polyp has maximum malignant potential?

(a) Sessile
(b) Penduculated
(c) Superficial spreading
(d) All of the above

Ans: (a) Sessile

- Sessile > Villous adenoma for malignant potentia

135. Strong correlation of Colorectal cancer is seen in:

(a) Peutz Jeghers syndrome
(b) FAP
(c) Juvenile pulposis
(d) Hyperplastic polyps

Ans: (b) FAP

- Though they form only <1% of all CRC
- Life time risk of CRC is almost 100%

136. Factor associated with CRC include:

(a) High fiber
(b) Low fiber
(c) Smoked fish
(d) Japanese race

Ans: (b) Low fiber

137. Amsterdam criteria includes all *except:*

(a) Atleast 3 relatives should be affected
(b) 2 successive generations affected
(c) All 3 should be 1st degree relatives
(d) FAP excluded

Ans: (c) All 3 should be 1st degree relatives

138. Colonic metastasis is most commonly related to:

(a) Depth of invasion
(b) Pre op CEA level
(c) Tumor size
(d) Circumferential involvement

Ans: (a) Depth of invasion

139. False about malignancy in Ulcerative colitis is:

(a) Poorly differentiated and higher stage
(b) Related to extent and duration of disease
(c) Poor prognosis as compared to sporadic at equal stage
(d) Evenly distributed

Ans: (c) Poor prognosis as compared to sporadic at equal stage

140. After undergoing surgery for carcinoma colon, a patient developed single liver metastasis of 2 cm. What is the best next step?

(a) RFA
(b) Chemoradiation
(c) Acetic acid injection
(d) Resection

Ans: (d) Resection

141. Ramu, a 60-year-old patient with Carcinoma descending colon presents with Acute intestinal obstruction. Patient is stable with BP-110/80. In Emergency department, treatment of choice is:

(a) Defunctioning transverse colostomy
(b) Hartman's procedure
(c) Total colectomy
(d) Left colectomy

Ans: (b) Hartman's procedure

142. Most common cause of disease related death in Crohn's disease is:

(a) Sepsis
(b) Cancer
(c) Bleeding
(d) Obstruction

Ans: (b) Cancer

- GI cancer is the most leading cause of disease related death in patients with Crohn's disease
- Long term survival studies suggested that Crohn's patients have death rate approximately 2-3 times higher than general population due to chronic wound complication and Sepsis

143. Cell of origin in GIST:

(a) Interstitial cells of Cajal
(b) Argentaffin cells
(c) Smooth muscle cells
(d) Epithelial cells

Ans: (a) Interstitial cells of Cajal

144. The following are true about GIST *except:*

(a) Cell of origin Inetrstitial cell of Cajal is found in myenteric plexus
(b) Very low incidence
(c) Predominant in male
(d) Does not occur in young children

Ans: (d) Does not occur in young children

145. Most common site of GIST:

(a) Esophagus
(b) Stomach
(c) Small intestine
(d) Colon

Ans: (b) Stomach

146. False about GIST is:

(a) Stomach is the most common site
(b) Can present with bleeding
(c) Commonly metastasize to lymph nodes
(d) Can present with peritoneal metastasis

Ans: (c) Commonly metastasize to lymph nodes

147. True about GIST all *except:*

(a) Most common in duodenum
(b) Necrosis and ulceration present
(c) PET is used to assess response to therapy
(d) Well circumscribed

Ans: (a) Most common in duodenum

148. All are mutations found in GIST *except:*

(a) KIT
(b) PDGFRA
(c) CD 117
(d) None of the above

Ans: (c) CD 117

149. SDH related tumors are:

(a) WT positive
(b) Carney's triad associated
(c) CD 117 negative
(d) All of the above

Ans: (d) All of the above

150. Wild type GIST– false statement:

(a) Negative for KIT mutation
(b) Negative for PGDFRA
(c) Rare
(d) DOG -1 positive

Ans: (d) DOG -1 positive

151. Most common symptomatic benign neoplasm of small bowel is:

(a) Adenoma
(b) GIST
(c) Lymphangioma
(d) Hemangoima

Ans: (b) GIST

152. Most common stomach tumor which bleeds:

(a) Adenocarcinoma
(b) SCC
(c) Leiomyosarcoma
(d) Fibrosarcoma

Ans: (c) Leiomyosarcoma

153. All are true about GIST *except:*

(a) Epitheloid and spindle cell variant
(b) Types have no clinical implication
(c) Mitosis is the most important prognostic factor
(d) Histopathology can predict metastatic potential

Ans: (d) Histopathology can predict metastatic potential

154. All are included in risk stratification *except:*

(a) Site
(b) Mitosis
(c) Size
(d) Stage

Ans: (d) Stage

155. All are imatinib resistant GIST *except:*

(a) WT GIST
(b) PDGFRA mutation in exon 18D842V
(c) KIT Mutation in Exon 9
(d) Secondary resistance

Ans: (c) KIT Mutation in Exon 9

156. A 35 years female underwent laparoscopic cholecystectomy and HPE revealed gallbladder cancer with tumor extension into perimuscular connective tissue. What is the next ideal management?

(a) Excision of port sites
(b) Wedge resection of liver, nodal dissection and resection of port sites
(c) Resection of Segment IV B and V, nodal dissection and resection of port sites
(d) Resection of segment IVB and V, nodal dissection

Ans: (b) Wedge resection of liver, nodal dissection and resection of port sites

157. Sunburst calcification is seen in:

(a) Serous cystadenoma of pancreas
(b) Mucinous cystadenoma of pancreas
(c) IPMN
(d) Solid pseudopapillary tumor

Ans: (a) Serous cystadenoma of pancreas

158. Mucinous cystic neoplasm of pancreas, false statement is:

(a) Less amylase in fluid
(b) Staining for ER and PR receptors positivity
(c) Enucleation is the treatment of choice
(d) It is the most common cystic neoplasm of pancreas

Ans: (c) Enucleation is the treatment of choice

159. First gene to be involved in developing pancreatic adenocarcinoma is:

(a) KRAS
(b) CDKN2A
(c) p53
(d) DPC4

Ans: (a) KRAS

160. Medial survival of patients who undergo surgery for pancreatic cancer is:

(a) 11 months
(b) 22 months
(c) 6 months
(d) 16 months

Ans: (b) 22 months

161. Most common complication following Whipple procedure is:

(a) Pancreatic fistula
(b) Wound infection
(c) Delayed gastric emptying
(d) Bile leak

Ans: (c) Delayed gastric emptying

162. Carcinoma gallbladder risk factors all *except:*

(a) Porcelain gallbladder
(b) Primary sclerosing cholangitis
(c) Choledochal cyst
(d) Multiple, more than 2 cm calculi in GB

Ans: (d) Multiple, more than 2 cm calculi in GB

163. Most common site for insulinoma:

(a) Tail
(b) Body
(c) Head
(d) Equally distributed

Ans: (d) Equally distributed

164. Which of the following form does not form by Gastrinoma triangle?

(a) Pylorus
(b) Junction of neck and body
(c) Cystic duct
(d) Duodenum 2nd and 3rd part

Ans: (a) Pylorus

165. Double duct sign seen in:

(a) Periampullary Carcinoma
(b) Chronic pancreatitis
(c) Cholangiocarcinoma
(d) Carcinoma Gallbladder

Ans: (a) Periampullary Carcinoma

166. Risk factor for cholangiocarcinoma:

(a) Liver fluke
(b) Hydatid disease
(c) OCP
(d) Anabolic Steroids

Ans: (a) Liver fluke

167. Aflatoxin is a carcinogen for which cancer?

(a) Hepatocellular carcinoma
(b) Mesothelioma
(c) Lung Cancer
(d) Pancreatic Cancer

Ans: (a) Hepatocellular carcinoma

PART 2

168. Which is not a risk factor for Gallbladder cancer:

(a) Mirrizi syndrome
(b) APBJ
(c) High fat diet
(d) Choledochal cyst

Ans: (c) High fat diet

169. Which of the following type of gallstones is commonly found in GBC patients?

(a) Large cholesterol stones
(b) Large Black pigment stones
(c) Large Brown pigment stones
(d) Large calcium stones

Ans: (a) Large cholesterol stones

- Type of stone doesn't correlate with increase in incidence of cancer
- ***But it was found incidentally that*** Large cholesterol stones ***is commonly found in GBC patients***

DON'T GET CONFUSED

170. Most common site of GBC is:

(a) Body
(b) Fundus
(c) Cystic duct
(d) Infundibulum

Ans: (c) Cystic duct

171. Which of the following tumor marker is more specific for GBC?

(a) CA 19-9
(b) CEA
(c) PIVKA
(d) CA 72-2

Ans: (b) CEA

- *CEA Elevation >4 ng/mL (50% sensitive and 93% specific)*
- *CA 19-9 Elevation >20 U/mL (79% Sensitive and 79% Specific)*

172. Incidence of gallstones in patients with Gallbladder cancer is:

(a) 10-20%
(b) 30-40%
(c) 50-60%
(d) 60-90%

Ans: (d) 60-90%

173. Which of the following statement is false regarding lymph node involvement of carcinoma gallbladder?

(a) > 10 mm ring like node in CT is considered positive
(b) Only 38% nodes are identified in CT
(c) Enlarged lymph nodes are most often metastatic
(d) Positive aortocaval lymph node is considered inoperable

Ans: (c) Enlarged lymph nodes are most often metastatic

- Enlarged lymph nodes are most often inflammatory
- N2 = M1
- Nodal metastasis outside hepatoduodenal ligament has same prognosis as distant metastatic disease

174. Which of the following is not a component of Extended cholecystectomy?

(a) Cholecystectomy + en bloc resection of segments IVB and V
(b) Inter aortocaval nodal frozen

(c) Hepatoduodenal lymphadenectomy

(d) Bile duct excision

Ans: (d) Bile duct excision

Bile duct excison if:

- Prior scarring of porta
- Infundibular tumor extending into porta
- Cystic duct margin positive
- Very obese patients

175. Subserosal plane of dissection during cholecystectomy is not violated by which of the following tumor?

(a) T3
(b) T4
(c) T2
(d) T1b

Ans: (d) T1b

- The likelihood of N1 disease is vanishingly small for patients with T1 tumors
- For this reason, simple cholecystectomy should be curative for patients with pathologically confirmed stage I disease
- Only situation when reoperation is required is – cystic duct margin positive

176. Standard treatment option for patients with T2 disease is:

(a) Open Cholecystectomy
(b) Laparoscopic Cholecystectomy
(c) Extended Cholecystectomy + Portal Lymphadenectomy
(d) Extended Cholecystectomy + Bile duct excision

Ans: (c) Extended Cholecystectomy + Portal Lymphadenectomy

- Subserosal plane of dissection violate T2 tumors
- T2 tumors resected by simple cholecystectomy have a 40% to 50% margin positivity
- Nodal metastases in T2 tumors – 50%
- For these reasons, extended cholecystectomy with portal lymphadenectomy is the procedure of choice for patients with stage II disease

177. Resection of Port site recurrence is beneficial in:

(a) Providing oncologic clearance
(b) Prevent pain and local cutaneous complications
(c) Improving survival
(d) Reduce mortality

Ans: (b) Prevent pain and local cutaneous complications

178. A radiographically suspicious gallbladder polyp includes all *except:*

(a) > 1cm
(b) Musocal invasion
(c) > 3 polyps
(d) Sessile polyps

Ans: (c) > 3 polyps

- Multiple polyps are usually cholesterol polyps and are not associated with malignancy
- **Sonography findings suspicious of malignancy include:**
  - Size greater than 1 cm
  - Polyp number less than 3
  - Sessile polyps
  - Polyps with evidence of possible gallbladder mucosal invasion

179. True statement about GBC is:

(a) GBC is associated with APBJ is common in females
(b) Majority of GBC follow adenoma carcinoma sequence
(c) Type 1 porcelian GB is a risk factor for GBC
(d) Active Typhoid infection is a risk factor for GBC

Ans: (d) Active Typhoid infection is a risk factor for GBC

- **Typhoid carrier is an important risk factor**
- *Patients with APBJ get cancer at a younger age than patients with sporadic GBC. Children with APBJ frequently have epithelial hyperplasia of the gallbladder*

180. A 40-year-old female underwent lap cholecystectomy for suspected gallstone disease. Final histopathology turned out to be GBC with invasion of muscularis propria. Cystic duct margin and cystic lymph node are –ve. Current recommended management is:

(a) No further surgery only observation
(b) Only segment 4b, 5 resection since cystic duct lymph node is –ve
(c) Segment 4b, 5 resection with radical lymphadenectomy and without CBD excision since cystic duct margin is –ve
(d) Segment 4b, 5 resection with radical lymphadenectomy and with CBD excision

Ans: (c) Segment 4b, 5 resection with radical lymphadenectomy and without CBD excision since cystic duct margin is –ve

181. All are true statements regarding GBC *except:*

(a) Port site recurrence can rarely occur as sole site of disease
(b) Lymph node +ve disease is associated with poor survival
(c) Jaundice is an indicator of unresectability
(d) Combination chemotherapy with Gemcitabine and Oxaliplatin is useful in adjuvant setting

Ans: (c) Jaundice is an indicator of unresectability

182. All of the following are risk factors for CA GB *except:*

(a) Gallstones
(b) Adenomyomatosis
(c) Porcelain gallbladder
(d) Choledochal cyst

Ans: (b) Adenomyomatosis

183. Risk factors associated with malignancy in GB polyp are all *except:*

(a) Age > 60 years
(b) Co-existence of gallstones
(c) Size > 5 mm
(d) Documented increase in size

Ans: (c) Size > 5 mm

184. Risk factors for malignant change in an asymptomatic patient with a gallbladder polyp on ultrasound include all of the following, *except:*

(a) Age > 60 years
(b) Rapid increase in size of polyp
(c) Size of polyp > 5 mm
(d) Associated gallstones

Ans: (c) Size of polyp > 5 mm

185. True about CA GB and gallstones:

(a) 3% association
(b) 30% association
(c) 50% association
(d) 90% association

Ans: (d) 90% association

186. Precancerous lesions of GB are all *except:*

(a) Porcelain GB
(b) Typhoid carrier
(c) ABPDJ
(d) Biliary ascariasis

Ans: (d) Biliary ascariasis

187. Organism associated with fish consumption and also causes carcinoma gallbladder:

(a) Gnathostoma
(b) Anglostrongyloidosis cantonensis
(c) Clonorchis sinensis
(d) H. dimunata

Ans: (c) Clonorchis sinensis

188. All are risk factors for CA GB *except:*

(a) Adenomyosis
(b) ABPDJ
(c) Gallstones
(d) Adenomatous polyps

Ans: (a) Adenomyosis

189. All of the following are risk factors for carcinoma gallbladder, *except:*

(a) Typhoid carriers
(b) Clonorchis
(c) Choledochal cyst
(d) Oral contraceptives

Ans: (d) Oral contraceptives

190. Precancerous lesion of gallbladder is:

(a) Porcelain gallbladder
(b) Mirizzi's syndrome
(c) Cholesterosis
(d) Acalculous Cholecystitis

Ans: A > B

191. In a male after laparoscopic cholecystectomy, specimen is sent for histopathology which shows carcinoma gallbladder stage T1a. Appropriate management is:

(a) Conservative and follow up
(b) Extended cholecystectomy
(c) Excision of all port sites
(d) Radiotherapy

Ans: (a) Conservative and follow up

192. After laparoscopic cholecystectomy, if biopsy reveals in situ cancer of gallbladder (Stage I), then the appropriate management is:

(a) Follow-up
(b) Extended cholecystectomy
(c) Excision of all port sites
(d) Radiotherapy

Ans: (a) Follow-up

193. Survival in unresectable GB carcinoma is:

(a) 4–6 months
(b) 8–10 months
(c) 1 year
(d) 12–24 months

Ans: (a) 4–6 months

194. T2N1 of CA GB represents which stage:

(a) IA
(b) IB
(c) II
(d) III

Ans: (d) III

195. True about CA GB:

(a) T1a can be treated and cured by laparoscopic cholecystectomy
(b) T1b needs radical operation in all cases
(c) Port site metastasis is localized disease
(d) Pre-operative diagnosis of CA GB has different survival according to stage

Ans: (a) T1a can be treated and cured by laparoscopic cholecystectomy

196. Most common gallbladder malignancy is:

(a) Adenocarcinoma
(b) Squamous cell carcinoma
(c) Mucinous cystadenocarcinoma
(d) Serous cystadenocarcinoma

Ans: (a) Adenocarcinoma

197. All are true about CA GB *except:*

(a) Redo surgery is radical or extended cholecystectomy increases significant survival advantage
(b) Inter-aortocaval node involvement potentially rule out cure
(c) <25% 5 years survival for all stages
(d) Pancreaticoduodenectomy has 5 years survival of 25%

Ans: (d) Pancreaticoduodenectomy has 5 years survival of 25%

198. Best prognosis in CA GB is seen in:

(a) Papillary
(b) Schirrhous
(c) Nodular
(d) Any of the above

Ans: (a) Papillary

199. Laparoscopic cholecystectomy was done, on histopathology, stage was T2. Next line of treatment:

(a) Observation
(b) Extended cholecystectomy
(c) Radiotherapy
(d) Chemotherapy

Ans: (b) Extended cholecystectomy

200. Most Common type of carcinoma gallbladder with gallstones is:

(a) Adenocarcinoma
(b) Anaplastic carcinoma
(c) Squamous cell carcinoma
(d) Transitional cell carcinoma

Ans: (a) Adenocarcinoma

201. A 40-year-old woman has undergone a cholecystectomy. Histopathology reveals that she has a 3 cm adenocarcinoma in the body of the gallbladder infiltrating up to the serosa. Which of the following further management would you advise her:

(a) Chemotherapy
(b) Radiotherapy
(c) Radical cholecystectomy
(d) Follow up with regular ultrasound examinations

Ans: (c) Radical cholecystectomy

202. Most Common association seen in carcinoma gallbladder:

(a) Peritoneal deposits
(b) Duodenal infiltration
(c) Secondaries to liver
(d) Cystic node involvement

Ans: (c) Secondaries to liver

203. Most common type of cancer gallbladder in a patient with gallstone:

(a) Adenocarcinoma
(b) Squamous carcinoma
(c) Sarcoma
(d) Melanoma

Ans: (a) Adenocarcinoma

204. In a male after laparoscopic cholecystectomy, specimen is sent for histopathology which shows carcinoma gallbladder stage IB. Appropriate management is:

(a) Conservative and follow up
(b) Extended cholecystectomy
(c) Excision of all port sites
(d) Radiotherapy

Ans: (b) Extended cholecystectomy

205. All of the following are false for carcinoma gallbladder *except:*

(a) Carries a good prognosis
(b) Gallstones may be a predisposing factor
(c) Commonly squamous cell carcinoma
(d) Jaundice is rare

Ans: (b) Gallstones may be a predisposing factor

206. Gallbladder carcinoma is M1 stage when which of the following lymph nodes are involved:

(a) Superior mesenteric lymph nodes
(b) Aortic lymph nodes
(c) Celiac lymph nodes
(d) Pancreato-duodenal lymph nodes

Ans: (b) Aortic lymph nodes

207. Ideal preferred treatment for carcinoma of the gallbladder in majority is:

(a) Radical resection that includes gallbladder in continuity with the right hepatic lobe and regional lymph node dissection
(b) Radiation therapy
(c) Chemotherapy
(d) Palliative

Ans: (d) Palliative

208. A 70-year-old man presents to an emergency department with a history of recent weight loss and persistent right upper quadrant pain. CT scan reveals a gallbladder stone and thickening of the anterior wall of the gallbladder. He undergoes a laparoscopic cholecystectomy. Pathology reveals a moderately differentiated 2 cm gallbladder adenocarcinoma invading perimuscular connective tissue. Margins of resection are negative for tumor. A follow-up CT scan 2 weeks after surgery shows mild periportal fullness.What would be the best approach at this time?

(a) Perform en bloc resection of the gallbladder, resection of segments IVb and V of the liver, and regional lymph node dissection
(b) No further therapy is warranted; surveillance with CT scans and lab tests every 3 months
(c) Requires second laparotomy to assess extent of remaining disease to guide further therapy
(d) Perform USG guided biopsy of periportal nodes; if positive, then fluoropyrimidine-based chemoradiation is indicated

Ans: (a) Perform en bloc resection of the gallbladder, resection of segments IVb and V of the liver, and regional lymph node dissection

209. A 55-year-old white female undergoes a laparoscopic cholecystectomy for symptomatic cholelithiasis. Operation went well, and patient was discharged home. One week later, she comes to your office for a routine postoperative follow-up. Final pathology report shows an incidental finding of a gallbladder carcinoma confined to the mucosa. In further advising patient, you should inform her that:

(a) She should undergo radiation therapy
(b) She should undergo right hepatectomy to remove locally infiltrating disease
(c) She should undergo regional lymphadenectomy
(d) She does not require any further therapy

Ans: (d) She does not require any further therapy

210. True about GBC is:

(a) Speckled cholesterol deposits are found on GB wall
(b) Thickened nodules of mucosa and muscle
(c) More likely accompanied by larger stone
(d) More common in males

Ans: (c) More likely accompanied by larger stone

211. After lap cholecystectomy foci of carcinoma that invades but doesn't penetrate through lamina propria is found on HPE. Further management will be:

(a) Lap resection of GB fossa
(b) Open extended chole (Segment 4b and 5+LN)
(c) Observation
(d) CBD excision

Ans: (c) Observation

212. CA 19-9 is useful marker for:

(a) Ca gallbladder
(b) Ca ovary
(c) HCC
(d) Choriocarcinoma

Ans: (a) Ca gallbladder

213. Prophylactic cholecystectomy is indicated in all except:

(a) Patient with pancreaticobiliary maljunction
(b) Northern Indian women
(c) Porcelain gallbladder
(d) Asymptomatic documented cholelithiasis

Ans: (d) Asymptomatic documented cholelithiasis

- Patients with pancreaticobiliary maljunction and a normal-size bile duct may benefit from prophylactic cholecystectomy and northern Indian women may also benefit

214. Indication for resection of CBD in CA gallbladder are all *except:*

(a) Tumor in GB neck
(b) Porcelain gallbladder
(c) Suspicious of mucosal spread of CBD
(d) Scarring causing compromised in skeletonization of porta hepatis

Ans: (b) Porcelain gallbladder

- *If the tumor is in the gallbladder neck and there is suspicion of mucosal spread into the common bile duct, or if inflammation and scarring compromise adequate skeletonization of the porta hepatis, then resection of the common bile duct with Roux-en-Y hepaticojejunostomy should be performed*

215. Tumor invasion of main portal vein/hepatic artery in gallbladder makes T status in TNM staging to:

(a) T4
(b) T3
(c) T2
(d) T1

Ans: (a) T4

216. Extended cholecystectomy involves excision of hepatic segments:

(a) V and IVa
(b) V and IVb
(c) VI and IVa
(d) VI and IVb

Ans: (b) V and IVb

217. Risk factors for malignant change in asymptomatic patient with gallbladder polyp on USG include all *except:*

(a) Age > 60 years
(b) Rapid increase in size
(c) Size > 5 mm
(d) Associated gallstones

Ans: (c) Size > 5 mm

218. Not a risk factor for gallbladder cancer:

(a) Gallstones
(b) Choledochal cyst
(c) Cholesterosis
(d) Estrogen

Ans: (c) Cholesterosis

219. Least common site of occurrence of cholangiocarcinoma is:

(a) Multifocal (b) Hilum

(c) Distal CBD (d) Intrahepatic bile duct

Ans: (a) Multifocal

Anatomic Site of Occurrence

- 40% to 60% develop in the hilum (hereafter referred to as hilar cholangiocarcinomas)
- 20% to 30% in the distal lower biliary tract (distal cholangiocarcinomas)
- 10% arise intrahepatically (the so-called peripheral or intrahepatic cholangiocarcinomas)
- Less than 10% develop in a diffuse or multifocal manner

220. Level of bilirubin consistent with diagnosis of malignant biliary obstruction is:

(a) 4 mg/dl (b) 6 mg /dl

(c) 8 mg/dl (d) 10 mg/dl

Ans: (d) 10 mg/dl

- Benign causes of obstructive jaundice typically produce bilirubin levels ranging from 2 to 4 mg/dL (rarely exceeding 15 mg/dL)
- ***Biliary obstruction from cholangiocarcinoma usually results in serum bilirubin levels greater than 10 mg/dL (with a mean level of approximately 18 mg/dL)***
- 30% rate of bactibilia has been observed among patients with extrahepatic cholangiocarcinoma

221. Which of the following modality is useful for evaluation of suspicious malignancy of the distal CBD?

(a) PTBD (b) PTC

(c) EUS (d) ERCP

Ans: (c) EUS

- Can visualise lesion less than 3 mm
- EUS guided biposy can be taken
- EUS guided biliary decompression for failed ERCP stenting
- Diagnostic test of choice is ERCP for distal bile duct tumors

222. Which of the following is not a criteria for unresectability of hilar cholangiocarcinoma?

(a) Portal hypertension (b) Main portal vein involvement

(c) N2 disease (d) Lobar atrophy with Ipsilateral portal vein involvement

Ans: (d) Lobar atrophy with Ipsilateral portal vein involvement

Criteria for Unresectability for Cholangiocarcinoma

- Medical contraindication to surgical intervention
- Advanced cirrhosis/portal hypertension
- Bilateral second-order biliary
- Main portal vein involvement
- Lobar atrophy with contralateral second-order biliary radical involvement
- Lobar atrophy with contralateral portal vein involvement
- N2 nodal involvement
- Distant metastases

223. Which of the following is a important factor determining survival in patient undergoing surgery for hilar cholangiocarcinoma?

(a) Longituidinal tumor extend (b) Lymph node involvement

(c) Positive surgical margin (d) Partial hepatectomy

Ans: (b) Lymph node involvement

- Predictors of improved survival
  - Well-differentiated tumors
  - Negative resection margin
  - Performance of a concomitant hepatic resection
- Patients with histologically positive margins of resection demonstrated survival outcomes indistinguishable from those with locally advanced tumors undergoing operative exploration without attempted resection
- 5-year actuarial survival partial hepatectomy was 37%, compared with 0% with bile duct excision alone

224. Which of the following is not an acceptable surgical procedure for the management of Extrahepatic cholangiocarcinoma?

(a) Hepatectomy (b) Whipple's pancreaticoduodenectomy

(c) Orthotopic liver transplantation (d) Excision of extra hepatic biliary apparatus

Ans: (d) Excision of extra hepatic biliary apparatus

225. All are true regarding Hilar cholangiocarcinoma *except:*

(a) Complete caudate lobe resection is required only in left sided hilar cholangiocarcinoma

(b) Limited involvement of main portal vein is not a contraindication of resection

(c) Local resection is associated with inferior survival compared to en bloc hepatectomy

(d) Histologically proven metastasis beyond hepatoduodenal ligament is considered as Distant metastasis

Ans: (a) Complete caudate lobe resection is required only in left sided hilar cholangiocarcinoma

226. Risk factor for developing cholangiocarcinoma is:

(a) PSC (b) Clonorchis

(c) Chronic portal bacteremia and portal phlebitis (d) All of the above

Ans: (d) All of the above

227. A 66-year-old man is noted to have painless jaundice on a routine follow up. Work up reveals biliary obstruction at the hilum. ERCP confirms a high-grade stricture predominantly involving left hepatic duct. Brushings reveal atypical cells and no malignancy. He is offered surgical management, an en bloc resection of left hepatic lobe and extrahepatic bile duct and complete periportal lymphadenectomy. Which is true about management of this patient with hilar cholangiocarcinoma?

(a) Surgical resection is associated with an operative mortality rate of 30%

(b) Recurrences occur most commonly at bed of resection followed by retroperitoneal nodes

(c) Less than 10% of patients have resectable cancer at the time of diagnosis

(d) Distant metastases occur in two third of cases

Ans: (b) Recurrences occur most commonly at bed of resection followed by retroperitoneal nodes

228. Which of the following statements about adjuvant therapy for biliary cancers is true?

(a) No clear evidence appears patients treated in the adjuvant setting have median survival of approximately 2 years

(b) Adjuvant radiation is superior to chemotherapy alone

(c) Adjuvant therapy can improve overall survival for patients with R0 resections

(d) Fluoropyrimidine-based chemoradiation is standard because it is superior to radiation alone

Ans: (a) No clear evidence appears patients treated in the adjuvant setting have median survival of approximately 2 years

229. A 67-year-old woman is evaluated for obstructive jaundice. Cholangiographic findings indicate cancer of the lower end of the CBD. Clinical examination would most likely reveal which of the following?

(a) Enlarged gallbladder
(b) Shrunken gallbladder
(c) Enlarged pancreas
(d) Shrunken pancreas

Ans: (a) Enlarged gallbladder

230. A 57-year-old previously healthy business executive presents with gradually increasing obstructive jaundice. An ultrasound of the liver shows dilated intrahepatic ducts, but CBD is normal. An ERCP shows a filling defect at level of the common hepatic duct. Endoscopic brush biopsies are taken, and histology confirms cholangiocarcinoma. In discussing these findings, the surgeon should inform the patient that:

(a) Affects men more commonly than women
(b) Tumor is a result of gallstones
(c) Tumor is best treated with a stent to relieve obstructive jaundice
(d) Weight loss is common in this condition

Ans: (a) Affects men more commonly than women

231. Best management of Localized Klatskin tumors is:

(a) Pancreaticoduodenectomy
(b) Resect entire extrahepatic biliary tree with hepatic resection if necessary
(c) Resect middle third of biliary tree with Hepaticojejunostomy
(d) Chemoradiation

Ans: (b) Resect entire extrahepatic biliary tree with hepatic resection if necessary

232. True regarding Cholangiocarcinoma is:

(a) Majority are Intrahepatic
(b) Type 1 cholangiocarcinoma lies above confluence of right and left hepatic ducts
(c) Most patients benefit from adjuvant chemoradiation after surgery
(d) Resection with enteric biliary bypass is considered appropriate in patients with early disease

Ans: (d) Resection with enteric biliary bypass is considered appropriate in patients with early disease

233. Contraindication to resection of adenocarcinoma of bile duct is:

(a) Tumor location in distal CBD
(b) Tumor location at bifurcation of bile duct
(c) Invasion of right and left portal vein
(d) Invasion of right portal vein and right hepatic artery

Ans: (c) Invasion of right and left portal vein

234. Appropriate treatment for a cholangiocarcinoma of the hepatic bifurcation?

(a) Right hepatic lobectomy
(b) Left hepatic lobectomy
(c) Pancreaticoduodenectomy (Whipple)
(d) Bile duct resection and hepaticojejunostomy plus partial hepatectomy

Ans: (d) Bile duct resection and hepaticojejunostomy plus partial hepatectomy

235. Non-resectability criteria in hilar cholangiocarcinoma are all *except:*

(a) Involvement of secondary biliary radicals bilaterally
(b) Metastasis to celiac nodes
(c) Involvement of right branch of portal vein
(d) Contralateral involvement of bile duct

Ans: (c) Involvement of right branch of portal vein

236. Type II cholangiocarcinoma involve:

(a) Division of both ducts and not extending outside (b) Common hepatic duct only

(c) Secondary hepatic duct (d) Extending beyond hilum

Ans: (a) Division of both ducts and not extending outside

237. All are true about prognosis of cholangiocarcinoma *except:*

(a) Scirrhous type has better prognosis than papillary

(b) Major prognostic factors are margin status and tumor stage

(c) Bile duct resection alone is associated with high chances of recurrence

(d) Curative resection includes hepatic resection + bile duct resection + lymphadenectomy

Ans: (a) Scirrhous type has better prognosis than papillary

238. Klatskin tumor is:

(a) Merkel cell carcinoma of skin (b) Primitive neuroectodermal tumor of chest wall

(c) Common hepatic duct tumor (d) Adenocarcinoma of anal canal

Ans: (c) Common hepatic duct tumor

239. Most common site of cholangiocarcinoma:

(a) Distal biliary duct (b) Hilum

(c) Intrahepatic duct (d) Multifocal

Ans: (b) Hilum

240. Cholangiocarcinoma histologically resembles:

(a) Squamous cell type (b) Colloid cell type

(c) Schirrhous type (d) Columnar cell type

Ans: (c) Schirrhous type

241. All are criteria of non-resectability in patients with hilar cholangiocarcinoma *except:*

(a) Hepatic duct involvement upto secondary radicals bilaterally

(b) Encasement or occlusion of main portal vein proximal to its bifurcation

(c) Atrophy of one lobe with encasement of contralateral portal vein branch

(d) Atrophy of one lobe with ipsilateral involvement of secondary biliary radicals

Ans: (d) Atrophy of one lobe with ipsilateral involvement of secondary biliary radicals

242. Contraindication of resection in cholangiocarcinoma are all *except:*

(a) Involvement of main trunk of portal vein (b) Hepatic atrophy with contralateral bile duct encasement

(c) Hepatic atrophy with contralateral portal vein encasement (d) Hepatic atrophy with ipsilateral bile duct involvement

Ans: (d) Hepatic atrophy with ipsilateral bile duct involvement

243. ERCP is indicated for the following *except:*

(a) Distal CBD tumor (b) Hepatic porta tumor

(c) Proximal cholangiocarcinoma (d) Gallstone pancreatitis

Ans: (c) Proximal cholangiocarcinoma

244. Not a risk factor for cholangiocarcinoma is:

(a) Thorotrast (b) Radon

(c) Dioxin (d) Aflatoxin

Ans: (d) Aflatoxin

245. Not a predisposing factor for cholangiocarcinoma:

(a) Asiatic cholangio-hepatitis (b) Cholelithiasis

(c) Ulcerative colitis (d) Choledochal cyst

Ans: (b) Cholelithiasis

246. APBDJ is associated with:

(a) Cholangiocarcinoma (b) Carcinoma GB

(c) Choledochal cyst (d) All of the above

Ans: (d) All of the above

247. Predisposing factor for cholangiocarcinoma is:

(a) PSC (b) Gallstones

(c) Ankylostomiasis (d) All of the above

Ans: (a) PSC

248. Cholangiocarcinoma has been associated with infection by:

(a) Paragonimus westermani (b) Clonorchis sinensis

(c) Loa Loa (d) Schistosoma haematobium

Ans: (b) Clonorchis sinensis

249. Which of the following does not predispose to cholangiocarcinoma?

(a) Ulcerative colitis (b) Clonorchis sinensis

(c) Choledochal cyst (d) Chronic pancreatitis

Ans: (d) Chronic pancreatitis

250. All of the following are known predisposing factors for cholangiocarcinoma *except:*

(a) Stones in gallbladder (b) Clonorchis sinensis

(c) Ulcerative colitis (d) Primary sclerosing cholangitis

Ans: (a) Stones in gallbladder

251. An increased incidence of cholangiocarcinoma is seen in all of the following except:

(a) Hydatid cyst of liver (b) Polycystic disease of liver

(c) Sclerosing cholangitis (d) Liver flukes

Ans: (a) Hydatid cyst of liver

252. All the following increase risk for cholangiocarcinoma *except:*

(a) Ulcerative colitis (b) Cholelithiasis

(c) Sclerosing cholangitis (d) Clonorchis

Ans: (b) Cholelithiasis

253. Bismuth classification is used for:

(a) Carcinoma GE junction (b) Hilar cholangiocarcinoma

(c) Carcinoma rectosigmoid (d) Distal pancreatic tumors

Ans: (b) Hilar cholangiocarcinoma

254. Carcinoid syndrome produces valvular disease primarily involving:

(a) Tricuspid valves (b) Pulmonary valves

(c) Mitral valves (d) Aortic valves

Ans: (a) Tricuspid valves

255. In which of the following carcinoid tumor is most common?

(a) Esophagus (b) Stomach

(c) Small bowel (d) Appendix

Ans: (c) Small bowel

256. Carcinoid tumor is most common in:

(a) Esophagus (b) Stomach

(c) Jejunum (d) Appendix

Ans: (d) Appendix

257. Kalloo, 25-year-old presented with mass in right iliac fossa. On laparotomy it was found to be carcinoid 2.5 cm in diameter. What is the next step in management?

(a) Segmental resection (b) Right hemicolectomy

(c) Appendicectomy (d) Yearly 5 HIAA

Ans: (b) Right hemicolectomy

258. Which site of carcinoid is least potential for malignancy?

(a) Lung (b) Stomach

(c) Small intestine (d) Appendix

Ans: (a) Lung

259. Most common neoplasm of appendix is:

(a) Carcinoid (b) Adenocarcinoma

(c) Lymphoma (d) Sarcoma

Ans: (a) Carcinoid

260. Most common site of carcinoid syndrome is:

(a) Bronchus (b) Adrenal

(c) Small intestine (d) Appendix

Ans: (c) Small intestine

261. Carcinoid tumors secrete all of the following *except:*

(a) Histamine (b) 5-hydroxytryptamine

(c) Bradykinin (d) 5-hydroxytryptophan

Ans: (c) Bradykinin

262. Carcinoid syndrome is associated with all *except:*

(a) Pellagra (b) Flushing

(c) Bronchospasm (d) Urine VMA

Ans: (d) Urine VMA

263. Most common site of carcinoid is:

(a) Appendix (b) Liver

(c) Stomach (d) Rectum

Ans: (d) Rectum

264. Least common valvular disease in carcinoids:

(a) TS
(b) PS
(c) TR
(d) PR

Ans: (d) PR

265. All of the following about carcinoids are true *except:*

(a) Most common malignant tumor of small intestine
(b) Extensive involvement of small intestine is associated with higher probability of lung metastasis
(c) 5-year survival for carcinoids is >60%
(d) Appendiceal carcinoids are more common in females

Ans: (b) Extensive involvement of small intestine is associated with higher probability of lung metastasis

266. Which of the following is true about small bowel carcinoids?

(a) Small bowel and appendix accounts for almost 60% of all GI carcinoids
(b) Rectum spared
(c) 5-year survival for carcinoids is >60%
(d) Appendiceal carcinoids are more common in females than males

Ans: (b) Rectum spared

267. All are seen in carcinoids *except:*

(a) Diarrhea
(b) Constipation
(c) Liver metastasis
(d) 5HT secretion

Ans: (b) Constipation

268. All are true about carcinoid *except:*

(a) Small bowel is the least common site
(b) Multifocal in 30% cases
(c) Associated with synchronous malignancy
(d) Associated with MEN 1

Ans: (a) Small bowel is the least common site

269. All are seen in carcinoids *except:*

(a) Diarrhea
(b) Cyanosis
(c) Acute appendicitis
(d) Flushing

Ans: (c) Acute appendicitis

270. True about small bowel carcinoids is:

(a) Most common site is duodenum
(b) Doesn't cause endocardial fibroelastosis
(c) Increased risk of CA lung
(d) Most common malignancy of small bowel

Ans: (d) Most common malignancy of small bowel

PART SEVEN: CHARTS AND TABLES FOR FINAL REVISION

CHAPTER 67

TABLES AND CHARTS FOR FINAL REVIEW

Named Staging/Grading	Organ
Duke staging	Ca colon
Jackson staging	Ca penis
Gleason score	Ca prostate
Robson staging	Renal cell Ca
Nevin staging	Ca Gallbladder
Noguchi classification	Adeno Ca lung
Chang staging	Medulloblastoma
Sullivan modification of Macfarlane system	Adrenocortical Ca
Bloom Richardson grading	Ca Breast
Masaoka staging	Thymomas
Shimida index	Neuroblastoma
Reese Elsworth classification and **Esson** prognostic index	Retinoblastoma
Bismuth Corlette classification	Perihilar cholangiocarcinoma
Lauren, Ming, Goseki, Borrmann classifications	Gastric Ca

Reversible	
Metaplasia	***One adult cell type is replaced by another***
	Often 2° to irritation and/or environment exposure (e.g., ***Most common is columnar to squamous metaplasia*** in bronchi of smokers)
Dysplasia	Abnormal growth with ***loss of cellular orientation and architectural organization***
	*Most common in **epithelial** cells*
	Commonly preneoplastic
Carcinoma in situ	When ***dysplasia involves the entire thickness*** of the epithelium, but does NOT penetrate the basement membrane
Irreversible	
Anaplasia	***Lack of differentiation*** is called anaplasia – It is a ***hallmark of malignancy***
Desmoplasia	***Fibrous tissue formation*** in response to neoplasm
Neoplasia	A clonal proliferation of cells that is ***uncontrolled and excessive***

Types of metastases
Skip metastases: • Bypassing of local lymph nodes with involvement of more distant lymph nodes; Also a tumor nodule that is located within the same bone as the main tumor BUT not in continuity with it – Examples are: Ca ***lung, Osteosarcoma,*** Ca ***esophagus;*** papillary Ca thyroid, ***Oral*** Ca, Breast Ca (rarely)
Retrograde metastases: • Due to obstruction of lymphatics by tumor cells, the lymph flow is disturbed and tumor cells spread against the flow of lymph causing retrograde metastases at unusual sites. Example are:

Contd.

Contd.

- Metastases of Ca prostate to supraclavicular N
- Metastases of Ca adrenals to lung
- Metastases of Ca lung to axillary lymph nodes

Drop metastases:

- Intradural but extramedullary spinal metastases that arise from intracranial lesions are called drop metastases (Most common in *children*). Examples are:
  - ***Medulloblastoma*** (Most common 50%)
  - Glioblastoma
  - Ependymoma
  - Germinoma
  - Pinealoblastoma
  - Astrocytoma

Disorder	Tumor/Cancer	Remarks
Chromosome 11p-WT1 gene	**W**ilms tumor	**A**niridia, **G**enitourinary anomalies, mental **R**etardation (WAGR)
Chromosome 13q-Rb1 gene; Knuton's two-hit hypothesis	Retinoblastoma, osteosarcoma	Associated metal retardation, skeletal malformation, AD or sporadic new mutation
Trisomy 21 (Down's)	Lymphocytic or nonlymphocytic leukemia	*Risk is 15 times normal*
Klinefelter's syn. (47 XXY)	Breast cancer, extragonadal germ cell tumors	
Gonadal dysgenesis (XO/XY)	Gonadoblastoma	Gonads must be removed; 25% chance of gonadal malignancy
	DNA fragility	
Xeroderma pigmentosum	Basal, squamous cell skin cancers	AR, *failure to repair solar damaged DNA*
Fanconi's anemia	Leukemia, AML	AR; *positive diepoxybutane test; chromosome fragility*
Bloom's syndrome	Leukemia, lymphoma	AR; *chromosome fragility*
Ataxia-telangiectasia	Lymphoma, leukemia	AR; sensitive to X-rays, radiomimetic drugs; chromosome fragility
Dysplastic nevus syndrome	Melanoma	AD
Immunodeficiency syndromes		
Wiskott-Aldrich syndrome	Lymphoma, leukemia	***XLR,*** Immunodeficiency
X-linked Immunodeficiency	Lymphoma (Duncan's syndrome)	EBV
X-linked agammaglobulinemia	Lymphoma, leukemia	Immunodeficiency
Servere combined immunodeficiency (SCID)	Lymphoma, leukemia	*Adenosine deaminaze (ADA) deficiency*
	Others	
Tuberous sclerosis	Fibroangiomatous nevi, myocardial rhabdomyoma	AD
Hemochromatosis	*Hepatoma*	Cirrhosis, AD/AR
Gardner syndrome	*Adenocarcinoma of colon, skull and soft tissue tumors*	AD, *APC* gene
Peutz-Jeghers syndrome	GI carcinoma, ovarian neoplasia	AD
Tyrosinemia, galactosemia	Hepatic carcinoma	Nodular cirrhosis, AR
MEN 1 (Wermer's syndrome)	**P**arathyroid adenoma, **P**ancreatic islet cell tumor, **P**ituitary adenoma, carcinoid	AD, Zollinger-Ellison syndrome **PPP**
MEN 2A (Sipple syndrome)	Medullary thyroid carcinoma pheochromocytoma, hyperparathyroidism	AD, monitor calcitonin and calcium levels
MEN 2B (MEN 3)	Medullary thyroid carcinoma, pheochromocytoma Mucosal neuroma Marfanoid habitus	

Virus	Associated cancers
DNA viruses	
Human Papilloma virus (HPV)	Genital (cervical, vulvar, penile) warts may progress to carcinoma
Epstein-Barr virus (EBV)	***Gastric cancer (Most common EBV*** associated cancer); Anaplastic ***nasopharyngeal carcinoma; Burkitt's*** lymphoma (African type); ***Hodgkin's*** lymphoma (Mixed cellularity type); ***CNS lymphoma in AIDS*** patients
Human Herpes Virus B (HHV B)	Kaposi's sarcoma
Hepatitis B virus (HBV)	Primary hepatocellular carcinoma
RNA viruses	
Human T cell leukemia virus (HTLV1)	T cell leukemia/lymphoma
Hepatitis C virus (HCV)	Primary hepatocellular carcinoma

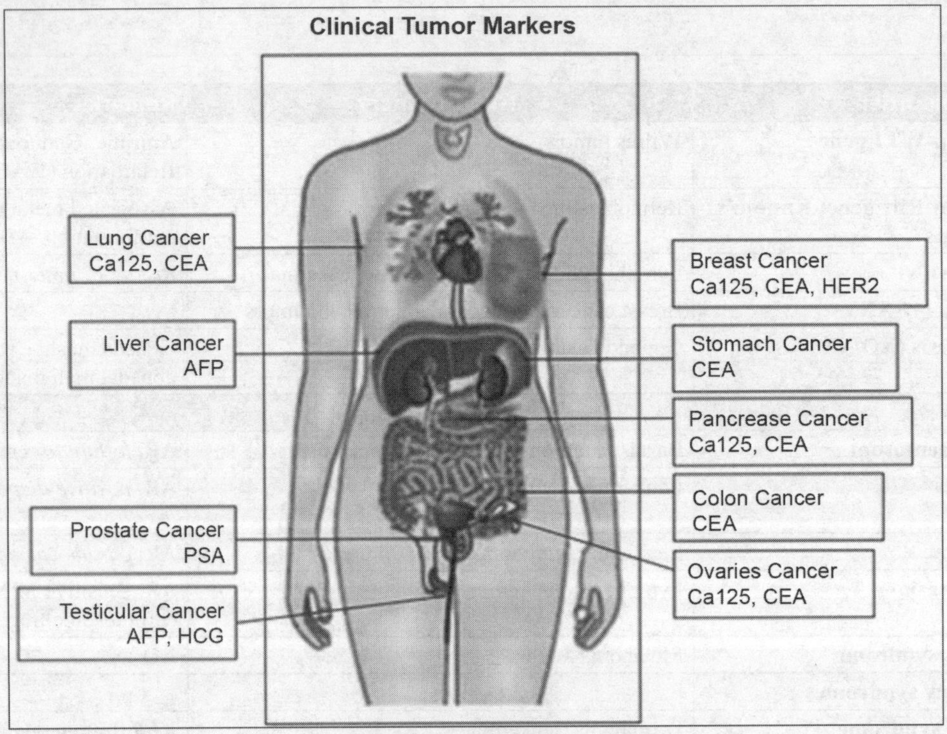

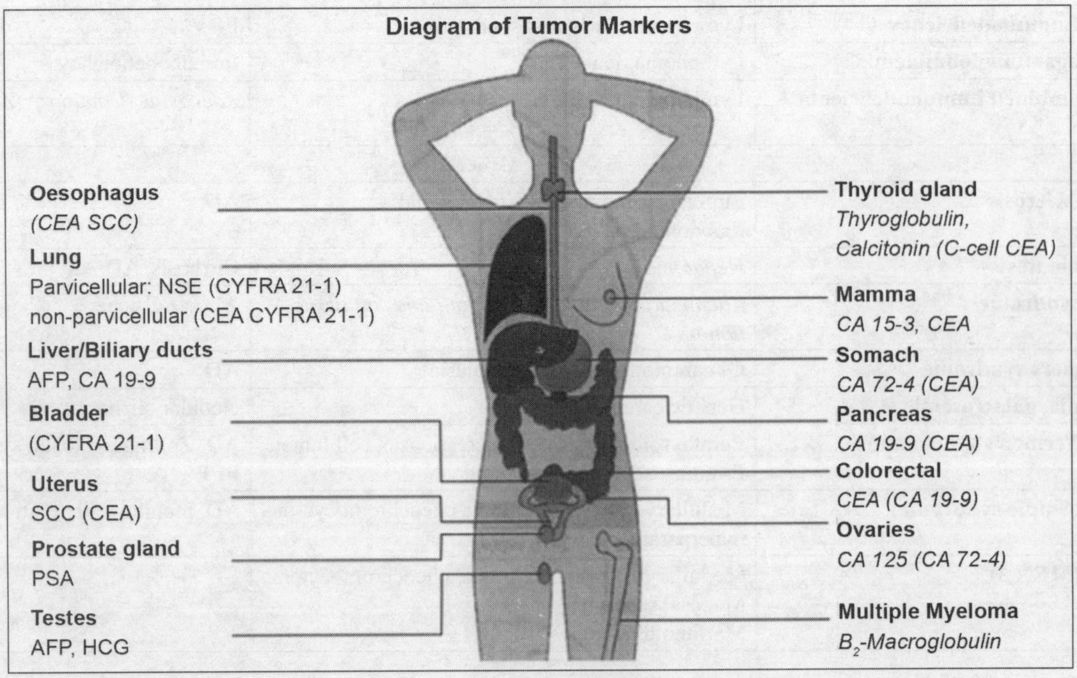

ECOG Performance Status Categories	
Grade	**Description**
0	Fully active, able to carry on all pre-disease performance without restriction
1	Restricted in physically strenuous activity, but ambulatory and able to carry out work of a light or sedentary nature, e.g., light house work, office work
2	Ambulatory and capable of all self care, but unable to carry out any work activities. Up and about more than 50% of waking hours
3	Capable of only limited self care, confined to bed or chair more than 50% of working hours
4	Completely disabled. Cannot carry on any self care. Totally confined to bed or chair
5	Dead

Karnofsky Performance Status Scale		
Able to carry on normal activity and to work; no special care needed	100	Normal with no complaints; no evidence of disease
	90	Able to carry on normal activity; minor signs or symptoms of disease
	80	Normal activity with efforts; some signs and symptoms of disease
Unable to work; able to live at home and care for most personal needs; varying amount of assistance needed	70	Cares for self; unable to carry on normal activity or do active work
	60	Requires occasional assistance, but able to care for most of his/her personal needs
	50	Requires considerable assistance and frequent medical care
Unable to care for self; requires equivalent of institutional or hospital care; disease may be progressing rapidly	40	Disabled; requires special care and assistance
	30	Severely disabled; hospital admission is indicated although death is not imminent
	20	Very sick; hospital admission necessary; active supprotive treatment necessary
	10	Moribund; fatal processes progressing rapidly
	0	Dead

Recommended Antiemetic Therapy for Single-day Intravenous Chemotherapy		
Emetic Risk Category	**Prevention of Acute Emesis (Day 1 Prechemotherapy)**	**Prevention of Delayed Emesis**
High	5-HT_3 receptor antagonist *plus* dexamethasone *plus* apreditant	Dexamethasone days 2-4 *plus* aprepitant, days 2 and 3
Moderate • AC • Non-AC	 5-HT_3 receptor antagonist *plus* dexamethasone *plus* aprepitant Palonosetron *plus* dexamethasone	 Aprepitant days 2 and 3 Dexamethasone days 2 and 3
Low	Dexamethasone or prochlorperazine	No preventive measures
Minimal	As needed	No preventive measures

ONCOTYPE DX ASSAY

Recurrence score	Risk	Benefit of chemotherapy
<18	**Low**	Small and will not outweigh the risks
18-30	**Intermediate**	Unclear
>31	**High**	Greater than the risks

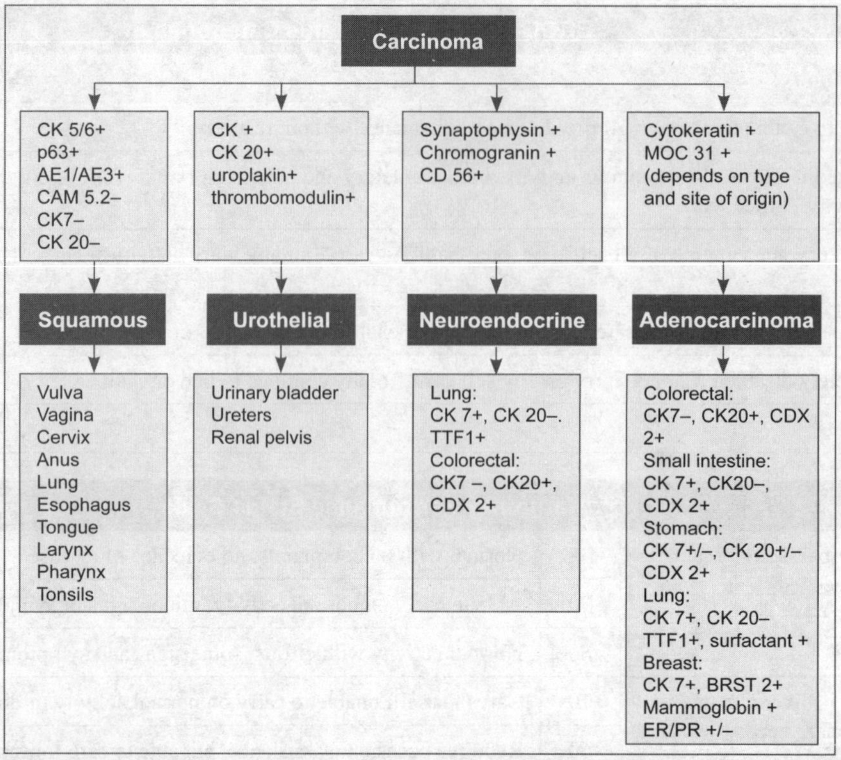

Tumor Lysis Syndrome

Complication	Etiology	Manifestations	Management
Hyperkalemia	Intracellular K^+ release rate exceeds renal clearance capacity; K^+ leakage secondary to failling ATP levels	• Electrocardiographic abnormalities • Muscle cramps, weakness and paresthesias • Nausea, vomiting and diarrhea	• Aggressive hydration • Cation exchange resins • Calcium gluconate • Sodium bicorbonate • Hypertonic dextrose + insulin • Loop diuretics
Hyperphosphatemia	Intracellular PO_4 release rate that exceeds renal clearance capacity	• Acute renal failure • Secondary hypocalcemia	• Aggressive hydration • Hypertonic dextrose + insulin • Oral phosphate binders
Hypocalcemia	Secondary to hyperphosphatemia and ensuing tissue precipitation of calcium phosphate	• Muscle twitches, cramps, tetany, carpopedal spasm, or paresthesia • Mental status changes, confusion, delirium, hallucinations • Rarely seuzures • Exacerbation of hyperkalemia	• Manage hyperphosphatemia
Hypercalcemia	Intracellular uric acid release rate exceeds renal clearance capacity	• Acute renal failure	• Aggressive hydration
Lactic acidosis	Hypovolemia and acute renal failure	• Acidemia	• Allopurinol • Urate oxidase • Conventional hemodialysis of acute renal failure develops • Volume replacement • Correct acidosis

American Society of Anesthesiologists General Classification of Physical Status	
Physical Satus	**Description**
1	Normal, healthy patient
2	Mild systemic disease without functional limitation
3	Severe systemic disease with functional limitation
4	Life-threatening severe systemic disease
5	Moribund, not expected to survive operation
6	Brain-dead organ donor
E	Emergency operation

Lauren Classification System	
Intestinal	**Diffuse**
Environmental	Familial
Gastric atrophy, intestinal metaplasia	Blood type A
Men > women	Women > men
Increasing incidence with age	Younger age group
Gland formation	Poorly differentiated, signed ring cells
Hematogenous spread	Transmural, lymphatic spread
Microsatellite instability	Decreased E-cadherin
APC gene mutations	
p53, p16 inactivation	*p53, p16* inactivation

Comparison of Esophageal Resection Techniques					
	EBE	**TTE**	**THE**	**VSE**	**MIE**
Incisions	Neck Chest Abdomen	Chest Abdomen	Neck Abdomen	Neck Abdomen	Neck (Chest) (Abdomen)
Anastomosis	Neck	Chest	Neck	Neck	Neck
Lymphadenectomy	Radical thoracic, abdominal	Available thoracic, abdominal	Available lower mediastinal, abdominal	None	Available thoracic, abdominal
Pyloroplasty	Yes	Yes	Yes	No	Yes
Preservation of vagus nerves	No	No	No	Yes	No

Early Gastric Cancer	
Type I	**Exophytic lesion extending into the gastric lumen**
Type II	Superficial variant
IIA	Elevated lesions with a height no more than the thickness of the adjacent mucosa
IIB	Flat lesions
IIC	Depressed lesions with an eroded but not deeply ulcerated appearance
Type III	Excavated lesions that may extent into the muscularis propria without invasion of this layer by actual cancer cells

Biopsy Techniques for Breast Lesions		
Technique	**Advantage**	**Disadvantages**
Fine-needle aspiration cytology	Rapid, painless, inexpensive, No incision prior to selection of local therapy	Does not distinguish invasive from *in situ* cancer. Markers (ER, PR, HER2) not routinely available Requires experienced cytopathologist. False-negative results and insufficient specimens occur

Contd.

Contd.

Core-cutting needle biopsy	Rapid, relatively painless, inexpensive. No incision. Can be read by any pathologist, markers routinely available	False-negative results, incomplete lesion characterization can occur
Excisional biopsy	False-negative results rare. Complete histology before treatment decisions. May serve as definitive lumpectomy	Expensive, more painful, Creates as incision to be incorporated into definitive surgery. Unnecessary surgery with potential for cosmetic deformity in patients with benign abnormalities

INDICATIONS FOR SURGICAL BIOPSY AFTER CORE NEEDLE BIOPSY

Failure to sample calcifications
Diagnosis of atypical ductal hyperplasia
Diagnosis of atypical lobular hyperplasia or lobular carcinoma *in situ*
Lack of concordance between imaging findings and histologic diagnosis
Radial scar
Papillary lesions

BI-RADS Category	Assessment	Clinical Recommendation
0	Assessment Incomplete	Need to review prior studies and/or complete additional imaging
1	Negative	Continue routine screening
2	Benign	Continue routine screening
3	Probably Benign Finding	Short-term follow-up at 6 months, then every 6 to 12 months for 1 to 2 years
4	Suspicious Abnormality	Perform biopsy, preferably needle biopsy
5	Highly Suspicious of Malignancy	Biopsy and treatment, as necessary
6	Known Biopsy–Proven Malignancy	Assure that treatment is completed

Inherited Genome Maintenance Defects with Cancer Predisposition

Maintenance Mechanism	Syndrome	Gene Defect
Checkpoint response	Li-Fraumeni, Familial breast cancer, Retinoblastoma Familial melanoma	*p53, CHK2 BRCA1, CHK2 RB* *p16^{INK4A}*
Mismatch repair	HNPCC/Lynch syndrome	*MLH1, MSH2, PMS2, MSH6*
Nucleotide excision repair	Xerodema pigmentosa	*XP genes*
DSB response/repair	Ataxia telangiectasia AT-like disorder Nijmegen breakage Fanconio anemia Familial breast cancer SCID, rare lymphoma SCID, rate leukemia	*ATM* *MRE 11* *NBS1* *Fanc genes* *BRCA1, BRCA2, CHK2, PALB2* *Artemis* *Ligase IV*
Helicase activity	Bloom Werner Rothmund Thomson	*BLM* *WRN* *RECQ4*
Mitotic checkpoint	Mosaic variegated aneuploidy	*BUB1B*

Hereditary Risk Factors Associated with Development of Pancreatic Cancer

Gene	Associated Syndrome	Clinical Significance
PRSS1	Familial pancreatitis	Mutation results in chronic pancreatitis and 40% lifetime risk of PDAC
STK11	Peutz-Jeghers syndrome	Mutation results in > 100-fold increase in the risk of PDAC

Contd.

Contd.

CDKN2A	Familial atypical mole and multiple melanoma syndrome	Mutation leads to increased risk of melanoma and >40-fold increase risk of PDAC
CTFR	Cystic fibrosis	Thick secretions result in chronic pancreatitis and 30-fold increase in risk of PDAC
BRCA2	Hereditary breast and ovarian cancer	Mutation results in elevated risk of breast and ovarian cancer and 10-fold increase in risk of PDAC
MLH1	Lynch syndrome	Mismatch repair gene mutation leads to increased risk of colon cancer and eight-fold increase in risk of PDAC
APC	Familial adenomatous polyposis	Mutation results in polyposis coli and colon cancer with four-fold increase in risk of PDAC

Gene/Locus	Associated Syndrome/Clinical Features	Breast Cancer Risk	Mutation/Minor Allele Frequency
High Penetrance Genes			
BRCA1 (17q21)	Hereditary breast/ovarian cancer; bilateral/mulifocal breast tumor, prostate, colon, liver, bone cancers	60-85% (lifetime); 15-40% risk of ovarian cancer	1/400
BRCA2 (13q 12.3)	Hereditary breast/ovarian cancer; male breast caner, pancreas, gallbladder, pharynx stomach, melanoma, prostate cancer. Also causes D1 Fanconi anemia (biallelic mutations)	60-85% (lifetime); 15-40% risk of ovarian cancer	1/400

Cancer Susceptibility Syndromes caused by Activation of Proto-Oncogenes

Syndrome	Gene	Protein Function
Costello syndrome	*HRAS*	Small GTPase; positive regulator of proliferation
Hereditary papillary renal cancer	*MET*	Receptor tyrosine kinase; positive regulator of proliferation
Multiple endocrine neoplasia type 2	*RET*	
Hereditary gastrointestinal stromal tumors	*KIT*	
Familial melanoma	*CDK4*	Cell cycle regulator

Immunohistochemical Studies Useful in the Differential Diagnosis of Carcinoma vs Another Neoplasm

Tumor Type	Immunoperoxidase Stains			
	Pan-Keratin	CD45 and Other Markers	S-100 Protein, HMB-45	Vimentin
Carcinoma	+	–	–	–/+
Malignant lymphoma	–	+	–	–/+
Malignant melanoma	–	–	+	+
Sarcoma	–	–	–	+

Immunohistochemical Markers	Tumors
Calcitonin	Medullary thyroid carcinoma
CK20	Carcinoma of gastrointestinal, pancreatobiliary tract, urothelium, mucinous ovarian tumor
CK7	Carcinomas of the lung, breast, endometrium, ovary, pancreas; mesothelioma; squamous cell carcinoma of the cervix
Napsin A	Lung adenocarcinoma; renal cell carcinoma
PAX-B	Differentiated thyroid carcinoma; lymphoma; ovarian carcinoma; renal cell carcinoma
Thyroglobulin	Highly specific for differentiated thyroid carcinoma
TTF-1	Differentiated thyroid carcinoma; adenocarcinomas of the lung, colon, breast and pancreas, meningioma; ovarian mucinous carcinoma; squamous cell carcinomas of the lung, head and neck and cervix

Most Useful Organ-Specific Markers	
Organ or Type of Cancer	**Antibody**
Breast	GCDFP-15, estrogen receptor
Lung	TTF-1, napsin A
Gastrointestinal carcinoma	CDX-2
Stomach	CDX-2 + Hep-Par
Colon	CDX-2 + CDK20
Liver	Hep-Par, arginase
Kidney	CD10 + PAX-2 + PAX-8
Prostate	Prostate-specific antigen + prostein
Urinary bladder	CK7, CK20, CK5/6, GATA3
Seminoma/embryonal carcinoma	OCT-4
Ovarian, serous	WT-1 + PAX-8
Mesothelioma	Calretinin, CK5/6, WT1
Thyroid	TTF-1 + thyroglobulin
Neuroendocrine	Chromogranin + synaptophysin

Cytokine Milieu and Effects in Cancer Cachexia	
Cytokine	**Effects**
TNF-α	Lipolysis, muscle degradation, increased glucose turnover
Interferon-γ	Potentiates lipolysis, decreases protein synthesis
Interleukin-1 (IL-1)	Induces anorexia, early satiety, peripheral proteolysis, potentiates release of IL-6
IL-6	Severe wasting
Proteolysis-inducing factor	Skeletal muscle degradation
Lipid mobilizing factor	Lipolysis

Carcinogens and Tobacco-Induced Cancers	
Cancer Type	**Likely Carcinogen Involvement***
Lung	PAH, NNK (major) 1, 3-butadiene, isoprene, ethylene oxide, ethyl carbamate, aldehydes, benzene, metals
Larynx	PAH
Nasal	NNK, NNN, other *N*-nitrosamines, aldehydes
Oral cavity	PAH, NNK, NNN
Esophagus	NNN, other *N*-nitrosamines
Liver	NNK, other *N*-nitrosamines, furan
Pancreas	NNK, NNAL
Cervix	PAH, NNK
Bladder	4-aminobiphenyl, other aromatic amines
Leukemia	Benzene
Colorectal	Heterocyclic aromatic amines

ONCOGENIC VIRUS

Virus	Taxon	Virion	Site of Persistance	Diseases in Normal Hosts	Diseases in Immuno compromised Hosts
High-risk human papillomavirus types (e.g. HPV16)	Alphapapilloma-virus	Nonenveloped	Anogenital mucosa, oral mucosa	Carcinomas of the cervix, penis, anus, vagina, vulva, tonsils, base of tongue	Increased incidence of same diseases
Hepatitis B virus (HBV)	Hepadnaviridae	Enveloped	Hepatocytes	Cirrhosis, hepatocellular carcinoma	Same diseases, increased incidence with AIDS

Contd.

Contd.

Hepatitis C virus (CV)	Flaviviridae	Enveloped	Hepatocytes	Cirrhosis, hepatacellular carcinoma, splenic marginal zone lymphoma	Same diseases, increased incidence with AIDS
Epstein-Barr virus (EBV, HHV-4)	Gammaherpes-virinae	Enveloped	B cells, pharyngeal mucosa	Mononucleosis, Burkitt lymphoma, other non-Hodgkin lymphoma, nasopharyngeal carcinoma	Increased incidence of same diseases, lymphoproliferative disease, other lymphomas, oral hairy leukoplakia leiomyosarcoma
Kaposi's sarcoma herpes-virus (KSHV, HHV-8)	Gammaherpes-virinae	Enveloped	Oral mucosa endothelium B cells	Kaposi's sarcoma (KS), multicentric Castleman disease (MCD)	Increased KS MCD incidence, primary effusian lymphoma
Merkel cell polyomavirus (MCPyV, MCV)	Orthopolyoma-virus	Nonenveloped	Skin (lymphocytes)	Merkel cell carcinoma (MCC)	Increased MCC incidence
Human T-cell leukemia virus (HTLV-1)	Deltaretrovirus	Enveloped	T and B cells	Adult T-cell leukemia/lymphoma, tropical spastic paraparesis, myelopathy, uveitis dermatitis	Unknown

Multiple Endocrine Neoplasia Syndromes and Familial Medullary Thyroid Cancer

Characteristics	MEN-1	MEN-2A	MEN-2B	Familial medullary thyroid carcinoma
Chromosome	11q12-13	Pericentromeric 10	Pericentromeric 10	Pericentromeric 10
Genetic defect	*MEN-1* mutation	*RET* mutation	*RET* mutation	*RET* mutation
MTC	No	Bilateral	Bilateral	Bilateral
Pheochromocytoma	No	70% bilateral	70% bilateral	No
Parathyroid disease	Hyperplasia	Hyperplasia	No	No
Phenotype	No	No	Bony abnormalities, mucosal neuromas, Marfanoid habitus, bumpy lips	No
Mode of inheritance	Autosomal dominant	Autosomal dominant	Autosomal dominant	Autosomal dominant
Course of MTC	No MTC	Variable, frequently indolent	More virulent	Most indolent
Pancreatic endocrine tumors	Yes: Pancreatic polypeptide, 80-100%; gastrinoma, 50%; insulinoma, 20%; growth hormone-releasing factor, vasoactive intestinal peptide (uncommon)	No	No	No

Types of Anesthetic Procedures Commonly Used in Cancer Pain

Type of procedure	Most common indications
Inhalation therapy with nitrous oxide	Breakthrough pain, incidental pain in patients with diffuse poorly controlled pain
Intravenous barbiturates (sodium pentobarbital)	Diffuse body pain and suffering inadequately controlled by systemic opioids
Local anesthetic by intravenous, subcutaneous, or transdermal application	Neuropathic pain in any site with local application to the area of hyperesthesia or allodynia
Trigger point injections	Focal muscle pain

Contd.

Contd.

Nerve Block	
Peripheral	Pain in discrete dermatomes in chest and abdomen or in distal extremities
Epidural	Unilateral lumbar or sacral pain, midline perineal pain, bilateral lumbosacral pain
Intrathecal	Midline perineal pain, bilateral lumbosacral pain
Autonomic	
Stellate ganglion	
Lumbar sympathetic vascular insufficiency of the lower extremity	
Celiac plexus	

Neuroablative and Neurostimulatory Procedures for Relief of Pain from Cancer

Site	Procedure	Indications
Neruroablative Procedures		
Nerve root	Rhizotomy	Useful in somatic and neuropathic pain from tumor infiltration of the cranial and, rarely, intercostal nerves
Spinal cord	Dorsal root entry zone lesion	Useful in unilateral neuropathic pain from brachial, intercostal, and lumbosacral plexopathy and postherpetic neuralgia
	Cordotomy	Useful in unilateral pain below the waist; often combined with local neurolytic blocks in perineal and bilateral lumbosacral plexopathy; may be performed bilaterally
	Myelotomy	Useful in midline pain below the waist but rarely used because it involves extensive surgery
Brainstem	Mesencephalic tractomy	Useful in pain in the nasopharynx and trigeminal region
Thalamus	Thalamotomy	Useful in unilateral neuropathic pain in the chest and lower extremity
Cortex	Cingulotomy	Useful through a stereotactic approach for diffuse pain
Pituitary	Transphenoidal hypophysectomy	Useful in pain control of bone metastases in endocrine-dependent tumors, breast and prostate
Neurostimulatory Procedures		
Peripheral nerve	Transcutaneous and percutaneous electrical nerve stimulation	Useful in reducing painful dysesthesias from tumor infiltration of nerve or trauma (e.g., neuroma)
Spinal cord	Dorsal column stimulation	Of limited use in neuropathic pain in the chest, midline and lower extremities
Thalamus	Thalamic stimulation	Of rare use in neuropathic pain in the chest, midline or lower extremity

Nerve	Site (Syndrome)
Median	
	Distal portion of the humerus
	Elbow (pronator syndrome)
	Elbow (anterior interosseous nerve syndrome, Kiloh Nevin syndrome)
	Wrist (carpal tunnel syndrome)
	Wrist (sublimis syndrome, pseudo-carpal tunnel syndrome)
Ulnar	
	Elbow (cubital tunnel syndrome, tardy ulnar palsy)
	Wrist (ulnar tunnel syndrome, Guyons canal syndrome)
Radial	
	Axilla (Saturday nigh palsy, sleep palsy)
	Distal end of humerus

Contd.

Contd.

	Eblow (posterior interosseous nerve syndrome)
Suprascapular	
	Shoulder
Plantar and interdigital	
	Foot (Mortons metatarsalgia)
Posterior tibial	
	Ankle (tarsal tunnel syndrome)
Common peroneal	
	Knee
Lateral femoral cutaneous	
	Anterior superior iliace spine (meralgia paraesthetica)

Patterns of Muscle Wasting in the Hand	
Thenar wasting	Median nerve palsy (C8)
Hypthenar wasting	Ulnar nerver palsy (T1)
Intrinsic wasting	Ulnar nerver palsy (T1)

Sensory Distribution of the Nerve Supply to the Hand

Nerve	**Sensory Distribution**
Ulnar	Little finger and ulnar half of the ring finger
Median	Thumb, index, middle and radial half of the ring finger
Radial	Base of the thumb on the dorsum of the hand

Special Hand Tests

Test	**Technique**	**Significance**
Allen's test	Elevate the hand and apply digital pressure on the radial and ulnar arteries to occlude them. Ask the patient to make a fist several times. The tips of the finger should go pale. Release each artery in turn and observe the return of colour	Tests the adequacy of the blood supply to the hand from the radial and ulnar arteries and the arcade between them
Tinel's test	Tap over the nerve of interest. Tingling may indicate nerve compression.	Identifies compression of a peripheral nerve
Phalen's test	Place the wrist in maximum flexion with the elblows extended	Compression of the medial nerve causes paraesthesia
Froment's sign	Ask the patients to grip a sheet of paper between the index finger and thumb of both hands. Grip the paper yourself similarly. Ask the patient to resist as you attempt to pull the paper away	A positive test indicated by flexion of the thumb interphalangeal joint suggests weakness of the adductor pollicis muscle supplied by the ulnar nerve. Recruitment of the median nerve-innervated flexor pollicis brevis explains the thumb posture

PART EIGHT: STATISTICS

CHAPTER

68 STATISTICS

REVIEW NOTES ON STATISTICS

Presentation of Statistical Data

Histogram

- It is a pictorial diagram of frequency distribution consisting of a series of blocks adjacent to each other with no intervening space and area of each block is proportional to the frequency
- Class intervals are given along the horizontal axis and frequencies along the vertical axis
- It represents categories of continuous and ordered data
- **Frequency polygon**–It is obtained by joining the mid-points of the histogram blocks

Frequency curve

- When number of observations is very large and group interval is reduced, frequency polygon loses its angulations resulting in a smooth curve known as Frequency curve

Line diagram

- Line diagrams are used to show the trend of events with the passage of time

Cumulative frequency curve or Ogive

- It is a Line diagram, representing cumulative frequency distribution of quantitative data
- The curve is plotted by taking the variable on the x axis and the cumulative frequency on y axis
- Median can be calculated from Ogive

Pie Charts

- Instead of comparing the length of a bar, the areas of segments of a circle are compared
- The area of each segment depends upon the angle
- Considered inferior to bar charts and often necessary to indicate percentages in segments

Pictogram [a form of bar chart]

- Method of presenting data to "man on street" and to those who cannot understand orthodox charts
- Small pictures or symbols are used to present data
- Fractions of picture can be used to represent numbers smaller than the value of a whole symbol

Types of Data

Ungrouped and grouped

- Ungrouped data is presented individually, e.g., Weight of 11 players of Indian cricket team. Dhoni–60 kg, Sachin–55 kg, Zaheer–65 kg etc
- Grouped data→presented as groups consisting of identical data by frequency. Weight of Indian players, weighing 40-50 kg, 50-60 kg, 60 and above

Qualitative and Quantitative

- Qualitative data → non numerical, based on categorical scale, e.g., Height in terms of short, medium and tall. It has no notion of magnitude or size of attribute
- Quantitative → numerical or based on numbers

Continuous and discrete

- Continuous → data for which unlimited number of possible values exist, e.g., Height, Weight etc
- Discrete → data for which distinct categories and a limited number of possible values exist, e.g., Number of children in a family. All qualitative data are discrete

Scales of Measurement
Nominal Scale:
Data is divided into qualitative categories or groups, e.g., Male/Female, or Urban/Semi Urban/Rural There is no order or ratio
Dichomatous Scale:
Where data is divided into only two categories or group, i.e., Male or Female
Ordinal Scale
Used when data can be placed in a meaningful order, e.g., 1st, 2nd and 3rd or mild, moderate or severe There is no information about size of the interval, i.e., difference between 1st and 2nd
Interval Scale
Used when data can be placed in a meaningful order and there is information about size of the interval It does not have an absolute Zero, so ratio of scores is not meaningful, e.g.,100 degree C is not twice as hot as 50 degree C
Ratio Scale
Data can be placed in a meaningful order and there is information about size of the interval It has an absolute Zero, so ratio of scores is meaningful, e.g., Weight in gram, time in second, BP in mm of Hg

Measure of Central Tendency
Imply a value in the distribution (central value), around which other values are distributed
Mean
• It is widely used and is the most useful of statistical averages • To obtain mean, individual observations are added together and divided by the number of observations • Advantage → Easy to calculate and understand • Disadvantage → It may be unduly influenced by abnormal or extreme values in the distribution
Median
• To obtain median, the data is arranged in an ascending or descending order of magnitude and then the value of the middle observation is located, which is called the median • If the number of items or values is even, the practice is to take the average of the two middle values • Advantages → Not unduly influenced by abnormal or extreme values in the distribution • Used for numeric data that is skewed and for ordinal data • Most preferred measure of central tendency
Mode
• It is the most frequently occurring value in a series of value or observation • Advantage: Easy to understand, and is not [or least] affected by extreme values in the distribution • It is the only average that can be applied to qualitative data **Mode= Mean – 3 (Mean – Median)**

There can be more than one mode for a series of data and even no mode in a series of data

In a frequency polygon, mode can be located from the point where the curve takes a turn from increase to decrease. Used primarily for bimodal distribution

Measures of Dispersion [Range, Mean Deviation and SD]
Range
• It is the simplest measure of dispersion • It is defined as difference between highest and lowest figures in a given sample • In grouped data, range is taken as the difference between the mid-points of the extreme categories • Range gives no details about the dispersion of values between the two extreme values
Mean Deviation
• It is the average of the deviations from the arithmetic mean • Mean deviation = $\Sigma (x - \bar{x}) / \eta$

Contd.

Contd.

Standard Deviation

- It is the best and most frequently used measure of deviation
- It is defined as "Root – Means Square – Deviation"
- It is denoted by the Greek letter sigma σ [SD of population] or by initials SD [SD of sample]

  SD (for Sample size > 30) = $\sqrt{[\Sigma(x-\bar{x})]/\eta}$

  SD (for Sample size ≤ 30) = $\sqrt{[\Sigma(x-\bar{x})^2]/(\eta-1)}$
- SD gives us an idea of 'spread' of dispersion → Larger the SD, greater the dispersion of values about mean

Coefficient of Variance [CV]

- It is a ratio, has no units of measurement
- $CV = \frac{SD}{Mean} \times 100$
- It is SD expressed as the "percentage of the mean".
- Advantage → Helps to compare the deviation or variability in two set of dissimilar measurements (BP, Height) in the same group or Compare variability of same character in two or more different groups

Normal Distribution: Standard Normal Curve or Guassian Curve

- Smooth, bell-shaped, perfectly symmetrical curve, based on an infinitely large number of observations
- Total area of the curve is 1; its mean is zero; and its standard deviation is 1
- The mean, median and mode all coincide. Mean divides the area under the curve into 2 equal halves
- A random variable (x) is standardized when it has been adjusted so that its mean= 0 and SD = 1
- **Standardization** is done by subtracting the mean of x, from x and dividing the resulting difference by SD of x. A standardized variable = $(x-\bar{x})/\sigma$

Skewed or Asymmetrical Distribution

- Frequency distribution curve is not symmetrical about the peak
- One tail of the curve is longer than other
- A relative measure of skewness as given by Karl Pearson is:

  Skewness = [3(Mean – Median)] / SD
- If the skewness so calculated is:
  - "+ve" → i.e., Mean > Median → *Skewness is to the right* (Tail is towards right side and there are large number of low scores, small number of high scores)
  - "–ve" → i.e., Mean < Median → *Skewness is to the left* (Tail is towards left side and there are large number of high scores, small number of low scores)

- **Relative deviate or Standard normal variate or *Z score*** → is the measure of distance of a value (x) from the mean ($\bar{x}$) of a normal distribution curve in units of SD

  $Z = (x-\bar{x})/\sigma$

Sampling Methods

Simple Random Sample:

- Each of the units (individuals or households) in the sampling frame is assigned a number
- A table of random numbers [E.g., Tippets Random Number Table], lottery method or computer software is used to determine which units are to be included in the sample
- Each unit has an equal chance of being drawn in the sample
- This technique provides the greatest number of possible samples
- Applicable when the population is small, homogenous and readily available

Contd.

Contd.

Systematic Random Sample:
• No pre numbering is necessary (Sampling frame not required) • If the sample to be drawn = n, The total population = N. Then quotient "r" = N/n • A unit is selected at random and other units are selected by adding "r" to previous selected number or every rth unit at regular intervals is picked • Each unit in sampling frame has same chance of being selected, but number of possible samples is greatly reduced • Preferred when population is large, scattered and not homogenous
Stratified Random Sample:
• Sample is drawn in a way that each portion of sample represents a corresponding strata of universe • Useful where population is heterogenous with regard to characteristic under study or when the characteristic is influenced by different sections of the population, viz., Religion [Hindus, Muslims], age-groups etc • Entire population is divided into homogenous sub groups [strata] depending on the characteristic to be studied and simple random sampling is done from each strata • Precision of the estimate of the characteristic under study is increased and due representation of population is maintained

Choice of Test of Significance

Attribute	Type	Test
Probability distribution	Normal	'Z' test
	Near normal	't' test , Chi square test, Fishers test
Number of samples to be compared	Two	't' test, Chi square test, 'Z' test
	More than two	ANOVA
Sample size	Small (≤ 30)	't' test, ANOVA, Non-parametric test
	Large (> 30)	Z test, Chi square test
Type of data	Qualitative	Chi square test, Kruskal Wallis test
	Quantitative	't' test, ANOVA, Z test

Student 'T' Test [Devised by WS Cassette]

- Based on *"t" distribution* [a continuous, symmetrical, bell shaped, unimodal distribution of infinite range similar in shape to normal distribution, but more spread out]
- It shows greater variation due to chance than normal distribution and is used to analyse small samples
- *As sample size increases,* t distribution closely resembles the normal distribution
- *As sample size decreases, t value decreases and probability that the difference is ascribed to chance increases and there is increased probability for accepting the null hypothesis*
  - **Student t test for single small sample** → compares a single sample mean with population mean
  - Student t test for independent samples **(Unpaired t test)** → compares mean of 2 small samples [< 30 size]
  - Student t test for paired samples **(Paired t test)** → compares mean of 2 small paired samples [< 30 size]. Each individual gives a pair of observation, may be before and after play of a factor, e.g., BP before and after drug intake
- Used to evaluate the null hypothesis for continuous (quantitative) variables (e.g., height, weight, BP)
- *Applied to find the significance of difference between two means, when sample size is less than 30*
- For each degree of freedom, a row of increasing t value corresponds to a row of decreasing probability for accepting the null hypothesis

Chi-square Test (χ^2) –Developed by Karl Pearson

- It is a type of non-parametric test used for qualitative data in form of proportions
- It is an alternate method of testing the significance of difference between two proportions
- Used as a test of goodness of fit: it determines whether the observed frequency distribution differs from the theoretical distribution [i.e., normal, binomial or Poisson] by chance or the sample is drawn from a different population
- Used to find whether any association between two events or discrete attributes is real or by chance
- Advantage: Can also be used when more than two groups are to be compared
- Yates correction → Applied when expected frequency in any cell of 2 × 2 contingency table is < 5

Standard Error [SE]

- When a number of random samples (with different sample means) are drawn from a population
- Frequency distribution of all the sample means drawn from the same population shows → Sample means are distributed normally about the population mean (μ)
- Variation of sample mean is measured in terms of SE [i.e. SD of sample mean from universe mean]
- 95% of sample means lie within limits of 2 SE on either side of the true or population mean
- Standard error [SE] = $\frac{SD}{\sqrt{\eta}}$, Normal deviate (N.D.) = $(\bar{x} - \mu) / \sigma / \sqrt{\eta}$

Confidence limits	Normal deviate (N.D.)	Significance
μ is outside the 95% confidence limits	N.D. > 2	$P < 0.05$; Significant at 5% level
μ is just within 95% confidence limits	N.D. = 2	$P = 0.05$; Just significant at 5% level
μ is within the 95% confidence limits	N.D. < 2	$P > 0.05$; Not significant at 5% level

Application: To calculate sample size, To work out limits of desired confidence within which population mean would lie and To determine if sample is drawn from a known population or not

McNemar's test is a non-parametric test used on nominal data. It is applied to 2 × 2 contingency table with a dichotomous trait, with matched pairs of subjects

Degree of Freedom [DF]

- In Chi square test, **DF = (c - 1) (r - 1);** c = Number of columns; n = Number of rows
- In unpaired 't' test, DF = n1+ n2 – 2, where n1 and n2 are number of observation in each series
- In paired 't' test, DF = n-1
- In testing the significance of correlation, DF = n – 2, n is the number of paired measurements

p value

- 'p' value is the actual probability of committing type 1 error. It is based on statistical calculation
- If, $p < \alpha$ [usually taken as 5% or 0.05], the association is statistically significant and null hypothesis is rejected

Null hypothesis: It assumes no significant difference between 2 samples, whatever difference that occurs is by chance

Null hypothesis	Accepted	Rejected
True	Correct conclusion	Type I (α) error
False	Type II (β) error	Correct conclusion

Type I error or α error

- Rejecting a null hypothesis when actually it is true (a statistically significant difference is found between two groups when actually there is no difference)
- If null hypothesis is false there can be no type I error
- Probability of a type I error is equal to alpha
- Multiple comparisons and repeated testing for significance increase likelihood of type I error

APPLICATION–Sample size determination and Statistical testing is based on **α** error **(α= 0.05)**

Type II error or β error

- Acceptance of a null hypothesis as true when actually it is false
- The study fails to find a statistically significant difference when actually there is a difference
- If null hypothesis is true there can be no type II error
- Probability of a type II error is equal to beta
- It is inversely related to type I error

APPLICATION – It is used to determine the **power of study** = 1 – β

Power of study (1–β): Is the probability that the study would reject a null hypothesis as false when it is actually false

Conventionally a study is required to have a power of 0.8 to be acceptable, i.e., a study that has less than 80% chance of detecting a false null hypothesis is unacceptable

Correlation coefficient [symbol "r"] → tends to lie between –1.0 and + 1.0

- "r" value near +1 → signals a strong positive association. [If one variable increases the other also increases]
- "r" value near - 1 → signals a strong negative association [when one variable increases the other decreases]
- r = 0 → signals no association between x and y

Probability

- **Probability of an event** is the likelihood that the event will occur. It can never be > 1 [100%] or < 0 [0%]
- **Probability of (A)** = No. of times event A actually occurs / Total no. of events during which event A occurs

Additive rule: [P(A or B) = P(A) + P(B)]

- Applied while considering the probability of one of at least *two mutually exclusive events occurring*
- One event excludes the probability of occurrence of other, e.g., on tossing a coin, getting head excludes the possibility of getting tails

Multiplicative rule: [P(A and B) = P(A) × P(B)]

- Applied while considering the probability of one of at least two independent events occurring together
- Mutually non exclusive, i.e., one event does not exclude the probability of occurrence of other, e.g., out of 100 smokers, development of cancer in one does not exclude possibility of having cancer in other

Poisson distribution

- Used to describe the occurrence of rare events in a large population. The probability of occurrence of event is indefinitely small and 'n' the number of observations is very large
- E.g., Probability distribution for count of events (earthquake) occurring randomly in a given period of time
- Here variance = mean

Binomial distribution

- Distribution of outcome from a series of data characterized by 2 mutually exclusive [Dichotomous] categories
- Population under observation can be divided into 2 groups, one with a certain characteristic and other without it
- If the probability of a person being male is "p" and not being male is "q" [1-p] in a group of "n" persons
- Then mean number of frequencies of males = np, SD= npq
- If p=q, the curve will be symmetrical or else skewed

Uniform distribution or rectangular distribution

- A distribution in which all events occur with equal frequency. It does not occur very often
- Uniform distribution divided into equally spaced intervals, will have equal number of members in each interval

Log normal distribution

- It is a skewed distribution when graphed using an arithmetic scale but a normal distribution when graphed using a logarithmic scale

Bland – Altman Analysis

- *It is a process used to assess agreement between 2 methods of measurement of the same characteristic*
- Important prerequisite is → 2 methods measuring same characteristic use same scale of measurement.
- Primary application → To compare a new measurement technique/method with a gold standard

Survival or Life Table Analysis

- It is used to measure a defined outcome in a population (or sample), followed over a variable time period
- Subjects are entered independently and observed at different time periods and for varying length of time
- Subjects lost to follow up are included in analysis for the time period they were observed
- Contribution of each subject is weighted by the time under observation (measured in person years)
- Types:
  - Demographic or population life table → based on application of national or other age specific mortality data to a theoretical population
  - Cohort or clinical life table → based on data obtained from an observed or studied sample. Each subject has a known initial point and a well defined endpoint of observation with dichotomous outcome (Alive or dead)

Kaplan Meier method of analysis of clinical Cohort–provides nonparametric estimate of cumulative incidence for defined outcomes based on incomplete observations

Cronbach's α (alpha) is a measure of *internal consistency or reliability.* Alpha varies from 0 to 1.

Cronbach's α	≥ 0.9	0.9 > α ≥ 0.8	0.8 > α ≥ 0.7	0.7 > α ≥ 0.6	0.6 > α ≥ 0.5	α < 0.5
Internal consistency	Excellent	Good	Acceptable	Questionable	Poor	Unacceptable

Spearman's Rank Correlation Coefficient [Rho]

It is used, if measurements are in terms of rank (not quantitative terms)

Rho = 1 – [(6x Σ d²) / n (n² – 1)] where d = difference in ranks of each pair of data, n= number of pairs of observation

- Value of **Rho** ranges between –1[Inverse or negative relationship] to + 1 [Positive relationship]
- Values between – 0.1 to – 0.3 and 0.1 to 0.3 indicate **weak relationship,** between – 0.3 to – 0.5 and 0.3 to 0.5 indicate **moderate relationship and** < – 0.5 and > 0.5 indicate **strong relationship**
- Application: To determine whether pairs formed for RCT are really matched

Regression Analysis

- is a mathematical model to describe the effect of ≥ 1 independent variable on a dependent variable
- **Linear regression:** Describes the effect of one independent variable on a dependent variable

  $y = a + bx$

  ['x' is independent and 'y' is dependent variable, b= regression coefficient, 'a' is y axis intercept (y for x=0)]
- **Multiple linear regression:** Describes effect of two or more independent variable on a dependent variable

  $y = a + b_1x_1 + b_2x_2 + b_nx_n$ [Here each dependent variable has its own regression coefficient]
- **Non linear:** Involves more complex mathematical forms, including logarithmic functions

Regression coefficient: Is average change in dependent variable for each unit of independent variable

Regression line: Approximation of relationship between independent variable and dependent variable

REVIEW QUESTIONS ON STATISTICS

1. **In a feedback survey patients rated a Hospital service as Very Satisfied/Satisfied/Dissatisfied/Very dissatisfied. Which Scale of measurement is used?**

(a) Nominal scale
(b) Ordinal scale
(c) Interval scale
(d) Ratio scale

Ans: (b) Ordinal scale

2. **All of the following are quantitative variables *except:***

(a) Serum Cholesterol
(b) Weight
(c) Blood pressure
(d) Gender

Ans: (d) Gender

3. **Blood group is an example for:**

(a) Interval scale data
(b) Ordinal scale data
(c) Categorical data
(d) None of the above

Ans: (c) Categorical data

4. **All of the following are measured in Ratio scale *except:***

(a) Serum HDL
(b) Temperature in Celsius
(c) Blood pressure
(d) Fasting Blood sugar

Ans: (b) Temperature in Celsius

5. **Platelet count is an example for:**

(a) Categorical variable (b) Discrete variable
(c) Continuous variable (d) Dichotomous variable

Ans: (b) Discrete variable

6. **Serum Potassium level is an example for:**

(a) Categorical variable (b) Discrete variable
(c) Continuous variable (d) Dichotomous variable

Ans: (d) Dichotomous variable

7. **Best method to plot the incidence of a disease over time is:**

(a) Histogram (b) Line Chart
(c) Scatter Diagram (d) Ogive

Ans: (b) Line Chart

8. **Graph that is used to correlate two Quantitative data is:**

(a) Histogram (b) Line Diagram
(c) Scatter Diagram (d) Frequency curve

Ans: (c) Scatter Diagram

9. **All of the following graphical methods can compare between two variables except:**

(a) Bar chart (b) Line Diagram
(c) Histogram (d) Scatter Diagram

Ans: (c) Histogram

10. **The following graph shows the number of dengue deaths in a district 'X' from the year 2001 to 2015. Identify the type of graph used for this data presentation:**

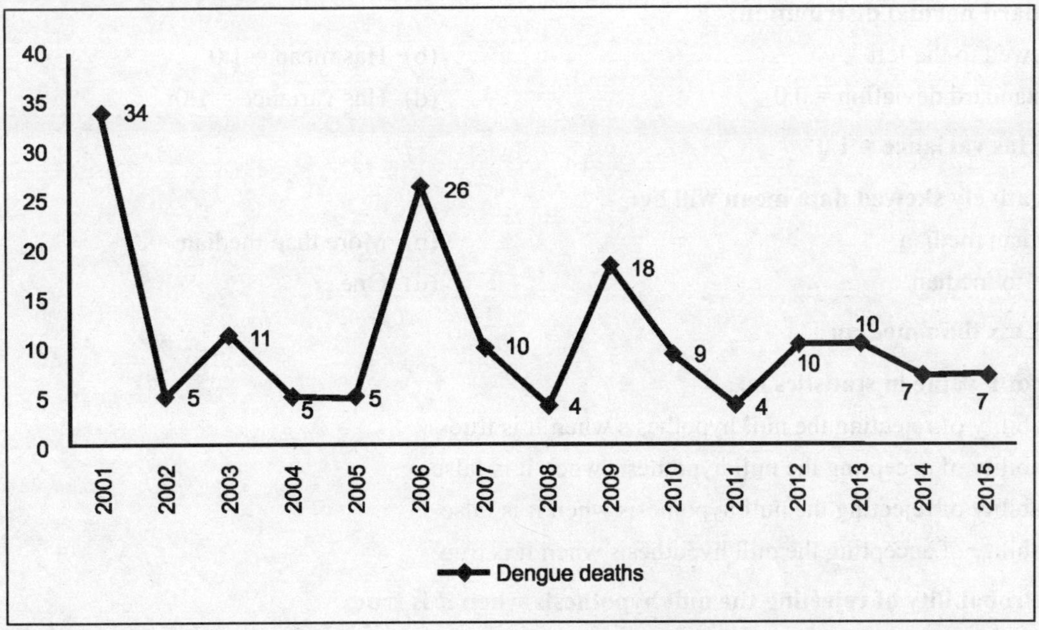

(a) Frequency polygon (b) Frequency curve
(c) OGIVE (d) Line diagram

Ans: (d) Line diagram

11. Median is useful in all the following variables *except:*

(a) BP (b) Survival

(c) Out of pocket expenditure (d) Type of Gastric carcinoma

Ans: (d) Type of Gastric carcinoma

12. Standard deviation is the measure of:

(a) Chance (b) Central tendency

(c) Deviation from mean value (d) None

Ans: (c) Deviation from mean value

13. While calculating the incubation period for measles in a group of 25 kids, standard deviation is 2 and the mean incubation period is 8 days, calculate standard error:

(a) 0.4 (b) 1.0

(c) 2.0 (d) 0.5

Ans: (a) 0.4

14. The Hb level in healthy women has mean 13.5 g/dl and standard deviation 1.5 g/dl, what is the Z score for a woman with Hb level 15.0 g/dl:

(a) 9.0 (b) 10.0

(c) 2.0 (d) 1.0

Ans: (d) 1.0

15. The mean Hb level of women in the reproductive age group was 11.5 g/dl. 95% confidence interval = 8.5 to 14.5 g/dl. Calculate the Standard Deviation:

(a) 1.5 (b) 2.0

(c) 2.5 (d) 3.0

Ans: (a) 1.5

16. The standard normal distribution:

(a) Is skewed to the left (b) Has mean = 1.0

(c) Has standard deviation = 0.0 (d) Has variance = 1.0

Ans: (d) Has variance = 1.0

17. For a negatively skewed data mean will be:

(a) Less than median (b) More than median

(c) Equal to median (d) One

Ans: (a) Less than median

18. Meaning of P value in statistics is:

(a) Probability of rejecting the null hypothesis when it is true

(b) Probability of accepting the null hypothesis when it is false

(c) Probability of rejecting the null hypothesis when it is false

(d) Probability of accepting the null hypothesis when it is true

Ans: (a) Probability of rejecting the null hypothesis when it is true

19. Type I sampling error is classified as:

(a) Alpha error (b) Beta error

(c) Gamma error (d) Delta error

Ans: (a) Alpha error

20. Type I Error statistical error occurs if:

(a) Rejecting the null hypothesis when it is true
(b) Accepting the null hypothesis when it is false
(c) Rejecting the null hypothesis when it is false
(d) Accepting the null hypothesis when it is true

Ans: (a) Rejecting the null hypothesis when it is true

21. Power of study can be increased by:

(a) Increasing alpha error
(b) Decreasing beta error
(c) Decreasing alpha error
(d) Increasing beta error

Ans: (b) Decreasing beta error

22. All are true about P-value *except:*

(a) Is the probability of committing Type-I error
(b) Is equal to 1–beta
(c) Is the chance that the presence of difference is concluded when actually there is none
(d) When P-value is less than a, the result is statistically significant

Ans: (b) Is equal to 1–beta

23. All are true *except:*

(a) Alpha is the maximum tolerable probability of type-I error
(b) Beta is the probability of type-II error
(c) When Null Hypothesis is true but is rejected, it is Type-II error
(d) P-value can be more or less than alpha

Ans: (c) When Null Hypothesis is true but is rejected, it is Type-II error

24. Statistical Power of a trial is equal to:

(a) 1 + alpha
(b) 1–beta
(c) Alpha + beta
(d) Alpha / beta

Ans: (b) 1–beta

25. The "P" value of a randomized controlled trial comparing operation A (new procedure) and Operation B (Gold standard) is 0.04. From this, we conclude that:

(a) Type II error is small and we can accept the findings of the study
(b) The probability of false negative conclusion that operation A is better than operation B, when in truth it is not, is 4%
(c) The power of study to detect a difference between operation A and B is 96%
(d) The probability of a false positive conclusion that operation 'Operation A is better that Operation B', when in truth it is not, is 4%

Ans: (d) The probability of a false positive conclusion that operation 'Operation A is better that Operation B', when in truth it is not, is 4%

26. After applying a statistical test, an investigator gets the 'P value' as 0.01. it means that:

(a) The probability of finding a significant difference is 1%
(b) The probability of declaring a significant difference is 1%
(c) The difference is not significant 1% times and significant 99% times
(d) The power of the test used is 99%

Ans: (c) The difference is not significant 1% times and significant 99% times

27. When we say that "the difference is significant", it means that:

(a) It is likely by chance and when P> 0.0.5
(b) It is unlikely by chance and when P > 0.05
(c) It is unlikely by chance and when P < 0.05
(d) It is likely by chance and when P < 0.05

Ans: (c) It is unlikely by chance and when P < 0.05

28. Pearson or Spearman coefficient is used for evaluation of:

(a) Differences in proportion
(b) Comparison of more than 2 means
(c) Comparison of variance
(d) Correlation

Ans: (d) Correlation

29. Appropriate statistical method to compare two means is:

(a) Chi-square test
(b) Student's t-test
(c) Odds Ratio
(d) Correlation Coefficient

Ans: (b) Student's t-test

30. Pearson or Spearman coefficient is used for evaluation of:

(a) Differences in proportion
(b) Comparison of more than 2 means
(c) Comparison of variance
(d) Correlation

Ans: (d) Correlation

31. In a study, variation in cholesterol was seen before and after giving a drug. The test which would give its significance is:

(a) Unpaired t-test
(b) Fischer test
(c) Paired t-test
(d) Chi-square test

Ans: (c) Paired t-test

32. A study was undertaken to assess the effect of a drug in lowering serum cholesterol levels. 15 obese women and 10 non-obese women formed the 2 limbs of the study. Which test would be useful to correlate the results obtained?

(a) ANOVA test
(b) Student's t-test
(c) Chi-square test
(d) Fischer test

Ans: (b) Student's t-test

33. Chi-square test is used to measure the degree of:

(a) Significance of difference between two proportions
(b) Regression between two variables
(c) Correlation between two variables
(d) Agreement between two observations

Ans: (a) Significance of difference between two proportions

34. Test of association between two qualitative variables is done by:

(a) Chi-square test
(b) Correlation
(c) Regression
(d) None

Ans: (a) Chi-square test

35. While applying a chi-square test, the degree of freedom was calculated to be 6. The possible contingency table could be a:

(a) 3 × 2 table
(b) 4 × 3 table
(c) 2 × 4 table
(d) 5 × 3 table

Ans: (b) 4 × 3 table

36. In a particular trial, the association of lung cancer with smoking is found to be 40% in one sample and 60% in another. What is the best test to compare the results?

(a) Chi-square test (b) Fischer test

(c) Paired t test (d) ANOVA test

Ans: (a) Chi-square test

37. ANOVA is used:

(a) To compare means in 2 groups (b) To compare means in 3 or more groups

(c) To compare means in 1 group before and after intervention (d) To find correlation

Ans: (b) To compare means in 3 or more groups

38. A study was done to compare the blood sugar levels of pan chewers and tobacco smokers. The mean blood sugar level of both the groups was more than their respective median. The appropriate test of significance to be used to compare the two groups would be:

(a) Independent t test (b) Paired t test

(c) Wilcoxons signed rank test (d) Wilcoxons rank sum test

Ans: (d) Wilcoxons rank sum test

39. The correlation between variables A and B in a study was found to be 1.1. This indicates:

(a) Very strong correlation (b) Moderately strong correlation

(c) Weak correlation (d) Computational mistake in calculating correlation

Ans: (d) Computational mistake in calculating correlation

40. Which of the following is not true about 'correlation'?

(a) It indicates degree of association between two characteristics

(b) Correlation coefficient of 1 means that the two variables exhibit linear relationship

(c) Correlation can measure risk

(d) Causation implies correlation

Ans: (c) Correlation can measure risk

41. If we know the value of one variable in an individual and wish to know the value of another variable, we calculate:

(a) Coefficient of correlation (b) Coefficient of regression

(c) SE of mean (d) Geometric mean

Ans: (b) Coefficient of regression

42. Which of the following is not true about 'correlation'?

(a) It indicates degree of association between two characteristics

(b) Correlation coefficient of 1 means that the two variables exhibit linear relationship

(c) Correlation can measure risk

(d) Causation implies correlation

Ans: (c) Correlation can measure risk

43. A coefficient of correlation value of "r = +0.8" indicates:

(a) Strong direct relationship between two variables (b) Strong inverse relationship between two variables

(c) Insignificant association between two variables (d) One variable is the cause of the other variable

Ans: (a) Strong direct relationship between two variables

44. Correlation in height and weight are measured by:

(a) Coefficient of variation (b) Range of variation

(c) Correlation coefficient (d) None

Ans: (c) Correlation coefficient

45. As the injected Insulin Units level increases the blood sugar level decreases. This is an example for:

(a) Positive correlation (b) Negative correlation

(c) Bidirectional (d) Zero correlation

Ans: (b) Negative correlation

46. Strong correlation is signified by a correlation coefficient of:

(a) Zero (b) 1

(c) Less than 1 (d) More than 1

Ans: (b) 1

47. Total Cholesterol level = a + b (calorie intake) + c (physical activity) + d (body mass index); is an example of:

(a) Simple linear regression (b) Simple curvilinear regression

(c) Multiple linear regression (d) Multiple logistic regression

Ans: (c) Multiple linear regression

48. An investigator finds out that 5 independent factors influence the occurrence of a disease. Comparison of multiple factors that are responsible for the disease can be assessed by:

(a) ANOVA (b) Multiple linear regression

(c) Chi-square test (d) Multiple logistic regression

Ans: (c) Chi-square test

49. Test used to compare Kaplan-Meier survival curve:

(a) ANOVA (b) Bland Altmann analysis

(c) Chi-square test (d) Cox proportional hazards test

Ans: (d) Cox proportional hazards test

50. A Gastro-surgeon wants to compare the survival data of colon cancer patients following three different surgical procedures. Which is the most appropriate statistical test for comparing the survival data of these 3 groups of patients?

(a) Log-Rank Test (b) Kruskal Wallis test

(c) Conditional proportional hazards regression model (d) Cox proportional hazards regression model

Ans: (d) Cox proportional hazards regression model

51. Sensitivity is defined as:

(a) True positive/True positive+True negative (b) True positive/True positive+False negative

(c) True negative/False positive+True negative (d) True negative/True negative+False negative

Ans: (b) True positive/True positive+False negative

52. Diagnostic power of test is reflected by:

(a) Sensitivity (b) Specificity

(c) Predictive value (d) Population attributable risk

Ans: (c) Predictive value

53. Predictive accuracy of screening test depends on:

(a) Sensitivity (b) Specificity
(c) Prevalence (d) All of the above

Ans: (d) All of the above

54. If the cutoff point in interpretation of test is raised one of the following may occur:

(a) Sensitivity decrease and Specificity increase (b) Sensitivity increase and Specificity decrease
(c) Sensitivity and Specificity both increase (d) Sensitivity and Specificity both decrease

Ans: (a) Sensitivity decrease and Specificity increase

55. Amount of previously unrecognized disease that is diagnosed as a result of screening effort is:

(a) Predictive value (b) Yield
(c) Prevalence (d) Surveillance

Ans: (b) Yield

56. Ideal screening test should have all except:

(a) High sensitivity (b) Low specificity
(c) High yield (d) High specificity

Ans: (b) Low specificity

57. Correlation between variables A and B in a study was found to be 1.1. This indicates:

(a) Very strong correlation (b) Moderately strong correlation
(c) Weak correlation (d) Computational mistake in calculating correlation

Ans: (d) Computational mistake in calculating correlation

58. Major purpose of randomization in a clinical trial is:

(a) Facilitates double blinding
(b) Help ensure study objects are representative of general population
(c) Ensure groups are comparable on base-line characteristics
(d) Reduce selection bias in allocation to treatment

Ans: (d) Reduce selection bias in allocation to treatment

59. In RCT, Single blind trial is so planned that:

(a) Participant is not aware whether he belongs to study group
(b) Participant is not aware whether he belongs to study group or control group
(c) Participant is aware whether he belongs to study group
(d) Participant is aware whether he belongs to study group or control group

Ans: (b) Participant is not aware whether he belongs to study group or control group

60. When a drug is evaluated for its usefulness in controlled conditions, it is termed as trial signifying?

(a) Efficacy (b) Effectiveness
(c) Efficiency (d) Effect modification

Ans: (a) Efficacy

61. Case control study is not characterized by:

(a) Cases with disease are compared to control without disease
(b) Assessment of past exposure may be biased
(c) Definition of cases may be difficult
(d) Incidence rates may be computed directly

Ans: (d) Incidence rates may be computed directly

62. First becoming sick in an epidemic is called as:

(a) Index case (b) Primary case
(c) First case (d) Contact case

Ans: (b) Primary case

63. In the context of epidemiology following are important criteria for making causal interference *except:*

(a) Strength of association (b) Consistency
(c) Coherence of association (d) Predictive value

Ans: (d) Predictive value

64. Denominator for calculating Positive predictive value is:

(a) True positive + False negative (b) False positive + True negative
(c) True positive + False positive (d) True negative + False negative

Ans: (c) True positive + False positive

65. Z score is used in:

(a) Nominal data (b) Normal distribution curve
(c) t test (d) Chi square test

Ans: (b) Normal distribution curve

66. Which of the following statements is correct with regard to confidence limits?

(a) Smaller the confidence level, wider the interval
(b) Lesser variable our data, wider is confidence interval
(c) Width of confidence interval is independent of sample size
(d) Confidence interval for 95% is wider than 80%

Ans: (d) Confidence interval for 95% is wider than 80%

67. Sampling method that provides greatest number of possible samples:

(a) Simple random sample (b) Systematic random sample
(c) Stratified random sample (d) Cluster sampling

Ans: (a) Simple random sample

68. Time interval between reception of infection and maximum infectivity of host is known:

(a) Generation time (b) Serial interval
(c) Latent period (d) Median incubation period

Ans: (a) Generation time

69. Which of the following denotes Pearsons skewness coefficient?

(a) Mode-Mean/SD (b) Mean-Mode/SD
(c) SD/Mode-Mean (d) Mean-Mode/SD

Ans: (b) Mean-Mode/SD

70. An investigator concluded that presence or absence of live factors determine disease condition. Which of the following would be most appropriate next study to determine if any of these five factors are independent precursors of disease?

(a) Multiple linear regression analysis
(b) Multiple logistic regression analysis
(c) ANOVA
(d) Kruskal Wallis Analysis of ranks

Ans: (a) Multiple linear regression analysis

71. A population is divided into relevant subgroups and random sample selection is done from each of the subgroups. This is which type of sampling method?

(a) Systematic random sampling
(b) Stratified random sampling
(c) Simple random sampling
(d) Cluster sampling

Ans: (b) Stratified random sampling

72. By giving equal time for interviewing control and cases which of following bias is avoided?

(a) Selection bias
(b) Berkesonian bias
(c) Measurement bias
(d) Confounding bias

Ans: (c) Measurement bias

73. Incidence can be calculated by:

(a) Case control study
(b) Prospective study
(c) Retrospective study
(d) Cross-sectional study

Ans: (b) Prospective study

74. Standard error is:

(a) SD/n
(b) SDxn
(c) SD/2n
(d) SD/square root of n

Ans: (c) SD/2n

75. Increase in confidence limit causes:

(a) No insignificant change
(b) Significant change
(c) No change
(d) Change from significant to non-significant

Ans: (d) Change from significant to non-significant

76. L-J chart is for:

(a) Accuracy
(b) Positivity
(c) Sensitivity
(d) Specificity

Ans: (a) Accuracy

77. If we reject hypothesis when it is actually true, it is known as:

(a) Type 1 error
(b) Type 2 error
(c) Power
(d) Specificity

Ans: (a) Type 1 error

78. A graphical presentation of frequency distribution for grouped data for a continuous variable is known as:

(a) Simple bar diagram
(b) Histogram
(c) Component bar diagram
(d) Line diagram

Ans: (b) Histogram

79. Time interval between first possible detection and final critical point is known as:

(a) Median incubation period
(b) Screening time
(c) Generation time
(d) Minimum incubation period

Ans: (b) Screening time

80. Comparision of value obtained and a predetermined objective is done by:

(a) Evaluation
(b) Monitoring
(c) Input-output analysis
(d) Network analysis

Ans: (a) Evaluation

81. Kaplan Meier method is for:

(a) Survival
(b) Incidence
(c) Prevalence
(d) Frequency

Ans: (a) Survival

82. Graph showing relationship between 2 variables is:

(a) Frequency polygram
(b) Histogram
(c) Scatter diagram
(d) Pictogram

Ans: (c) Scatter diagram

83. Non-parametric test used to compare three/more independent groups of sampled data:

(a) Chi-square test
(b) F test
(c) Kruskal Wallis test
(d) McNemar test

Ans: (c) Kruskal Wallis test

84. Difference between mean of two samples is tested by:

(a) Chi-square test
(b) Pie test
(c) T test
(d) F Test

Ans: (c) T test

85. Measure of central tendency that is most affected by extreme score in a sample distribution is:

(a) Median
(b) Mode
(c) Standard deviation
(d) Mean

Ans: (d) Mean

86. Area under 2SD of normal curve is:

(a) 66%
(b) 95%
(c) 97%
(d) 99%

Ans: (b) 95%

87. Measurement of blood pressure is which type of data:

(a) Nominal
(b) Ordinal
(c) Interval
(d) Continuous

Ans: (d) Continuous

88. Method used for comparison of a new test with an available gold standard test is:

(a) Regression analysis/Likelihood test
(b) Correlation analysis/Bland and Altmann test
(c) Baltin and Altimore method
(d) Kimorov and Samletor technique

Ans: (b) Correlation analysis/Bland and Altmann test

89. For a negatively skewed data mean will be:

(a) Less than median
(b) More than median
(b) Equal to median
(d) One

Ans: (a) Less than median

90. Matching is done for removal of:

(a) Bias
(b) Known confounding
(c) Unknown confounding
(d) Known confounding + Unknown confounding

Ans: (b) Known confounding

91. The most important measure to establish a causal relationship is:

(a) Consistency
(b) Temporality
(c) Biological plausibility
(d) Dose-response relationship

Ans: (b) Temporality

92. Hawthorne effect is seen in:

(a) Case-control study
(b) Cohort study
(c) Cross-sectional study
(d) Retrospective cohort study

Ans: (b) Cohort study

93. Mammography has 90% sensitivity and 98% specificity for breast carcinoma. What is probability that a woman breast carcinoma remains undiagnosed for 2 consecutive years (examination)?

(a) 1/10
(b) 2/10
(c) 1/100
(d) 2/100

Ans: (c) 1/100

94. Which of the following statements regarding research is not true?

(a) A cross-sectional study is one where a series of patients with a particular disease or condition are compared with matched control patients
(b) Type 1 error is when benefit is perceived when really there is none (false positive)
(c) Randomised trials are essential for testing new drugs
(d) It is a common practice to set the level of power for the study at 80 per cent with 5 percent significance level

Ans: (a) A cross-sectional study is one where a series of patients with a particular disease or condition are compared with matched control patients

95. Retrospective evaluation of medical performance is known as:

(a) Medical audit
(b) Medical evaluation
(c) Performance evaluation
(d) Professional screening

Ans: (a) Medical audit

96. All are methods of survival analysis *except:*

(a) Kaplan Meier
(b) Kruskal Wallis
(c) Actuarial method
(d) Survival rate

Ans: (b) Kruskal Wallis

97. In a population of 10,000 people, prevalence of disease is 20%. Sensitivity of screening test is 95%. Specificity is 80%. Positive predictive value of test is:

(a) 54.3%
(b) 47%
(c) 17%
(d) 98.3%

Ans: (a) 54.3%

98. There are 10,000 cases studied with 20% diseased. Sensitivity is 85% and specificity is 80% What will be the positive predictive value?

(a) 51.5%
(b) 47%
(c) 17%
(d) 97%

Ans: (a) 51.5%

99. The fundamental principles of leadership are:

(a) Vision and willingness
(b) Command and control
(c) Time management and mentoring
(d) Coaching, pacesetting and democratic

Ans: (a) Vision and willingness

100. Which of the following measures doesn't contribute to frailty?

(a) Impaired cognition
(b) One or more falls in past 6 months
(c) Osteoporosis
(d) Hematocrit <35%

Ans: (a) Impaired cognition

PART NINE: LATEST PATTERN QUESTIONS

CHAPTER 69 LATEST PATTERN QUESTIONS AND MISCELLANEOUS

1. **A patient had several episodes of syncope, blurred vision, profuse sweating, lethargy. Blood test show hypoglycemia and USG shows mass in epigastrium. Most likely diagnosis is:**

   (a) Metastatic brain tumor (b) Insulinoma
   (c) Pheochromocytoma (d) Meningioma

   Ans: (b) Insulinoma

2. **A 55-year-old male with prostate cancer is treated with goserelin. Which of the following agents is the best choice for adjunctive therapy in this patient's treatment regimen?**

   (a) Dexamethasone (b) Estrogen
   (c) Dutasteride (d) Flutamide

   Ans: (d) Flutamide

3. **A 33-year-old female presents with pain in the lower abdomen. She says the pain has been ongoing for the past 2 months and she feels full in the lower pelvic area. At times, she has had difficulty holding urine and has been constipated. X-rays and bloodwork are unremarkable. Needle aspiration of the mass reveals clear fluid from the left ovary, which measures 7 cm. The fluid has no evidence of malignancy. She most likely has which of the following conditions?**

   (a) Endometrioma (b) Tubo-ovarian abscess
   (c) Serous cystadenoma (d) Cystic teratoma

   Ans: (c) Serous cystadenoma

4. **A 17-year-old male presents with a tender mass in his leg. He has had general malaise for 3 months. A leg X-ray reveals a mass with an "onion layering" pattern. A biopsy shows a small, round, blue cell tumor. What is the best treatment for this patient?**

   (a) Surgical resection alone (b) Surgery followed by radiation
   (c) Preoperative chemotherapy followed by surgery (d) Chemotherapy alone

   Ans: (c) Preoperative chemotherapy followed by surgery

5. **A 75-year-old male presents with gross hematuria which has been a recurrent problem for the last 6 months. The patient has a history of prostate cancer treated with external radiation therapy 5 years ago. The hematuria has been so severe that the patient has required blood transfusion and was treated with formalin chemical fulguration of the bladder. On cystoscopy, a diagnosis of radiation cystitis has been documented. What is the best next treatment?**

   (a) Recommend cystectomy with diverting urostomy
   (b) Alum cauterization of the bladder
   (c) Irrigation catheter with instilling of cold normal saline at zero degree–Celsius
   (d) Hyperbaric oxygen therapy at 2.4 ATA for 90 minutes for 30 to 40 treatments

   Ans: (d) Hyperbaric oxygen therapy at 2.4 ATA for 90 minutes for 30 to 40 treatments

6. **A 71-year-old female presents with a 2-month history of weight loss, jaundice, vague abdominal pain and itching. She has recently been diagnosed with diabetes mellitus type 2. Physical exam reveals vague abdominal pain, skin excoriations, and a positive Courvoisier sign. Which one of the following would contraindicate surgery in this patient?**
(a) Age greater than 70 years
(b) Positive nodes adjacent to head of the pancreas
(c) Invasion of superior mesenteric vein
(d) An unknown 2 cm satellite lesion in the liver

Ans: (d) An unknown 2 cm satellite lesion in the liver

7. **A 65-year-old male with no significant past medical history present with complaints of a 6-week history of diarrhea and abdominal cramping. He denies nausea, vomiting, or hematochezia, but endorses a 12-pound weight loss. The physical examination is remarkable for flushing of the face, bilateral expiratory wheezes and a right-sided systolic murmur. Twenty-four-hour urine testing reveals elevated levels of 5-hydroxyindoleacetic acid. Abdominal CT reveals a mass in the tip of the appendix. What is indicated by the presence of these findings?**
(a) Presence of tumor in the appendix only
(b) Tumor invasion through the serosa of the appendix
(c) Metastasis of tumor to the liver
(d) Tumor production of dopamine

Ans: (c) Metastasis of tumor to the liver

8. **A 49-year-old male with fatigue and easy bruising is found to have terminal deoxynucleotidyl transferase (TdT) positive cells in the blood. He may have which of the following conditions?**
(a) Acute myelogenous leukemia
(b) Hodgkin lymphoma
(c) Hairy cell leukemia
(d) Acute lymphoblastic leukemia

Ans: (d) Acute lymphoblastic leukemia

9. **Select the true statement about prostate cancer:**
(a) Surgery is better suited to younger patients without spread
(b) Metastatic disease is not treatable
(c) Radical prostatectomy has a much higher cure rate than radiation therapy
(d) Radiation therapy has a much higher cure rate than radical prostatectomy

Ans: (a) Surgery is better suited to younger patients without spread

10. **A 36-year-old man with colon cancer was treated with a chemotherapy regimen consisting of leucovorin, fluorouracil, oxaliplatin and a drug with side effects of impaired wound healing, hemorrhage, and gastrointestinal perforation. Which of the following drugs best fit this description?**
(a) Irinotecan
(b) Panitumumab
(c) Bevacizumab
(d) Trastuzumab

Ans: (c) Bevacizumab

11. **A 77-year-old male presents with a weakened urinary stream, weight loss and fatigue. A rectal exam is done which reveals a 2 cm hard nodule. Biopsy shows a transitional cell malignancy. What feature in the patient's medical history may be a clue to this particular malignancy?**
(a) A male who has anal sex with another male
(b) Prior pelvic radiation
(c) Hormonal therapy
(d) Living in Asia

Ans: (b) Prior pelvic radiation

12. **A 33-year-old female presents with significant abdominal distension over the past 3 months. She also has become short of breath and has no exercise endurance. She has no idea how all this happened. Her health was excellent before. She is single, does not smoke, drink alcohol, or use illicit drugs. Ultrasound of the pelvis reveals large, solid mass in the left ovary and ascites. A chest X-ray reveals a large, right-sided pleural effusion. The fluid cytology is negative for a malignancy. What is the most likely diagnosis?**
(a) Ovarian fibroma
(b) Ovarian thecoma
(c) Brenner tumor
(d) Ovarian adenocarcinoma

Ans: (a) Ovarian fibroma

13. A 68-year-old woman being treated for stage three ovarian cancer is referred to the hyperbaric oxygen treatment facility by her oncologist. She has hemorrhagic cystitis secondary to radiation treatment and her oncologist feels that hyperbaric oxygen would facilitate healing. Part of her current treatment strategy includes doxorubicin. How soon can she start hyperbaric oxygen therapy?

(a) Immediately

(b) She must wait at least 3 days from her last dose of doxorubicin

(c) She must wait 6 months

(d) She is no longer a candidate for hyperbaric oxygen therapy due to doxorubicin use

Ans: (b) She must wait at least 3 days from her last dose of doxorubicin

14. A 49-year-old female notices a red, scaly rash on her left breast, which has been present for the past eight weeks. She denies any symptoms and reports applying a hydrocortisone cream. The exam reveals no mass. However, a biopsy reveals large, clear cells at the dermal-epidermal junction. The mucin staining is positive. Which of the following is true?

(a) Similar condition may be located on the vulva or penis
(b) Lesions are usually not painful
(c) Lesions usually ulcerate
(d) Rarely associated with ductal carcinoma

Ans: (a) Similar condition may be located on the vulva or penis

Paget's disease

15. A 77-year-old male presents with low back pain. Lumbar spine X-rays reveals a combination of blastic and lytic lesions at L3-L4. Which of the following should be done next for this patient?

(a) MRI of spine
(b) Digital rectal exam
(c) Complete blood count and calcium
(d) Bone scan

Ans: (b) Digital rectal exam

16. A 55-year-old male presents after a course of radiation therapy for squamous cell carcinoma of the tongue with a non-healing oral lesion and exposed bone. When gathering information, what is a highly influential factor for an increased incidence of osteoradionecrosis of the mandible?

(a) Prophylactic antibiotics were held during radiotherapy
(b) Total radiation dose less than 6,000 rads (cGy)
(c) A tooth extraction one month before starting radiotherapy
(d) Total radiation dose greater than 7,000 rads (cGy)

Ans: (d) Total radiation dose greater than 7,000 rads (cGy)

17. A male patient present with flushing and diarrhea. Physical exam shows nodular hepatomegaly that is demonstrated by CT to be multiple metastases with a 2 cm mass in the ileum. A 24-hour collection for 5-HIAA is elevated. Which of the following treatments is not appropriate?

(a) Octreotide
(b) Iterferon-alpha
(c) Phenoxybenzamine
(d) Diphenhydramine

Ans: (c) Phenoxybenzamine

18. Which of the following is evidence of extracapsular spread of cancer on MRI of the prostate?

(a) Focal capsular bulge

(b) Irregular capsular bulge

(c) Asymmetry or frank invasion of neurovascular bundles

(d) All of the above

Ans: (d) All of the above

19. A patient with bone cancer is being treated with a long-acting morphine formula. He presents with vague complains of abdominal distension, nausea, hard stools and straining. The working diagnosis is that he may have developed opioid-induced constipation. The Bristol stool form scale is used to characterize his constipation. What criteria does it use to assess constipation?

(a) Stool size
(b) Stool color
(c) Stool shape
(d) Stool weight

Ans: (c) Stool shape

British stool scale

20. Acrokeratosis neoplastica most commonly is associated with which condition?

(a) Systemic lupus erythematosus
(b) Diabetes mellitus type 1
(c) Squamous cell carcinoma of the upper respiratory and digestive tracts
(d) Previous diagnosis of malignant melanoma

Ans: (c) Squamous cell carcinoma of the upper respiratory and digestive tracts

21. You are on the oncology floor and a patient with renal failure is being treated with several chemotherapeutic agents. The oncologist asks you to order the drug, glucarpidase, after the cancer medications have been given. What is the reason for administering glucarpidase?

(a) It prevents hemorrhagic cystitis
(b) It reduces cardiomyopathy
(c) Inactivates methotrexate
(d) Replenishes the bone marrow

Ans: (c) Inactivates methotrexate

Glucarpidase inactivates methotrexate

22. A 70-year-old white male status post radiation therapy (6600 cGy) for prostate cancer 5 years previously has developed rectal bleeding and discomfort thought to be secondary to radiation proctitis. The patient has not responded to sucralfate or sulfasalazine. What is the most appropriate next step in this patient's evaluation and treatment?

(a) Colonscopy
(b) Rectal biopsy
(c) Hyperbaric oxygen therapy
(d) Diverting colostomy

Ans: (c) Hyperbaric oxygen therapy

23. A child presents with a yellow-orange, hairless scalp lesion with a pebbly surface. Which of the following secondary carcinomas may develop in the lesion later in life?

(a) Basal cell carcinoma
(b) Squamous cell carcinoma
(c) Merkel cell carcinoma
(d) Melanoma

Ans: (a) Basal cell carcinoma

Basal cell carcinoma–Pebbly surface

24. A 47-year-old male presents to the clinic with symptoms of episodic hypertension, palpitations, headaches, tachycardia and sweating. His symptoms are not present at the time of examination. The metabolites of which of the following are most likely to be present following a 24-hour urine sample?

(a) Serotonin
(b) Insulin
(c) Metanephrine
(d) Vasoactive intestinal peptide

Ans: (c) Metanephrine

25. A 65-year-old male was treated for acute lymphocytic leukemia with multiple chemotherapeutic agents. One month after the therapy was stopped, he presents to the emergency department with complaints of abdominal pain, nausea, vomiting and fatigue. His blood work reveals elevated levels of amylase and lipase. The ultrasound is unremarkable. What is the agent most likely responsible for his condition?

(a) 6-mercaptopurine
(b) Doxorubicin
(c) Methotrexate
(d) Asparaginase

Ans: (d) Asparaginase

26. **A 3-year-old child who had a hematopoietic stem cell transplant 3 months ago and now has a right septic knee joint. The fungal culture grew Fusarium. What is the antifungal of choice?**

(a) Ketoconazole
(b) Griseofulvin
(c) Nystatin
(d) Amphotericin

Ans: (d) Amphotericin

Amphotericin intravenous–Broad Spectrum

27. **Examination of a 53-year-old female with alcohol use disorder reveals cirrhosis and mild ascites (Child-Pugh A). She has an alpha-fetoprotein level of 1340 mg/mL. An MRI identified multinodular, enhancing lesion in the liver of more than 50% with characteristic features of a hepatocellular carcinoma and portal vein thrombosis. The patient is classified as grade 1 on the Eastern Cooperative Oncology Group (ECOG) scale and stage N1. What should be the initial approach?**

(a) Consider hepatobiliary surgery referral for partial liver resection
(b) Consider transplant surgery referral for orthotopic liver transplantation
(c) Consider interventional radiology referral for transarterial chemoembolization
(d) Consider oncology referral for sorafenib

Ans: (d) Consider oncology referral for sorafenib

28. **A 56-year-old female is found to have an asymptomatic thyroid nodule and is euthyroid. Fine needle biopsy shows follicles that resemble normal thyroid tissue but after excision, a fibrous capsule with focal invasion is identified. The tumor cells show PAX-PPAR gamma fusion gene. What is the most probable diagnosis?**

(a) Follicular carcinoma
(b) Medullary thyroid carcinoma
(c) Papillary thyroid carcinoma
(d) Anaplastic thyroid carinoma

Ans: (a) Follicular carcinoma

29. **Birt-Hogg-Dube syndrome has been associated with carcinoma of which of the following?**

(a) Liver
(b) Pancreas
(c) Kidney
(d) Thyroid

Ans: (c) Kidney

30. **A 65-year-old male presented with a cough and hemoptysis for 4 weeks. CT showed 1.5 cm right upper lobe lesion and normal-sized lymph nodes. PET-CT showed fludeoxyglucose (FDG) uptake in the mass and right hilar lymph node. What is the next step in his care?**

(a) Do preoperative clearance for surgery
(b) Refer to oncology
(c) Perform convex probe endobronchial ultrasound sampling of hilar lymph node
(d) Perform convex probe endobronchial ultrasound sampling of mediastinal and hilar lymph nodes

Ans: (d) Perform convex probe endobronchial ultrasound sampling of mediastinal and hilar lymph nodes

31. **A 22-year-old female presents to the dermatology office with the concern of multiple firm, white papules clustered on her low back that she first notices several months ago. They are asymptomatic and not changing. She has no other medical conditions but does report that her father has similar lesions on his nose and neck as well as a family history of renal cell carcinoma. Which of the following genes may possible be responsible for her condition?**

(a) TSC2
(b) PTEN
(c) FLCN
(d) CYLD

Ans: (c) FLCN

Birt Hugg Dube syndrome

32. A patient is started on a chemotherapeutic agent for a malignancy. The patient develops a hemolytic anemia with uremic syndrome. Which of the following is the most likely drug that caused these conditions?

(a) Mitomycin
(b) Cyclosporine
(c) Cyclophosphamide
(d) Azathioprine

Ans: (a) Mitomycin

33. A patient is being evaluated for a nonhealing wound in an irradiated field. He had squamous cell carcinoma of the neck and received 8000 Gy of radiation along with chemotherapy 12 months ago. Which historical chemotherapy agent would be most concerning for the development of pulmonary fibrosis during a course of hyperbaric oxygen therapy?

(a) Adriamycin
(b) Bleomycin
(c) Cis-platinum
(d) Doxyrubicin

Ans: (b) Bleomycin

34. A 15-year-old female presents with increased snoring and difficulty articulating, which she attributes to her tongue. She states that her tongue has slowly enlarged over the last 5 weeks. Her tongue appears to be enlarged, although it does not protrude from her mouth and has no visually obvious lesions. She denies trauma to the tongue. Given her presentation, which of the following is the most likely etiology for her enlarging tongue?

(a) Down syndrome
(b) Hyperthyroidism
(c) Lymphagioma
(d) Lymphoma

Ans: (c) Lymphagioma

Cystic Hygroma

35. A 67-year-old female complains of a pruritic rash of her genitals. Exam shows an erythematous, well-demarcated lesion that involves most of the labia majora. Biopsy shows clusters of large, anaplastic cells infiltrating the epidermis with increased cytoplasm separating them from normal cells. The anaplastic cells stain for mucin. What is the most probable diagnosis?

(a) Sarcoma botryoides
(b) Extramammary Paget disease
(c) Clear cell adenocarcinoma
(d) Bowen disease

Ans: (b) Extramammary Paget disease

36. A woman whose mother was diagnosed with breast cancer in her 50's undergoes initial screening mammogram and calcifications associated with a single unilateral BI-RADS 4 lesion are identified. She elects to undergo stereotactic biopsy, and the breast biopsy cores are sent to pathology for examination. A solitary focus of atypical ductal hyperplasia with associated calcifications is the only abnormality reported. What would be the most likely recommended subsequent treatment due to this finding?

(a) Bilateral radical mastectomy
(b) Surveillance only
(c) Repeat mammogram in one to three years
(d) Excisional lumpectomy

Ans: (d) Excisional lumpectomy

37. A 55-year-old female presents with lower abdominal pain, bloating, and pain during sexual intercourse. She has had spotty bleeding for a few months but believed it was just a part of her postmenopausal phase. She undergoes a pelvic ultrasound which reveals a solid ovarian mass with well-defined margins. A needle biopsy reveals large cells shaped like a signet ring and mucoid degeneration. What is the next step in her management?

(a) Upper endoscopy
(b) Bilateral oophorectomy and hysterectomy
(c) Chemotherapy followed by radiation
(d) Danazol

Ans: (a) Upper endoscopy

38. Carcinoembryonic antigen (CEA) describes glycoproteins involved in cell adhesion. CEA is produced in grastrointestinal tissue during fetal development, and production stops before birth. CEA is low in healthy adults blood. The serum levels are elevated in some types of cancer, which means that it can be used as a tumor marker. Which of the following is not true in regards CEA?

(a) Well-differentiated tumors secrete more CEA

(b) CEA is more elevated in organ-confined tumors than in those involving lymph node and distant metastasis

(c) Tumors that cause bowel obstruction produce higher CEA levels

(d) CEA can help distinguish between adenocarcinoma of the lung and mesothelioma

Ans: (b) CEA is more elevated in organ-confined tumors than in those involving lymph node and distant metastasis

39. Which of the following is true in regards to the carcinoembryonic antigen?

(a) CEA is used as a screening test for early detection of caner

(b) CEA is elevated in hypothyroidism

(c) Left-sided tumors have higher CEA levels

(d) Diploid tumors have higher levels of CEA than aneuploid tumors

Ans: (c) Left-sided tumors have higher CEA levels

40. A 60-year-old farmer presents with several lesions on his head, neck and nose. He says he has had these skin lesions for many years but they do not seem to be going away. He has been a farmer all his life and has no other pertinent medical history. On physical exam you note two lesions that appear waxy and have a central depression. The edges have a pearly appearance. Excisional biopsy reveals a malignancy. If this lesion occurred on the eye, which is the most common site of involvement?

(a) Upper eyelid

(b) Lateral canthus

(c) Medial canthus

(d) Conjunctiva

Ans: (c) Medial canthus
Basal Cell Carcinoma–Pearly Appearance

41. Which of the following is not an indication for a prostate MRI?

(a) Staging of biopsy-proven prostate cancer

(b) Previously treated prostate cancer with rising prostate-specific antigen (PSA) to assess for recurrence

(c) Screening for prostate cancer in patients with elevated PSA

(d) Elevated PSA and negative biopsy

Ans: (c) Screening for prostate cancer in patients with elevated PSA

42. A 54-year-old housewife discovered a lump in her left breast accidentally when she was showering. Clinically, it is a 2 × 3 cm lump that is mobile and firm. No palpable axillary swellings. Mammography reveals granular microcalcifications with normal architecture. True-cut biopsy shows fibroadenosis with areas of large abnormal nuclei with no basement membrane invasion. What is the appropriate treatment?

(a) Modified radical mastectomy

(b) Breast-conserving surgery (BCS) with sentinel lymph node biopsy (SLNB)

(c) Follow up with tamoxifen

(d) Simple mastectomy followed by radiotherapy

Ans: (b) Breast-conserving surgery (BCS) with sentinel lymph node biopsy (SLNB)

43. Based on the National Comprehensive Cancer Network (NCCN) guidelines, which of the following patients should not be offered genetic testing for hereditary breast and ovarian cancer syndrome?

(a) A 61-year-old woman who develops infiltrating ductal carcinoma which is triple negative

(b) A 44-year-old woman who develops infiltrating ductal carcinoma which is estrogen and progresterone receptor positive

(c) A 61-year-old woman who was previously diagnosed with ovarian cancer and who develops infiltrating ductal carcinoma

(d) A 44-year-old woman with whose father had breast cancer and who develops infiltrating ductal carcinoma which is estrogen receptor positive

Ans: (a) A 61-year-old woman who develops infiltrating ductal carcinoma which is triple negative

44. A 49-year-old female presents with complaints of a mass just below her ear. She noticed it this past weekend while showering. She denies any trauma and is on no medications. On exam, the mass is firm but feels irregular on the surface. A fine needle aspiration biopsy is read as pleomorphic adenoma. Which of the following is considered to be a risk factor for this malignancy?

(a) Diet (b) Radiation exposure

(c) Alcohol (d) Smoking

Ans: (b) Radiation exposure

Pleomorphic adenoma has risk of malignant transformation on radiation exposure (risk factor)

45. An 85-year-old female is brought to the emergency department for confusion. Her family reports she has become depressed and is talking to her long-dead husband. She complains of abdominal, back and hip pain with constipation. The neurological exam is non-focal. The cardiopulmonary exam is unremarkable. There is a 3-centimeter, fixed breast mass. What is the most likely ECG finding?

(a) Flattened T waves (b) Prolonged QT interval

(c) Shortened QT interval (d) Peaked T waves

Ans: (c) Shortened QT interval

Breast cancer leads to hyperclacemia- Shortened QT interval

46. A patient undergoes a workup for low-grade fever, weight loss and general malaise. Blood studies reveal the presence of cells positive for tartrate-resistant acid phosphatase. He most likely has which of the following conditions?

(a) Hodgkin lymphoma (b) Multiple myeloma

(c) Acute lymphoblastic leukemia (d) Hairy cell leukemia

Ans: (d) Hairy cell leukemia

47. Which is not a feature of prostate cancer with bony metastases?

(a) Elevated alkaline phosphatase (b) Elevated prostate-specific antigen

(c) Elevated acid phosphatase (d) Elevated levels of parathyroid hormone

Ans: (d) Elevated levels of parathyroid hormone

48. A young female who has always been shy about participating in sports because of her body appearance presents to the plastic surgeon. She states that ever since she was a child, her right upper arm and breast were not well developed compared to the left side. She denies any major functional ability but feels very conscious of the fact that her right breast is much smaller than the left breast. Examination reveals that she has marked hypoplasia of the right upper chest and breast and also has upper limb abnormalities. The chest X-ray reveals ipsilateral hyperlucent hemithorax. During follow-up of this patient, which type of malignancy can occur?

(a) Breast cancer (b) Osteogenic sarcoma

(c) Lymphoma (d) Basal cell cancer

Ans: (c) Lymphoma

Hematological syndromes occur at high rate in Poland syndrome

49. A 65-year-old G2P2 female with a past medical history of hypertension presents to the breast clinic for evaluation of an "itchy rash" involving her right breast. She has been on hormone replacement therapy for symptomatic management of hot flashes since 49 years of age. She has no family history of breast or ovarian cancer and has received annual mammograms since 50 years of age. Her last breast imaging was 10 months ago and was negative for suspicious findings. On further questioning, she admits to the presence of a coarse-textured, itchy rash of her right nipple for the past four months that has now spread to the areola. She was treated for eczema with topical steroids by her primary care provider with no relief, so has now been referred to the breast clinic for evaluation. She denies nipple discharge but occasionally notes some blood inside her bra that she attributes to the skin irritation. On examination, the right nipple and entire areola are reddened, with a dry, thickened, peeling appearance. A small, 1 cm fixed mass in the ten O'clock position approximately 1 cm from the edge of the areola is present. A small amount of bloody fluid can be expressed from the nipple. Which of the following is the most likely diagnosis?

(a) Refractory atopic dermatitis (b) Paget disease of the breast

(c) Benign fibroadenoma (d) Breast cellulitis

Ans: (b) Paget disease of the breast

50. An 84-year-old male presents with an eyelid lesion that was diagnosed as a seborrheic keratosis. When you ask him if he has any other skin lesion on his body, he tells you that over the past few months he has developed about 50 similar lesions on his abdomen. What is this finding called?

(a) Troisier-sign (b) Leser-Trelat sign

(c) Trousseau sign (d) Levine sign

Ans: (b) Leser Trelat sign

Paraneoplastic sign associated with Gastric adenocarcinoma

51. What does the presence of AR-V7 (androgen receptor splice variant-7 messenger RNA) detected in circulating tumor cells in patients with castrate-resistant prostate cancer indicate?

(a) Resistance to enzalutamide (b) Resistance to abiraterone acetate

(c) Resistance to both enzalutamide and abiraterone acetate (d) Sensitivity to both enzalutamide and abiraterone acetate

Ans: (c) Resistance to both enzalutamide and abiraterone acetate

52. The late development of malignancy in wounds and scars has been found to occur in which situation?

(a) Burn scar (b) Solar radiation

(c) X-ray injury (d) Hand fracture

Ans: (a) Burn scar

Marjolin's Ulcer

53. Which of the following is a viral protein that induces tumors by binding to a cellular tumor suppressor protein?

(a) Epstein-Barr nuclear antigen proteins (b) Hepatitis B virus e protein

(c) Adenovirus E1A (d) Human immunodeficiency virus gas protein

Ans: (c) Adenovirus E1A

54. Which of the following medications is found to be helpful in patients with familial adenomatous polyposis?

(a) Indomethacin (b) Celecoxib

(c) Diclofenac (d) Naproxen

Ans: (b) Celecoxib

COX2 INHIBITOR

55. A patient starts a chemotherapeutic agent. He later develops a "pins and needles" feeling in his legs. Which medication is most likely to have caused this effect?

(a) Chlorhexidine (b) Cyclophosphamide
(c) Prednisone (d) Vincristine

Ans: (d) Vincristine

Peripheral Neuropathy

56. A 3-year-old boy is brought in by his mother after she was giving him a bath and noticed a mass in his abdomen. She reports no significant past medical history. The child is quiet on examination. There is a palpable abdominal mass in the left quadrant, which does not cross the midline. It is not pulsatile but firm. Tenderness is elicited on deep palpation. Urine shows a trace amount of blood. What is the most likely diagnosis?

(a) Pheochromocytoma (b) Wilms' tumor
(c) Neuroblastoma (d) Lymphoma

Ans: (b) Wilms' tumor

Hematuria and Doesn't Cross Midline

57. To lower the risk of neutropenia and infection induced by alkylating agents and platinum-containing chemotherapeutic agents, what drug do oncologists often administer to patients at the same time?

(a) Allopurinol (b) Folinic acid
(c) Vitamin C (d) Amifostine

Ans: (d) Amifostine

58. After undergoing a mastectomy, a 55-year-old female is found to have injury to the long thoracic nerve. Which of the following is the most common result?

(a) Inability to shrug her shoulders (b) Inability to comb her hair
(c) Winging of scapula (d) Shortness of breath

Ans: (c) Winging of scapula

59. A 44-year-old female is found to have a very large left breast that has been increasing in size over the past 3 months. Biopsy reveals a huge mass measuring 8 cm. The microscopy reveals fibrous stromal proliferation with an epithelial lining. What is the most likely diagnosis?

(a) Intraductal carcinoma (b) Fat necrosis
(c) Papilloma (d) Phyllodes tumor

Ans: (d) Phyllodes tumor

60. What is the most common side effect of anti-endothelial growth factor receptor (EGFR) agents?

(a) Gastrointestinal distress (b) Hair loss
(c) Fatigue and muscle weakness (d) Skin rash

Ans: (d) Skin rash

Photosensitivity

61. What is the mechanism of action of vinca alkaloids?

(a) Inhibition of DNA synthesis (b) Inhibition of RNA synthesis
(c) Inhibition of purine synthesis (d) Inhibition of function of microtubules

Ans: (d) Inhibition of function of microtubules

62. Which of the following is treated with bupropion?

(a) Smoking cessation (b) Multiple personality disorder
(c) Bipolar disorder (d) Alcohol withdrawal

Ans: (a) Smoking cessation

63. Which is not a risk factor for lung cancer?

(a) Radon
(b) Asbestos
(c) Tobacco
(d) Alcohol

Ans: (d) Alcohol

64. Which layer of bowel must colon cancer cross in order to spread?

(a) Mucosa
(b) Muscularis mucosa
(c) Adventitia
(d) Endothelial layer

Ans: (b) Muscularis mucosa

65. Which of the following statements about cystadenoma of the ovary is false?

(a) Increases risk for cystadenoma of the pancreas
(b) Is a common benign tumor
(c) Are unilocular and contain straw-colored fluid
(d) Is totally different from serous carcinoma of the ovary

Ans: (a) Increases risk for cystadenoma of the pancreas
No relation to pancreas (Cystadenoma means Serous cystadenoma)

66. Which of the following about glioblastoma multiforme is FALSE?

(a) Men are affected more than women
(b) Seizures occur as presenting symptoms in many patients
(c) Prognosis with treatment has remained unchanged over the last decade
(d) Hemorrhagic transformation is not uncommon within tumors

Ans: (c) Prognosis with treatment has remained unchanged over the last decade

67. Which of the following molecular abnormalities is associated with anaplastic astrocytoma?

(a) p53 suppressor on 17p 13.1
(b) Neurofibromin
(c) N-myc oncogene
(d) CDKN2 suppressor

Ans: (d) CDKN2 suppressor

68. A 54-year-old presents with a history of deep seated burning pain around his wrists, hands, knees and ankles. On examination, he is most tender around his wrists and ankles. X-rays of distal lower extremities reveal hypertrophic osteoarthropathy. Which of the following is the most likely diagnosis?

(a) Rheumatoid arthritis
(b) Osteoarthritis
(c) Cancer of the lung
(d) Syphilis

Ans: (c) Cancer of the lung
HPOA–Paraneoplastic syndrome of Carcinoma Lung

69. Which factor is not associated with an increased risk of gastric cancer?

(a) Salt-preserved, smoked and cured foods
(b) N-nitroso compounds in cigarette-tobacco smoke
(c) Alcohol consumption
(d) Rubber, tin and coal exposure

Ans: (c) Alcohol consumption

70. What is the most common mass in the minor salivary glands?

(a) Warthin tumor
(b) Basal cell carcinoma
(c) Adenoid cystic carcinoma
(d) Pleomorphic adenoma

Ans: (c) Adenoid cystic carcinoma

71. **Which of the following is a specific clinical sign suggestive of renal cell carcinoma?**
(a) Deep vein thrombosis (b) Right varicocele
(c) Lower extremity edema (d) Flank pain

Ans: (b) Right varicocele

72. **Which of the following is most commonly used to treat metastatic prostate cancer?**
(a) Surgery (b) Leuprolide
(c) Spironolactone (d) Steroids

Ans: (b) Leuprolide

73. **Which of the following is not an absolute contraindication for conservative breast therapy?**
(a) Estrogen/progresterone receptor-positive tumor (b) Two tumors are located in different quadrants
(c) Diffuse microcalcifications that appear malignant (d) Prior breast radiation

Ans: (a) Estrogen/progresterone receptor-positive tumor

74. **Which of the following viruses is implicated as a cause of nasopharyngeal carcinoma?**
(a) Cytomegalovirus (b) Epstein-Barr virus
(c) Human herpes virus 8 (d) Varicella zoster virus

Ans: (b) Epstein-Barr virus

75. **Where are psammoma bodies are seen?**
(a) Glioblastoma (b) Pituitary adenoma
(c) Ependymoma (d) Meningioma

Ans: (d) Meningioma

76. **A 66-year-old female presents with increasing bilateral shoulder and hip weakness that has been progressing over the last 3 months. Relevant medical history includes a diagnosis of breast cancer six months prior. What is her most likely diagnosis?**
(a) Myasthenia gravis (b) Metastatic breast cancer
(c) Post-polio syndrome (d) Dermatomyositis

Ans: (d) Dermatomyositis
Paraneoplastic Syndrome Associated with Breast Cancer

77. **Which of the following has not been implicated as a cause of liver cancer?**
(a) Smoking (b) Primary biliary cirrhosis
(c) Androgen steroids (d) Oral contraceptives

Ans: (a) Smoking

78. **What is the most common heart tumor in patients with tuberous sclerosis?**
(a) Myxoma (b) Rhabdosarcoma
(c) Fibroma (d) Rhabdomyoma

Ans: (d) Rhabdomyoma

79. **A 17-year-old male presents with continuous pain in his right leg for about 3 months. He has lost some weight and has constant pain. An X-ray reveals a mass with a "moth-eaten" appearance in the distal femur. What is the likely diagnosis?**
(a) Giant cell (b) Osteogenic sarcoma
(c) Ewing sarcoma (d) Prostate metastases

Ans: (c) Ewing sarcoma

Moth eaten/Onion skin appearance–Ewing's sarcoma

80. Which of the following types of cancer has the worst prognosis if it spreads to the brain?

(a) Kidney
(b) Breast
(c) Malignant melanoma
(d) Uterus

Ans: (c) Malignant melanoma

81. Which is true about gastric lymphomas?

(a) It is most common extra nodal size
(b) It is never associated with H. Pylori
(c) Radical surgery is preferred treatment
(d) Diagnosis can be made by CT scan

Ans: (a) It is most common extra nodal size

82. Which of the following clinical syndromes is most commonly associated with a thymoma?

(a) Myasthenia gravis
(b) Aplastic crises
(c) Carcinoid syndrome
(d) Cushing's syndrome

Ans: (a) Myasthenia gravis

83. Of all the following, which has the best response to radiation therapy?

(a) Mesothelioma
(b) Non-small cell carcinoma of the lung
(c) Squamous cell carcinoma of the esophagus
(d) Cervical carcinoma of the esophagus

Ans: (d) Cervical carcinoma of the esophagus

84. Which of the following women is least likely to develop a second primary breast cancer?

(a) Premenopausal women
(b) Women with initial diagnosis of lobular carcinoma *in situ*
(c) Women over the age of 80
(d) Women with a BRCA gene

Ans: (c) Women over the age of 80
Younger female higher chance of 2nd primary

85. A 53-year-old female with a history of migraines with aura presents with numbness on the left side of her chin for 3 weeks. Which diagnostic test is most likely to provide the diagnosis?

(a) Echocardiogram
(b) Mammogram
(c) MRI of the cervical spine
(d) Serum calcium

Ans: (c) MRI of the cervical spine
Leptomeningeal Metastasis of Carcinoma Breast

86. What is the most common malignancy causing inferior vena cava syndrome?

(a) Melanoma
(b) Renal cell carcinoma
(c) Colon cancer
(d) Liver adnocarcinoma

Ans: (b) Renal cell carcinoma
Obstruction of IVC

87. What is the most serious complication of multiple myeloma?

(a) Fractures
(b) Hypercalcemia
(c) Renal failure
(d) Spinal cord compression

Ans: (d) Spinal cord compression

88. A 56-year-old female complains of general malaise and headaches. She says she has palpitations, diaphoresis, and is very anxious all the time. She has noticed that her headaches can be very severe at times and are throbbing in nature. Her past medical history is unremarkable. She says her deceased sister had very high blood pressure. On physical exam, you discover that she has a blood pressure of 230/110 mm Hg and a pulse of 110 beats per minute. On her oral mucosa you also discover a number of soft nodules which are non-tender. Further work reveals that she has a white blood cell count of 7, hemoglobin of 11.2, platelet count of 325,000, and a calcium of 11.9. You become concerned and decide to further evaluate the patient. Which of the following is most appropriate for further evaluation of this patient?

(a) Renal scan
(b) Calcitonin levels
(c) Endoscopy to look for ulcer disease
(d) CT scan of the abdomen

Ans: (b) Calcitonin levels

MEN 2 Syndrome

89. Lymphatic drainage from cancer of the esophagus does not usually spread to which group of lymph nodes?

(a) Axillary
(b) Cervical
(c) Mediastinal
(d) Celiac

Ans: (a) Axillary

90. A papillary lesion of the shaft of the penis is excised. Histology shows epithelial cells with clear vacuolization that extend into underlying tissue broadly. Select the most probable diagnosis:

(a) Verrucous carcinoma
(b) Condyloma acuminatum
(c) Pyoderma vegetans
(d) Squamous cell carcinoma

Ans: (a) Verrucous carcinoma

91. The anti-cancer drug, doxorubicin, is associated with which of the following?

(a) Cardiomyopathy
(b) Pulmonary fibrosis
(c) Tuberculosis
(d) Renal cyst

Ans: (a) Cardiomyopathy

92. The translocation of the myc gene (t8:14) is usually seen in:

(a) Mycosis fungoides
(b) Nodular sclerosis B lymphoma
(c) Burkitt lymphoma
(d) Multiple myeloma

Ans: (c) Burkitt lymphoma

93. Which of the following is a component of the Li Fraumeni syndrome?

(a) Sarcoma
(b) Breast cancer
(c) Leukemia
(d) All of them

Ans: (d) All of them

94. Which of the following statements about squamous cell cancers is false?

(a) Only about 10 percent arise in the periphery
(b) Forms large pools of keratin
(c) Can often be diagnosed by sputum cytology
(d) Superior sulcus tumors are always squamous cell in origin

Ans: (d) Superior sulcus tumors are always squamous cell in origin

95. Which of the following neoplastic drug often used to treat seminomas works by inhibiting topoisomerase II?

(a) Cisplatin (b) Ciprofloxacin

(c) Etoposide (d) Cyclophosphamide

Ans: (c) Etoposide

96. Retroperitoneal leiomyosarcoma:

(a) Is the most common primary retroperitoneal malignancy (b) Is more common in men

(c) Peaks in the 50-60 years age group (d) Can originate from the wall of the IVC

Ans: (d) Can originate from the wall of the IVC

97. Which is NOT a risk factor for colon cancer?

(a) Family history (b) Excess fat consumption

(c) Inadequate folate intake (d) High fiber diet

Ans: (d) High fiber diet

98. Which anti-cancer drug is frequently applied topically for actinic keratosis and superficial skin cancers?

(a) Interferon (b) Azathioprine

(c) Fluorouracil (d) Cyclophosphamide

Ans: (c) Fluorouracil

99. Fine needle aspiration can confirm a diagnosis in all thyroid disorders *except* which of the following?

(a) Hurthle cell cancer (b) Pupillary cancer

(c) Anaplastic cancer (d) Medullary cancer

Ans: (a) Hurthle cell cancer

100. What is a common presentation of post-transplant lymphoproliferative disorder?

(a) Fever (b) Weight loss

(c) Cervical node enlargement (d) Anorexia

Ans: (c) Cervical node enlargement

101. What is the second most common histology of prostate cancer?

(a) Transitional (b) Squamous cell

(c) Adenocarcinoma (d) Melanoma

Ans: (a) Transitional

102. Which tumor is known to produce Schiller-Duval bodies?

(a) Seminoma (b) Leydig cell tumor

(c) Medullary cancer (d) Endodermal sinus tumor

Ans: (d) Endodermal sinus tumor

103. A female has been complaining of vague abdominal pain for a few weeks. She has been taking a laxative to relieve her constipation but now has severe bone pain. In the emergency room she is found to have a first-degree heart block and her stools are positive for blood. An upper gastrointestinal series reveals multiple shallow ulcers in the antrum. Further testing should be directed at which part of the body?

(a) Neck (b) Chest

(c) Abdomen (d) Urine

Ans: (a) Neck

Bones...stones…groans,….moans

Parathyroid Adenoma

104. Which of the following cancers has the worst prognosis?

(a) Hodgkin lymphoma
(b) Choriocarcinoma
(c) Basal cell carcinoma
(d) Actinic keratosis

Ans: (b) Choriocarcinoma

105. A 42-year-old Chinese man present with several months history of aural fullness and decreased hearing in the left ear. The patient relocated to the United States from Hong Kong at age 12 years. He is otherwise healthy, but he smokes approximately half a pack of cigarettes each day and drinks socially. Examination is significant for decreased mobility in the left tympanic membrane and a bulging mass in the left lateral nasopharyngeal wall behind the torus. Which of the following tests or procedures is NOT appropriate at this initial workup?

(a) Blood test for immunoglobulin A (IgA) antibodies to viral capsid antigen
(b) Biopsy of the nasopharyngeal mass obtained in the office
(c) Positron emission tomography (PET) scan
(d) MRI with gadolinium and fat suppression of the nasopharynx

Ans: (b) Biopsy of the nasopharyngeal mass obtained in the office

106. What is the most ominous significance of leukocoria?

(a) Fungal infection
(b) HIV
(c) Retinoblastoma
(d) Melanoma

Ans: (c) Retinoblastoma

107. A 65-year-old female diabetic reports a 6 months history of right upper quadrant pain decreased by leaning forward. She has recurrent superficial thrombophlebitis and jaundice. What is the most probable diagnosis?

(a) Pancreatic carcinoma
(b) Cirrhosis secondary to viral hepatitis
(c) Carcinoma of the ampulla of Vater
(d) Choledocholithiasis

Ans: (a) Pancreatic carcinoma

108. Which tumor in adults is most likely to metastasize to the brain?

(a) Melanoma
(b) Lung cancer
(c) Breast cancer
(d) Genitourinary cancers

Ans: (b) Lung cancer

109. Which of the following statements about criteria in Duke classification of colorectal cancer is FALSE?

(a) Liver metastases
(b) Tumor not extending through the submucosa
(c) Tumor penetrating the bowel wall without lymph node involvement
(d) Tumor is highly differentiated

Ans: (d) Tumor is highly differentiated

110. Which of the following disorders is associated with increased risk of breast cancer?

(a) Chronic mastitis
(b) Intraductal papilloma
(c) Atypical hyperplasia
(d) Phyllodes tumor

Ans: (c) Atypical hyperplasia

111. A 45-year-old male presents with a small, elevated lesion on his scalp. The lesion appears red with a smooth shiny surface and a central crater that appears like a horn. He reports that the lesion developed rather quickly over the past few weeks and is painless. What is the most likely diagnosis?

(a) Squamous cell cancer
(b) Keratoacanthoma
(c) Melanoma
(d) Actinic keratosis

Ans: (b) Keratoacanthoma

Central Crater

112. Onion skinning on a bone radiograph is indicative of which condition?

(a) Osteogenic sarcoma
(b) Chondroma
(c) Ewing's sarcoma
(d) Osteoma

Ans: (c) Ewing's sarcoma

113. Cytogenetic analysis reveals that patients with primitive neuroectodermal tumors have which of the following translocations that involve the EWS gene?

(a) t(22;11)
(b) t(21;22)
(c) t(7;22)
(d) All of the above

Ans: (a) t(22;11)

114. In glioblastoma multiforme, what is the most consistent chromosomal abnormality?

(a) Gain of chromosome 17p
(b) Gain of chromosome 7
(c) Loss of chromosome 1p
(d) Loss of chromosome 11p

Ans: (b) Gain of chromosome 7

115. What is the most common type of bladder cancer after infection with Schistosomiasis haematobium?

(a) Transitional cancer
(b) Squamous cells
(c) Adenocarcinoma
(d) Carcinoma *in situ*

Ans: (b) Squamous cells

116. Which is not a gastric cancer protective factor?

(a) Wine consumption
(b) High consumption of fiber, fruit and vegetables
(c) Aspirin and non-steroidal anti-inflammatory drugs
(d) Histamine-2-receptors antagonist and proton pump inhibitors

Ans: (d) Histamine-2-receptors antagonist and proton pump inhibitors

Wine has no proven association with Gastric cancer. Few studies of UK showed there is reduction of gastric cancer relatively

117. Chemoprevention is a proven strategy in which of the following conditions?

(a) Prostate cancer
(b) Breast cancer
(c) Head and neck cancer
(d) Lung cancer

Ans: (b) Breast cancer

118. A 58-year-old male is admitted with a resectable non-small cell carcinoma of the lung. Metastatic workup revealed a large, localized left adrenal mass. A needle biopsy of the adrenal gland was inconclusive for tumor. What is the next step?

(a) Proceed with surgery of the lung
(b) Proceed with removal of adrenal
(c) Send the patient for chemotherapy
(d) Resect both the lung and adrenal mass

Ans: (d) Resect both the lung and adrenal mass

119. Which is the most common hormone or hormone-like substance produced by pulmonary carcinoma?

(a) Adrenocorticotropic hormone (ACTH) or ACTH-like substance
(b) Antidiuretic hormone
(c) Gonadotropin
(d) Parathormone

Ans: (a) Adrenocorticotropic hormone (ACTH) or ACTH-like substance

120. A 24-year-old male presents with multiple painless, rubbery, enlarged cervical nodes. For the past few weeks, he has also been complaining of fever, night sweats, weight loss and generalized itching. Biopsy of the nodes reveals cellular infiltrates with large nuclei. Which of the following is the most likely diagnosis?

(a) Multiple myeloma
(b) Sarcoid
(c) Hodgkin disease
(d) Tuberculosis

Ans: (c) Hodgkin disease

121. A 66-year-old male with a history of chronic cigarette smoking presents with weight loss and frequent chest infections. Chest X-ray and CT scan reveal a centrally located lung mass. Laboratory test show hyponatremia. Which lung cancer is the most likely cause?

(a) Small cell
(b) Squmous
(c) Adenocarcinoma
(d) Bronchial carcinoid

Ans: (a) Small cell

Small Cell Carcinoma–Highest Smoking Association and Secretes ADH

122. A young male presents with osteogenic sarcoma and metastates to the lung. What is the most appropriate treatment?

(a) Complete radical resection
(b) Complete research followed by chemotherapy
(c) Chemotherapy
(d) Chemotherapy followed by complete resection

Ans: (d) Chemotherapy followed by complete resection

123. Which of the following molecular abnormalities is associated with WHO Grade II astrocytoma?

(a) Tubulin
(b) p53 suppressor on 17p13.1
(c) N-myc oncogene
(d) Neurofibromin

Ans: (b) p53 suppressor on 17p13.1

124. An elderly, febrile patient suffering from weight loss and fatigue has small, firm violaceous nodules, which are shown on biopsy to contain myelogenous blasts. These findings suggest which hematologic conditions?

(a) Acute monocytic leukemia
(b) Hodgkin lymphoma
(c) Non-Hodgkin lymphoma
(d) Chronic myeloid leukemia

Ans: (a) Acute monocytic leukemia

Leukemia Cutis–Most commonly associated with AML

125. Which finding is least characteristic of complete hydatidiform moles?

(a) Hypertension
(b) Dark vaginal bleeding
(c) Hyperemesis
(d) Hypothyroidism

Ans: (d) Hypothyroidism

126. Which is true about thyroid cancer?

(a) Usually will present with hyperthyroidism

(b) Fine needle aspiration biopsy is adequate to make diagnosis of all thyroid cancers

(c) Mass is always hard and palpable

(d) Can present with a cold nodule

Ans: (d) Can present with a cold nodule

127. Which of the following is a risk factor for prostate cancer?

(a) A blood relative affected with the disease (b) Smoking

(c) Alcoholism (d) Benign prostatic hyperplasia

Ans: (a) A blood relative affected with the disease (Highest risk)

128. Which of the following modalities offers the highest cure rate for recurrent non-melanoma skin cancers of the lip?

(a) Cryotherapy (b) Excision

(c) Mohs micrographic surgery (d) Radiation

Ans: (c) Mohs micrographic surgery

129. What is the recommended treatment for stage II adenocarcinoma of the lung?

(a) Surgical resection (b) Chemoradiotherapy

(c) Hospice (d) All of the above

Ans: (a) Surgical resection

130. Which of the following medications is typically avoided in patients with pheochromocytoma due to the risk of hypertensive crisis?

(a) Promethazine (b) Metoclopramide

(c) Haloperidol (d) Ondansetron

Ans: (b) Metoclopramide

131. Penile cancer generally occurs on which area of the penis?

(a) Prepuce (b) Foreskin

(c) Glans (d) Shaft

Ans: (c) Glans

132. Which of the following is produced by arrhenoblastoma?

(a) Estrogens (b) Androgens

(c) Follicle stimulating hormone (d) Luteinizing hormone

Ans: (b) Androgens

133. Which of the following choices is true of familial polyposis coli?

(a) Polyps are present at birth (b) Polyps are not found in small bowel

(c) Colon cancer usually develops by age 35-40 (d) Upper endoscopy is not used to detect polyps

Ans: (c) Colon cancer usually develops by age 35-40

134. Which parotid gland tumor has a tendency to invade along nerves?

(a) Pleomorphic adenoma (b) Warthin's

(c) Lymphomas (d) Adenoid cystic

Ans: (d) Adenoid cystic

135. Which of the following malignancies is not associated with asbestosis exposure?

(a) Colon cancer
(b) Testicular cancer
(c) Mesothelioma
(d) Esophageal cancer

Ans: (b) Testicular cancer

136. Which of the following is true about juvenile nasopharyngeal angiofibroma (JNAs)?

(a) JNAs commonly present with epistaxis and almost never clacify
(b) JNAs almost never present with epistasis or classify
(c) JNAs commonly present with epistaxis and commonly calcify
(d) JNAs almost never present with epistaxis and commonly clacify

Ans: (a) JNAs commonly present with epistaxis and almost never clacify

137. What is the most common presentation of a patient with uterine cancer?

(a) Pain
(b) Vaginal bleeding
(c) Dysuria
(d) Painful intercourse

Ans: (b) Vaginal bleeding

138. A 65-year-old male retired pipefitter is concerned about the prior long history of asbestos exposure. He has smoked a pack a day for 45 years. His physical exam is essentially normal. There are pleural plaques but no other findings on the chest radiograph. Pulmonary function tests are normal. Select the incorrect statement:

(a) The patient is at no increased risk of mesothelioma due to smoking
(b) The patient is a higher risk for emphysema from smoking because of the asbestos exposure
(c) He has asbestosis
(d) The plaques on the chest radiograph indicate asbestos

Ans: (c) He has asbestosis

139. A 48-year-old man presents to the oncology clinic after biopsy proven gastric adenocarcinoma of the cardia with endoscopic ultrasound with invasion of the muscularis propia and negative fine needle aspiration of a suspicious 20 mm lymph node at the lesser curvature. What further recommendations will be considered not appropriate?

(a) Perform chest abdomen and pelvis computerized tomography to rule out metastatic disease and proceed with surgical resection if negative
(b) Perform chest, abdomen and pelvis computerized tomography to rule out metastatic disease and proceed with biopsy or paracentesis confirmation of solitary mass or ascites for malignancy suspicion
(c) Perform chest, abdomen and pelvis computerized tomorgraphy to rule out metastatic disease and proceed positron emission tomography combined with computerized tomography for resectale tumors
(d) Perform chest, abdomen and pelvis positron emission tomography combined with computerized tomography to rule out metastatic disease and proceed with staging laparoscopy with peritoneal cytology prior surgery

Ans: (a) Perform chest, abdomen and pelvis computerized tomography to rule out metastatic disease and proceed with surgical resection if negative

140. Which tumor markers are elevated with pure testicular seminomas?

(a) Beta-human chorionic gonadotropin (beta-hCG)
(b) Alpha-fetoprotein
(c) Lactate dehydrogenase (LDH)
(d) Beta-hCG and LDH

Ans: (d) Beta-hCG and LDH

141. Cerebrospinal fluid alpha-fetoprotein may be elevated in which of the following?

(a) Choroid plexus tumors
(b) Ependymomas
(c) Germ cell tumors
(d) Medulloblastomas

Ans: (c) Germ cell tumors

142. A 32-year-old male with AIDS has headaches followed right hemiparesis. MRI shows a left frontal white matter lesion that homogeneously enhances. What is the most likely tumor?

(a) Kaposi sarcoma
(b) Primary central nervous system lymphoma
(c) Metastatic carcinoma
(d) Glioblastoma multiforme

Ans: (b) Primary central nervous system lymphoma

143. In a patient with fibrous dysplasia, malignant transformation is most likely to occur when the lesion occurs in what part of the body?

(a) Femur
(b) Pelvis
(c) Craniofacial
(d) Tibia

Ans: (c) Craniofacial

144. What is the most common feature of bladder cancer?

(a) Dysuria
(b) Hematuria
(c) Flank pain
(d) Urgency of urination

Ans: (b) Hematuria

145. Which of the following is a tumor marker for nonseminoma testicular cancer?

(a) Alkaline phosphatase
(b) CA-125
(c) Carcinoembryonic antigen
(d) Alpha-fetoprotein

Ans: (d) Alpha-fetoprotein

146. Select the correct statement about primary central nervous system lymphoma imaging in patients with HIV:

(a) It is likely to show enhancement on MRI
(b) Initial imaging on MRI is likely to show multiple lesions
(c) Brain biopsy is very rarely needed to make the diagnosis
(d) The gold standard for diagnosis is magnetic resonance spectroscopy

Ans: (a) It is likely to show enhancement on MRI

147. Which of the following neoplastic drug is used in the treatment of seminomas and works by inhibiting topoisomerase II?

(a) Cisplatin
(b) Ciprofloxacin
(c) Etoposide
(d) Cyclophosphamide

Ans: (c) Etoposide

148. Which is true of human chorionic gonadotropin (hCG) levels after treatment of a molar pregnancy?

(a) Serum hCG levels rapidly drop and do not need to be followed
(b) Normal levels are usually reached in a week
(c) If hCG levels rise, then one may have metastatic disease
(d) Intervention is required when the hCG levels continue to fall

Ans: (c) If hCG levels rise, then one may have metastatic disease

149. What percent of prostatic carcinoma is found in the gland's posterior lobe?

(a) 25% (b) 40%

(c) 60% (d) 75%

Ans: (d) 75%

150. Which of the following clinical features of breast cancer is not associated with a poor prognosis?

(a) Erythema of skin (b) Peau d'orange

(c) Dermal lymphatic invasion (d) Nipple inversion

Ans: (d) Nipple inversion

151. Hereditary kidney cancers account for about 5 to 8 percent of all renal malignancies. Which of the following is not a disorder associated with hereditary renal cancer?

(a) Granulomatosis with polyangiitis syndrome (b) Von Hippel-Lindau

(c) Tuberous sclerosis (d) Lynch syndrome

Ans: (a) Granulomatosis with polyangiitis syndrome

152. Which of the following medications is less likely to cause significant bone marrow suppression?

(a) Cisplatin (b) Vincristine

(c) Cyclophosphamide (d) Methotrexate

Ans: (b) Vincristine

153. Where does renal cell cancer most commonly metastasize?

(a) Lungs (b) Bone

(c) Liver (d) Brain

Ans: (a) Lungs

154. A 24-year-old female with von Hippel-Lindau syndrome has a CT showing a right cerebellar cyst. Select the best management:

(a) Repeat CT in 3 months (b) Radiation therapy

(c) Surgical resection (d) Lumbar puncture to evaluate for parasitic infection

Ans: (c) Surgical resection

155. A patient present with a 3 cm lesion in the left upper lobe, which proved to be an adenocarcinoma. Since the patient had also been complaining of headaches, a CT scan revealed a 2 cm mass in the parietal lobe. Additional work up for metastatic disease was negative. What is the best management of this patient?

(a) Simultaneous radiation to the lung and cranial lesion

(b) Craniotomy followed by a lobectomy

(c) Lobectomy followed by a craniotomy

(d) Chemotherapy and radiation therapy

Ans: (b) Craniotomy followed by a lobectomy

156. Which condition is associated with aflatoxins?

(a) GI bleeding (b) Ovarian cancer

(c) Hepatocellular cancer (d) Esophageal cancer

Ans: (c) Hepatocellular cancer

157. A 50-year-old female with chronic hepatitis B presents with weight loss and jaundice. There is ascites and peripheral edema. Transaminases are 4 times normal and alkaline phosphatase is 250 U/L. Alpha fetoprotein is 7200 ng/mL and ultrasound shows a 4 × 5 cm mass in the lever. CT guided biopsy was done. What is the most probable diagnosis?

(a) Hepatocellular adenoma
(b) Hepatocellular carcinoma
(c) Metastatic colon cancer
(d) Hydatid cyst

Ans: (b) Hepatocellular carcinoma

158. Which of the following malignancies with bone metastases has the best 5-year survival rate?

(a) Lung
(b) Breast
(c) Thyroid
(d) Prostate

Ans: (c) Thyroid

159. Which of the following antineoplastic drugs is most likely responsible for peripheral neuropathy?

(a) Bleomycin
(b) Cisplatin
(c) Cyclophosphamide
(d) Vincristine

Ans: (d) Vincristine

160. A 71-year-old female with a history of smoking undergoes a CT scan, which reveals a 3-centimeter by 3-centimeter peripheral lesion in the lung. Biopsy reveals tall columnar cells which have invaded the normal lung tissue. What is the most likely diagnosis?

(a) Carcinoid
(b) Squamous cell
(c) Adenocarcinoma
(d) Metastic breast cancer

Ans: (c) Adenocarcinoma

161. A CT head of a 72-year-old man shows a right hemispheric mass with hyperostosis of the skull adjacent to the mass. He most likely has which of the following tumors?

(a) Glioblastoma multiforme
(b) Pituitary adenoma
(c) Metastatic lung cancer
(d) Meningioma

Ans: (d) Meningioma

162. Carcinoembryonic antigen is most likely to be significantly elevated in the serum of patients with:

(a) Pancreatitis
(b) Hepatitis
(c) Small cell lung cancer
(d) Colorectal cancer

Ans: (d) Colorectal cancer

163. A patient complaining of severe right hand and finger pain presents to you with an apical lung mass. Diagnosis of a superior sulcus tumor is made. Which nerve is most commonly associated with this syndrome?

(a) Median nerve
(b) Upper brachial plexus
(c) Radial nerve
(d) Ulnar nerve

Ans: (d) Ulnar nerve

164. From which of the following does a rhabdomyosarcoma originate?

(a) Fat tissue
(b) Subcutaneous tissue
(c) Striated muscle
(d) Smooth muscle

Ans: (c) Striated muscle

165. What is the principal etiologic factor of basal cell carcinoma (BCC)?

(a) UV-A radiation
(b) UV-B radiation
(c) UV-C radiation
(d) Ionizing radiation

Ans: (b) UV-B radiation

166. Which of the following is not found in neurofibromatosis type 2?

(a) Ependymoma (b) Optic glioma
(c) Meningioma (d) Schwannoma

Ans: (b) Optic glioma

167. For what medical disorder is a neurolytic celiac plexus block often performed?

(a) Peripheral vascular disease (b) Buerger disease
(c) Acute pancreatitis (d) Pancreatic cancer

Ans: (d) Pancreatic cancer

168. Which of the following cancers is associated with reciprocal translocation t(x: 18)?

(a) Osteogenic sarcoma (b) Ewing's sarcoma
(c) Multiple myeloma (d) Synovial sarcoma

Ans: (d) Synovial sarcoma

169. Which of the following is not a poor prognosticator for patients with breast cancer?

(a) Edema (b) Skin ulceration
(c) Peau d'orange (d) Bloody nipple discharge

Ans: (d) Bloody nipple discharge

170. Exposure to which heavy metal is known to increase risk of prostate cancer?

(a) Chromium (b) Cadmium
(c) Calcium (d) Cobalt

Ans: (b) Cadmium (NEET SS 2018)

171. Which of the following is the MOST common histology for a hypopharyngeal tumor?

(a) Adenocarcinoma (b) Lymphoma
(c) Squamous cell carcinoma (d) Verrucous carcinoma

Ans: (c) Squamous cell carcinoma

172. A 54-year-old smoker presents with a history of burning, deep-seated pain around his hands, wrists, knees and ankles. On examination, he is most tender around his wrists and ankles. X-ray of his distal lower extremities reveals hypertrophic osteoarthropathy. What is the most likely diagnosis?

(a) Rheumatoid arthritis (b) Osteoporosis
(c) Cancer of lung (d) Buerger disease

Ans: (c) Cancer of lung

173. A 45-year-old female noticed a lump in the lower, lateral quadrant of her right breast. The lump was removed and a frozen section showed it to be a carcinoma. The most likely pathway of spread of the lesion by lymphatics would be first to which of the following?

(a) Lymph nodes in the posterior triangle of the neck
(b) Lymph nodes in the anterior mediastinum
(c) The anterior or pectoral group of axillary lymph nodes
(d) The posterior or subscapular group of axillary lymph nodes

Ans: (c) The anterior or pectoral group of axillary lymph nodes

174. A 65-year-old non-smoking male present with 7-pound weight loss and profuse voluminous water sputum. He says he has only a dry cough and feels weak. Which of the following pathology may be responsible for his symptoms?

(a) Esophageal cancer (b) Achalasia
(c) Bronchoalveolar lung cancer (d) Carcinoid

Ans: (c) Bronchoalveolar lung cancer

175. In a female with breast cancer, it is decided to treat her with trastuzumab. What does this medication block?

(a) Estrogen receptors (b) Kras

(c) Her 2 (d) P52

Ans: (c) Her 2 (DNB SS 2016)

176. Which is true regarding multiple endocrine neoplasia syndromes (MEN syndromes)?

(a) Parathyroid tumors are more common in MEN 2A than in MEN 1

(b) Medullary cell carcinoma is the most common finding in patients with MEN 2A

(c) Lipomas are not associated with MEN 1

(d) Collagenomas are uncommon with MEN 1

Ans: (b) Medullary cell carcinoma is the most common finding in patients with MEN 2A

177. In telangiectatic osteosarcoma, which of the following morphologic changes suggests a good response to the preoperative neoadjuvant chemotherapy?

(a) Presence of osteoid and blood-filled lacunae

(b) Necrosis in more than 60 percent of the tumor cells

(c) Necrosis in more than 75 percent of the tumor cells

(d) Necrosis in more than 95 percent of the tumor cells

Ans: (d) Necrosis in more than 95 percent of the tumor cells

178. Which systemic syndrome least often accompanies mediastinal masses?

(a) Cushing syndrome (b) Myasthenia gravis

(c) Hypothyroidism (d) Hypertension

Ans: (c) Hypothyroidism

179. A 37-year-old undergoes a colonoscopic removal of a 3 cm sigmoid polyp. The pathology reveals a poorly differentiated carcinoma limited to the stalk with no lymphatic or vascular invasion. What is the next step in the management of this patient?

(a) Perform a sigmoid colectomy (b) Observation

(c) Chemotherapy followed by surgery (d) Radiation therapy

Ans: (a) Perform a sigmoid colectomy

180. For a malignant ulcerative lesion 1 cm in greatest dimension located in the floor of the mouth, what treatment modality provides the best outcome based on functional results?

(a) Chemotherapy (b) Electrodesiccation

(c) Radiation therapy (d) Surgical excision

Ans: (d) Surgical excision

181. For primary small cell carcinoma of the lung, what is the most common site for recurrence?

(a) Brain (b) Liver

(c) Bone (d) Mediastinum

Ans: (d) Mediastinum

182. Which of the following is the most common radiologic finding in postradiation sarcoma?

(a) Cortical bone destruction (b) Osteosclerosis

(c) Osteopenia (d) Mineralized soft-tissue mass

Ans: (a) Cortical bone destruction

183. Which medication is associated with pulmonary fibrosis?

(a) Aspirin
(b) Bleomycin
(c) Colchicine
(d) Isoniazid

Ans: (b) Bleomycin

184. In a 65-year-old with a ductal carcinoma *in situ* of left breast, what other treatment is administered besides a lumpectomy?

(a) Chemotherapy
(b) Radiation
(c) Axillary nodes dissection
(d) Bilateral mastectomy

Ans: (b) Radiation

185. Hormone replacement therapy is associated with which type of cancer?

(a) Ovarian
(b) Cervical
(c) Lung
(d) Breast

Ans: (d) Breast

186. Which of the following is not associated with intraepidermal carcinoma of the penis?

(a) Human papillomavirus
(b) Phimosis
(c) Aniline dye
(d) Smoking

Ans: (c) Aniline dye

187. Reduced ability to taste food is a common complaint in patients who take which drug?

(a) Aspirin
(b) Heparin
(c) Bleomycin
(d) Lithium

Ans: (c) Bleomycin

188. A 70-year-old male has biopsy of prostatic nodule that shows small glands with a single layer of epithelial cells and prominent, enlarged nucleoli. Which portion of the prostate has the highest incidence of the findings?

(a) Transitional zone
(b) Peripheral zone
(c) Central zone
(d) Anterior fibro-muscular zone

Ans: (b) Peripheral zone

189. With which of the following lesions is Cowden syndrome associated?

(a) Multiple harmartomas
(b) Multiple sebaceous cysts
(c) Multiple bullae
(d) Multiple subcutaneous abscess

Ans: (a) Multiple harmartomas

190. Which of the following has been associated with penile cancer?

(a) Phimosis
(b) Paraphimosis
(c) Balanitis
(d) Posthitis

Ans: (a) Phimosis

191. A 60-year-old man who smokes presents with a large, 4.5 cm tongue lesion. He has palpable lymph node in the right submandibular triangle. Which of the following is NOT part of the workup for this lesion?

(a) Biopsy of the lesion
(b) Chest radiograph
(c) Bone scan
(d) CT scan of the neck and oral cavity

Ans: (c) Bone scan

192. A young female presents with gross hematuria and weight loss. Work up reveals that she has a genetic disorder that makes her susceptible to several malignancies. Which of the following syndromes is associated with a high-risk of renal cell cancer?

(a) Tuberous sclerosis
(b) Von Hippel-Lindau
(c) Fitz-Hugh-Curtis
(d) Down syndrome

Ans: (b) Von Hippel-Lindau

193. Which is FALSE about brain tumors?

(a) Glioblastoma multiforme is an aggressive cancer
(b) Most common childhood brain tumor is medulloblastoma
(c) Brain tumors frequently spread to the systemic circulation
(d) In childhood, brain tumors typically are found in posterior fossa

Ans: (c) Brain tumors frequently spread to the systemic circulation (Best possible answer)

194. A 48-year-old female has a 3-month history of unilateral nipple discharge. Excisional biopsy shows nipple infiltration with large cell having clear cytoplasm. The cells occur in clusters and singly in the epidermis. Staining is diastase-resistant and PAS-positive. What is the most probably diagnosis?

(a) Inflammatory breast cancer
(b) Intraductal papilloma
(c) Mammary Paget's disease
(d) Mucinous carcinoma

Ans: (c) Mammary Paget's disease

195. A tumor between the celiac trunk and the superior mesenteric artery is most likely to compress which structure?

(a) Neck of pancreas
(b) Transverse colon
(c) Sigmoid colon
(d) Body of pancreas

Ans: (a) Neck of pancreas

196. A 60-year-old man presents with a 2-month history of an enlarged lymph node in the right neck. He is a longtime smoker of cigarettes and denies fever, nigh sweats, fatigue, or cough. On physical examination, there is a 1.5 cm hard, fixed mass below the angle of the mandible in the right neck. Which of the following is the most likely cause of an enlarged lymph node in the neck?

(a) Thyroglossal duct cyst
(b) Dermoid tumor
(c) Carotid body tumor
(d) Metastatic squamous cell carcinoma

Ans: (d) Metastatic squamous cell carcinoma

197. Which of the following gene mutations is implicated in familial or hereditary breast cancer?

(a) RET proto-oncogene
(b) RAS gene
(c) BRCA gene
(d) P53 gene

Ans: (c) BRCA gene

198. A 54-year-old male underwent to routine screening colonoscopy and found to have an invasive carcinoma with lymphovascular invasion at the base of one of three polyps removed. What is not recommended for his colon cancer evaluation?

(a) RAS/NRAS/BRAF mutational testing
(b) DNA mismatch repair (dMMR)/microsatellite instability (MSI) testing
(c) Carcinoembryonic antigen (CEA)
(d) Baseline CT of the chest, abdomen and pelvis with intravenous and oral contrast

Ans: (a) RAS/NRAS/BRAF mutational testing

199. Which is true regarding lentigo maligna?

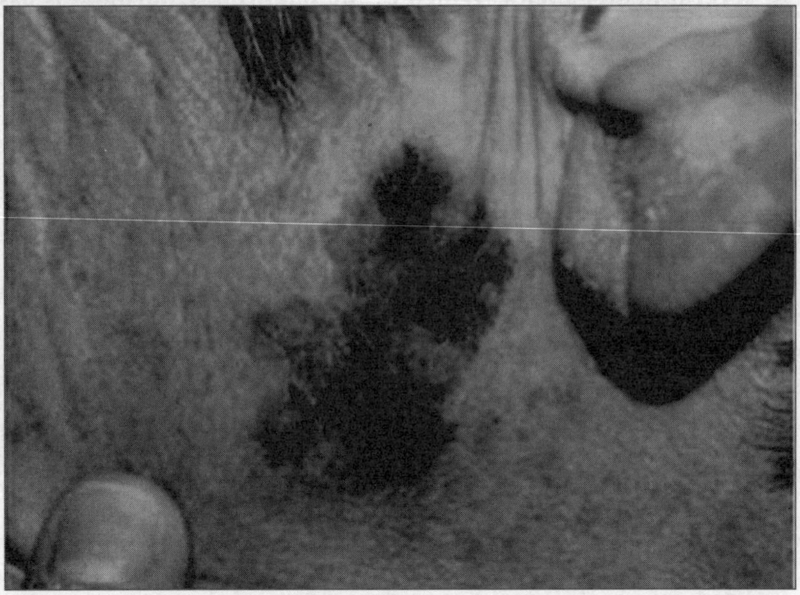

(a) Is a precursor for cervical cancer
(b) Is a precursor lesion for melanoma
(c) Is associated with human papillomavirus
(d) Usually gives rise to basal cell cancers

Ans: (b) Is a precursor lesion for melanoma

200. What is the most common risk factor for bladder cancer?

(a) Alcohol
(b) Smoking
(c) Diabetes
(d) Medications

Ans: (b) Smoking

201. Which feature is not true about BRCA 1 mutation breast cancers?

(a) Carry a risk for ovarian cancer also
(b) Are high grade
(c) Are triple positive
(d) 40% are at risk for developing colon cancer

Ans: (c) Are triple positive

202. A 73-year-old male has had metastatic prostate cancer for 9 months and has lost 13 kg. He has had some anorexia but is still eating. Select the mediator that may be causing the weight loss:

(a) Interleukin 3
(b) Tumor necrosis factor alpha
(c) Complement 3a protein
(d) Interferon alpha

Ans: (b) Tumor necrosis factor alpha

203. A 34-year-old with colon cancer was treated with a chemotherapy regimen consisting of leucovorin, fluorouracil, oxaliplatin and bevacizumab. Soon after, the patient reported that he has been experiencing excessive bleeding and wounds were not healing as expected. Which drug was likely to be responsible for these side effects?

(a) Leucovorin
(b) Fluorouracil
(c) Oxaliplatin
(d) Bevacizumab

Ans: (d) Bevacizumab

204. BRCA 1 mutation follows which pattern of inheritance?

(a) Autosomal dominant
(b) Autosomal recessive
(c) X-linked dominant
(d) X-linked recessive

Ans: (a) Autosomal dominant

205. Which of the following congenital disorders can increase the risk of cancer in males?

(a) Turner syndrome
(b) Cryptorchidism
(c) Klinefelter syndrome
(d) Moebius sydrome

Ans: (b) Cryptorchidism

206. Which of the following visual field defects results from a pituitary gland tumor?

(a) Bitemporal hemianopsia
(b) Binasal hemianopsia
(c) Left homonymous hemianopsia
(d) Scotoma

Ans: (a) Bitemporal hemianopsia

207. Which of the following is the most likely cause of migratory thrombophlebitis in a 66-year-old jaundiced individual?

(a) Pancreatic adenocarcinoma
(b) Acute cholangitis
(c) Primary biliary cirrhosis
(d) Sclerosing cholangitis

Ans: (a) Pancreatic adenocarcinoma

208. Your patient's daunorubicin infusion has infiltrated. You will discontinue the infusion and treat the extravasation site with which of the following?

(a) Warm compresses
(b) Direct pressure
(c) The appropriate antidote
(d) Ice packs

Ans: (d) Ice packs

209. Which malignancy is not associated with acanthosis nigricans?

(a) Stomach
(b) Uterus
(c) Lung
(d) Skin

Ans: (d) Skin

210. A patient with newly diagnosed colorectal cancer has immunohistochemical testing on the tumor sample after resection showing MLH1 and PSM2 staining present, but MSH2 and MSH6 absent. What is the next step in confirming the diagnosis of Lynch syndrome?

(a) No further testing is required as there is a high likelihood this patient has Lynch syndrome
(b) Test for EPCAM mutation
(c) Proceed to germline mutation testing for MSH2
(d) Proceed to germline mutation testing for MSH6

Ans: (c) Proceed to germline mutation testing for MSH2

211. Which statement is false concerning radiation-induced esophageal pathology?

(a) Radiation-induced acute esophagitis occurs early 2 to 4 weeks after radiation is initiated
(b) Radiation-induced stricture is a common complication
(c) Esophageal motility is commonly affected, dysmotility occurring 4 to 8 weeks post radiation initiation
(d) Radiation-induced strictures of the esophagus occur about 6 months after radiation is completed

Ans: (b) Radiation-induced stricture is a common complication

212. Which is true about cancer?

(a) Nitrosamines are known to cause colon cancer
(b) Ovarian cancer has been associated with human papillomavirus
(c) Naphthylamine is associated with bladder cancer
(d) Chest X-rays predispose to lung cancer

Ans: (c) Naphthylamine is associated with bladder cancer

213. Which abdominal surgery has been linked to an increased risk of colorectal cancer?

(a) Appendectomy (b) Cholecystectomy

(c) Laparoscopic hernia repair (d) Antrectomy with vagotomy

Ans: (b) Cholecystectomy

214. A 55-year-old female is evaluated for abdominal and back pain. Blood work and physical exam are normal. Computed scan of abdomen reveals a 6 cm cystic lesion in tail region of pancreas. Histology reveals internal septations and papillary projections from its walls. What is the most likely diagnosis in this patient?

(a) Lymphoma (b) Retroperitoneal sarcoma

(c) Pancreatic pseudocyst (d) Mucinous cystoadenoma

Ans: (d) Mucinous cystoadenoma

215. Which of the following is the best biochemical marker to follow after total thyroidectomy for papillary carcinoma?

(a) Melatonin (b) Calcium

(c) Serum thyroid-stimulating hormone (d) Thyroglobulin

Ans: (d) Thyroglobulin

216. Which of the following does not imply poor prognosis in a female with intraductal breast cancer?

(a) A tumor size > 3 cm (b) Microscopic tumor in > 4 nodes

(c) Presence of HER2 (d) Young female

Ans: (a) A tumor size > 3 cm

217. Which of the following is not a microscopic characteristic of papillary thyroid carcinoma?

(a) Branching papillae with a central fibrovascular core

(b) Ground-glass appearance of nuclei

(c) Fusiform cells in a whirling pattern

(d) Psammoma bodies

Ans: (c) Fusiform cells in a whirling pattern

218. Which of the following is not true of neuroblastomas?

(a) They are masses which originate from the parasympathetic chain

(b) They can present with an abdominal mass

(c) Metastases to lungs can occur when treatments is delayed

(d) They can be difficult to differentiate from Wilms tumor on examination

Ans: (a) They are masses which originate from the parasympathetic chain

219. Which of the following medications is used to treat metastatic non-small cell lung cancer?

(a) Tositumomab (b) Erlotinib

(c) Bevacizumab (d) Bortezomib

Ans: (b) Erlotinib

220. A 65-year-old male with no significant past medical history presents to with a chief complaint of pruritus and new onset "bumps" all over his back, chest and abdomen. He admits to some recent unintentional weight loss and fatigue. There is the concern the patient may be displaying the sign of Leser-Trelat, characterized by an abrupt eruption of multiple seborrheic keratoses. What underlying malignancy is the most common in patients with the sign of Leser-Trelat?

(a) Prostate cancer (b) Lung cancer

(c) Gastric cancer (d) Bladder cancer

Ans: (c) Gastric cancer

221. A 36-year-old man has painless bilateral parotid enlargement and adenopathy in the neck. What's most likely?

(a) Warthin tumor
(b) Mumps
(c) Benign lymphoepithelial cysts
(d) Sjogren syndrome

Ans: (c) Benign lymphoepithelial cysts

222. A 56-year-old female is found to have painless, unilateral, slow growing tumor of the parotid gland. What is the best treatment?

(a) Radiation therapy
(b) Enucleation
(c) Total removal or the parotid gland with preservation of the facial nerve
(d) Superficial removal of the parotid gland with preservation of the facial nerve by dissection

Ans: (d) Superficial removal of the parotid gland with preservation of the facial nerve by dissection

223. A 17-year-old has a CT scan following a bout of acute pancreatitis. A 2 cm right adrenal mass is seen. He is asymptomatic. What is the next step in the management of this patient?

(a) Biochemical evaluation for hormone secretion
(b) Adrenalectomy
(c) CT-guided biopsy
(d) Reassurance, no follow up needed

Ans: (a) Biochemical evaluation for hormone secretion

224. Which type of bladder cancer is commonly seen in individuals exposed to rubber and organic chemicals?

(a) Transitional cell carcinoma
(b) Squamous cell carcinoma
(c) Adenocarcinoma
(d) Lymphoma

Ans: (a) Transitional cell carcinoma

225. A hemiplegic male had a long history of an indwelling Foley catheter. He underwent a cystoscopy for microscopic hematuria and was found to have exophytic mucosal projections on fibrous stalks. Histology revealed inflammatory cells covered by normal appearing epithelial cells. What is the most likely diagnosis?

(a) Cystitis
(b) Inverted papilloma
(c) Transitional cell cancer
(d) Carcinoma *in situ*

Ans: (b) Inverted papilloma

226. A 60-year-old male presents with a one year history of progressive abdominal enlargement. Physical exam shows ascites and no hepatomegaly. CT of the abdomen reveals a nodular, small liver with a 7 cm mass in the left lobe. Albumin is 2.6 g/dL and hepatitis B serology is positive. The patient does not use alcohol. What is the most probable cause of the patient's deterioration?

(a) Low fiber diet
(b) Aflatoxin
(c) Lack of vitamin A
(d) Acute pancreatitis

Ans: (b) Aflatoxin

227. A 55-year-old patient with metastatic colorectal cancer with KRAS wild-type started treatment with cetuximab. Which electrolyte may become abnormal in this patient?

(a) Sodium
(b) Magnesium
(c) Chloride
(d) Bicarbonate

Ans: (b) Magnesium

228. Which of the following medications affects microtubule formation?

(a) Methotrexate
(b) Procarbazine
(c) Cyclophosphamide
(d) Paclitaxel

Ans: (d) Paclitaxel

229. Which is true of endometrial hyperplasia?

(a) It commonly becomes malignant
(b) It is associated with vaginal bleeding
(c) Can be diagnosed with ultrasound
(d) It is common during puberty

Ans: (b) It is associated with vaginal bleeding

230. During esophageal surgery, which route of conduit placement is not acceptable?

(a) Transpleural
(b) Posterior mediastinal
(c) Retrosternal
(d) Presternal

Ans: (d) Presternal

231. Which tumor marker is highly specific to epithelial ovarian cancer?

(a) CEA
(b) CA 125
(c) CA 15-3
(d) CA 19-9

Ans: (b) CA 125

232. What is Stewart Treves syndrome?

(a) Ewing tumor of the femur
(b) Hodgkin tumor of the mediastinum
(c) Angiosarcoma after chronic lymphedema
(d) Infection of bile duct with C. sinensis

Ans: (c) Angiosarcoma after chronic lymphedema

233. Which of the following about cancer in achalasia is FALSE?

(a) Cancer may occur in 5-10 percent of patients
(b) Tumor is usually bulky and rarely resectable
(c) Tumor is most common in the distal esophagus
(d) Stasis and esophagitis may be contributory conditions

Ans: (c) Tumor is most common in the distal esophagus

234. The majority of esophageal cancer are histologically divided into squamous cell carcinoma and adenocarcinoma. Which risk factors are not related to squamous cell carcinoma?

(a) History of smoking, alcohol consumption and diets low in fruits and vegetables
(b) History of smoking, high body mass index and gastroesophageal reflux disease
(c) Human papillomavirus infection has been correlated with an increased incidence of squamous cell cancers of the aerodigestive tract
(d) Preexisting esophageal anatomical diseases

Ans: (b) History of smoking, high body mass index and gastroesophageal reflux disease

235. Which condition is associated with amyloid?

(a) Hashimoto disease
(b) Riedel thyroiditis
(c) Medullary cancer
(d) Anaplastic cancer

Ans: (c) Medullary cancer

236. What is the most common cause of metastasis causing epidural spinal cord compression?

(a) Prostate
(b) Lung
(c) Lymphoma
(d) Breast

Ans: (d) Breast

237. Elevated levels of calcitonin are most likely to be seen in patients with which condition?

(a) Papillary thyroid cancer
(b) Medullary thyroid cancer
(c) Anaplastic thyroid cancer
(d) Follicular thyroid cancer

Ans: (b) Medullary thyroid cancer (DNB SS 2015)

238. What is the most frequent location of intracranial meningiomas?

(a) Parasagittal/falcine
(b) Olfactory groove
(c) Sphenoidal ridge
(d) Optic sheath

Ans: (a) Parasagittal/falcine

239. What is the best treatment for a patient with chemotherapy induced nausea and vomiting?

(a) Diphenhydramine
(b) Ondansetron
(c) Dopamine
(d) Lorazepam

Ans: (b) Ondansetron

240. Which of the following is the most likely cause of morbidity and mortality associated with desmoid tumors seen with Gardner syndrome?

(a) Potential for metastasis
(b) Local invasion or obstruction
(c) Operative errors
(d) Potential malignancy

Ans: (b) Local invasion or obstruction

241. Lymphangitic metastases are characterized by the following imaging findings?

(a) Centrilobular peribronchial thickening or beaded peripheral interlobular septa on high resolution CT
(b) Halo sign on high resolution CT
(c) Endobronchial pattern on chest radiograph
(d) Consolidative pattern on chest radiograph

Ans: (a) Centrilobular peribronchial thickening or beaded peripheral interlobular septa on high resolution CT

242. When polyps are discovered, which groups of patients would be at the highest risk for cancer?

(a) A 65-year-old with anemia
(b) A 55-year-old with a single 1 cm polyp in the sigmoid colon
(c) A 14-year-old with multiple 1 cm polyps in the right colon and a family history
(d) A 22-year-old with ulcerative colitis

Ans: (c) A 14-year-old with multiple 1 cm polyps in the right colon and a family history

243. Which of the following pulmonary lymph node drainage systems is incorrect?

(a) Right upper lobe drains to right paratracheal and then to neck
(b) Right middle lobe drains to subcarinal and then to right paratracheal
(c) Right lower lobe drains to subcarinal and then to right paratracheal
(d) Left lower lobe drains subcarinal and then to left paratracheal

Ans: (d) Left lower lobe drains subcarinal and then to left paratracheal

244. What is not true about endometrial cancer?

(a) Endometrial cancer most often presents as postmenopausal bleeding in the sixth and seventh decades
(b) Only ten percent of patients with postmenopausal bleeding, when investigated, will have endometrial cancer
(c) Uterine cancer is the fourth most common cancer in women
(d) A risk factor for endometrial cancer is an early menopause

Ans: (d) A risk factor for endometrial cancer is an early menopause

245. A 69-year-old heavy smoker has been diagnosed with lung cancer. He has been told that he has a T4 lesion. Invasion of which of the following structures is usually not characterized as a T4 lesion?

(a) Superior vena cava
(b) Esophagus
(c) Pericardium
(d) Carina

Ans: (c) Pericardium

246. What is the radiological hallmark of a craniopharyngioma on a plain radiograph?

(a) Calcified cyst
(b) Bony erosion
(c) Codman triangle
(d) Periosteal swelling

Ans: (a) Calcified cyst

247. A 37-year-old presents with a large left breast mass. There are no significant external findings but biopsy reveals a well-circumscribed mass that has a large epithelial and cellular stromal component. She may have which of the following conditions?

(a) Cystosaroma phyllodes
(b) Fat necrosis
(c) Paget's disease
(d) Hamnartoma

Ans: (a) Cystosaroma phyllodes

248. A patient presents with a 1.5 cm Merkel cell carcinoma in the periorbital region and no evidence of lymphadenopathy. Which treatment is definitely not indicated?

(a) Wide local excision
(b) Neck dissection
(c) Radiation therapy to the primary site
(d) Chemotherapy

Ans: (d) Chemotherapy

249. What is the most common histology of oral cavity cancer?

(a) Melanoma
(b) Basal cell
(c) Squamous cell
(d) Ameloblastic

Ans: (c) Squamous cell

250. Which of the following patients has an increased risk of endometrial cancer?

(a) Women younger than age 40
(b) Multiparous women
(c) Hypothyroid women
(d) Women taking tamoxifen

Ans: (d) Women taking tamoxifen

251. Invasion of which nerve from lung cancer could cause facial or eye pain?

(a) Intercostal nerve
(b) Vagus nerve
(c) Phrenic nerve
(d) Auriculotympanic nerve

Ans: (b) Vagus nerve

252. Which of the following is NOT a diagnostic criterion for postradiation sarcoma?

(a) The tumor is located in the field of irradiation
(b) The latent period between irradiation for index lesion and development of PRS is more than 4 years
(c) Histologic features of the index lesion and PRS are completely different
(d) The index lesion for which the patient received irradiation is a sarcoma

Ans: (d) The index lesion for which the patient received irradiation is a sarcoma

253. From which location does pheochromocytoma originate?

(a) Adrenal cortex
(b) Renal cortex
(c) Adrenal medulla
(d) Renal medulla

Ans: (c) Adrenal medulla

254. Which of the following diagnostic methods are not used to monitor patients with well-differentiated thyroid cancer for signs of recurrence?

(a) Measurement of unstimulated and stimulated triglycerides serum levels
(b) High-resolution ultrasonography
(c) Radioactive iodine whole-body scanning
(d) High-resolution, contrast-enhanced CT scanning

Ans: (d) High-resolution, contrast-enhanced CT scanning

255. Where do the majority of tumors of the salivary glands occur?

(a) Parotid gland
(b) Minor salivary glands
(c) Submandibular gland
(d) Hard palate

Ans: (a) Parotid gland

256. A female has been found to have a 3 cms cancerous breast lesion. At surgery, no lymph nodes are identified. The mass is found to be positive for HER2/neu and negative for both estrogen and progesterone receptions. Which of the following is the best treatment for this patient?

(a) Radiation therapy
(b) Chemotherapy
(c) Trastuzumab
(d) Mastectomy

Ans: (c) Trastuzumab

257. An adult female with a breast mass has a mammogram which is reported as breast imaging reporting and data system (BI-RADS) 4. What is recommended?

(a) Continue routine screening because the lesion is benign
(b) Do additional diagnostic testing because the testing is incomplete
(c) Perform a biopsy because the lesion is suspicious for breast cancer
(d) Repeat mammography in 6 months because the lesion is probably benign

Ans: (c) Perform a biopsy because the lesion is suspicious for breast cancer

258. Which of the following risk factor is most strongly associated with ductal adenocarcinoma of the pancreas?

(a) Chronic pancreatitis
(b) Diabetes mellitus
(c) Smoking
(d) Alcohol

Ans: (a) Chronic pancreatitis

259. A 52-year-old male presents with a slowly growing mass of the hard palate. It is asymptomatic and measures 0.75 × 0.75 cm. No other abnormalities are found. Needle biopsy shows a pleomorphic adenoma. Select the best management.

(a) Observation
(b) Enucleation
(c) Complete excision ensuring clear margins
(d) Wide excision with lymph node dissection

Ans: (c) Complete excision ensuring clear margins

260. Which of the following lung lobes is involved in cancer of the cardiac notch?

(a) Superior lobe of the left lung
(b) Inferior lobe of the left lung
(c) Superior lobe of the right lung
(d) Inferior lobe of the right lung

Ans: (a) Superior lobe of the left lung

261. A patient present with an 8 mm papule that has changed considerably in size and color over the past couple of months. There is no personal or family history of skin cancer. Which of the following would be most appropriate for the management of this patient?

(a) Observe the lesion over the next 3 months

(b) Perform a full-body examination at that visit

(c) Consider CT to investigate possible internal malignancies

(d) Perform a CA-125 for possible evidence of malignancy

Ans: (b) Perform a full-body examination at that visit

262. Malignant mesothelioma is known to have a strong association with asbestos exposure. Which of the following exposures is also associated with the development of malignant mesothelioma?

(a) Coal dust

(b) Respiratory syncytial virus

(c) Empyema

(d) Radiation exposure

Ans: (d) Radiation exposure

263. What is the most common histology bladder cancer with Schistosoma haematobium infection?

(a) Adenocarcinoma

(b) Columnar cell

(c) Squamous cell

(d) Transitional cell

Ans: (c) Squamous cell

264. A 63-year-old patient presented with a palpable mass in her right breast. Diagnostic mammogram showed a spiculated mass measuring 1.7 cm. Ultrasound demonstrated a hypoechoic mass measuring 1.8 cm × 0.9 cm. Biopsy revealed a well-differentiated mucinous carcinoma that was ER/PR positive and HER2/neu negative. Lumpectomy and sentinel node biopsy revealed 1.8 cm mucinous carcinoma with widely negative margins. No associated ductal carcinoma *in situ* or lymphovascular invasion was noted. Two sentinel nodes were negative. Oncotype score was 3. Which is your treatment recommendation?

(a) Radiation therapy to the breast and endocrine therapy

(b) Radiation therapy to the breast and nodes and endocrine therapy

(c) Chemotherapy, then radiation therapy to the breast

(d) Mastectomy and endocrine therapy

Ans: (a) Radiation therapy to the breast and endocrine therapy

265. What is the most common presentation of a prolactinoma in men?

(a) Galactorrhea

(b) Headache

(c) Azoospermia

(d) Priapism

Ans: (b) Headache

266. A 50-year-old man has worked outside without his shirt for most of his life. He has a raised, irregular bordered, skin lesion with multiple colors. Pathologic analysis shows invasion into the dermis of malignant cells. Which of the following is the most likely diagnosis?

(a) Cherry angioma

(b) Malignant melanoma

(c) Basal cell carcinoma

(d) Squamous cell carcinoma

Ans: (b) Malignant melanoma

267. Which of the following is an expected finding in a 55-year-old with central pain syndrome?

(a) Malignancy

(b) Radiation myelopathy

(c) Spinal stenosis

(d) Traumatic compression

Ans: (b) Radiation myelopathy

268. A male with a 4-year history of headaches developed generalized seizures and bilateral leg weakness. CT shows calvarial hyperostosis and a mass. Biopsy of the mass shows whorls and psammoma bodies. What is the most probable diagnosis?

(a) Glioblastoma multiforme
(b) Metastatic prostate cancer
(c) Astrocytoma
(d) Meningioma

Ans: (d) Meningioma

269. Hormonal assays indicate that most meningiomas express receptors to which of the following?

(a) Androgen
(b) Glucocorticoid
(c) Progesterone
(d) Estrogen

Ans: (c) Progesterone

270. Which is not a risk factor for ovarian cancer?

(a) Nulliparity
(b) Use of contraceptive
(c) Family history
(d) Presence of BRCA gene

Ans: (b) Use of contraceptive

271. A 58-year-old man was diagnosed with rectal adenocarcinoma by rectal sigmoidoscopy after bright red blood per rectum clinical presentation. Transrectal ultrasound stage was T2N1 at 5 cm from the anal verge and no metastatic evidence by computed tomography. Which of the following is the most appropriate next step?

(a) Upfront not-sphincter paring by abdominal perineal resection (APR)
(b) Upfront not-sphincter sparing by abdominal perineal resection (APR) including total mesorectal excision (TME)
(c) Neoadjuvant therapy followed by restaging tumor response prior to surgical resection decision
(d) Upfront surgical resection followed with adjuvant therapy for node-positive rectal cancer

Ans: (c) Neoadjuvant therapy followed by restaging tumor response prior to surgical resection decision

272. A 52-year-old male was recently diagnosed with mediastinal germ cell tumor of embryonal carcinoma type that is infiltrating into the medial lobe of his right lung. He has 80 pack-year history of smoking and has Gold Stage III COPD. He also has history of chronic pancreatitis. His performance status is Eastern Cooperative Oncology Group (ECOG) 1. His PFT shows a predicted forced expiratory volume (FEV)1 of 1.5 liters. What should the treatment plan for this patient include?

(a) Four cycles of cisplatin, bleomycin and etoposide (BEP) for 2 cycles alone.
(b) Four cycles of cisplatin, ifosfamide and etoposide (VIP) alone
(c) Four cycles of cisplatin, bleomycin and etoposide (BEP) followed by resection of residual tumor with lobectomy (if indicated)
(d) Four cycles of cisplatin, ifosfamide and etoposide (VIP) followed by resection of residual tumor with lobectomy (if indicated)

Ans: (d) Four cycles of cisplatin, ifosfamide and etoposide (VIP) followed by resection of residual tumor with lobectomy (if indicated)

273. In which of the following parts of the body does adenocarcinoma rarely develop?

(a) Tongue
(b) Prostate
(c) Lung
(d) Bladder

Ans: (a) Tongue

274. Which is not a high-risk feature of stage II colon cancer that supports adjuvant therapy after surgical resection?

(a) Lymphovascular invasion
(b) Insufficient node sampling (<12)
(c) Poor (high-grade) histological differentiation
(d) High levels of microsatellite instability (MSI-H)

Ans: (d) High levels of microsatellite instability (MSI-H)

275. Which of the following is not true of a testicular seminoma?

(a) The majority occur in young men in their twenties and thirties

(b) It is sensitive to radiotherapy

(c) Metastases to the lung rarely occur

(d) It has a very poor prognosis

Ans: (d) It has a very poor prognosis

276. Select the malignancy that is most often associated with pericardial effusions.

(a) Mesothelioma
(b) Breast
(c) Lung
(d) Lymphoma

Ans: (c) Lung

277. A patient with a 3 centimeter non-small cell lung cancer has positive contralateral supraclavicular nodes. Which of the following is the correct management of this patient?

(a) Give chemotherapy for 4 weeks followed by surgery

(b) Surgery followed by combination chemotherapy and radiation

(c) Chemotherapy and radiation only

(d) Surgery followed by adjuvant immunotherapy

Ans: (c) Chemotherapy and radiation only

278. What is the definitive treatment of intraductal papillary mucinous neoplasm (IPMN)?

(a) Surgery
(b) Chemotherapy
(c) Radiation therapy
(d) Chemoradiation therapy

Ans: (a) Surgery

279. A patient reports headaches and palpitations. There is mild hypertension, increased levels of plasma norepinephrine and epinephrine and urinary catecholamines. MRI shows an adrenal mass. What kind of cell type is most likely to be found in the tumor?

(a) Neuron
(b) Chromaffin cell
(c) Thyroid cell
(d) Lymphoid cell

Ans: (b) Chromaffin cel

280. What malignancy is most common in patients with chronic celiac disease?

(a) Carcinoid
(b) T-cell lymphoma of gut
(c) Gastric adenocarcinoma
(d) Kaposi sarcoma

Ans: (b) T-cell lymphoma of gut

281. A 55-year-old lady of Chinese decent attends the clinic complaining of pigmentation of the nail on her great toe. The medial border of the nail is colored brown-black. It has been present for six months and gradually increasing in size. More recently she has noticed the discoloration starting to spread onto the surrounding skin. What is this sign called?

(a) Stain sign
(b) Hutchinson sign
(c) Boyer sign
(d) Hutchinson freckle

Ans: (b) Hutchinson sign

282. Which is NOT a common finding in a patient with von Hippel-Lindau syndrome?

(a) Hemangioblastoma
(b) Ependymoma
(c) Retinal angiomatoses
(d) Renal cysts

Ans: (b) Ependymoma

283. What phase of the cell cycle is most resistant to chemotherapeutic agents?

(a) G1 phase
(b) G0 phase
(c) S phase
(d) M phase

Ans: (b) G0 phase

284. Which of the following is not a characteristic of Hereditary Nonpolyposis Colorectal Cancer (Lynch syndrome)?

(a) Proximal colon cancer involvement
(b) Family history of colon cancer
(c) Onset before age 45
(d) Extracolonic cancers do not occur

Ans: (d) Extracolonic cancers do not occur

285. Which is false about melanoma?

(a) Melanomas can occur on an unexposed area of skin
(b) Vertical growth of melanoma is associated with worse prognosis than radial growth
(c) Acral lentiginous melanomas are the most common form of melanoma in black people
(d) Superficial spreading melanomas have the highest risk of spread among all melanomas

Ans: (d) Superficial spreading melanomas have the highest risk of spread among all melanomas

286. An 18-year-old female presents with new onset seizures and an MRI shows a temporal lobe mass. The craniotomy pathology shows the diagnosis to be pleomorphic xanthoastrocytoma (PXA). Which of the following is true?

(a) PXA is a World Health Organization grade III astrocytic neoplasm
(b) Prognosis is poor
(c) The usual lesion is a heterogeneous cystic mass close to the cerebral surface with calcifications
(d) Metastases are likely in this age group

Ans: (c) The usual lesion is a heterogeneous cystic mass close to the cerebral surface with calcifications

287. Which of the following is a common complication of cisplatin use?

(a) Hepatotoxicity
(b) Ophthalmopathy
(c) Bone marrow suppression
(d) Nephrotoxicity

Ans: (d) Nephrotoxicity

288. What is the first test utilized to investigate the etiology of a solid thyroid mass?

(a) Thyroid function test
(b) Fine needle aspiration
(c) Ultrasound
(d) Nuclear scan

Ans: (b) Fine needle aspiration

289. Liver cancer is associated with which of the following?

(a) Nitrosamines
(b) Smog
(c) Benzopyrene
(d) Aflatoxin

Ans: (d) Aflatoxin

290. Which patient should be screened for microsatellite instability/mismatch repair deficiency/Lynch syndrome?

(a) Only patients fitting Amsterdam and/or Bethesda criteria
(b) Only patients who are diagnosed with colorectal cancer before age 50
(c) Only patients with family history of colorectal cancer
(d) All patients with colorectal cancer

Ans: (d) All patients with colorectal cancer

291. Which of the following is a correct statement about the treatment for malignant mesothelioma?

(a) Radical extrapleural pneumonectomy provides the best survival

(b) Radical pleurectomy is only a palliative procedure

(c) Radiation therapy given preoperatively yields long-term survival

(d) Multimodality chemotherapy combined with surgery prevents recurrence

Ans: (b) Radical pleurectomy is only a palliative procedure

292. A patient with mild dysphagia undergoes endoscopy, which reveals a squamous cell carcinoma. The patient has stage 1 esophageal cancer. What is the present day recommended treatment?

(a) Preoperative chemotherapy and radiation

(b) Postoperative radiation

(c) Surgery

(d) Preoperative chemotherapy, followed by surgery and radiation

Ans: (c) Surgery

293. Which finding is NOT associated with MEN 2A?

(a) Medullary carcinoma of the thyroid
(b) Mucosal neuromas
(c) Parathyroid tumors
(d) Pheochromocytomas

Ans: (b) Mucosal neuromas

294. A person found working in a factory where aniline exposure is common might develop what malignancy?

(a) Prostate cancer
(b) Benign prostate hypertrophy
(c) Bladder cancer
(d) Renal ell cancer

Ans: (c) Bladder cancer

295. Which breast cancer has the highest tendency for invasion of dermal lymphatics?

(a) Paget
(b) Infiltrating ductal carcinoma
(c) Inflammatory breast
(d) Cystosarcoma phyllodes

Ans: (c) Inflammatory breast

296. What is the most common lesion seen in asbestos related disease?

(a) Noncaseating granulomas
(b) Bronchogenic carcinoma
(c) Malignant mesothelioma of the pleura
(d) Benign pleural plaques

Ans: (d) Benign pleural plaques

297. Which of the following is the MOST common location for mucosal melanoma of the sinonasal tract?

(a) Superior turbinate
(b) Middle turbinate
(c) Olfactory region
(d) Anterior portion of the nasal septum

Ans: (d) Anterior portion of the nasal septum

298. What is the most common posterior mediastinal tumor?

(a) Lymphoma
(b) Thymoma
(c) Seminoma
(d) Neurogenic

Ans: (d) Neurogenic

299. What is the best procedure in a patient with a malignant pleural effusion with a trapped lung?

(a) Pleurectomy (b) Pleuro-peritoneal shunt

(c) Thoractomy with decortications and pleurodesis (d) Thoracoplasty

Ans: (b) Pleuro-peritoneal shunt

300. Which of the following is true regarding vaginal cancer?

(a) Most patients with vaginal caner are 20-50 years old

(b) HPV, smoking, early age at onset of first sexual intercourse are risk factors

(c) Multiple sexual partners is not a risk

(d) Abnormal vaginal bleeding is not a symptom

Ans: (b) HPV, smoking, early age at onset of first sexual intercourse are risk factors

301. Which of the following is false regarding esophageal leiomyoma?

(a) May present on a stalk

(b) Carries a very low malignancy-risk

(c) Intramural and generally requires esophageal resection

(d) Equal gender and race distribution

Ans: (c) Intramural and generally requires esophageal resection

302. Which of these is a risk factor for pleomorphic adenoma?

(a) Smoking (b) Alcohol

(c) Radiation (d) Sun exposure

Ans: (c) Radiation

303. Which is not associated with early prostate cancer?

(a) Usually seen in the posterior lobe

(b) Can be palpated on a rectal exam

(c) Can be associated with an elevated prostate acid phosphatase

(d) Can cause urinary retention

Ans: (d) Can cause urinary retention

304. A patient is diagnosed with carcinoma of the skin of penis. Cancer cells are likely to metastasize directly to which of the following lymph nodes?

(a) Axillary nodes (b) Superficial inguinal nodes

(c) Deep inguinal nodes (d) Lumbar nodes

Ans: (b) Superficial inguinal nodes

305. Which is not a symptom associated with hypercalcemia of malignancy?

(a) Lethargy (b) Muscle weakness

(c) Seizure (d) Depression

Ans: (c) Seizure

306. Which of the following is not a feature of adenocarcinoma of the lung?

(a) Desmoplastic reaction (b) Extensive necrosis

(c) Rapid growth (d) Cavitation

Ans: (d) Cavitation

307. Which of the following malignancies is more common in patients with von Hippel-Lindau syndrome?

(a) Glioblastoma multiforme (b) Hypernephroma

(c) Hepatoma (d) Lymphoma

Ans: (b) Hypernephroma

308. A 63-year-old female presents with a rapidly growing neck mass. She has now been complaining of dysphagia and neck pain. All the blood work is normal. Needle biopsy reveals malignant cells with severe dysplasia. No treatment is offered to her because the mass is rapidly growing. The patient most likely has which of the following conditions?

(a) Follicular thyroid mass (b) Anaplastic tumor

(c) Lymphoma (d) Actinomycosis

Ans: (b) Anaplastic tumor

309. What is the best way to make a diagnosis of a hepatocellular adenoma?

(a) Fine needle aspiration (b) Open surgical biopsy

(c) Angiography (d) ERCP cytology

Ans: (b) Open surgical biopsy

310. Expression of which of the following in breast cancer would indicate probable response to trastuzumab?

(a) Estrogen receptors (b) Progesterone receptors

(c) Her2/neu receptors (d) Androgen receptor

Ans: (c) Her2/neu receptors

311. Which of the following disease is characterized by development of angiofibromas in the skin and hamartomas in the brain?

(a) Neurofibromatosis (b) Tuberous sclerosis

(c) Sturge-Weber syndrome (d) Von-Hippel-Lindau disease

Ans: (b) Tuberous sclerosis

312. What is the most common presentation of mesothelioma on chest radiographs?

(a) Pneumothorax (b) Large pleural effusion

(c) Unilateral pleural thickening (d) Mediastinal adenopathy

Ans: (c) Unilateral pleural thickening

313. Which cancer is associated with prolonged uncontrolled use of tamoxifen?

(a) Breast (b) Skin

(c) Uterine (d) Ovary

Ans: (c) Uterine

314. Which of the following is not a risk factor for cervical squamous cell carcinoma?

(a) Early age of sexual intercourse (b) Obesity

(c) History of human papilloma virus infection (d) Multiple sex partners

Ans: (b) Obesity

315. Which of the following is the most common malignancy of the female pelvic region?

(a) Endometrial (b) Vaginal

(c) Cervical (d) Fallopian tube

Ans: (a) Endometrial

316. Which is true about lung cancer?

(a) Pleural malignancy is associated with asbestosis

(b) Pancoast tumors involve the base of the lung

(c) A small cell lung cancer is generally found in the periphery of the lung

(d) Adenocarcinoma is a type of small cell lung cancer

Ans: (a) Pleural malignancy is associated with asbestosis

317. Renal cell carcinoma (RCC) in Von Hippel-Lindau disease may be distinguished from spontaneous RCC by:

(a) Older age at presentation (b) Bilaterality in a majority

(c) Multicentricity in a minority (d) None of the above

Ans: (d) None of the above

318. In which of the following tumors is human chorionic gonadotrophin levels NOT elevated?

(a) Seminoma (b) Choriocarcinoma

(c) Islet cell tumors (d) Thymoma

Ans: (d) Thymoma

319. Which of the following statements is true about HIV associated CNS lymphoma?

(a) There will be enhancement of primary CNS lymphoma

(b) On MRI there is likely to be multiple lesions at presentation

(c) The diagnostic gold standard is MRS

(d) There is a strong association with human papilloma virus (HPV)

Ans: (a) There will be enhancement of primary CNS lymphoma

320. What is the most common malignancy in post-transplant patients?

(a) B-cell lymphoma (b) Skin cancers

(c) Cervical cancers (d) T-cell lymphomas

Ans: (b) Skin cancers

321. The risk factor commonly associated with renal cancer is:

(a) Alcohol (b) Smoking

(c) Schistosomiasis (d) Medications

Ans: (b) Smoking

322. An 18-month-old boy is seen in the clinic for his routine examination. On examination, the boy has a solid mass in his right testis. The mother claims that the boy has been feeling fine and eating well. She denies any trauma. Blood work reveals elevated levels of alpha-fetoprotein. What is the most likely mass in this child?

(a) Teratoma (b) Neuroblastoma

(c) Choriocarcinoma (d) Yolk sac tumor

Ans: (d) Yolk sac tumor

323. In a patient with a mediastinal non-seminomatous germ cell tumor with elevated levels of human chorionic gonadotropin (HCG) and a-fetoprotein (AFP), multimodality chemotherapy reduces both HCG and AFP levels to normal. The CT scan reveals a residual mass in the chest. On exploration of the patient, what is the most likely histology of the remnant?

(a) Non-seminomatous germ cell (b) Teratoma

(c) Seminoma (d) Thymoma

Ans: (b) Teratoma

324. The use of diethylstilbestrol has been linked to which of the following cancer?

(a) Uterine cancer
(b) Vaginal cancer
(c) Bladder cancer
(d) Breast cancer

Ans: (b) Vaginal cancer

325. Which of the following medications works on the S phase of the cell cycle?

(a) Bleomycin
(b) Cytarabine
(c) Paclitaxel
(d) Vincristine

Ans: (b) Cytarabine

326. What should be the treatment for a patient with a confirmed pituitary mass and acromegaly symptoms?

(a) Radiation to the pituitary gland
(b) Growth hormone injections
(c) Surgical removal of the mass
(d) Frequent follow-up assessments for worsening of symptoms

Ans: (c) Surgical removal of the mass

327. A patient is found to have a 2.2 cm speculated mass in the tail of the pancreas found on screening CT scan. There is no local extension or lymphadenopathy. CA 19-9 level and bilirubin are normal. What is the next best step in the management of this patient?

(a) CT guided biopsy
(b) Chemotherapy
(c) Endoscopic ultrasound to assess respectability and perform biopsy
(d) Magnetic resonance cholangiopancreatography

Ans: (b) Chemotherapy

328. A 27-year-old patient is found to have diarrhea, weakness and signs of malabsorption. Endoscopy reveals flattened mucosa and presence of antigliadin antibody. The patients are prone to develop what disorder in the long run?

(a) Crohn's disease
(b) Lymphoma
(c) Parkinson disease
(d) Normal pressure hydrocephalus

Ans: (b) Lymphoma

329. What is the recommended treatment for a confirmed diagnosis of dermatofibrosarcoma protuberans?

(a) Cryosurgery
(b) Chemotherapy
(c) Mohs micrographic surgery
(d) Radiation

Ans: (c) Mohs micrographic surgery

330. Which of the following is false about an intraductal papilloma?

(a) They are commonly associated with bilateral bloody nipple discharge
(b) They can be diagnosed with a ductogram
(c) Local excision is adequate treatment
(d) It is a benign lesion

Ans: (a) They are commonly associated with bilateral bloody nipple discharge

331. What is the MOST common complication when I131 is used to treat patients with residual thyroid cancer?

(a) Hyperthyroidism
(b) Hypothyroidism
(c) Graves disease
(d) Cancer

Ans: (b) Hypothyroidism

332. A 59-year-old presents with jaundice and is found to have pancreatic cancer. Which of the following is true about this malignancy?

(a) The majority of pancreatic cancers occur in the head of the pancreas
(b) The incidence of pancreatic cancer has been declining in the last two decades
(c) There is no relationship between diabetes mellitus and pancreatic cancer
(d) A palpable gallbladder often results because of mass invasion into the cystic duct

Ans: (a) The majority of pancreatic cancers occur in the head of the pancreas

333. Which of the following adrenal masses can one safely observe?

(a) A 2 cm adrenal lesion with positive urinary metanephrine
(b) A 3 cm non-funcational cystic lesion
(c) A 7 cm asymptomatic mass
(d) A 3 cm non-functional lesion that is PET avid

Ans: (b) A 3 cm non-funcational cystic lesion

334. What agent has been proven partially effective as an adjuvant treatment for colorectal cancer in a patient with unresectable metastases?

(a) Bevacizumab
(b) Cyclophosphamide
(c) Methotrexate
(d) Aspirin

Ans: (a) Bevacizumab

335. Select the incorrect statement about familial adenomatous polyposis:

(a) There is autosomal dominant inheritance
(b) Without treatment, all patients will develop colon cancer
(c) Polyps never involve the duodenum
(d) 20 percent of patients develop desmoids tumor after colectomy

Ans: (c) Polyps never involve the duodenum

336. A female notices discharge from her nipples and amenorrhea. The pregnancy test is negative. Her exam otherwise is normal except suggestion of a possible slight left temporal quadrantanopsia. What is the most likely diagnosis?

(a) Prolactin secreting pituitary adenoma
(b) FSH pituitary tumor
(c) ACTH pituitary tumor
(d) Hypothyroidism

Ans: (a) Prolactin secreting pituitary adenoma

337. What other tumor does Merkel cell carcinoma most closely resemble on histopathologic analysis?

(a) Keratoacanthoma
(b) Basal cell carcinoma
(c) Metastatic small cell carcinoma of the lung
(d) Squamous cell carcinoma

Ans: (c) Metastatic small cell carcinoma of the lung

338. Acceptable treatment for localized prostate cancer includes which of the following?

(a) Brachytherapy (prostatic seed implication)
(b) External beam radiotherapy
(c) Radical prostatectomy
(d) All of the above

Ans: (d) All of the above

339. What is the most appropriate therapy for non-metastatic renal cell carcinoma?

(a) Chemotherapy
(b) Radiation therapy
(c) Radical nephrectomy
(d) Nephrectomy

Ans: (c) Radical nephrectomy

340. A 45-year-old patient undergoes laparoscopy for bilateral ovarian masses. Each mass has a unilocular cyst and has multiple papillary excrescences. The fluid in the cysts is clear. Select the most likely diagnosis.

(a) Polycystic ovarian syndrome
(b) Serous cystadenocarcinoma
(c) Mucinous cystadenocarcinoma
(d) Teratoma

Ans: (b) Serous cystadenocarcinoma

341. Kaposi sarcoma has been linked to which infection?

(a) Lyme
(b) Syphilis
(c) Herpes
(d) Mumps

Ans: (c) Herpes

342. What is the most appropriate first-time treatment option for a RAS/BRAF wild-type metastatic rectal adenocarcinoma in a fit 56-year-old patient?

(a) Sequential capecitabine, irinotecan and oxaliplatin (CAPOX)
(b) Folinic acid, fluorouracil and oxaliplatin (FOLFOX) plus bevacizumab
(c) FOLFOX plus cetuximab
(d) Irinotecan with fluorouracil and folinic acid (FOLFIRI) plus bevacizumab

Ans: (c) FOLFOX plus cetuximab

343. A patient with pheochromocytoma induced hypertension will have which of the following?

(a) High systolic pressure
(b) High diastolic pressure
(c) High MAP
(d) Episodic pressure elevation

Ans: (d) Episodic pressure elevation

344. A patient and her mother are diagnosed with neurofibromatosis. The mother reports her mother had neurofibromatosis and died of a tumor. What was the most likely diagnosis of the grandmother?

(a) Malignant plexiform neurofibroma
(b) Squamous cell carcinoma
(c) Malignant neurofibroma
(d) Melanoma

Ans: (a) Malignant plexiform neurofibroma

345. What is the most common testicular malignancy?

(a) Leydig cell tumor
(b) Sertoli cell tumor
(c) Nonseminomatous germ cell tumor
(d) Seminomatous germ cell tumor

Ans: (c) Nonseminomatous germ cell tumor

346. A patient present with a lung mass of unknown etiology. Biopsy reveals a well-defined germinal center with regional lymph nodes showing only reactive changes. Which of the following is not a feature of this disorder?

(a) Completely benign lesion
(b) Treatment is resection
(c) Malignant transformation can occur
(d) Lymph nodes are generally not involved

Ans: (a) Completely benign lesion

347. Which is false about the histology of breast cancer?

(a) Prognosis is related to type of histology
(b) Majority are squamous cell malignancies
(c) May arise from the ducts or the lobules
(d) Intraductal cancer is the most common

Ans: (b) Majority are squamous cell malignancies

348. A 72-year-old female smoker with type 2 diabetes and alcoholic cirrhosis dies of complications from her chronic illnesses. Autopsy shows a mass in the pancreas that is hard and infiltrative. The rest of the pancreas shows fibrosis with acinar loss, dilation of ducts, moderate infiltration of lymphocytes, but normal islets. Select the most likely findings for the pancreatic mass.

(a) Dense, fibrotic stroma with moderately differentiated cells that secrete mucus
(b) Fibrosis with acinar loss, dilation of ducts, moderate infiltration of lymphocytes
(c) Necrosis with neutrophilic infiltrate
(d) Atrophy of exocrine gland, fibrosis and plugging of ducts

Ans: (a) Dense, fibrotic stroma with moderately differentiated cells that secrete mucus

349. Of the following choices, which is the most common malignant bone tumor?
(a) Osteosarcoma
(b) Osteoid osteoma
(c) Ewing's sarcoma
(d) Osteochondroma

Ans: (a) Osteosarcoma

350. The test of choice for making diagnosis of renal cell cancer is:
(a) PET
(b) Renal angiography
(c) Abdominal CT
(d) Excretory urography

Ans: (c) Abdominal CT

351. Post-transplantation lymphoproliferative disorder is associated with which of the following viruses?
(a) Epstein-Barr virus
(b) Human immunodeficiency virus
(b) Herpes simplex virus
(d) Parvovirus

Ans: (a) Epstein-Barr virus

352. The use of alpha-fetoprotein and des gamma carboxy prothrombin have been used as markers for:
(a) Down syndrome
(b) Syringomyelia
(c) Liver cancer
(d) Seminoma

Ans: (c) Liver cancer

353. Which of the following is not true of surgery for thyroid malignancies?
(a) Most patients become hypothyroid immediately
(b) There is a risk of transient hypoparathroidism
(c) Hyperthyroid patients may require beta blockade prior to surgery
(d) Venous congestion after surgery may present with tracheal compression

Ans: (a) Most patients become hypothyroid immediately

354. Which of the following is not an early symptom in a patient with gestational trophoblastic disease?
(a) Hyperemesis gravidarum
(b) Painless vaginal bleeding
(c) Uterine size greater than dates
(d) Muffled fetal heart tones on Doppler exam

Ans: (d) Muffled fetal heart tones on Doppler exam

355. Which of the following statements about lung cancer is true?
(a) The majority are small cell
(b) Incidence is increasing in females
(c) Lymph node involvement is rare
(d) Most common cause of lung cancer is environmental pollution

Ans: (b) Incidence is increasing in females

356. C cells (parafollicular cells) are involved with which of the following?

(a) Papillary carcinoma
(b) Hurthle cell carcinoma
(c) Medullary carcinoma
(d) Anaplastic cancer

Ans: (c) Medullary carcinoma

357. What non-steroidal agent is used in the treatment of prostate cancer?

(a) Tamoxifen
(b) Clomiphene
(c) Flutamide
(d) Fluoxetine

Ans: (c) Flutamide

358. A Fitzpatrick type IV patient presents for treatment of a 5 mm superficial basal cell carcinoma on the face. He elects to underdo cryotherapy using liquid nitrogen from a spray can for treatment. Which of the following is a common complication about which the patient should be counseled before the procedure?

(a) Bleeding
(b) Hypopigmentation
(c) Water avoidance
(d) Need for suturing

Ans: (b) Hypopigmentation

359. A 46-year-old female has several nodules palpated in the left lobe of the thyroid gland. There is no lymphadenopathy and on pathologic analysis each nodule show papillary structures with small, scattered, laminated, round calcifications. Select the other finding most likely seen in the tumors:

(a) Normal appearing follicles with fibrous capsule showing foal invasion
(b) Clear nuclei having longitudinal nuclear grooves
(c) Small round cells in sheets having cytoplasmic glycogen
(d) Anaplastic and giant cells

Ans: (b) Clear nuclei having longitudinal nuclear grooves

360. What is the most common cause of death in a patient with untreated bladder cancer?

(a) Pulmonary embolism
(b) Myocardial infarct
(c) Uremia
(d) Hemorrhage

Ans: (c) Uremia

361. Which is false about surgery for thyroid cancers?

(a) Total thyroidectomy can be curative
(b) Should always be performed with regional lymph node dissection
(c) Papillary cancer has a favourable prognosis
(d) Can lead to damage to parathyroid glands

Ans: (b) Should always be performed with regional lymph node dissection

362. Which of these conditions does not predispose to esophageal cancer?

(a) Achalasia
(b) Scleroderma
(c) Plummer Vinson syndrome
(d) Zenker diverticulum

Ans: (d) Zenker diverticulum

363. Which is an absolute contraindication to breast radiotherapy?

(a) Psoriasis
(b) Coronary artery disease (CAD)
(c) Scleroderma
(d) Chronic obstructive pulmonary disease (COPD)

Ans: (c) Scleroderma

364. Which of the following is not associated with the incidence of Barrett esophagus and esophageal adenocarcinoma?

(a) Increased by central obesity

(b) Decreased incidence with Helicobacter pylori gastritis

(c) Increased instance with cigarette smoking

(d) Increased with the use of aspirin and NSAIDs

Ans: (d) Increased with the use of aspirin and NSAIDs

365. What is the advantage of Gleason group compared to Gleason score?

(a) Gleason groups are easier for patients to understand

(b) Gleason groups correlate better with prognosis

(c) Gleason group is more accurate

(d) Gleason group is easier for pathologist to determine

Ans: (a) Gleason groups are easier for patients to understand

366. Which of following forms of lung cancer is most likely to present as large, central mass without distant metastases?

(a) Squamous cell carcinoma
(b) Adenocarcinoma
(c) Small cell carcinoma
(d) Large cell carcinoma

Ans: (a) Squamous cell carcinoma

367. Which of the following is the least likely presentation of thrombosis of the inferior vena cava?

(a) Ascites
(b) Lower extremity edema bilaterally
(c) Upper extremity edema bilaterally
(d) Pulmonary embolism

Ans: (c) Upper extremity edema bilaterally

368. A patient presents with weight loss and nausea. She has lost 10 lbs over 2 months and has altered bowel movements. Work up reveals that she has a sigmoid colon cancer. What is the first site where the colony cancer usually spreads?

(a) Liver
(b) Lymph nodes
(c) Ureter
(d) Rectum

Ans: (b) Lymph nodes

369. A 59-year-old male with gross hematuria. Kidney biopsy reveals enlarged nuclei, with prominent nucleoli and abnormal nuclei. Staining reveals presence of mucin the cytoplasm. The patient may have which of the following?

(a) Adenocarcinoma
(b) Melanoma
(c) Squamous cell cancer
(d) Transitional cell cancer

Ans: (a) Adenocarcinoma

370. What virus is associated with Kaposi sarcoma?

(a) HIV
(b) Herpes simplex
(c) Human herpesvirus type 8
(d) Hepatitis C

Ans: (c) Human herpesvirus type 8

371. An elderly diabetic male presents with jaundice and weight loss. The gallbladder is palpable. What is the most likely diagnosis?

(a) Duodenal ulcer
(b) Cirrhosis
(c) Ascending cholangitis
(d) Pancreatic cancer

Ans: (d) Pancreatic cancer

372. A 29-year-old male with HIV for 4 years complains of a 2-month history of visual changes with distortion of a portion of the left visual field. MR shows a 3 cm right occipital lobe lesion that shows enhancement of the rim. Select the tumor that is rare other than in patients with AIDS.

(a) Astrocytoma
(b) Primary lymphoma of the CNS
(c) Metastatic lymphoma
(d) Kaposi sarcoma

Ans: (b) Primary lymphoma of the CNS

373. Which of the following medications is the best initial choice to treat pheochromocytoma associated hypertension?

(a) Clonidine
(b) Propranolol
(c) Captopril
(d) Phenoxybenzamine

Ans: (d) Phenoxybenzamine

374. Which of the following is not a feature of penile cancer?

(a) Risk is increased with chemical exposure
(b) Commonly arises on glans penis
(c) May be associated with human papillomavirus
(d) May spread to inguinal lymph nodes

Ans: (a) Risk is increased with chemical exposure

375. After radiation therapy to the chest, a patient develops a necrotic skin ulcer, which has failed to heal with conservative medical management for the past 3 months. What is the best treatment option?

(a) Local excision with skin graft
(b) Hyperbaric oxygen treatment
(c) Application of growth factor to wound
(d) Myocutaneous flap

Ans: (d) Myocutaneous flap

376. Dumping syndrome is most commonly observed after which procedure?

(a) Colon resection
(b) Cholecystectomy
(c) Gastric resection
(d) Cholecystectomy

Ans: (c) Gastric resection

377. Bile duct obstruction can occur due to a carcinoma of which of the following?

(a) Body of pancreas
(b) Tail of pancreas
(c) Stomach
(d) Head of pancreas

Ans: (d) Head of pancreas

378. A 17-year-old male complaining of bone pain undergoes a biopsy. The biopsy reveals small round blue cells that appear like pseudorosettes. Which of the following conditions does this patient have?

(a) Osteogenic sarcoma
(b) Ewing's sarcoma
(c) Osteomyelitis
(d) Chondroma

Ans: (b) Ewing's sarcoma

379. Which of the following is false about testicular tumors?

(a) May be bilateral
(b) May mimic orchitis
(c) Could be associated with a hydrocele
(d) Usually spread to para-aortic lymph nodes

Ans: (d) Usually spread to para-aortic lymph nodes

380. By what mechanism does bleomycin cause lung fibrosis?

(a) Increasing capillary permeability
(b) Free radicals
(c) Reperfusion injury
(d) Increasing calcium influx

Ans: (b) Free radicals

381. A 56-year-old has pancreatic cancer. Which of the following is false about the disorder?

(a) Can present with painless jaundice
(b) May present with the Budd-Chiari syndrome
(c) Diagnosis sometimes can only be made at surgery
(d) The Whipple procedure can be used to treat cancers of the tail of the pancreas

Ans: (d) The Whipple procedure can be used to treat cancers of the tail of the pancreas

382. What is the most likely diagnosis in a 64-year-old female wit bloody nipple discharge from the right nipple?

(a) Paget disease of nipple
(b) Intraductal papilloma
(c) Phyllodes tumor
(d) Lobular carcinoma

Ans: (b) Intraductal papilloma

383. Which of the following drugs acts on topoisomerase II?

(a) Methotrexate
(b) Cyclophosphamide
(c) Azathioprine
(d) Etoposide

Ans: (d) Etoposide

384. Which of the following drugs is an alkylating agent?

(a) Bleomycin
(b) Vincristine
(c) Tamoxifen
(d) Busulfan

Ans: (d) Busulfan

385. What is the underlying pathology in cystic hygromas?

(a) Failure of lymphatic sacs to develop connections
(b) Atrophy of lymphatic channels
(c) Neoplastic growth of normal lymphatics
(d) Inflammation of lymphatic ducts

Ans: (a) Failure of lymphatic sacs to develop connections

386. Which subtype of basal cell cancer is the most difficult to diagnose?

(a) Nodular
(b) Morpheaform
(c) Cystic
(d) Infiltrative

Ans: (b) Morpheaform

387. A 78-year-old white man present with a 0.5 cm erythematous plaque on his arm. Skin biopsy results reveal a nodular basal cell carcinoma. Which of the following is the best treatment option?

(a) Referral for Mohs surgery
(b) Radiation therapy
(c) Clinical observation
(d) Surgical excision or curettage

Ans: (d) Surgical excision or curettage

388. Which is not associated with gastric cancer?

(a) Acanthosis nigricans
(b) Blumer shelf
(c) Krukenberg tumor
(d) Grey Turner sign

Ans: (d) Grey Turner sign

389. What is the most common initial presentation of a patient with Peutz-Jeghers syndrome?

(a) Nose bleed
(b) GI bleed
(c) Intussusception
(d) Diarrhea

Ans: (c) Intussusception

390. What is the most common primary tumor of the liver?

(a) Hepatoma
(b) Hydatid cyst
(c) Hamartoma
(d) Hemangioma

Ans: (a) Hepatoma

391. Which of the following malignancies with bone metastasis has the worst 5-year survival rate?

(a) Lung
(b) Breast
(c) Thyroid
(d) Prostate

Ans: (a) Lung

392. Ototoxicity is most likely to occur with which of the following medications?

(a) Doxorubicin
(b) Cisplatinum
(c) 5-FU
(d) Bleomycin

Ans: (b) Cisplatinum

393. Which of the following biomarkers is considered to be useful in diagnosing prostate cancer?

(a) Carcinoembryonic antigen (CEA)
(b) Cancer antigen 125 (CA-125)
(c) Alpha-fetoprotein (AFP)
(d) Prostate-specific antigen (PSA)

Ans: (d) Prostate-specific antigen (PSA)

394. Which malignancy is not hormone dependent?

(a) Breast cancer
(b) Prostate cancer
(c) Uterine cancer
(d) Bronchial carcinoma

Ans: (d) Bronchial carcinoma

395. What is the appropriate treatment for stage II/III small cell carcinoma of the lung?

(a) Resection
(b) Preoperative chemotherapy and resection
(c) Chemotherapy and radiation
(d) Resection and postoperative chemotherapy

Ans: (c) Chemotherapy and radiation

396. What is the most common type of posterior mediastinal neurogenic tumor in adults?

(a) Pheochromocytoma
(b) Carcinoid
(c) Neurilemmoma
(d) Neuroblastoma

Ans: (c) Neurilemmoma

397. What is the most common histology of bladder cancer in a patient with a Schistosoma haematobium infection?

(a) Adenocarcinoma
(b) Columnar cell
(c) Squamous cell
(d) Transitional cell

Ans: (c) Squamous cell

398. The depth of penetration of esophageal cancer is best assessed with:

(a) CT scan
(b) Endoscopic ultrasound
(c) MRI
(d) Manometry

Ans: (b) Endoscopic ultrasound

399. What treatment for basal cell carcinomas has the highest cure rate?

(a) Electrodesiccation and curettage
(b) Cryotherapy
(c) Mohs micrographic surgery
(d) Surgical excision

Ans: (c) Mohs micrographic surgery

400. Which of the following is the major risk factor for pancreatic cancer?

(a) Alcohol
(b) Smoking
(c) High protein diet
(d) Excess caffeine-containing beverages

Ans: (b) Smoking

401. What does breast imaging reporting and data system (BI-RADS) 6 mean?

(a) The assessment in incomplete
(b) Negative study
(c) Benign finding
(d) Known biopsy-proven cancer

Ans: (d) Known biopsy-proven cancer

402. A patient had several syncopes preceded by blurred vision and profuse diaphoresis. Work up revealed hypoglycemia and discovery of a pancreatic mass. What is the most likely diagnosis?

(a) Glucagonoma
(b) Insulinoma
(c) Gastrinoma
(d) Somatostatinoma

Ans: (b) Insulinoma

403. Which of the following is not typically associated with von Hippel-Lindau disease?

(a) Islet cell tumors
(b) Pancreatic cysts
(c) Renal artery stenosis
(d) Renal cell carcinoma

Ans: (c) Renal artery stenosis

404. Which medication has been found to lower the risk of colorectal cancers?

(a) Omeprazole
(b) Aspirin
(c) Azathioprine
(d) Misoprostol

Ans: (b) Aspirin

405. Which tumor is often associated with Rathke pouch?

(a) Melanoma
(b) Craniopharyngioma
(c) Pituitary adenoma
(d) Nasal carcinoma

Ans: (b) Craniopharyngioma

406. Which of the following cancers is most common in patients who undergo transplants or receive chemotherapy?

(a) Colon cancer (b) Lung cancer

(c) Skin cancer (d) Blood cancer

Ans: (c) Skin cancer

407. Which is true of Pancoast tumor?

(a) Produces superior vena cava syndrome (b) Most often caused by small cell cancer

(c) Affects upper brachial plexus (d) Can involve subclavian artery

Ans: (d) Can involve subclavian artery

408. What usually causes post-transplant lymphomas?

(a) Cytomegalovirus (b) Epstein-Barr virus

(c) Herpes (d) HIV

Ans: (b) Epstein-Barr virus (NEET SS 2019)

409. Unopposed estrogen therapy can result in endometrial hyperplasia and carcinoma. What type of cancer can result?

(a) Clear cell carcinoma (b) Adenocarcinoma

(c) Adenosquamous carcinoma (d) Papillary serous carcinoma

Ans: (b) Adenocarcinoma

410. Which of the following lesions most closely resembles a squamous cell cancer?

(a) Condyloma lata (b) Keratoacanthoma

(c) Seborrhea (d) Lichen planus

Ans: (b) Keratoacanthoma

411. What is the most common malignancy in women that is associated with a malignant pleural effusion?

(a) Breast (b) Ovary

(c) Uterus (d) Colon

Ans: (a) Breast

412. After colorectal cancer, what is the next most common cancer in patients with Lynch syndrome?

(a) Gastric (b) Endometrial

(c) Ovarian (d) Transitional cell

Ans: (b) Endometrial

413. What is the most common histological type of oral cavity carcinoma?

(a) Squamous cell (b) Basal cell

(c) Transitional cell (d) Melanotic

Ans: (a) Squamous cell

414. Which of the following cancer is NOT found to be associated with paraneoplastic cerebellar degeneration?

(a) Breast cancer (b) Renal cancer

(c) Ovarian cancer (d) Small cell lung cancer

Ans: (b) Renal cancer

415. What is the most common primary neoplasm of the liver?

(a) Cholangiocarcinoma
(b) Hepatocellular carcinoma
(c) Hepatic adenoma
(d) Hepatoblastoma

Ans: (b) Hepatocellular carcinoma

416. Which of the following genetic conditions is autosomal recessive and associated with the development of skin cancer?

(a) Peutz-Jeghers
(b) Seminoma
(c) Neurofibromatosis
(d) Xeroderma pigmentosa

Ans: (d) Xeroderma pigmentosa

417. Which cancer is most often associated with Lambert-Eaton syndrome?

(a) Adenocarcinoma of the lung
(b) Malignant thymoma
(c) Small cell cancer of the lung
(d) Lymphosarcoma

Ans: (c) Small cell cancer of the lung

418. Which substance is thought to be a causative factor in mesothelioma?

(a) Agent Orange
(b) Nicotine
(c) Radon gas
(d) Asbestos

Ans: (d) Asbestos

419. Which of the following is NOT a risk factor for esophageal cancer?

(a) Tylosis
(b) Barrett's
(c) Achalasia
(d) Leiomyoma

Ans: (d) Leiomyoma

420. What is the second most common site for metastasis from sigmoid colon cancer?

(a) Liver
(b) Lymph nodes
(c) Lungs
(d) Brain

Ans: (a) Liver

421. Which of the following molecular abnormalities is associated with neuroblastoma?

(a) p53 suppressor on 17p13.1
(b) CDKN2 suppressor
(c) Neurofibromin
(d) N-myc oncogene

Ans: (d) N-myc oncogene

422. During a routine work up a male is found to have a prostate nodule on a digital rectal exam. Work up reveals that it is prostate cancer. The lesion is localized and after discussion with the patient, it is determined that active surveillance is that ideal method to treat him. Which of the following is not a criterion generally used to manage patients for "active surveillance"?

(a) Gleason score of 3 to 6
(b) PSA levels less than 10
(c) T1-2a disease
(d) Patient age less than 60

Ans: (d) Patient age less than 60

423. Which is a presenting feature of Leydig cell tumors?

(a) Urinary retention
(b) Gynecomastia
(c) SVC syndrome
(d) Priapism

Ans: (b) Gynecomastia

424. A 28-year-old white male presents to the office with a chief complaint of sensitive "bumps" on his arms that have been present for 5 years. Based on your history and physical examination, you suspect the patient has multiple piloleiomyomas. What genetic syndrome might this patient have?

(a) Cowden syndrome
(b) Tuberous sclerosis
(c) Birt-Hogg Dube syndrome
(d) Hereditary leiomyomatosis and renal cell carcinoma

Ans: (d) Hereditary leiomyomatosis and renal cell carcinoma

425. Which type of breast cancer has the best prognosis?

(a) Paget's
(b) Inflammatory breast cancer
(c) Mucinous
(d) Medullary

Ans: (c) Mucinous

426. A 37-year-old man presents to your clinic with a history of a pigmented skin lesion on his back. His dermatologist performed biopsy demonstrating a 1.4 mm thick melanoma. He has no palpable axillary or inguinal adenopathy. Next step in management is:

(a) Staging PET/CT scan
(b) Wide local excision with 1 cm margin
(c) Wide local excision with 1 cm margin and sentinel node biopsy
(d) Wide local excision with 2 cm margin and sentinel node biopsy

Ans: (d) Wide local excision with 2 cm margin and sentinel node biopsy

427. A 45-year-old woman presents with a new diagnosis of a 3.5 mm thick melanoma of foot. On examination, she has palpable inguinal adenopathy. What is the next step in management?

(a) Fine-needle aspiration biopsy of the palpable inguinal node
(b) Wide local excision with 2 cm margin and sentinel node biopsy
(c) Wide local excision with 2 cm margin and inguinal node dissection
(d) Systemic immunotherapy alone

Ans: (a) Fine-needle aspiration biopsy of the palpable inguinal node

428. Sentinel node biopsy should be considered on all melanoma patients with:

(a) Primary melanoma > 0.5 mm thick
(b) Primary melanoma 0.75–1 mm thick with high-risk features
(c) Lymphedema
(d) Palpable adenopathy

Ans: (b) Primary melanoma 0.75–1 mm thick with high-risk features

429. Completion lymph node dissection is:

(a) Has a 5% risk for lymphedema
(b) Will demonstrate additional nodal disease in 50% of patients
(c) Confers a survival benefit in patients with node-positive disease
(d) Should be recommended after a positive sentinel node biopsy

Ans: (d) Should be recommended after a positive sentinel node biopsy

430. Overall survival in metastatic melanoma is NOT improved with treatment with which medication?

(a) Interferon-alpha
(b) Ipilimumab
(c) Vemurafenib
(d) Dabrafenib

Ans: (a) Interferon-alpha

431. All of the following characteristics regarding BCC are true *except:*

(a) Induced by UV radiation
(b) Frequently metastasize to distant sites
(c) Associated with a known mutation in hedgehog signaling
(d) Surgical therapy is often curative

Ans: (b) Frequently metastasize to distant sites

432. Regarding NMSCs, incisional biopsies or definitive wide excisions should be performed:

(a) Transversely on extremities
(b) Longitudinally on extremities
(c) With no consideration for the next step
(d) In the easiest manner to close

Ans: (b) Longitudinally on extremities

433. A 38-year-old, red-headed woman who has an extensive history of tanning presents with raised, pearly white lesion on her shoulder. The immediate next step in management is:

(a) Close follow-up
(b) Wide excision with 3 mm margins
(c) Radiation therapy
(d) Full-thickness biopsy

Ans: (d) Full-thickness biopsy

434. Features that are associated with a worse prognosis in SCC include all of the following *except:*

(a) Poorly differentiated histology
(b) Evidence of perineural invasion
(c) Lymph node metastasis
(d) Noninvasive or *in situ* disease at time of presentation

Ans: (d) Noninvasive or *in situ* disease at time of presentation

435. Which of the following is a true statement regarding MCC:

(a) Associated with Merkel cell polyomavirus
(b) Less common in immunosuppressed populations
(c) Radiation resistant
(d) Can be distinguished as cutaneous in origin by TTF-1 staining

Ans: (a) Associated with Merkel cell polyomavirus

436. DFSPs are accurately characterized by each of the following statements *except:*

(a) Associated with a distinct chromosomal translocation
(b) Commonly spreads to lymph nodes
(c) May be treated with tyrosine kinase inhibitors
(d) Clear surgical margins are generally curative

Ans: (b) Commonly spreads to lymph nodes

437. A 35-year-old woman in her 16th week of an uncomplicated pregnancy presents with a new left breast mass during a routine prenatal visit. On physical examination, there is a 3 cm palpable mass, at the 4 O'clock position of the left breast. There are no palpable lymph nodes in the left axilla. Most appropriate next step of management is:

(a) Diagnostic mammography
(b) Breast ultrasound
(c) Excisional biopsy of the mass
(d) Observation until third trimester

Ans: (b) Breast ultrasound

438. A 33-year-old woman in her 19th week of an uncomplicated pregnancy develops a right breast mass that measures 2 cm, at the 2 O'clock position. Imaging reveals a suspicious mass in the same area and is categorized as BIRADS 4. There are no palpable lymph nodes in the right axilla. Most appropriate next step of management is:

(a) Modified radical mastectomy (MRM)
(b) Observation until postpartum
(c) Core needle biopsy of the mass
(d) Excisional biopsy of the mass

Ans: (c) Core needle biopsy of the mass

439. A 30-year-old woman in her 10th week of an uncomplicated pregnancy presents with new 2 cm right breast mass that is biopsyproven infiltrating ductal carcinoma. There are no palpable lymph nodes in the axilla. Imaging reveals no other lesions in either breast. Most appropriate next step of management is:

(a) MRM

(b) Neoadjuvant chemotherapy, followed by MRM

(c) Neoadjuvant chemotherapy, followed by PM + axillary lymph node dissection

(d) PM followed by external beam radiation

Ans: (a) MRM

440. A 34-year-old woman in her 20th week of an uncomplicated pregnancy develops an infiltrating ductal carcinoma of the left breast that is 3.5 cm in size. There are no other lesions in either breast on imaging. There is a palpable lymph node in the left axilla. She is interested in preserving her breast. The most appropriate next step of management is:

(a) MRM
(b) Neoadjuvant chemotherapy
(c) Termination of pregnancy
(d) SLNB

Ans: (b) Neoadjuvant chemotherapy

441. A 35-year-old woman who developed left breast cancer during pregnancy has been treated with PM + ALND. The tumor size was 2.3 cm; surgical margins were negative; 2/15 lymph nodes were involved with tumor. Tumor was ER+/PR+/Her-2-. She is now in her 30th week of pregnancy. Fetus is doing well. Which of the following is the most appropriate management?

(a) Early induction of labor

(b) Termination of pregnancy

(c) Cessation of chemotherapy 3 weeks prior to labor

(d) Cesarean section should be performed instead of vaginal delivery

Ans: (c) Cessation of chemotherapy 3 weeks prior to labor

442. Regarding the use of sentinel lymph node biopsy during pregnancy, which of the following is true?

(a) Sentinel lymph node biopsy is contraindicated

(b) The accuracy of sentinel lymph node biopsy during pregnancy is unknown

(c) Lymphazurin blue is safe

(d) Methylene blue is safe

Ans: (b) The accuracy of sentinel lymph node biopsy during pregnancy is unknown

443. Which of the following adjuvant therapies is safe during pregnancy?

(a) Tamoxifen
(b) Methotrexate
(c) Paclitaxel
(d) Cyclophosphamide

Ans: (d) Cyclophosphamide

444. Preferred treatment regimen for resectable stage II–III esophageal cancer:

(a) Surgery alone
(b) Concurrent chemoradiation
(c) Surgery followed by concurrent chemoradiation
(d) Neoadjuvant chemoradiation followed by surgery

Ans: (d) Neoadjuvant chemoradiation followed by surgery

445. A 68-year-old male with stage T4N0M0 unresectable esophageal cancer is seen brought to you for consultation. The recommended treatment is:

(a) Chemotherapy followed by radiation therapy alone
(b) Chemotherapy followed by concurrent chemoradiation
(c) Dose-escalated radiation using external beam or brachytherapy
(d) Concurrent chemoradiation to standard doses

Ans: (d) Concurrent chemoradiation to standard doses

446. Adenocarcinoma and squamous cell carcinoma of the esophagus represent:

(a) One disease with the same etiologic factors and treatments
(b) A strong case can be made that they represent different diseases, but with same treatment options
(c) A strong case can be made that they represent different diseases, with different treatment options
(d) Etiologic factors and epidemiologic trends have not been clearly identified for esophageal cancer

Ans: (c) A strong case can be made that they represent different diseases, with different treatment options

447. A 75-year-old male with asymptomatic metastatic adenocarcinoma is scheduled to undergo chemotherapy with cisplatin and continuous infusion 5-FU. He asks if there are any other therapies he should be considering and you recommend:

(a) Trastuzumab, a monoclonal antibody against HER2/neu
(b) Cetuximab, a monoclonal antibody against EGFR
(c) Everolimus, an mTOR inhibitor
(d) Bevacizumab, a monoclonal antibody against VEGF

Ans: (a) Trastuzumab, a monoclonal antibody against HER2/neu

448. Lymphatic drainage of the esophagus is correct in all below *except:*

(a) Cervical esophagus drains to the neck and supraclavicular nodes
(b) Upper thoracic esophagus drains to nodes on the innominate artery and ligamentum arteriosum, paraesophageal and paratracheal nodes
(c) Middle thoracic drains to the tracheobronchial, paraesophageal and pulmonary hilar nodes
(d) Lower thoracic esophagus drains to paraesophageal, diaphragmatic and pancreaticoduodenal nodes

Ans: (d) Lower thoracic esophagus drains to paraesophageal, diaphragmatic and pancreaticoduodenal nodes

449. Advantages of a transhiatal esophagectomy include all the following *except:*

(a) Avoidance of a thoracotomy
(b) Improved safety of a cervical anastomosis
(c) Decreased pulmonary complications
(d) Completeness of lymphadenectomy

Ans: (d) Completeness of lymphadenectomy

450. Which surgical technique can be technically challenging when resecting a cT3N1 squamous cell carcinoma of esophagus measured at 24 cm from incisors?

(a) Transhiatal esophagectomy
(b) Transthoracic esophagectomy
(c) Three-field esophagectomy
(d) Ivor-Lewis esophagectomy

Ans: (a) Transhiatal esophagectomy

451. Which of the following tumors can be treated with EMR?

(a) A 2 cm poorly differentiated tumor without ulceration
(b) A 2.5 cm with ulceration and submucosal invasion
(c) A 3 cm moderately differentiated tumor that is superficially elevated
(d) A 2.5 cm moderately differentiated tumor with ulceration

Ans: (c) A 3 cm moderately differentiated tumor that is superficially elevated

452. Which of the following is NOT true in differentiating diffuse-and intestinal-type cancers?

(a) Diffuse type is usually found in the cardia but can arise anywhere in the stomach
(b) Intestinal type carries a worse prognosis
(c) H. pylori is linked to both intestinal and diffuse subtypes of cancers
(d) Intestinal type is usually found in older patients and associated with atrophic gastritis

Ans: (b) Intestinal type carries a worse prognosis

453. What is the minimum number of lymph nodes needed for pathology in order to accurately stage a tumor N0?

(a) 8
(b) 10
(c) 12
(d) 15

Ans: (d) 15

454. Which of the following statements concerning gastric adenocarcinoma is TRUE?

(a) Predisposition is primarily genetic rather than environmental
(b) Incidence peaks at age 40
(c) Approximately 40% patients present with an early lesion (no muscularis propria invasion)
(d) *H. pylori,* chronic gastritis, and gastric adenomatous polyps are all risk factors for development of gastric adeno carcinoma

Ans: (d) *H. pylori,* chronic gastritis, and gastric adenomatous polyps are all risk factors for development of gastric adenocarcinoma

455. A 66-year-old male with a distant history of gastric ulcers comes to your office complaining of vague abdominal pain and a 5 pound weight loss over the last month. He takes over-the-counter Nexium which usually controls his heartburn. What would your *initial* work up entail?

(a) Reassurance and follow-up in 6 months as long as he has no family history of gastric cancer
(b) Instruction to continue his PPI and avoid salted and chemically preserved foods with follow-up in 6 months
(c) Outpatient CT scan of the abdomen and pelvis with PO and IV contrast
(d) Outpatient EGD, endoscopic ultrasound with biopsy

Ans: (d) Outpatient EGD, endoscopic ultrasound with biopsy

456. Most common cause of gastric outlet obstruction in adults is:

(a) Hypertrophic pyloric stenosis
(b) Duodenal stricture secondary to peptic ulceration
(c) Gastric adenocarcinoma
(d) Gastric lymphoma

Ans: (c) Gastric adenocarcinoma

457. For tumors of the distal stomach, a subtotal gastrectomy is preferred over total gastrectomy for all of the following reasons *except:*

(a) Subtotal gastrectomy confers a significantly better 5-year survival rate
(b) Total gastrectomy is a technically more difficult surgery
(c) Subtotal gastrectomy allows for a better nutritional status
(d) There is less perioperative morbidity and mortality

Ans: (a) Subtotal gastrectomy confers a significantly better 5-year survival rate

458. A 61-year-old woman has a partial gastrectomy with a D2 dissection and is found to have a pathologic staging of T2N1M0 (Stage IIA). Which of the following is the best postoperative management for this patient?

(a) Screening endoscopy and CT abdomen pelvis every 6 months to check for recurrence
(b) Chemotherapy before and after surgery or adjuvant chemoradiation therapy

(c) Screening PET scan every 6 months to check for recurrence and/or distant metastasis

(d) Postoperative radiation alone

Ans: (b) Chemotherapy before and after surgery or adjuvant chemoradiation therapy

459. A 48-year-old man was diagnosed with cT3N1 adenocarcinoma of the distal stomach. Staging CT imaging did not reveal any evidence of distant metastases. Diagnostic laparoscopy confirmed the absence of peritoneal spread. Which of the following is the best treatment strategy for this patient?

(a) D2 gastric resection followed by 5FU/LV-based chemoradiation

(b) Preoperative chemotherapy with epirubicin cisplatin and 5-FU (ECF) X 3 cycles followed by surgery followed by 3 more cycles of ECF

(c) D2 gastric resection followed by 1 year of oral S-1 where available

(d) All of the above are appropriate options

Ans: (d) All of the above are appropriate options

460. Which of the following is true regarding D2 dissection in gastric cancer?

(a) Removal of nodes along the lesser and greater curvatures of the stomach

(b) Removal of (a) plus para-aortic nodes

(c) Removal of (a) plus nodes along the left gastric artery, common hepatic artery, celiac trunk and splenic artery and hilum

(d) Removal of (a) plus left supraclavicular nodes

Ans: (c) Removal of (a) plus nodes along the left gastric artery, common hepatic artery, celiac trunk and splenic artery and hilum

461. A 65-year-old man presents with GI bleeding to the emergency department (Hgb 6.8 mg/dL) and is slightly tachycardic. After initial resuscitation and blood transfusion, the vital signs improve and repeat hemoglobin is 8.6 mg/dL. Endoscopy revealed a 0.9 cm submucosal lesion noted in the third portion of duodenum. Biopsy reveals carcinoid tumor and staging CT scan is negative for liver metastasis. Surgical plan should include:

(a) Pancreaticoduodenectomy

(b) Endoscopic mucosal resection

(c) Duodenectomy with primary anastomosis

(d) LAR somatostatin therapy

Ans: (b) Endoscopic mucosal resection

462. Factors that decrease the risk of malignancy in the small bowel include:

(a) Slow transit time

(b) Decreased IgA secretion

(c) High pH (alkaline) of contents

(d) Low amount of lymphoid tissue

Ans: (c) High pH (alkaline) of contents

463. Most frequently diagnosed small bowel malignancy is:

(a) Hemangioma

(b) Lymphoma

(c) GIST

(d) Intestinal neuroendocrine tumors

Ans: (d) Intestinal neuroendocrine tumors

464. A 51-year-old woman presents with abdominal bloating, pelvic discomfort and lower limb edema. Physical examination reveals a right-sided pelvic fullness. Ultrasound examination reveals a complex cystic lesion associated with the right ovary. Three years earlier the woman was treated for breast cancer, which was triple-negative (HER2/ER/PR negative), invasive ductal carcinoma. Her family history is significant for high-grade serous ovarian carcinoma diagnosed in a maternal aunt. In which of these genes does this woman most likely carry a germline mutation?

(a) BRCA2

(b) BRCA1

(c) XRCC2

(d) TP53

Ans: (b) XRCC2

465. Routine screening colonoscopy in a 50-year-old otherwise healthy man identifies 19 polyps. Histologic examination reveals multiple pathologies including tubular adenomas, villous adenomas and hyperplastic polyps. The family history is negative for colorectal polyposis. What autosomal-recessive condition could this presentation potentially represent?

(a) Attenuated familial adenomatous polysis (b) Hereditary mixed polyposis syndrome
(c) Peutz-Jeghers syndrome (d) MUTYH-associated polyposis

Ans: (d) MUTYH-associated polyposis

466. A 56-year-old woman diagnosed with follicular thyroid cancer has a history significant for invasive ductal breast carcinoma at age 42 years and endometrial cancer at age 45 years. What feature(s) on examination might you expect to see that can be associated with a potential cause of her multiple primary tumors?

(a) Ash leaf spots (b) Macrocephaly
(c) Polydactyly (d) Sebaceous neoplasms

Ans: (b) Macrocephaly
Cowden syndrome–Thyroid, Breast and Endometrial cancer, Macrocephaly
Gorlin syndrome–Polydactyly
Muir Torre syndrome–Sebaceous adenoma

MISCELLANEOUS

467. Which of the following is most common inherited malignancy?

(a) Infant leukemia (b) Wilm's tumour
(c) Retinoblastoma (d) Neuroblastoma

Ans: (c) Retinoblastoma

468. Mother of one-and-half-year-old child gives history of white reflex from one eye for past 1 month. On CT Scan orbit there is calcification seen within the globe. Most likely diagnosis:

(a) Congenital cataract (b) Retinoblastoma
(c) Endophthalmos (d) Coats' disease

Ans: (b) Retinoblastoma

469. A 1-year-old child having leucocoria was detected to be having a unilateral large retinoblastoma filling half the globe. Current therapy would be:

(a) Enucleation (b) Chemotherapy followed by local dyes
(c) Laser photodynamic therapy (d) Scleral radiotherapy followed by chemotherapy

Ans: (a) Enucleation

470. A 2-year-old child presented with leucocoria in right eye since 2 months. On examination, total retinal detachment was present in same eye. Ultrasound B scan revealed heterogenous subretinal mass with calcification with retinal detachment. Most likely diagnosis is:

(a) Coats' disease (b) Retinoblastoma
(c) Toxocariasis (d) Retinal tuberculoma

Ans: (b) Retinoblastoma

471. After removal of retinoblastoma, which tissue is sectioned to find distant metastasis?

(a) Optic nerve
(b) Vortex vein
(c) Central retinal vein
(d) Scleral and choroidal tissue

Ans: (a) Optic nerve

472. Retinoblastoma can present with all *except:*

(a) Leucocoria
(b) Squint
(c) Microphthalmos
(d) Cataract

Ans: (c) Microphthalmos

473. Most common orbital tumor in children:

(a) Choroidal melanoma
(b) Retinoblastoma
(c) BCC
(d) Adenoma lacrimal gland

Ans: (b) Retinoblastoma

474. Retinoblastoma differs from pseudoglioma by:

(a) Decreased intraocular tension
(b) Blurring of vision
(c) Enlargement of optic foramen
(d) All of the above

Ans: (c) Enlargement of optic foramen

475. Most common secondary malignancy in survivors of retinoblastoma is:

(a) CA thyroid
(b) NPC
(c) Optic glioma
(d) Osteosarcoma

Ans: (d) Osteosarcoma

476. As regards to intraocular retinoblastoma, which one of following statements is false?

(a) 94% of cases are sporadic
(b) Patients with sporadic retinoblastoma don't pass their genes to their offsprings
(c) Calcification in the tumor can be detected on USG scan
(d) Reese-Ellsworth classification is useful in predicting visual prognosis following radiotherapy

Ans: (b) Patients with sporadic retinoblastoma don't pass their genes to their offsprings

477. Knudson's 2 hit hypothesis is for:

(a) Glaucoma
(b) Retinoblastoma
(c) Optic glioma
(d) Meningioma

Ans: (b) Retinoblastoma

478. A patient with known mutation in Rb gene is disease free from Retinoblastoma. Patient is at highest risk of developing which of the following malignancies?

(a) Renal cell carcinoma
(b) Osteosarcoma
(c) Pinealoblastoma
(d) Chondrosarcoma

Ans: (b) Osteosarcoma

479. Increased LDH in aqueous humour suggests diagnosis of:

(a) Galactosemia
(b) Retinoblastoma
(c) Glaucoma
(d) Gyrate atrophy

Ans: (b) Retinoblastoma

...ment of choice for metastatic disease in retinoblastoma is:

(a) Chemotherapy (b) Enucleation

(c) Radiotherapy (d) Cryotherapy

Ans: (a) Chemotherapy

481. Treatment of choice for bilateral retinoblastoma:

(a) Chemotherapy (b) Enucleation

(c) Radiotherapy (d) Cryotherapy

Ans: (a) Chemotherapy

482. Most multifocal bilateral retinoblastomas require:

(a) Chemotherapy (b) Enucleation

(c) Radiotherapy (d) Combined modality

Ans: (d) Combined modality

483. Fibro-epithelioma of Pinkus, a rare variant of BCC presents typically on:

(a) Head and neck region (b) Torso and extremities

(c) Sun exposed areas of face (d) Trunk

Ans: (b) Torso and extremities

484. In TNM classification of melanoma, T4 is:

(a) >4 mm thickness without ulceration (b) 2-4 mm thickness with ulceration

(c) >4 mm thickness with ulceration (d) 2-4 mm thickness without ulceration

Ans: (a) >4 mm thickness without ulceration

485. Assertion: CDKN2A mutation causes loss of function of p16 and ARF and hereditary melanoma

Basis: p16 protein inhibits phosphorylation and inactivation of RB protein while ARF inhibits degradation of p53:

(a) Statement A and B are both correct; B is basis of A

(b) Statement A and B are both correct; B is not the basis of A

(c) Statement B is true but A is false

(d) Statement A is true but B is false

Ans: (a) Statement A and B are both correct; B is basis of A

486.

A	**SCC Only**	Actinic keratosis is a premalignant condition and UV exposure is a risk factor
B	**BCC Only**	Hedgehog pathway gene and clinically visible tortuous overlying telangiectatic vessels on the surface
C	**Both**	P53 and N-RAS, increased risk with increasing latitude
D	**Neither**	Radioresistant and keratoacanthoma is a variant

True match regarding BCC and SCC and associated features:

(a) C is correct (b) B is correct

(b) A is correct (d) D is correct

Ans: (b) B is correct